Insurance Handbook
FOR THE Medical Office

Insurance Handbook
FOR THE Medical Office

12 EDITION

MARILYN TAKAHASHI FORDNEY
CMA-AC (AAMA)

Formerly Instructor of Medical Insurance, Medical Terminology,
Medical Machine Transcription, and Medical Office Procedures
Ventura College
Ventura, California

3251 Riverport Lane
St. Louis, Missouri 63043

INSURANCE HANDBOOK FOR THE MEDICAL OFFICE ISBN: 978-1-4377-2256-7

ISBN 978-1-4377-2256-7

Publishing Director: Andrew Allen
Executive Editor: Susan Cole
Associate Developmental Editors: Elizabeth Fergus and Karen Baer
Publishing Services Manager: Catherine Jackson
Senior Project Manager: David Stein
Design Direction: Kim Denando

Printed in the United States

Last digit is the print number: 9 8 7 6 5 4 3 2 1

This twelfth edition is dedicated to my husband,
Sándor Havasi,
with love, respect, and gratitude;
to his wonderful family and their wonderful families;
and to all the beautiful people—friends, relatives, insurance billers, coders,
instructors, and new and former students—who, for more than 35 years,
have inspired and motivated me with their support to continue writing
in this challenging and ever-changing career field.

"I hear and I forget, I see and I remember, I do and I understand."
CHINESE PROVERB

About the Author

A dedicated professional, Marilyn Takahashi Fordney worked as a medical assistant for 14 years in various settings. During her 19-year teaching career, she taught courses in administrative medical assisting, medical insurance, and medical terminology at many community colleges and in adult education schools. Fordney is a Certified Medical Assistant. In 1977 she was named Woman of the Year by the Business and Professional Women's Club of Oxnard, California. In June 2005 Fordney was inducted into the Council of Fellows by the Text and Academic Authors Association in Las Vegas, Nevada.

Fordney's books have won national awards. This textbook, *Insurance Handbook for the Medical Office*, won the William Holmes McGuffey Award in Life Sciences for its excellence and longevity in the field. *Medical Insurance Billing and Coding: An Essentials Worktext*, a spin-off of the *Handbook*, won the Texty Excellence Award in its first edition.

The success of Fordney's books has allowed her to establish two foundations. The Fordney Foundation for DanceSport is a nonprofit foundation for amateur ballroom dancers ages 6 to 25. The foundation's objective is to help children and young adults to realize their dreams of artistic expression through ballroom dancing. The Havasi Wilderness Foundation is a nonprofit foundation to assist in the preservation and protection of the earth's most precious places for future generations. It gives opportunities to disadvantaged schools and children so that they can visit and learn about the wilderness in state and national or private parks.

Preface

WELCOME TO THE TWELFTH EDITION

When this textbook was first published in 1977, few people were aware of how important the subject of health insurance would become. *Insurance Handbook for the Medical Office* now celebrates its thirty-fifth year. I have told others around me, "I don't think I ever dreamed I would be writing this long," and sometimes I pinch myself to see if it is really true. Through the years this textbook has become the leader in its field because of its interactive learning system. The *Handbook* has gained wide acceptance across the nation among educators and working insurance billers and coders.

On account of the many legislative mandates and technologic advances that have occurred since the previous edition, putting the twelfth edition together has been challenging and exciting. Because changes occur daily in the insurance industry, *Insurance Handbook for the Medical Office* will be revised every 2 years to keep the information current.

PURPOSE

The goals of this textbook are to prepare students to excel as insurance billers and to increase efficiency and streamline administrative procedures for one of the most complex tasks of the physician's business: insurance coding and billing.

Why Is This Book Important to the Profession?

In the past 16 years, health care professionals and the community have witnessed the emergence of an administrative medical specialty known variously as insurance billing specialist, medical biller, or reimbursement specialist. Several national organizations offer certification in the field, which is quickly achieving recognition and professionalism. Thus the *Handbook* has been written to address this specialty as another branch of the administrative medical assistant profession. Health care reform has led to an explosion of jobs in the medical field, especially for those trained in coding and processing insurance claims both electronically and manually. Training in this area is necessary because, as a result of a lack of knowledge among office personnel, it is common to find medical practices either undercharging or not charging for billable services.

Insurance claims are being submitted for patients on recommendation of management consultants to control cash flow, obtain correct reimbursement amounts, honor insurance contracts, compete with other medical practices, and maintain a good relationship with patients. Even offices that do not routinely complete insurance claims for patients make exceptions for elderly patients or patients with mental incompetence, illiteracy, diminished eyesight, or a poor command of the English language. When the amount of the bill is hundreds or thousands of dollars or when a surgical report is required, the physician's office should submit the bill to obtain maximum reimbursement. Individuals who administer the federal government's Medicare program increasingly promote electronic transmission of insurance claims for medium and large medical practices. Because of these factors, as well as federal mandates to document care electronically, the amount of knowledge and skills that one must have has substantially increased. This textbook addresses all clerical functions of the medical biller, and illustrations throughout the textbook feature generic forms created to help simplify billing procedures.

Who Will Benefit From This Book?

Numerous schools and colleges have established 1-year certificate programs for those interested in a career as an insurance billing specialist, and many programs offer medical insurance as a full-semester, 18-week course. Community college extension divisions also offer community service classes and short courses in this subject. Some schools include it as part of a medical assisting program's curriculum, so the individual has knowledge in all administrative functions of a physician's office. The textbook may be used as a learning tool and resource guide in all of those programs, as well as in vocational or commercial training institutes and welfare-work programs. *Insurance Handbook for the Medical Office* also serves as a text for in-service training in the private medical office. The *Handbook* may be used for independent home study, if no formal classes are available in the community. The lay reader who is not pursuing a career in the medical field will find the textbook useful when working with a claims assistance professional or for billing his or her insurance plans. Insurance companies and their agents have found the *Handbook* to be a valuable reference tool when answering clients' questions.

The textbook is designed primarily for students who plan to seek employment in an outpatient setting (e.g., physician's office or clinic) or who wish to establish an independent billing business and need a thorough understanding of the reimbursement process. Many types of insurance coverage are available in the United States. The types most commonly encountered in physicians' offices and clinics have been emphasized in this textbook in simple, nontechnical explanations and tables. Documentation in the medical record is the key to substantiating procedure and diagnostic code selections for proper reimbursement. Thus, in this edition, Chapter 4, Medical Documentation and the Electronic Health Record, has been further updated and enhanced. In recent years, the federal government targeted this issue with the introduction of Medicare compliance policies related to documentation and confidentiality; such issues are therefore covered to help physicians comply with possible reviews or audits of their billing practices. Because of the implementation by 2013 of the *International Classification of Diseases, Tenth Revision, Clinical Modification*, this diagnostic code system information has been greatly expanded throughout the textbook and workbook. It will help ease the transition to this larger more specific code system. Since the health care reform impacts federal programs, employers, and health insurance companies, information about the legislation and when it phases in is explained throughout various chapters. Finally, the textbook may be used as a stand-alone reference source or as an educational tool to increase the knowledge of someone currently working as an insurance billing specialist in a private medical office.

CONTENT

General Features

Each chapter has been updated to reflect 2012 policies and procedures.

- All chapters have been completely restructured for better organization and flow of content, with legal information included where applicable to insurance billing and coding. The information presented is not a substitute for legal advice, and the physician and his or her insurance billing specialist should always seek legal counsel about specific questions of law as they relate to medical practice.
- "Service to Patients" boxes: A color-screened box at the beginning of each chapter highlights patient service with regard to the topic being discussed.

Service to Patients

Procedure codes must reflect the services rendered to the patient so that optimal payment is generated by an insurance plan based on selection of the correct code. Codes are chosen dependent on supporting documentation in the patient's medical record.

- HIPAA Compliance Alerts are interspersed throughout all of the chapters for emphasis.

- Objectives are provided at the beginning of each chapter, sequenced to match the technical content, and help guide instructors in preparing lecture material and inform readers about what material is presented.
- By reviewing the key terms introducing each chapter, students are alerted to important words for the topic. Key abbreviations follow the key terms; spellouts of the abbreviations are provided in a section that follows the glossary near the back of the textbook.
- Boxed examples are shown throughout each chapter.
- Key points are presented at the end of each chapter, summarizing and emphasizing the most important technical information for the chapter.

Many experts in the field reviewed the chapters in the eleventh edition so that improvements in content, clarity of topics, and deletions could be considered. A unique color-coded icon feature used throughout the textbook denotes and clarifies information specific to each type of payer. This system makes the learning process more effective by helping students identify each insurance payer with a specific color and graphic. These icons follow:

 All Payers: All payer guidelines, including all private insurance companies and all federal and state programs.

 All Private Payers: All private insurance companies.

 Medicaid: State Medicaid programs.

 Medicare: Federal Medicare programs, Medicare/Medicaid, Medicare/Medigap, and Medicare Secondary Payer (MSP).

TRICARE: TRICARE Standard (formerly CHAMPUS), TRICARE Prime, TRICARE Extra.

 CHAMPVA: Civilian Health and Medical Program of the Department of Veterans Affairs.

Workers' Compensation: State workers' compensation programs.

ORGANIZATION

Chapters 1 through 6: basic health insurance information and coding examples are shown for persons who are studying for a certification examination. Special emphasis is placed on correct and incorrect procedural codes and appropriate documentation—the keys to obtaining maximum reimbursement.

Example 6-8	Office Emergency
Incorrect Coding	
99212	Office visit, level 2, established patient
12005	Simple repair of scalp laceration, 12.6 cm
99070	Surgical tray (itemized)
Correct Coding	
99212	Office visit, level 2, established patient
99058	Office services provided on an emergency basis
12005	Simple repair of scalp laceration, 12.6 cm

- Chapter 2, HIPAA Compliance and Privacy in Insurance Billing, focuses on the Health Insurance Portability and Accountability Act (HIPAA). The chapter explains HIPAA's impact on insurance reform and administrative simplification.
- Chapter 7, The Paper Claim: CMS-1500 (08-05), uses a unique block-by-block approach specific to each different payer that denotes and clarifies information about the recently revised CMS-1500 (08-05) insurance claim form. The icons and graphics system is used to help students retain information. Templates illustrate placement of information on the form.

- Chapter 8, Electronic Data Interchange: Transactions and Security, has been updated. It contains additional HIPAA information on requirements for electronic transmission of insurance claims and explains the security rules.
- Chapters 9 through 16: Many specific quick-action solutions for insurance problems and information about tracing delinquent claims and appealing denied claims are provided. Thorough up-to-date information is presented for Medicare, Medicaid, TRICARE, private plans, workers' compensation, managed care plans, disability income insurance, and disability benefit programs. Helpful billing tips and guidelines for submitting insurance claims are given for each type of insurance program covered.
- Chapter 17, Hospital Billing, is intended especially for those students interested in pursuing a career in the hospital setting. Information about the revised UB-04 claim form is presented.
- Chapter 18, Seeking a Job and Attaining Professional Advancement, provides information pertinent to seeking a position as an insurance billing specialist, a self-employed claims assistance professional, or an electronic claims processor. The chapter explains the impact of HIPAA compliance policies for a business associate when hired by a medical practice to do insurance claim submission.
- The appendix aids the insurance billing specialist in locating audiotapes, books, newsletters, periodicals, software, and videotapes from various resources. It lists names, addresses, toll-free telephone numbers, and websites.
- An extensive glossary of basic medical and insurance terms and a comprehensive list of all the technical abbreviations within each chapter, along with their spellouts, is included.

ANCILLARIES

Workbook

Users of the *Workbook* that accompanies this edition of the textbook will find the following features:

- Competency-based education: A point system has been applied to code and claims completion for *Workbook* assignments for instructors who need to document and gather statistics for competency-based education. The

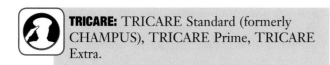

25. FEDERAL TAX I.D. NUMBER	SSN EIN	26. PATIENT'S ACCOUNT NO.	27. ACCEPT ASSIGNMENT? (For govt. claims, see back)	28. TOTAL CHARGE	29. AMOUNT PAID	30. BALANCE DUE
74 10640XX	☐ ☒	010	☒ YES ☐ NO	$ 70 92	$	$ 70 92

| 31. SIGNATURE OF PHYSICIAN OR SUPPLIER INCLUDING DEGREES OR CREDENTIALS (I certify that the statements on the reverse apply to this bill and are made a part thereof.)

CONCHA ANTRUM MD 030320XX

SIGNED *Concha Antrum MD* DATE | 32. SERVICE FACILITY LOCATION INFORMATION

a.   b. | 33. BILLING PROVIDER INFO & PH # (555) 486 9002
COLLEGE CLINIC
4567 BROAD AVENUE
WOODLAND HILLS XY 12345 0001
a. 3664021CC   b. |

reference initials

worksheets for each assignment are available on the Evolve website. *Handbook* learning objectives, *Workbook* performance objectives for all assignments, use of the tutorial software with reinforcement by *Workbook* assignments, the test section at the end of the *Workbook*, the quizzes of key terms featured on the website, and incorporation of classroom activities and suggestions from the *TEACH Instructor's Resource Manual* and the *Instructor's Electronic Resource Guide on CD-ROM* provide a complete competency-based educational program.

- Patient records and ledgers have been updated and reworded to correspond with the 2011 procedural and diagnostic code books.
- All chapters have fill-in-the-blank, multiple choice, mix and match, and true/false review questions. New review questions have been added. Answers have been put into the *TEACH Instructor's Resource Manual*.

General Features

For students, the *Workbook* that accompanies the textbook is a practical approach to learning insurance billing. It progresses from easy to more complex issues within each chapter and advances as new skills are learned and integrated. Chapter outlines serve as a lecture guide. Each chapter has performance objectives for assignments that indicate to students what will be accomplished. Key terms are repeated for quick reference when studying. Key abbreviations followed by blank lines are listed alphabetically so that students can assemble their own reference list for each chapter, thus reinforcing the abbreviations' spellouts. Patients' medical records, financial accounting statements, and encounter forms are presented as they might appear in the physician's files, so students may learn how to abstract information to complete claim forms properly and accurately. Patient records and ledgers have been completely updated for technical clinical content and reworded to correspond with the 2011 procedural and diagnostic code books. Easily removable forms and other sample documents are included in the *Workbook* for completion and to enhance keying skills. Insurance claim forms and letterheads are available on the Evolve website. Some assignments give students hands-on experience in keying forms for optical character recognition (OCR) computer equipment, which is used in all states for insurance claims processing and payment. Current procedural and diagnostic code exercises are used throughout the *Workbook* to facilitate and enhance coding skills for submitting a claim or posting to a patient's financial account statement. Critical thinking problems are presented in each chapter. Special appendixes are included at the end of the *Workbook*. These include a simulated practice, the College Clinic, with a group of physicians who employ the student; a mock fee schedule with codes and fees (including

Medicare); and an abbreviated Medicare Level II HCPCS alphanumeric code list. The appendixes may be used as reference tools to complete the procedural code problems. These appendixes include the following:

- Appendix A details information for a simulated practice called College Clinic. Information is provided about the group of physicians, and a mock fee schedule is included with codes and fees (including Medicare).
- Appendix B provides an abbreviated Medicare Level II HCPCS alphanumeric code list with a list of modifiers.

Student Software Challenge (Located on Evolve)

The Student Software Challenge located on Evolve is user-friendly software that provides students with another opportunity for hands-on learning. This software simulates a realistic experience by having students gather necessary documents and extract specific information to complete the CMS-1500 (08-05) insurance claim form. All source documents appear on screen and may be viewed simultaneously in a separate window. The Student Software Challenge also allows users to print the claim form for evaluation and edit it to correct errors.

The main objective is to complete CMS-1500 (08-05) forms for each case and insert accurate data, including diagnostic and procedural code numbers. Instructors may want their students to work through the first case or basic cases 1 through 4 strictly for learning and to use Case 5 for testing and grading. Cases 6 through 10, which are advanced and insurance specific (e.g., Medicare, TRICARE), may be used for practice or testing. This simulated learning methodology makes possible an easier transition from classroom to workplace.

Additional features of the Student Software Challenge for the twelfth edition of this textbook include the following:

- Blank interactive forms that can be typed into and printed or saved to be turned in to the instructor. This creates clean claims that are easier to read and grade.
- Complete fee schedule to simplify the insertion of fees on the CMS-1500 (08-05) claim form or financial accounting record.

TEACH Instructor's Resource Manual

The *TEACH Instructor's Resource Manual* is available in printed form and on the Evolve site; it contains lesson plans, *Workbook* answer keys, a test bank, and PowerPoint slides. This resource allows instructors the flexibility to quickly adapt the textbook for their individual classroom needs and to gauge students' understanding. The *TEACH Instructor's Resource Manual* features the following:

- Guidelines for establishing a medical insurance course
- Answer keys to the *Workbook* and Student Software Challenge assignments and tests with rationales, optional codes, and further explanations for most of the code problems
- Lesson plans for each chapter
- Suggested classroom activities and games
- Ideas on how to use the text as an adjunct to an administrative medical assisting or medical office procedures course
- Pretests for each chapter

Evolve Companion Website

Evolve is an interactive learning environment that works in coordination with the textbook. It provides Internet-based course management tools that instructors can use to reinforce and expand on the concepts delivered in class. It can be used for the following:

- To publish the class syllabus, outline, and lecture notes
- To set up "virtual office hours" and e-mail communication
- To share important dates and information through the online class calendar
- To encourage student participation through chat rooms and discussion boards

Evolve also provides online access to free Learning Resources designed specifically to give students and instructors the information they need to quickly and successfully learn the topics covered in this textbook. These Learning Resources include the following:

- Self-assessment quizzes to evaluate students' mastery through multiple choice, true/false, fill-in-the-blank, and matching questions. Instant scoring and feedback are available at the click of a button.
- Weblinks: Hundreds of websites have been carefully gathered to supplement the content of the textbook. The weblinks are regularly updated, with new ones added as they are developed.
- Technical updates to keep up with changes in government regulations and codes, as well as other industry changes.
- An image collection of forms and summaries of important chapter concepts from the textbook for use as overheads or as PowerPoint slides. A PowerPoint presentation will capture attention and create lively lectures to assist in learning and retention.
- A test bank with more than 1000 questions to assist instructors in test construction. The questions are provided in various formats, such as multiple choice,

true/false, mix and match, completion of blanks, and labeling of illustrations. Questions are rated for difficulty (i.e., easy, moderate, or hard) to help instructors with test construction for the topic being taught. The tests can be customized, revised, and printed.

Medical Insurance Online

Medical Insurance Online is an exciting resource for instructors and students. The new and improved *Medical Insurance Online* has been completely revamped to align more closely with the *Handbook*. The course consists of 18 modules that correspond with the flow and organization of each chapter in the book. The modules have been designed as short segments ("lessons") followed by interactive exercises and activities that reinforce key concepts. Each module is followed by a scored quiz that allows both students and instructors to evaluate comprehension and identify weak areas. The course ends with an examination that is automatically scored and reported to the instructor.

Key features of the *Medical Insurance Online* course for the twelfth edition of this text include the following:

- Interactive exercises and self-assessment activities provide students with frequent opportunities to recall and recognize important concepts.
- Weblinks direct students to websites for additional resources and study.
- Quizzes and examinations allow students to evaluate their comprehension and know their grade at any time as they progress through the course.
- Key terms have been linked to an extensive glossary that provides students with definitions when they are needed.

SUMMARY

The *Handbook* and its ancillaries provide a complete competency-based educational program. *Handbook* learning objectives, *Workbook* performance objectives, assignments, tests, Student Software Challenge, the virtual externship available on *Medical Insurance Online*, and incorporation of lesson plans and suggested classroom activities from the *TEACH Instructor's Resource Manual* ensure that students know everything they need to succeed in the workforce. Escalating costs of medical care, the impact of technology, and the explosion of managed care plans have affected insurance billing procedures and claims processing and have necessitated new legislation for government and state programs. Therefore it is essential that all medical personnel who handle claims continually update their knowledge. This may be accomplished by reading bulletins from state agencies and regional insurance carriers, speaking with insurance representatives, or attending insurance workshops offered at local colleges or local chapters of professional associations, such as those mentioned in Chapters 1 and 18. It is hoped that this textbook will resolve any unclear issues pertaining to current methods and become the framework on which the insurance billing specialist builds new knowledge as understanding and appreciation of the profession are attained.

ACKNOWLEDGMENTS

During my 14 years as a medical assistant, 19 years of teaching, and more than 35 years of writing, hundreds of students, physicians, friends, colleagues, and instructors have contributed valuable suggestions and interesting material for this textbook. I thank all of them, especially the following individuals:

- Lois C. Oliver, retired professor, Pierce College, Woodland Hills, California, helped me organize my first medical insurance class in 1969 and offered assistance and encouragement throughout the preparation of the first edition of the *Handbook*.
- Marcia O. "Marcy" Diehl, CMA-A (AAMA), CMT, a former co-author and retired instructor, Grossmont Community College, El Cajon, California, generously shared her knowledge, ideas, and class materials. Marcy motivated me to submit my first manuscript to several publishers, and without her urging I probably would not have taken action in that direction.
- Members of the California Association of Medical Assistant Instructors (CAMAI) contributed suggestions for improving the textbook and gave me motivation from time to time to continue the project.
- Mary E. Kinn, CPS, CMA-A (AAMA), author and retired assistant professor, Long Beach City College, Long Beach, California, provided a perspective review of my syllabus. Without her positive endorsement, the first edition of this book might not have been published.
- Special thanks to the students of Linda French's former classes at Simi Valley Adult School and Career Institute in Simi Valley, California, who contributed their criticisms, lent technical subject matter, offered suggestions, and through voluntary participation helped to enhance and create *Workbook* assignments for one of the previous editions.

- Karen Levein, CPC, CPC-I, instructor at Burbank Adult School and The Coding Source, who offered clarification suggestions for the *Handbook*, gave technical assistance for the *Workbook* assignments, and updated many codes in the *TEACH Resource Manual* answer keys. Her input is due to current classroom experiences with students.

I gratefully acknowledge the work of Kim Denando, Art and Design, Elsevier, for the design of this edition. Sun West Studio of Ventura, California, took the photograph for "About the Author." Jack Foley, photographer, and Nick Kaufmann Productions took the photographs found throughout the textbook. I acknowledge and thank them all.

I also thank the print shop staff, Publications Department, Ventura College, Ventura, California, who printed the first California syllabus of this text.

I am indebted to many individuals on the staff at Elsevier for encouragement and guidance. I express particular appreciation to Susan Cole, *Executive Editor*; Karen Baer and Elizabeth Fergus, *Associate Developmental Editors*; David Stein, *Project Manager*; and Catherine Jackson, *Publication Services Manager*, for coordination of the entire project.

Numerous supply companies were kind enough to cooperate by providing forms and descriptive literature of their products, and their names are found throughout the textbook and *Workbook* figures.

But colleagues, production staff, and editors working as a team do not quite make a book; there are others to whom I must express overwhelming debt and enduring gratitude, and these are the consultants who reviewed some of the chapters or who provided vital information about private, state, and federal insurance programs. Without the knowledge of these advisers, the massive task of compiling an insurance textbook truly national in scope might never have been completed. Although the names of all those who graciously assisted me are too numerous to mention, I take great pride in listing my principal consultants for this twelfth edition.

Marilyn Takahashi Fordney, CMA-AC (AAMA)
Oxnard, California

Principal Consultants and Reviewers

Conejo Chapter of the American
Association of Professional Coders
Thousand Oaks, California

George S. Conomikes and Staff
President, Conomikes Associates, Inc., Los Angeles,
California

Deborah Emmons, CMA (AAMA)
President, S.T.A.T. Transcription Service, Port
Hueneme, California

Sandy Gutt
Instructor, Southern California Regional Occupational
Center, Torrance, California

Lucille M. Loignon, MD, FACS
Diplomate, American Board of Ophthalmology,
Oxnard, California

Kathy A. McCall, CMA-AC (AAMA), BS, MA
Retired Professor of Allied Health, Community College
of Allegheny County, Pittsburgh, Pennsylvania

Griff Stelzner
Assistant Claims Manager, State Compensation
Insurance Fund, Oxnard, California

Carolyn Talesfore
Advertising and Promotions Manager, Bibbero Systems,
Inc., Petaluma, California

EDITORIAL REVIEW BOARD

Char Bates, CMA
Instructor
Gurnee, Illinois

Nancy Cross, M.Ed., RHIA, CPC
Accounts and Records Supervisor
Bordeaux Long Term Care
Adjunct Faculty
Nashville State Community College
Nashville, Tennessee

Amy DeVore, CPC, CMA (AAMA)
Medical Coding and Medical Assisting
Butler County Community College
Butler, Pennsylvania

Mary Kay Driscoll, MBA, RHIA, RMC, CMBS
Lead Faculty/Program Director
Advanced Medical Coding and Billing Program
Lincoln College Online
West Orange, New Jersey

Cindy Glewwe, M.Ed., RHIA
Health Science Curriculum Manager
Rasmussen College
Eden Prairie, Minnesota

Sally Heiderman
Instructor
Inner Office, Inc.
Brookfield, Ohio

Carolyn Helms, BS, RMA
Medical Assisting Program Director
Atlanta Technical College
Atlanta, Georgia

Carol Hendrickson, Masters and CCS-P
Adjunct Professor
Pasco Hernando Community College
New Port Richey, Florida

Judy Hurtt, Master of Education
Instructor
East Central Community College
Decatur, Mississippi

Karen Levein, CPC, CPC-I
Instructor
Medical Billing and Coding
Burbank Adult School
Burbank, California
The Coding Source
Los Angeles, California

Loretta M. McDonald, BA, MPS, CPC, CHI, CBCS, CMAA
Healthcare Information Management Instructor
New Horizons CLC
Nashville, Tennessee

Regine Monfette, CMBS
Assistant Manager
Allied Business Schools
Laguna Hills, California

Mary Kay Muir, BS, CPC
HCIM Program Manager
Online Live Virtual Training
New Horizons Computer Learning Centers
San Antonio, Texas

Stephanie K. Pratap, M.A. in English and B.A. in English
Course Maintenance Specialist
Allied Business Schools
Laguna Hills, California

Angela P. Rein, RMA, AS, BSHM, CPC, MAHS, CPC-H
Medical Billing and Coding Department Chair
Sanford Brown College
Collinsville, Illinois

Nina Scott, MSEd, RHIA, CCS, CCSP
Program Director
Health Information Technology
Itawamba Community College
Tupelo, Mississippi

Dorothy D. Steed, CPC-H, CHCC, CPUM, CPHM, CCS-P, ACS-OP, RCC, CPC-I, CEMC, CFPC, CPMA, PCS, FCS, RMC, CPAR
Consultant/Educator
Atlanta, Georgia

Patricia A. Stich, Masters of Education
Assistant Professor
Waubonsee Community College
Sugar Grove, Illinois

Nina Thierer, CMA (AAMA), BS, CPC, CCAT
Associate Professor
Ivy Tech Community College
Fort Wayne, Indiana

Sally Tumminelli, CPC, CGSC, CHI, CBCS
Instructor
Advantage Career Institute
West Long Branch, New Jersey

Stacey F. Wilson, BS Biology, Registered Medical Technologist (ASCP), Certified Phlebotomist (ASCP), Masters in Health Administration, Certified Medical Assistant (AAMA)
Program Chair, Medical Assistant Program
Cabarrus College of Health Sciences
Concord, North Carolina

Contents

UNIT 2
The Claims Process

UNIT 3
Health Care Payers

Insurance Handbook
FOR THE Medical Office

UNIT 1
Career Role and Responsibilities

KEY TERMS*

American Health Information
  Management Association
American Medical Association
cash flow
claims assistance professional

ethics
etiquette
insurance billing specialist
list service (listserv)
medical billing representative

multiskilled health practitioner
reimbursement specialist
respondeat superior
senior billing representative

KEY ABBREVIATIONS*

AAMA	ASHD	HIPAA	NPP
ACA	CAP	listserv	
AHIMA	e-mail	MSHP	
AMA	GED	MSO	

*Definitions for the key terms and key abbreviations are located near the back of this textbook in the glossary.

Role of an Insurance Billing Specialist

OBJECTIVES

After reading this chapter, you should be able to:

- Identify the background and importance of accurate insurance claims submission, coding, and billing.
- Assess responsibilities assigned to insurance billing and coding specialists and electronic claims processors.
- Name the office procedures performed during a work day that may affect billing.
- Specify the educational requirements for a job as an insurance billing specialist and a coder.
- Describe the variety of career advantages and areas of specialization open to those trained as insurance billing specialists.
- List qualifications and skills to be acquired by an insurance billing specialist.

- State the personal image to be projected as an insurance billing specialist.
- Describe professional behavior when working as an insurance billing specialist.
- Differentiate between medical ethics and medical etiquette.
- Specify instances when an employer and/or an employee can be liable when billing for medical services.
- Explain how insurance knowledge and medical knowledge can be kept current.

Service to Patients

When choosing a career as an insurance billing specialist, match your talents to the job. An attitude directed at serving the patient's needs should be your priority. Be alert to discover ways you can serve the patient while carrying out your job duties. A medical insurance billing specialist's primary goal is to assist in the revenue cycle, both helping the patient in obtaining maximum insurance plan benefits and ensuring a cash flow to the health care provider. Revenue is regular income, and the cycle is the regularly repeating set of events that produces it. The insurance billing specialist's responsibility is to conduct business in an ethical manner. Service to patients gives the opportunity to show high values, principles, and moral character, which will be appreciated and noticed.

BACKGROUND OF INSURANCE CLAIMS, CODING, AND BILLING

Welcome to the world of insurance billing, an exciting, ever-changing, and fast-growing career field. To help you focus on important terms and definitions, some of the basic words in this and subsequent chapters appear in **bold** or *italic* type. See the glossary at the end of this textbook for a comprehensive list of key abbreviations and key terms, with detailed definitions to broaden your knowledge.

A physician may have many problems that can affect obtaining maximum payment for services. He or she relies on professionals to handle billing, electronic

---

Performance objectives, testing and review material, and hands-on practical exercises for this chapter are available in these resources:

 The Insurance Handbook Student Workbook   The Insurance Handbook Evolve Site

transmission, and follow-up of claims. The health care industry is one of the most heavily regulated industries in the United States.

A number of billing and payment mechanisms are associated with third-party health insurance payers, and a number of health insurance policy issues pertaining to compliance are connected with each payer.

Two billing components exist: facility billing and professional billing. Facility billing is done for hospitals, acute care hospitals, skilled nursing or long-term care facilities, rehabilitation centers, or ambulatory surgical centers. Professional billing is done for physicians or *nonphysician practitioners* (NPPs). An NPP is an individual, such as a physician assistant, nurse practitioner, advanced registered nurse practitioner, certified nurse anesthetist, physical therapist, speech therapist, licensed clinical social worker, or certified registered nurse practitioner, who has not obtained a medical degree but is allowed to see patients and prescribe medications. These people are sometimes referred to as *physician extenders.* An insurance billing specialist must realize that NPPs should have a provider number and are permitted to submit claims to third-party payers. There may be occasions when the patient does not see a physician but is directed to the NPP. Proper authorization and documentation is required, and then a financial record source document called an *encounter form* is generated for the NPP. Hence this course is designed for professional billing.

Payment schedules for payment of professional services are based on the payer type (e.g., managed care, workers' compensation, or Medicare). Under Medicare, physicians are paid according to relative value units, which are based on three things: (1) the cost (overhead) of delivering care, (2) malpractice insurance, and (3) the physician's work. A fee schedule is published by the Centers for Medicare and Medicaid Services (CMS), a federal organization that sets the mandates for financing and delivery of care to Medicare and Medicaid beneficiaries in the United States. Managed care organizations establish their own physician fee schedules. Their rates are close to what Medicare pays.

Whether you are employed to perform hospital or professional billing functions, the basic setup of a business office encompasses the following units or combined departments: reception of the patient, rendering of medical services, documentation of the services, and financial accounting. You must understand their functions in relation to the business office and the practice as a whole and how they affect payment for services. The flow of information is one of the most vital components of an organization. Knowing the job duties within the organization can assist in the effective flow of information such as by written documents, telephone calls, oral communication among co-workers, or electronic mail (e-mail).

Office procedures performed throughout a workday include the following:

- *Scheduling appointments* involves assigning time slots for patients' visits. Canceling and rescheduling may also be involved. If the time is not properly assigned, there may be an influx or low volume of patients at a given time. Paperwork required for the visit must be obtained. It is important to record why the patient requires a visit.
- *Registering patients* may involve preregistration for visits by using a questionnaire referred to as a *patient registration form.* Financial and personal data are collected and accurately recorded (input) in a timely manner. Incorrect information affects the back office procedures and submission and payment of claims.
- *Documenting* pertinent clinical notes and assigning a diagnosis and service code to the patient's condition and visit is done by the provider of service. The notes in the patient's medical record include the reason for the visit, history, physical examination, diagnostic tests, results, diagnosis, and plan of treatment. Other forms pertaining to treatment requests by secondary providers are recorded by this team. The insurance billing specialist may be required to contact the insurance company to obtain authorization for treatment by secondary providers. He or she must also ensure that forms are properly completed and data are input into the system. Both proper documentation and assignment of the correct code for service affect reimbursement.
- A *charge entry* pertains to inputting (posting) charges for patient care service rendered into the system. The insurance biller must ensure that the insurance is correctly sequenced in the system (e.g., primary versus secondary health insurance, workers' compensation, or automobile insurance versus primary health insurance). This person must ensure that the diagnosis coincides with the service rendered. For example, an obstetrics/gynecology visit should not have a diagnosis related to ophthalmology. Many times, individuals have the same names, so billing service dates and the name of the patient seen must be accurate. Charge entry staff must ensure that the correct charge is assigned to the correct patient. Proper charge entry ensures timely billing and reimbursement.
- *Filing* and maintaining health information records and distributing the mail to various departments within the office is done by a file clerk. He or she pulls health records and works with various internal and external forms required by the billing department.
- *Bookkeeping and accounting* is the posting of payments received (cash, checks, electronic funds transfer, or

debit and credit cards) to patients' financial accounts. The bookkeeper or accountant must pay special attention to adjustments, denials, and write-offs. These entries may require investigation for validation. He or she may also receive insurance third-party payer remittance advices and may be assigned to follow up on denials.

ROLE OF THE INSURANCE BILLING SPECIALIST

In the past, administrative front office staff working in a physician's office performed both administrative and clinical duties. As decades passed, staff members' duties entailed either one or the other. Currently, because of changes in government regulations and standards for the insurance industry, specific medical assisting job tasks have become specialized. In a medical practice, it is commonplace to find administrative duties shared by a number of employees (e.g., administrative medical assistant, bookkeeper, file clerk, insurance billing specialist, office manager, receptionist, or transcriptionist). Several job title names are associated with medical billing personnel. The professional title used may depend on the region within the United States. Some of the most popular titles include **insurance billing specialist,** electronic claims processor, medical biller, **reimbursement specialist, medical billing representative,** and **senior billing representative.** Hence the title suggests that the employee is proficient in all aspects of medical billing. In this handbook, the title "insurance billing specialist" is used throughout. In clinics and large practices, it is common to find a billing department made up of many people, and within the department, each position is specialized such as Medicare billing specialist, Medicaid billing specialist, coding specialist, insurance counselor, collection manager, and medical and financial records manager.

Some medical practices and clinics contract with management services organizations (MSOs), which perform a variety of business functions, such as accounting, billing, coding, collections, computer support, legal advice, marketing, payroll, and management expertise. An insurance billing specialist may find a job working for an MSO as a part of this team.

An independent billing company may be a suitable organization for an insurance billing specialist.

Cost pressures on health care providers are forcing employers to be more efficient, and hiring **multiskilled health practitioners (MSHPs)** may achieve this. An MSHP is a person cross-trained to provide more than one function, often in more than one discipline. Knowledge of insurance claims completion and coding enhances skills so that he or she can offer more flexibility to someone hired in a medical setting.

People called **claims assistance professionals (CAPs)** work for the consumer. They help patients organize, file, and negotiate health insurance claims of all types; assist the consumer in obtaining maximum benefits; and tell the patient how much to pay the providers to make sure there is no overpayment. It is possible for someone who has taken a course on insurance billing to function in this role.

Job Responsibilities

Whether employed by the medical practice of an academic medical center or hospital or by a self-employed biller, you should be able to perform any and all duties assigned pertaining to the business office. Front and back office personnel work together to ensure a strong billing cycle and enhanced reimbursement. Examples of generic job descriptions are shown in Figures 1-1 and 1-2 to illustrate the job duties, skills, and requirements that might be encountered for various insurance billing and coding positions. Job descriptions for claims assistance professionals and hospital coders may be found on the Evolve website. Job descriptions are used as tools by assisting managers, supervisors, and employers in recruiting, supervising, and evaluating individuals in these positions for salary upgrades. Companies have had to modify their job descriptions to address individuals with physical impairments who may be affected by the Americans with Disabilities Act.

Administrative front office duties have gained in importance for the following reasons. Documentation is vital to good patient care. It must be done comprehensively for proper reimbursement. Diagnostic and procedural coding must be reviewed for its correctness and completeness. Insurance claims must be promptly submitted, ideally within 1 to 5 business days, to ensure continuous cash flow. **Cash flow** is the amount of actual money available to the medical practice. Without money coming in, overhead expenses cannot be met and a practice will face financial difficulties. Data required for billing must be collected from all health care providers, as well as from hospitals, outpatient clinics, and laboratories involved in a case.

An insurance billing specialist in a large medical practice may act as an insurance counselor, taking the patient to a private area of the office to discuss the practice's financial policies and the patient's insurance coverage, as well as to negotiate a reasonable payment plan. The insurance billing specialist discusses claims processing with contracted and noncontracted third-party payers,

Text continued on page 10.

GENERIC JOB DESCRIPTION FOR ENTRY LEVEL INSURANCE BILLING SPECIALIST

Knowledge, skills, and abilities:
1. Minimum education level consists of certificate from one-year insurance billing course, associate degree, or equivalent in work experience and continuing education.
2. Knowledge of basic medical terminology, anatomy and physiology, diseases, surgeries, medical specialties, and insurance terminology.
3. Ability to operate computer, printer, photocopy, and calculator equipment.
4. Written and oral communication skills including grammar, punctuation, and style.
5. Ability and knowledge to use procedure code books.
6. Ability and knowledge to use diagnostic code books.
7. Knowledge and skill of data entry.
8. Ability to work independently.
9. Certified Professional Coder (CPC) or Certified Coding Specialist (CCS) status preferred.

Working conditions:
Medical office setting. Sufficient lighting.

Physical demands:
Prolonged sitting, standing and walking. Use of word processor or computer equipment. Some stooping, reaching, climbing, and bending. Occasional lifting of _____lbs. to a height of 5 feet. Hearing and speech capabilities necessary to communicate with patients and staff in person and on telephone. Vision capable of viewing computer monitors, calculators, charts, forms, text, and numbers for prolonged periods.

Salary:
Employer would list range of remuneration for the position.

Job responsibilities:	**Performance standards:**
1. Abstracts health information from patient records.	1.1 Uses knowledge of medical terminology, anatomy and physiology, diseases, surgeries, and medical specialties. 1.2 Consults reference materials to clarify meanings of words. 1.3 Meets accuracy and production requirements adopted by employer. 1.4 Verifies with physician any vague information for accuracy.
2. Exhibits an understanding of ethical and medicolegal responsibilities related to insurance billing programs.	2.1 Observes policies and procedures related to federal privacy regulations, health records, release of information, retention of records, and statute of limitations for claim submission. 2.2 Meets standards of professional etiquette and ethical conduct. 2.3 Recognizes and reports problems involving fraud, abuse, embezzlement, and forgery to appropriate individuals.

FIGURE 1-1 Generic job description for an insurance billing specialist.

3. Operates computer to transmit insurance claims.

    3.1 Operates equipment skillfully and efficiently.

    3.2 Evaluates condition of equipment and reports need for repair or replacement.

4. Follows employer's policies and procedures.

    4.1 Punctual work attendance and is dependable.

    4.2 Answers routine inquiries related to account balances and dates insurance forms submitted.

5. Transmits insurance claims accurately.

    5.1 Updates insurance registration and account information.

    5.2 Processes payments and posts to accounts accurately.

    5.3 Handles correspondence related to insurance claims.

    5.4 Reviews encounter forms for accuracy before submission to data entry.

    5.5 Inserts data for generating insurance claims accurately.

    5.6 Codes procedures and diagnoses accurately.

    5.7 Telephones third-party payers with regard to delinquent claims.

    5.8 Traces insurance claims.

    5.9 Files appeals for denied claims.

    5.10 Documents registration data from patients accurately.

    5.11 Maintains separate insurance files.

6. Enhances knowledge and skills to keep up-to-date.

    6.1 Attends continuing education activities.

    6.2 Obtains current knowledge applicable to state and federal programs as they relate to insurance claim submission.

    6.3 Keeps abreast and maintains files of current changes in coding requirements from Medicare, Medicaid, and other third-party payers.

    6.4 Assists with updating fee schedules and encounter forms with current codes.

    6.5 Assists in the research of proper coding techniques to maximize reimbursement.

7. Employs interpersonal expertise to provide good working relationships with patients, employer, employees, and third-party payers.

    7.1 Works with employer and employees cooperatively as a team.

    7.2 Communicates effectively with patients and third-party payers regarding payment policies and financial obligations.

    7.3 Executes job assignments with diligence and skill.

    7.4 Assists staff with coding and reimbursement problems.

    7.5 Assists other employees when needed.

    7.6 Assists with giving fee estimates to patients when necessary.

FIGURE 1-1, cont'd

GENERIC JOB DESCRIPTION FOR
AN ELECTRONIC CLAIMS PROCESSOR

Knowledge, skills, and abilities:
1. Minimum education level consists of certificate from one-year insurance billing course, associate degree, or equivalent in work experience and continuing education.
2. Knowledge of basic medical terminology, anatomy and physiology, diseases, surgeries, medical specialties, and insurance terminology.
3. Ability to operate computer and printer, as well as photocopy and calculator equipment.
4. Written and oral communication skills including grammar, punctuation, and style.
5. Ability and knowledge to use procedure code books.
6. Ability and knowledge to use diagnostic code books.
7. Knowledge and skill of data entry.
8. Ability to work independently.
9. Certified Electronic Claims Processor (CECP) status preferred.

Working conditions:
Medical office setting. Sufficient lighting.

Physical demands:
Prolonged sitting, standing and walking. Use of computer equipment. Some stooping, reaching, climbing, and bending. Occasional lifting of _____ lbs. to a height of 5 feet. Hearing and speech capabilities necessary to communicate with patients and staff in person and on telephone. Vision capabilities necessary to view computer monitors, calculators, charts, forms, text, and numbers for prolonged periods.

Salary:
Employer would list range of remuneration for the position.

Job responsibilities:	**Performance standards:**
1. Acts as a link between the medical provider or facility and third-party payers.	1.1 Uses knowledge of medical terminology, anatomy and physiology, diseases, surgeries, and medical specialties.
	1.2 Understands computer applications and equipment required to convert and transmit patient billing data electronically.
	1.3 Consults reference materials to clarify meanings of words.
	1.4 Meets accuracy and production requirements adopted by employer.
	1.5 Verifies with physician any vague information for accuracy.
	1.6 Reduces volume of paperwork and variety of claim forms providers need to submit claims for payment.
2. Converts patient billing data into electronically readable formats.	2.1 Inputs data and transmits insurance claims accurately, either directly or through a clearinghouse.
	2.2 Answers routine inquiries related to account balances and dates insurance data transmitted to third-party payers.

FIGURE 1-2 Generic job description for an electronic claims processor.

3. Uses software that eliminates common claim filing errors, provides clean claims to third-party payers, expedites payments to providers or facilities, and follows up on delinquent or denied claims.

2.3 Updates and maintains software applications with requirements of clearinghouses and third-party payers.

3.1 Codes procedures and diagnoses accurately.
3.2 Telephones third-party payers about delinquent claims.
3.3 Traces insurance claims.
3.4 Files appeals for denied claims.

4. Exhibits an understanding of ethical and medicolegal responsibilities related to insurance billing programs and plans.

4.1 Observes policies and procedures related to federal privacy regulations, health records, release of information, retention of records, and statute of limitations for claim submission.
4.2 Meets standards of professional etiquette and ethical conduct.
4.3 Recognizes and reports problems involving fraud, abuse, embezzlement, and forgery to appropriate individuals.

5. Operates computer equipment to complete insurance claims.

5.1 Operates equipment skillfully and efficiently.
5.2 Evaluates condition of equipment and reports need for repair or replacement.

6. Follows employer's policies and procedures.

6.1 Must have punctual work attendance and be dependable.

7. Enhances knowledge and skills to keep up-to-date.

7.1 Attends continuing education skills activities.
7.2 Obtains current knowledge applicable to state and federal programs as they relate to transmission of insurance claims.
7.3 Keeps abreast and maintains files of current changes in coding requirements from Medicare, Medicaid, and other third-party payers. Assists in the research of proper coding techniques to maximum reimbursement.

8. Employs interpersonal expertise to provide good working relationships with patients, employer, employees, and third-party payers.

8.1 Works with employer and employees cooperatively as a team.
8.2 Communicates effectively with patients and third-party payers regarding payment policies and financial obligations.
8.3 Executes job assignments with diligence and skill.
8.4 Assists staff with coding and reimbursement problems.
8.5 Assists other employees when needed.
8.6 Assists with giving fee estimates to patients when necessary.

FIGURE 1-2, cont'd

the billing of secondary insurance payers and patients once the third-party payer pays its portion, self-pay billing, and time payment plans. Federal and state programs require the provider to submit claims for the patient. In other plans, it is the patient's obligation, rather than the provider's, to send the claim to the third-party payer. However, most providers submit claims for patients as a courtesy. Any copayments or deductible amounts should be collected from the patient at each visit. Also, self-pay patients should be reminded that payment is due at the time of service. This is done to ensure that the physician will be paid for services rendered and to develop good communication lines. Patients who are informed are patients who pay their bills. The counselor learns the deductible amount and verifies with the insurance company whether any preauthorization, precertification, or second-opinion requirements exist. Credit counseling helps obtain payment in full when expensive procedures are necessary. In some offices the insurance biller may act as a collection manager who answers routine inquiries related to account balances and insurance submission dates; assists patients in setting up a payment schedule that is within their budget; follows up on delinquent accounts; and traces denied, "adjusted," or unpaid claims (Figure 1-3).

Having large accounts receivables (total amount of money owed for professional services rendered) in a health care practice is often a direct result of failure to verify insurance plan benefits, obtain authorization or precertification, or collect copayments and deductibles or inadequate claims filing. The rush to get a claim "out the door" cannot be justified when a practice has thousands or millions of dollars in unpaid or denied claims. Accounts receivables will be low and revenue high if a practice takes the extra time to ensure the claim is 100% accurate, complete, and verified.

FIGURE 1-3 Insurance biller talking to a patient on the telephone about copayment required for an office visit under the patient's insurance plan.

In 1997 the American Association of Medical Assistants (AAMA) developed a role delineation study analyzing the many job functions of the medical assistant; it was updated in 2002 and 2007 and renamed and published in 2008. Table 1-1 shows the 2007-2008 Occupational Analysis of the CMA (AAMA), with arrows indicating material covered in this textbook. The topics shown on the occupational analysis must be studied to pass the certification examination offered by the AAMA. Further information about many types of certification and registration is discussed in Chapter 18.

Educational and Training Requirements

Generally, a high school diploma or general equivalency diploma (GED) is required for entry into an insurance billing or coding specialist accredited program. The accredited program usually offers additional education in medical terminology, insurance claims completion, procedural and diagnostic coding, anatomy and physiology, computer skills, ethics and medicolegal knowledge, and general office skills. Completion of an accredited program for coding certification or an accredited health information technology program is necessary for a job as a coder.

Experience in coding and insurance claim processing or management, completion of a 1-year insurance specialist certificate program at a community college, or both are usually required for a job as an insurance billing specialist. The curriculum that might be offered in a 1-year certificate program is shown in Figure 1-4. You might find that the courses in your locale may be labeled with different titles and time frames; the information in Figure 1-4 is specifically from a community college in Pennsylvania. Courses should cover medical terminology, anatomy and physiology, introduction to computer technology, procedural and diagnostic coding, and comprehensive medical insurance billing. A 2-year educational course can result in obtaining an associate's degree. Training prepares an individual for a wide range of employment opportunities. Knowledge of computer hardware and software, electronic data transmission requirements, and health care claim reimbursement is recommended for people planning to become electronic claims processors. Many accredited programs include an externship (on-the-job) period of training that may be paid or unpaid.

The **American Health Information Management Association (AHIMA)** has published diagnostic and procedure coding competencies for outpatient services and diagnostic coding and reporting requirements for physician billing. Refer to these competencies for a more inclusive list of educational and training requirements by visiting the Evolve website listed in the Internet Resources at the end of this chapter. It has an active link to the AHIMA.

Table 1-1 General, Clinical, and Administrative Skills* of the CMA (AAMA)

General Skills

COMMUNICATION	LEGAL CONCEPTS	INSTRUCTION	OPERATIONAL FUNCTIONS
Recognize and respect cultural diversity	Perform within legal (including federal and state statutes, regulations, opinions, and rulings) and ethical boundaries	Function as a health care advocate to meet individual's needs	Perform inventory of supplies and equipment
Adapt communications to individual's understanding	Document patient communication and clinical treatments accurately and appropriately	Educate individuals in office policies and procedures	Perform routine maintenance of administrative and clinical equipment
Use professional telephone and interpersonal techniques	Maintain medical records	Educate the patient within the scope of practice and as directed by supervising physician in health maintenance, disease prevention, and compliance with patient's treatment plan	Apply computer and other electronic equipment techniques to support office operations
Recognize and respond effectively to verbal, nonverbal, and written communications	Follow employer's established policies dealing with the health care contract	Identify community resources for health maintenance and disease prevention to meet individual patient needs	Perform methods of quality control
Utilize and apply medical terminology appropriately	Comply with established risk management and safety procedures	Maintain current list of community resources, including those for emergency preparedness and other patient care needs	Receive, organize, prioritize, store, and maintain transmittable information using electronic technology
Receive, organize, prioritize, store, and maintain transmittable information utilizing electronic technology	Recognize professional credentialing criteria	Collaborate with local community resources for emergency preparedness	Serve as patient advocate professional and health coach in a team approach in health care
Serve as "communication liaison" between the physician and patient	Identify and respond to issues of confidentiality	Educate patients in their responsibilities relating to third-party reimbursements	
Serve as patient advocate professional and health coach in a team approach in health care			
Identify basics of office emergency preparedness			

Clinical Skills

FUNDAMENTAL PRINCIPLES	DIAGNOSTIC PROCEDURES	PATIENT CARE
Identify the roles and responsibilities of the medical assistant in the clinical setting	Collect and process specimens	Perform initial-response screening following protocols approved by supervising physician
Identify the roles and responsibilities of other team members in the medical office	Perform CLIA-waived tests	Obtain, evaluate, and record patient history using critical thinking skills
Apply principles of aseptic technique and infection control	Perform electrocardiography and respiratory testing	Obtain vital signs
Practice standard precautions, including handwashing and disposal of biohazardous materials	Perform phlebotomy, including venipuncture and capillary puncture	Prepare and maintain examination and treatment areas
Perform sterilization techniques	Use knowledge of principles of radiology	Prepare patient for examinations, procedures, and treatments
Comply with quality assurance practices		Assist with examinations, procedures, and treatments
		Maintain examination/treatment rooms, including inventory of supplies and equipment
		Prepare and administer oral and parenteral (excluding IV) medications and immunizations (as directed by supervising physician and as permitted by state law)
		Use knowledge of principles of IV therapy
		Maintain medication and immunization records
		Screen and follow up on test results
		Recognize and respond to emergencies

Continued

Table 1-1 General, Clinical, and Administrative Skills* of the CMA (AAMA)—cont'd

Administrative Skills	
ADMINISTRATIVE PROCEDURES	**PRACTICE FINANCES**
Schedule, coordinate, and monitor appointments	→ Perform procedural and diagnostic coding for reimbursement
Schedule inpatient/outpatient admissions and procedures	→ Perform billing and collection procedures
→ Apply third-party and managed care policies, procedures, and guidelines	→ Perform administrative functions, including bookkeeping and financial procedures
Establish, organize, and maintain patient medical record	→ Prepare submittable ("clean") insurance forms
File medical records appropriately	

AAMA, American Association of Medical Assistants; *CLIA,* Clinical Laboratories Improvement Act; *CMA,* certified medical assistant; *IV,* intravenous.

*All skills require decision making based on critical thinking concepts.

MEDICAL INSURANCE SPECIALIST CERTIFICATE PROGRAM

PROGRAM DESCRIPTION: The Medical Insurance program prepares you for employment in the area of medical insurance and health care claims processing. This program also serves the needs of health care personnel interested in upgrading their professional skills. Training in computerized medical billing, CPT-4 and ICD-9-CM coding, and processing medical insurance claims are included in the curriculum. Students may be enrolled on a full-time or part-time basis, and may complete the program by attending either day or evening classes. Accelerated or fasttrack courses are also available for those wishing to complete this program within a short time period. The program graduates students with marketable skills that are in demand. They are employed in hospitals, insurance companies, private medical laboratories, billing bureaus, and doctors' offices. Graduates may apply credits toward other certificate or associate degree programs.

The following courses are included in this program:

First Semester

Medical Terminology	3 Credits
Administrative Medical Office Management	4 Credits
Biology	3 Credits
Keyboarding	3 Credits
Computer I	2 Credits
	TOTAL 15 Credits

Second Semester

Principles and Applications of Medical Insurance	3 Credits
Current Issues of Medical Insurance	3 Credits
Medical Financial Management	3 Credits
Word Processing	3 Credits
Basic Principles of Composition	3 Credits
	TOTAL 15 Credits

FIGURE 1-4 Example of a 1-year medical insurance specialist certificate program offered at a community college. Basic coding is taught as a part of the course in Administrative Medical Office Management, and advanced coding is covered in Principles and Applications of Medical Insurance. Biology may be titled Anatomy and Physiology in some colleges. (Reprinted with permission from Community College of Allegheny County, Pittsburgh, PA.)

A moderate to high degree of knowledge of the health insurance business is necessary if your goal is to become a self-employed insurance billing specialist or claims assistance professional. In addition to insurance terminology, claims procedures, and coding, you must know commercial third-party payers' requirements, as well as Medicare and state Medicaid policies and regulations. You also need human relations skills and proficiency in running a business including marketing and sales expertise.

To reach a professional level, certification is available from many national associations, depending on the type of certification desired. Refer to Chapter 18 for more information on this topic.

Career Advantages

Jobs are available in every state, ranging from nonmanagement to management positions. Insurance billing specialists can receive a salary of $8000 part-time to $50,000 full-time or more per year, depending on knowledge, experience, duties, responsibilities, locale, and size of the employing institution. Jobs are available in consulting firms, insurance and managed care companies, clinics, hospitals, multispecialty medical groups, and private physicians' practices. You can also be an instructor, a lecturer, or a consumer advocate. You can be your own boss by either setting up an in-home billing service or establishing an office service for billing.

Self-Employment or Independent Contracting

After gaining some experience, many people establish independently owned and self-operated businesses within their communities as medical insurance billing specialists, coders, claim assistance professionals, or collectors. However, the responsibilities are greater in this area because such work demands a full-time commitment, a lot of hard work, long hours to obtain clients, and the need to advertise and market the business. This means you are responsible for everything: advertising, billing, bookkeeping, and so on. Some billers work from their homes, and others rent or lease an office. If you eventually plan on self-employment and you are weak in an area, such as accounting, then take a bookkeeping course. Chapter 18 discusses setting up your own business.

Flexible Hours

Another advantage of this career field is the opportunity to have flexible hours. Most other employees in the physician's office must adhere to the physician's schedule. However, the medical insurance billing specialist may want to come in early to transmit electronic claims during off-peak hours or stay late to make collection calls. It may be advantageous to both the physician and insurance specialist to vary his or her schedule according to the needs of the practice. In-home or office billing services save a medical practice valuable time, money, and overhead costs because the physician does not have to cover benefits or equipment.

Disabled Workers

A career as an insurance billing specialist or a collector of delinquent accounts can be rewarding for persons with disabilities. These jobs are for individuals who have current knowledge of health care insurance billing, as well as state and federal collection laws. Interacting well with people both in person and by telephone is essential in these roles. The financial management responsibilities and other jobs involving telephone communications are an opportunity for someone who is visually impaired because he or she is usually a good listener when properly and specifically trained. Special equipment may be necessary to enhance job performance such as a Braille keyboard, magnified computer screen, audible scanner, or digital audio recorder.

Working independently from a home office may appeal to a physically disabled person when there is no need to commute to a physician's office on a daily basis. Accessing information remotely via the computer and fax machine is a manageable method for success. However, it is important first to gain experience before trying to establish a home office business.

The government amended the Rehabilitation Act in 1998 to "require Federal agencies to make their electronic and information technology accessible to people with disabilities" because inaccessible technology may obviously interfere with one's ability to obtain and use information quickly and easily. Section 508 was enacted to diminish barriers in information technology. This makes new opportunities available for people with disabilities. You can learn more by visiting the Section 508 website listed in the Internet Resources at the end of this chapter.

Inquire at your local vocational rehabilitation center for training disabled individuals. Specific to being a delinquent account collector, you may contact ACA International (formerly known as the American Collectors Association [ACA]) in Minneapolis (the website is http://www.acainternational.org), which has developed a training program for the visually impaired. Chapter 10 is devoted to the topic of collections.

Qualifications

Attributes

An individual must have a variety of characteristics or qualities to function well as an insurance billing specialist. Strong critical thinking and reading skills with good comprehension are a must. Being a logical and practical thinker, as well as a creative problem solver, is important. Being meticulous and neat makes it easier to get the job done at the workstation. A person with good organizational skills who is conscientious and loyal is always an asset to the employer. Because a large amount of specific data must be obtained, this work requires an individual who is detail oriented. A person with a curious nature will dig deeper into an issue and not be satisfied with an answer unless the "whys" and "whats" are defined. This also helps one to grow while on the job and not become stagnant. This list is by no means complete; perhaps you can think of additional attributes that might lead to a more successful career.

Skills

A person who completes insurance claims must have many skills. One needs the following skills to be proficient:

- Solid foundation and working knowledge of medical terminology, including anatomy, physiology, disease, and treatment terms, as well as the meanings of abbreviations.
   Application: Interpretation of patient's chart notes and code manuals.
   Incorrect: Final diagnosis: ASHD.
   Correct: Final diagnosis: Arteriosclerotic heart disease.
   Locating the diagnostic code using an abbreviation is difficult; therefore you must be able to translate it.
- Expert use of procedural and diagnostic code books and other related resources.
   Application: Code manuals and other reference books are used to assign accurate codes for each case billed.
- Precise reading skills.
   Application: Differentiate between technical descriptions of two different but similar procedures.
   Procedure (CPT) Code No. 43352 Esophagostomy (fistulization of esophagus, external; cervical approach).
   Procedure (CPT) Code No. 43020 Esophagotomy (cervical approach, with removal of foreign body).
   Note that the additional letter "s" to the surgical procedure in the first part of the example changes the entire procedure.
- Basic mathematics.
   Application: Calculate fees and adjustments on the insurance claim forms and enter into the patient accounts. It is essential that these figures be accurate.
- Knowledge of medicolegal rules and regulations of various insurance programs.
   Application: Avoid filing of claims considered fraudulent or abusive because of code selection and program policies.
- Knowledge of compliance issues.
   Application: Federal Privacy, Security, Transaction rules in addition to Fraud, Waste, and Abuse. For further information, see Chapter 2.
- Basic keyboarding and computer skills.
   Application: Good keyboarding and data entry skills and knowledge of computer programs are essential because the industry increasingly involves practice management software and electronic claims submission; handwritten claims are a format of the past.

- Proficiency in accessing information through the Internet.
   Application: Obtain federal, state, and commercial insurance regulations and current information as needed through the Internet. Sign on as a member of a **list service (listserv),** which is a service run from a website where questions may be posted. Find one composed of working coders to obtain answers on how to code complex, rare, or difficult medical cases.
- Knowledge of billing and collection techniques.
   Application: Use latest billing and collection ideas to keep cash flow constant and avoid delinquent accounts.
- Expertise in the legalities of collection on accounts.
   Application: Avoid lawsuits by knowing state and federal collection laws as they apply to medical collection of accounts receivable.
- Generate insurance claims with speed and accuracy.
   Application: If you develop your own business as a medical claims and billing specialist, you may be paid according to the amount of paid claims the health care practice is reimbursed. Because you will rely on volume for an income, the more expeditious you become, the more money you earn. Therefore accuracy in selecting the correct codes and data entry and motivation in completing claims also become marketable skills. Measure your correct claim productivity for precision and time when you complete the insurance claim forms for this course and see how many accurate claims you can generate.

Personal Image

To project a professional image, be attentive to apparel and grooming (Figure 1-5). If a person works at home, the tendency is to dress casually (e.g., blue jeans, sneakers, shorts, and tank tops). In a work setting, however, a uniform may be required, or you might be expected to wear business attire that is conservative and stylish but not trendy. For women, this includes a business suit, dress, or skirt of appropriate length; slacks; sweaters; blouses; and dress shoes. For men, a business suit or dress slacks and jacket, shirt, tie (optional), and dress shoes are appropriate.

When hired, it is important to discuss appropriate dress code with the supervisor. Keep in mind that fragrances can be offensive or cause allergies to some clients and patients; therefore use good judgment. Fingernails should be carefully manicured and appropriate to the dress code. For a woman, subdued eye makeup is appropriate for day use. Consult the employer for office policy regarding body piercing and tattoos.

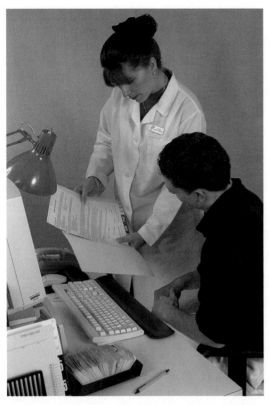

FIGURE 1-5 Male and female medical personnel who project a clean, fresh, and professional image.

Remember that you are in a professional environment and must present yourself in such a way.

Behavior

Many aspects make an individual a true professional: getting along with people rates high on the list, as does maintaining confidentiality of patients' medical histories and ongoing medical treatment. An insurance billing specialist depends on many co-workers for information needed to bill claims (e.g., the receptionist who collects the patient information). Therefore it is necessary to be a team player and treat patients and co-workers with courtesy and respect. Consider all co-workers' duties as important because they are part of the team helping you reach the goal of processing the billing and obtaining maximum reimbursement for the patient and physician. Communicate effectively. Be honest, dependable, and on time. Never take part in office gossip or politics. Be willing to do the job and be efficient in how you carry it out.

MEDICAL ETIQUETTE

Before beginning work as an insurance billing specialist, it is wise to have a basic knowledge of medical **etiquette** as it pertains to the medical profession, the insurance industry, and the medical coder (Figure 1-6). Medical

FIGURE 1-6 Interaction of insurance billing specialist with patient, depicting medical etiquette.

etiquette has to do with how medical professionals conduct themselves. Customs, courtesy, and manners of the medical profession can be expressed in three simple words: *consideration for others.*

In every business that interacts with customers or clients, the focus begins with good customer service. The Service to Patients box in this chapter emphasizes this point; if you did not read it, go back and do so now. If you work in an office in which patients go by your desk, acknowledge them with a smile, a nod, or a greeting. Patients may arrive for their appointments ill or injured and suffering from a lot of negativity. If a mistake is made, there is power in an apology given at the first sign of trouble. Attentiveness and a helpful, friendly atmosphere can smooth out the kinks and wrinkles of stressful and negative situations. All people have the need to feel special, and they go toward individuals who make them feel that way. All of these personal skills mean good customer service and satisfaction and can lead to professional success for you and the medical practice.

Several points about medical etiquette bear mentioning, as follows:

1. Never keep another physician who wants to talk about a medical case to your physician/employer waiting longer than necessary in the reception room. Usher him or her into the physician's office as soon as it is unoccupied.
2. Always connect another physician who is calling on the telephone to your physician immediately, asking as few questions as possible. The only exception is if you know the physician calling is treating one of your patients and you wish to verify the name to pull the chart or other data for your physician.
3. Follow the basic rules of etiquette with co-workers while working in the office such as acknowledging

people who enter your office or come to your desk by saying, "I'll be with you in a moment."

4. Identify yourself to callers and people you call.
5. Do not use first names until you know it is appropriate to do so.
6. Maintain a professional demeanor and a certain amount of formality when interacting with others. Remember to be courteous and always project a professional image.
7. Observe rules of etiquette when sending e-mail messages and placing or receiving cell phone calls. These rules fall under the Health Insurance Portability and Accountability Act (HIPAA) and are stated in detail in Chapters 2 and 4.

MEDICAL ETHICS

Medical **ethics** are not laws but standards of conduct generally accepted as moral guides for behavior by which an insurance billing or coding specialist may determine the propriety of his or her conduct in a relationship with patients, the physician, co-workers, the government, and insurance companies. You are entrusted with holding patients' medical information in confidence, collecting money for your physician, and being a reliable resource for your co-workers. Acting with ethical behavior means carrying out responsibilities with integrity, decency, honesty, competence, consideration, respect, fairness, trust, and courage.

The earliest written code of ethical principles and conduct for the medical profession originated in Babylonia about 2500 BC and is called the *Code of Hammurabi*. Then, about the fifth century BC, Hippocrates, a Greek physician who is known as the "Father of Medicine," conceived the Oath of Hippocrates.

In 1980 the **American Medical Association (AMA)** adopted a modern code of ethics, called the *Principles of Medical Ethics*, for the benefit of the health professional and to meet the needs of changing times. The Principles of Medical Ethics of the AMA (Box 1-1) guide physicians' standards of conduct for honorable behavior in the practice of medicine.

It is the coder's responsibility to inform administration or his or her immediate supervisor if unethical or possibly illegal coding practices are taking place. Illegal activities are subject to penalties, fines, and/or imprisonment and can result in loss of morale, reputation, and the good will of the community. Standards of ethical coding developed by the AHIMA are available at its website (see Internet Resources at the end of this chapter).

The following are principles of ethics for the insurance billing specialist:

- Never make critical remarks about a physician to a patient or anyone else. Maintain dignity; never belittle patients.
- In certain circumstances, it may be unethical for two physicians to treat the same patient for the same condition. Always notify your physician if you discover that a patient in your practice may have questionable issues of care, conduct, or treatment with your office or another physician's practice.
- Maintain a dignified, courteous relationship with all persons in the office—patients, staff, and the physician—as well as with insurance adjusters, pharmaceutical representatives, and others who come into or telephone the office.
- Do not make critical statements about the treatment given a patient by another physician.

Box 1-1   Principles of Medical Ethics of the American Medical Association

Preamble

The medical profession has long subscribed to a body of ethical statements developed primarily for the benefit of the patient.

As a member of the profession, a physician must recognize responsibility not only to patients, but also to society, to other health professionals, and to self. The following principles adopted by the American Medical Association are not laws but standards of conduct that define the essentials of honorable behavior for the physician.

I. A physician shall be dedicated to providing competent medical service with compassion and respect for human dignity.

II. A physician shall deal honestly with patients and colleagues, and strive to expose those physicians deficient in character or competence, or who engage in fraud or deception.

III. A physician shall respect the law and also recognize a responsibility to seek changes in those requirements that are contrary to the best interests of the patient.

IV. A physician shall respect the rights of patients, of colleagues and of other health professionals, and shall safeguard patient confidences within the constraints of the law.

V. A physician shall continue to study, apply, and advance scientific knowledge; make relevant information available to patients, colleagues, and the public; obtain consultation; and use the talents of other health professionals when indicated.

VI. A physician shall, in the provision of appropriate patient care, except in emergencies, be free to choose whom to serve, with whom to associate, and the environment in which to provide medical services.

VII. A physician shall recognize a responsibility to participate in activities contributing to an improved community.

Anyone who uses the Internet for health-related reasons has a right to expect that organizations that provide health products, services, or information online will uphold ethical principles. The Internet Healthcare Coalition has developed an eHealth Code of Ethics, which is available at its website (see Internet Resources at the end of this chapter).

It is *illegal* to report incorrect information to government-funded programs such as Medicare, Medicaid, and TRICARE. Federal legislation has been passed on fraud and abuse issues that relate to federal health care programs. Chapter 2 explains in detail the Criminal False Claims Act and HIPAA mandates. However, private third-party payers operate under different laws, and it is *unethical but may not be illegal, depending on state laws,* to report incorrect information to private third-party payers. Incorrect information may damage the individual and the integrity of the database, allow reimbursement for services that should be paid by the patient, or deny payment that should be made by the insurance company.

Examples of illegal and unethical coding follow:

1. Violating guidelines by using code numbers or modifiers to increase payment when the case documentation does not warrant it.

2. Coding services or procedures that were not performed for payment.
3. Unbundling services provided into separate codes when one code is available and includes all the service.
4. Failing to code a relevant condition or complication when it is documented in the health record, or vice versa, assigning a code without documentation from the provider.
5. Coding a service in such a way that it is paid when usually it is not covered.
6. Coding another condition as the principal or primary diagnosis when most of the patient's treatment is for the preexisting condition.

The AHIMA has established a code of ethics. This code is appropriate for persons handling health information, whether they are health information specialists, insurance billing specialists, or coders (Figure 1-7).

In the final analysis, most ethical issues can be reduced to right and wrong, with the main focus being the moral dictum to do no harm.

EMPLOYER LIABILITY

As mentioned, insurance billing specialists can be either self-employed or employed by physicians, clinics, or hospitals. Physicians are legally responsible for their own

Preamble
This Code of Ethics sets forth ethical principles for the health information management profession. Members of this profession are responsible for maintaining and promoting ethical practices. This Code of Ethics, adopted by the American Health Information Management Association, shall be binding on health information management professionals who are members of the Association and all individuals who hold an AHIMA credential.

  I. Health Information management professionals respect the rights and dignity of all individuals.
  II. Health information management professionals comply with all laws, regulations, and standards governing the practice of health information management.
  III. Health information management professionals strive for professional excellence through self-assessment and continuing education.
  IV. Health information management professionals truthfully and accurately represent their professional credentials, education, and experience.
  V. Health information management professionals adhere to the vision, mission, and values of the Association.
  VI. Health information management professionals promote and protect the confidentiality and security of health records and health information.
  VII. Health information management professionals strive to provide accurate and timely information.
  VIII. Health information management professionals promote high standards for health information management practice, education, and research.
  IX. Health information management professionals act with integrity and avoid conflicts of interest in the performance of their professional and AHIMA responsibilities.

FIGURE 1-7 AHIMA Code of Ethics, revised and adopted by AHIMA House of Delegates, October 4, 1998. (From American Health Information Management Association *Journal of AHIMA* 70(1): p. 1 of insert before p. 17, 1999. Copyright 1999 by the American Health Information Management Association. All rights reserved. No part of this may be reproduced, reprinted, stored in a retrieval system, or transmitted, in any form or by any means, electronic, photocopying, recording, or otherwise, without the prior written permission of the association.)

conduct and any actions of their employees performed within the context of their employment. This is referred to as *vicarious liability*, also known as **respondeat superior,** which literally means "let the master answer." However, this does not mean that an employee cannot be sued or brought to trial. Actions of the insurance biller may have a definite legal ramification on the employer, depending on the situation. For example, if an employee knowingly submits a fraudulent Medicare or Medicaid claim at the direction of the employer and subsequently the business is audited, both the employer and employee can be brought into litigation by the state or federal government. An insurance biller always should check with his or her physician-employer to determine whether he or she is included in the medical professional liability insurance policy, otherwise known as *malpractice insurance.* If not included, he or she could be sued as an individual. It is the physician's responsibility to make certain all staff members are protected.

CONFIDENTIALITY

An insurance billing specialist must be held responsible for maintaining confidentiality when working with patients and their records. The next chapter presents information related to the privacy issues of the Health Insurance Portability and Accountability Act (HIPAA).

EMPLOYEE LIABILITY

Billers and coders can be held personally responsible under the law for billing errors and have been listed as defendants in billing-fraud lawsuits. If you knowingly submit a false claim or allow such a claim to be submitted, you can be liable for a civil violation. If you conceal information or fail to disclose it to obtain payment, you can be held liable. If you are not the person preparing a false claim, but you mail or electronically file it, you can be implicated in mail or wire fraud.

Errors and omissions insurance is protection against loss of money caused by failure through error or unintentional omission on the part of the individual or service submitting the insurance claim. Some physicians may contract with a billing service to handle claims submission, and some agreements contain a clause stating that the physician will hold the company harmless from "liability resulting from claims submitted by the service for any account." This means the physician is responsible for mistakes made by the billing service. Thus errors and omissions insurance would not be necessary in this instance. If a physician asks the insurance biller to do something that is the least bit questionable, such as

writing off patient balances for certain patients automatically, make sure you have a legal document or signed waiver of liability relieving you of the responsibility for such actions. If you notice a problem, it is your responsibility to correct it and to document your actions in writing.

SCOPE OF PRACTICE

An individual who works as a CAP acts as an informal representative of patients (policyholders and Medicare beneficiaries), helping them to obtain insurance reimbursement. A CAP reviews and analyzes existing or potential policies, renders advice, and offers counseling, recommendations, and information. A CAP may not interpret insurance policies or act as an attorney. The legal ability of a CAP to represent a policyholder is limited. When a claim cannot be resolved after a denied claim has been appealed to the insurance company, the CAP must be careful in rendering a personal opinion or advising clients that they have a right to pursue legal action. Always check in your state to see whether there is a scope of practice. In some states, a CAP could be acting outside the scope of the law by giving advice to clients on legal issues, even if licensed as an attorney but not practicing law full time. If the client wishes to take legal action, it is his or her responsibility to find a competent attorney specializing in contract law and insurance. In some states, giving an insured client advice on purchase or discontinuance of insurance policies is construed as being an insurance agent.

A number of states require CAPs to be licensed, depending on the services rendered to clients. CAPs who perform only the clerical function of filing health insurance claims do not have to be licensed. Check with your state's department of insurance and insurance commissioner (see Chapter 9) to determine whether you should be licensed.

If working as a CAP who does not handle checks or cash, inquire about an errors and omissions insurance policy by contacting the Alliance of Claims Assistance Professionals (ACAP).* When employed as a medical assistant who is submitting insurance claims, information on professional liability insurance may be obtained from the American Association of Medical Assistants, Inc.†

FUTURE CHALLENGES

As you begin your study to become an insurance billing specialist, remember that you are expected to profitably manage a medical practice's financial affairs or patient

---

*ACAP, 25500 Hawthorne Blvd., Suite 1158, Torrance, CA 90505.
†AAMA, 20 North Wacker Drive, Suite 1575, Chicago, IL 60606.

accounts, otherwise, you will not be considered qualified for this position. In subsequent chapters, you will learn the important information and skills to help you achieve this goal. You will be expected to do the following:

- Know billing regulations for each insurance program and managed care plan in which the practice is a participant.
- Know the aspects of compliance rules and regulations.
- State various insurance rules about treatment and referral of patients.
- Become proficient in computer skills and use of various medical software packages.
- Learn electronic billing software and the variances of each payer.
- Develop diagnostic and procedural coding expertise.

- Know how to interpret third-party remittance advice summary reports, explanation of benefit documents, or both.
- Attain bookkeeping skills necessary to post, interpret, and manage patient accounts.
- Keep current and stay up-to-date by reading the latest health care industry association publications, participating in e-mail listserv discussions, joining a professional organization for networking, and attending seminars on billing and coding.
- Cross-train so that you become familiar with other aspects of the medical practice.
- Strive toward becoming certified as an insurance billing specialist and/or coder, and once certified, seek continuing education credits to become recertified. Chapter 18 has more information about the professional organizations that offer certification.

KEY POINTS

This is a brief chapter review or summary of the key issues presented. To further enhance your knowledge of the technical subject matter, review the key terms and key abbreviations for this chapter by locating the meanings in the glossary at the end of this book, which appears in a section before the index.

1. The person who does billing for physicians has become a proficient specialist known by a number of job titles such as insurance billing specialist or reimbursement specialist.
2. Individuals who help patients organize and file claims are called claims assistance professionals.
3. Insurance claims must be promptly submitted to ensure continuous cash flow for a medical practice. If not, overhead expenses cannot be met, and a practice will face financial difficulties.
4. Because of the increased technical knowledge that a biller must have, education and training must be more comprehensive and skills must be developed in coding and claims completion. When proficiency is reached, a person can work for a medical practice or may possibly set up his or her own billing service. In this career, jobs can be rewarding for persons with disabilities.
5. Individuals who do billing and complete insurance claims must have many skills such as knowledge of

medical terminology and abbreviations, expert use of procedural and diagnostic code books, precise reading skills, ability to perform basic mathematic calculations, knowledge of medicolegal rules and regulations of various insurance programs, ability to understand and apply compliance issues, basic computer skills (keyboarding and software applications), proficiency in accessing information via the Internet, ability to carry out billing and collection techniques, expertise in the legalities of collection on accounts, and ability to generate insurance claims expediently and accurately.

6. Becoming a professional is a gradual process, and one must project an appropriate image and develop as a courteous and respectful team player.
7. Etiquette in a medical setting must be adhered to routinely, and one must behave ethically at all times.
8. A physician who employs an insurance billing specialist is legally responsible for any actions his or her employees performed within the context of their employment. This is referred to as vicarious liability, also known as *respondeat superior*.
9. Remember, ignorance of the law is not a protection for anyone working in the medical office, so one must stay up-to-date and well-informed on state and federal statutes.

℮volve INTERNET RESOURCES

For active links to the following resources, visit the Evolve website at
http://evolve.elsevier.com/fordney/handbook

- A list of educational and training requirements of the AHIMA diagnostic and procedure coding competencies for outpatient services and diagnostic coding and reporting requirements for physician billing.
- Standards of ethical coding developed by the American Health Information Management Association.

- eHealth Code of Ethics developed by the Internet Healthcare Coalition Organization.
- Section 508 of the Rehabilitation Act in 1998, which makes electronic and information technology accessible to people with disabilities.
- To join a professional organization for networking such as the American Academy of Professional Coders (AAPC).

STUDENT ASSIGNMENT

Read the Introduction in the *Workbook*, which explains how you will be working as an insurance billing specialist during this course.

✓ Study Chapter 1.

✓ Answer the fill-in-the-blank, multiple choice, and true/false questions in the *Workbook* to reinforce the theory learned in this chapter and help prepare for a future test.

✓ Complete the assignments in the *Workbook* to help develop critical thinking and writing skills. As you proceed through the assignments in the *Workbook*, you will broaden your knowledge of medical terminology and gain an entry-level skill in diagnostic and procedural coding and insurance claim completion.

✓ Turn to the glossary at the end of this textbook for a further understanding of the key terms and key abbreviations used in this chapter.

KEY TERMS*

abuse
authorization
authorization form
breach of confidential
   communication
business associate
clearinghouse
code set
compliance
compliance plan
confidential communication
confidentiality
consent

consent form
covered entity
disclosure
e-health information
   management
electronic media
embezzlement
fraud
health care provider
individually identifiable health
   information
nonprivileged information
Notice of Privacy Practices

phantom billing
privacy
privacy officer, privacy official
privileged information
protected health information
security officer
Security Rule
standard
state preemption
transaction
use

KEY ABBREVIATIONS*

CCI	EDI	HL7	OIG
CD	eHIM	IIHI	ORT
CDT	FBI	MIP	OSHA
CLIA	FCA	NCVHS	P&P
CMS	FDIC	NDC	PHI
CPT	FTP	NHII	PO
DHHS	HCFAP	NPP	TCS
DOJ	HIPAA	OCR	TPO

*Definitions for the key terms and key abbreviations are located near the back of this textbook in the glossary.

CHAPTER 2

HIPAA Compliance and Privacy in Insurance Billing

OBJECTIVES

After reading this chapter, you should be able to:

- Define e-health information management (eHIM).
- Describe the initiative that is working toward development of a personal health record created and controlled by the individual or family.
- Name the two provisions of the Health Insurance Portability and Accountability Act (HIPAA) that relate most to health care.
- Explain the difference between Title I Insurance Reform and Title II Administrative Simplification.
- Describe the federal standards under HIPAA.
- Define protected health information (PHI).
- Identify the difference between disclosure and use of PHI.
- Illustrate the difference between privileged and nonprivileged information.

- Explain the Privacy Rule as it pertains to PHI.
- Explain the differences between a Notice of Privacy Practices (NPP), a consent, and an authorization when disclosing PHI.
- List the three major categories of security safeguards under HIPAA.
- State the guidelines for HIPAA privacy compliance.
- List the civil and criminal penalties of noncompliance with HIPAA regulations.
- List various types of insurance fraud.
- Define abuse as it relates to the subject of billing insurance claims.

Service to Patients

The insurance billing specialist has many opportunities to serve patients' needs. When presenting the Notice of Privacy, greet the patient with a smile and a helpful and caring attitude. Be ready to answer questions regarding the notice. Have the notice available in those languages spoken by a significant portion of the medical practice's patient population. Serve patients by respecting their privacy and keeping protected health information confidential, disclosing it only according to the medical practice's correct policies and procedures that comply with federal regulations.

Communicate your physician's commitment to improve quality of care and to ensure patient safety by avoiding errors.

Use of electronic formats in the health care industry is a driving force behind electronic communications that will make a full circle to complete the patient care process. It is your duty to understand how health information and electronic technologies tie together. As an educated and informed employee, you can better serve the patients who visit your office.

Performance objectives, testing and review material, and hands-on practical exercises for this chapter are available in these resources:

 The Insurance Handbook Student Workbook   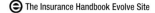 The Insurance Handbook Evolve Site

COMPLIANCE DEFINED

Compliance in the health care industry is the process of meeting regulations, recommendations, and expectations of federal and state agencies that pay for health care services and regulate the industry. Health care compliance encompasses the claims reimbursement processes, managed care procedures, Occupational Safety and Health Administration (OSHA), Clinical Laboratory Improvement Amendments (CLIA), licensure, and due diligence in obeying the law.

Any business that is involved with the health care industry must conform its practices to follow the principles and practices as identified by state and federal agencies. The professional elements of the principles and practices include the following:

- Regulations and recommendations to protect individuals
- Streamline processes
- Supporting system-wide stability

A compliance strategy provides a standardized process for handling business functions, much like a "user's manual." This will enable consistent and effective management and staff performance. Failure to comply with mandates leads to sanctions and fines from state and federal agencies. Failure to follow guidelines potentially results in more fraud and abuse in the claims reimbursement cycle.

HEALTH INFORMATION USING ELECTRONIC TECHNOLOGIES

Over the past decade, the United States (US) health care system has undergone rapid change with regard to the separate issues of privacy, security, and claims processing. A number of organizations have participated to help standardize and improve the delivery and quality of health care.

Some code systems and additional terminology have been created by the adoption of the many federal statutes. In this chapter, you will learn some important key terms related to health information as it pertains to compliance and its role in electronic technology. You will also get acquainted with important initiatives that control the use of health information. In subsequent chapters, you will learn many more terms and read more in-depth discussions on certain subjects related to compliance with government regulations that affect health care. These appear as color-screened sections titled "HIPAA Compliance Alert."

e-Health Information Management

e-Health information management, more commonly seen as eHIM, is a term coined by the American Health Information Management Association's eHealth Task Force to describe any and all transactions in which health care information is accessed, processed, stored, and transferred using electronic technologies.

National Health Information Infrastructure

The National Health Information Infrastructure (NHII) is an initiative set forth to improve patient safety and the quality of health care, as well as to better inform individuals regarding their own health information and to help them understand health care costs. It has also encouraged the use of computers and standardized electronic financial transactions.

NHII is overseen by the US Department of Health and Human Services (DHHS) with the National Committee on Vital and Health Statistics (NCVHS) serving as a public advisory committee (Box 2-1).

Health Level Seven

Health Level Seven (HL7) is a standards developing organization whose mission is "to provide standards for the exchange, management, and integration of data that support clinical patient care and the management, delivery, and evaluation of health care services. Specifically, to

---

Box 2-1   **National Health Information Infrastructure**

- An initiative to improve effectiveness, efficiency, and overall quality of health and health care in the United States
- A comprehensive knowledge-based network of interoperable systems of clinical, public health, and personal health information that would improve decision-making by making health information available when and where it is needed
- The set of technologies, standards, applications, systems, values, and laws that support all facets of individual health, health care, and public health
- Voluntary
- Not a centralized database of medical records or a government regulation
- The scope of the initiative, in addition to health care research, is as follows:
  - Personal health, which includes a personal health record created and controlled by the individual or family, plus nonclinical information, such as self-care trackers and directories of health care providers
  - Health care delivery, which includes information such as provider notes, clinical orders, decision-support programs, digital prescribing programs, and practice guidelines. Health care providers retain responsibility for their own patients' medical records.
  - Public health, which enables sharing of information to improve the clinical management of populations of patients such as vital statistics, population health risks, and disease registries

create flexible, cost-effective approaches, standards, guidelines, methodologies, and related services for interoperability between health care information systems." A **standard** means a rule, condition, or requirement.

Data exchanged between systems must share a well-defined knowledge of the meaning behind the data transferred; therefore part of HL7 focuses on efforts to manage vocabulary terms used in its messages. For example, this can be thought of as electronic (digital) supporting documentation. This collection of data is a stream of encoded information that translates into understandable language when it is received. For years, the insurance biller has been making a copy of a patient's paper chart note and attaching it to the CMS-1500 paper claim form. The health care industry's future looks to HL7 to expand the capabilities of submitting claims and to enable the transfer of the data contained within the health record without using paper at all! To get a general idea of HL7 in use, see Example 2-1.

Systematized Nomenclature of Human and Veterinary Medicine (SNOMED) International

SNOMED, a uniform lexicon system used for managing patient electronic health records (EHRs)—that is, medical records, teaching medical information science (informatics), indexing and managing research data, and billing for laboratory medicine procedure—is found in the book *Systematized Nomenclature of Human and Veterinary Medicine (SNOMED) International*, volumes I through IV. This code system is important because it helps standardize the terminology used in medical documentation. The Systematized Nomenclature of Medicine–Clinical Terminology

(SNOMED-CT) is a medical terminology classification system designed and created by the College of American Pathologists. It is used to code text data in EHRs and helps in standardizing clinical medical terminology. This topic is discussed in more detail in Chapter 5.

HEALTH INSURANCE PORTABILITY AND ACCOUNTABILITY ACT

The Health Insurance Portability and Accountability Act of 1996 (HIPAA), Public Law 104-191, has significant impact on both individuals and health care providers. Among five titles, two provisions of HIPAA relate most to health care, *Title I: Insurance Reform* and *Title II: Administrative Simplification*. HIPAA projects long-term benefits that include lowered administrative costs, increased accuracy of data, increased patient and customer satisfaction, and reduced revenue cycle time, ultimately improving financial management.

Title I: Health Insurance Reform

The primary purpose of HIPAA *Title I: Insurance Reform* is to provide continuous insurance coverage for workers and their insured dependents when they change or lose jobs. This aspect of HIPAA affects individuals as consumers, not particularly as patients. Previously, when an employee left or lost a job and changed insurance coverage, a "preexisting" clause prevented or limited coverage for certain medical conditions. HIPAA now limits the use of preexisting condition exclusions, prohibits discrimination for past or present poor health, and guarantees certain employers and individuals the right to purchase new health insurance coverage after losing a job. Additionally, HIPAA allows renewal of health insurance coverage regardless of an individual's health condition that is covered under the particular policy.

Title II: Administrative Simplification

The goals of HIPAA *Title II: Administrative Simplification* focus on the health care practice setting and aim to reduce administrative costs and burdens. Standardizing electronic transmissions of administrative and financial information reduces the number of forms and methods used in the claims processing cycle and reduces the nonproductive effort that goes into processing paper or nonstandard electronic claims. Additional provisions are meant to ensure the privacy and security of an individual's health data.

Two parts of the Administrative Simplification provisions are as follows:

1. Development and implementation of standardized electronic transactions using common sets of

---

Example 2-1 Health Level Seven Format of Date and Time of Birth

To determine the date and time of a patient's birth date (e.g., for a neonate, for whom the age in hours might be relevant), the time of the birth, using military time, can be recorded with the birth date. From this, the age can be generated from the date of birth (DOB). Baby Jane was born on March 24, 2012, at 8:26 am.

When the required Health Level Seven (HL7) format is YYYYMMDDHHMM, Baby Jane's date and time of birth will be entered for transmission as: 201203240826

YYYY	MM	DD	HH	MM
2012	03	24	08	26
Year	Month	Day	Hour	Minute

descriptors (i.e., standard code sets). These must be used to represent health care concepts and procedures when performing health-related financial and administrative activities electronically (i.e., standard transactions) (Box 2-2). HIPAA has been part of a great shift in processing electronic data. Transaction standards apply to the following, which are called covered entities under HIPAA: health care third-party payers, health care providers, and health care clearinghouses. A **clearinghouse** is an independent organization that receives insurance claims from the physician's office, performs software edits, and redistributes the claims electronically to various third-party payers.

2. Implementation of privacy and security procedures to prevent the misuse of health information by ensuring the following:
   ● Privacy and confidentiality
   ● Security of health information

Administrative simplification has created uniform sets of standards that protect and place limits on how confidential health information can be used. For years, health care providers have locked medical records in file cabinets and refused to share patient health information. Patients now have specific rights regarding how their health information is used and disclosed because federal and state laws regulate the protection of an individual's privacy. Knowledge and attention to the rights of patients are important to the compliance endeavor in a health care practice. Providers are entrusted with health information and are expected to recognize when certain health information can be used or disclosed.

Patients have the legal right to request (1) access and amendments to their health records, (2) an accounting of those who have received their health information, and (3) restrictions on who can access their health records. Understanding the parameters concerning these rights is crucial to complying with HIPAA.

Health care providers and their employees can be held accountable for using or disclosing patient health information inappropriately. HIPAA regulations will be enforced, as clearly stated by the US government. The revolution of HIPAA will take time to understand and implement correctly, but as the standards are put into action, both within the practice setting and across the many different fields comprising the health industry, greater benefits will be appreciated by the health care provider, staff, and patients.

Defining Roles and Relationships: Key Terms

HIPAA legislation required the *US Department of Health and Human Services* (DHHS or HHS*) to establish national standards and identifiers for electronic transactions, as well as implement privacy and security standards. In regard to HIPAA, *Secretary* refers to the HHS Secretary or any officer or employee of HHS to whom the authority involved has been delegated.

The Office of E-Health Standards and Services within the *Centers for Medicare and Medicaid Services* (CMS), previously known as the Health Care Financing Administration (HCFA), enforces the insurance portability and transaction and code set requirements of HIPAA for Medicare and Medicaid programs.

The *Office for Civil Rights* (OCR) enforces privacy and security rules.

Electronic media refers to the mode of electronic transmission, including the following:

● Internet (online mode—wide open)
● Extranet or private network using Internet technology to link business parties
● Leased telephone or dial-up telephone lines, including fax modems (speaking over telephone is not considered an electronic transmission)
● Transmissions that are physically moved from one location to another using magnetic tape, disk, or compact disk media

A **transaction** refers to the transmission of information between two parties to carry out financial or administrative activities related to health care. These data transmissions include information that completes the health care insurance claim process and are discussed further in Chapter 8.

Refer to Box 2-3 for titles of additional entities that oversee the HIPAA-related functions.

Box 2-2	Examples of Administrative and Financial Data	
Administrative Information	**Financial Information**
Referral certification and authorization for services	Health care claim submission for services
Enrollment/disenrollment of individual into health plan	Process health plan premium payment
Health plan eligibility	Check status of a previously submitted claim
	Health care payment and remittance advice
	Coordination of benefits

---

*Both DHHS and HHS are used throughout the textbook as abbreviations for Department of Health and Human Services.

Box 2-3 Overseers of HIPAA Functions

A **covered entity** transmits health information in electronic form in connection with a *transaction* covered by HIPAA. The covered entity may be (1) a health care coverage carrier such as Blue Cross/Blue Shield, (2) a health care clearinghouse through which claims are submitted, or (3) a health care provider such as the primary care physician.

A **business associate** is a person who, on behalf of the covered entity, performs or assists in the performance of a function or activity involving the use or disclosure of individually identifiable health information, including claims processing or administration, data analysis, processing or administration, utilization review, quality assurance, billing, benefit management, practice management, and repricing. For example, if a provider's practice contracts with an outside billing company to manage its claims and accounts receivable, the billing company would be a business associate of the provider (the covered entity).

A **health care provider** is a person trained and licensed to provide care to a patient and also a place that is licensed to give health care such as a hospital, skilled nursing facility, inpatient/outpatient rehabilitation facility, home health agency, hospice program, physician, diagnostic department, outpatient physical or occupational therapy, rural clinic, or home dialysis supplier.

Privacy and security officers oversee the HIPAA-related functions. These individuals may or may not be employees of a particular health care practice. A **privacy officer** or **privacy official (PO)** is designated to help the provider remain in compliance by setting policies and procedures (P&P) and by training and managing the staff regarding HIPAA and patient rights, and the PO is usually the contact person for questions and complaints.

A **security officer** protects the computer and networking systems within the practice and implements protocols such as password assignment, backup procedures, firewalls, virus protection, and contingency planning for emergencies.

Box 2-4 HIPAA Help

If a health care provider either transmits directly or uses a "business associate" (e.g., billing company or clearinghouse) to send information electronically for any of the transactions listed, the health care provider is a "covered entity" and must comply with HIPAA.

HIPAA requires the designation of a privacy officer or privacy official (PO) to develop and implement the organization's policies and procedures (P&P). The PO for an organization may hold another position within the practice or may not be an employee of the practice at all. Often, the PO is a contracted professional and available to the practice through established means of contact.

The business associate is often considered an extension of the provider practice. If an office function is outsourced with use or disclosure of individually identifiable health information, the organization that is acting on behalf of the health care provider is considered a business associate. For example, if the office's medical transcription is performed by an outside service, the transcription service is a business associate of the covered entity (the health care provider/practice). See Box 2-4.

HIPAA privacy regulations as a federal mandate apply unless the state laws are contrary or more stringent with regard to privacy. A state law is contrary if it is impossible to comply with the state law while complying with federal requirements or if the state law stands as an obstacle to the purposes of the federal law. **State preemption,** a complex technical issue not within the scope of the health care provider's role, refers to instances when state law takes precedence over federal law. The PO determines when the need for preemption arises.

HIPAA in the Practice Setting

The individuals mentioned in Box 2-3 create relationships that guide the health care provider and the practice. A health care provider can be a physician's assistant, nurse practitioner, social worker, chiropractor, radiologist, or dentist; HIPAA does not affect only medical physicians. The health care provider is designated as a HIPAA-mandated covered entity under certain conditions. It is important to remember that health care providers who transmit any health information in electronic form in connection with a HIPAA transaction are covered entities. Electronic form or media can include floppy disk, compact disk (CD), or file transfer protocol (FTP) over the Internet. Voice-over-modem faxes, meaning a telephone line, are not considered electronic media, although a fax from a computer (e.g., WinFax program) is considered an electronic medium.

THE PRIVACY RULE: CONFIDENTIALITY AND PROTECTED HEALTH INFORMATION

What I may see or hear in the course of the treatment or even outside of the treatment in regard to the life of men, which on no account one must spread abroad, I will keep to myself holding such things shameful to be spoken about.

Hippocrates, 400] G

The Hippocratic Oath, federal and state regulations, professional standards, and ethics all address patient privacy. Because current technology allows easy access to health care information, HIPAA imposes new requirements for health care providers. Since computers have become indispensable for the health care office, confidential health data have been sent across networks, e-mailed over the Internet, and even exposed by hackers, with few safeguards taken to protect data and prevent information from being intercepted or lost. With the implementation of standardizing electronic transactions of health care information, the use of technologies poses new risks for privacy and security. These concerns were addressed under HIPAA, and regulations now closely govern how the industry handles its electronic activities.

Privacy is the condition of being secluded from the presence or view of others. **Confidentiality** is using discretion in keeping secret information. Integrity plays an important part in the health care setting. Staff members of a health care organization need a good understanding of HIPAA's basic requirements and must be committed to protecting the privacy and rights of the practice's patients.

Disclosure means the release, transfer, provision of access to, or divulging in any other manner of information outside the entity holding the information. An example of a disclosure is giving information to the hospital's outpatient surgery center about a patient you are scheduling for a procedure.

Consent is the verbal or written agreement that gives approval to some action, situation, or statement. A **consent form** is not required before physicians use or disclose protected health information (PHI) for treatment, payment, or routine health care operations (TPO).

Treatment includes coordination or management of health care between providers or referral of a patient to another provider. PHI can be disclosed to obtain reimbursement. Other health care operations include performance reviews, audits, training programs, and certain types of fundraising (Figures 2-1 through 2-4).

Keep in mind that a HIPAA privacy consent is not the same as a consent to treat. Exceptions may occur based on specific state law requirements, an emergency situation, or a language barrier that makes consent impossible to obtain or when treating prison inmates.

Under the HIPAA Privacy Rule, **authorization** is an individual's formal, written permission to use or disclose his or her personally identifiable health information for purposes other than treatment, payment, or health care operations. For some "extra" activities, including marketing, research, and psychotherapy notes, an **authorization form** is necessary for use and disclosure of PHI that is not included in any existing consent form agreements. Documentation pertaining to psychiatric counseling is kept with the patient's medical records, but psychotherapy notes should be kept separate.

Individually identifiable health information (IIHI) is any part of an individual's health information, including demographic information (e.g., address, date of birth), collected from the individual that is created or received by a covered entity. This information relates to the individual's past, present, or future physical or mental health or condition; the provision of health care to the individual; or the past, present, or future payment for the provision of health care. IIHI data identify the individual or establish a reasonable basis to believe the information can be used to identify the individual. For example, if you as a health care provider are talking to an insurance representative, you will likely give information such as the patient's date of birth and last name. These pieces of information would make it reasonably easy to identify the patient. If you are talking to a pharmaceutical representative about a drug assistance program that covers a new pill for heartburn and you say that your practice has a patient living in your town who is indigent and has stomach problems, you are not divulging information that would identify the patient.

Protected health information (PHI) is any information that identifies an individual and describes his or her health status, age, sex, ethnicity, or other demographic characteristics, whether that information is or is not stored or transmitted electronically. It refers to IIHI that is transmitted by electronic media, maintained in electronic form or transmitted, or maintained in any other form or medium. PHI does not include IIHI in education records covered by the Family Educational Right and Privacy Act.

Traditionally, the focus was on protecting paper medical records and documentation that held patient's health information such as laboratory results and radiology reports. HIPAA Privacy Regulation expands these protections to apply to PHI. The individual's health information is protected regardless of the type of medium in which it is maintained. This includes paper, the health care provider's computerized practice management and billing system, spoken words, and x-ray films.

Use means the sharing, application, utilization, examination, or analysis of IIHI within an organization that holds such information. When a patient's billing record is accessed to review the claim submission history, the individual's health information is in "use."

HIPAA imposes requirements to protect not only disclosure of PHI outside of the organization but also for internal uses of health information. PHI may not be used or disclosed without permission of the patient or someone authorized to act on behalf of the patient, unless the use or disclosure is specifically required or permitted by the regulation (e.g., TPO). The two types of disclosure required by HIPAA Privacy Rule are to the individual who is the subject of the PHI and to the Secretary of DHHS to investigate compliance with the rule.

**REQUIRED ELEMENTS
OF HIPAA AUTHORIZATION**

Identification of person (or class) authorized to request

Identification of person (or class) to whom covered entity is to use/disclose

Description of information to be released with specificity to allow entity to know which information the authorization references

Description of each purpose of the requested use or disclosure

Expiration date, time period, or event

Statement that is revocable by written request

Individual's (patient's) signature and date

Statement of representative's authority

Authorization for Release of Information

PATIENT NAME: ___Levy_____Chloe_____E._____
                          LAST   FIRST   MI   MAIDEN OR OTHER NAME
DATE OF BIRTH: _02_ - _12_ - _1950_ SS# _320_ - _21_ - _3408_ MEDICAL RECORD #: _____3075_____
                          MO DAY YR
ADDRESS: _____3298 East Main Street_____ CITY: __Woodland Hills___ STATE: _XY_ ZIP: _12345-0001_

DAY PHONE: _____013-340-9800_____ EVENING PHONE: _____013-549-8708_____

I hereby authorize _____Gerald Practon, MD_____ **(Print Name of Provider) to release information from my medical record as indicated below to:**
NAME: _____Margaret L. Lee, MD_____
ADDRESS: _____328 Seward Street_____ CITY: ____Anytown____ STATE: _XY_ ZIP: _45601-0731_

PHONE: _____013-219-7698_____ FAX: _____013-290-9877_____

INFORMATION TO BE RELEASED:
                          DATES:
☒ History and physical exam   __6-8-20XX__
☐ Progress notes   _____
☐ Lab reports   _____
☐ X-ray reports   _____
☐ Other:_____   _____
_____   _____

| I specifically authorize the release of information relating to: |
| ☐ Substance abuse (including alcohol/drug abuse) |
| ☐ Mental health (including psychotherapy notes) |
| ☐ HIV related information (AIDS related testing) |
| X_____ |
| SIGNATURE OF PATIENT OR LEGAL GUARDIAN   DATE |

PURPOSE OF DISCLOSURE: ☐ Changing physicians   ☒ Consultation/second opinion   ☐ Continuing care
☐ Legal   ☐ School   ☐ Insurance   ☐ Workers Compensation
☐ Other (please specify):_____

1. I understand that this authorization will expire on _09/01/20XX_ (Print the Date this Form Expires) days after I have signed the form.

2. I understand that I may revoke this authorization at any time by notifying the providing organization in writing, and it will be effective on the date notified except to the extent action has already been taken in reliance upon it.

3. I understand that information used or disclosed pursuant to this authorization may be subject to redisclosure by the recipient and no longer be protected by Federal privacy regulations.

4. I understand that if I am being requested to release this information by _____Gerald Practon, MD_____ (Print Name of Provider) for the purpose of:
   _____

   a. By authorizing this release of information, my health care and payment for my health care will not be affected if I do not sign this form.
   b. I understand I may see and copy the information described on this form if I ask for it, and that I will get a copy of this form after I sign it.
   c. I have been informed that _____Gerald Practon, MD_____ (Print Name of Provider) will/will not receive financial or in-kind compensation in exchange for using or disclosing the health information described above.

5. I understand that in compliance with _____XY_____ (Print the State Whose Laws Govern the Provider) statute, I will pay a fee of $ _5.00_ (Print the Fee Charged). There is no charge for medical records if copies are sent to facilities for ongoing care or follow up treament.

___*Chloe E. Levy*_____ __*6/1/XX*__ OR _____
SIGNATURE OF PATIENT   DATE   PARENT/LEGAL GUARDIAN/AUTHORIZED PERSON   DATE

                                             ☐
_____ _____ _____
RECORDS RECEIVED BY   DATE   RELATIONSHIP TO PATIENT

| FOR OFFICE USE ONLY |
| DATE REQUEST FILLED_____ BY: _____ |
| IDENTIFICATION PRESENTED_____ FEE COLLECTED $_____ |

FIGURE 2-1 Completed authorization for release of information form for a patient relocating to another city. The figure indicates the required elements for HIPAA authorization. Note: This form is used on a one-time basis for reasons other than treatment, payment, or health care operations. When the patient arrives at the new physician's office, a consent for treatment, payment, or health care operations form will need to be signed. (From *Federal Register* 64(212): Appendix to Subpart E of Part 164: Model Authorization Form, November 3, 1999.)

NAME OF FACILITY
Consent for Release of Information

Date _May 16, 20XX_

1. I hereby authorize _College Hospital_ to release the following information from the
   <u>Name of Institution</u>
   health record(s) of _Martha T. Jacobson_
   <u>Patient name</u>

   52 East Rugby Street, Woodland Hills, XY 12345
   <u>Address</u>

   covering the period(s) of hospitalization from:
   Date of Admission _January 3, 20XX_
   Date of Discharge _January 5, 20XX_
   Hospital # _278-1200_   Birthdate _June 27, 1960_
2. Information to be released:
   ☐ Copy of (complete) health record(s)   ☑ Discharge summary
   ☐ History and physical   ☐ Operative report
   ☐ Other _____
3. Information is to be released to: _Michael Hotta, MD_
   260 West Main Street, Woodland Hills, XY 12345
4. Purpose of disclosure _June 14, 20XX consultation_

5. I understand this consent can be revoked at any time except to the extent that disclosure
   made in good faith has already occurred in reliance to this consent.
6. Specification of the date, event, or condition upon which this consent expires:
   December 31, 20XX
7. The facility, its employees and officers, and attending physician are released from legal
   responsibility or liability for the release of the above information to the extent indicated and
   authorized herein.

Signed _Martha T. Jacobson_
<u>(Patient or Representative)</u>

<u>(Relationship to Patient)</u>
May 16, 20XX
<u>(Date of Signature)</u>

FIGURE 2-2 Consent for Release of Information form to a hospital. (Reprinted with permission from the American Health Information Management Association. Copyright 2010 by the American Health Information Management Association. All rights reserved.)

Confidential Information

The insurance billing specialist must be responsible for maintaining confidentiality of patients' health information when working with patients and their medical records. Example 2-2 lists some of the PHI that is typical in a medical office that falls under HIPAA compliance regulations.

The patient record and any photographs obtained are confidential documents and require an authorization form that must be signed by the patient to release information (see Figures 2-1 through 2-4). If the form is a photocopy, it is necessary to state that the photocopy is approved by the patient, or write to the patient and obtain an original signed document.

Example 2-2 Protected Health Information in a Medical Office

Intake forms	Encounter sheets
Laboratory work requests	Physician's notes
Physician-patient conversations	Prescriptions
Conversations that refer to patients by name	Insurance claim forms
Physician dictation tapes	X-rays
Telephone conversations with patients	E-mail messages

COLLEGE CLINIC
4567 Broad Avenue
Woodland Hills, XY 12345-0001
Phone: 555/486-9002
Fax: 555/487-8976

CONSENT TO THE USE AND DISCLOSURE OF HEALTH INFORMATION

I understand that this organization originates and maintains health records which describe my health history, symptoms, examination, test results, diagnoses, treatment, and any plans for future care or treatment. I understand that this information is used to:

- plan my care and treatment
- communicate among health professionals who contribute to my care
- apply my diagnosis and services, procedures, and surgical information to my bill
- verify services billed by third-party payers
- assess quality of care and review the competence of healthcare professionals in routine healthcare operations

I further understand that:

- a complete description of information uses and disclosures is included in a *Notice of Information Practices* which has been provided to me
- I have a right to review the notice prior to signing this consent
- the organization reserves the right to change their notice and practices
- any revised notice will be mailed to the address I have provided prior to implementation
- I have the right to object to the use of my health information for directory purposes
- I have the right to request restrictions as to how my health information may be used or disclosed to carry out treatment, payment, or health care operations
- the organization is not required to agree to the restrictions requested
- I may revoke this consent in writing, except to the extent that the organization has already taken action in reliance thereon.

☐ I request the following restrictions to the use or disclosure of my health information.

_____

_____   _____
Date   Notice Effective Date

_____   _____
Signature of Patient or Legal Representative   Witness

_____   _____
Signature   Title

Date _____   __ Accepted __ Rejected

FIGURE 2-3 An example of a consent form used to disclose and use health information for treatment, payment, or health care operations. This is not required under HIPAA, but you may find that some medical practices use it. (From Fordney MT, French L: *Medical insurance billing and coding: a worktext*, Philadelphia, 2003, Elsevier.)

Exceptions to HIPAA

Unauthorized release of information is called **breach of confidential communication** and is considered a HIPAA violation, which may lead to fines.

Confidentiality between the physician and patient is automatically waived in the following situations:

1. When the patient is a member of a managed care organization (MCO) and the physician has signed a contract with the MCO that has a clause that says "for quality care purposes, the MCO has a right to access the medical records of their patients, and for utilization management purposes," the MCO has a right to audit those patients' financial records. Other managed care providers need to know about the patients if

FIGURE 2-4 Patient signing a consent form.

involved in the care and treatment of members of the MCO.

2. When patients have certain communicable diseases that are highly contagious or infectious and state health agencies require providers to report, even if the patient does not want the information reported.
3. When a medical device breaks or malfunctions, the Food and Drug Administration requires providers to report certain information.
4. When a patient is suspect in a criminal investigation or to assist in locating a missing person, material witness, or suspect, police have the right to request certain information.
5. When the patient's records are subpoenaed or there is a search warrant. The courts have the right to order providers to release patient information.
6. When the patient is suing someone, such as an employer, and wishes to protect herself or himself.
7. When there is a suspicious death or suspected crime victim, providers must report cases.
8. When the physician examines a patient at the request of a third party who is paying the bill, as in workers' compensation cases.
9. When state law requires the release of information to police that is for the good of society such as reporting cases of child abuse, elder abuse, domestic violence, or gunshot wounds.

For information on confidentiality as it relates to computer use, refer to Chapter 8.

The purpose of the Privacy Rule is to ensure that patients who receive medical treatment may have control in the manner in which specific information is used and to whom it is disclosed. **Confidential communication** is a privileged communication that may be disclosed only with the patient's permission. Everything you see, hear, or read about patients remains confidential and does not leave the office. Never talk about patients or data

contained in medical records where others may overhear. Some employers require employees to sign a confidentiality agreement (Figure 2-5). Such agreements should be updated periodically to address issues raised by the use of new technologies.

Privileged Information

Privileged information is related to the treatment and progress of the patient. The patient must sign an authorization to release this information or selected facts from the medical record. Some states have passed laws allowing certain test results (e.g., disclosure of the presence of the human immunodeficiency virus [HIV] or alcohol or substance abuse) and other information to be placed separate from the patient's medical record. A special authorization form is used to release this information.

Nonprivileged Information

Nonprivileged information consists of ordinary facts unrelated to treatment of the patient, including the patient's name, city of residence, and dates of admission or discharge. This information must be sensitized against unauthorized disclosure under the privacy section of HIPAA. The patient's authorization is not necessary for the purposes of treatment, payment, or health care operations, unless the record is in a specialty hospital (e.g., alcohol treatment) or a special service unit of a general hospital (e.g., psychiatric unit). Professional judgment is required. The information is disclosed on a legitimate need-to-know basis, meaning that the medical data should be revealed to the attending physician because the information may have some effect on the treatment of the patient.

Patients' Rights
Right to Privacy

All patients have a right to privacy. It is important never to discuss patient information other than with the physician, an insurance company, or an individual who has been authorized by the patient. If a telephone inquiry is made and you need to verify that callers are who they say they are, you should do the following:

● Ask for one or more of the following items: patient's full name, home address, date of birth, Social Security number, mother's maiden name, or dates of service.
● Ask for a call-back number and compare it with the number on file.
● Ask the patient to fax a sheet with his or her signature on it so that you can compare it with one on file.
● Some hospitals may assign a code word or number that may be a middle name or date that is easy for patients

EMPLOYEE CONFIDENTIALITY STATEMENT

As an employee of _____ABC Clinic, Inc._____ (employer), having been trained as an insurance billing specialist with employee responsibilities and authorization to access personal medical and health information, and as a condition of my employment, I agree to the following:

A. I recognize that I am responsible for complying with the Health Insurance Portability and Accountability Act (HIPAA) of 1996 policies regarding confidentiality of patients' information, which, if I violate, may lead to immediate dismissal from employment and, depending on state laws, criminal prosecution.

B. I will treat all information received during the course of my employment, which relates to the patients, as confidential and privileged information.

C. I will not access patient information unless I must obtain the information to perform my job duties.

D. I will not disclose information regarding my employer's patients to any person or entity, other than that necessary to perform my job duties, and as permitted under the employer's HIPAA policies.

E. I will not access any of my employer's computer systems that currently exist or may exist in the future using a password other than my own.

F. I will safeguard my computer password and will not show it in public.

G. I will not allow anyone, including other employees, to use my password to access computer files.

H. I will log off of the computer immediately after I finish using it.

I. I will not use e-mail to transmit patient information unless instructed to do so by my employer's HIPAA privacy officer.

J. I will not take patient information from my employer's premises in hard copy or electronic form without permission from my employer's HIPAA privacy officer.

K. Upon termination of my employment, I agree to continue to maintain the confidentiality of any information learned while an employee and agree to relinquish office keys, access cards, or any other device that provides access to the provider or its information.

Mary Doe
_____
Signature

September 14, 20XX
_____
Date

Mary Doe
_____
Print name

Brenda Shield
_____
Witness

FIGURE 2-5 An example of an employee confidentiality agreement that may be used by an employer when he or she is hiring an insurance billing specialist.

to remember. If a patient does not know the code word, then ask for personal identifying information as mentioned.

If a telephone inquiry is made about a patient, ask the caller to put the request in writing and include the patient's signed authorization. If the caller refuses, have the physician return the call. If a relative telephones asking about a patient, have the physician return the call. When you telephone a patient about an insurance matter and reach voice mail, use care in the choice of words when leaving the message in the event the call was inadvertently received at the wrong number. Leave your name, the office name, and the return telephone number. Never attempt to interpret a report or provide information about the outcome of laboratory or other diagnostic tests to the patient. Let the physician do it (Figure 2-6).

Do's and Don'ts of Confidentiality

Don't: Discuss a patient with acquaintances, yours or the patient's.

Don't: Leave patients' records or appointment books exposed on your desk. If confidential documents are on your desk and patients can easily see them as they walk by, either turn the documents over or lock them in a secure drawer when you leave your desk, even if you are gone for only a few moments.

FIGURE 2-6 Insurance billing specialist consulting with the supervisor/office manager about office policies regarding release of a patient's medical record.

Don't: Leave a computer screen with patient information visible, even for a moment, if another patient may see the data. If patient information is on your computer, either turn the screen off or save it on disk, lock the disk in a secure place, and clear the information from the screen.

Do: Properly dispose of notes, papers, and memos by using a shredding device.

Do: Be careful when using the copying machine because it is easy to forget to remove the original insurance claim or medical record from the document glass.

Do: Use common sense and follow the guidelines mentioned in this chapter to help you keep your professional credibility and integrity.

Privacy Rules: Patient Rights Under HIPAA

Patients are granted the following six federal rights that allow them to be informed about PHI and to control how their PHI is used and disclosed:

1. *Right to **Notice of Privacy Practices (NPP),*** a document in plain language that is usually given to the patient at the first visit or at enrollment. The staff must make a reasonable "best effort" to obtain a signature from the patient acknowledging receipt and this must be done once only. If the patient cannot or will not sign, this should be documented in the patient's health record. The NPP must be posted at every service delivery site and available in paper form for those who request it. A provider's website must have the NPP placed on the site and must deliver a copy electronically on request.

2. *Right to request restrictions on certain uses and disclosures of PHI.* Patients have the right to ask for restrictions on how a medical office uses and discloses PHI for TPO (e.g., a patient had a successfully treated sexually transmitted disease many years before and requests that, whenever possible, this material not be disclosed). A provider is not required to agree to these requests but must have a process to review the requests, accept and review any appeal, and give a sound reason for not agreeing to the request. Restrictions must be documented and followed. See Box 2-5, which details the regulations for disclosing the minimum necessary PHI, de-identification of PHI, marketing related to the patient, and fundraising activities related to patients.

3. *Right to request confidential communications* by alternative means or at an alternative location (e.g., call at work rather than at the residence or test results sent in writing instead of by telephone). The patient does not need to explain the reason for the request. The health care office must have a process in place to both evaluate requests and appeals and respond to the patient. Patients may be required by the office to make their request in writing. Such a document protects the practice's compliance endeavors.

4. *Right to access (inspect and obtain a copy of) PHI.* Privacy regulations allow the provider to require the patient make the request for access in writing. Generally, a request must be acted on within 30 days. A reasonable, cost-based fee for copies of PHI may only include the costs for supplies and labor for copying, postage when mailed, and preparing a summary of the PHI if the patient has agreed to this instead of complete access. If a digital office copier is used, be sure precautions are taken to digitally shred information after every copy, print scan, or fax job so that information is kept secure.

Under HIPAA Privacy Regulation, patients do not have the right to access the following:

● Psychotherapy notes (Box 2-6)
● Information compiled in reasonable anticipation of, or for use in, legal proceedings
● Information exempted from disclosure under the Clinical Laboratory Improvement Amendments (CLIA)

The office may deny patient access for the previously mentioned reasons without giving the patient the right to review the denial.

If the health care provider has determined that the patient would be endangered (or cause danger to another person) from accessing the confidential health information, access may be denied. In this case, the patient has the right to have the denial reviewed by another licensed professional who did not participate in the initial denial decision.

Box 2-5 HIPAA Help

These key terms are addressed in the Notice of Privacy Practices (NPP) that apply to the patient's right to request restrictions on certain uses and disclosures of protected health information (PHI).

- **Minimum Necessary.** Privacy regulations require that use or disclosure of only the minimum amount of information necessary to fulfill the intended purpose be permitted. There are some exceptions to this rule. You do not need to limit PHI for disclosures in regard to health care providers for treatment, the patient, DHHS for investigations of compliance with HIPAA, or as required by law.

  Minimum Necessary determinations for *uses of PHI* must be determined within each organization, and reasonable efforts must be made to limit access to only the minimum amount of information needed by identified staff members. In smaller offices, employees may have multiple job functions. If a medical assistant helps with the patient examination, documents vital signs, and then collects the patient's copayment at the reception area, the assistant will likely access clinical and billing records. Simple procedure and policy (P&P) about appropriate access to PHI may be sufficient to satisfy the Minimum Necessary requirement. Larger organizations may have specific restrictions on who should have access to different types of PHI because staff members tend to have a more targeted job role. Remain knowledgeable about your office's policy regarding Minimum Necessary. If you are strictly scheduling appointments, you may not need access to the clinical record. An x-ray technician will likely not need to access the patient billing records.

  Minimum Necessary determinations for *disclosures of PHI* are distinguished by two categories within the Privacy Rule:
  1. For disclosures made on a routine and recurring basis, you may implement policies and procedures, or standard protocols, for what will be disclosed. These disclosures would be common in your practice. Examples may include disclosures for workers' compensation claims or school physical forms.
  2. For other disclosures that would be considered nonroutine, criteria should be established for determining the Minimum Necessary amount of PHI and to review

each request for disclosure on an individual basis. A staff member (e.g., privacy officer [PO], medical records supervisor) will likely be assigned to determine this situation when the need arises.

As a general rule, remember that you must limit your requests to access PHI to the Minimum Necessary to accomplish the task for which you will need the information.

- **De-identification of Confidential Information.** Other requirements relating to uses and disclosures of PHI include health information that does not identify an individual or leaves no reasonable basis to believe that the information can be used to identify an individual. This "de-identified" information is no longer individually identifiable health information (IIHI). Most providers will never have the need to de-identify patient information, and the requirements for de-identifying PHI are lengthy. The regulations give specific directions on how to ensure all pieces of necessary information are removed to fit the definition. De-identified information is not subject to the privacy regulations because it does not specifically identify an individual.

- **Marketing.** When communicating about a product or service, the goal is to encourage patients to purchase or use the product or service. For example, a dermatologist may advertise for a discount on facial cream when you schedule a dermabrasion treatment. You will likely not be involved in marketing, but keep in mind the general rule that PHI (including names and addresses) cannot be used for marketing purposes without specific authorization of the patient. Sending appointment reminders and general news updates about your organization and the services you provide would not be considered marketing and would not require patient authorization.

- **Fundraising.** Again, you will likely not be involved in fundraising activities, but HIPAA allows demographic information and dates of care to be used for fundraising purposes without patient authorization. The disclosure of any additional information requires patient authorization. Your organization's NPP will state that patients may receive fundraising materials and are given the opportunity to opt out of receiving future solicitations.

Box 2-6 HIPAA Help

According to the HIPAA Privacy Rule, the term *psychotherapy notes* means notes that are recorded (in any medium) by a health care provider who is a mental health professional documenting or analyzing the contents of conversation during a private counseling session or a group, joint, or family counseling session and that are separated from the rest of the individual's medical record.

professional, not all information gathered and recorded in the health record of the mental health provider is considered psychotherapy notes. The law lists the following specific items that are excluded from such notes:

- Medication prescription and monitoring
- Counseling session start and stop times
- Modalities and frequencies of treatment furnished
- Results of clinical tests
- Any summary of the following items: diagnosis, functional status, treatment plan, symptoms, prognosis, and progress to date

In general, the major difference between what are and are not considered psychotherapy notes is the information that is the *recorded (in any manner) documentation and/or analysis of conversation.* This information should also be kept separate from the medical section of the patient

Regarding psychotherapy notes, HIPAA gives special protection to PHI. Disclosure of a patient's mental health records requires specific patient permission. This means that when an insurance payer requests the health records to review the claim, a patient authorization is required.

Certain clinical data are excluded from the definition of psychotherapy notes. In other words, when an individual is using the services of a mental health

health record to be distinguished as psychotherapy notes. For example, Jane Doe tells her psychologist the details of her childhood trauma. The documented conversation specific to her trauma (e.g., what occurred, how she felt) is considered the psychotherapy notes and cannot be released without specific permission from Jane Doe.

It is also important to understand that patients do not have the right to obtain a copy of psychotherapy notes under HIPAA. However, the treating mental health provider may decide when a patient may obtain access to this health information.

State law must always be considered. Some states allow patients access to their psychotherapy notes; therefore state law would take precedence over HIPAA as a result of the state preemption allowance.

5. *Right to request an amendment of PHI.* Patients have the right to request that their PHI be amended. As with the other requests, the provider may require the request to be in writing. The provider must have a process to accept and review both the request and any appeal in a timely fashion. The health care provider may deny this request in the following circumstances:
   - The provider who is being requested to change the PHI is not the creator of the information (e.g., office has records sent by referring physician).
   - The PHI is believed to be accurate and complete as it stands in the provider's records.
   - The information is not required to be accessible to the patient (see item 4: *Right to access (inspect and obtain a copy of) PHI*).

Generally, the office must respond to a patient's request for amendment within 60 days. If a request is denied, the patient must be informed in writing of the reason for the denial. The patient must also be given the opportunity to file a statement of disagreement.

6. *Right to receive an accounting of disclosures of PHI.* Providers should maintain a log of disclosures of PHI, either on paper or within the organization's computer system, of all disclosures other than those made for TPO, facility directories, and some national security and law enforcement agencies. The process for providing an accounting should be outlined in the practice's policy manual. Patients may request an accounting (or tracking) of disclosures of their confidential information and are granted the right to receive this accounting once a year without charge. Additional accountings may be assessed a cost-based fee.

These accountings started on April 14, 2003, when privacy regulations became enforceable. Items to be documented must include the following:

- Date of disclosure
- Name of the entity or person who received the PHI, including their address, if known

- Brief description of the PHI disclosed
- Brief statement of the purpose of the disclosure

The patient is entitled to one accounting per year free of charge. Additional accountings may be assessed a cost-based fee. See Boxes 2-7 and 2-8.

Verification of Identity and Authority

Before any disclosure, you must verify the identity of persons requesting PHI if they are unknown to you. You

---

Box 2-7 HIPAA Help

In summary, **patients have the right to** the following:
- Be informed of the organization's privacy practices by receiving a Notice of Privacy Practices (NPP).
- Have their information kept confidential and secure.
- Obtain a copy of their health records.
- Request to have their health records amended.
- Request special considerations in communication.
- Restrict unauthorized access to their confidential health information.

   Patients cannot keep their confidential health information from being used for treatment, payment, or health care operations (TPO) nor may they force amendments to their health record. As you become more acclimated to your organization's policies and procedures regarding the handling of protected health information (PHI), you will be better able to recognize how your position is an important part in HIPAA compliance.

Box 2-8 HIPAA Help

Health care providers and staff will likely not be reading the *Federal Register* and thus will want to familiarize themselves with the general forms used in their practice setting. They should be aware of the following:
- **Written acknowledgment:** After providing the patient with the Notice of Privacy Practices (NPP), a "good faith" effort must be made to obtain written acknowledgment of the patient receiving the document. If the patient refuses to sign or is unable to sign, this must be documented in the patient record.
- **Authorization forms:** Use and disclosure of protected health information (PHI) is permissible for treatment, payment, or health care operations (TPO) because the NPP describes how PHI is used for these purposes. The health care provider is required to obtain signed authorization to use or disclose health information for situations beyond the TPO. This is a protection for the practice. Providers must learn about the particular "authorization" forms used in their office. Psychotherapy notes are handled separately under HIPAA. Such notes have additional protection, specifically that an authorization for any use of disclosure of psychotherapy notes must be obtained.

   Your organization will be expected to handle requests made by patients to exercise their rights. You must know your office's process for dealing with each specific request. With your understanding of HIPAA and your organization's policy manual, you will be guided in procedures specific to your health care practice.

may request identifying information such as date of birth, Social Security number, or even a code word stored in your practice management system that is unique to each patient. Public officials may present badges, credentials, official letterheads, and other legal documents of authority for identification purposes.

Additionally, you must verify that the requestor has the right and the need to have the PHI. Exercising professional judgment fulfills your verification requirements for most disclosures because you are acting on "good faith" in believing the identity of the individual requesting PHI. It is good practice when making any disclosure to note the "authority" of the person receiving the PHI and how this was determined. This evidence of due diligence on your part would enforce a needed structure on your staff and dampen any complaints that might arise.

Validating Patient Permission

Before making any uses or disclosures of confidential health information other than for the purposes of TPO, your office must have appropriate patient permission. Always check for conflicts between various permissions your office may have on file for a given patient (Table 2-1). This information should be maintained either in your practice management system or in the medical chart, where it can be easily identified and retrieved.

For example, if a covered entity has agreed to a patient's request to limit how much of the PHI is sent to a consulting physician for treatment, but then received the patient's authorization to disclose the entire medical record to that physician, this would be a conflict. In general, the more restrictive permission would be the deciding factor. Privacy regulations allow resolving conflicting permissions by either obtaining new permission from the patient or communicating orally or in writing with the patient to determine the patient's preference. Be sure to document any form of communication in writing.

Training

Under HIPAA regulations, a covered entity must train all members of its workforce. This training must include the practice's P&P with respect to PHI as "necessary and appropriate for the members of the workforce to carry out their function within the covered entity." This training will address how your role relates to PHI in your office, and you will be instructed on how to handle confidential information. The PO for your health care practice will likely be the instructor for this type of training. HIPAA training focuses on how to handle confidential information securely in the office, as discussed later.

Safeguards: Ensuring That Confidential Information Is Secure

Every covered entity must have appropriate safeguards to ensure the protection of an individual's confidential health information. Such safeguards include administrative, technical, and physical measures that will "reasonably safeguard" PHI from any use or disclosure that violates HIPAA, whether intentional or unintentional (Box 2-9).

Complaints to Health Care Practice and Workforce Sanctions

Individuals, both patients and staff, must be provided with a process to make a complaint concerning the P&P of the covered entity. If a violation involves the misuse of PHI, this incident should be reported to the practice's PO. Should there be further cause, the OCR may also be contacted.

Workforce members are subject to appropriate sanctions for failure to comply with the P&P regarding PHI set forth in the office. Types of sanctions applied vary, depending on factors involved with the violation. Sanctions can range from a warning to suspension to termination. This information should be covered in the P&P manual. Written documentation of complaints and sanctions must be prepared with any disposition.

Mitigation

Mitigation means to "alleviate the severity" or "make mild." In reference to HIPAA, the covered entity has an affirmative duty to take reasonable steps in response to breaches. If a breach is discovered, the health care provider is required to mitigate, to the extent possible, any harmful effects of the breach. For example, if you learn you have erroneously sent medical records by fax to an incorrect party, steps should be taken to have the recipient destroy the PHI. Mitigation procedures also include activities of the practice's business associates. Being proactive and responsible by mitigating reduces the potential for a more disastrous outcome from the breach or violation.

Refraining From Intimidating or Retaliatory Acts

HIPAA privacy regulations prohibit a covered entity from intimidating, threatening, coercing, discriminating against, or otherwise taking retaliatory action against the following:

● Individuals for exercising HIPAA privacy rights
● Individuals for filing a complaint with HHS; for testifying, assisting, or participating in an investigation

Table 2-1   Title II Administrative Simplification: Uses and Disclosures of Protected Health Information

PERMITTED DISCLOSURES (NO AUTHORIZATION REQUIRED)	WHAT IT MEANS FOR YOUR PRACTICE
Disclose PHI to patient	You may discuss the patient's own medical condition with him or her. **Doing so does not require signed authorization from the patient.**
Disclose PHI for treatment	Treatment includes speaking with the patient, ordering tests, writing prescriptions, coordinating his or her care, and consulting with another health care provider about the patient. **"Treatment" does not require signed authorization from the patient.**
Disclose PHI for payment	Payment includes obtaining the patient's eligibility or benefits coverage information from the insurance payer, obtaining preapproval for treatment, and billing and managing the claims process. **"Payment" does not require signed authorization from the patient.**
Disclose PHI for health care operations	Do not confuse this with performing surgery. The term *health care operations* refers to the business activities in which your organization participates. Examples include case management, certification, accreditation, medical reviews, and audits to detect fraud and abuse. **"Operations" do not require signed authorization from the patient.**
Disclose PHI for public purposes	PHI may be disclosed for public health purposes such as reporting a communicable disease, injury, child abuse, domestic violence, judicial and administrative proceedings, law enforcement, coroner or medical examiner, or research purposes if PHI is "de-identified." This is not an all-inclusive list, but **these examples do not require signed authorization from the patient.**
Disclose PHI for workers' compensation	You may disclose PHI as authorized by the laws relating to workers' compensation. Such disclosures to programs that provide benefits for work-related injuries or illness **do not require signed authorization from the patient.**
DISCLOSURES THAT REQUIRE PATIENT'S OPPORTUNITY TO AGREE OR OBJECT	**WHAT IT MEANS FOR YOUR PRACTICE**
Disclose PHI to persons involved with the patient	You must provide patients with an opportunity to object to sharing PHI with family, friends, or others involved with their care. The health care provider can use professional judgment when disclosing PHI to a person involved with the patient's care when the patient is not present. **This requires the patient to have the opportunity to agree or object.**
DISCLOSURES (AUTHORIZATION REQUIRED)	**WHAT IT MEANS FOR YOUR PRACTICE**
Disclose psychotherapy	Psychotherapy notes may not be disclosed without authorization except for use by the notes' originator (therapist) for treatment. **Signed authorization IS required.**
Disclose PHI to a child's school for permission to participate in sports	You may not disclose a child's PHI to the school to permit the student's participation in a sports activity. **Signed authorization IS required.**
Disclose PHI to employer	You may not disclose PHI to a patient's employer unless the information is necessary to comply with Occupational Safety and Health Administration (OSHA), Mine Safety and Health Administration (MSHA), or other state laws. **With certain exceptions, signed authorization IS required.**
Disclose PHI to insurer	You may not disclose PHI to an insurer for underwriting/eligibility without authorization from the patient (e.g., if the patient is trying to obtain a life insurance policy). **Signed authorization IS required.**
Disclose PHI for fundraising	If your health care practice does fundraising or marketing, you may not disclose PHI without prior authorization from the patient. **Signed authorization IS required.**

PHI, Protected health information.

Box 2-9   Examples of Safeguards

Administrative	Technical	Physical
Verifying the identity of an individual picking up health records	User name/password required to access patient records from computer	Locked, fireproof filing cabinets for storing paper records

about the covered entity's privacy practices; or for reasonably opposing any practice prohibited by the regulation

TRANSACTION AND CODE SET REGULATIONS: STREAMLINING ELECTRONIC DATA INTERCHANGE

Under Title II Administrative Simplification, the HIPAA *Transaction and Code Set* (TCS) regulation was developed to introduce efficiencies into the health care system. The purposes and objectives are to achieve a higher quality of care and to reduce administrative costs by streamlining the processing of routine administrative and financial transactions. HHS has estimated that by implementing TCS, almost $30 billion over 10 years would be saved. A **code set** is any set of codes with their descriptions used to encode data elements such as tables of terms, medical concepts, medical diagnostic codes, or medical procedure codes.

Technology and the use of *electronic data interchange* (EDI) have made the processing of transactions more efficient and reduced administrative overhead costs in other industries. EDI is the exchange of data in a standardized format through computer systems. Standardizing transactions and code sets is required to use EDI effectively, with the implementation of standard formats, procedures, and data content.

TCS regulation required the implementation of specific standards for transactions and code sets by October 16, 2003. The intent of TCS requirements is to achieve a single standard. As an example in the pre-HIPAA environment, when submitting claims for payment, health care providers did business with insurance payers who required the use of their own version of local code sets (e.g., state Medicaid programs) or identifiers and paper forms. Before HIPAA, more than 400 versions of a *National Standard Format* (NSF) existed to submit a claim

for payment. HIPAA will streamline the standards and enable greater administrative efficiencies throughout the health care system. As these methods are adapted, health care provider offices will benefit from less paperwork, and standardizing data will result in more accurate information and a more efficient organization (Table 2-2).

Medical code sets are data elements used uniformly to document why patients are seen (diagnosis, ICD-9-CM) and what is done to them during their encounter (procedure, CPT-4, and HCPCS). Each covered entity organization is responsible for implementing the updated codes in a timely manner, using the new HIPAA-mandated TCS codes and deleting old or obsolete ones (Table 2-3).

HIPAA also provides standards for the complete cycle of administrative transactions and electronic standard formats, which are presented in detail in Chapter 8 (Box 2-10).

Standard Unique Identifiers

The use of standard unique identifiers improves efficiency in the management of health care by simplifying administration systems. This enables the efficient electronic transmission of certain health information used across the industry, as follows:

- *Standard Unique Employer Identifier* (use employer identification number [EIN] to identify employers; compliance was required on July 30, 2004). The EIN will be used to identify employers rather than input the actual name of the company. Employers can use their EINs to identify themselves in transactions involving premium payments to health plans on behalf of their employees or to identify themselves or other employers as the source or receiver of information about eligibility. Employers can also use EINs to identify themselves in transactions when enrolling or disenrolling employees in a health plan.

Table 2-2	Title II Administrative Simplification: Recognized Benefits of TCS and EDI
BENEFIT	**RESULT**
More reliable and timely processing	Fast eligibility evaluation; reduced accounts receivable cycle; industry averages for claim turnarounds are 9 to 15 days for electronic versus 30 to 45 days for paper claims
Quicker reimbursement from payer	Improves cash flow for the health care organization
Improved accuracy of data	Decreases processing time, increases data quality, and leads to better reporting
Easier and more efficient access to information	Improves patient support
Better tracking of transactions	Assists tracking of transactions (i.e., when sent and received), allowing for monitoring (e.g., prompt payments)
Reduction of data entry/manual labor	Electronic transactions assist automated processes (e.g., automated labor payment posting)
Reduction in office expenses	Reduces office supplies, postage, and telephone charges

EDI, Electronic data interchange; *TCS,* transaction and code set.

Table 2-3	Medical Code Sets	
CODE SET	**ORGANIZATION**	**UPDATE**
Current Procedural Terminology (CPT)	American Medical Association (AMA)	Annually; changes go into effect each January 1; Category III codes update in January and July.
Code on Dental Procedures and Nomenclature (CDT)	American Dental Association (ADA)	
National Drug Codes (NDC)	Food and Drug Administration (FDA)	Daily; see www.fda.gov/cder for quarterly updates.
Health Care Common Procedure Coding System (HCPCS)	Centers for Medicare and Medicaid Services (CMS)	Major update January 1; periodic updates throughout the year as needed.
International Classification of Diseases Clinical Modification (ICD-9-CM and ICD-10)	Department of Health and Human Services (DHHS)	Annually; changes go into effect each October 1 for Medicare claims.

Box 2-10 HIPAA Help

When a patient comes into your office and is treated, his or her confidential health information is collected and put into the computerized practice management system. The services rendered are assigned a standard code from the HIPAA-required code sets (e.g., CPT), and the diagnosis is selected from another code set (e.g., ICD-9-CM), much the same as before HIPAA.

When claims are generated for electronic submission, all data collected are compiled and constructed into a HIPAA standard transaction. This electronic data interchange (EDI) is recognized across the health care sector in computer systems maintained by providers, the clearinghouses, and insurance payers. The harmony among the covered entities results in a more efficient claim life cycle.

- *Standard Unique Health Care Provider Identifier.* This is a 10-digit number for the health care provider and is assigned permanently—a lifetime number. It is known as the National Provider Identifier (NPI) number and providers began applying for this number on May 23, 2005.
- *Standard Unique Health Plan Identifier.* The Final Rule was published January 23, 2004 and became effective May 23, 2005.
- *Standard Unique Patient Identifier.* The intention to create a standard for a uniform patient identifier prompted protest among public interest groups, who saw a universal identifier as a civil liberties threat. Therefore the issue of a universal patient identifier is on hold indefinitely.

THE SECURITY RULE: ADMINISTRATIVE, PHYSICAL, AND TECHNICAL SAFEGUARDS

The **Security Rule** comprises regulations related to the security of *electronic* protected health information (ePHI) along with regulations related to electronic transactions and code sets, privacy, and enforcement, which make up the Administrative Simplification HIPAA provisions. Security measures encompass all the administrative, physical, and technical safeguards in an information system. The Security Rule addresses only ePHI, but the concept of preserving PHI that will become ePHI makes attention to security for the entire office important. The policies and procedures required by the Security Rule must be maintained for 6 years. The Security Rule is divided into three main sections: administrative safeguards, technical safeguards, and physical safeguards.

Administrative safeguards prevent unauthorized use or disclosure of PHI through administrative actions and P&P to manage the selection, development, implementation, and maintenance of security measures to protect ePHI.

Technical safeguards are technologic controls in place to protect and control access to information on computers in the health care organization.

Physical safeguards also prevent unauthorized access to PHI. These physical measures and P&P protect a covered entity's electronic information systems and related buildings and equipment from natural and environmental hazards and unauthorized intrusion.

More about the Security Rule is discussed in Chapter 8.

Guidelines for HIPAA Privacy Compliance

As an insurance billing specialist, you will likely answer the telephone and speak during the course of your business, and there will be questions about what you can and cannot say. Reasonable and appropriate safeguards must be taken to ensure that all confidential health information in your office is protected from unauthorized and inappropriate access, including both verbal and written forms.

Some of the following situations may be referred to as incidental disclosures, and this topic is discussed in further detail with additional examples later in this chapter.

1. Consider that conversations occurring throughout the office could be overheard. The reception area and waiting room are often linked, and it is easy to hear the scheduling of appointments and exchange of confidential information. It is necessary to observe areas and maximize efforts to avoid unauthorized disclosures. Simple and affordable precautions include using privacy glass at the front desk and having conversations away from settings where other patients or visitors are present. Health care providers can move their dictation stations away from patient areas or wait until no patients are present before dictating. Telephone conversations by providers in front of patients, even in emergency situations, should be avoided. Providers and staff must use their best professional judgment.

2. Be sure to check in the patient medical record and in your computer system to determine whether there are any special instructions for contacting the patient regarding scheduling or reporting test results. Follow these requests as agreed by the office.

3. Patient sign-in sheets are permissible, but limit the information you request when a patient signs in and change it periodically during the day. A sign-in sheet must not contain information such as reason for visit or the patient's medical condition because some providers specialize in treating patients with sensitive issues. Thus showing that a particular individual has an appointment with your practice may pose a breach of patient confidentiality.

4. Make sure you have patients sign a form acknowledging receipt of the NPP. The NPP allows you to release the patient's confidential information for billing and other purposes. If your practice has other confidentiality statements and policies besides HIPAA mandates, these must be reviewed to ensure they meet HIPAA requirements.

5. Formal policies for transferring and accepting outside PHI must address how your office keeps this information confidential. When using courier services, billing services, transcription services, or e-mail, you must ensure that transferring PHI is done in a secure and compliant manner. Identifying data that must be removed from e-mail before being sent are name of patient; address information other than city, state, and ZIP code; telephone and fax numbers; e-mail address; Social Security number; medical record number; health plan beneficiary number; account number; certificate/license numbers; vehicle identifier; device identifiers; device serial number; website address; biometric identifiers; full-face photograph;

geographic subdivisions smaller than state; dates (except for years) related to birth, death, admission, and discharge; and any other unique identifying number, code, or characteristic, unless otherwise permitted.

6. Computers are used for a variety of administrative functions, including scheduling, billing, and managing medical records. Computers are typically present at the reception area. Keep the computer screen turned so that viewing is restricted to authorized staff. Screen savers should be used to prevent unauthorized viewing or access. The computer should automatically log off the user after a period of being idle, requiring the staff member to reenter his or her password.

7. Keep your user name and password confidential and change them often. Do not share this information. An authorized staff member, such as the PO, will have administrative access to reset your password if you lose it or if someone discovers it. Also, practice management software can track users and follow their activity. Do not set yourself up by giving out your password. Safeguards include password protection for electronic data and storing paper records securely.

8. Safeguard your work area; do not place notes with confidential information in areas that are easy to view by nonstaff. Cleaning services will access your building, usually after business hours; ensure that you safeguard PHI.

9. Place medical record charts face down at reception areas so that the patient's name is not exposed to other patients or visitors to your office. Also, when placing medical records on the door of an examination room, turn the chart so that identifying information faces the door. If you keep medical charts in the office on countertops or in receptacles, it is your duty to ensure that nonstaff persons will not access the records. Handling and storing medical records will certainly change because of HIPAA guidelines.

10. Do not post the health care provider's schedule in areas viewable by nonstaff individuals. The schedules are often posted for convenience of the professional staff, but this may be a breach in patient confidentiality.

11. Fax machines should not be placed in patient examination rooms or in any reception area where nonstaff persons may view incoming or sent documents. Only staff members should have access to the faxes.

12. If you open your office mail or take telephone calls pertaining to medical record requests, direct these issues to the appropriate staff member.

13. If you are involved in coding and billing, be sure to recognize, learn, and use HIPAA TCS.

14. Send all privacy-related questions or concerns to the appropriate staff member.

15. Immediately report any suspected or known improper behavior to your supervisor or the PO so that the issue may be documented and investigated.

16. If you have questions, contact your supervisor or the PO.

Health care organizations face challenges in implementing the HIPAA requirements; do not let these overwhelm you. Your office is required to take reasonable steps to build protections specific to your health care organization. Compliance is an ongoing endeavor involving teamwork. Understand your office's established P&P. Monitor your own activities to ensure you are following the required procedures. Do not take shortcuts when your actions involve patient privacy and security.

Be alert to other activities in your office. Help your co-workers change work habits that do not comply with HIPAA. Do not ignore unauthorized uses and disclosures of PHI, and do not allow unauthorized persons to access data. You have an obligation to your employer and the patients you serve.

CONSEQUENCES OF NONCOMPLIANCE WITH HIPAA

The prosecution of HIPAA crimes is handled by different governing bodies. HHS handles issues regarding TCS and security. Complaints can be filed against a covered entity for not complying with these rules. The OCR oversees privacy issues and complaints, referring criminal issues to the Office of Inspector General (OIG). The OIG provides the workup for referral cases, which may involve the Federal Bureau of Investigation (FBI) and other agencies.

Civil Monetary Penalties Law (42 US Code §320a-27a)

The US Congress enacted the Civil Monetary Penalty (CMP) statute to provide administrative remediation to combat health care fraud and abuse. HIPAA's Final Rule includes civil monetary penalties when there is a pattern of upcoded claims or billing for medically unnecessary services. CMP imposes civil monetary penalties and assessments against a person or organization for making false or improper claims against any federal health care program.

Serious civil and criminal penalties apply for HIPAA noncompliance. A civil penalty is a fine assessed for violation of a law or regulation, whereas a criminal penalty is a fine and imprisonment for criminal violation of a federal or state law. General noncompliance with the privacy, security, and transaction regulations results in a $100 fine per violation and up to $25,000 per person for identical violations in a given calendar year. Specific to the Privacy Rule is a $50,000 fine and imprisonment for 1 year if one knowingly obtains or discloses IIHI. The person who obtains or discloses such health information under false pretenses is subject to a $100,000 fine. If one obtains or discloses PHI with the intent to sell, transfer, or use it for commercial advantage, personal gain, or malicious harm, a maximum fine of $250,000 and up to 10 years' imprisonment may be applied.

OFFICE OF INSPECTOR GENERAL

The mission of the OIG is to safeguard the health and welfare of the beneficiaries of HHS programs and to protect the integrity of HHS programs (Medicare and Medicaid). The OIG was established to identify and eliminate fraud, abuse, and waste and "to promote efficiency and economy in departmental operations." HIPAA legislation has radically changed the focus and mission within the OIG. HIPAA pushed the OIG into a new era, guaranteeing funds for the OIG programs and mandating initiatives to protect the integrity of all health care programs. The OIG undertakes nationwide audits, as well as investigations and inspections to review the claim submission processes of providers and reimbursement patterns of the programs. Recommendations are made to the HHS Secretary and the US Congress on correcting problematic areas addressed in the federal programs according to the OIG.

Efforts to combat fraud were consolidated and strengthened under Public Law 104-191, the Health Insurance Portability and Accountability Act of 1996 (HIPAA). The act established a comprehensive program to combat fraud committed against all health plans, both public and private. The legislation required the establishment of a national Health Care Fraud and Abuse Control Program (HCFAP), under the joint direction of the Attorney General and the Secretary of the Department of Health and Human Services (HHS) acting through the Department's Inspector General (HHS/OIG). The HCFAP program is designed to coordinate federal, state, and local law enforcement activities with respect to health care fraud and abuse. The act requires HHS and the Department of Justice (DOJ) to detail in an annual report the amounts deposited and appropriated to the Medicare Trust Fund, as well as the source of such deposits.

Health care providers must be aware of the potential liabilities when submitting claims for payment that are deemed to be "fraudulent" or inappropriate by the government. The government may impose significant financial and administrative penalties when health care claims are not appropriately submitted, including criminal prosecution against the offending party. Fraud, according to the OIG, can result from deliberate unethical behavior or simply from mistakes and miscues that cause excessive reimbursement. The OIG is the professional health care provider's (and his or her agents') "partner" in fighting fraud and abuse.

Compliance Program Guidance recommendations from the OIG must be the guiding principles of a health care practice in regard to the potential for unethical behavior or the mistakes that may occur within the organization. The *OIG Compliance Program for Individual and Small Group Physician Practices* and the *OIG Compliance Program Guidance for Third-Party Medical Billing Companies* are two publications in a series for the health care industry that provide guidance and acceptable principles for business operations (see Internet Resources at the end of this chapter).

If you are involved in the claims processing procedures in your organization, note the importance and urgency in following the legal and ethical path when performing your duties. Your "honest mistake" could lead to a situation that puts the health care provider at risk for investigation of fraud, waste, or abuse if it continues and is not corrected.

Fraud and Abuse Laws

Fraud can occur when deception is used in a claim submission to obtain payment from the payer. Individuals who knowingly, willfully, and intentionally submit false information to benefit themselves or others commit fraud. Fraud can also be interpreted from mistakes that result in excessive reimbursement. No proof of "specific intent to defraud" is required for fraud to be considered. Fraud usually involves careful planning. Examples are listed in Box 2-11.

Abuse means incidents or practices by physicians, not usually considered fraudulent, that are inconsistent with accepted sound medical business or fiscal practices. Examples are listed in Box 2-12.

In subsequent chapters about various insurance programs, additional information about fraud and abuse pertinent to each program is given.

Federal False Claims Act (31 US Code §3729-33)

"A false claim is a claim for payment for services or supplies that were not provided specifically as presented or for which the provider is otherwise not entitled to payment." Presenting a claim for an item or service based on a code known to result in greater payment or to submit a claim for services not medically necessary is also a violation of the False Claims Act (FCA). The government uses the FCA as a primary enforcement tool.

Although no proof of specific intent to defraud is required, liability can occur when a person knowingly presents or causes to present such a claim or makes, uses, or causes a false record or statement to have a false or fraudulent claim paid or approved by the federal government.

Box 2-11   Examples of Fraud

- Bill for services or supplies not provided (**phantom billing** or invoice ghosting) or for an office visit if a patient fails to keep an appointment and is not notified ahead of time that this is office policy.
- Alter fees on a claim form to obtain higher payment.
- Forgive the deductible or copayment.
- Alter medical records to generate fraudulent payments.
- Leave relevant information off a claim (e.g., failing to reveal whether a spouse has health insurance coverage through an employer).
- Upcode (e.g., submitting a code for a complex fracture when the patient had a simple fracture).
- Shorten (e.g., dispensing less medication than billed for).
- Split billing schemes (e.g., billing procedures over a period of days when all treatment occurred during one visit).
- Use another person's insurance card in obtaining medical care.
- Change a date of service.
- Post adjustments to generate fraudulent payments.
- Solicit, offer, or receive a kickback, bribe, or rebate in return for referring a patient to a physician, physical therapist, or pharmacy or for referring a patient to obtain any

item or service that may be paid for in full or in part by Medicare or Medicaid.
- Restate the diagnosis to obtain insurance benefits or better payment.
- Apply deliberately for duplicate payment (e.g., billing Medicare twice, billing Medicare and the beneficiary for the same service, or billing Medicare and another insurer in an attempt to get paid twice).
- Unbundle or explode charge (e.g., billing a multichannel laboratory test as if individual tests were performed).
- Collusion between a physician and an employee of a third-party payer when the claim is assigned (if the physician deliberately overbilled for services, overpayments could be generated with little awareness on the part of the Medicare beneficiary).
- Bills based on gang visits (e.g., a physician visits nursing home and bills for 20 visits without furnishing any specific service to or on behalf of individual patients).
- Knowingly bill for the same item or service more than once or when another party bills the federal health care program for an item or service also billed by the physician.

Box 2-12 **Examples of Medical Billing Abuse**

- Refer excessively to other providers for unnecessary services.
- Charge excessively for services or supplies.
- Perform a battery of diagnostic tests when only a few are required for services.
- Violate Medicare's physician participating agreement.
- Call patients for repeated and unnecessary follow-up visits.
- Bill Medicare beneficiaries at a higher rate than other patients.
- Submit bills to Medicare instead of to third-party payers (e.g., claims for injury from an automobile accident, in a store, or the workplace).
- Breach assignment agreement.
- Fail to make required refunds when services are not reasonable and necessary.

- Require patients to contract to pay their physician's full charges, in excess of the Medicare charge limits.
- Require a patient to waive rights to have the physician submit claims to Medicare and obligate a patient to pay privately for Medicare-covered services.
- Require patients to pay for services not previously billed, including telephone calls with the physician, prescription refills, and medical conferences with other professionals.
- Require patients to sign a global waiver agreeing to pay privately for all services that Medicare will not cover, and using these waivers to obligate patients to pay separately for a service that Medicare covers as part of a package or related procedures.

A coder or biller who has knowledge of fraud or abuse should take the following measures:

1. Notify the provider both personally and with a dated, written memorandum.
2. Document the false statement or representation of the material fact.
3. Send a memorandum to the office manager or employer stating your concern if no change is made.
4. Maintain a written audit trail with dated memoranda for your files.
5. Do not discuss the problem with anyone who is not immediately involved.

Qui Tam Provision

Qui tam in the FCA provisions allows a private citizen to bring a civil action suit for a violation on behalf of the federal government (Example 2-3). This involves fraud by government contractors and other entities that receive or use government funds. The individual who files a qui tam suit is known as a "relator" and is also referred to as a "whistleblower." The whistleblower shares in any money recovered from a successful qui tam action.

Example 2-3 **Qui Tam Action**

A qui tam relator alleged that a hospital violated the False Claims Act by bundling tests when billing nursing homes and unbundling those charges when billing Medicare, double billing, and submitting multiple and excessive bills.

Criminal False Claims Act (18 US Code)

The Criminal False Claims Act did not apply specifically to the health care industry before HIPAA. HIPAA amendments to the criminal code include the following:

- Theft or Embezzlement (18 US Code §669). This law brings fines and imprisonment against any individual who "knowingly and willfully embezzles, steals, or otherwise without authority converts to the use of any person other than the rightful owner, or intentionally misapplies any of the moneys, funds, securities, premiums, credits, property, or other assets of a health care benefit program." This law does not just affect Medicare and Medicaid programs. **Embezzlement** means stealing money that has been entrusted in one's care. In many cases of insurance claims embezzlement, the physician is held as the guilty party and has to pay huge sums of money to a third-party payer when false claims are submitted by an employee. If an undiscovered embezzler leaves the employer and you are hired to replace that person, you could be accused some months down the line of doing something that you did not do. Take precautions as an employee to protect the medical practice. These precautions are discussed in Chapter 10.
- False Statement Relating to Health Care Matters (18 US Code §1035). Any individual who knowingly and willfully "falsifies, conceals, or covers up by any trick, scheme, or device a material fact; or makes any materially false, fictitious, or fraudulent statements or representations, or makes or uses any materially false writing or document knowing the same to contain any materially false, fictitious, or fraudulent statement or entry, in connection with the delivery of or payment for health care benefits, items, or services" is subject to fines and imprisonment.
- Health Care Fraud (18 US Code §1347). Any individual who knowingly and willfully "executes, or attempts to execute, a scheme or artifice to defraud any health care benefit program; or to obtain, by means of false or fraudulent pretenses, representations, or promises, any of the money or property owned by, or under the custody or control of, any health care benefit program, in connection with the delivery of or payment for health care benefits, items, or services" is subject to fines and

imprisonment. If serious bodily injury or even death occurs, the person may face life imprisonment.

● Obstruction of Criminal Investigations of Health Care Offenses (18 US Code §1518). An individual is subject to fines and imprisonment when the person "willfully prevents, obstructs, misleads, delays or attempts to prevent, obstruct, mislead, or delay the communication of information or records relating to a violation of a Federal health care offense to a criminal investigator."

Stark I and II Laws (42 US Code §1395)

Stark II laws prohibit the submission of claims for "designated services" or referral of patients if the referring physician has a "financial relationship" with the entity that provides the services. This differs from anti-kickback laws because it deals with self-referral instead of referral to another physician. Originally named "Stark I," this law pertained only to clinical laboratories that prohibited physicians from referring a patient to a clinical laboratory in which the doctor or a member of his or her family had a financial interest. Stark laws carry exceptions, so it is important to understand the referral processes and in-office ancillary services used by your health care organization.

Anti-Kickback Statute

According to CMS, discounts, rebates, or other reductions in price may violate the Anti-Kickback statute because such arrangements induce the purchase of items or services payable by Medicare or Medicaid. However, some arrangements are clearly permissible if they fall within a "safe harbor." One safe harbor protects certain discounting practices. For purposes of this safe harbor, a "discount" is the reduction in the amount a seller charges a buyer for a good or service based on an "arms-length" transaction. In addition, to be protected under the discount safe harbor, the discount must apply to the original item or service purchased or furnished; that is, a discount cannot be applied to the purchase of a different good or service than the one on which the discount was earned. A "rebate" is defined as a discount that is not given at the time of sale. A "buyer" is the individual or entity responsible for submitting a claim for the item or service that is payable by the Medicare or Medicaid programs. A "seller" is the individual or entity who offers the discount.

Safe Harbors

Safe harbors specify various business and service arrangements that are protected from prosecution under the Anti-Kickback statute. These include certain investments, care in underserved areas, and other arrangements.

Additional Laws and Compliance

Other laws pertaining to fraud and abuse include the Federal Deposit Insurance Corporation (FDIC) Mail and Wire Fraud provisions, as follows:

● §1341. Frauds and swindles. An individual is subject to both fines and imprisonment when having "devised or intending to devise any scheme or artifice to defraud, or for obtaining money or property by means of false or fraudulent pretenses" by use of the U.S. Postal Service, whether sent by or delivered to the Postal Service.

● §1343. Fraud by wire, radio, or television. An individual will be fined and/or imprisoned "for obtaining money or property by means of false or fraudulent pretenses, representations, or promises, transmits or causes to be transmitted by means of wire, radio, or television communication."

The US government is clearly committed to the investigation and prosecution of health care fraud. As with HIPAA policies and procedures, it is imperative that health care entities develop their own compliance program to identify and prevent fraud.

Operation Restore Trust

Launched in 1995, Operation Restore Trust (ORT) was designed to coordinate the activities of the OIG along with CMS and other HHS entities in identifying and preventing fraud. An established hotline (1-800-HHS-TIPS) for the public allows reporting issues that might indicate fraud, abuse, or waste. ORT has been successful because of planning with the DOJ and other law enforcement agencies, training state and local organizations to detect fraud and abuse, and implementing statistical methods to identify providers for audits and investigations.

Medicare Integrity Program

The goals of the Medicare Integrity Program (MIP) are to identify and reduce Medicare overpayments through a series of audits and reviews of provider claims and cost report data. Initiatives of MIP include identifying plan beneficiaries with additional insurance and educating health care providers. Program integrity contractors help expand the scope of the MIP. This endeavor has recovered several billions of dollars in the fight against fraud, waste, and abuse in the Medicare program.

Correct Coding Initiative

The Correct Coding Initiative (CCI) was developed to detect improperly coded claims through the use of computer edits. Services that should be grouped together and paid as one item rather than billed separately to obtain higher reimbursement are identified with the computer system.

Increased Staffing and Expanded Penalties for Violations

A significant increase in staffing among the OIG, DOJ, and FBI over the past decade has included prosecutors (a more than 400% increase since 1993) and FBI agents (more than 300% since 1993). With additional employees, the industry has seen the promotion of compliance endeavors across the health care sector. Penalties for violations have increased.

Special Alerts, Bulletins, and Guidance Documents

Special Fraud Alerts are published by the OIG to alert the industry concerning specific patterns or trends related to fraudulent or abusive activities regarding the Medicare and Medicaid programs. *Special Advisory Bulletins* report industry practices and arrangements that may indicate fraud and abuse. Other guidance documents include updates, response letters, and alerts important to more specifically targeted matters. All notices are available at the OIG website, and you can sign up for their mailing list.

Exclusion Program

According to OIG:

> *No program payment will be made for anything that an excluded person furnishes, orders, or prescribes. This payment prohibition applies to the excluded person, anyone who employs or contracts with the excluded person, any hospital or other provider where the excluded person provides services, and anyone else. The exclusion applies regardless of who submits the claims and applies to all administrative and management services furnished by the excluded person.*

Excluded persons/facilities are convicted for program-related fraud and patient abuse, actions from licensing boards, and defaulting on Health Education Assistance Loans.

Your health care organization must not conduct business with any health care provider or subcontract with any agent who has been listed as an Excluded Individual. Be sure to check the updated listings at the OIG website.

APPLICATION TO PRACTICE SETTING

HIPAA affects all areas of the health care office, from the reception area to the provider. In conjunction with being educated and trained in job responsibilities, every staff member must be educated about HIPAA and trained in the P&P pertinent to the organization.

Reasonable safeguards are measurable solutions based on accepted standards that are implemented and periodically monitored to demonstrate that the office is in compliance. Reasonable efforts must be made to limit the use or disclosure of PHI. If you are the front desk receptionist and you close the privacy glass between your desk and the waiting area when you are making a call to a patient, this is a reasonable safeguard to prevent others in the waiting room from overhearing.

Incidental uses and disclosures are permissible under HIPAA only when reasonable safeguards or precautions have been implemented to prevent misuse or inappropriate disclosure of PHI. When incidental uses and disclosures result from failure to apply reasonable safeguards or adhere to the minimum necessary standard, the Privacy Rule has been violated. If you are in the reception area and you close the privacy glass when having a confidential conversation and you are still overheard by an individual in the waiting room, this would be "incidental." You have applied a reasonable safeguard to prevent this from happening. The OCR has addressed what is permissible regarding incidental disclosures such as the following:

1. Health care professionals may discuss a patient's condition in a treatment area or over the telephone with the patient, a provider, or a family member. However, when telephoning a patient about an insurance matter and reaching voice mail, use care in the choice of words when leaving the message in the event the call was inadvertently received at the wrong number. Leave your name, the office name, and return telephone number. Never provide information about the results of diagnostic tests to the patient. Let the physician do it.
2. Health care professionals may discuss laboratory test results with a patient or other provider in a joint treatment area. A *health care professional* is an individual who has been trained in a health-related field, whether clinical or administrative. The professional may be licensed, certified, or registered by a state or government agency or professional organization.
3. A physician may discuss a patient's condition or treatment regimen in the patient's hospital room.
4. A pharmacist may discuss a prescription with a patient over the pharmacy counter or with a physician or the patient by telephone.
5. A physician may give instructions to a staff member to bill a patient for a certain procedure even if it may be overheard by persons in the reception room.
6. A patient's name may be called out in the reception room; however, some offices prefer to use first names and not call out last names.

ORGANIZATION AND STAFF RESPONSIBILITIES IN PROTECTING PATIENT RIGHTS

The covered entity must implement written P&P that comply with HIPAA standards. P&P are tailored guidelines established to accommodate each health care practice and designed to address PHI. HIPAA requires each practice to implement P&P that comply with privacy and security rules. The office should have a policy and procedures manual to train providers and staff and to serve as a resource for situations that need clarification. Revisions in P&P must be made as needed and appropriate to comply with laws as they change. Documentation must be maintained in written or electronic form and retained for 6 years after its creation or when it was last in effect, whichever is later.

COMPLIANCE PROGRAM GUIDANCE FOR INDIVIDUAL AND SMALL GROUP PHYSICIAN PRACTICES

The OIG published the *Individual and Small Group Physician Practices* in September 2000. This guidance recommended by the OIG is voluntary; however, an effective plan reduces the risk of legal action and creates a "good faith" effort in combating fraud, waste, and abuse. A **compliance plan** requires that a health care practice review all billing processes through audits and establish controls that will correct weaknesses and prevent errors.

A well-designed compliance program can (1) speed the claims processing cycle, (2) optimize proper payment or claims, (3) minimize billing mistakes, (4) reduce the likelihood of a government audit, (5) avoid conflict with Stark laws and the Anti-Kickback statute, (6) show a "good faith" effort that claims will be submitted appropriately, and (7) relay to staff that there is a duty to report mistakes and suspected or known misconduct.

If you are a claims processing staff member, your organization's claims processing supervisor should research industry sector program guidance to help with specific concerns regarding the specialty/facility setting. Check the OIG website to view addenda, comments, and drafts of additional compliance guidance subjects.

Increased Productivity and Decreased Penalties With Plan

The presence of an OIG compliance program can significantly mitigate imposed penalties in the event of an OIG audit or other discovery of fraudulent billing activities. These P&P can be found in the provider's P&P manual. For those not currently in the role of a Privacy/Security/Compliance Officer, knowledge of P&P as they pertain to both HIPAA and OIG is invaluable.

Because health care providers rely on the expertise of their billing and coding staff to process claims accurately and promptly, they also look to these staff members for advice and guidance. If you are directly involved in this area of your organization, you will likely be expected to understand the complexities of the various laws and regulations governing the medical claims process.

Compliance plans effectively become a "meeting of the minds" among the players; providers, claims processing staff, and payers all agree to process claims in accordance with shared values. Consider your organization's OIG compliance program as a way to integrate regulatory requirements directly into your claims processing procedures. OIG views the experienced claims processing staff as the critical screen for the health care provider's claims. The common denominators in the key benefits identified by OIG are efficiency, consistency, and integrity.

Seven Basic Components of a Compliance Plan

OIG outlines the following seven components of an effective program guidance plan specifically for the individual and small group physician practices:

1. Conducting internal monitoring and auditing
2. Implementing compliance and practice standards
3. Designating a compliance officer or contact
4. Conducting appropriate training and education
5. Responding appropriately to detected offenses and developing corrective action
6. Developing open lines of communication
7. Enforcing disciplinary standards through well-publicized guidelines

Conducting Internal Monitoring and Auditing

A comprehensive auditing and monitoring program will not eliminate misconduct within an organization but will minimize the risk of fraud and abuse by identifying the risk areas. OIG does not provide a specific set of guidelines on conducting audits or ongoing monitoring. The compliance officer, with the committee's assistance, should identify problem areas and should have established auditing priorities and procedures as part of the organization's compliance program.

Special attention should be made to the risk areas associated with claims submission and processing. Also, a thorough review of the organization's standards and written P&P should be conducted to ensure proper guidelines for complying with state and federal laws and insurance payer requirements.

Implementing Compliance and Practice Standards

Written standards and procedures address risk areas that an office needs to monitor and follow. Specific risk areas* identified by OIG include the following:

- Billing for items or services not rendered or not provided as claimed
- Submitting claims for equipment, medical supplies, and services that are not reasonable and necessary
- Double billing resulting in duplicate payment
- Billing for noncovered services as though covered
- Knowing misuse of provider identification numbers, which results in improper billing
- Unbundling, or billing for each component of the service instead of billing or using an all-inclusive code
- Failure to use coding modifiers properly
- Clustering
- Upcoding the level of service provided

In addition to these risk areas, policies should be developed that address the following:

- Definition of reasonable and necessary
- Proper medical documentation
- Federal sentencing guidelines
- Record retention

You should be able to access your organization's P&P manual to review the standards and protocol for these issues involving your practice.

Designating a Compliance Officer or Contact

As with the HIPAA PO, the compliance officer is the key individual overseeing your organization's compliance program monitoring with the support of the Compliance Committee. Again, as with HIPAA, policies and procedures need to be drafted. These established guidelines identify and prevent fraud and abuse activities as described by OIG.

The number of members on your compliance committee is not important, and prospective staff members from human resources, claims auditing, billing, legal, and medicine departments can ensure a comprehensive mix. You may currently participate on your office's

compliance committee or may be asked to do so in the future. The compliance committee acts as a review board. Some committees consist of provider-client office staff and billing company staff. Some committees are simply the provider-client and the billing company staff or a combination of the provider-client, their practice manager, and the billing company staff. The committee, empowered by management, legitimizes the compliance strategy within your organization. In addition to possessing professional experience in claims processing and auditing, committee members are expected to use good judgment and high integrity to fulfill committee obligations.

Conducting Appropriate Training and Education

Because OIG compliance program guidelines are based on Federal Sentencing Guidelines, significant elements of an effective compliance program involve proper education and training of staff. Every employee and individual who interacts with your health care organization and may be accountable for potential misconduct should be considered in the organization's training sessions.

You should be required to attend training in a "general" compliance training session at least annually. For staff members involved in claims processing (coding and billing), a separate training session should be held to cover internal procedures, federal and state laws regarding fraud and abuse, and specific government and other payer reimbursement policies. Periodic professional courses in continuing education should be available. Coding and billing personnel should receive training at least annually to remain updated on CPT/HCPCS and ICD-9-CM codes for each year. You will attend training on site, at a remote location, or both.

Effective training can reduce potential errors, penalties, and fines. An educated staff makes fewer errors, reduces your organization's risks, and requires less micromanagement.

Responding Appropriately to Detected Offenses and Developing Corrective Action

When faced with the discovery of an offense or an error, inaction may be interpreted as indifference. This could impose a potential jeopardy to the reputation of the health care provider's practice. Your office should have a process for investigating problems and taking necessary corrective action. Issues that would raise concern include significant change in claims that are rejected; software edits that show a pattern of misuse of codes or fees; unusually high volume of charges, payments, or

*Data from *Federal Register* 65(194):59439, 2000.

rejections; and notices from insurance payers regarding claims submitted by your office.

You and your fellow staff members should be encouraged to report concerns for any suspected or known misconduct, with an established chain of command in the reporting path. Some incidences of misconduct may violate criminal, civil, or administrative law. If the situation warrants, the compliance officer should report the misconduct promptly to the appropriate government authority.

Report fraud and abuse. Contact the HHS OIG as follows:

- Telephone hotline 1-800-HHS-TIPS (1-800-447-8477)
- TTY 1-800-377-4950
- Fax 1-800-223-8164
- Website http://www.oig.hhs.gov/fraud/hotline

Developing Open Lines of Communication

Effective lines of communication provide a channel for employees to report suspected or known misconduct without immediately resorting to an external agency. In this way, your health care organization can resolve issues internally. "Open door" policies ensure an environment where staff members feel secure to ask about the organization's existing P&P and to report questionable activities. Your role as a conscientious employee allows you to know the steps to take in reporting any suspicious business activity.

You will learn your office's procedure for reporting misconduct. It is important to follow these guidelines to protect your reputation and credibility within the workplace. Depending on the size of the practice, the methods for contacting managerial staff may include anonymous telephone calls through a "hotline" or written report forms.

Enforcing Disciplinary Standards Through Well-Publicized Guidelines

The unfortunate downside to compliance is that misconduct does occur. For this reason, health care organizations must have established disciplinary guidelines and must make these well known to employees and other agents who contract with the organization. We all want to know what will happen if we "make a mistake" and what progressive forms of discipline await situations involving misconduct. Disciplinary standards include the following:

- Verbal warning
- Written warning
- Written reprimand
- Suspension or probation
- Demotion
- Termination of employment
- Restitution of any damages
- Referral to federal agencies for criminal prosecution

Whether the misconduct was intentional or negligent, all levels of employees need to know what is expected of them. Your office must publish this information and disseminate it to all employees.

WHAT TO EXPECT FROM YOUR HEALTH CARE PRACTICE

Although every health care organization or practice is different in regard to policies and procedures, you now know what to expect in the workplace, as follows:

- Practice adherence to HIPAA and OIG mandates and recommendations
- Privacy/Security/Compliance Officer (even if one person)
- P&P manual
- Employee training and education (at least annually and whenever there are changes in business operations that affect staff members directly)

KEY POINTS

This is a brief chapter review or summary of the key issues presented. To further enhance your knowledge of the technical subject matter, review the key terms and key abbreviations for this chapter by locating the meanings in the glossary at the end of this book that appear in a section before the index.

1. The Health Insurance Portability and Accountability Act (HIPAA) has affected confidentiality and disclosure of protected health information (PHI), completion and electronic transmission of insurance claims, fraud and abuse in claims submission, and implementation of compliance and practice standards.

2. While employed by a medical practice, the insurance billing specialist's duty is to have complete knowledge and understanding of HIPAA mandates, carry out policies and procedures that comply with federal regulations, and keep up to date with these statutes. This will assist both the physician and the patients.

3. The National Health Information Infrastructure (NHII) is an initiative set forth to improve patient safety and the quality of health care, as well as to better inform individuals regarding their own health information and to help them understand health care costs.

4. *e-Health information management* (eHIM) is a phrase that describes any and all transactions in which health care information is accessed, processed, stored, and transferred using electronic technologies.

5. The primary purpose of HIPAA *Title I: Insurance Reform* is to provide continuous insurance coverage for workers and their insured dependents when they change or lose jobs. *Title II: Administrative Simplification* focuses on the health care practice setting and aims to reduce administrative costs and burdens.

6. Serious civil and criminal penalties such as fines and imprisonment apply for HIPAA noncompliance.

7. PHI refers to data that identify an individual and describe his or her health status, age, sex, ethnicity, or other demographic characteristics, whether that information is or is not stored or transmitted electronically.

8. Under HIPAA, PHI may not be used or disclosed without permission of the patient or someone authorized to act on behalf of the patient, unless the use or disclosure is specifically required or permitted by the regulation (e.g., treatment, payment, or health care operations [TPO]). The two types of disclosure required by HIPAA Privacy Rule are to the individual who is the subject of the PHI and to the Secretary or DHHS to investigate compliance with the rule.

9. When comparing privileged and nonprivileged information, privileged information is related to the treatment and progress of the patient. The patient must sign an authorization to release this information or selected facts from the medical record. Nonprivileged information consists of ordinary facts unrelated to treatment of the patient, including the patient's name, city of residence, and dates of admission or discharge.

10. Under HIPAA, a Notice of Privacy Practices (NPP) document must be given to the patient at the first visit or at enrollment explaining the individual's rights and the physician's legal duties in regard to PHI. Use and disclosure of PHI is permissible for TPO because the NPP describes how PHI is used for these purposes. Thus a consent form is not required. The health care provider is required to obtain a signed authorization form to use or disclose health information for situations beyond the TPO. This is a protection for the practice. Psychotherapy notes are handled separately under HIPAA. Such notes have additional protection, specifically that an authorization for any use of disclosure of psychotherapy notes must be obtained.

11. *Disclosure* means the release, transfer, provision of access to, or divulging in any other manner of information outside the entity holding the information. *Use* means the sharing, employment, application, utilization, examination, or analysis of IIHI within an organization that holds such information. When a patient's billing record is accessed to review the claim submission history, the individual's health information is in "use."

12. The three major categories of security safeguards include administrative, technical, and physical measures that will reasonably protect PHI from any use or disclosure that is in violation of HIPAA.

13. The difference between *fraud* and *abuse* is that fraud can occur when deception is used in a claim submission to obtain payment from the payer. Individuals who knowingly, willfully, and intentionally submit false information to benefit themselves or others commit *fraud*. Abuse means incidents or practices by physicians, not usually considered fraudulent, that are inconsistent with accepted sound medical business or fiscal practices.

You must strongly consider the lessons learned from the privacy, transaction, and security rules in conjunction with OIG compliance recommendations. The most important points are to read your organization's P&P manual and to ask questions about the many aspects of HIPAA or the general operations of your organization. Always use your ethical and "best practice" approach to be an informed and effective employee.

℮volve INTERNET RESOURCES

For active links to the following resources, visit the Evolve website at
http://evolve.elsevier.com/fordney/handbook

- American Health Information Management Association
- American Medical Association
- Centers for Medicare and Medicaid Services
- Department of Health and Human Services, Office of Inspector General
- Federal Bureau of Investigation
- Medicaid program current information on fraud
- Medicare or Medicaid programs current information on fraud
- National Health Information Infrastructure
- National Health Information Structure
- Office of Civil Rights
- Office of the Inspector General Red Book
- OIG Compliance Program Guidance for Third-Party Medical Billing Companies
- OIG Compliance Program for Individual and Small Group Physician Practices
- Phoenix Health Systems: HIPAA Advisory
- US Government Printing Office
- Workgroup for Electronic Data Interchange

STUDENT ASSIGNMENT

✓ Study Chapter 2.
✓ Answer the fill-in-the-blank, multiple choice, and true/false questions in the *Workbook* to reinforce the theory learned in this chapter and help prepare you for a future test.
✓ Complete the assignments in the *Workbook* to give you experience in making decisions regarding situa-

tions of fraud, abuse, incidental disclosures or compliance violations, consents, or authorizations.
✓ Turn to the glossary at the end of this textbook for a further understanding of the key terms and key abbreviations used in this chapter.

UNIT 2
The Claims Process

KEY TERMS*

accounts receivable
  management
applicant
assignment
blanket contract
cancelable
capitation
Civilian Health and Medical
  Program of the Department
  of Veterans Affairs
claim
coinsurance
competitive medical plan
conditionally renewable
contract
coordination of benefits
daysheet
deductible
disability income insurance
electronic signature
eligibility
emancipated minor
encounter form
exclusions

exclusive provider organization
expressed contract
extended
financial accounting record
foundation for medical care
guaranteed renewable
guarantor
health insurance
health maintenance
  organization
high risk
implied contract
indemnity
independent or individual
  practice association
insured
major medical
Maternal and Child Health
  Program
Medicaid
Medicare
Medicare/Medicaid
member
noncancelable policy

nonparticipating provider
optionally renewable
participating provider
patient registration form
personal insurance
point-of-service plan
posted
preauthorization
precertification
predetermination
preexisting conditions
preferred provider organization
premium
running balance
State Disability Insurance
subscriber
TRICARE
Unemployment Compensation
  Disability
Veterans Affairs outpatient
  clinic
Workers' compensation
  insurance

KEY ABBREVIATIONS*

AAMB	EPO	MAB	PMS
AAPC	FMC	MCD	POS
ADSM	FSA	MCHP	POS plan
A/R	HBMA	Medi-Medi	PPO
CHAMPVA	HDHP	MGMA	ROA
CMP	HFMA	MSA	SDI
COB	HMO	nonpar	SOF
COBRA	HRA	NPP	UCD
DoD	HSA	PAHCOM	VA
DOS	IPA	par	WC

*Definitions for the key terms and key abbreviations are located near the back of this textbook in the glossary.

CHAPTER 3

Basics of Health Insurance

OBJECTIVES

After reading this chapter, you should be able to:

- Describe the history of insurance in the United States.
- List changes brought about by the health care reform of 2010.
- State four concepts of a valid insurance contract.
- Explain the difference between an implied and an expressed physician-patient contract.
- Define common insurance terms.
- State the types of health insurance coverage.
- Describe in general terms the important federal, state, and private health insurance plans.
- Explain the administrative life cycle of a physician-based insurance claim from completion to third-party payer processing and payment.
- Determine the appropriate questions to ask a patient for a complete patient registration form.

- List the types of computerized signatures for documents and insurance claims.
- Demonstrate how to track submitted insurance claims.
- List the functions of an aging accounts receivable report in a computerized practice management system or a "tickler" file in a paper environment.
- Explain how insurance billing and coding information can be kept up to date.
- Describe the proper information to post to the patient's financial account after claims submission and payment received.

Service to Patients

Good customer service is emphasized in most industries that serve the consumer, and when processing insurance matters, it is equally important. Some suggestions are as follows:

- You must be friendly and courteous to each patient when handling insurance claims to maintain a harmonious physician-patient relationship. Collections often can be significantly improved and simplified if the patient feels free to discuss personal financial problems at any time and is educated regarding the physician's fees.
- Quickly obtain precertification, preauthorization, or predetermination so that the patient's treatment plan may be carried out without delay.
- Assist and instruct the patient in filling out a patient information form so that data are accurate and complete.

- Explain and answer the patient's questions about your office's Notice of Privacy Practices (NPP). Remember, it is important for you to understand what the NPP states.
- Promptly transmit accurate insurance claim data to the third-party payer so that reimbursement is received in a timely manner on behalf of the patient.
- As an insurance biller, you should be able to answer complex billing and insurance questions for patients. However, to save time and help patients, all business or clinical team members (not just those in the billing department) should be able to give general information correctly.

Performance objectives, testing and review material, and hands-on practical exercises for this chapter are available in these resources:

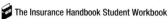

The Insurance Handbook Student Workbook   The Insurance Handbook Evolve Site

HISTORY

The insurance industry is among the world's largest businesses. In the 1800s, life insurance came to be widely offered. Health insurance began to be available in the early part of the twentieth century because anyone can have an accident or become ill unexpectedly, leading to large expenses. **Health insurance** is a contract between a policyholder and a third-party payer or government program to reimburse the policyholder for all or a portion of the cost of medically necessary treatment or preventive care on the basis of the contract purchased. Its main purpose is to help offset some of the high costs accrued during sickness or when an injury occurred.

During the Renaissance, when Italian traders insured valuable cargo to be shipped across the Mediterranean, they recorded the insurance agreement on a piece of folded paper called a "polizza." English merchants adapted the term to their insurance practices, modifying the pronunciation to suit the Anglo-Saxon tongue, resulting in the word "policy."

INSURANCE IN THE UNITED STATES

In 1850 the Franklin Health Assurance Company of Massachusetts began offering insurance for nonfatal injury. About 10 years later, the Travelers Insurance Company of Hartford marketed a plan that is similar to today's health insurance. Many other companies began writing health insurance policies, and in 1911 Montgomery Ward and Company offered benefits to its ill or injured employees. This was the first group plan. These commercial plans paid only when an individual was sick or received an injury.

By the 1960s, most private insurance companies sold policies that included hospital care, surgical fees, and physicians' services. In addition to those benefits, many plans now offer catastrophic health insurance coverage, preventive care, dental insurance, disability income insurance, and long-term care and home health care insurance for the chronically ill, disabled, and developmentally disabled. State insurance laws regulate the way policies are written and minimum requirements of coverage.

Medical care costs continuously escalate, forcing insurance companies to reduce the benefits of individual subscribers. Rising costs have caused the federal government to adopt cost-containment policies for the Medicare, Medicaid, and TRICARE programs. Although managed care began in the 1930s when Kaiser Industries provided health care to their employees, it was not until the 1980s that many types of plans arose across the nation to control the cost of medical care and help those who could not afford health insurance. Because individual needs vary, each patient may have a different type of health insurance policy with various benefits. Patients may be covered under individual policies or have several plans and be insured under different types of private, state, or federal programs.

Health Benefit Exchanges

Under the Patient Protection and Affordable Care Act and the Health Care and Education Reconciliation Act of 2010, state-based American Health Benefit Exchanges and Small Business Health Options Program (SHOP) Exchanges will be established and must open on January 1, 2014. These exchanges can be regional and will be administered by a governmental agency or nonprofit organization. The exchanges will be a central clearinghouse in which an individual can compare prices and select plans from different tiers of coverage. Those who buy insurance through the individual plan must purchase plans through the exchange to take advantage of federal subsidies. Those who receive coverage through their employers will continue to select and purchase their plans as they do now. Individuals and small businesses of up to 100 employees can purchase qualified coverage. States are permitted to allow businesses with more than 100 employees to purchase coverage in the SHOP Exchange beginning in 2017.

With the advent of health care reform in 2010, additional changes occurred that affect the uninsured; pre-existing conditions; prescription drugs; employers' responsibilities; and programs such as Medicare, Medicaid, and ERISA (Employee Retirement Income Security Act). In this chapter and Chapters 11, 12, 13, and 15, further explanation of this reform is given in more detail.

LEGAL PRINCIPLES OF INSURANCE

The role of a medical insurance billing specialist is to complete the insurance claim accurately and assist claims submission so that optimal accurate reimbursement is received quickly. However, before developing the skill of coding and completing insurance claim forms, it is necessary to know frequently encountered legal problems and how to handle them. Legal situations occur daily in the performance of these job duties and involve confidentiality of medical records, accurate insurance claim transmission, fraud and abuse issues, credit and collection laws, and so on. An insurance biller cannot escape liability by pleading ignorance. It cannot be overemphasized that keeping up to date on health care plan policies and procedures is essential. Most legal issues of private health insurance claims fall under civil law, and Medicare, Medicaid, and TRICARE programs fall under federal laws. Insurance is regulated by state law and is not considered a federally regulated industry, except that Health

Insurance Portability and Accountability Act (HIPAA) and Office of Inspector General (OIG) federal regulations help govern the entire industry.

It is important for an insurance billing specialist to know some basic insurance terms, understand basic insurance concepts, and have a working knowledge of medical terminology.

Insurance Contracts

The first legal item in the business of handling medical insurance is the insurance contract (also known as a policy), which is a legally binding document. There is no standard health insurance contract. Individuals who take out a policy receive an original document composed by the insuring company.

The following four considerations are involved in drawing up a valid insurance contract:

1. The person must be a mentally competent adult and not under the influence of drugs or alcohol when signing the contract.
2. The insurance company must make an offer (the signed application), and the person must accept the offer (issuance of the policy), without concealment or misrepresentation of facts on the application.
3. An exchange of value (the first premium payment) submitted with the application, known as a *consideration*, must be present.
4. A legal purpose must exist, which is an insurable interest in the case of a health insurance policy. This means that the policyholder expects to continue in good health, but the insurance policy will provide something of value if an accident or illness strikes.

A policy can be challenged when a fraudulent statement is made by the subscriber. A challenged policy means that coverage may not be in effect. After a policy has been in force for 2 years (3 years in some states), a policy becomes incontestable (may not be challenged). If the time limit has passed and a policy is guaranteed renewable, the policy becomes incontestable even if false statements were made on the application.

PHYSICIAN-PATIENT CONTRACTS AND FINANCIAL OBLIGATION

Implied or Expressed Contracts

A physician and his or her staff must be aware of the physician's obligations to each patient, as well as his or her liabilities in regard to service, and the patient's obligations to the physician. The physician-patient contract begins when the physician accepts the patient and agrees to treat him or her. This action can be either an implied

or expressed contract. An **implied contract** is defined as not manifested by direct words but implied or deduced from the circumstance, the general language, or the conduct of the patient. For example, if Mary Johnson goes to Dr. Doe's office and Dr. Doe gives Ms. Johnson professional services that she accepts, this is an implied contract. If the patient is unconscious when treatment is rendered, treatment is based on an implied-in-fact contract. An **expressed contract** can be verbal or written. However, most physician-patient contracts are implied.

Private Patients

For a patient who carries private medical insurance, the contract for treatment is between the physician and the patient. The patient is liable for the entire bill. The insurance is meant to help offset the expense. However, for patients who belong to a preferred provider organization (PPO), the patient is not liable for the bill if the physician does not follow his or her contract with the payer.

Guarantor

A **guarantor** is an individual who promises to pay the medical bill by signing a form agreeing to pay or who accepts treatment, which by this act constitutes an expressed promise. Usually, a patient is the guarantor and must be of legal age (18 or 21 years, depending on state law). However, if the patient is a child of a divorced parent, the custodial parent bears the responsibility of the child's medical expenses unless the divorce decree states otherwise. An adoptive parent may be the custodial parent (guarantor) and, therefore, solely liable for the child's bill. A father is ordinarily responsible for his children's debts if they are minors and are not emancipated (Figure 3-1).

Emancipated Minor

An **emancipated minor** is a person younger than 18 years of age who lives independently, is totally self-supporting, is married or divorced, is a parent even if not married, or is in the military and possesses decision-making rights. College students living away from home even when financially dependent on their parents are considered emancipated. Parents are not liable for the medical expenses incurred by an emancipated minor. The patient record should contain the minor's signed statement that he or she is on his or her own.

Managed Care Patients

A physician under contract to a managed care plan may or may not periodically receive an updated list of current enrollees. The physician is obligated to see those individuals who are enrolled if one of them calls for an

FIGURE 3-1 Receptionist explaining where a guarantor's signature goes on a patient registration form for the medical services rendered to a family member.

appointment. However, the contract for treatment occurs when the patient is first seen. If the primary care physician no longer wishes to treat a patient on a managed care plan, termination is handled according to the contract. Generally, approval must be obtained from the third-party administrator of the plan to have the patient reassigned.

An insurance specialist should be able to read and explain managed care plan contracts that the office participates with, but if the specialist is unable to interpret these matters, professional assistance from the physician's attorney, the medical practice's accountant, or the managed care plan should be sought. He or she should understand billing and collection requirements and track payments made by the managed care plan.

Employment and Disability Examinations

Courts in most jurisdictions have ruled that there is no physician-patient relationship in an employment or disability examination and the doctor does not owe a duty of care to the person being examined, mainly because the insurance company is requesting the examination and the patient is not seeking the medical services of the physician.

Workers' Compensation Patients

Workers' compensation cases involve a person being injured on the job. These cases may be referred to as *industrial accidents* or *illnesses*. In these types of cases, the contract exists between the physician and the insurance company. When there is a dispute as to whether the injured party was hurt at work, a Patient Agreement form (see Figure 15-11) must be signed by the patient who agrees to pay the physician's fees if the case is declared to be non–work related.

THE INSURANCE POLICY

Insurance policies are complex and contain a great deal of language that is difficult to understand. This can cause misunderstanding by patients or anyone trying to obtain information from the policy. Basic health insurance coverage includes benefits for hospital, surgical, and other medical expenses. **Major medical** or *extended benefits* contracts are designed to offset large medical expenses caused by prolonged illness or serious injury. Some of these policies include coverage for *extended care* or *skilled nursing facility* benefits. The **insured** is known as a **subscriber** or in some insurance programs, a **member,** *policyholder,* or *recipient* and may not necessarily be the patient seen for the medical service. The subscriber may or may not be the guarantor. The insured is the individual (enrollee) or organization protected in case of loss under the terms of an insurance policy. In group insurance, the employer is considered the insured, and the employees are the risks. However, when completing an insurance claim form, the covered employee is listed as the insured. A policy might also include *dependents* of the insured. Generally, this term refers to the spouse and children of the insured, but under some contracts, parents, other family members, and domestic partners may be covered as dependents. Under the health care reform legislation of 2010, health plans must allow employees to keep their children on their plans until the children are 26 years old.

Policy Application

Before a policy is issued, the insurance company decides whether it will enter into a contract with the **applicant** who is applying for the insurance coverage. Information is obtained about the applicant so that the company can decide whether to accept the risk. Generally, the application form has two sections: the first part contains basic information about the application, and the second part concerns the health of the individual.

An insurance policy is a legally enforceable agreement, or **contract.** If a policy is issued, the applicant becomes part of the insurance contract or plan. The policy becomes effective only after the company offers the policy and the person accepts it and then pays the initial premium. If a premium is paid at the time the application is submitted, then the insurance coverage can be put into force before the policy is delivered. Depending on the laws in some states, the applicant also can have temporary conditional insurance if the agent issues a specific type of receipt.

Policy Renewal Provisions

Health insurance policies may have renewal provisions written into the policy stating the circumstances when the company may refuse to renew, may cancel coverage, or may increase the premium. It is important for the biller to understand that coverage may change from the last time the physician saw the patient for an appointment. It is always a good routine to verify insurance information each time the patient comes for an appointment. Eligibility verification means to check and confirm that the patient is a member of the insurance plan and that the member identification number is correct. It may seem redundant, but it may avoid a lot of future confusion and delays in payment.

In private health insurance, there are five classifications: (1) cancelable, (2) optionally renewable, (3) conditionally renewable, (4) guaranteed renewable, and (5) noncancelable.

A renewable provision in a **cancelable** policy grants the insurer the right to cancel the policy at any time and for any reason. The company notifies the insured that the policy is canceled and refunds any advance premium the policyholder has paid. In some states, this type of policy is illegal.

In an **optionally renewable** policy, the insurer has the right to refuse to renew the policy on a date (premium due or anniversary date) specified in the contract and may add coverage limitations or increase premium rates.

Conditionally renewable policies grant the insurer a limited right to refuse to renew a health insurance policy at the end of a premium payment period. Reasons stated in the policy may be due to age, employment status, or both, but not because of the insured's health status.

The **guaranteed renewable** classification is desirable because the insurer is required to renew the policy as long as premium payments are made. However, these policies may have age limits of 60, 65, or 70 years, or they may be renewable for life.

In a **noncancelable policy,** the insurer cannot increase premium rates and must renew the policy until the insured reaches the age specified in the contract. Some disability income policies have noncancelable terms.

Policy Terms

To keep the insurance in force, a person must pay a monthly, quarterly, or annual fee called a **premium.** If the premium is not paid, a *grace period* of 10 to 30 days is usually given before insurance coverage ceases. Many states have laws that allow the insurance company to apply the provider's payment to the patient's insurance premium. This forces the provider to recoup payment from the patient. In addition, usually a **deductible** (a specific amount of money) must be paid each year before

the policy benefits begin. Generally, the higher the deductible, the lower the cost of the policy. Most policies, as well as Part B of the Medicare program, have a **coinsurance** or *cost-sharing* requirement, which means the insured will assume a percentage of the fee (e.g., 20%) or pay a specific dollar amount (e.g., $5 or $10) for covered services.

Managed care plans use the term *copayment* (copay) when referring to the amount the patient pays at the point of arriving in the office and before he or she sees the physician. It is not advisable to routinely waive copayments because the health care provider has agreed to accept a patient portion. Many insurance companies do not tolerate this practice. Not only would it be a loss of income to the provider, but also the federal government can assess penalties for not collecting coinsurance for patients seen under the Medicare program if the provider is audited. Generally, deductibles, coinsurance, and copayments should be collected at the time of service with the exception of the Medicare program, which does not recommend collecting the deductible in advance from the beneficiary. In cases of financial hardship, a discount or waiver may be considered. Be sure to document this and obtain the patient's signature and any document that verifies the patient's financial status.

Health insurance policies consider an *accident* to be an unforeseen and unintended event. Some policies cover accidents occurring from the first day the policy is in force. Others may contain an *elimination period* or a *waiting period* before benefits for sickness or accident become payable.

Generally, it is the patient's responsibility to give a written notice of **claim** to the insurance company within a certain number of days, known as a *time limit*. However, Blue Cross and Blue Shield plans, some managed care plan contracts, and Medicare guidelines require that the provider of service be obligated to submit the claim. Usually as a courtesy, the claim is filed for the patient by the provider of professional services. The insurance billing specialist must be able to abstract proper information from the patient record, which is used to code the diagnoses and services rendered; to complete an insurance claim form; to make entries (post) to a patient's financial accounting record (ledger); and to follow-up on unpaid claims. If any one of these procedures is not done properly, correct reimbursement or payment (also called **indemnity**) from the third-party payer will not be generated.

Follow-up on unpaid claims is made by contacting the claims representative, called a *claims adjudicator* or an *adjuster*. If the payment is to go directly from the insurance company to the physician, then the patient must sign a document granting permission.

Coordination of Benefits

A **coordination of benefits (COB)** statement is included in most policies and contracts with providers.

When the patient has more than one insurance policy (dual coverage or duplication of coverage), this clause requires insurance companies to coordinate the reimbursement of benefits to determine which carrier is going to be primary and which secondary, thus preventing the duplication or overlapping of payments for the same medical expense. The combination of payments from the primary and secondary carrier cannot be more than the amount of the provider's charges (Example 3-1).

Example 3-1   Coordination of Benefits for Dual Coverage Case

Mr. Smith has Insurance A and Insurance B. The claim is for $100. The claim is sent to Insurance A. Insurance A allows $80 for the procedure and pays $80. The claim is then sent to Insurance B. Insurance B also allows $80 for the procedure. The claim that was sent to Insurance B was not for $100 but for the remaining $20. The $20 is within the amount allowed by Insurance B, therefore Insurance B pays the $20. Some carriers try to play by their own rules by stating that because Insurance A paid $80 and the $80 equals the amount Insurance B pays, then Insurance B will pay no more for the claim. These rules were established by the National Association of Insurance Commissioners and approved by every State Insurance Commissioner. Therefore be observant of insurance claims like this.

Most state legislatures have adopted the *birthday law*, which is a change in the order of determination of coordination of benefits regarding primary and secondary carriers for dependent children. Rather than the father's insurance being primary, the father's or mother's carrier may be primary. The health plan of the person whose birthday (month and day, *not* year) falls earlier in the calendar year pays first, and the plan of the other person covering the dependent is the secondary payer. If both mother and father have the same birthday, the plan of the person who has had coverage longer is the primary payer. If one of the two plans has not adopted this birthday rule (i.e., if one plan is in another state), the rules of the plan without the birthday rule determine which plan is primary and which secondary. In cases of divorce, consider that you are not an enforcer of court laws and the divorce decree is between the parents of the child. Have the parent accompanying the child pay the bill at the time of service. He or she can be reimbursed by the responsible party. Keep issues of divorce a matter of decisions made within the court system. If a copy of the court decision is presented, bill the insurance of the parent deemed responsible.

Unions and companies that self-insure their employees do not fall under this birthday law. The states that do not have birthday laws are Georgia, Hawaii, Idaho, Massachusetts, Mississippi, Vermont, Virginia, and Washington, DC. Some plans may use the "general rule" for dependent children and identify the father's coverage as the primary carrier.

Finally, a carrier may delay a claim, stating that the carrier is attempting to coordinate benefits with the other carrier. This process can be time-consuming and may take 90 days or more to resolve. As a biller, you should be diligent in following up on this situation so that the stalled cash flow issue can be resolved. In some situations the patient may be ultimately responsible for the bill; if you help the patient understand that, this will bring payment and help resolve the account balance quicker.

General Policy Limitations

Health insurance policies contain **exclusions**—some more than others. If a person has an injury or illness that is excluded in his or her policy, then there is no insurance coverage for that injury or illness. These exclusions or limitations of the policy could be losses resulting from military service, attempted suicide, or self-inflicted injuries; losses caused by an injury on the job; pregnancy; and so on. Be aware that some insurance policies may state that a procedure or service is not covered (excluded) when the state law says the procedure is a "mandated benefit." Some examples are reconstructive breast surgery after mastectomy, surgical procedures affecting the upper and lower jawbones, and infertility coverage under group policies. Thus further investigation is necessary beyond reading the policy.

Many policies do not provide benefits for conditions that existed and were treated before the policy was issued; these are called **preexisting conditions.** In some instances, such conditions might be covered after a specified period of time (12 to 18 months) after the issuance of the policy. Some policies have a *waiver* or *rider,* which is an attachment to a policy that modifies clauses and provisions of the policy by either adding coverage or excluding certain illnesses or disabilities that would otherwise be covered. Generally, waivers are used to eliminate benefits for specific preexisting conditions. Under the health care reform legislation of 2010, insurance companies cannot deny coverage to children with preexisting medical problems. In 2014, insurers are barred from denying coverage to those with preexisting conditions or charging them more or from charging more for women.

Case Management Requirements

Preapproval

Many private third-party payers and prepaid health plans have certain requirements that must be met before they approve hospital admissions, inpatient or outpatient surgeries, and elective procedures. First, **eligibility** requirements must be obtained. These are conditions or qualifying factors that must be met before the patient receives benefits (medical services) under a specified insurance plan, government program, or managed care plan. The carrier can refuse to pay part or the entire fee if these requirements are not met. **Precertification** refers to discovering whether a treatment (surgery, hospitalization, tests) is covered under a patient's contract. **Preauthorization** relates not only to whether a service or procedure is covered, but also to finding out whether it is medically necessary. **Predetermination** means discovering the maximum dollar amount that the carrier will pay for surgery, consulting services, radiology procedures, and so on.

Obtain precertification or predetermination when a procedure is tentatively scheduled. The information that may be required to obtain precertification approval by fax or telephone is shown in Figure 3-2. Use the form shown in Figure 3-3 to obtain predetermination by mail. Figure 11-2 is an example of a preauthorization form. This form also can be used to document the information received when verifying the patient's insurance coverage by telephone. It should become part of the patient's record and used for reference when billing future insurance claims.

After the information is received from the third-party payer, give the patient an estimate of fees for the proposed surgery. An example of suggested wording for a letter is given in Figure 3-4. This written estimate makes collection quicker and easier.

CHOICE OF HEALTH INSURANCE

A person can obtain health insurance in three ways: (1) take out insurance through a group plan (contract or policy), (2) pay the premium on an individual basis, or (3) enroll in a prepaid health plan.

Group Contract

A *group contract* is any insurance plan by which a group of employees (and their eligible dependents) or other homogeneous group is insured under a single policy issued to their employer or leader, with individual certificates given to each insured individual or family unit. A group policy usually provides better benefits and offers lower premiums. However, the coverage for each person in the group is the same. If a new employee declines enrollment, he or she must sign a waiver stating this fact. Under the health care reform legislation of 2010, employers may change the kind of medical benefits they offer their employees (e.g., increase copayments and deductibles or reduce what the plans cover).

Conversion Privilege

Many physicians can obtain comprehensive group coverage through plans sponsored by the professional organizations to which they belong. Sometimes this is called a **blanket contract.** If the person leaves the employer or organization or the group contract is terminated, the insured may continue the same or lesser coverage under an individual policy if the group contract has a *conversion privilege.*

Usually, conversion from a group policy to an individual policy increases the premium and could reduce the benefits. However, if the person has a condition that would make him or her ineligible for coverage or is a case considered at **high risk,** it is advantageous to convert to an individual policy because no physical examination is required; therefore a preexisting condition cannot be excluded.

Income Continuation Benefits

According to the Consolidated Omnibus Budget Reconciliation Act of 1985 (COBRA), when an employee is laid off from a company with 20 or more workers, federal law requires that the group health insurance coverage be extended to the employee and his or her dependents at group rates for up to 18 months. This also applies to those workers who lose coverage because of reduced work hours. In the case of death of a covered employee, divorced or widowed spouse, or employee entitled to Medicare, the extension of coverage may be for 36 months. However, the employee must pay for the group policy; this is known as *income continuation benefits.* See the section on COBRA in Chapter 12 for additional information on this topic.

Medical Savings Accounts

The Health Insurance Portability and Accountability Act (HIPAA) of 1996 was federal legislation created to (1) expand efforts to combat fraud and abuse, as learned in the previous chapter, (2) protect workers and their families so that they can obtain and maintain health insurance if they change or lose their jobs, and (3) establish a medical savings account pilot project. An Archer *medical savings account* (MSA) is a type of tax-free savings account that allows individuals and their employers to set aside money to pay for health care expenses. An employer can set up an MSA for his or her employees and make an

COLLEGE CLINIC
4567 Broad Avenue
Woodland Hills, XY 12345-0000

Phone: 555/486-9002   Fax: 555/590-2189

Insurance Precertification Form

Date: 5/4/XX
To: Insurance Carrier ___Cal-Net Care___   From: ___Janet___ Office Mgr.
     Address ___9900 Baker Street___
     ___Los Angeles, CA 90067___

Check those that apply: Admission certification ✔   Outpatient___ Inpatient ✔
                            Surgery certification ✔   Emergency situation ✔

Patient's name ___Ronald Stranton___   Date of Birth: 4-14-49
Patient's address ___639 Cedar Street___   Sex: Male ✔ Female ___
     ___Woodland Hills, XY 12345___   Social Security No. 527-XX-7250
Insured's Name ___Same___   Policy Group ID No. A59
Insured's Address___   Employer: Aerostar Aviation

Treating physician ___Clarence Cutler, M.D.___   NPI #: 430 500 47XX
Primary Care Physician ___Gerald Practon, M.D.___ NPI #: 462 7889 7XX

Name of Hospital ___College Hospital___   Admission Date: 5/4/XX
                                                   Estimated Length of Stay: 3-5 d
Admitting Diagnosis ___Volvulus___   Diagnosis Code: 560.2
Complicating conditions to substantiate need for inpatient hospitalization___
          ___Complete bowel obstruction___
Date current illness or injury began ___5/2/XX___
Procedure/surgery to be done ___Reduction of Volvulus___   Procedure code ___44050___

Second opinion needed   Yes ___ No ✔ Date performed ___

Telephone precertification: ___Emergency Cert. 5/4/XX___
Name of representative certifying___McKenzie Kwan___
Direct-dial telephone number of representative ___1-800-463-9000 ext. 227___

Reason(s) for denial ___
Certification approved   Yes ✔ No ___ Certification approval No. 69874
Authorization for services Yes ✔ No ___ Authorization No. 69874E

Note: The information contained in this facsimile message is confidential and privileged information intended only for the use of the individual or entity named above. If the reader of this message is not the intended recipient, you are hereby notified that any dissemination, distribution, or copying of this communication is strictly prohibited. If you have received this communication in error, please immediately notify me by telephone and return the original facsimile to me via the U.S. Postal Service. Thank you.

FIGURE 3-2 Insurance precertification form. This form can be faxed to the insurance company or used when telephoning to obtain approval for hospitalization under a patient's insurance policy or managed care plan.

annual contribution to the MSA, which is tax-deductible for both employer and employee. MSA balances accumulate from year to year tax-free, but unused funds may not be carried over in a *flexible spending account* (FSA) (another type of MSA). Earned interest is not taxed. MSAs are portable, allowing individuals to take their MSA with them when they change jobs or relocate. When health care services are provided, the patient files a claim to receive reimbursement from these funds and uses the explanation of benefits (EOB) from the insurance company as documentation. Processing of the explanation of benefits for insurance claims with large deductibles (e.g., more than $1000), even though you know the insurance company will not be paying for the services, is necessary so that the patient/employee may submit documentation and recoup funds from the MSA. It also may be necessary to provide EOB documents from the insurance company to patients who do not receive them for

COLLEGE CLINIC
4567 Broad Avenue
Woodland Hills, XY 12345-0001

Phone: 555/486-9002   Fax: 555/487-8976

INSURANCE PREDETERMINATION FORM

Perry Cardi, MD
Physician

Patient: Leslee Austin
Address: 209 Refugio Road
City: Woodland Hills   State: XY
Social Security #: 629-XX-9260
Insurance Company: American Insurance
Insurance Co. Address: 4040 Broadway Ave
Valley Vista, XY 12345
Policy holder: Leslee Austin
Relationship to insured: Self X Spouse___ Child___ Other___
Type of coverage: HMO X PPO___ 80/20___ 70/30___ Other:___
Procedure/Service: Cardioversion (CPT 92960)
Diagnosis: Atrial fibrillation (ICD–9–CM 427.31)

Telephone #: (555) 486-8452
Date of Birth: 04-07-44
ZIP: 12345-0001
Accident Yes___ No X
Member #: Am 45692
Group #: 123P
Telephone #: (555) 238-5000

BENEFITS:
Coverage effective date: From 02/01/XX To 01/31/XX
Pre-existing exclusions: Lupus erythematosus
Major medical   Yes X No___
Deductible   Yes___ No X Amount $___
Per family: Yes___ No X Amount $___
Deductible paid to date: Amount $___
Out of pocket expense limit: Amount $___
Per:___

Maximum benefit or benefit limitation: $1,000,000 lifetime
Second opinion requirements: Yes___ No X
Precertification/Preauthorization Yes X No___
Reference #: 432786
Authorized by: Lucille Vasquez

COVERAGE: COVERAGE DETAILS AND LIMITS
Procedures/Services
Office visits   YES X NO___   Physical exam; one per year
Consultations   YES X NO___
ER visits   YES X NO___
X-ray   YES X NO___
Laboratory   YES X NO___   Need authorization
Office surgery   YES X NO___   Need authorization
Hospital surgery   YES X NO___
Anesthesia   YES X NO___   Need authorization
DME   YES X NO___
Physician payment schedule: RVS___ RBRVS___ UCR___ Other X

Payment sent to: Provider X Patient___ Time limit after submission? 30 days
Verification by: Karen Reynolds   Date: 07-14-XX

FIGURE 3-3 Insurance predetermination form. This form can be sent to the insurance company to find out the maximum dollar amount that will be paid for primary surgery, consulting services, postoperative care, and so on.

this same purpose. Medicare beneficiaries are eligible to enroll in a similar tax-advantaged savings account, which may be referred to as a *Medicare medical savings account.*

Health Savings Accounts

The Medicare reform act was signed into law in December 2003, giving Americans a tool for defraying medical costs called *health savings accounts* (HSAs). HSAs are open

to anyone younger than 65 years of age who enrolls in a high-deductible (e.g., more than $1050/individual or $2100/family in 2006) health plan (HDHP). Annual out-of-pocket expenses (deductibles and copays) apply and may not exceed $5150 for self-only coverage ($10,200 for family coverage). Employers pay the monthly premiums. Employees pay the deductibles when they receive health care treatment and may share some of the costs of the plan via payroll deductions. These accounts are a

COLLEGE CLINIC
4567 Broad Avenue
Woodland Hills, XY 12345-0000

Phone: 555/486-9002   **Fax: 555/487-8976**

Current date

Patient's name
Address
City, State, ZIP code

Dear

This letter gives you an estimate of the fees for your proposed surgery. Verification of coverage and benefit information has been obtained from your insurance company. Listed are your benefits for the proposed surgical expenses and the estimated balance after your insurance carrier pays.

Surgical procedure	Craniotomy
Date of surgery	February 21, 20XX
Name of hospital	College Hospital
Hospital address	4500 Broad Ave., Woodland Hills, XY 12345

		Insurance pays	Estimated balance
Surgeon's fee	2548.09	1344.24	1203.85
Preoperative visit			
Preoperative tests			

You have a policy deductible of $1000 which___ has ✓ has not been met.

The surgery requires the use of an anesthesiologist, assistant surgeon, and a pathologist. These physicians will bill you separately for their services. The hospital will also bill you separately.

This office will file your insurance claim for the surgical procedure, so the insurance payment should come directly to us. If the insurance carrier sends you the payment, then you are responsible to get the payment to this office within five days. Your balance after surgery should be approximately $1203.85. You are responsible for any remaining balance after our office receives the insurance payment.

Thank you for choosing our medical practice. If you have any questions, please call me.

Sincerely,

Karen Martinez, CMA
Administrative Medical Assistant

FIGURE 3-4 Sample letter to a patient supplying an estimate of the fees for proposed surgery.

tax-favored savings plan in which a working person can deposit money in an HSA and deduct the amount of the deposits from taxable income. Withdrawals from HSAs are tax-free when used for qualifying medical expenses. Money left unspent in an HSA may be rolled over year after year.

Health Reimbursement Arrangements

An alternative plan is a *health reimbursement account* (HRA), which has a high deductible and may be better than an HSA for a chronically ill person (e.g., a person with diabetes). However, only employers can contribute to the account, and it can be used to fund the first part of a high deductible. Workers do not put their own funds in HRAs. Employers may keep the money if a worker quits. These funds can be carried over year to year.

Healthcare Flexible Spending Accounts

Another option is a healthcare flexible spending account (HFSA). HFSAs are employer sponsored and allow a specific amount of wages to be put aside for qualified medical expenses and childcare. The funds in HFSAs cannot be rolled over from year to year. Under the health care reform of 2010, a written prescription is required for over-the-counter medications to ensure that only the cost of the drugs is deducted from the patient's taxable income.

High-Deductible Health Plans

High-deductible health plans (HDHPs), also known as consumer-directed health plans, are combined with an HSA or HRA and give insurance coverage that has tax advantages to assist in saving for future medical expenses. They have annual out-of-pocket limits and a higher annual deductible than traditional health insurance plans.

Individual Contract

Any insurance plan issued to an individual (and dependents) is called an *individual contract*. Usually, this type of policy has a higher premium, and often the benefits are less than those obtainable under a group health insurance plan. Sometimes this is called **personal insurance.**

Prepaid Health Plan

This is a program of health care in which a specified set of health benefits is provided for a subscriber or enrolled group of subscribers who pay a yearly fee or fixed periodic payments. Providers of services are paid by capitation. **Capitation** is a system of payment used by managed care plans in which physicians and hospitals are paid a fixed, per capita amount for each patient enrolled over a stated period of time, regardless of the type and number of services provided. For additional information on this topic, refer to Chapter 11.

TYPES OF HEALTH INSURANCE COVERAGE

Many forms of health insurance coverage are currently in effect in the United States. These are referred to as third-party payers (private insurance, government plans, managed care contracts, and workers' compensation). A brief explanation of the programs to be discussed in this text is given here, but for an in-depth study, refer to the appropriate chapters that follow.

 CHAMPVA: The Civilian Health and Medical Program of the Department of Veterans Affairs **(CHAMPVA)** is administered by the Department of Veterans Affairs. This federal program shares the medical bills of spouses and children of veterans with total, permanent, service-connected disabilities or of the surviving spouses and children of veterans who died as a result of service-connected disabilities (see Chapter 14).

 Competitive Medical Plan: A **competitive medical plan (CMP)** is a type of managed care organization created by the 1982 Tax Equity and Fiscal Responsibility Act (TEFRA). This federal legislation allows for enrollment of Medicare beneficiaries into managed care plans (see Chapter 12).

 Disability Income Insurance: **Disability income insurance** is a form of health insurance that provides periodic payments to replace income when the insured is unable to work as a result of illness, injury, or disease (see Chapter 16). This type of insurance should not be confused with workers' compensation because those injuries must be work related.

 Exclusive Provider Organization: An **exclusive provider organization (EPO)** is a type of managed health care plan in which subscriber members are eligible for benefits only when they use the services of a limited network of providers. EPOs combine features of both HMOs and PPOs. Employers agree not to enter into an agreement with any other plan for coverage of eligible employees. EPOs are regulated under state health insurance laws (see Chapter 11).

Foundation for Medical Care: A foundation for medical care (FMC) is an organization of physicians, sponsored by a state or local medical association, concerned with the development and delivery of medical services and the cost of health care (see Chapter 11).

 Health Maintenance Organization: A **health maintenance organization (HMO)** is an organization that provides a wide range of comprehensive health care services for a specified group at a fixed periodic payment. The emphasis is on preventive care. Physicians are reimbursed by capitation. An HMO can be sponsored by the government, medical schools, hospitals, employers, labor unions, consumer groups, insurance companies, or hospital medical plans (see Chapter 11).

 Independent or Individual Practice Association: An **independent or individual practice association (IPA)** is a type of managed care plan in which a program administrator contracts with a number of physicians who agree to provide treatment to subscribers in their own offices or clinics for a fixed capitation payment per month. Subscribers to IPA plans have limited or no choice of physician. IPA physicians continue to see their fee-for-service patients (see Chapter 11).

 Maternal and Child Health Program: A **Maternal and Child Health Program (MCHP)** is a state and federal program for children who are younger than 21 years of age and have special health care needs. It assists parents with financial planning and may assume part or all of the costs of treatment, depending on the child's condition and the family's resources (see Chapter 13).

 Medicaid: Medicaid (MCD) is a program sponsored jointly by federal, state, and local governments to provide health care benefits to medically indigent persons on welfare (public assistance), aged individuals who meet certain financial requirements, and the disabled. Some states have expanded coverage for other medically needy individuals who meet special state-determined criteria. Coverage and benefits vary widely from state to state. In California, this program is known as Medi-Cal (see Chapter 13).

 Medicare: Medicare is a national four-part program. It consists of a hospital insurance system (Part A), supplementary medical insurance (Part B), Medicare Plus Choice Program (Part C), and the Medicare Prescription Drug benefits (Part D). It is for individuals who are at least 65 years of age. It was created by the 1965 Amendments to the Social Security Act and is operated under the provisions of the act. Benefits are also extended to certain disabled people (e.g., totally disabled or blind), and coverage and payment are provided for those requiring kidney dialysis and kidney transplant services (see Chapters 12 and 13).

 Medicare/Medicaid: Medicare/Medicaid (Medi-Medi) is a program that covers those persons eligible for both Medicare and Medicaid (see Chapters 12 and 13).

 Point-of-Service Plan: A **point-of-service (POS) plan** is a managed care plan consisting of a network of physicians and hospitals that provides an insurance company or employer with discounts on its services. Patients can refer themselves to a specialist or see a nonprogram provider for a higher copayment (see Chapter 11).

Preferred Provider Organization: A variation of a managed care plan is a **preferred provider organization (PPO).** This is a form of contract medicine by which a large employer (e.g., hospitals or physicians) or any organization that can produce a large number of patients (e.g., union trusts or insurance companies) contracts with a hospital or a group of physicians to offer medical care at a reduced rate (see Chapter 11).

TRICARE: A government-sponsored program called **TRICARE** provides military and nonmilitary hospital and medical services for spouses of active service personnel, dependents of active service personnel, retired service personnel and their dependents, and dependents of members who died on active duty. Active duty service members (ADSMs) are not eligible for TRICARE but have benefits like TRICARE Prime in which the Department of Defense (DoD) covers all allowable charges for medically necessary care (see Chapter 14).

Unemployment Compensation Disability: **Unemployment Compensation Disability (UCD)** or **State Disability Insurance (SDI)** is insurance that covers off-the-job injury or sickness and is paid for by deductions from a person's paycheck. This program is administered by a state agency in only six states (see Chapter 16).

Veterans Affairs Outpatient Clinic: A **Veterans Affairs (VA) outpatient clinic** renders medical and dental services to a veteran who has a service-related disability (see Chapter 14).

Workers' Compensation Insurance: **Workers' compensation (WC) insurance** is a contract that insures a person against on-the-job injury or illness. The employer pays the premium for his or her employees (see Chapter 15).

EXAMPLES OF INSURANCE BILLING

Sometimes it is difficult to comprehend the full scale of insurance billing. As an example of total medical billing, six cases are presented to help you understand the entire billing picture from simple to complex.

CASE 1: A new patient comes in with complaints of a sore throat and an infected nail. Evaluation and management (E/M) services are discussed in detail in Chapter 6.

The physician's office bills for:

Evaluation and management services
Penicillin injection
Office surgery for infected nail
Sterile surgical tray (may or may not be billed, depending on third-party payer)

CASE 2: A patient comes in because of an accident and has complaints that require evaluation and management services, x-ray films, and laboratory studies (urinalysis) performed in the physician's office.

The physician's office bills for:

E/M services
X-ray studies (including interpretation) and laboratory tests (urinalysis, including interpretation)

CASE 3: A patient is seen by the family physician after office hours in the hospital emergency department.

The physician's office bills for E/M services.

The hospital bills for hospital (outpatient) emergency department services (use and supplies).

CASE 4: A physician sends a patient's Papanicolaou smear to a private clinical laboratory.

The physician's office bills for:

E/M services
Handling of specimen

The laboratory bills for the Papanicolaou smear.

CASE 5: A patient is sent to a local hospital for an upper gastrointestinal radiographic series. An x-ray technician obtains the films in the hospital, and a privately owned radiologic group does the interpretation.

The hospital bills for the technical component of the upper gastrointestinal x-ray series (use of equipment).

The radiologic group bills for the professional component of the upper gastrointestinal x-ray series (the interpretation).

CASE 6: A patient is seen in the office and is immediately hospitalized for surgery.

The physician's office bills for initial hospital admission (E/M services) and surgical procedure (e.g., hysterectomy). (The physician is a surgeon.)

The assistant surgeon bills for assisting the surgeon during hysterectomy. (Some third-party payers do not allow payment.)

The anesthesiologist bills for anesthesia administered during hysterectomy.

The hospital (inpatient) bills for hospital room, operating room, anesthesia supplies, medications, x-ray films, laboratory tests, and medical and surgical supplies (dressings, intravenous lines). The hospital (inpatient) might also bill for blood for transfusions, electrocardiogram, radiation therapy, and respiratory therapy.

An insurance billing specialist in the offices of the attending physician, assistant surgeon, anesthesiologist, radiologic group, and private clinical laboratory submits an itemized statement and/or insurance claim form for reimbursement from the insurance payer or gives the patient the necessary information to submit his or her own claim to the insurance company. **EXCEPTION** Medicare patients by federal law may not submit their own claims for physician or hospital services. Exceptions are mentioned in Chapter 12.

In the hospital and hospital emergency department, a member of the hospital staff inputs services into a central computer system that produces an itemized statement and completed insurance claim form via computer to be submitted to the third-party payer. Hospital billing is explained in Chapter 17.

PROCEDURE 3-1: HANDLING AND PROCESSING INSURANCE CLAIMS

Most offices today are computerized and use practice management software (PMS) for scheduling, **accounts receivable management** (coding and billing) and patient statements, electronic health records, and other administrative functions such as generating patient reminders and letters. However, some smaller offices thrive in the paper environment and will continue to do so.

A computerized office may still generate paper insurance claim forms and send them to the insurance payer; however, this chapter differentiates health care practices that have computerized operations from those that are simply using paper ledgers and generating paper-only claims and do not use the computer for any administrative practice management functions.

To help you better understand the differences in methodologies used by paper-based offices versus the computerized office, use the icons as a guide.

Different methods exist for processing insurance claims for the health care practice. The most common ones follow:

1. Posting charges and submitting to the insurance payer on the legacy paper CMS (formerly HCFA) 1500 (08-05) claim form. This form has been used in the industry since 1975. The CMS 1500 (08-05) can be prepared manually by filling in the claim information with a pen or it can be generated by the computer.

2. Electronic claims transmitted from in-office computers.
3. Contracting with an outside billing service company to prepare and electronically transmit claims on behalf of the health care provider's office.
4. Direct data entry (DDE) into the payer's system. The billing specialist logs into the insurance company's system and keys in the data required to process the claim.

Keep in mind that HIPAA regulations will determine whether a health care provider is a covered entity and whether it is required to submit claims electronically.

When using any of these methods, the administrative life cycle of an insurance claim showing the basic steps (Figure 3-5) in handling and processing insurance claims in a physician's office, to the insurance carrier, and after payment is received is as follows:

1. **Preregistration—Patient Registration Information Form:** Some medical practices preregister a new patient during the initial telephone call, have a designated staff member contact the patient before the appointment time, or send a letter confirming appointment with an informative brochure about the medical practice and a patient registration form. This form may be printed off the website, completed online, or completed when the patient arrives for his or her appointment. It is a good idea to give directions and/or a map of how to get to the office and to

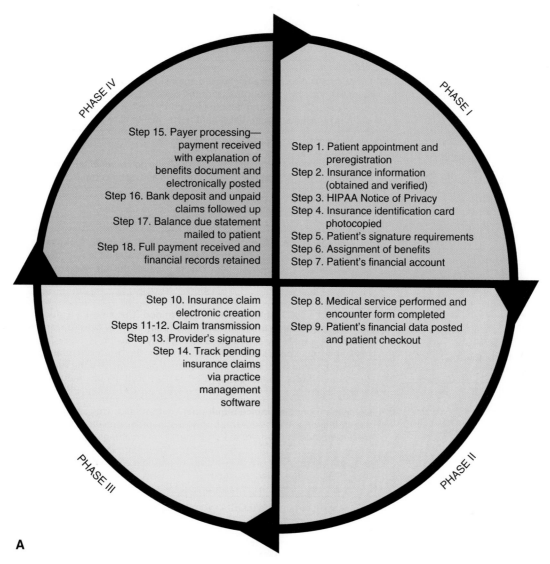

FIGURE 3-5 A, Revenue cycle overview showing the basic steps in processing an insurance claim in a physician's office, to the third-party payer, and after payment is received.

Continued

ask the patient to arrive early. An average window of time is approximately 15 to 20 minutes before the scheduled appointment. This allows time to collect vital statistics and insurance information and to discuss the patient's responsibility with respect to payment policies. Medical practices that see children should have a statement on the form that states "For pediatric patients, the parent, relative, or person escorting the patient is responsible for any payments due at the time of service." A **patient registration form** also may be called a *patient information form* or *intake sheet* (Figures 3-6 and 3-7). It may be developed by the physician and personalized for his or her own use or may be a generic form purchased from a medical supply company. If the patient has a medical problem that makes it difficult to complete the form such as rheumatoid arthritis of the hands or limited vision, then the insurance billing specialist should interview the patient and fill in the necessary data. Instruct the patient to fill in all spaces and indicate N/A (not applicable) if an item does not apply. Read the form carefully after completion to make sure *complete* and *accurate* personal and financial information have been obtained from the patient. If the form is returned with blank spaces, assist the patient in completing the form. The patient registration form should contain the following facts:

● Name: first, middle initial, and last. The name must match that shown on the insurance identification card. (Some pediatric patients do not have the same last name as their parents or stepparents.) Insurance payments show the policyholder's name, and it is time-consuming to find and give credit to the patient's account without this information

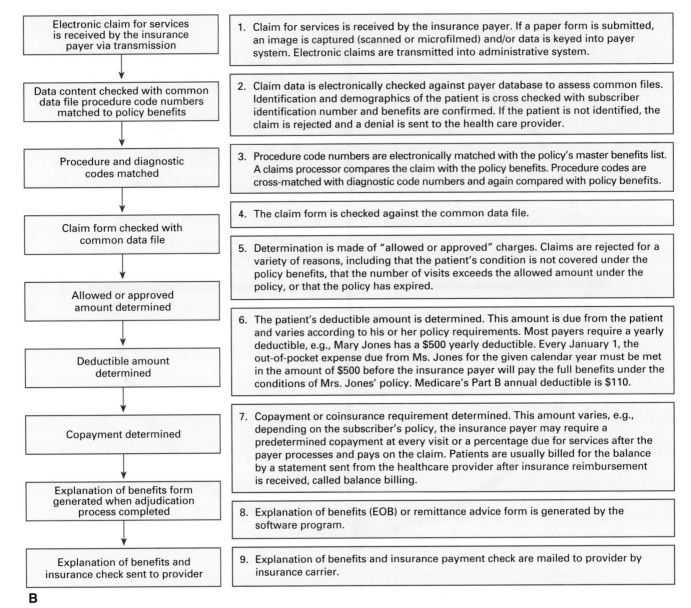

Electronic claim for services is received by the insurance payer via transmission	1. Claim for services is received by the insurance payer. If a paper form is submitted, an image is captured (scanned or microfilmed) and/or data is keyed into payer system. Electronic claims are transmitted into administrative system.
Data content checked with common data file procedure code numbers matched to policy benefits	2. Claim data is electronically checked against payer database to assess common files. Identification and demographics of the patient is cross checked with subscriber identification number and benefits are confirmed. If the patient is not identified, the claim is rejected and a denial is sent to the health care provider.
Procedure and diagnostic codes matched	3. Procedure code numbers are electronically matched with the policy's master benefits list. A claims processor compares the claim with the policy benefits. Procedure codes are cross-matched with diagnostic code numbers and again compared with policy benefits.
Claim form checked with common data file	4. The claim form is checked against the common data file.
Allowed or approved amount determined	5. Determination is made of "allowed or approved" charges. Claims are rejected for a variety of reasons, including that the patient's condition is not covered under the policy benefits, that the number of visits exceeds the allowed amount under the policy, or that the policy has expired.
Deductible amount determined	6. The patient's deductible amount is determined. This amount is due from the patient and varies according to his or her policy requirements. Most payers require a yearly deductible, e.g., Mary Jones has a $500 yearly deductible. Every January 1, the out-of-pocket expense due from Ms. Jones for the given calendar year must be met in the amount of $500 before the insurance payer will pay the full benefits under the conditions of Mrs. Jones' policy. Medicare's Part B annual deductible is $110.
Copayment determined	7. Copayment or coinsurance requirement determined. This amount varies, e.g., depending on the subscriber's policy, the insurance payer may require a predetermined copayment at every visit or a percentage due for services after the payer processes and pays on the claim. Patients are usually billed for the balance by a statement sent from the healthcare provider after insurance reimbursement is received, called balance billing.
Explanation of benefits form generated when adjudication process completed	8. Explanation of benefits (EOB) or remittance advice form is generated by the software program.
Explanation of benefits and insurance check sent to provider	9. Explanation of benefits and insurance payment check are mailed to provider by insurance carrier.

B

FIGURE 3-5, cont'd B, Adjudication: Insurance payer life cycle of an insurance claim shows the basic steps of a third-party payer to pay an insurance claim and the documents generated.

- Practice management systems allow a cross-reference of the patient, subscriber, and guarantor's names, as well as Social Security number, so that when you recall the policyholder's name, the patient's name also appears.
- In a paper or manual system, keep an alphabetic card index of parental or billing names that also lists each patient's name.
- Street address, including apartment number, ZIP code, and telephone numbers with area code (cell and landline).
- Business address, telephone number with extension, and occupation.
- E-mail address.

- Date of birth (HIPAA requires eight digits [year/month/day] to be submitted to payers; for example, the eight-digit format of January 2, 1936, is 19360102). Your practice management system may collect these data in a different format but transmit in the required eight-digit format.
- Person responsible for account (guarantor) or insured's name
- Social Security number
- Spouse's name and occupation
- Referring physician's name or other referral source
- Driver's license number
- Emergency contact (close relative or friend with name, address, and telephone number)

Insurance cards copied ☒
Date: __JAN. 20, 20XX__

Patient Registration
Information
Please PRINT AND complete ALL sections below!

Account # : __84516__
Insurance # : __H-550-64-5172-02__
Co-Payment: $ __OV $10 ER $50__

Is your condition a result of a work injury? YES (NO) An auto accident? YES (NO)   Date of injury: _____

PATIENT'S PERSONAL INFORMATION   Marital Status ☐ Single ☒ Married ☐ Divorced ☐ Widowed   Sex: ☐ Male ☒ Female

Name: _____FUHR_____ (last name) _____LINDA_____ (first name) __L.__ (initial)
Street address: __3070 Tipper Street__   (Apt. # __4__) City: __Oxnard__   State: __CA__ Zip: __93030__
Home phone: (_555_) __276-0101__   Work phone: (_555_) __372-1151__   Cell phone: (_555_) __243-1777__
Date of Birth: _11_ / _05_ / _65_   Driver's Lic.: (State & #) __G0075012__   SSN _550_ – _XX_ – _5172_
How do you wish to be addressed? __LINDA__   E-mail: __fuhrL@yahoo.com__   Fax # (_____)
Employer/Name of School: __Electronic Data Systems__   ☒ Full Time ☐ Part Time
Spouse's Name: _FUHR_ (last) _GERALD_ (first) _T._ (initial)   Spouse's Work # (_555_) _921-0075_   SSN _545_ – _XX_ – _2771_

PATIENT'S/RESPONSIBLE PARTY INFORMATION

Responsible party: __GERALD T. FUHR__   Date of Birth: _06_ / _15_ / _64_
Relationship to Patient: ☐ Self ☒ Spouse ☐ Other _____   SSN _545_ – _XX_ – _2771_
Responsible party's home phone: (_555_) __276-0101__   Work phone: (_555_) _921-0075_
    Address: __3070 Tipper Street__   (Apt. # _4_) City: __Oxnard__   State: __CA__ Zip: __93030__
Employer's name: __General Electric__   Phone number: (_555_) _485-0121_
    Address: __317 East Main__   City: __Oxnard__   State: __CA__ Zip: __93030__
    Your occupation: __Technician__
Spouse's Employer's name: __Electronic Data Systems__   Spouse's Work phone: (_555_) _372-1151_
    Address: __2700 West 5th Street__   City: __Oxnard__   State: __CA__ Zip: __93030__

PATIENT'S INSURANCE INFORMATION   Please present insurance cards to receptionist.

PRIMARY insurance company's name: __ABC Insurance Company__
Insurance address: __P.O. Box 12340__   City: __Fresno__   State: __CA__ Zip: __93765__
Name of insured: __Linda L. Fuhr__   Date of Birth: _11_ / _05_ / _65_   Relationship to insured: ☒ Self ☐ Spouse ☐ Other ☐ Child
Insurance ID number: __H-550-XX-5172-02__   Group number: __17098-020-00004__
SECONDARY insurance company's name: __None__
Insurance address: _____   City: _____   State: ___ Zip: ___
Name of insured: _____   Date of Birth: __ / __ / ___   Relationship to insured: ☐ Self ☐ Spouse ☐ Other ☐ Child
Insurance ID number: _____   Group number: _____
Check if appropriate: ☐ Medigap policy ☐ Retiree coverage

PATIENT'S REFERRAL INFORMATION   (please circle one)

Referred by: __Margaret Taylor (Mrs. W.T.)__   If referred by a friend, may we thank him or her? (YES) NO
Name(s) of other physician(s) who care for you: __Jason Smythe, MD__

EMERGENCY CONTACT

Name of person not living with you: __Hannah Gildea__   Relationship: __Aunt__
Address: __4621 Lucretia Avenue__   City: __Oxnard__   State: __CA__ Zip: __93030__
Phone number (home): (_555_) __274-0132__   Phone number (work): (____) _____

Assignment of Benefits • Financial Agreement
I hereby give lifetime authorization for payment of insurance benefits to be made directly to __Gerald Practon, MD__, and any assisting physicians, for services rendered. I understand that I am financially responsible for all charges whether or not they are covered by insurance. In the event of default, I agree to pay all costs of collection, and reasonable attorney's fees. I hereby authorize this healthcare provider to release all information necessary to secure the payment of benefits.
I further agree that a photocopy of this agreement shall be as valid as the original.
Date: __Jan 20, 20XX__   Your Signature: *Linda L Fuhr*
Method of Payment: ☐ Cash ☒ Check ☐ Credit Card
FORM # 58-8423 • BIBBERO SYSTEMS, INC. • PETALUMA, CA. • TO ORDER CALL TOLL FREE : 800-BIBBERO (800-242-2376) • FAX (800) 242-9330   (REV. 9/06)

FIGURE 3-6 Patient registration information form showing a comprehensive listing of personal and financial information obtained from the patient on his or her first visit to the office. (Courtesy Bibbero Systems, Inc., Petaluma, CA. Telephone: 800-242-2376; fax: 800-242-9330; website: www.bibbero.com.)

• Insurance billing information: all insurance company names, addresses, policy numbers, and group numbers. This is important because of the coordination of benefits clause written into some health insurance policies. Older patients are given the option of joining managed care programs and are allowed to switch every 30 days. Always ask each older patient whether he or she is covered by traditional Medicare or a Medicare HMO. A good patient information sheet has space where this information can be written in by the patient.

2. **Verification of Insurance:** Verify insurance and all other information that may have changed at each visit because patients may transfer from one insurance plan to another, move, or change jobs. This may be done by giving the patient a copy of the previously completed patient registration form and asking him or her to correct any incorrect data in red. Established

FIGURE 3-7 Receptionist giving instructions to a patient on how to complete the patient registration form.

patients may have changed employers or may have married or divorced.

3. **Notice of Privacy Practices:** Each patient is given a Notice of Privacy Practice (NPP) that explains how his or her health information is used. Obtain patient's acknowledgment of receipt of the NPP. If the patient refuses or is unable to sign, document this in his or her health record. An NPP is mandatory under federal law through HIPAA.

4. **Insurance Identification Card:** Photocopy front and back sides of all of the patient's insurance identification cards (Figure 3-8). A copy produces error-free insurance data and can be used in lieu of completing the insurance section of the patient registration form. Ask for a photo identification, such as a driver's license, to verify the person has not used someone else's card. If the insurance plan requires referral or precertification for any services, call the insurance company to verify coverage and applicable deductible or copayment. On a return visit, ask to see the card and check it with the data on file (Figure 3-9). If it differs, photocopy both sides and write the date on the copy, using this as the base for revising data on file.

RELEASE OF INFORMATION

If the physician is submitting an insurance claim for the patient, the patient is not required to sign a release of information form before information can be given to an insurance company for obtaining payment for professional services. However, some medical practices prefer to operate at a higher level of privacy and continue to obtain patients' signatures on release of information forms.

5. **Patient's Signature Requirements:** Under HIPAA regulations, a patient's signed authorization is not required for treatment, payment, or health care operations (TPO). There may be circumstances when the patient would like to give authorization for reasons beyond TPO; therefore the Authorization for Release of Information form should be available and presented to the patient.

 Electronic environment: Patient signatures cannot be submitted electronically. Use the signature-on-file (SOF) provision to satisfy Medicare's patient signature requirements. Electronic billers are permitted to obtain a lifetime authorization from the beneficiary and retain it in a file for future use on all electronic claims. This authorization allows the office to submit assigned and unassigned claims on the beneficiary's behalf. To use this procedure, the patient should sign a brief statement that reads as follows:

(Name of Beneficiary) (Health Insurance Claim Number)
"I request that payment of authorized Medicare benefits be made either to me or on my behalf to (name of physician or supplier) for any services furnished me by physician or supplier. I authorize any holder of medical information about me to release to the Centers for Medicare & Medicaid Services (CMS) and its agents any information needed to determine these benefits or the benefits payable for related services."
Signature Indicator: Patient signature source. Must not be blank. If invalid value is reported, a claim level rejection will occur.

Valid Values:
C = Signed CMS-1500 (08-05) claim form on file
M = Signed signature authorization form for Block 13 on file
B = Signed signature authorization form for both Blocks 12 and 13 on file
P = Signature generated by provider because the patient was not physically present for service
S = Signed signature authorization form for Block 12 on file
NSF—All versions
ANSI—Versions 30.32 and 30.51
ANSI—Version 5010 (HIPAA)

Most patient registration forms include a statement to sign regarding these two authorizations (see bottom of Figure 3-6).

Paper environment: Since the enforcement of HIPAA regulations, a patient's signature for the release of information in Block 12 is no longer required. The signature requirement for the assignment of benefits is included in Block 13 of the CMS-1500 (08-05) insurance claim form (Figure 3-10). If a signature is obtained on a separate form, it may be filed in the

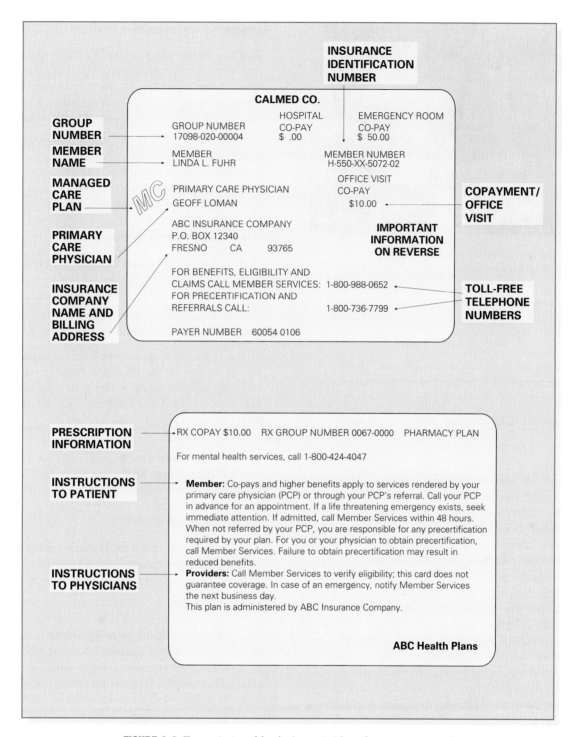

FIGURE 3-8 Front *(top)* and back *(bottom)* sides of an insurance card.

patient's health record and the abbreviation "SOF" or the preferred spelled-out notation "signature on file" may be used on the insurance claim form.

For a patient on a federal program, such as Medicare or TRICARE (see Chapters 12 and 14), acceptance of assignment means not only that the payment will come to the physician but also that the physician will accept

what the federal program designates as the "allowed amount." The federal program pays a percentage of the allowed amount, and the patient pays a remaining coinsurance (cost-sharing) percentage.

6. **Assignment of Benefits:** For the health care provider to receive reimbursement directly from the insurance payer, the patient must sign an assignment of benefits

FIGURE 3-9 Patient presenting an insurance identification card to the receptionist for photocopying.

> 13. INSURED'S OR AUTHORIZED PERSON'S SIGNATURE I authorize payment of medical benefits to the undersigned physician or supplier for services described below.
>
> SIGNED _____

FIGURE 3-10 Section 13 from the health insurance claim form CMS-1500 (08-05), illustrating authorization for assignment of benefits.

statement for each insurance company. However, before explaining an assignment, it is important to define the difference between participating and nonparticipating providers. A **participating provider (par)** has a contractual agreement with an insurance plan to render care to eligible beneficiaries and bills the third-party payer directly (Example 3-2). The third-party payer pays its portion of the allowed amount, and the provider bills the patient for the balance not paid by the insurer after the disallowed portion is adjusted off of the account. However, in Blue Plans, the provider is referred to as a *member physician* and may accept the payment as payment in full or bill the patient for any unpaid balance, depending on the contract. Managed care plans also refer to participating providers as member physicians. If the amount of the patient's responsibility can be determined, collect it at the time of the visit.

A **nonparticipating provider (nonpar)** is a physician without a contractual agreement with an insurance plan to accept an allowed amount and to render care to eligible beneficiaries (Example 3-3). The provider may or may not file an insurance claim as a courtesy to the patient and may obtain full payment at the time of service. The patient should be made aware that his or her insurance plan will cover a considerable amount less on the claim when receiving services from a nonpar provider.

Example 3-2 Participating Provider

Dr. Gomez accepts assignment and is a participating (par) provider for the Liberty Health Insurance Plan. Pedro Nunez, a new patient, is seen in the office with complaints of a sore throat and infected nail for which a $150 fee is charged for office surgery, penicillin injection, and E/M services. The patient has met his deductible for the year.

Provider fee (total billed amount)	$150
Provider contracted rate (allowable charge)	$140
Patient coinsurance or copayment amount	$10
Insurance claims payment	$130
Provider's adjusted (write-off) amount	$10

Dr. Gomez collects $10 from the patient and is paid a total of $140.

Example 3-3 Nonparticipating Provider

Dr. Warner does not accept assignment and is a nonparticipating (nonpar) provider for the XYZ Health Insurance Plan. Estelle Cutter, an established patient, is seen in the office complaining that her ears are full of earwax that needs to be removed. A $60 fee is charged.

Provider fee (total billed amount)	$60
Usual and customary rate (UCR)	$55
Patient coinsurance or copayment amount	$10
Insurance claims payment	$44
Provider may bill patient over UCR	$6

Dr. Warner collects $16 from the patient and is paid a total of $60 because he can collect the difference between his fee and the patient's copayment plus the insurance payment.

The general definition of **assignment** is the transfer, after an event insured against, of an individual's legal right to collect an amount payable under an insurance contract. Most of the time an agreement is obtained by having the patient sign an assignment of insurance benefits document directing payment to the physician. However, the paper CMS-1500 (08-05) claim form contains a provision that, when signed by the insured, directs the insurance company to pay benefits directly to the provider of care on whose charge the claim is based. An assignment of benefits becomes a legally enforceable document but must refer to specific hospitalization, course of treatment, or office visits. Each course of treatment needs to have an assignment document executed by the patient unless an annual or lifetime signature authorization is accepted and in the patient's financial file, except when automobile or homeowners' liability insurance is involved.

Private Carriers: For private insurance companies with whom the provider does not have a contractual agreement, accepting assignment means that the insurance check will be directed to the provider's office instead of to the patient. Because there is no signed agreement with the carrier, the difference between the billed amount and the carrier's allowed amount is not written off but collected from the patient as is any copayment or deductible. In private third-party liability cases, the physician needs to negotiate with the insurance company to make sure benefits are paid to him or her directly.

Managed Care: In managed care plans, a participating provider (also called a *preferred provider*) is a physician who has contracted with a plan to provide medical services to plan members. A nonparticipating provider refers to a physician who has not contracted with a managed care plan to provide medical services to plan members. The assignment is automatic for individuals who have signed with managed care contracts.

Medicaid: For Medicaid cases, there is no assignment unless the patient has other insurance in addition to Medicaid. The Medicaid fiscal intermediary pays the provider directly.

Medicare: The words *participating*, *nonparticipating*, and *assignment* have slightly different meanings in the Medicare program. A physician who accepts assignment on Medicare claims is called a *participating (par) physician* and may not bill or accept payment for the amount of the difference between the submitted charge and the Medicare allowed amount. However, an attempt must be made to collect 20% of the allowed charge (coinsurance) and any amount applied to the deductible. A physician who does not participate is called a *nonparticipating (nonpar) physician* and has an option regarding assignment. The physician either may not accept assignment for all services or may exercise the option of accepting assignment for some services and collecting from the patient for other services performed at the same time and place. The physician collects the fee from the patient but may bill no more than the Medicare-limiting charge. The check is sent to the patient. When treating federal or state government employees or a Medicare recipient, the physician may lose the fee if government guidelines are not followed.

TRICARE: A provider who accepts TRICARE standard assignment (participates) agrees to accept the allowable charge as the full fee and cannot charge the patient the difference between the provider's charge and the allowable charge. The exception to this is when the provider does not accept assignment on the claim. A provider that participates or does not participate with TRICARE can submit a claim and not accept assignment on a claim-by-claim basis. In the event the provider does not accept assignment, TRICARE sends the sponsor all payments. TRICARE does not communicate with the provider if the provider has questions about the claim. It is up to the provider to bill the sponsor for payment. The provider can collect 115% of the TRICARE allowable from the patient when a CMS-1500 (08-05) claim form is marked "no" in the accepting assignment block.

Workers' Compensation: There is no assignment for industrial cases. The workers' compensation carrier pays the fee for services rendered according to its fee schedule, and the check automatically goes to the physician. The patient is not responsible for payment of services for any work-related injury or illness.

FIGURE 3-11 Encounter form: Procedural codes for professional services are taken from the *Current Procedural Terminology* (CPT) book, and diagnostic codes are taken from the *International Classification of Diseases, Ninth Revision, Clinical Modification* (ICD-9-CM) book. (Courtesy Bibbero Systems, Inc., Petaluma, CA. Telephone: 800-242-2376; fax: 800-242-9330; website: www.bibbero.com.)

7. **Patient's Financial Account:** Patient information is entered into the practice management software program. Accuracy is crucial because the data will be used to construct the claim for transmission to the insurance company. If the medical practice is not computerized, a manual system includes paper daysheets and patient ledger cards.

8a. **Encounter Form:** An **encounter form** (also called a *charge slip, multipurpose billing form, patient service slip, routing form, superbill,* or *transaction slip*) is attached to the patient's health record during the visit (Figure 3-11). This contains the patient's name, the date, and in some instances, the previous balance due. It also contains the procedural and diagnostic codes and the date the patient should return for an appointment. This two- or three-part form is a combination bill, insurance form, and routing document used in both computer- and paper-based systems. This also can be a computerized multipurpose billing form that may be scanned to input charges and diagnoses into the patient's computerized account. Time is saved, and fewer errors occur because no keystrokes are involved. Medical practices use the encounter form as a communications tool (routing sheet) and as an invoice to the patient. When used as a routing sheet, it becomes a source document for insurance claim data. The encounter form is completed by the provider. Both a procedural code for services performed and a diagnostic code are chosen by the provider of services. In some situations, a certified coder may review the patient's health record to assign a proper code on the basis of the documentation. The encounter form's procedure and diagnostic code sections should be updated and reprinted biannually with correct descriptions because changes, additions, and deletions occur that may affect the practice. Remove all codes not used or seldom used and revise and add current, valid, commonly used codes for the practice. Because there is no grace period, update encounter forms twice a year: by October 1 for changes in diagnostic codes and by January 1 for changes in procedural codes. Some practices develop encounter forms for different services (e.g., surgical services, office services [within the facility], and out-of-office service [hospital visits, emergency, outpatient facility, nursing home, or house calls]). Examples of encounter forms are shown in Figures 8-3 and 10-8.

8b. **Physician's Signature:** After examination and treatment, the physician or health care provider rendering services completes the encounter form by checking off the procedure (services and treatments) codes and diagnostic codes (Figure 3-12). The physician signs the encounter form and indicates whether the patient needs another appointment.

8c. **Determine Fees:** Some medical practices may have patients carry the encounter form to the reception desk, where fees are determined and input for billing (Figure 3-13). He or she is given the opportunity to pay and make a future appointment.

9. **Bookkeeping—Financial Accounting Record and Accounts Receivable Management:** The value of maintaining careful records of all insurance matters cannot be overemphasized. Accounts receivable (A/R) management breathes life into the practice's cash flow. Encompassed in A/R management is establishing the patient **financial accounting record** and carrying out the claims process. For compilation of claim data, services are entered into the computer by either front desk personnel or the in-office billing

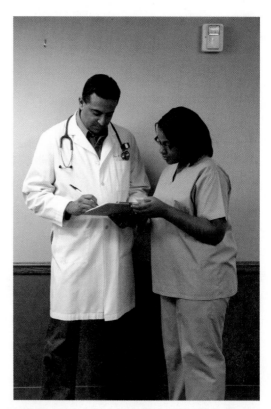

FIGURE 3-12 Physician checking off procedures on the encounter form at the conclusion of a patient's office visit.

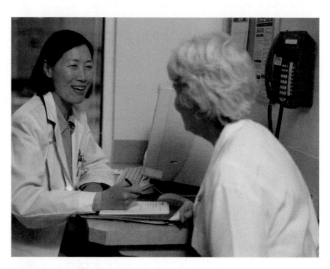

FIGURE 3-13 Insurance billing specialist discussing the encounter form with the patient at the medical office's checkout station.

department. If the practice outsources this function, an off-site billing company retrieves the data and processes the claims. All charges and patient payments are posted to their respective accounts.

 Electronic environment: A financial account is set up in the practice management system. Data obtained from the patient registration

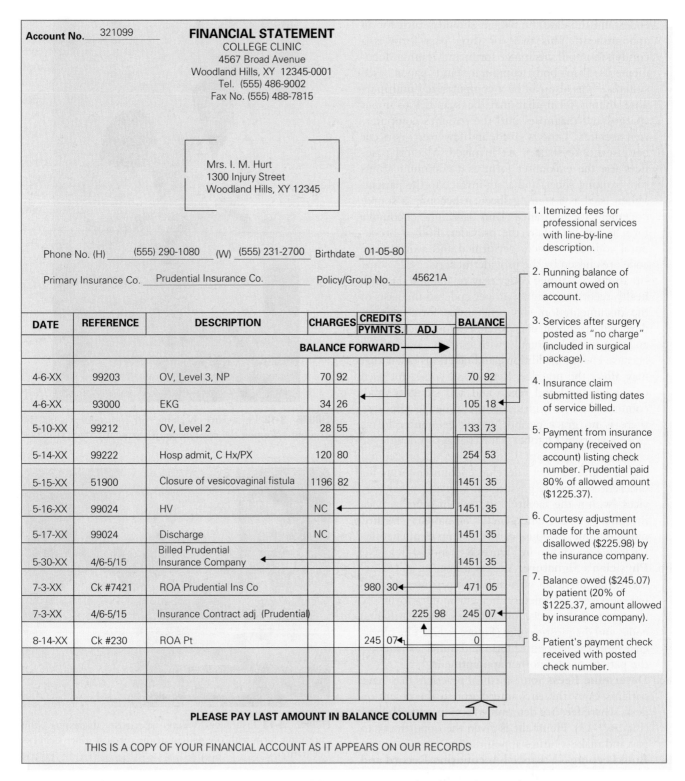

FIGURE 3-14 Financial accounting record illustrating posting of professional service descriptions, fees, payments, adjustments, and balance due.

process are keyed into the program, and a patient account is established. Usually, an account number is automatically assigned by the program and used for tracking and reporting. All items posted to each patient account are housed in the computer database for accurate and easy retrieval.

Paper environment: In the paper environment, a ledger card is maintained for each patient who receives professional services (Figure 3-14). An established private patient who is injured on the job requires two ledgers, one for private care and one for posting workers' compensation insurance.

Using the encounter form, daily transactions are **posted** (recorded) by the billing staff. Professional fees (charges), payments (cash, check, or credit card), adjustments, and balance due are also posted in the practice management software program. Accuracy is especially important when keying data into the computer because this is where the movable data start to build an insurance claim.

At the end of each day, a daysheet is generated and printed. A **daysheet,** or daily record sheet, is a register for recording daily business transactions. The totals from this can be compared with the encounter forms to ensure all charges, payments, and adjustments were properly posted. Also, the daysheet is a useful tool for "checks and balances" when assessing the bank deposit slip for accuracy.

Paper environment: The paper environment allows transactions to be recorded on the patient ledger cards. All patients seen on one day have their charges (debits) recorded on the daysheet, along with all payments and adjustments (credits). Each day the totals are carried forward and a new daysheet is set up to receive posting for that day (Figure 3-15). The ledger card should show an entry of the date an insurance claim is sent, including the date of services that were billed. Each service must be posted on a single line, and a **running balance** is calculated in the right column. When the ledger is completely filled, the account balance is brought forward (also known as **extended**) to a new card.

Step-by-step instructions for completing a ledger card are given at the end of this chapter in Procedure 3-2.

10. **Insurance Claim:** Under HIPAA guidelines, providers who are not small providers (institutional organizations with fewer than 25 full-time employees or physicians with fewer than 10 full-time employees) must send all claims electronically in the approved format.

FIGURE 3-15 Medical office employee posting to a patient's financial accounting record or daysheet.

Generally, the insurance billing specialist in the physician's office completes the claim information for the following cases: (1) all hospitalized (both surgical and medical) patients, (2) all claims in which the benefits are assigned to the physician, and (3) special procedures (minor surgery or extensive testing). In these cases, the insurance billing specialist generates an accurate claim to be submitted by using exact procedural and diagnostic codes, including the use of any appropriate documents (operative report or invoice), and mails it to the correct third-party payer when circumstances call for it to be sent in hardcopy.

The minimum information required by third-party payers is as follows:

- What was done? (services and procedures using procedure codes and appropriate modifiers discussed in Chapter 6)
- Why was it done? (diagnoses using diagnostic codes discussed in Chapter 5)
- When was it performed? (date of service [DOS])
- Where was it received? (place of service [POS])
- Who did it? (provider name and identifying number)

A helpful hint is to group together or batch all outstanding charges to the same type of insurance at one time. This cuts down on errors; allows easier trackability; and in the paper environment, makes manual completion of the forms less tedious.

It is preferable to electronically transmit claims as soon as possible after professional services are rendered. Time limits range from 30 days to $1\frac{1}{2}$ years for filing an insurance claim from the date of service. This can vary, depending on the commercial carrier, federal or state program, or whether the claim is for an illness or accident. Claims filed after the time limit will be denied, and a detailed appeal process may be required to have the claim reconsidered. This topic is discussed further within the chapters on Medicare, Medicaid, TRICARE, and workers' compensation.

Financial losses from delay can occur in the following instances. If a patient has had a long-term illness, insurance benefits can expire before a claim is processed. If several physicians treat the same patient, some insurance companies pay only one of the physicians. (Typically, whoever files the claim first is paid first.) In this scenario, the other physicians may have to wait for disbursement by the physician who received the check. Submit hospitalized patients' insurance claim forms promptly on discharge or on a regular schedule (weekly or twice a month depending on the office protocol) regardless of the discharge date for long-term inpatients.

For patients who pay at time of service and who wish to submit their own insurance claims, they are given two copies of the encounter form. The patient retains one copy for personal records and attaches the second copy to the insurance claim form and forwards it to the insurance company.

11. **Submitting the Paper Claim:** If a paper claim is submitted, a copy of the CMS-1500 (08-05) form is placed in the office's pending file or the patient's health record chart, depending on office protocol. The date the claim is mailed is noted on the patient's ledger card and recorded on the insurance claims register.

Mail claims in batches to each carrier to save on postage. You may use a large manila envelope, depending on the quantity of claims being submitted or use a window envelope in which the insurance address shows through the front so that there is no need to address by hand.

12. **Transmitting the Electronic Claim:** When filing claims electronically (details discussed in Chapter 8), a batch is created, and a digital file is stored in a predetermined directory. These files are either transmitted directly to the insurance payer or transmitted to a clearinghouse over a dial-up modem, digital subscriber line (DSL) modem, or via the Internet.

Claims are transmitted electronically as required by HIPAA or in cases of exemption or waiver, on a paper CMS-1500 (08-05) form. When sending paper claims, make a copy for office records and create an insurance claims register or spreadsheet to track and follow-up claims.

Refer to Figure 3-5, *B*, for the phases of adjudication (claim settlement) by the third-party payer for payment, partial payment, denial, or rejection.

13. **Provider's Signature:** Providers rarely sign the CMS-1500 (08-05) insurance claim form. However, when a signature is required, it can be accepted in several formats—handwritten, facsimile stamp, or electronic signature. State and government programs require a signature. In the Medicare program, certificates of medical necessity require an original signature.

Physician's Representative. Sometimes a physician gives signature authorization to one person on the staff to sign insurance claims; that person then becomes known as the physician's representative, referred to in Figure 3-16 as the "attorney-in-fact." For an authorization of this type, a document should be typed and signed before a notary public. This means that whoever signs the form is attesting to it because it is a legal document. If the medical practice is ever audited and fraud or embezzlement is discovered, then the person who had signature authorization, as well as the physician, can be brought into the case. The federal government will prosecute if this involves a Medicare patient; the state government will prosecute if a Medicaid patient is involved.

Computerized Signatures. There are three levels of computerized signatures: Level 1—digitized signature; Level 2—button, PIN, biometric, or token; and Level 3—digital signature. An **electronic signature** looks like the signer's handwritten signature. The signer authenticates the document by key entry or with a pen pad using a stylus to capture the live signature.

Example

David Smith, MD

It also can be defined as an individualized computer access and identification system (e.g., a unique personal identification number [PIN], series of letters, electronic writing, voice, computer key, token, or fingerprint transmission [biometric system]).

Example

Electronically signed:
David Smith, MD
07/12/2008   10:30:08

A *digital signature* may be lines of text or a text box stating the signer's name, date, and time and a statement indicating a signature has been attached from within the software application. Level 3 is the strongest signature because it protects the signature by a type of

PROVIDER'S NOTARIZED SIGNATURE AUTHORIZATION

State of ___Iowa___)
)ss
County of ___Des Moines___)

Know all persons by these presents:

  That I ___John Doe, MD___ have made, constituted, and appointed and by these presents do make, constitute and appoint ___Mary Coleman___ my true and lawful attorney-in-fact for me and in my name place and stead to sign my name on claims, for payment for services provided by me submitted to the ___Blue Cross and Blue Shield of Iowa___ . My signature by my said attorney-in-fact includes my agreement to abide by the full payment concept and the remainder of the certification appearing on all ___CMS-1500___ claim forms. I hereby ratify and confirm all that my said attorney-in-fact shall lawfully do or cause to be done by virtue of the power generated herein.

  In witness whereof I have hereunto set my hand this ___20th___ day of ___January___ 20_XX_ .

_____
John Doe, MD
(Signature)

Subscribed and sworn to before me this _20th_ day of _January_ 20 _XX_

_____
Notary Public

My commission expires _____ .

FIGURE 3-16 Example of a provider's signature authorization form that can be completed, notarized, and sent to the third-party payer after a copy is retained for the physician's records.

tamper-proof seal that breaks if the message content is altered. Refer to Chapter 8 for additional information on computerized signatures.

Signature Stamp. Paper environment: Some medical practices use a signature stamp so that the staff can process insurance forms and other paperwork without interrupting the physician by waiting for her or his signature. For an authorization of this type, a document should be typed and signed before a notary (Figure 3-17).

However, use of this stamp can lead to problems because it is possible to stamp unauthorized checks, transcribed medical reports, prescriptions, or credit card charge slips. Discontinue the practice if such a stamp is used infrequently. If one is used regularly, prevent problems by doing the following:

● Make only one stamp.
● Allow only long-term, trusted, bonded staff members to have access to the stamp.

● Keep the stamp in a location with a secure lock.
● Limit access to the stamp.

State laws may require that insurance claims or other related documents have an original signature or otherwise bars the use of signature stamps. You must follow those rules regardless of any carrier manual regulations. For information on state laws, contact your state legislature at your state capitol. For data about signatures on hospital medical records, see Chapter 17.

14. **Track Pending Insurance Claims:** In the computerized practice management system, a date is noted each time a claim is generated for submission, whether it is sent electronically or is printed on a paper claim form from the computer. An aging A/R report to determine outstanding balances can be generated using the date the claim was filed as a point to assess how many days old the claim is. The *aging report* is used to obtain the total A/R amount, which shows a snapshot of how much money is due to the practice from each patient account.

PROVIDER'S NOTARIZED FACSIMILE OR STAMP SIGNATURE AUTHORIZATION

State of ___Florida___)

County of ___Jacksonville___)ss
)

___John Doe, MD___ being first duty sworn, deposes and says:

I hereby authorize the ___Blue Cross of Florida___
                          (Name of Fiscal Administrator)
to accept my facsimile or stamp signature shown below

___*John Doe, MD*___
(Facsimile or Stamp Signature)

as my true signature for all purposes under the ___Medicare___
                                                 (Name of Insurance Program)
in the same manner as if it were my actual signature, including
my agreeing to abide by the full payment concept and the
remainder of the certification normally signed by the source of
care as it appears on all ___CMS-1500___ claim forms.

___*John Doe, MD*___
(Signature)

Subscribed and sworn to before me this ___3rd___ day
of ___January___ 20XX.

_____
Notary Public in and for
_____ County, State of_____
(SEAL)
My commission expires _____ .

FIGURE 3-17 Example of a provider's facsimile or stamp signature authorization form that can be completed, notarized, and sent to the third-party payer after a copy is retained for the physician's records.

Paper environment: When submitting paper claims, keep a duplicate of the claim in the office pending file or in the computer system files in the event payment is not received within a predetermined amount of time and the claim must be followed up. This file also may be referred to as a suspense, follow-up, or "tickler" file. The term *tickler* came into existence because it tickles or jogs the memory at certain dates in the future. You may be accustomed to hearing the term "aging report" as discussed earlier.

If a computerized system is not being used, establish an insurance claims register (tracing file) to keep track of the status of each case that has been billed. Record to whom the claim was sent and the submission date on the insurance claims register and the patient's ledger card. The insurance billing specialist handling the insurance forms can see at a glance which claims are becoming delinquent and the amounts owed to the physician. This is an efficient method used for 30- to 60-day follow-up. Figure 3-18 shows a document generated by a practice management system to assist in following up on electronically transmitted claims.

Keep two copies of each claim for the physician's records, one to be filed by patient name and the other by carrier name. Or simply record the name of the insurance company on each patient's ledger card and keep a file for each carrier by date of service. Filing by carrier allows all

Outstanding Claims
Primary Insurance
August 10, 2010

Billing No.	Patient Name	Primary Insurance	Claim Sent	Bill Balance
1002	Simpson, Teri E	United Western Benefit		47.50
1003	Lee, Michael	United Western Benefit		83.55
1005	Bortolussi, Jabe	ABC Insurance Company	05/25/2007	465.00
1006	Blackwood, Crystal L	TRICARE	05/25/2007	16.07
1007	Helms, Clinton A	Medicare Health Systems Corporation	05/25/2007	33.25
1008	Jameson, Richard D	Royal Pacific Insurance Company	05/25/2007	41.07
1010	Kelsey, Ron	XYZ Insurance	06/09/2007	66.23
1011	Simpson, Teri E	United Western Benefit		16.07
1012	Simpson, Teri E	United Western Benefit		40.20
1013	Simpson, Teri E	United Western Benefit		16.07
1014	Simpson, Teri E	United Western Benefit		8.00
1015	Lee, Michael	United Western Benefit		16.07
1016	Lee, Michael	United Western Benefit		28.55
1017	Lee, Michael	United Western Benefit		40.20
1018	Martin, John R	Medicare Health Systems Corporation		149.86
1019	Jameson, Richard D	Royal Pacific Insurance Company		86.42
1020	Nunez, Margaret A	Aetna Health Plan		18.25
	Report Count: 17			1172.36

FIGURE 3-18 Practice management software screen showing outstanding claims, patients' balances due, and names of insurance companies to follow-up on claims.

inquiries to be included in a single letter to the insurance company to eliminate having to write to the same company three or four times.

15. **Insurance Payments:** After the claim is processed by the insurance payer, a remittance statement is generated and either sent on paper or transmitted electronically. Payment is accompanied by an explanation of the amounts disbursed or determined not payable. Payment is posted to the patient's financial account (ledger card and daysheet for the paper environment).

16. **Bank Deposit:** After the insurance payer determines reimbursement, a check and corresponding explanation of benefits (EOB)/remittance advice (RA) are sent to the health care provider. Electronic funds transfer (EFT) may be used in place of a mailed paper check. EFT allows the automatic deposit of funds from the payer into the provider's bank account, just as you may have set up with your own paycheck. Electronic EOBs and RA may also be received by modem, downloaded, and printed.

A payment (check) from the third-party payer should be received in 2 to 8 weeks, accompanied by an EOB or RA document. The duplicate claim form is pulled from the file to verify the payment received against the amount billed.

The payment is posted (credited) to the patient's account and current daysheet indicating the date posted, name of insurance company, check or voucher number, amount received, contracted adjustment, and outstanding balance. After proper payment is received, the duplicate copy of the insurance claim is attached to the EOB form. These are filed in an annual alpha file according to insurance type, date of service, or patients' names. A date file using the posting date as reference is another option. Some medical practices file claim forms at the back section of the patient's medical record after payment is received and accepted; this is an optional but not preferred system.

In either electronic or paper office environments, all checks and cash are entered onto the bank deposit slip and deposited at the bank. In the paper-driven office, a copy of the claim form is placed in the patient's health record chart or in a "paid" folder depending on office protocol. A monthly review of outstanding claims, also known as aged receivables, determines further collection activity.

For further information on improper payments received and tracing delinquent claims, see Chapter 9.

17. **Monthly Statement:** The claim transaction is completed when the claim generated for each date of service has been processed by all responsible parties and the patient's financial account is at zero. For the patient who has insurance, a monthly statement for any outstanding balance should be sent indicating that insurance has been billed and the amount due is the patient's responsibility. The patient statement should always reflect the same fee as that submitted to the insurance company minus the amount paid by the patient copayment and/or the insurance amount reimbursed. Patients who do not have insurance should receive a monthly statement indicating all outstanding balances due minus any payments or adjustment applied since the last billing statement.

Some companies offer services to enable patients to pay their bills online securely through the medical practice's website. They also have electronic or eStatements that reduce processing and mailing costs by delivering patient statements securely or leave balance due reminders. Online bill payment may be set up to automatically draft patients' debit/credit cards; this eliminates checks and postage and speeds payments.

18. **Financial Records Retained:** Whether your office is computerized or still operates in a paper-based environment, you will not escape the volumes of paperwork that business produces! Financial records must be retained and may include the following (not an all-inclusive list):

- Copy of the completed patient information form, patient authorization or signature-on-file for assignment of benefits form, copies of insurance identification cards, responsible-party authorization, insurance correspondence.
- Explanation of benefits or remittance advice documents sent from insurance payers.
- Logs of all telephone conversations and actions taken regarding insurance disputes or collection activities. If you do not store these notes in the corresponding patient health record, then you will likely have a master file set up where all logs are kept.
- Encounter forms, referral, and authorization slips.
- Daysheets and deposit slips.

KEEPING UP TO DATE

- Make a folder or binder of pertinent insurance information. Obtain information booklets and policy manuals from the local offices of the various insurance companies. Obtain sample copies of all the forms required for the insurance plans most used in your physician's office. Keep samples of completed claim forms.
- Changes occur daily and monthly, so keep well informed by reading your Medicaid, Medicare, TRICARE, and

local medical society bulletins. Maintain a chronologic file on each of these bulletins for easy reference, always keeping the latest bulletin on top.

- Attend any workshops offered in your area on insurance in the medical practice. Network with other insurance specialists to compare policies and discuss common problems. The American Association of Medical Assistants has chapters in many states that feature educational workshops and lectures.

- Become a member of the American Academy of Professional Coders (AAPC), American Association of Medical Billers (AAMB), Medical Association of Billers (MAB), Medical Group Management Association (MGMA), Healthcare Financial Management Association (HFMA), Healthcare Billing and Management Association (HBMA), Professional Association of Health Care Office Management (PAHCOM), and/or American Health Information Management Association (AHIMA). Each of these associations distributes journals or newsletters on a monthly basis featuring current information.

- Make good use of the Internet!

- For addresses of the professional associations mentioned in this chapter, refer to Table 18-2.

PROCEDURE 3-2

Prepare and Post to a Patient's Financial Accounting Record

OBJECTIVES: To prepare, insert descriptions, and post fees, payments, credit adjustments, and balances due to a patient's ledger card

EQUIPMENT/SUPPLIES: Typewriter or computer, patient accounts or ledger cards, and calculator

DIRECTIONS: Follow these steps to post charges, payments, adjustments, and balances to a patient's ledger/account (see Figure 3-14) and practice this skill by completing the assignments in the *Workbook*.

1. Personal data: Insert the patient's name and address to prepare the ledger card. Some ledgers may require additional information (attending physician's name; type of insurance; insurance company's name with policy and group numbers; patient's home and work telephone numbers; birth date; Social Security number; driver's license number; spouse's and/or dependents' names; and name, address, and telephone number of nearest relative), depending on the style of card chosen for a medical practice.

2. Date: Post the date of service (DOS) in the date column, description of the services in the professional service description column, and charge amount in the charge column. The posting date is the actual date the transaction is recorded. If the DOS differs from the posting date, reference the DOS in the description column. This date column should never be left blank.

3. Reference: List a *Current Procedural Terminology* (CPT) procedure code number in the reference column.

4. Description: Write a brief description of the transaction that is being posted, such as OV for office visit or HV for hospital visit. Indicate the Evaluation and Management service levels (1 through 5) using the last digit of the E/M code (e.g., 99205 = Level **5**). List the name of other services or surgical procedures (e.g., ECG, vaccination, tonsillectomy).

- Charges: Add the charge to the running current balance and enter the current balance in the right column.

- Payments: Post the current date the payment is received and indicate ROA (received on account) and who made the payment (e.g., pt [patient] or name of insurance company) in the description column. List the type of payment (cash, check, debit card, money order, or credit card) and voucher or check number (e.g., ck #430) in the reference column.

- Adjustments: Post the date the adjustment is being made and indicate the type of adjustment (e.g., insurance plan adj., contract adj., courtesy adj.).

- Billing comments: Indicate when the insurance company was billed by posting the current date and name of the insurance company. Include the dates of service being billed in the reference column (e.g., 4/20/XX through 5/1/XX). Indicate when the patient statement was sent and amount due if different from the current balance (e.g., Patient billed $45.00 balance after insurance payment).

- Other comments: Indicate other comments that pertain directly to the account (e.g., account sent to ABC Collection Agency, account scheduled for small claims court).

5. Charges: Refer to the fee schedule and post each fee (charge) on a separate line in the "charge" column. Charges are debited (subtracted) from the account balance.

6. Payments: Enter the amount paid in the "payment" column and credit (subtract) the payment received from the amount in the running current balance column and enter the current balance.

7. Adjustments: Post the contracted insurance plan discount in the "Adjustment" column by referencing the DOS, insurance company name, and type of

PROCEDURE 3.2—cont'd

Prepare and Post to a Patient's Financial Accounting Record

contract discount (e.g., HealthNet PPO discount or Medicare courtesy adjustment). Adjustments are credited to the account balance.

8. Current balance: Line by line, credit and debit by adding and subtracting postings to the running balance to determine the amount for the current balance column as shown in Figure 3-14. If a line is used to indicate a date an action was taken (e.g.,

insurance company or patient billed, account sent to collection), bring down the running balance from the previous line. This column must always contain an amount and should never be left blank. Optional: Post the adjustment on the same line as the payment.

9. Submit an itemized billing statement to the patient for the balance due.

DATE	DESCRIPTION	CHARGE	PAYMENT	ADJUSTMENT	BALANCE
					1346.17
7-3-XX	ROA Prudential Ins #7421		980.30	120.80	245.07

KEY POINTS

This is a brief chapter review or summary of the key issues presented. To further enhance your knowledge of the technical subject matter, review the key terms and key abbreviations for this chapter by locating the meanings in the glossary at the end of this book that appear in a section before the index.

1. An insurance contract (policy or agreement) is a legal document in which the insured (policyholder or subscriber) receives coverage that helps offset when medical services are necessary. The four concepts of a valid insurance contract follow. (1) The person must be a mentally competent adult and not under the influence of drugs or alcohol when signing the contract. (2) The insurance company must make an offer (the signed application), and the person must accept the offer (issuance of the policy), without concealment or misrepresentation of facts on the application. (3) An exchange of value (the first premium payment) submitted with the application, known as a consideration, must be present. (4) A legal purpose must exist, which is an insurable interest in the case of a health insurance policy. This means that the policyholder expects to continue in good health but the insurance policy will provide something of value if an accident or illness strikes.

2. The insurance biller must understand insurance terminology and policy provisions as they relate to billing and claims submission. An implied contract is defined as not manifested by direct words but implied or deduced from the circumstance, the general

language, or the conduct of the patient. On the other hand, an expressed contract can be verbal or written. However, most physician-patient contracts are implied.

3. There are many types of private and federal insurance programs, such as managed care, workers' compensation, Medicare, Medicaid, and TRICARE.

4. Establish an insurance claims register or log (tracing file) to keep track of the status of each case that has been billed. Record to whom the claim was sent and the submission date on the insurance claims register and the patient's ledger card.

5. The patient registration form must be reviewed for accuracy and completeness of the content. This information becomes critical when completing and following up on claims.

6. Verifying an insured's eligibility to receive benefits and obtaining prior approval from the insurance company to give a specific treatment are vital issues for collecting payment when medical services are provided.

7. An aging accounts receivable report to determine outstanding balances can be generated using the date claim was filed as a point to assess how many days old the claim is. This report is used to understand how much money is due to the practice from each patient account.

8. Each type of insurance has different time limits for claims submission, and if electronically transmitted after the designated time, they will be denied.

9. After insurance payments are received, they must be posted to each patient's account and any necessary adjustments made with the outstanding balance billed to the patient.
10. Because federal program regulations have ongoing changes and new diagnostic and procedural codes are adopted annually, it is imperative that the insurance biller keep up to date on technical information and have access to current reference books.
11. With the advent of health care reform in 2010, health benefit exchanges were created and changes occurred that affect the uninsured; preexisting conditions; prescription drugs; employers' responsibilities; and programs such as Medicare, Medicaid, and ERISA (Employee Retirement Income Security Act).

Ǝvolve INTERNET RESOURCES

For active links to the following resources, visit the Evolve website at
http://evolve.elsevier.com/fordney/handbook
Websites for government health insurance programs such as Medicare, TRICARE, and CHAMPVA; state and federal Medicaid and disability benefit programs; and workers' compensation insurance are listed at the end of chapters discussing those topics. Specific health insurance plans may be located by using an Internet search engine and inserting their names.

- America's Health Insurance Plans
  Custom forms such as patient instruction forms, history forms, report forms, patient reminder cards, and others may be designed by office staff and ordered or designed by the medical stationery/supply company after assembling the necessary information. Some of these forms may be available over the Internet from the following suppliers' websites:
- Bibbero Systems, Inc.
- Histacount Medical Practice Web
- Medical Arts Press Web

STUDENT ASSIGNMENT

✓ Study Chapter 3.

✓ Answer the fill-in-the-blank, multiple choice, and true/false questions in the *Workbook* to reinforce the theory learned in this chapter and to help prepare you for a future test.

✓ Complete the assignments in the *Workbook* to help reinforce the basic steps in submitting an insurance claim form.

✓ Turn to the glossary at the end of this textbook for a further understanding of the key terms and key abbreviations used in this chapter.

KEY TERMS*

acute
attending physician
chief complaint
chronic
comorbidity
comprehensive
concurrent care
consultation
consulting physician
continuity of care
counseling
critical care
detailed
documentation
electronic health record
emergency care
eponym

established patient
expanded problem focused
external audit
facsimile
family history
health record/medical record
high complexity
history of present illness
internal review
low complexity
medical decision making
medical necessity
medical report
moderate complexity
new patient
non-physician practitioner
ordering physician

past history
physical examination
primary care physician
problem focused
prospective review
referral
referring physician
resident physician
retrospective review
review of systems
social history
straightforward
subpoena
subpoena duces tecum
teaching physician
treating or performing physician

KEY ABBREVIATIONS*

ARRA
C
CC
CCU
CHEDDAR
D
dx, Dx
ED or ER
EHR
E/M service
EMR
EPF level of history or
    examination

ESI
fax
FH
HC medical decision
    making
HIM
HIV
HPI
ICU
imp
LC medical decision
    making
LLQ

LUQ
MC medical decision
    making
MDM
NLP
NP
NPP
PCP
PE or PX
PF level of history
    or examination
PFSH
PH

PO
POR system
RCU
RLQ
R/O
ROS
RUQ
SF medical decision
    making
SH
SOAP style
SOR system
WNL

*Definitions for the key terms and key abbreviations are located near the back of this textbook in the glossary.

CHAPTER
4

Medical Documentation and the Electronic Health Record

OBJECTIVES

After reading this chapter, you should be able to:

- Explain reasons legible documentation is required.
- Identify principles of documentation.
- State contents of a medical report.
- Define common medical, diagnostic, and legal terms.
- List documents required for an internal review of health records.
- Describe the difference between prospective and retrospective review of records.
- State reasons why an insurance company may decide to perform an external audit of medical records.

- Explain techniques used for fax confidentiality.
- Respond appropriately to the subpoena of a witness and records.
- Identify principles for retention of health records.
- Formulate a procedure for termination of a case.
- State guidelines for insurance billing specialists for preventing lawsuits.

Service to Patients

It is essential that all medical staff who work with health records serve patients by the following:
- Keeping their personal health information private and confidential.
- Following federal Health Insurance Portability and Accountability Act (HIPAA) guidelines for consent and disclosure of information to keep a medical practice compliant and patients confident.
- Sending written reports or "thank you" letters to communicate and document good patient care if a patient is sent to another doctor for a consultation, is seen in consultation, or is referred to a specialist for the transfer of total or specific care.
- Helping them manage their online electronic personal records by keeping patients informed of the provider's role in access, update, and exchange of data.

THE DOCUMENTATION PROCESS

Health Record

The connection between insurance billing and the health record, also known for decades as the *medical record*, should be explained to better understand its importance as the foremost tool of clinical care and communication. A **health record** can be defined as written or graphic information documenting facts and events during the rendering of patient care. It may be kept in either a paper or an electronic format. However, paper-based offices are becoming a part of the past and the electronic format is gradually becoming the norm. Federal legislation established by the American Recovery and Reinvestment Act of 2009 (ARRA) encourages implementation by offering five annual financial incentives for qualifying offices that

---

Performance objectives, testing and review material, and hands-on practical exercises for this chapter are available in these resources:

 The Insurance Handbook Student Workbook   ⊝ The Insurance Handbook Evolve Site

convert to an electronic format beginning in 2011 and ending in 2015 or 2016.

Contents of a health record vary from case to case but some of the most common medical office documents are as follows:

- Patient registration (demographic information)
- Medication record
- History and physical examination notes or report
- Progress or chart notes
- Consultation reports
- Imaging and x-ray reports
- Laboratory reports
- Immunization record
- Consent and authorization forms
- Operative report
- Pathology report

In a hospital setting, in addition to the aforementioned, there are attending physician's orders, date of admission, hospital stay dates, discharge date, and discharge summary. As discussed in Chapter 2, the federal government has set standards to protect the confidentiality, security, and integrity of a patient's protected health information (PHI). Any one of several systems may be used in a medical practice. They are problem-oriented record (POR) system, source-oriented record (SOR) system, or integrated record system. An electronic health record (EHR) system can be kept as a POR or SOR system.

A POR system consists of flow sheets, charts, or graphs that allow a physician to quickly locate information and compare evaluations. These data sheets are commonly used to record blood sugar levels for diabetic patients, blood pressure readings for hypertensive patients, weight for obese patients, immunizations, medication refills, and so on.

In the SOR system, documents are arranged according to sections (e.g., history and physical section, progress notes, laboratory tests, radiology reports, or surgical operations). The integrated record system files all documents in reverse chronologic order; thus it may be more difficult to locate data because they are scattered throughout the record.

Electronic Health Record System

In an EHR system, networked computers use practice management software and patient medical information software that interface together. The medical information software uses either free-text or built-in templates to help structure documentation through a process of answering a series of questions and entering data. Thus

an **electronic health record (EHR)** is a collection of medical information about the past, present, and future of a patient that resides in a centralized electronic system. This system receives, stores, transmits, retrieves, and links data for giving health care services from many information systems such as laboratory test results, radiology reports and x-ray images, pathology reports, and financial documents. However, the difference between an EHR and an *electronic medical record* (EMR) is that an EMR is an individual physician's EMR for the patient, including medical history, allergies, and appointment information, and the EHR is all patient medical information from many information systems, including all components of the EMR.

An EHR system has several advantages over a paper-based system. It requires no physical space because the files remain in an electronic database and are available online. Abstracting data is eliminated because data are automatically captured for various documents via dictation or templates except when free-form documentation, such as narrative notes, dictations, and natural language processing (NLP), is used. The free-text approach encourages use of abbreviations or fewer spelled out words that may result in scant or undecipherable documents. NLP is a field of computer science that deals with converting information from databases into readable human language. Cloning occurs when each entry in the medical record is worded similar to the previous entries. Cloned documentation is considered a misrepresentation of the medical necessity requirement for coverage of services. It is foreseen that use of Systematized Nomenclature of Medicine for Clinical Terminology (SNOMED-CT), which is a medical terminology classification system that codes text data in an EHR system, will assist in standardizing clinical medical terminology. Health care data may be used for developing protocols and critical pathways for disease management. Electronic signatures or codes are applied to documents when they are reviewed and authenticated by the creator. Procedure and diagnostic coding may be computer assisted or automated. Insurance verification may be completed automatically during the preregistration process. Insurance claims are compiled and transmitted in batches to a clearinghouse or to the insurance carriers. The revenue cycle is managed completely online.

ELECTRONIC SECURITY STANDARDS

The Medicare Modernization Act created the Commission on Systemic Interoperability to develop a strategy to make health care information available at all times to

ELECTRONIC SECURITY STANDARDS—cont'd

patients and physicians. To reach a goal of having electronic records for all Americans by 2014, adoption of health information standards and increase of funding demonstration projects has begun.

One provision of the Health Insurance Portability and Accountability Act (HIPAA) directs the adoption of national electronic standards for automatic transfer of certain health care data among health care payers, plans, and providers. This provision encourages medical practices to convert to an electronic record-keeping system or paperless office because this will help transition insurance claim attachments from the paper world into the electronic world. Another provision is that information systems have security safeguards to protect against improper disclosure, unauthorized access, or unintended alteration of information for both the data and the system. The American Recovery and Reinvestment Act (ARRA) of 2009 requires covered entities to notify individuals if their protected health information was accessed or disclosed in an unauthorized manner or by unauthorized individuals unless accidentally accessed.

An electronic **medical report** is part of the health record and is a permanent legal document that formally states the outcomes of the patient's examination or treatment in letter or report form. It is this record that provides the information needed to complete the insurance claim form. When billing the insurance company, the date of service (DOS), place of service (POS), diagnosis (dx or Dx), and procedures are recorded and transmitted in electronic format. The codes are used for interpretation by the insurance company when processing a claim.

The key to substantiating procedure and diagnostic code selections for appropriate reimbursement is supporting documentation in the EHR. Proper documentation can prevent penalties and refund requests in case the physician's practice is reviewed or audited. Some states or facilities use different terminology when referring to the health record such as medical information, medical record, progress or chart note, hospital record, or health care record.

Documenters

All individuals providing health care services may be referred to as *documenters* because they chronologically record pertinent facts and observations about the patient's health. This process is called **documentation** (charting) and may be electronically handwritten, dictated and transcribed, or downloaded from a personal digital assistant (PDA) or smartphone using an electronic template. It is the health care physician's responsibility to either handwrite the medical information or dictate it for transcription. Some documenters use a speech recognition system, which is a computerized voice recognition system that makes it possible for a computer system to respond to spoken words. Two basic categories are (1) navigation or command control, which allows an individual to launch and operate software applications with spoken directions, and (2) *dictation software*, which makes it possible for a computer system to recognize spoken words and automatically convert them into text.

When a dictation software speech recognition system is used, many practices use a medical editor (*correctionist*) who proofreads and edits the computer-generated documents. Some practices use printed checklists for typical examinations. The physician notes his or her findings on the checklists and gives this document to an employee for input to the EMR system. The EMR system has access to these checklists to minimize typing costs.

The receptionist obtains the first document completed by the patient, called the *patient registration information form*, as shown in Figure 3-7. The medical assistant or a front desk staff member is often the one to record entries for no-show appointments, prescription refills, and telephone calls in the patients' health records. The insurance billing specialist uses the information in the health record for billing purposes, and it is his or her responsibility to bring any substandard documentation to the physician's or office manager's attention depending on office policy. In the hospital setting, a trained health information management (HIM) professional maintains the health record for completeness.

When referring to guidelines for documentation of the health record and completion of the insurance claim form, a physician's title may change, depending on the circumstances of each patient encounter. This can get confusing at times, so to clarify the physician's various roles and the roles of the practitioners who work for the physician, some of these titles are defined as follows:

- **Attending physician** refers to the hospital staff member who is legally responsible for the care and treatment given to a patient.
- **Consulting physician** is a provider whose opinion or advice regarding evaluation or management of a specific problem is requested by another physician.

- **Non-physician practitioner (NPP)** is a nurse practitioner, clinical nurse specialist, licensed social worker, nurse midwife, physical therapist, speech therapist, audiologist, or physician assistant who furnishes a consultation or treats a patient for a specific medical problem, pursuant to state law, and who uses the results of a diagnostic test in the management of the patient's specific medical problem.
- **Ordering physician** is the individual in the hospital directing the selection, preparation, or administration of tests, medication, or treatment.
- **Primary care physician (PCP)** oversees the care of patients in a managed health care plan and refers patients to see specialists for services as needed.
- **Referring physician** is a provider who sends the patient for tests or treatment.
- **Resident physician** is a physician who has finished medical school and is performing one or more years of training in a specialty area on the job at a hospital (medical center). Residents perform the elements required for an evaluation and management (E/M) service in the presence of or, jointly with, the teaching physician, and residents document the service.
- **Teaching physician** is a doctor who has responsibilities for training and supervising medical students, interns, or residents and who takes them to the bedsides of patients in a teaching hospital to review course and treatment. Teaching physicians must document that they supervised and were physically present at the time during key portions of the service provided to the patient when performed by a resident.
- **Treating or performing physician** is the provider who renders a service to a patient. In the Medicare program, the definition of a treating physician is a physician who furnishes a consultation or treats a beneficiary for a specific medical problem and who uses the results of a diagnostic test in the management of the beneficiary's specific medical problem. A radiologist performing a therapeutic intervention procedure is considered a treating physician. A radiologist performing a diagnostic intervention or diagnostic procedure is not considered a treating physician.

LEGIBLE DOCUMENTATION

If handwritten, entries in the patient's record must be legible. Such entries should be returned to the physician for clarification and/or rewritten.

Reasons for Legible Documentation

It is important that all patients seen by a provider have comprehensive legible documentation about what occurred during the visit for the following reasons:

1. Avoidance of denied or delayed payments by insurance carriers investigating the medical necessity of services.
2. Enforcement of medical record-keeping rules by insurance carriers requiring accurate documentation that supports procedure and diagnostic codes.
3. Subpoena of health records by state investigators or the court for review.
4. Defense of a professional liability claim.
5. Execution of the physician's written instructions by a patient's caregiver.

GENERAL PRINCIPLES OF HEALTH RECORD DOCUMENTATION

In the early 1990s the American Medical Association (AMA) modified the terminology "office visits" and used "office and other outpatient services" when coding for those services; the AMA also adopted the phrase "evaluation and management" (E/M) for the name of the section of Current Procedural Terminology (CPT) in which those codes appear. This wording better reflects the components involved when performing an office visit. However, E/M services are also performed in other settings such as inpatient hospital facilities and nursing homes. The AMA and Centers for Medicare and Medicaid Services (CMS) developed documentation guidelines for CPT E/M services. These were released to Medicare carriers by CMS in 1995 and then modified and released again in 1997. The guidelines were developed because Medicare has an obligation to those enrolled to ensure that services paid for have been provided and are medically necessary. Auditors determined that some medical practices should improve their quality of documentation.

Physicians are not required to use these guidelines but are encouraged to do so for the four reasons as stated for legible documentation. Some physicians have adopted the 1995 guidelines, and others use those introduced in 1997. A modification of the 1997 guidelines is under consideration but has not been released as of this edition. Insurance claims processors and auditors may use the 1995 or 1997 guidelines when doing an internal or external chart audit to determine whether the reported services were actually rendered and the level of service was warranted. A variety of formats of documentation are accepted by Medicare administrative contractors (also called fiscal intermediaries, fiscal agents, and fiscal carriers) as long as the information is understood. When significant irregular reporting patterns are detected, a review is conducted.

MEDICALLY NECESSARY

Third-party payers and federal programs have a responsibility to ensure that professional services provided to patients were medically necessary. Documentation must support the level of service and each procedure rendered.

Medical Necessity

Payment may be delayed, downcoded, or denied if the medical necessity of a treatment is questioned. As a rule, **medical necessity** is a criterion used by insurance companies, as well as federal programs such as Medicare, when making decisions to limit or deny payment. Some medical practices use electronic medical necessity software that checks to verify the medical services or procedures are justified by the patient's symptoms and diagnosis. Medical treatment must be done in accordance with standards of good medical practice and the proper level of care provided in the most appropriate setting. However, insurers differ on this definition and may or may not cover the services, depending on the benefits of the plan. Inform the patient of this situation with a letter, as shown in Figure 4-1. Chapter 12 discusses more about the Advance Beneficiary Notice of Noncoverage (ABN), also known as a *waiver of liability agreement* or *responsibility statement*, that is used in this type of situation.

External Audit Point System

As learned in Chapter 2, if a provider has submitted insurance claims for payments that are deemed to be fraudulent or inappropriate by the government, then an investigation may be conducted in the form of an audit of the practice's financial records. A point system is used while reviewing each patient's health record during the performance of an audit. Points are awarded only if documentation is present for elements required in the health record. Because every health record is documented differently by each provider of service, a patient's history may contain details for more than one body area or organ system. Thus when gathering points, it is possible the auditor may shift the points from the history of present illness to those required for the review of the patient's body systems. In addition, when sufficient points have been reached within a section for the level of code used in billing, no further documentation is counted for audit purposes, even though there may be additional comments for other body systems. This point system is used to show where deficiencies occur in health record documentation. It is also used to evaluate and substantiate proper use of diagnostic and procedural codes.

Health maintenance organizations, preferred provider organizations, and all private carriers have the right to claim refunds in the event of accidental (or intentional) miscoding. However, Medicare has the power to levy fines and penalties and exclude providers from the Medicare program. If improper coding patterns exist and are not corrected, then the provider of service will be penalized. Insurance carriers go by the rule "If it is not documented, then it was not performed," and they have the right to deny reimbursement.

Legalities of Health Record Billing Patterns

Insurance carriers have become stricter in enforcing accurate coding substantiated by documentation. It is not uncommon for prepayment and postpayment random audits or reviews by Medicare carriers to occur that monitor the accuracy of physicians' use of medical services and procedure codes. Medicare administrative contractors (fiscal intermediaries) have "walk-in rights" (access to a medical practice without an appointment or search warrant) that they may invoke to conduct documentation reviews, audits, and evaluations. Billing patterns that may draw attention to a medical practice for possible audit are as follows:

- Billing intentionally for unnecessary services
- Billing incorrectly for services of *physician extenders* (NPPs) (e.g., nurse practitioner, midwife, physician assistant)
- Billing for diagnostic tests without a separate report in the health record
- Changing dates of service on insurance claims to comply with policy coverage dates
- Waiving copayments or deductibles, or allowing other illegal discounts
- Ordering excessive diagnostic tests (e.g., laboratory tests, x-ray studies)
- Using two different provider numbers to bill the same services for the same patient
- Misusing provider identification numbers, resulting in incorrect billing
- Using improper modifiers for financial gain
- Failing to return overpayments made by the Medicare program

DOCUMENTATION GUIDELINES FOR MEDICAL SERVICES

The following is a brief overview of documentation guidelines for medical services:

1. The health record should be accurate, complete (detailed), and legible.

COLLEGE CLINIC
4567 Broad Avenue
Woodland Hills, XY 12345-0001
Phone: 555/486-90020
Fax: 555/487-8976

September 20, 20XX

Dear ABC Managed Care Plan Participant:

This is a quick fact sheet to help our patients understand that some services may not be paid by ABC Managed Care Plan unless there is a *medical* reason to perform them.

The coverage provided by ABC Managed Care Plan, in most instances, includes payment for medically necessary services provided to treat a problem or illness. However, patients who wish their health care providers to perform services outside of those considered a "medical necessity" will be responsible for paying for those services out-of-pocket.

For example, many patients come to our office for the purpose of removing noncancerous facial moles. Although this procedure may be desired by the patient, ABC Managed Care Plan will not pay for the removal without a medical reason for it.

The patient's cost for noncancerous facial mole removal at our practice is approximately $75.

Please understand that, legally, we are required to submit our bill to ABC Managed Care Plan using accurate information about all of the services you received. Using a false medical reason to try to get insurance to pay for a service it otherwise would not cover is considered fraud, and our doctors will not do this. We regret that ABC Managed Care Plan may not wish to pay for a service you desire, but we must follow insurance regulations.

If you would like additional information about payment coverage for these services, you may refer to your ABC Managed Care Plan benefits handbook or call your ABC Managed Care Plan customer service representative at 555-271-0311.

Thank you for choosing us to assist you with your health care needs. As always, providing high-quality health care to you is and remains our primary purpose. If you have any questions about this information, please do not hesitate to telephone and ask our front office staff for more information.

Sincerely,

Mary Anne Mason, CPC

FIGURE 4-1 Letter to a patient who is a member of a managed care plan that provides important information about medical procedures or services that are not covered for payment unless there is a medical necessity.

2. The documentation of each patient encounter should include or provide reference to the following:
   a. Chief complaint or reason for the encounter
   b. Relevant history
   c. Examination
   d. Findings
   e. Prior diagnostic test results
   f. Assessment, clinical impression, or diagnosis
   g. Plan for care
   h. Date and legible identity of the health care professional

3. The reason for the encounter or chief complaint should be stated, and the rationale should be documented or inferred for ordering diagnostic and other ancillary services (x-rays or laboratory tests).
4. Past and present diagnoses including those in the prenatal and intrapartum period that affect the newborn should be accessible to the treating or consulting physician.
5. Appropriate health risk factors should be identified.
6. The patient's progress, response to and changes in treatment, planned follow-up care and instructions, and diagnosis should be documented.

7. Patient refusal to follow medical advice should be documented and a letter sent to the patient about this noncompliance. Information on termination of a case is found at the end of this chapter.

8. Procedure and diagnostic codes reported on the health insurance claim form or billing statement should be supported by the documentation in the health record and be at a level sufficient for a clinical peer to determine whether services have been coded accurately.

9. The confidentiality of the health record should be fully maintained consistent with the requirements of medical ethics and the law.

10. Each chart entry must have a date and signature or electronic validation including the title or position of the person verifying the documentation. If a signature log has been established for paper-based records, then initials are acceptable, because these would be defined in the log (Figure 4-2). A *signature log* is a list of all staff members' names, job titles, signatures, and initials. In regard to paperless documents, if passwords are used for restricted access, electronic or digital signatures may be acceptable.

11. Charting procedures for progress notes should be standardized. For office visits, many physicians in a paper-based system use either a method called the SOAP style (Figure 4-3) or the CHEDDAR style (Figure 4-4). Some physicians prefer to document using a narrative or more detailed descriptive style, which is also commonly used when creating a medical report such as history and physical report, operative report, radiologic report, or pathology report (see Figures 4-7 and 4-8). However, whatever method is used, make sure it is detailed enough to support current documentation requirements.

FIGURE 4-2 Example of a signature log for paper-based records.

FIGURE 4-3 In a paper-based system, explanation of the acronym "SOAP" used as a format for progress notes defining subjective and objective information, the assessment, and the treatment plan.

FIGURE 4-4 In a paper-based system, explanation of the acronym "CHEDDAR" used as a format for progress notes.

12. Treatment plans should be written. Include patient/family education and specific instructions for follow-up. Treatment must be consistent with the working diagnosis.

13. Medications prescribed and taken should be listed, specifying frequency and dosage.

14. *Request* for a consultation from the attending or treating physician and the *need* for consultation must be documented. The consultant's opinion and any services ordered or performed must be documented and communicated to the requesting physician. Remember the four Rs: There must be a *requesting* physician, and the consultant must *render* an opinion and send a *report*. The requesting physician must document the *reason* for a consult in the patient's medical record. A possible fifth R of consultations is *return*. The consulting physician must return the patient to the requesting physician for treatment of the problem so that no transfer of care is shown.

15. Record a patient's failure to return for needed treatment by noting it in the health record, in the appointment book, and on the financial record or ledger card. Follow up with a telephone call or send a letter to the patient advising him or her that further treatment is indicated.

16. Corrections: For electronic health records, the software program should make an electronic record entry permanent when originally completed and authenticated. To make a correction, note that a section is in error with the date and time and enter the correct information with a notation of when and why the physician changed the entry. Authenticate the correction via electronic signature and date. Never delete or key over incorrect data in a computerized file. Another method for correcting a health record is to flag it as amended or obsolete and create an addendum either typed as a separate document or for a chart note inserted below in the next space available. Another option is to move it to a limited-access section of the electronic record. An addendum is discussed later in this chapter. For paper-based records, use a permanent, not water-soluble, ink pen (legal copy pen) to cross out an incorrect entry on a patient's record. Mark it with a single line and write the correct information, then date and initial the entry. Never erase, white out, or use self-adhesive paper over any information recorded on a patient record (Example 4-1).

17. Document all laboratory tests ordered in the health record. When the report is received, the physician should initial the report, indicating that it has been read. Each documentation is considered an element and allows a point if the record undergoes an external audit.

18. Ask the physician for approval for a different code before transmitting the claim to the insurance carrier if the insurance biller questions any procedure or diagnostic codes marked on the encounter form (Figure 4-5).

Example 4-1

Incorrect	BP 1~~$0~~/~~9~~0
	190/70
Correct	BP ~~150/70~~ *mtf*
Incorrect	right leg is ~~markedly~~ *slightly* edematous...
Correct	right leg is ~~markedly~~ *slightly* edematous... *1/2/20XX* *mtf*
Correctly typed	right leg is slightly edematous... 1–2–20XX mtf

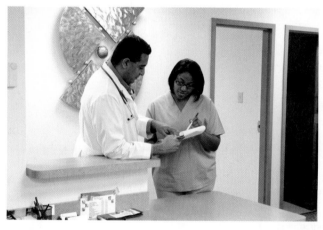

FIGURE 4-5 Insurance billing specialist checking information with physician before recording it on the insurance claim.

19. Retain all records until you are positive they are no longer necessary by conforming to federal and state laws, as well as the physician's wishes. Retention of records is discussed at the end of the chapter and shown in Table 4-2.

SIGNATURE LOG

Make sure all health record entries are signed or electronically verified by the physician (author) with his or her title or position. This provides clear evidence that the physician reviewed the note and/or ensures he or she is aware of all test results (normal and abnormal). Documented physician review of test results can be factored when determining appropriate coding levels for services.

CONTENTS OF A MEDICAL REPORT

The degree of documentation depends on the complexity of the service and the specialty of the physician. For example, a "normal chest examination" may have a different meaning to a cardiologist than it does to a family physician as far as the details of the examination and documentation.

The first time a new patient is seen, a family and social history is taken and updated as needed in subsequent visits. When a new or an established patient comes to see the physician with a new injury or illness, the documentation should also include the patient's health history, the physical examination, results from any tests that are performed, the medical decision-making process, the diagnosis, and the treatment plan.

Documentation of History

The following documentation information for the history and physical examination is based on the 1997 Medicare guidelines. The history includes the chief complaint (CC); history of present illness (HPI); review of systems (ROS); and past history, family, or social history (PFSH).* The extent of the history depends on clinical judgment and the nature of the presenting problems. Each history includes some or all of the following elements (Figure 4-6).

Chief Complaint

The **chief complaint (CC)** is a concise statement usually in the patient's own words describing the symptom, problem, condition, diagnosis, physician-recommended return, or other factor that is the reason for the encounter. *The CC is a requirement for all levels of history*: problem focused, expanded problem focused, detailed, and comprehensive; these are described at the end of the next section.

History of Present Illness

The **history of present illness (HPI)** is a chronologic description of the development of the patient's present illness from the first sign or symptom or from the previous encounter to the present. If the physician is unable to obtain a sufficient diagnosis for the patient's condition, the health record documentation must reflect this. The history may include one or more of the following eight descriptive elements:

---

*These abbreviations in the history portion of the report may vary, depending on the physician who is dictating (e.g., PI for present illness, PH for past history, FH for family history).

Hospital number: 00-83-06

Scott, Aimee

Rex Rumsey, MD

HISTORY

CHIEF COMPLAINT: Pain and bleeding after each bowel movement for the past 3 to 4 months.

PRESENT ILLNESS: This 68-year-old white female says she usually has three bowel movements a day in small amounts, and there has been a change in the last 3 to 4 months in frequency, size, and type of bowel movement. She has slight burning pain and irritation in the rectal area after bowel movements. The pain lasts for several minutes, then decreases in intensity. She has had no previous anorectal surgery or rectal infection. She denies any blood in the stool itself or associated symptoms. Bright red blood occurs after stools have passed.

PAST HISTORY:
ILLNESSES: The patient had polio at age 8 from which she has made a remarkable recovery. Apparently, she was paralyzed in both lower extremities and now has adequate use of these. She has no other serious illnesses.

ALLERGIES: ALLERGIC TO PENICILLIN. She denies any other drug or food allergies.
MEDICATIONS: None.
OPERATIONS: Right inguinal herniorrhaphy 25 years ago.

SOCIAL HISTORY: She does not smoke or drink. She lives with her husband who is an invalid and for whom she cares. She is a retired former municipal court judge.

FAMILY HISTORY: One brother died of cancer of the throat (age 59), and another has cancer of the kidney (age 63).

REVIEW OF SYSTEMS:
SKIN: No rashes or jaundice.
HEENT: Head normocephalic. Normal TMs. Normal hearing. Pupils equal, round, reactive to light. Deviated septum. Oropharynx clear.
CR: No history of chest pain, shortness of breath, or pedal edema. She has had some mild hypertension in the past but is not under any medical supervision nor is she taking any medication for this.
GI: Weight is stable. See present illness.
OB-GYN: Gravida II Para II. Climacteric at age 46, no sequelae.
EXTREMITIES: No edema.
NEUROLOGIC: Unremarkable.

mtf
D: 5-17-20XX
T: 5-20-20XX

_____
Rex Rumsey, MD

FIGURE 4-6 Example of a medical report done in modified block format showing the six components of a history.

1. Location—Area of the body where the symptom is occurring.
2. Quality—Character of the symptom/pain (burning, gnawing, stabbing, fullness).
3. Severity—Degree of symptom or pain on a scale from 1 to 10. Severity also can be described with terms such as severe, slight, and persistent.
4. Duration—How long the symptom/pain has been present and how long it lasts when the patient has it.
5. Timing—When the pain/symptom occurs (e.g., morning, evening, after or before meals).
6. Context—The situation associated with the pain/symptom (e.g., dairy products, big meals, activity).

7. Modifying factors—Things done to make the symptom/pain worse or better. (For example, "If I eat spicy foods I get heartburn, but if I drink milk afterward the pain is not as bad.")
8. Associated signs and symptoms—The symptom/pain and other things that happen when the symptom/pain occurs (e.g., chest pain leads to shortness of breath).

Medicare Conditions for HPI for E/M Services

Brief HPI		Documentation of 1-3 of the 8 elements
Extended HPI	1995	Documentation of 4 or more elements
	1997	Documentation of 4 or more elements or the status of at least 3 chronic or inactive conditions

Review of Systems

A **review of systems (ROS)** is an inventory of body systems obtained through a series of questions that is used to identify signs or symptoms that the patient might be experiencing or has experienced. Checklists are permitted, but if a body system is not considered, then it should be crossed out. For an ROS, the following systems are recognized: constitutional symptoms (e.g., fever, weight loss), eyes, ears, nose, mouth, throat, cardiovascular, respiratory, gastrointestinal, genitourinary, musculoskeletal, integumentary (skin or breast), neurologic, psychiatric, endocrine, hematologic/lymphatic, and allergic/immunologic.

Medicare Conditions for ROS for E/M Services

Problem pertinent ROS		Positive and pertinent negatives for the system related to the problem
Extended ROS		Positive and pertinent for 2 to 9 systems
Complete ROS	1995	Review 10 or more systems, or a problem pertinent ROS plus a notation that all other systems appear negative
	1997	Review of at least 10 systems

Past, Family, and Social Histories

The past, family, and social histories (PFSH) consists of a review of three areas:

1. **Past history (PH)**—The patient's past experiences with illnesses, operations, injuries, and treatments
2. **Family history (FH)**—A review of medical events in the patient's family including diseases that may be hereditary or place the patient at risk
3. **Social history (SH)**—An age-appropriate review of past and current activities (e.g., smokes, consumes alcohol)

Medicare Conditions for PFSH for E/M Services

Pertinent PFSH		Specific information for 1 of the history areas directly related to the problem identified in the HPI
Complete PFSH	1995	Specific information for 2 or 3 history areas
	1997	Specific information for 1 specific item from 2 of the 3 history areas for established patient services (office, home care) and ER services. One specific item from each of the 3 history areas for new patient services (office, home care); hospital observation, inpatient services, initial care; consults; comprehensive nursing facility assessments

Documentation Review/Audit Worksheet

The documented history elements are counted and totaled (Figure 4-7, *A*). The health record should describe one to three elements of the present illness for a brief level of HPI. At least four elements of the HPI or the status of at least three chronic or inactive conditions is required for the extended level of HPI. Only two of three history elements are required for certain types of cases such as newborns or subsequent hospital care. Figure 4-7, *B*, shows Section I of the review/audit sheet that depicts the history containing the HPI, ROS, and PFSH. The check marks and circled element in the HPI (Section I) of the figure relate to the case illustrated.

The types of E/M services for the history are based on four levels of history. However, the ROS and PFSH must be totaled before the final decision on the level of service is assigned. The four levels of history may be defined as follows:

1. **Problem focused (PF)**—Chief complaint; brief history of present illness or problem
2. **Expanded problem focused (EPF)**—Chief complaint; brief HPI; problem-pertinent system review
3. **Detailed (D)**—Chief complaint; extended history of present illness; problem-pertinent system review extended to include a review of a limited number of additional systems; *pertinent* past, family, or social history directly related to the patient's problems.
4. **Comprehensive (C)**—Chief complaint; extended HPI; ROS that is directly related to the problem identified in the history of the present illness, plus a review of all additional body systems; *complete* PFSH.

In the ROS, the body systems are counted and totaled. The health record should describe one system of the ROS for a *pertinent to problem level*. For an *extended level*, two to nine systems are required. For a *complete level*, at least 10 organ systems must be reviewed and documented.

10-21-20XX

HISTORY OF PRESENT ILLNESS: This new patient is an 80-year-old — **Location**
white male who has had problems with voiding difficulty since 9-5 — **Duration**
2000. During the night, the patient had only 50 cc output and was — **Context**
Severity — catheterized this morning because of his poor urinary output (200 cc). — **Genitourinary (ROS)**
He was thought to have a distended bladder. He has not had any
Genitourinary (ROS) — gross hematuria. He has voiding difficulty, especially when lying down — **Modifying factor**
and voiding in the supine position. His voiding pattern is improved
while standing and sitting, however, the patient has developed a
Integumentary (ROS) — wound to his left lateral malleolus and is only able to ambulate with
assistance.

PAST MEDICAL HISTORY: Unremarkable. He does have some slowing
of his urinary stream and nocturia three to five times.

Notice that there is no family or social history for this new patient.

MEDICATIONS: He was on amitriptyline which may affect his bladder.

ALLERGIES: He has no known allergies.

PHYSICAL EXAMINATION: Shows the abdomen to be soft, nontender,
and not distended. His bladder was nonpalpable and nondistended.

Notice that the examination of the wound is missing.

GENITOURINARY: Normal penis. Testes descended bilaterally. His
prostate is 10 gm and benign in feeling.

IMPRESSION: Benign prostatic hypertrophy with some mild voiding
difficulty exacerbated by the patient's poor ambulatory status.

I suspect that as his ambulatory status improves, that his voiding
pattern will also improve. I will try him on Hytrin 5 mg/day by mouth. I will
follow him as needed.

Gene Ulibarri, MD

A mtf

---

1. History

Refer to data section (table below) in order to quantify. After referring to data, circle the entry farthest to the *RIGHT* in the table, which best describes the HPI, FOS and PFSH. If one column contains three circles, draw a line down that column to the bottom row to identify the type of history. If no column contains three circles, the column containing a circle farthest to the *LEFT*, identifies the type of history.

After completing this table which, classifies the history, circle the type of history within the appropriate grid in Section 5.

Descriptive elements of history	**HPI: Status of chronic conditions:** ☐ 1 condition ☐ 2 conditions ☐ 3 conditions **OR** **HPI (history of present illness) elements:** ☑ Location ☑ Severity ☐ Timing ☐ Modifying factors ☐ Quality ☑ Duration ☑ Context ☐ Associated signs and symptoms	☐ Status of 1-2 chronic conditions ☐ Brief (1-3)		☐ Status of 3 chronic conditions ☑ Extended (4 or more)
Systems of history	**ROS (review of systems):** ☐ Constitutional (wt loss, etc) ☐ Ears, nose, mouth, throat ☐ GI ☐ Integumentary (skin, breast) ☐ Endo ☐ Eyes ☐ Card/vasc ☐ GU ☐ Neuro ☐ Hem/lymph ☐ Resp ☐ Musculo ☐ Psych ☐ All/immuno ☐ All others negative	☐ None	☐ Pertinent to problem (1 system)	☑ Extended (2-9 systems)	☐ *Complete
Review of history	**PFSH (past medical, family, social history) areas:** ☑ Past history (the patient's past experiences with illnesses, operation, injuries and treatments) ☐ Family history (a review of medical events in the patent's family, including diseases which may be hereditary or place the patient at risk) ☐ Socal history (an age appropriate review of past and current activities)		☐ None	☑ Pertinent (1 history area)	☐ **Complete (2 or 3 history areas)
		PROBLEM FOCUSED	EXP.PROB. FOCUSED	DETAILED	COMPRE-HENSIVE

Levels of history

B

FIGURE 4-7 A, Documentation from a health record highlighting elements required for the history. B, Review/audit sheet Section I with check marks and circled elements show how the history in the example is declared as detailed. This shows two of three history components *(arrow)* used for the purpose of determining the assignment of a procedure code at the appropriate level of service.

| Elements Required for Each Level of History ||||
Present History	Review of Systems	Past, Family, or Social History	Levels of History
Brief	N/A	N/A	Problem focused
Brief problem	Problem pertinent	N/A	Expanded focused
Extended	Extended	Pertinent	Detailed
Extended	Complete	Complete	Comprehensive

FIGURE 4-8 Elements required for each type of history. One to three elements must be met to qualify for a given level of history.

Refer to Figure 4-7, *B*, for a visual understanding of Section I of the review/audit sheet. The check marks and circled element in the ROS (Section I) of the figure relate to the case illustrated.

The PFSH review areas are counted and totaled. The health record must contain at least one history area for a *detailed extended level* and specific items from two of the three history areas for a *comprehensive level* of PFSH. Refer to Figure 4-7, *B*, for a visual guide of the PFSH in Section I of the review/audit sheet. Note the difference in the number of required elements for new versus established patients and the circled element for the case in question.

A vertical line is drawn down the right four columns that contain the most elements to determine the history level. The elements of HPI, ROS, and PFSH must at least be met or may exceed the criteria determined for a PF, EPF, D, or C history level.

Figure 4-8 shows a gradual advancement of the elements that are required for each level of history. One to three elements must be met to qualify for a given level of history.

Documentation of Examination
Physical Examination

The **physical examination (PE or PX)** is objective in nature; that is, it consists of the physician's findings by examination or test results. Figure 4-9 is an illustration of a multiorgan system examination from the CMS Documentation Guidelines for 1997 that shows the details (elements) of examination for each body area within the genitourinary system. The three circled elements of the genitourinary system and one circled element of the gastrointestinal system relate to the case shown in Figure 4-7, *A*. For purposes of examination, the following body areas and organ systems are recognized.

Organ Systems/Body Areas—Elements of Examination.

Constitutional (vital signs, general appearance)
Eyes
Ears, nose, mouth, and throat
Neck
Respiratory
Cardiovascular
Chest, including breasts and axillae
Gastrointestinal (abdomen)
Genitourinary (male)
Genitourinary (female)
Lymphatic
Musculoskeletal
Skin
Neurologic
Psychiatric

NOTE: In addition, any reasons for not examining a particular body area or system should be listed.

Types of Physical Examination. When performing an internal review of a patient's health record, the number of elements identified by bullets is counted for each system and a total is obtained. The total is circled on Section II of the review/audit sheet as shown for the case illustrated (Figure 4-10).

The levels of evaluation and management services are based on four types of physical examination (PE):

1. Problem focused (PF)—A limited examination of the affected body area or organ system. The health record should describe one to five elements identified by a bullet in Figure 4-10 for a problem-focused level of PE.
2. Expanded problem focused (EPF)—A limited examination of the affected body area or organ system and other symptomatic or related organ systems. At least six elements identified by a bullet in Figure 4-10 are required for an expanded problem-focused level of PE.
3. Detailed (D)—An extended examination of the affected body areas and other symptomatic or related organ systems. At least two elements identified by a bullet in Figure 4-10 from each of six areas/body systems OR at least 12 elements identified by a bullet in two or more areas/body systems are required for a detailed level of PE.
4. Comprehensive (C)—A general multisystem examination or complete examination of a single organ system. For a comprehensive level of PE, all elements must be identified by a bullet in Figure 4-10 and documentation must be present for at least two elements identified by a bullet from each of nine areas/body systems.

MULTIORGAN SYSTEM EXAMINATION REQUIREMENTS (SHADED)
CONTENT and DOCUMENTATION

Level of Exam	Perform and Document
Problem focused	One to five elements identified by a bullet.
Expanded Problem Focused	At least six elements identified by a bullet.
Detailed	At least twelve elements identified by a bullet.
Comprehensive	Perform all elements identified by a bullet; document every element in every shaded box and at least one element in every unshaded box.

Genitourinary

System/Body Area	Elements of Examination
Constitutional	• Measurement of **any three of the following seven** vital signs: 1) sitting or standing blood pressure, 2) supine blood pressure, 3) pulse rate and regularity, 4) respiration, 5) temperature, 6) height, 7) weight (may be measured and recorded by ancillary staff) • General appearance of patient *e.g.development, nutrition, body habitus, deformities, attention to grooming*
Neck	• Examination of neck *e.g. masses, overall appearance, symmetry, tracheal position, crepitus* • Examination of thyroid *e.g. enlargement, tenderness, mass*
Respiratory	• Assessment of respiratory effect *e.g. intercostal retractions, use of accessory muscles, diaphragmatic movement* • Auscultation of lungs *e.g. breath sounds, adventitious sounds, rubs*
Cardiovascular	• Auscultation of heart with notation of abnormal sounds and murmurs • Examination of peripheral vascular system by observation *e.g. swelling, varicosities* and palpation *e.g. pulses, temperature, edema, tenderness*
Chest (breasts)	See genitourinary (female)
Gastrointestinal (abdomen)	⊙ Examination of abdomen with notation of presence of masses or tenderness • Examination for presence or absence of hernia • Examination of liver and spleen • Obtain stool sample for occult blood test when indicated
Genitourinary (male)	• Inspection of anus and perineum Examination (with or without specimen collection for smears and cultures) of genitalia including: • Scrotum *e.g. lesions, cysts, rashes* • Epididymides *e.g. size, symmetry, masses* ⊙ Testes *e.g. size, symmetry, masses* • Urethral meatus *e.g. size, location, lesions, discharge* ⊙ Penis *e.g. lesions, presence or absence of foreskin, foreskin retractability, plaque, masses, scarring, deformities* Digital rectal examination including: ⊙ Prostate gland *e.g. size, symmetry, nodularity, tenderness* • Seminal vesicles *e.g. symmetry, tenderness, masses, enlargement* • Sphincter tone, presence of hemorrhoids, rectal masses
Genitourinary (female) Includes at least seven of the eleven elements to the right identified by bullets:	• Inspection and palpation of breasts *e.g. masses or lumps, tenderness, symmetry, nipple discharge* • Digital rectal examination including sphincter tone, presence of hemorrhoids, rectal masses Pelvic examination (with or without specimen collection for smears and cultures) including: • External genitalia *e.g. general appearance, hair distribution, lesions* • Urethral meatus *e.g. size, location, lesions, prolapse* • Urethra *e.g. masses, tenderness, scarring* • Bladder *e.g. fullness, masses, tenderness* • Vagina *e.g. general appearance, estrogen effect, discharge, lesions, pelvic support, cystocele, rectocele* • Cervix *e.g. general appearance, lesions, discharge* • Uterus *e.g. size, contour, position, mobility, tenderness, descent or support* • Adnexa/parametria *e.g. masses, tenderness, organomegaly, nodularity* • Anus and perineum

Genitourinary (continued)

System/Body Area	Elements of Examination
Lymphatic	• Palpation of lymph nodes in neck, axillae, groin and/or other location
Skin	• Inspection and/or palpation of skin and subcutaneous tissue *e.g. rashes, lesions, ulcers*
Neurological/psychiatric	Brief assessment of mental status including: • Orientation to time, place and person • Mood and affect *e.g. depression, anxiety, agitation*

Skin

System/Body Area	Elements of Examination
Constitutional	• Measurement of **any three of the following seven** vital signs: 1) sitting or standing blood pressure, 2) supine blood pressure, 3) pulse rate and regularity, 4) respiration, 5) temperature, 6) height, 7) weight (may be measured and recorded by ancillary staff) • General appearance of patient *e.g. development, nutrition, body habitus, deformities, attention to grooming*
Eyes	• Inspection of conjunctivae and lids
Ears, nose, mouth and throat	• Inspection of lips, teeth and gums • Examination of oropharynx *e.g. oral mucosa, hard and soft palates, tongue, tonsils, and posterior pharynx*
Neck	• Examination of thyroid *e.g. enlargement, tenderness, mass*
Gastrointestinal (abdomen)	• Examination of liver and spleen • Examination of anus for condyloma and other lesions
Lymphatic	• Palpation of lymph nodes in neck, axillae, groin and/or other location
Extremities	• Inspection and palpation of digits and nails *e.g. clubbing, cyanosis, inflammation, petechiae, ischemia, infections, nodes*
Skin	• Palpation of scalp and inspection of hair of scalp, eyebrows, face, chest, pubic area (when indicated) and extremities • Inspection and/or palpation of skin and subcutaneous tissue *e.g. rashes, lesions, ulcers, susceptibility in and presence of photo damage* in **eight of the following ten areas:** 1) head including face, 2) neck, 3) chest including breasts and axilla, 4) abdomen, 5) genitalia, groin, buttocks, 6) back, 7) right upper extremity, 8) left upper extremity, 9) right lower extremity, 10) left lower extremity Note: For the comprehensive level, the examination of all eight anatomic areas must be performed and documented. For the three lower levels of examination, each body area is counted separately. For example, inspection and/or palpation of the skin and subcutaneous tissue of the head and neck extremities constitutes two areas. • Inspection of eccrine and apocrine glands of skin and subcutaneous tissue with identification and location of any hyperhidrosis, chromhidroses or bromhidrosis
Neurological/psychiatric	Brief assessment of mental status including: • Orientation to time, place and person • Mood and affect *e.g. depression, anxiety, agitation*

FIGURE 4-9 Review/audit worksheet of a general multiorgan system physical examination that shows the details (elements) of examination for each body area/system. Circled bullets relate to the example case shown in Figure 4-7, A. (From the Iowa Medical Society, IMS Services, West Des Moines, IA, 1998.)

SECTION II

Four elements identified

	General Multisystem Exam		Single Organ System Exam
E X A M	1-5 elements identified by ●	PROBLEM FOCUSED	1-5 elements identified by ●
	≥6 elements identified by ●	EXPANDED PROBLEM FOCUSED	≥6 elements identified by ●
	≥2 elements identified by ● from 6 areas/systems OR ≥12 elements identified by ● from at least 2 areas/systems	DETAILED	≥12 elements identified by ● EXCEPT ≥9 elements identified by ● for eye and psychiatric exams
	≥2 elements identified by ● from 9 areas/systems	COMPREHENSIVE	Perform all elements identified by ● ; document all elements in shaded boxes; document ≥1 element in unshaded boxes.

FIGURE 4-10 Review/audit worksheet Section II for a general multisystem physical examination and single organ system examination. The circled item relates to a problem-focused examination for the example case (see Figure 4-8, A) for coding purposes. (From the Iowa Medical Society, IMS Services, West Des Moines, IA, 1998.)

The extent of the examination and what is documented range from limited examinations of single body areas to general multisystem or complete single-organ system examinations, depending on clinical judgment and the nature of the presenting problem.

1995 Medicare Conditions for the Physical Examination for E/M Services

Problem focused	Documentation of only 1 body area or organ system
Expanded problem focused or detailed	Documentation of up to 7 systems (the affected body area or system plus up to 6 additional systems)
Comprehensive	Documentation of 8 or more systems

1997 Medicare Conditions for General Multisystem Examination

Problem focused	One to 5 elements identified by a bullet in 1 or more body or system areas
Expanded problem focused	At least 6 elements identified by a bullet in 1 or more body or system areas
Detailed	At least 2 elements identified by a bullet from each of 6 body areas or systems or at least 12 elements in 2 or more body or system areas
Comprehensive	Perform all elements for each selected system or body area; document at least 2 elements identified by a bullet from each of at least 9 body or system areas

Documentation of Medical Decision Making Complexity

Medical decision making (MDM) is a health care management process done after performing a history and physical examination on a patient that results in a plan of treatment. It is based on establishing one or more diagnoses and/or selecting a management or treatment option, amount or complexity of data reviewed, and risk of complications or associated morbidity or mortality. *Morbidity* is a diseased condition or state, whereas *mortality* has to do with the number of deaths that occur in a given time or place.

Number of diagnoses or management options is based on the number and types of problems addressed during the visit, the complexity of establishing a diagnosis, and the number of management options that must be considered by the physician. For the case illustrated, the number of problems is 1, which equals 3 points (Figure 4-11, *top section*).

Amount or complexity of data to be reviewed is based on the types of diagnostic tests ordered or reviewed. A decision to obtain and review old health records or obtain history from sources other than the patient increases the amount and complexity of data to be analyzed. For the case illustrated, no points apply (see Figure 4-11, *middle section*).

Risk of complications, morbidity, or mortality is based on other conditions associated with the presenting problem known as the risk of complications, morbidity, or mortality, as well as comorbidities, the

COMPLEXITY

SECTION III A AND B

A — NUMBER OF DIAGNOSES OR TREATMENT OPTIONS

Problems to exam physician	Number X points = Result		
Self-limited or minor (stable, improved or worsening)	Max = 2	1	
Est. problem (to examiner); stable, improved		1	
Est. problem (to examiner); worsening		2	
New problem (to examiner); no additional workup planned	Max = 1 / 1	3	3
New prob. (to examiner); add. workup planned		4	
		TOTAL	3

Bring total to line A in final result for complexity

B — AMOUNT AND/OR COMPLEXITY OF DATA TO BE REVIEWED

Data to be reviewed	Points
Review and/or order of clinical lab tests	1
Review and/or order of tests in the radiology section of CPT	1
Review and/or order of tests in the medicine section of CPT	1
Discussion of test results with performing physician	1
Decision to obtain old records and/or obtain history from someone other than patient	1
Review and summarization of old records and/or obtaining history from someone other than patient and/or discussion of case with another health care provider	2
Independent visualization of image, tracing or specimen itself (not simply review of report)	2
TOTAL	0

Bring total to line B in final result for complexity

Draw a line down the column with 2 or 3 circles and circle decision making level OR draw a line down the column with the center circle and circle the decision making level.

A	Number diagnoses or treatment options	≤1 Minimal	2 Limited	3 Multiple	≥4 Extensive
B	Amount and complexity of data	≤1 Minimal or low	2 Limited	3 Moderate	≥4 Extensive
C	Highest risk	Minimal	Low	Moderate	High
	Type of decision making	Straight-foward	Low complex	Moderate complex	High complex

Note: The wound was not a considering factor in the medical decision making.

FIGURE 4-11 Section III of the review/audit worksheet. *Part A:* Number of diagnoses or treatment options. *Part B:* Amount or complexity of data to be reviewed. *Lower one third:* Used to compile the results obtained from Parts A, B, and C (see Figure 4-10) to determine the level of medical decision making. In Figure 4-7, **A** and **B** for the example case, circled points and words relate to a moderately complex level of decision making for coding and billing purposes. (From the Iowa Medical Society, IMS Services, West Des Moines, Iowa, 1998.)

diagnostic procedures, or the possible management options (treatment rendered—surgery, therapy, drug management, services, and supplies). **Comorbidity** means underlying disease or other conditions present at the time of the visit. In determining the level of risk, the element (presenting problem, diagnostic procedure ordered, or management options selected) that has the highest level (minimal, low, moderate, or high) is used.

To discover whether the level of risk is minimal, low, moderate, or high, bulleted elements are marked on the review/audit sheet (Figure 4-12, *Section III, Part C*). For the case illustrated, the elements fall within the moderate level of risk category.

To conclude the internal review of a patient's health record, a level must be determined by the health care provider from one of four types of medical decision making: **straightforward (SF), low complexity (LC), moderate complexity (MC),** and **high complexity (HC).** The bottom portion of Figure 4-12, *Section III,* shows the results obtained from Parts A, B, and C highlighted. For the case illustrated, the number of diagnoses is declared *multiple*, there are no *data to review*, and the risk of complications is *moderate*; therefore a *moderately complex* level of decision-making has been assigned to be used for coding and billing purposes.

DOCUMENTATION TERMINOLOGY

Terminology for Evaluation and Management Services

While learning the complexities of medical documentation and how important it is as it relates to coding and billing, you have discovered that you must have a good foundation of medical terminology. To use the diagnostic and procedure code books efficiently, you must become familiar with their language, abbreviations, and symbols. The first terms introduced are most commonly used for E/M services.

New Versus Established Patient

In coding E/M services, two categories of patients are considered: the new patient and the established patient. A **new patient (NP)** is one who *has not received* any professional services from the physician or another physician of the same specialty who belongs to the same group practice *within the past 3 years.* An **established patient** is one who *has received* professional services from the physician or another physician of the same specialty who belongs to the same group practice *within the past 3 years.* Refer to the decision tree in Figure 4-13 to help you

make a decision as to whether a patient is considered new or established.

A physician may provide a course of action to evaluate and manage a patient who is seeking medical care (i.e., refer to a specialist for consultation, see a referral from another physician, give concurrent care as one of several physicians, render continuity of care for a doctor who is out of town, administer critical care, direct emergency care, or furnish counseling discussion to a patient's family).

Consultation

A **consultation** includes services rendered by a physician whose opinion or advice is requested by another physician or agency in the evaluation or treatment of a patient's illness or a suspected problem. The requesting physician must document the request in the patient's health record and the consulting physician should state: "Patient is seen at the request of Dr. John Doe for a ... reason." Consultations may occur in a home, office, hospital, extended care facility, or other location. A physician consultant recommends diagnostic or therapeutic services and may initiate these services if requested by the referring physician. The opinion must be in writing, documented in a consultation report, and communicated to the referring physician. The consultant may order a diagnostic or therapeutic service to formulate the opinion at an initial or subsequent visit.

Reimbursement is significantly more than for an equivalent office visit.

Referral

A **referral** is the transfer of the total or specific care of a patient from one physician to another for known problems. It is not a consultation. For example, a patient is sent by a primary care physician to an orthopedist for care of a fracture.

However, when dealing with managed care plans, the term *referral* is also used when requesting an authorization for the patient to receive services elsewhere (e.g., referral for laboratory tests, radiology procedures, specialty care). As a courtesy, the physician may send a thank-you note to the referring physician with comments about the patient's condition.

Concurrent Care

Concurrent care is the providing of similar services (e.g., hospital visits) to the same patient by more than one physician on the same day. Usually, such cases involve the presence of a physical disorder (e.g., diabetes) at the

SECTION III

C

RISK OF COMPLICATIONS AND/OR MORBIDITY OR MORTALITY

Level of risk	Presenting problem(s)	Diagnostic procedure(s) ordered	Management options selected
MINIMAL	• One self-limited or minor problem (e.g., cold, insect bite, tinea corporis)	• Laboratory tests requiring venipuncture • Chest x-rays • KOH prep • EKG/EEG • Urinalysis • Ultrasound e.g. echo	• Rest • Gargles • Elastic bandages • Superficial dressings
LOW	• Two or more self-limited or minor problems • One stable chronic illness (e.g., well-controlled hypertension, non-insulin dependent diabetes, cataract, BPH) • Acute uncomplicated illness or injury (e.g., cystitis, allergic rhinitis, simple sprain)	• Physiologic test not under stress (e.g., pulmonary function tests) • Non-cardiovascular imaging studies with contrast (e.g., barium enema) • Superficial needle biopsies • Clinical laboratory tests requiring arterial puncture • Skin biopsies	• Over-the-counter drugs • Minor surgery with no identified risk factors • Physical therapy • Occupational therapy • IV fluids without additives
MODERATE	• One or more chronic illnesses with mild exacerbation, progression or side effects of treatment • Two or more stable chronic illnesses • Undiagnosed new problem with uncertain prognosis (e.g., lump in breast) • Acute illness with systemic symptoms (e.g., pyelonephritis, pneumonitis, colitis) • Acute complicated injury (e.g., head injury with brief loss of consciousness)	• Physiologic test under stress (e.g., cardiac stress test, fetal contraction stress test) • Diagnostic endoscopies with no identified risk factors • Deep needle or incisional biopsy • Cardiovascular imaging studies with contrast and no identified risk factors (e.g., arteriogram, cardiac cath) • Obtain fluid from body cavity (e.g., lumbar puncture, thoracentesis, culdocentesis)	• Minor surgery with identified risk factors • Elective major surgery (open percutaneous or endoscopic) with no identified risk factors • Prescription drug management • Therapeutic nuclear medicine • IV fluids with additives • Closed treatment of fracture or dislocation without manipulation
HIGH	• One or more chronic illnesses with severe exacerbation, progression or side effects of tx • Acute or chronic illnesses or injuries that may pose a threat to life or bodily function (e.g., multiple trauma, acute MI, pulmonary embolus, severe respiratory distress, progressive severe rheumatoid arthritis, psychiatric illness with potential threat to self or others, peritonitis, acute renal failure) • An abrupt change in neurological status (e.g., seizure, TIA, weakness, sensory loss)	• Cardiovascular imaging studies with contrast with identified risk factors • Cardiac electrophysiological tests • Diagnostic endoscopies with identified risk factors • Discography	• Elective major surgery (open, percutaneous or endoscopic) with identified risk factor • Emergency major surgery (open, percutaneous or endoscopic) • Parenteral controlled substances • Drug therapy requiring intensive monitoring for toxicity • Decision not to resuscitate or de-escalate care because of poor prognosis

FIGURE 4-12 Section III, *Part C*, of the review/audit worksheet used for determining the level of risk. The highlighted areas relate to a moderate level of risk for the example case (see Figure 4-7, A) for coding purposes. (From the Iowa Medical Society, IMS Services, West Des Moines, IA, 1998.)

same time as the primary admitting diagnosis, and this may alter the course of treatment or lengthen recovery time for the primary condition. For example, two internists (a general internist and a cardiologist) see the same patient in the hospital on the same day. The general internist admitted the patient for diabetes and requested that the cardiologist also follow the patient's periodic chest pain and arrhythmia. If the second doctor is not identified in carrier records as a cardiologist, the claim may be denied. This is because the services appear to be

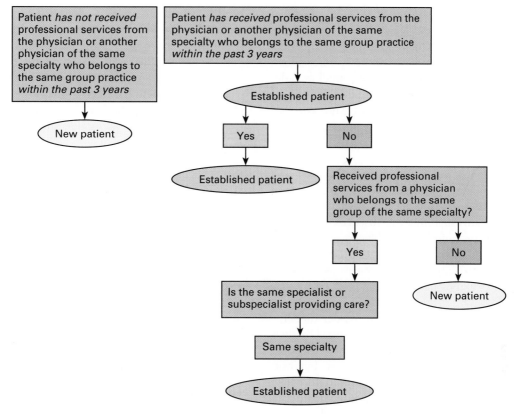

FIGURE 4-13 Decision tree for new patient versus established patient when selecting a CPT evaluation and management code.

duplicated by physicians of the same specialty. When billing insurance companies, physicians providing concurrent care may be cross-referenced on the claim form. Medicare has a list that includes 62 specialties and subspecialties to help carriers more accurately judge whether concurrent care is necessary. Periodically, the physician should check with the carrier's provider service representative to determine whether the provider has updated its subspecialty status so that claims for concurrent care are not denied.

Continuity of Care

If a case involves **continuity of care** (e.g., a patient who has received treatment for a condition and is then referred by the physician to a second physician for treatment for the same condition), both physicians are responsible for providing arrangements for the patient's continuing care. In such a case, records must be provided by the referring physician and the insurance billing specialist must obtain summaries or records of the patient's previous treatment. Obtain hospital reports before coding if the patient was seen in the hospital, emergency department, or outpatient department. Contact the hospital's health record department for copies of reports after outpatient treatment or after a patient's discharge. In some cases, coding from hospital reports can increase reimbursement but

can delay submission of claims because reports may not be available in a timely manner.

Critical Care

Critical care means the intensive care provided in a variety of acute life-threatening conditions requiring constant "full attention" by a physician. It can be provided in the critical care unit or emergency department (ED) of a hospital. A critical illness or injury acutely impairs one or more vital organ systems such that there is a high probability of imminent or life-threatening deterioration in the patient's condition. Examples of vital organ system failure include, but are not limited to, central nervous system failure, circulatory failure, shock, and renal, hepatic, metabolic, or respiratory failure. Critical care may sometimes, but not always, be rendered in a critical care area such as a coronary care unit (CCU), intensive care unit (ICU), respiratory care unit (RCU), or ED (also called the emergency room [ER]).

Emergency Care

Emergency care differs from critical care in that it may be given by the physician in a hospital ED or in a physician's office setting. Emergency care is that provided to acutely ill patients and may or may not involve organ system failure but does require immediate medical attention. In physician-directed emergency care, advanced life support, the physician is located in a hospital emergency or critical care department and is in two-way voice communication with ambulance or rescue personnel outside the hospital. The physician directs the performance of necessary medical procedures. Physicians who work in the ED of a hospital are not employees of the hospital and bill separately for the services they perform.

In the Medicare program, an emergency medical condition is currently defined as a medical condition manifesting itself by acute symptoms of sufficient severity (including severe pain) such that the absence of immediate medical attention could reasonably be expected to result in placing the patient's health in serious jeopardy, serious impairment to body functions, or serious dysfunction of any body organ or part.

Many states have adopted the prudent lay person definition of an emergency as defined in the Balanced Budget Act of 1996. This is similarly stated as "any medical condition of recent onset and severity, including but not limited to severe pain, that would lead a prudent lay person, possessing an average knowledge of medicine and health, to believe that his or her condition, sickness, or injury is of such a nature that failure to obtain immediate medical care could result in placing the patient's health in serious jeopardy, serious impairment to bodily functions, or serious dysfunction of bodily organ or part."

Counseling

Counseling is a discussion with a patient, family, or both concerning one or more of the following: diagnostic results, impressions, or recommended diagnostic studies; prognosis; risks and benefits of treatment options; instructions for treatment or follow-up; importance of compliance with chosen treatment options; risk factor reduction; and patient and family education.

Diagnostic Terminology and Abbreviations

Problems can occur with documentation because of missing or misused essential words. For example, if an entry says "diastolic dysfunction" instead of "heart failure due to diastolic dysfunction" you have more complete documentation of the medical condition with the second statement. Always query the physician if in doubt about the documentation to obtain the most specific, accurate terminology into the record.

Some physicians document "imp" (impression) or "Dx" (diagnosis), which usually serves as the diagnosis when completing the claim. If the diagnosis is not in the health record and there is doubt about the diagnosis, always ask the physician to review it. Physicians often document laboratory results and stop documenting before giving a diagnosis. Attach a note to the insurance claim for the physician to read before transmitting the claim. If the patient has been in the hospital, request the electronic file of the discharge summary, which contains the admitting and discharge diagnoses.

Official American Hospital Association policy states that "abbreviations should be totally eliminated from the more vital sections of the health record, such as final diagnosis, operative notes, discharge summaries, and descriptions of special procedures." Many physicians are not aware of this policy, and the final diagnosis may appear as an abbreviation in the patient's record. Frequently, an abbreviation translates to several meanings. Use your medical dictionary (most list abbreviations alphabetically with the unabbreviated words) to interpret the abbreviation or ask the physician when clarification is necessary.

Refer to Figure 4-14, which indicates commonly used abbreviations that appear in office progress notes. Most medical practices create and retain a list of acceptable abbreviations with translations in their office policy manual to avoid misinterpretation. In the *Workbook*, refer to the detailed list of common medical abbreviations in Appendix A. Additional knowledge will be obtained when you complete each assignment involving a patient's health record in the *Workbook* because you must define all of the abbreviations.

If a lay term appears in a patient record, the correct medical term should be substituted to locate the correct diagnostic code (e.g., "contusion" for "bruise").

An **eponym** (term including the name of a person [e.g., Graves' disease]) should not be used when a comparable anatomic term can be used in its place (Example 4-2).

Example 4-2

EPONYM	COMPARABLE MEDICAL TERM
Buerger's disease	Thromboangiitis obliterans
Graves' disease	Exophthalmic goiter
Wilks' syndrome	Myasthenia gravis

The word *acute* refers to a condition that runs a short (typically 3 to 5 days) but relatively severe course. The word *chronic* means a condition persisting over a long period of time. When the terms "acute" or "chronic" are listed in the diagnostic statement, always

GIOVANNI, CARLOS A.

DATE	PROGRESS NOTES
11-11-xx	Pt referred to College Hospital ER by employer for workers' compensation injury. I was called in as on-call
	neurosurgeon to evaluate the pt. Pt states that today at 2 p.m. he fell from the roof of a private home while
	installing an antenna at 2231 Duarte St., Woodland Hills, XY 12345 in Woodland Hills County. He describes the
	incident as follows: "When I was attaching the base of an antenna, the weight of the antenna shifted and knocked
	me off the roof." Pt complains of head pain and indicates brief loss of consciousness. I performed a C HX/PX.
	Complete skull x-rays showed fractured skull. CT of head/brain (without contrast) indicates well-defined R.
	subdural hematoma. Pt suffering from cerebral concussion; no open wound. Tr plan: Adm pt to College
	Hospital (5 p.m.) and schedule R infratentorial craniotomy to evacuate hematoma. (H/MDM). Obtained
	authorization and prepared Dr.'s First Report.
	AP/llf *Astro Parkinson, MD*
11-12-xx	Performed R infratentorial craniotomy and evacuated subdural hematoma. Pt stable and returned to room; will be
	seen daily. TD: Estimated RTW 1-15-xx. Possible cranial defect & head disfigurement resulting. Pt to be
	hospitalized for approx 2 weeks.
	AP/llf *Astro Parkinson, MD*
11-13-xx	HV (EPF HX/PX M/MDM). Pt improving; recommend consult with Dr. Graff for cranial defect. Authorization
	obtained from adjuster (Steve Burroughs) at State Comp.
	AP/llf *Astro Parkinson, MD*
11-14-xx	Pt seen in cons by Dr. Cosmo Graff who stated he does not recommend correcting PO cranial defect. Both
	Dr. Graff and I explained how the defect resulted from the injury; there may be some improvement over time.
	Pt states he is grateful to be alive (EPF HX/PX M/MDM).
	AP/llf *Astro Parkinson, MD*
11-15-xx	Daily HV (EPF HX/PX M/MDM). Pt progressing appropriately; no complications have occurred.
thru	
11-29-xx	AP/llf *Astro Parkinson, MD*
11-30-xx	DC from hosp. Permanent cranial defect resulting from fracture and surgery. RTO 1 wk.
	AP/llf *Astro Parkinson, MD*
12-7-xx	OV (EPF HX/PX LC/MDM) Pt doing very well. No HA or visual disturbances, BP 120/80, alert and oriented.
	He is anxious to return to work. Pt cautioned about maintaining low activity level until released. RTO 2 wks.
	AP/llf *Astro Parkinson, MD*
12-21-xx	OV (PF HX/PX SF/MDM). Pt continues to improve. Suggested he start a walking program 3 x wk and monitor
	symptoms. May do light activity and lifting (10 lbs). Adv to call if any symptoms return. RTO 10 days.
	AP/llf *Astro Parkinson, MD*
12-29-xx	OV (PF HX/PX SF/MDM). Pt did not experience any symptoms with increased activity. No further trt necessary.
	Pt will increase activity and call if any problems occur. Pt scheduled to resume reg W on 1-15-xx. Final report
	submitted to workers' compensation carrier.
	AP/llf *Astro Parkinson, MD*

FIGURE 4-14 Medical office progress notes indicating some common medical abbreviations and symbols used in a patient's health record. Meanings of these abbreviations and symbols are listed in the *Workbook*, Appendix A.

search for these terms in the code description. If the same condition is described as both acute (subacute) and chronic and separate subentries exist in the diagnostic code book alphabetic index at the same indentation level, code both and sequence the acute (subacute) code first. For proper documentation to support chronic conditions, two criteria are that the documentation actually states something about the chronic condition and that the conditions are pertinent to the patient's current treatment. For example, if a physician states "controlled diabetes," this is a fact. If the physician asks the patient about his or her sugar level and diet and documents the findings, then something specific has been identified about the chronic condition and this would pass an audit for correct documentation.

Whenever the words "question of," "suspected," "rule out," or the abbreviation "R/O" are used in connection with a disease or illness, do not code these conditions as if they existed or were established. Instead, code the chief complaint, sign, or symptom. These are only a few of the many terms used in documentation.

An abnormal or unexpected finding without elaboration in the health record is insufficient documentation and should be described. Commonly used phrases or abbreviations that may not support billing of services are "WNL" (within normal limits), "noncontributory," "negative/normal," "other than the above, all systems were normal," and so on. For example, phrases used to document findings, such as "all extremities are within normal limits," do not indicate how many extremities or which ones were examined. Documentation must indicate exactly which limb was examined, and abbreviated wording would not pass an external audit. If it is determined such phrases are "canned" notes that can mean no assessment was actually performed, this is fraud.

Another word commonly used when examining a patient and the findings are within normal limits is "negative" (e.g., "ears, nose, and throat negative," "chest x-rays negative"). The physician needs to document that there were no abnormalities in the system being examined. Detailed documentation justifies billed services by providing verification and allows points when an external audit is performed. Thus it should be dictated "Chest film (or report) was reviewed" or "Chest x-ray report was read."

Directional Terms

The following terms are commonly used to describe location of pain and injuries to areas of the abdomen, as shown in Figure 4-15, *A* (four quadrants) and *B* (nine regions):

Right upper quadrant (RUQ) or right hypochondriac: Liver (right lobe), gallbladder, part of the pancreas, parts of the small and large intestines

Epigastric: Upper middle region above the stomach

Left upper quadrant (LUQ) or left hypochondriac: Liver (left lobe), stomach, spleen, part of the pancreas, parts of the small and large intestines

Right and left lumbar: Middle, right, and left regions of the waist

Umbilical: Central region near the navel

Right lower quadrant (RLQ) or right inguinal: Parts of the small and large intestines, right ovary, right uterine (fallopian) tube, appendix, and right ureter

Hypogastric: Middle region below the umbilical region contains urinary bladder and female uterus

Left lower quadrant (LLQ) or left inguinal: Parts of the small and large intestines, left ovary, left uterine tube, and left ureter

Surgical Terminology

Two frequently used terms are preoperative and postoperative (e.g., preoperative diagnosis or postoperative care). Preoperative (preop) pertains to the period before a surgical procedure. Commonly, the preoperative period begins with the first preparation of the patient for surgery and ends with the introduction of anesthesia in the operating suite, whereas postoperative (PO) pertains to the period of time after surgery. It begins with the patient's emergence from anesthesia and continues through the time required for the acute effects of the anesthetic and surgical procedures to decrease.

Surgical procedures of the integumentary system, such as repair of lacerations, are listed in the procedure code book as *simple, intermediate,* or *complex* repairs. Simple lacerations are superficial, requiring one-layer closure. Intermediate lacerations require layered closure of one or more of the deeper layers of the skin and tissues. Complex lacerations require more than layered closure and may require reconstructive surgery. Documentation should list the length (in centimeters) of all incisions and layers of involved tissues (subcutaneous, fascia, muscle, and grafts) so that correct procedure codes for excision of lesions and type of repair can be determined.

If time is a factor in coding for reimbursement, then documentation should list the length of time spent on the procedure, especially if of unusual duration such as prolonged services, counseling, or team conferences. This should be stated somewhere in the report.

If state-of-the-art instruments or equipment are used, document the equipment, as well as the time spent using it.

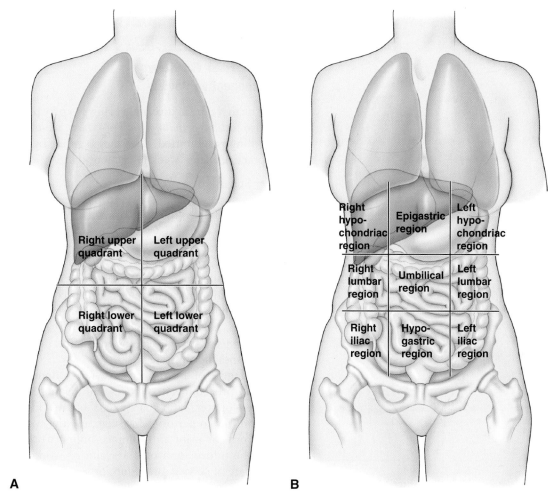

FIGURE 4-15 Regions of the abdomen. **A,** Four quadrants. **B,** Nine regions. (From Herlihy B, Maebius NK: *The human body in health and illness*, ed 3, St Louis, 2007, Elsevier Science.)

Therapeutic or cosmetic surgical procedures should be broken down into two categories—state how much of the procedure was functional and how much was cosmetic or therapeutic. Generally, the insurance carrier pays for the functional portion of the procedure even if there is no coverage for cosmetic or therapeutic procedures.

If you type reports to be submitted with insurance claims to help justify the claim, you should also become familiar with the terms for various operational incisions (Figure 4-16). Terms such as *undermining* (cut in a horizontal fashion), *take down* (to take apart), or *lysis of adhesions* (destruction of scar tissue) appear in many operations but should not be coded separately. Note the *position* (e.g., lithotomy, dorsal) of the patient during the operation and the *surgical approach* (e.g., vaginal, abdominal). These help determine the proper code selection. Major errors can occur when an insurance biller is not familiar with the medical terms being used. Ask the physician to clarify the case if there is a question because medical

terminology is technical and can puzzle even the most knowledgeable insurance billing specialist. Additional key words to look for that may affect code selection and reimbursements, in addition to the terminology listed in Table 4-1, along with brief definitions, are as follows:

Bilateral: Pertaining to both sides
Blood loss of more than 600 mL: Severe bleeding
Complete or total: Entire or whole
Complicated by: Involved with other situations at the same time
Hemorrhage: Escape of blood from vessels; bleeding
Initial: First procedure or service
Multiple: Affecting many parts of the body at the same time
Partial: Only a part, not complete
Prolonged procedure due to: Series of steps extended in time to get desired result
Simple: Single and not compound or complex
Subsequent: Second or more procedures or services
Surgical: Pertaining to surgery

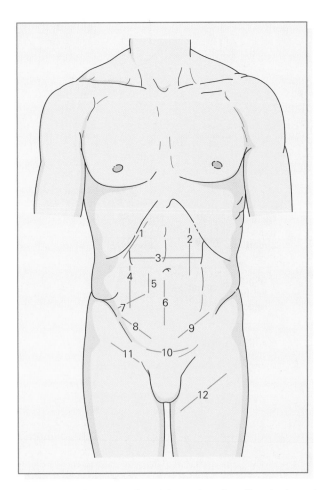

FIGURE 4-16 Operational incisions. Anterior (front) view: *1*, subcostal incision; *2*, paramedian incision; *3*, transverse incision; *4*, upper right rectus incision; *5*, midrectus incision; *6*, midline incision; *7*, lower right rectus incision; *8*, McBurney or right iliac incision; *9*, left iliac incision; *10*, suprapubic incision, *11*, hernia incision; *12*, femoral incision.

Uncomplicated: Not intricately involved; straightforward (procedure)

Unilateral: Pertaining to one side

Unusual findings or circumstances: Rare or not usual conclusion

Very difficult: Hard to do, requiring extra effort and skill

Additional words used to detail accidents and injuries are shown in Figures 15-5 through 15-9.

Many good books are available for a more thorough discussion of medical terminology.*

*Chabner D-E: *The language of medicine*, ed 8, St Louis, 2007, Saunders; Leonard PC: *Building a medical vocabulary*, ed 9, St Louis, 2010, Elsevier.

REVIEW AND AUDIT OF HEALTH RECORDS

Internal Reviews
Prospective Review

The first type of **internal review** is a **prospective review,** also termed *prebilling audit* or *review,* which is done *before* billing is submitted. This may be done by some medical practices daily, weekly, or monthly.

● Stage 1 of a prospective review is done to verify that completed encounter forms match patients seen according to the appointment schedule and have been posted on the daysheet. A prospective review is begun by obtaining the encounter forms and locating the dates in question for the review in the appointment schedule, printing the schedule as verification. The appointment schedule is then compared with the encounter forms to match patients for the date in question. Next, check to see if all charges (procedures or services) have been posted on the daysheet or daily transaction register.

● Stage 2 of a prospective review is done to verify that all procedures or services and diagnoses listed on the encounter form match data on the insurance claim form. To perform this stage, use the completed claim form or print an insurance billing worksheet. Match the information on the claim or worksheet with the date of service, procedure or service, and diagnosis on the encounter form. It is possible that one or more diagnoses may not match. A common reason is because an active diagnosis has not been entered into the computer system and the computer defaults to the last diagnosis given for an established patient. Another problem occurs when the diagnosis is not linked to the procedure. Such problems must be found before billing and corrected before claims are printed.

Retrospective Review

The second type of internal review is called a **retrospective review,** which is done after billing insurance carriers. A coder or insurance biller may be asked to perform a retrospective review to determine whether there is a lack of documentation. To accomplish this, pull 15 to 20 health records per provider from the past 2 to 4 months at random. The following are recommended internal audit tools:

● Pencil
● Internal record review worksheets
● Current procedure code book
● Current diagnostic code book
● Current Healthcare Common Procedures Coding System (HCPCS) code book
● Medical dictionary

Table 4-1	Terminology Used in Coding Procedures
MEDICAL TERM	**DEFINITION**
Ablation	Surgical removal of a body part, as by incision
Acquired	Condition or disorder contracted after birth; not hereditary or innate
Amputation	Removal of a body part, limb, or organ
Anastomosis	Surgical or pathologic connection of two tubular structures
Anomaly	Congenital or developmental defect; deviation from normal
Arthrocentesis	Surgical puncture of a joint to remove fluid
Arthrodesis	To surgically immobilize a joint; fusion
Aspiration	To draw in by inhaling or draw out by suction
Biopsy	Removal of living tissue for microscopic examination
Cauterization	Means of destroying tissue, treating infectious wounds, or stopping bleeding with use of chemicals (silver nitrate), heat, freezing, or electrical current
Chemosurgery	Use of chemicals to destroy tissue
Chemotherapy	Use of chemicals to treat disease
Closed treatment	To treat a condition (e.g., a fracture) without surgically opening the location closure to bring together the edges of a wound
Congenital	Condition present from birth; believed to be inherited
Curettage	Scraping of a cavity to remove tissue, growths, or debris
Débridement	Excision of dead or damaged tissue and foreign matter from a wound
Decompression	Removal of pressure
Decortication	Removal of external layer (beneath the capsule) from any organ or structure
Defect	Imperfection, malformation, dysfunction, or absence
Destructive	Causing ruin; opposite of constructive
Dialysis	To separate from the blood harmful waste products normally secreted in the urine
Dilation	Enlargement of a hollow structure or opening
Discission	Incision or cutting into
Dissection	Cutting of parts for the purpose of separation and study
Drainage	Continuous withdrawal of fluid from a wound, sore, or cavity
Endoscopy	Visual examination of the interior of a canal or hollow internal organ by means of a special instrument
Evacuation	Removal of waste material
Excision	The act of cutting out
Exploration	An active examination, usually involving endoscopy or a surgical procedure, to aid in diagnosis
Fixation	The act of holding or fastening; immobilize; make rigid
Foreign body	Any substance or particle in the body that does not appear, form, or grow naturally
Fulguration	Destruction by means of high-frequency electric sparks
Graft	Any organ, tissue, or object used for implanting or transplanting to encourage healing, improve function, safeguard against infection, improve appearance, or replace a diseased body organ
Immunoassay	Any of several methods used for measuring chemical substances such as hormones, drugs, and specific proteins
Implant	Tissue or substance inserted or grafted into body
Incision	To cut into
Indwelling	Located or implanted inside the body such as a catheter or tube for drainage or administration of drugs
In situ	Localized; in one specific location without disturbing or invading surrounding tissue
Instrumentation	Application or use of instruments or tools
Internal	Within the body
Insertion	To place or implant; site of attachment
Introduction	Device for controlling and directing; to insert into the body via tube, needle, oral, or anal entrance
Ligation	The process of binding or tying a body structure
Lysis	Destruction, decomposition, breakdown, or separation
Manipulation	Use of hands to produce a desired movement or effect in the body
Marsupialization	Surgical conversion of a closed cavity (abscess or cyst) into an open pouch to allow healing
Obstruction	Blockage of a structure that prevents it from functioning normally
Occlusion	Blockage of any passage, canal, opening, or vessel in the body; acquired or congenital
Open treatment	To lay open internal parts to administer treatment
Paring	Surgical removal of foreign material or dead or damaged tissue by cutting or scraping
Percutaneous	Through the skin
Qualitative	Referring to the quality, value, or nature of something
Quantitative	A measurable amount or portion
Radical	Extreme or drastic treatment or surgery aimed at eliminating a major disease by removing all affected tissue and any surrounding tissue that might be diseased
Reconstitution	Returning a substance that has been changed to its original state for preservation and storage
Reconstruction	Repair, mold, change, or alter to effect recovery
Reduction	To restore to a normal position
Repair	To remedy, replace, or heal; restore to a healthy state
Replantation	Surgical replacement of a body part
Revision	To amend or alter; to correct or improve
Resection	Partial excision of a body structure
Shunt	An artificial passage constructed to divert flow from one route to another
Suture	Material (wire, thread, or staples) used in closing or attaching body tissue; to unite body tissue by stitching together; the seam formed by stitching body tissue together; line of union (border or joint) such as between the skull bones
Therapy	Treatment of disease or pathologic conditions
Transection	A cross section; division by cutting transversely
Transposition	Displacement of an organ from one side of the body to the other; congenital anomaly in which a part of the body normally appearing on the right side is located on the left side of the body
Traumatic	Physical or psychologic wound or injury

- Abbreviation reference book
- Drug reference book (e.g., *Physicians' Desk Reference* or drug reference for nurses)
- Laboratory reference book
- Provider's manual for insurance program or plan
- Insurance carrier's newsletters

Forms similar to the Internal Record Review Form shown in Figures 4-7 through 4-12 may be used as tools to gather information from the patient's record, laboratory reports, pathology reports, radiology reports, operative reports, and other diagnostic tests. If the physician's documentation is inadequate, errors or deficiencies will appear as the review is being conducted. You will discover that doing an internal review of this type is not an exact science and critical thinking skills are put into use. Because documentation guidelines and code policies are updated and refined periodically, it is extremely important to read and keep bulletins from all insurance carriers, especially from the local fiscal Medicare intermediary. Advise the physician of any new requirements. This resource may be the only notification of changes unless you routinely attend local or national workshops.

EXTERNAL AUDIT

An **external audit** is a retrospective review of medical and financial records at the request of a physician, an outside contractor, an insurance company, or external reviewer as part of the practice's compliance plan. It may be done by a Medicare representative to investigate suspected fraud or abusive billing practices.

In 1984, Michigan signed into law the Health Care Claim Act with felony penalties ranging to 10 years in prison and fines of up to $50,000 per count for attempting to defraud an insurance company. Other states are following suit in establishing such laws. Another federal law to prevent overuse of services and to spot Medicare fraud is the Federal False Claims Amendment Act of 1986, which is discussed in detail in Chapter 12.

Most insurance companies perform routine audits on unusual billing patterns, such as the same diagnosis code for every visit, or billing the same procedure code repeatedly. Additional red flags to auditors are lack of documentation for hospital admissions, canned template documentation, illegible documentation, blank documentation, or tests documented but not performed. Insurance companies have computer software programs capable of editing and screening insurance claims to identify billing excesses or potential abuses before payment is rendered. Insurance carriers may hire undercover agents who visit physicians' offices if overuse and abuse of procedure codes are suspected. Physicians who charge excessive fees are routinely audited by most carriers. Carriers spot-check by sending questionnaires to patients and asking them if they received medical care from Dr. Doe to verify the services rendered. The answers are then compared with what the physician billed. Many insurance companies have installed antifraud telephone hotlines or billing question telephone lines for patients. Investigations can result from such calls, depending on the circumstances. Tips also come from peer review organizations, state licensing boards, whistle-blowing physicians, former staff members, and patients. If there is any suspicion of fraud, the insurance company will notify the medical practice, specify a date and time at which they will come to the office, and indicate which records they wish to audit (Figure 4-17).

Investigators question the patient, look at the documentation in the medical record, and interview the staff and all physicians who have participated in the care of the patient. Points are awarded if documentation is present. Auditors also look at appointment books and add up the hours the physician sees patients on any given day when a medical practice uses time-based procedure codes when submitting insurance claims.

Audit Prevention
Health Insurance Portability and Accountability Act Compliance Program

As mentioned in Chapter 2, HIPAA was created in 1996 by the Department of Health and Human Services (HHS) Office of the Inspector General (OIG) to combat fraud and abuse, to protect workers so that they could obtain and

FIGURE 4-17 Insurance billing specialist searching for a patient's chart in the files to pull records for an external audit.

EXTERNAL AUDIT—cont'd

maintain health insurance if changing or losing a job, and establish a medical savings account. The act also developed the concept of compliance planning as related to clinical documentation. OIG and HHS, as well as the Health Care Compliance Association (HCCA), and many other health care agencies have asked physicians to voluntarily develop and implement compliance programs. OIG published guidelines to assist a physician and his or her staff in establishing a medical practice's compliance program to enhance documentation for Medicare cases, as well as all patients seen by the physician. Purposes of a compliance program are to reduce fraudulent insurance claims and to provide quality care to patients.

A *compliance program* is composed of policies and procedures to accomplish uniformity, consistency, and conformity in medical record keeping that fulfills official requirements. If a medical practice experiences an external Medicare audit, HHS OIG and the Department of Justice consider that the medical practice made a reasonable effort to avoid and detect misbehavior if a compliance plan has been in place. When errors are found and a determination is made that fraud did occur, an existing compliance program shows a good faith effort that the medical practice is committed to ethical and legal business. There is no

single best compliance program because every medical practice is different. However, there are some elements that lead to a successful compliance program:

- Written standards of conduct
- Written policies and procedures
- Compliance officer and/or committee to operate and monitor the program
- Training program for all affected employees
- Process to give complaints anonymously
- Internal audit performed routinely
- Investigation and remediation plan for problems that develop
- Response plan for improper or illegal activities

A compliance program must be tailored to fit the needs of each medical practice depending on its corporate structure, mission, size, and employee composition. The statutes, regulations, and guidelines of the federal and state health insurance programs, as well as the policies and procedures of the private health plans, should be integrated into every medical practice's compliance program. The ultimate goals are to improve quality of services and control of claims submission and reduce fraud, waste, abuse, and the cost of health care to federal, state, and private health insurers.

Software Edit Checks

An *edit check* is a good audit prevention measure to have in place because the software program automatically screens transmitted insurance claims and electronically examines them for errors and/or conflicting code entries. Carriers accept a variety of levels of service; however, if only one or two levels are consistently listed, this is usually not realistic and will attract attention and, possibly, an audit. If services are downcoded and the physician neglected to document the correct level of services performed, an addendum to a medical record must be made to justify the level of service reported (Figure 4-18). Amended chart notes must be labeled "Addendum" or "Late entry," dated on the day of the amendment, and signed by the physician.

There must be correct use of diagnostic and procedural codes with modifiers. Modifiers are two digits added onto CPT codes for procedures and services and are not used in diagnostic coding. These are further discussed in Chapter 6. If the diagnosis does not match the service provided, the claim will be thrown out by the edit check of the computer program. It is equally important

that everything involved in patient care be well documented so that selected diagnostic and procedural codes are supported.

In subsequent chapters, you will obtain further knowledge on what needs to be documented in relationship to diagnostic and procedure codes. Information on the Civil Monetary Penalties Law to prosecute cases of Medicare and Medicaid fraud can be found in Chapter 12.

Once an individual has been found guilty of committing a Medicare or Medicaid program-related crime, 5 to 15 years or lifetime exclusion from program participation is mandatory under Section 1128(a) of the Social Security Act. An individual can be anyone who participates in fraud or abuse including the physician, nurse, home health aide, insurance billing specialist, claims assistance professional, electronic claims processor, and medical assistants. Being an excluded individual is a serious matter and requires a reinstatement process to work in those environments again. Recovering from your loss of credibility and trustworthiness may be a monumental task. Do not jeopardize your future in the medical field!

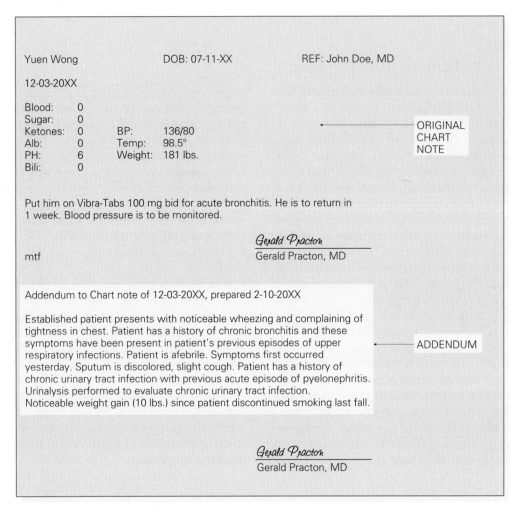

Yuen Wong   DOB: 07-11-XX   REF: John Doe, MD

12-03-20XX

Blood: 0
Sugar: 0
Ketones: 0   BP: 136/80   ORIGINAL
Alb: 0   Temp: 98.5°   CHART
PH: 6   Weight: 181 lbs.   NOTE
Bili: 0

Put him on Vibra-Tabs 100 mg bid for acute bronchitis. He is to return in
1 week. Blood pressure is to be monitored.

                                  Gerald Practon
mtf   Gerald Practon, MD

Addendum to Chart note of 12-03-20XX, prepared 2-10-20XX

Established patient presents with noticeable wheezing and complaining of
tightness in chest. Patient has a history of chronic bronchitis and these
symptoms have been present in patient's previous episodes of upper
respiratory infections. Patient is afebrile. Symptoms first occurred   ADDENDUM
yesterday. Sputum is discolored, slight cough. Patient has a history of
chronic urinary tract infection with previous acute episode of pyelonephritis.
Urinalysis performed to evaluate chronic urinary tract infection.
Noticeable weight gain (10 lbs.) since patient discontinued smoking last fall.

                                  Gerald Practon
                              Gerald Practon, MD

FIGURE 4-18 Example of an addendum to a patient's health record to justify the level of service reported. The insurance carrier downcoded the services from level 99213 to 99212.

Faxing Documents

The common term "fax" is derived from the word **facsimile,** which means transmission of written and graphic matter by electronic means. Faxes are a communication tool, but as more documents become electronic they are securely transmitted via the Internet instead of by fax. Faxing is used to transmit insurance claims data directly to an electronic claims processor, resubmit an unpaid insurance claim, send further documentation on a claim to insurance carriers, obtain preauthorization for surgery on a patient, network with other insurance billers, and send medical reports between offices and to other medical facilities across the country. Unless otherwise prohibited by state law, information that is transmitted by fax is acceptable and may be filed with the patient's health record. Documents to be faxed can be a graphic illustration, typewritten, or handwritten with pen. Pencil does not fax to recipient as clearly as does pen. To prevent deterioration of documents faxed on thermal paper (when the machine is not a plain paper fax), photocopy the document onto regular paper before it is filed with health records.

Fax transmission of PHI falls under the HIPAA privacy rules. Therefore it is important to prevent PHI from access by other members of the household or visitors to the household. Always properly dispose of fax log reports and any fax toner reels that may maintain images of PHI.

FAXING PROTECTED HEALTH INFORMATION

Under the Privacy Rule, providers may disclose (or fax) protected health information for treatment, payment, or health care operations. However, you may need to have a patient sign an authorization for release of information before faxing protected health information for other situations. Therefore be sure to refer to the HIPAA Privacy Rules in Chapter 2 to refresh your knowledge about protected health information.

Sensitive Information

From the legal standpoint, protecting the patient's confidentiality in the fax process is critical. If, because of circumstances, health records or a medical report must be faxed, you should have the patient sign an authorization to release information via fax equipment. The American Health Information Management Association (AHIMA) advises that fax machines should not be used for routine transmission of patient information. AHIMA recommends that documents should be faxed only when (1) hand or mail delivery will not meet the needs of immediate patient care or (2) required by a third party for ongoing certification of payment for a hospitalized patient.

Documents containing information on sexually transmitted diseases, drug or alcohol treatment, or human immunodeficiency virus (HIV) status should not be faxed. Psychiatric records and psychotherapy notes should not be faxed except for emergency requests. Psychotherapy notes may be defined as notes recorded in any medium that document or analyze the contents of conversation during a private, group, joint, or family counseling session. Psychotherapy notes exclude medication prescription and monitoring, counseling session start and stop times, modalities and frequencies of treatment furnished, results of clinical tests, and any summary of the following items: diagnosis, functional status, treatment plan, symptoms, prognosis, and progress to date.

Fax machines should be located in secure or restricted access areas. Do not fax to machines in mail rooms, office lobbies, or other open areas unless they are secured with passwords. To ensure protection, a cover sheet should be used for all transmissions. This can be a half sheet, full sheet, or small self-adhesive form attached to the top of the first page. It should contain the following information:

- Name of recipient
- Name of sender
- Date
- Total number of pages, including the cover sheet
- Fax and telephone numbers of recipient and sender in case of transmittal problems (e.g., lost page or dropped line)
- A statement that it is personal, privileged, and confidential medical information intended for the named recipient only (Figure 4-19).

Transmittal Destination

Noise or interference from telephone lines can be severe enough to distort a fax transmission, so when it is necessary, verify receipt. The following options are available to ensure that a faxed document has reached the correct destination:

- Place a telephone call to the requesting physician's office 10 to 15 minutes after faxing patient records to verify their receipt.
- Request that the authorized receiver sign and return an attached receipt form at the bottom of the cover sheet on receipt of the faxed information.
- Make arrangements with the recipient for a scheduled time for transmission.
- Send the fax to a coded mailbox. Coded mailboxes require the sender to punch in a code indicating the individual to whom the fax is addressed and the receiver to then punch in his or her own code to activate the printer.
- Ask the receiving party for a patient reference number (e.g., the patient's Social Security number). Blank out the patient's name and write in the reference number on the document before faxing it. Also ask other providers to fax records by reference number rather than by patient name.
- Run a fax transmission confirmation report from your own fax machine. Most current fax machines have this capability. The report will show what number was dialed and whether or not the transmission was successful.

If a fax is sent to the wrong destination, either telephone or complete a misdirected fax form online and fax it to the original phone number (Figure 4-20). Such incidents need to be investigated and possibly reported. Note the incident, along with the misdialed number, in the patient's health record and in a HIPAA disclosure log. Program frequently used numbers into the fax machine to avoid misdirecting faxed communications. Edit your release of records authorization form to allow for fax transmission because it is acceptable to honor an authorization sent via this method.

Medicare Guidelines

Check with the Medicare fiscal intermediary to find out whether faxing of claims and documents is acceptable for Medicare patients. The use of a fax transmittal system requires that the physician retain the original facsimile with the signature on it.

Financial Data

Never fax a patient's financial data. In court, faxing medical information can be justified on the basis of medical necessity, but faxing financial information cannot be justified.

Legal Documents

Consult an attorney to make sure that documents (e.g., contracts, proposals, or insurance claims) requiring

FAX TRANSMITTAL SHEET

To: _College Hospital (outpatient surgery)_   Date _10-21-20XX_

Fax Number: _(555) 486-8900_ Telephone Number _(555) 487 6789_ Time _10:00 a.m._

Number of pages (including this one): _3_

From: _Raymond Skeleton, MD_   Phone _(555) 486-9002_

Note: This transmittal is intended only for the use of the individual or entity to which it is addressed, and may contain information that is privileged, confidential, and exempt from disclosure under applicable law. If you are not the intended recipient, any dissemination, distribution, or photocopying of this communication is strictly prohibited. If you have received this communication in error, please notify this office immediately by telephone and return the original FAX to us at the address below by U.S. Postal Service. Thank you.

Remarks: _Enclosed are Margaret Yont's radiology reports on her L. tibia/fibula and L. foot fractures_

If you cannot read this FAX or if pages are missing, please contact:

COLLEGE CLINIC
4567 Broad Avenue
Woodland Hills, XY 12345-0001
Phone: 555/486-9002
Fax: 555/487-8976

INSTRUCTIONS TO THE AUTHORIZED RECEIVER: PLEASE COMPLETE THIS STATEMENT OF RECEIPT AND RETURN TO SENDER VIA THE ABOVE FAX NUMBER.

- -

I, _Cheryl Watson, CMA_ , verify that I have received _3_ (no. of pages including cover sheet)

from _Raymond Skeleton, MD_ (sending facility's name)

FIGURE 4-19 Example of a fax cover sheet for medical document transmission.

signatures are legally binding if faxed. To ensure legality, do the following:

- Transmit the entire document, front and back, to be signed and not only the page that requires a signature so that the receiver has full disclosure of the agreement.
- As mentioned earlier, obtain confirmation that the receiver is in receipt of all pages sent because an incomplete document may be invalid.
- Insert a clause in the contract stating that faxed signatures will be treated as originals.
- Follow up and obtain the original signature in hard copy form as soon as possible.

Subpoena

Subpoena literally means "under penalty." In legal language, it is a writ requiring the appearance of a witness at a trial or other proceeding. Strictly defined, a ***subpoena duces tecum*** requires the witness to appear and bring or send certain records "in his possession." For a *subpoena duces tecum* for health information to be valid under the HIPAA privacy rule, it must be accompanied by court order or the covered entity must receive satisfactory assurance from the party seeking the information that reasonable efforts have been made to ensure that the individual who is the subject of the PHI requested has been given notice of the request or that the party seeking the information has made reasonable efforts to secure a qualified protective order that meets the requirements of the HIPAA privacy rule. Some issues affecting electronically stored information (ESI) is that they may be altered, overwritten without leaving any evidence, or stored in several computer systems. ESI includes *metadata* or supportive data that is information on the computer system about the medical data, such as the following:

College Clinic
4567 Broad Avenue
Woodland Hills, XY 12345-0001
Telephone: 555/486-9002
Fax: 555/487-8976

Misdirected Fax of Protected Health Information

To: <u>Name of recipient</u>
Fax number: <u>555/580-0544</u>

Re: Misdirected fax

Confidential Notice Concerning Protected Health Information

We have discovered that protected health information of _____
Name of patient

concerning _____
Statement of misdirected data

was transmitted to you in error. Because this is sensitive and protected health information, please contact me immediately at the above telephone number so that I may provide you with instructions for the return of these confidential documents.

Comments:
The documents faxed to you are confidential. Information contained in the fax transmission is intended only for the use of the individual (or facility) identified as "recipient." If you are not the intended recipient of this information, you are prohibited from using, disclosing, copying, or distributing this information to any other party. Such information must be returned to the sender.

FIGURE 4-20 Example of a misdirected fax form that may be completed online and faxed to the wrong fax recipient.

- Substantive data is application based and may contain modifications, edits, or comments.
- System-based data includes author, date and time when the entry was created, and date of modification.
- Embedded data is text, numbers, content directly input but not visible on output (e.g., spreadsheet formulas or hyperlinks).

The subpoena party may want access to review and analyze the metadata. A subpoena is a legal document signed by a judge or an attorney in the name of a judge. In cases in which a pretrial of evidence or deposition is set up, the subpoena may be issued by a notary public, in which event it is called a *notary subpoena*. If an attorney signs it, he or she must attest it in the name of a judge, the court clerk, or other proper officer.

It is possible for a state investigator to subpoena patient records and then file administrative charges against the physician, not because of the practice of shoddy medicine but rather because the case was inadequately documented for the treatment provided. Health records also may be subpoenaed as proof in a medical malpractice case. Complete documentation and well-organized patient records help establish a strong defense in a medical professional liability claim.

Subpoena Process. A subpoena must be personally served or handed to the prospective witness or keeper of the health records. Neither civil nor criminal subpoenas can be served via the telecopier (fax) machine. The acceptance of a document by someone authorized to accept it is the equivalent of personal service. The subpoena cannot be left on a counter or desk. In a state civil case, a "witness fee" and payment for travel to and from court are given, if demanded, at the time a subpoena is served. The fee is discretionary in criminal cases. In some states, provision is made for substitute service by mail or through newspaper advertisements. This is permitted only after all reasonable efforts to effect personal service have failed.

Never accept a subpoena or give records to anyone without the physician's prior authorization. The medical office should designate one person as keeper of the health records. If the subpoena is only for health records or financial data, the representative for the specific doctor can usually accept it and the physician will not be called to court.

If a physician is on vacation and there is no designated keeper of the records, tell the deputy that the physician is not in and cannot be served. Suggest the deputy contact the physician's attorney and relay this information.

When the "witness fee" has been received and the subpoena has been served, notify the physician and the physician's legal counsel. In a paper-based office, pull the chart and place it and the subpoena on the physician's desk for review. Willful disregard of a subpoena is punishable as contempt of court.

The medical office is given a prescribed time in which to produce the records. It is not necessary to show them at the time the subpoena is served unless the court order so states. For electronic records, consult state and federal laws for guidance for setting up an office policy.

The attorney usually employs a person or copy service to copy records that are under subpoena. At the time the subpoena is served, a date is usually agreed on in which the representative will return and copy the portion of the record that is named in the subpoena. Often only the portion of the health record requested is removed from the original chart and put in a copy folder. Items such as the patient registration information sheet, encounter form, and explanation of benefits should not be included. You may also telephone the attorney who sent the subpoena and ask whether the records can be mailed. If so, mail them by certified mail with return receipt requested. Retain a copy of the records released. You will have to appear in court if specified in the subpoena. Verify with the court that the case is actually on the calendar. If you do not appear, you are in contempt of court and subject to a penalty, possibly several days in jail.

If original records are requested, move them to a safe place, preferably under lock and key, so that they cannot be taken away or tampered with before the trial date. Make photocopies of the original records because this prevents total loss of the records and assists in discovery of any altering or tampering while they are out of your custody. Number the pages of the records so that you will know if a page is missing. If later the plaintiff's attorney says there was an item in the record but this is missing from your original photocopied set, the physician's attorney may be able to have the case thrown out.

On the day of your court appearance, comply with all instructions given by the court. Do not give up possession of the records unless instructed to do so by the judge. Do not permit examination of the records by anyone before their identification in court. Do not leave the chart in the court unless it is in the possession of the judge or jury and a receipt for it has been obtained.

When you have questions, call the physician's attorney or the court's information and assistance staff.

Retention of Records

In an electronic system, health records are stored in the computer. Paper-based records are either stored in color-coded file folders containing a collection of paper documents or they reside in multiple electronic databases displayed in a variety of formats via computer access. Regardless of the system used, there are general guidelines that must be followed to record information correctly, use it according to law, and retain it.

Health Records

Preservation of health records is governed by federal, state, and local laws. The law that is the most stringent is the law that is adhered to. Individual states generally set a minimum of 6 to 10 years for keeping records, but it is the policy of most physicians to retain health records of all living patients indefinitely. With enactment of the Federal False Claims Act, proof materials for the establishment of evidence such as x-ray films, laboratory reports, and pathologic specimens probably should be kept indefinitely in the event of a legal inquiry. Calendars, appointment books, and telephone logs also should be filed and stored. Cases that involve radiologic injury claims (e.g., leukemia from radiation) may begin running the statute of limitations after discovery of the injury, which may occur 20 or 30 years after radiation exposure. Recommended retention periods for paper files are shown in Table 4-2. EHRs may have different retention periods, depending on state law. Effective December 1, 2006, changes to the Federal Rules of Civil Procedure make requests for electronic data a standard part of the discovery process during federal lawsuits. This includes not only health records but accounting documents, cell phone records, instant messaging, and electronic mail that might be needed for future litigation.

A person's health record may be of value not only to himself or herself in later years but also to the person's children. In some states a minor may file suit, after he or she has attained legal age, for any act performed during childhood that the person believes to be wrong or harmful. Sometimes a suit may be permitted even 2 to 3 years after the child has reached legal age. Thus it is important to keep records until patients are 3 to 4 years beyond the age of majority.

Deceased patients' charts should be kept for at least 5 years. In a paper-based system, shred documents that are no longer needed. Some practices prefer to use medical record storage companies. If records are disposed of by a professional company, be sure to obtain a certificate of destruction verifying method of disposal. This document should be kept on file indefinitely by the office manager. Maintain a log of destroyed records showing the patient's

Table 4-2 Records Retention Schedule

TEMPORARY RECORD	RETENTION PERIOD (YR)	PERMANENT RECORD (RETAINED INDEFINITELY)
Accounts receivable (patient ledger)	7	
Appointment sheets	3	Accounts payable records
Bank deposit slip (duplicate)	1	Bills of sale for important purchases (or until you no longer own them)
		Canceled checks and check registers
Bank statements and canceled checks	7	Capital asset records
		Cash books
Billing records (for outside service)	7	Certified financial statements
Cash receipt records	6	Contracts
		Correspondence, legal
Contracts (expired)	**7**	Credit history
Correspondence, general	6	Deeds, mortgages, contracts, leases, and property records
Daysheets (balance sheets and journals)	5	Equipment guarantees and records (or until you no longer own them)
Employee contracts	6	Income tax returns and documents
Employee time records	5	Insurance policies and records
Employment applications	4	Journals (financial)
Insurance claim forms (paid)	3	
Inventory records	3	
Invoices	6	Health records (active patients)
Health records (expired patients)	5	Health records (inactive patients)
Medicare financial records	7	
Remittance advice documents	8	Mortgages
Payroll records	7	Property appraisals and records
Petty cash vouchers	3	Telephone records
Postal and meter records	1	X-ray films
Tax worksheets and supporting documents	7	Year-end balance sheets and general ledgers

name, Social Security number, date of last visit, and treatment.

Financial Documents

According to income tax regulations on record retention, accounting records should be kept a minimum of 4 years (following the due date for filing the tax return or the date the tax is paid, whichever is later). Always contact an accountant before discarding records that may determine tax liability. Suggested retention periods are listed in Table 4-2.

A federal regulation mandates that assigned claims for Medicaid and Medicare be kept for 7 years; the physician is subject to auditing during that period. The Federal False Claims Amendment Act of 1986 allows a claim of fraud to be made up to 10 years from the date a violation was committed. Documentation must be available for inspection and copying by the investigator of the false claim (31 US Code §3729–3733).

HIPAA Documents

Under HIPAA guidelines, Notice of Privacy Practices (NPP) acknowledgements signed by patients must be kept on file for at least 6 years from the date of the creation or the date it was last in effect. For example, for an NPP effective beginning on December 1, 2009, the patients' acknowledgements may be disposed of in 6 years (December 1, 2015).

Termination of a Case

A physician may wish to withdraw formally from further care of a patient because of patient noncompliance (e.g., the patient discharged the physician, did not follow instructions, did not take the recommended medication, failed to return for an appointment, discontinued payment on an overdue account). A physician may terminate a contract by the following:

- Sending a letter of withdrawal (Figure 4-21) to the patient by certified mail with return receipt (Figure 4-22) so that proof of termination is in the patient's health record.
- Sending a letter of confirmation of discharge when the patient states that he or she no longer desires care (Figure 4-23). This should also be sent certified mail with return receipt requested.
- Sending a letter confirming that the patient left the hospital against medical advice or the advice of the physician. If there is a signed statement in the patient's hospital records to this effect, it is not necessary to

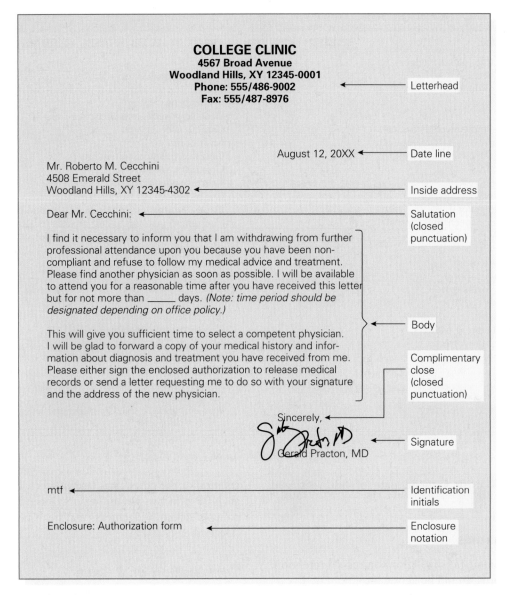

COLLEGE CLINIC
4567 Broad Avenue
Woodland Hills, XY 12345-0001
Phone: 555/486-9002
Fax: 555/487-8976   ◄────── Letterhead

August 12, 20XX ◄────── Date line

Mr. Roberto M. Cecchini
4508 Emerald Street
Woodland Hills, XY 12345-4302 ◄──────────── Inside address

Dear Mr. Cecchini: ◄──────────────────── Salutation
                                          (closed
                                          punctuation)

I find it necessary to inform you that I am withdrawing from further
professional attendance upon you because you have been noncompliant and refuse to follow my medical advice and treatment.
Please find another physician as soon as possible. I will be available
to attend you for a reasonable time after you have received this letter
but for not more than _____ days. *(Note: time period should be
designated depending on office policy.)*

                                          Body

This will give you sufficient time to select a competent physician.
I will be glad to forward a copy of your medical history and information about diagnosis and treatment you have received from me.   Complimentary
Please either sign the enclosed authorization to release medical   close
records or send a letter requesting me to do so with your signature   (closed
and the address of the new physician.   punctuation)

                    Sincerely, ◄────────

                    Gerald Practon, MD ◄────── Signature

mtf ◄──────────────────────────────────── Identification
                                          initials

Enclosure: Authorization form ◄──────────── Enclosure
                                          notation

FIGURE 4-21 Example of letter of withdrawal from a case that is typed in modified-block style
with closed punctuation and special notations (placement of parts of letter).

send a letter. If a letter is sent, a copy of the letter and
return signature card from the post office must be filed
with the patient's records.

If a noncompliant patient refuses a certified dismissal
letter and it is returned unopened, file the returned letter
and refusal notice in the patient's chart. Then in a plain
envelope send another copy of the letter to the patient.
Document the date and time it was posted and the location of the mailbox used. Place these data and initial them
in the patient's chart; after 10 days telephone the patient
to confirm receipt of the correspondence. If the patient

denies receiving it, then read it over the telephone. In
most regions, this will provide immunity against aban-
donment of a case, which is the discontinuance of medical
care by a provider without proper notice.

Prevention of Legal Problems

After reading Chapters 1 through 4, you have discovered
there are many instances in which an insurance biller
must be careful in executing job duties to avoid the possibility of a lawsuit. A summary of guidelines for prevention of lawsuits is shown in Box 4-1.

A

UNITED STATES POSTAL SERVICE

First-Class Mail
Postage & Fees Paid
USPS
Permit No. G-10

• Sender: Please print your name, address, and ZIP+4 in this box •

COLLEGE CLINIC
4567 BROAD AVENUE
WOODLAND HILLS, XY 12345 0001

B

SENDER: *COMPLETE THIS SECTION*

■ Complete items 1, 2, and 3. Also complete item 4 if Restricted Delivery is desired.
■ Print your name and address on the reverse so that we can return the card to you.
■ Attach this card to the back of the mailpiece, or on the front if space permits.

1. Article Addressed to:

Mr. John Doe
2761 Fort Street
Woodland Hills, XY 12345

COMPLETE THIS SECTION ON DELIVERY

A. Signature
X
☐ Agent
☐ Addressee

B. Received by (Printed Name)   C. Date of Delivery

D. Is delivery address different from item 1? ☐ Yes
   If YES, enter delivery address below: ☐ No

3. Service Type
☒ Certified Mail   ☐ Express Mail
☐ Registered   ☐ Return Receipt for Merchandise
☐ Insured Mail   ☐ C.O.D.

4. Restricted Delivery? (Extra Fee)   ☐ Yes

2. Article Number
   (Transfer from service label)   7005 1160 0003 8827 7393

PS Form 3811, February 2004   Domestic Return Receipt   102595-02-M-1540

C

7005 1160 0003 8827 7393

PLACE STICKER AT TOP OF ENVELOPE TO THE RIGHT OF RETURN ADDRESS. FOLD AT DOTTED LINE

CERTIFIED MAIL™

7005 1160 0003 8827 7393

U.S. Postal Service™
CERTIFIED MAIL™ RECEIPT
(Domestic Mail Only: No Insurance Coverage Provided)

For delivery information vist our website at www.usps.com®

OFFICIAL USE

Postage $

Certified Fee

Return Receipt Fee
(Endorsement Required)

Restricted Delivery Fee
(Endorsement Required)

Total Postage & Fees $

Postmark
Here

Sent To: Mr. John Doe
Street, Apt. No.;
or PO Box No.   2761 Fort Street
City, State, ZIP+ 4   Woodland Hills, XY 12345

PS Form 3800, June 2002   See Reverse for Instructions

FIGURE 4-22 A and **B** (front and back), A domestic return receipt Postal Service Form 3811. **C,** Receipt for certified mail Postal Service Form 3800 (U.S. Government Printing Office) shown completed.

COLLEGE CLINIC
4567 Broad Avenue
Woodland Hills, XY 12345-0001
Phone: 555/486-9002
Fax: 555/487-8976

September 3, 20XX

Mrs. Gregory Putnam
4309 North E Street
Woodland Hills, XY 12345-4398

Dear Mrs. Putnam:

This will confirm our telephone conversation today during which you discharged me from attending you as your physician in your present illness. In my opinion, your medical condition requires continued treatment by a physician. If you have not already obtained the services of another physician, I suggest you do so without further delay.

You may be assured that, upon your written authorization, I will furnish your new physician with information regarding the diagnosis and treatment you have received from me.

Very truly yours

Gerald Procton, MD

mtf

FIGURE 4-23 Letter to confirm discharge by patient. Letter typed in modified block style (dateline, complimentary close, and signature indented) with open punctuation (no commas after salutation or complimentary close).

Box 4-1   Prevention of Lawsuits—Guidelines for Insurance Billing Specialists

1. Keep information about patients strictly confidential.
2. Obtain proper instruction and carry out responsibilities according to the employer's guidelines.
3. Keep abreast of general insurance program guidelines, annual coding changes, and medical and scientific progress to help when handling insurance matters.
4. Secure proper written consent in all cases before releasing a patient's protected health information for purposes other than treatment, payment, or health care operations (TPO).
5. Do not refer to consent or acknowledgment forms as "releases." Use the word "consent" or "authorization" forms as required by law. This also produces a better understanding of the document to be signed.
6. Make sure documentation of patient care in the health record corresponds with billing submitted on the insurance claim.
7. Exercise good judgment in what you write and how you word electronic mail because it does not give security against confidentiality.
8. Make every effort to reach an understanding with patients in the matter of fees by explaining what services will be received and what the "extras" may be. For hospital cases, it is advisable to explain that the fee the physician charges is for his or her services only and that charges for the bed or ward room, operating room, laboratory tests, and anesthesia will be billed separately in addition to the physician's charges.
9. Do not discuss other physicians with the patient. Patients sometimes invite criticism of the methods or results of former physicians. Remember that you are hearing only one side of the story.
10. Tell the physician immediately if you learn that a new patient is still under treatment by another physician and did not give this information to the physician during the initial interview.
11. Do not compare the respective merits of various forms of therapy and refrain from discussing patients' ailments with them. Patients come to talk to the physician about their symptoms, and you may give them incorrect information. Let the physician make the diagnosis. Otherwise, you may seriously embarrass the physician, yourself, or both of you.
12. Report a physician who is doing something illegal that you are aware of. You can be held responsible for being silent and failing to report an illegal action.

Box 4-1 Prevention of Lawsuits—Guidelines for Insurance Billing Specialists—cont'd

13. Say nothing to anyone except as required by the attorney of the physician or by the court if litigation is pending.
14. Be alert to hazards that may cause injury to anyone in the office and report such problems immediately.
15. Consult the physician before turning over a delinquent account to a collection agency.
16. Be courteous in dealing with patients and always act in a professional manner.

PROCEDURE 4-1

Abstract Data From a Health Record

OBJECTIVE: To abstract data from a health record for composing a letter or completing an insurance claim form or other related billing document

EQUIPMENT/SUPPLIES: Patient's health record, form to insert abstracted data, and pen or pencil

DIRECTIONS: Follow these steps including rationales to learn this skill and practice it by completing the *Workbook* assignment.

1. What is the patient's diagnosis? This gives the reason for the visit.
2. What professional services were provided?
3. Did the patient undergo surgery? What surgical procedure was performed?
4. Read and review the patient's health record thoroughly to learn all parts of the case. In the *Workbook* assignment, use the checkoff list and answer the questions to assist you in understanding all aspects of the patient's health record.
5. What medication was prescribed, if any?
6. Does the patient have any past history indicating anything of importance?
7. Does the patient have any food or drug allergies? If so, what are they?
8. What is the etiology (cause) of the present disease, injury, or illness?
9. What is the prognosis (prediction) for this patient's medical condition?
10. What laboratory tests were ordered or performed?
11. What x-rays were ordered or obtained?
12. Define every abbreviation listed in the patient's chart notes or history and physical examination.
13. What documents assisted you in locating the answers to these questions?

PROCEDURE 4-2

Compose, Format, Key, Proofread, and Print a Letter

OBJECTIVE: To compose, format, key, proofread, and print a letter using common business letter style guidelines

EQUIPMENT/SUPPLIES: Computer, printer, letterhead stationery, envelope, attachments (documents if necessary), thesaurus, English dictionary, medical dictionary, and pen or pencil

DIRECTIONS: Follow these steps including rationales to learn this skill and practice it by completing the *Workbook* assignments.

1. Assemble materials, determine the recipient's address, and decide on modified or full block letter style or format.
2. Turn on the computer and select the word processing program. Open a blank document.
3. Key the date line beginning at least three lines below the letterhead and make certain it is in the proper location for the chosen style.
4. Double-space down and insert the inside address and make certain it is in the proper location for the chosen style. Select a style to insert an attention line, if necessary.
5. Double-space and key the salutation. Use either open or mixed punctuation. A business letter should include a title and the person's last name.
6. Double-space and enter the reference line ("Re:" or "Subject:") in the location for the chosen letter style. This assists the recipient in identifying the contents of the letter immediately.
7. Double-space and key the body (content) of the letter in single-space. Make certain the paragraph style is proper for the format chosen. Double-space between paragraphs. Save the letter to the computer hard drive every 15 minutes.
8. Proofread the letter on the computer screen for composition and format.

Continued

PROCEDURE 4-2—cont'd

Compose, Format, Key, Proofread, and Print a Letter

9. Proofread the letter on the computer screen for typographic, spelling, grammatical, and mechanical errors. Use the spell-check feature of the word processing program and reference books to check for correct spelling, meaning, or usage.

10. Key the second page heading (name, page number, and date) in vertical or horizontal format if a second page is necessary.

11. Key a complimentary close and make certain it is in the proper location for the chosen style.

12. Drop down four spaces and key the sender's name and title or credentials as printed on the letterhead because handwritten signatures may be difficult to read.

13. Double-space and insert the sender's reference initials in UPPERCASE and typist's initials in lowercase letters, separating the two sets of initials with either a colon or slash (e.g., DLJ:md or DLJ/md).

14. Single- or double-space to insert copy ("CC"), or enclosure ("Enclosure" or "En"), or attachment notations.

15. Double-space to insert a postscript ("PS"), if necessary.

16. Save the file before printing a hard copy and proofread the letter once more. Make corrections, if necessary.

17. Print the final copy to be sent and proofread. Make a copy to be retained in the files in case it is necessary for future reference.

18. Save the file to a CD-ROM to be stored for future reference.

19. Prepare an envelope and use the format for optical scanning recommended by the U.S. Postal Service. Insert special mailing instructions in the correct location on the envelope if sending by certified mail.

20. Clip attachments to the letter and give it to the physician for review and signature.

KEY POINTS

This is a brief chapter review or summary of the key issues presented. To further enhance your knowledge of the technical subject matter, review the key terms and key abbreviations for this chapter by locating the meanings in the glossary at the end of this book that appear in a section before the index.

1. Every patient seen by the physician must have comprehensive legible documentation about what occurred during the visit for the following reasons: (1) avoidance of denied or delayed payments by insurance carriers investigating the medical necessity of services; (2) enforcement of medical record-keeping rules by insurance carriers requiring accurate documentation that supports procedure and diagnostic codes; (3) subpoena of health records by state investigators or the court for review; (4) defense of a professional liability claim.

2. The foremost tool of clinical care and communication is the electronic health record.

3. Medical records are evolving into electronic media. HIPAA directs the adoption of national electronic standards for automatic transfer of certain health care data among health care payers, insurance plans, and providers.

4. In 1995 and 1997, CMS introduced documentation guidelines to Medicare carriers to ensure that services paid for have been provided and were medically necessary. Documentation must support the level of service and each procedure rendered.

5. External and internal audit of medical records shows where deficiencies occur in health record documentation and substantiates proper use of diagnostic and procedural codes.

6. Under HIPAA, all medical records must be signed or electronically verified by the provider to show that the note was reviewed and test results were acknowledged.

7. The levels of E/M services are based on four types of physical examination: problem focused, expanded problem focused, detailed, and comprehensive.

8. The 4 Rs for documentation for both the referring and consulting physicians are written or verbal *request* and medical *reason*, *render* opinion and document findings, and *report* to requesting physician.

9. Health record abbreviations should be eliminated from the more vital sections such as final diagnosis, operative notes, discharge summaries, and descriptions of special procedures.

10. An eponym should not be used when a comparable anatomic term can be used in its place.

11. The two types of internal review of records are prospective review (before billing insurance carrier) and retrospective review (after billing insurance carrier).

12. An edit check is a good audit prevention measure because the software program automatically screens transmitted insurance claims and electronically examines them for errors and/or conflicting code entries.

13. When health records are subpoenaed, produce only the records requested and nothing more. Retain a copy of the records released.

14. Individual states generally set a minimum of 6 to 10 years for keeping records, but it is the policy of most physicians to retain health records of all living patients indefinitely.

15. When a patient does not comply with physician or office policy, the physician may wish to withdraw formally from further care of the patient. The physician must send a formal letter of termination or withdrawal by certified mail with return receipt to the patient.

16. Patients' health information must be kept private and confidential. HIPAA guidelines for consent and disclosure of information will keep a medical practice compliant and the patients confident.

⊖volve INTERNET RESOURCES

For active links to the following resources, visit the Evolve website at
http://evolve.elsevier.com/fordney/handbook

- A model compliance plan for third-party billing companies

- American Hospital Association for policy about medical abbreviations

STUDENT ASSIGNMENT

✓ Study Chapter 4.
✓ Answer the fill-in-the-blank, multiple choice, and true/false questions in the *Workbook* to reinforce the theory learned in this chapter and help prepare you for a future test.
✓ Complete the assignments in the *Workbook* to give you experience in reviewing patients' medical reports and records.

✓ Turn to the glossary at the end of this textbook for a further understanding of the key terms and key abbreviations used in this chapter.

KEY TERMS*

adverse effect
benign tumor
chief complaint
combination code
complication
computer-assisted coding
conventions
E codes
eponym
etiology
in situ
International Classification of
    Diseases, Ninth Revision,
    Clinical Modification

International Classification of
    Diseases, Tenth Revision,
    Clinical Modification
International Classification of
    Diseases, Tenth Revision,
    Procedural Coding System
intoxication
italicized code
late effect
malignant tumor
metastasis
neoplasm
not elsewhere classifiable
not otherwise specified

physician's fee profile
poisoning
primary diagnosis
principal diagnosis
secondary diagnosis
slanted brackets
syndrome
V codes

KEY ABBREVIATIONS*

AHA
AHIMA
ASCVD
ASHD
CAC
CC

CM
CPT
DRG
DSM-IV
E codes
ICD-9-CM

ICD-10-CM
ICD-10-PCS
IDDM (type I diabetes)
MRI
NCHS
NEC

NIDDM
NOS
SNOMED
V codes

---

*Definitions for the key terms and key abbreviations are located near the back of this textbook in the glossary.

Diagnostic Coding

OBJECTIVES

After reading this chapter, you should be able to:

- Explain the reasons and importance of coding diagnoses.
- Describe the importance of matching the correct diagnostic code to the appropriate procedural code.
- Differentiate between primary (first listed), principal, and secondary diagnoses.
- Discuss the history of diagnostic coding.
- Identify reasons to use computer-assisted coding.

- Define and demonstrate an understanding of diagnostic code conventions, symbols, and terminology.
- Apply coding guidelines to translate written descriptions of conditions into diagnostic codes.
- Demonstrate the ability to abstract medical conditions from the medical record and accurately assign diagnostic codes by completing the problems in the *Workbook*.

Service to Patients

Good customer service to the patient is to know the diagnostic coding guidelines in both the inpatient and outpatient settings to obtain the proper payment from third-party payers.

Two basic principles are as follows:
- Diagnostic coding must be accurate because payment for inpatient services rendered to a patient may be based on the diagnosis.
- In the outpatient setting, the diagnosis code must correspond to the treatment or services rendered to the patient or payment may be denied.

THE DIAGNOSTIC CODING SYSTEM

This chapter deals with diagnostic coding for outpatient professional services, and the next chapter relates to coding of procedures for medical services. By 2013, diagnostic codes will transition from *International*

Classification of Diseases, Ninth Revision, Clinical Modification (ICD-9-CM) codes to *International Classification of Diseases, Tenth Revision, Clinical Modification* (ICD-10-CM) codes. This chapter helps you prepare for this transition. The first part of the chapter discusses ICD-9-CM coding procedures because the method you use to you locate a code is similar when using ICD-10-CM. Physicians will not use *International Classification of Diseases, Tenth Revision, Procedural Coding System* (ICD-10-PCS) coding, which is discussed in Chapter 17.

Proper coding can mean the financial success or failure of a medical practice. In addition to knowledge of current approved diagnostic coding guidelines, a working knowledge of medical terminology including familiarization of anatomy and physiology, clinical disease processes, and pharmacology is essential to becoming a top-notch coder

Performance objectives, testing and review material, and hands-on practical exercises for this chapter are available in these resources

 The Insurance Handbook Student Workbook　　 The Insurance Handbook Evolve Site

129

of diagnoses. The coding must be accurate because in many instances payment for outpatient services is related to the procedure codes but must be supported and justified by the diagnosis and the medical necessity of the service or treatment provided. Payment for services is based on diagnostic coding in the inpatient setting only. All documented diagnoses that affect the current status of the patient may be assigned a code. This includes conditions that exist at the time of the patient's initial contact with the physician, as well as conditions that develop subsequently and affect the treatment received. Diagnoses that relate to a patient's previous medical problem but have no bearing on the patient's present condition are not coded. The American Health Information Management Association (AHIMA) and American Hospital Association (AHA) diagnostic coding guidelines for outpatient services and diagnostic coding and reporting requirements for physician billing may be found by visiting the Evolve website listed in the Internet Resources at the end of this chapter. The website has an active link to AHIMA.

Sequencing of Diagnostic Codes

Codes must be sequenced correctly on an insurance claim so that the chronology of patient care events (main reason for the office visit) and severity of disease can be understood. The primary surgical procedure code must always be listed first on the claim form for full reimbursement, and the secondary procedures, which are paid at less than 100% of allowable, must be listed in succession. The correct diagnostic code must be matched to the appropriate surgical or medical procedure code for third-party reimbursement.

When submitting insurance claims for patients seen in a physician's office or an outpatient hospital setting, the **primary diagnosis** (first listed condition) is the main reason for the encounter. In an office setting, this is related to the **chief complaint (CC)**. The **secondary diagnosis**, listed subsequently, may contribute to the condition or define the need for a higher level of care but is not the underlying cause. The underlying cause of a disease is referred to as the **etiology** and is sequenced in the first position. The **principal diagnosis**, used in inpatient hospital coding, is the diagnosis obtained after study that prompted the hospitalization. It is possible for the primary and principal diagnosis codes to be the same. The concept of a "principal diagnosis" is only applicable to inpatient hospital claims or cases. Box 5-1 outlines the important considerations whenever you come across the same or similar phrases related to the diagnosis because they represent two very different coding scenarios in the outpatient versus inpatient settings.

Medicare administrative contractors (MACs) may accept and process up to a maximum of eight diagnoses

---

> ### Box 5-1   Primary Versus Principal Diagnosis
>
> **Primary Diagnosis**
>
> **Definition:** Main reason (diagnosis, condition, chief complaint) for the encounter/visit in the health record that is responsible for services provided.
> List first:
> **Location:** Outpatient setting only (physician office visits and hospital-based outpatient services).
> **Diagnosis Code:** Code the condition, sign, or symptom to the highest degree of certainty for the encounter/visit. May code signs, symptoms, abnormal test results, or other reason for the visit when a diagnosis has not been confirmed.
> May not code diagnosis documented as "probable," "suspected," "questionable," "rule out," or "working diagnosis."
>
> **Principal Diagnosis**
>
> **Definition:** Condition established after study that prompted the hospitalization.
> **Location:** Inpatient setting only.
> **Diagnosis Code:** Code the condition as if it existed or was established if at time of discharge documentation lists "probable," "suspected," "likely," "questionable," "possible," or "still to be ruled out."
> **Diagnosis-Related Group (DRG):** Assignment of DRG number to the principal diagnosis for hospital reimbursement.

---

on an electronic claim. Because paper claims have only four lines for listing diagnostic codes, check with the regional MAC to learn the procedure for submitting more than four codes. As of the printing of this edition, the CMS-1500 claim form is being revised to allow listing more lines and additional room for seven characters to accommodate ICD-10-CM coding.

Reasons for the Development and Use of Diagnostic Codes

Diagnostic coding was developed for the following reasons:

1. Tracking of disease processes
2. Classification of causes of mortality
3. Medical research
4. Evaluation of hospital service utilization

Medical practices use diagnostic codes on insurance claims to explain the visit and are not required to write out the diagnostic description on the claim form. The consequences of not using ICD-9-CM codes are many. For example, claims can be denied, fines or penalties can be levied, sanctions can be imposed, and the physician's level of reimbursement for inpatient claims may be affected. Diagnostic codes must be used on all claims; processing is accurate and prompt if coding is correctly done. When insurance claim reimbursement records are comprehensive, statistics can be gathered to make future payments more realistic for the physicians in private practice.

STANDARD TRANSACTION CODE SETS

As learned in Chapter 2, a code set is any set of codes with their descriptions used to encode data elements such as tables of terms, medical concepts, medical diagnostic codes, or medical procedure codes. Each transaction must include the use of medical and other code sets. The ICD-9-CM official guideline for coding and reporting is the standard code set outlined under HIPAA and must be used when assigning diagnostic codes. HIPAA does not require insurance health plans to change their business rules regarding payment based on the codes. However, insurance payers cannot reject an insurance claim because it includes a valid HIPAA standard code that the payer system does not yet recognize.

Occasionally, an insurance company replies to a claim with an explanation of benefits or remittance advice stating, "This procedure or item is not payable for the diagnosis as reported for lack of medical necessity." For example, a patient has undergone magnetic resonance imaging (MRI) of the brain. Medicare will not reimburse for MRI for the diagnosis of transient ischemic attack or Alzheimer's disease but will pay for it with the diagnosis of cerebral insufficiency. The procedures that are diagnosis related include most imaging services (e.g., radiography, computed tomography, or MRI), cardiovascular services (e.g., electrocardiograms, Holter monitors, echocardiography, Doppler imaging, or stress testing), neurologic services (e.g., electroencephalography, noninvasive ultrasonography), many laboratory services, and vitamin B_{12} injections. It is important to know which procedures are diagnosis related and exactly which diagnosis relates to the procedure being billed. A reference book may be helpful in this situation, and a number of manuals are available from commercial publishers. For cases dealing with the Centers for Medicare and Medicaid Services (CMS), consult the regional fiscal intermediary's website for local coverage determinations (LCDs) and the federal government's website for national coverage determinations (NCDs), or download the manual that is updated quarterly.

Physician's Fee Profile

A **physician's fee profile** is a compilation of each physician's charges and the payments made to him or her over a given period of time for each specific professional service rendered to a patient. Each insurance company keeps a profile on every provider for services that are processed for statistical and reimbursement purposes. As charges are increased, so are payments, and the profile is then updated through the use of statistical computer data gathered from submitted processed claims. Every claim form filed by a third-party payer is entered into permanent computerized records. The compiled data (fees charged, procedure and diagnostic codes) may be used in the future as the basis for the physician's fee profile. To ensure accuracy of future profiles, the insurance billing specialist should be sure all diagnoses are coded to the highest degree of specificity on a routine basis.

Two types of profiles exist: *individual customary profile* and *prevailing profile*. Depending on office policy, either the office manager or insurance biller should ask each third-party payer whether they will update the physician's fee profile on an annual basis.

HISTORY OF CODING DISEASES

From the earliest days of medical treatment, people have tried to name and classify diseases. Although many attempts have been made to systematize and clarify disease terminology, no one method has ever been accepted by the entire medical community.

Around 1869, the American Medical Association prepared the *American Nomenclature of Diseases*. In 1903 the *Bellevue Hospital Nomenclature of Diseases* was published; it was subsequently replaced by the *Standard Nomenclature of Diseases and Operations*. In the 1960s the American Medical Association published *Current Medical Information and Terminology* (CMIT), which used a computer format to make frequent revisions easier. Medical terms were alphabetically arranged and included detailed descriptions of the diseases and two- and four-digit code numbers. Publication of the book ceased in 1991.

Institutions (within a facility), pathologists, and those involved with generating medical reports and billing for laboratory medicine procedures use a system for retrieving types of diagnoses. As mentioned in Chapter 2, these codes are found in a comprehensive multilingual clinical terminology book entitled *Systematized Nomenclature of Medicine for Clinical Terminology* (SNOMED-CT), Volumes I through IV.*

In addition, this system is used for managing patient records, teaching medical information science (informatics), and indexing and managing research data. SNOMED-CT is also used to compare terminology context or classification description principles with the

*Available from the College of American Pathologists, 325 Waukegan Road, Northfield, IL, 60093-2750.

ICD-9-CM system. The United States (US) federal government licensed SNOMED-CT as a standard clinical reference terminology under HIPAA legislation. This process of linking content from one terminology or classification scheme to another is called *mapping*. This helps minimize duplicating data entry and patient data integration and helps with development of a "crosswalk." For example, when new codes are biannually introduced (April 1 and October 1), a crosswalk is made creating a map between the old and new codes.

Computer-Assisted Coding

Computer-assisted coding (CAC) is computer software that automatically generates a set of medical codes for review, validation, and use based on clinical documentation provided by health care practitioners. Many factors have pushed medical practices to adopt CAC, and some of these factors are as follows:

- Shortage of coders throughout the US
- Financial need to reduce the cost of filing insurance claims
- Increased complexity of coding systems, such as implementation of ICD-10-CM by 2013
- Adoption of electronic health records (EHR)
- Advancement in natural language processing (NLP) technology
- Constant changes in code numbers and coding rules and regulations
- Compliance liability for increased erroneous claims

CAC uses two technology options: structured input and NLP. In structured input, the physician inputs information on a data entry screen that has point-and-click fields, pull-down menus, structured templates, or macros. The system prompts the physician for detailed information. Words and phrases selected are linked to diagnostic and procedural codes that are automatically generated when all the fields are completed. Input of the detailed information results in a completed document with the appropriate level of detail. Recommended diagnostic and procedural codes are then checked and/or edited by a coder.

The NLP system uses artificial medical intelligence. The physician dictates a report, hand writes a note, or inputs a picture file. The document is sent to an NLP engine that scans the health record and chooses important, relevant words and converts them into suggested codes. A coder searches and validates the diagnostic and procedural codes and makes any changes, and the codes are transmitted to billing. NLP systems must be regularly updated to address new medical terminology and conform to changes in coding guidelines.

Automated coding software uses a statistics-based method, rules-based method, or both methods to assign codes. In a statistics-based program, also called a data-driven method, the software predicts the code for a word or phrase based on statistics from the past. A rules-based or knowledge-driven method applies coding rules such as those used in logic or rules-based encoders, groupers, and imaged coding applications to electronic clinical documents. The codes are processed through associated established rules for refinement and code assignment.

Another feature of CAC is called a *crosswalk* or *data mapping*. This aid gives a coder the ability to input a discontinued code and find a new replacement code. It also allows locating a code in ICD-9-CM to find a number of equivalent or suggested ICD-10-CM codes.

Sometimes, professional coders may disagree about which codes to apply to a specific case, thus checking and editing codes may be needed when using CAC. Usually, repetitive procedures are quick for coders to approve, but complex procedures may need more time for validation. CAC technology helps coders do their jobs faster and more efficiently and does not diminish the need for coders.

INTERNATIONAL CLASSIFICATION OF DISEASES

History

The *International Classification of Diseases* (ICD) had its beginnings in England during the seventeenth century. The US began using the ICD to report causes of death and prepare mortality statistics in the latter half of the nineteenth century. Hospitals began using the ICD in 1950 to classify and index diseases. The ninth revision of the *International Classification of Diseases* (ICD-9), published by the World Health Organization (WHO), is currently being used by state health departments and the US Public Health service (USPHS) for mortality reporting.

Organization and Format

In 1979 the ICD-9-CM was published by the US Department of Health Services. It is updated annually and has three volumes. Volume 1 is a Tabular List of Diseases, each having an assigned number. Volume 2 is an Alphabetic Index of Diseases. Volume 3 is a Tabular List and Alphabetic Index of Procedures used primarily in the hospital setting. The systematized arrangement in these books makes it possible to encode, computerize, store, and retrieve large volumes of information from the patient's medical record. ICD-9-CM is used by hospitals, physicians, and other health care providers to code and report clinical information necessary for participation in various government programs such as Medicare, Medicaid, and quality improvement organizations/professional review organizations.

Volumes 1 and 2 are used in physicians' offices and other outpatient settings to complete insurance claims. These two volumes are almost completely compatible with the original international version (ICD-9). The code numbers have from three to five digits. Although abbreviated versions of the ICD-9-CM are available, it is preferable to obtain the complete ninth revision of Volumes 1 and 2.

Annual updates of the ICD-9-CM are published in three publications: *Coding Clinic*, published by the American Hospital Association; the *American Health Information Management Association Journal*, published by the AHIMA; and the *Federal Register*, published by the US Government Printing Office. Coding from an out-of-date manual can delay payment, result in denied claims, or cause costly mistakes that can lead to financial disaster. Annual ICD-9-CM code revisions must be in place and in use by October 1 each year. There is no longer a 3-month grace period to implement these changes and revisions.

Beginning in 2005, changes occur April 1 and October 1 annually. Thus it is more important than ever to make sure updated codes are used. Refer to the Appendix for the names and addresses of several companies that publish the ICD-9-CM.

Psychiatric disorders are coded using the *Diagnostic and Statistical Manual of Mental Disorders, Fourth Edition* (DSM-IV). Refer to the Appendix for information regarding where to obtain this code book.

Contents

Table 5-1 is an outline of Volumes 1 and 2 of the ICD-9-CM.

● Volume 1 chapter headings with associated codes are listed.
● The Supplementary Classifications list V and E codes, which are discussed later.
● Sections A, B, C, and D of the appendices are not used in physician outpatient billing.
● Section E of the appendix may be used as a quick method of finding three-digit code categories.

Table 5-1	Outline of Volumes 1 and 2 of ICD-9-CM	
VOLUME 1	CHAPTER HEADINGS	CODES
1	Infectious and Parasitic Diseases	001-139
2	Neoplasms	140-239
3	Endocrine, Nutritional, and Metabolic Diseases and Immunity Disorders	240-279
4	Diseases of the Blood and Blood-Forming Organs	280-289
5	Mental Disorders	290-319
6	Diseases of the Nervous System and Sense Organs	320-389
7	Diseases of the Circulatory System	390-459
8	Diseases of the Respiratory System	460-519
9	Diseases of the Digestive System	520-579
10	Diseases of the Genitourinary System	580-629
11	Complications of Pregnancy, Childbirth, and the Puerperium	630-677
12	Diseases of the Skin and Subcutaneous Tissue	680-709
13	Diseases of the Musculoskeletal System and Connective Tissue	710-739
14	Congenital Anomalies	740-759
15	Certain Conditions Originating in the Perinatal Period	760-779
16	Symptoms, Signs, and Ill-Defined Conditions	780-799
17	Injury and Poisoning	800-999
SUPPLEMENTARY CLASSIFICATIONS		
Classification of Factors Influencing Health Status and Contact with Health Service		V01-V89
Classification of External Causes of Injury and Poisoning		E000-E999
APPENDICES		
A	Morphology of Neoplasms	
C	Classification of Drugs by American Hospital Formulary Service List Number and Their ICD-9-CM Equivalents	
D	Classification of Industrial Accidents According to Agency	
E	List of Three-Digit Categories	
VOLUME 2		
Section 1	Index to Diseases, alphabetic	
Section 2	Table of Drugs and Chemicals	
Section 3	Alphabetic Index to External Causes of Injuries and Poisoning (E Code)	

Volume 2 contains three sections: an Alphabetic Index for Diseases and Injuries, a Table of Drugs and Chemicals, and an Alphabetic Index to External Causes of Injuries and Poisonings (E codes). Some publishers place ICD-9-CM Volume 2 (alphabetic) before Volume 1 (tabular) to help the user expedite finding the correct code.

An outline and information on how to find codes in Volume 3 are provided in Chapter 17. This reference is used primarily in the hospital setting. Volume 3 will be replaced by ICD-10-PCS by 2013.

DIAGNOSTIC CODE BOOK CONVENTIONS

To become a proficient coder, it is important to develop an understanding of the conventions and terminology of ICD-9-CM. These conventions are used with ICD-10-CM with a few exceptions and a few additional ones. **Conventions** are rules or principles for determining a diagnostic code when using diagnostic code books such as each space, typefaces, indentations, punctuation marks, symbols, instructional notes, abbreviations, cross-reference notes, and specific usage of the words *and*, *with*, and *due to*. These rules assist in the selection of correct codes for the diagnoses encountered. Read all of the information at the introduction or beginning of Volumes 1 and 2 before coding. Volume 1, the Tabular List for disease classifications, makes use of certain abbreviations, punctuation, symbols, and other conventions, as shown in Box 5-2.

In Volume 2, the Alphabetic Index for disease classification, the symbol of **slanted brackets** (*[]*) is used to indicate the need for another code. A code is given after a listing followed by slanted brackets enclosing an additional code. Record both of these codes in the same sequence as indicated in the index.

An **italicized code** in the Tabular List may never be sequenced as principal or primary diagnoses.

General Coding Guidelines

The procedures for the basic steps in selecting ICD-9-CM and ICD-10-CM diagnostic codes is presented at the end of this chapter. Following are some general rules. Code only the conditions or problems that the physician is actively managing at the time of the visit. First, always use Volume 2, the Alphabetic Index, and second go to Volume 1, the Tabular (numerical) List before assigning a code. Never use just one volume and never code from the index. Begin with the Alphabetic Index to locate the main term of the diagnosis. The main term is the condition. The primary arrangement of the Alphabetic Index, the disease index, is by *condition*. If you cannot find the

condition listed, consider rearranging the word roots (e.g., crypt orchid/o or orchido crypt/o). Then, substitute a similar suffix.

Using a medical dictionary aids in accurate coding. Research any unfamiliar terminology, for example, amaurotic idiocy with severe mental retardation; impaludism. Look up the word(s) you do not know in your medical dictionary.

Organization and Format of Volume 2

Volume 2 elements are structured as follows:

- Main terms are classifications of diseases and injuries and appear as headings in bold type.
- Subterms are listings under main terms and are indented two spaces to the right under main terms.
- Modifiers (often referred to as nonessential modifiers because their presence or absence does not affect the code assigned) provide additional description and are enclosed in parentheses.
- Carryover lines continue the text and are indented more than two spaces from the level of the preceding line.
- Subterms of subterms are additional listings and are indented two spaces to the right under the subterm (Box 5-3; see also Figure 5-14).

Always code to the highest level of specificity. The more digits a code has, the more specific the description. A three-digit code may be used only when the diagnostic statement cannot be further subdivided. When a three-digit code has subdivisions, the appropriate subdivision must be coded. Some third-party payer computer systems kick out the lower-level codes (three-digit codes) and hold these claims for medical review, thereby delaying payment. Do not arbitrarily use a zero as a filler character when typing a diagnostic code number because this may be interpreted as indicating a different disease. The addition of a zero to a code number that does not require an additional digit also can cause a claim to be denied (Example 5-1).

Example 5-1	**Valid Codes and Invalid Codes Caused by Added Zero**
Valid code	**Invalid code caused by zero added**
373.2	373.20
496	496.0

Fifth-digit codes can appear as follows:

1. At the beginning of a chapter
2. At the beginning of a section
3. At the beginning of a three-digit category
4. In a four-digit subcategory

| **Box 5-2** | **Official ICD-9-CM Code Book Conventions*** |

Abbreviations

NEC
Not Elsewhere Classifiable (in the coding books). The category number for the term including NEC is to be used with ill-defined terms and only when the coder lacks the information necessary to code the term in a more specific category.
Example:
Fibrosclerosis Familial multifocal
NEC 710.8

NOS
Not Otherwise Specified (by the physician). This abbreviation is the equivalent of "unspecified." It refers to a lack of sufficient detail in the diagnosis statement to be able to assign it to a more specific subdivision within the classification.
Example:
153.9 Colon, unspecified
Large intestine NOS.

Punctuation

[ ]
Brackets are used to enclose synonyms, alternative wordings, or explanatory phrases.
Example: 482.2 Pneumonia due to *Haemophilus influenzae* [*H. influenzae*]
Brackets that appear beneath a code indicate the fifth digits that are considered valid fifth digits for the code. This convention is applied for those situations wherein not all common fifth digits are considered valid for each subcategory within a category.
Example: 715.0 Osteoarthrosis, generalized
[0, 4, 9]

[code]
Italicized (slanted) brackets enclosing a code, used in Volume 2, the Alphabetic Index, indicates the need for another code. Record both codes in the order as indicated in the index.
Example: Tachycardia
ventricular (paroxysmal)
psychogenic 316

⌐
Large bracket may signal a new or revised code.

( )
Parentheses are used to enclose supplementary words that may be present or absent in the statement of a disease or procedure without affecting the code number to which it is assigned.
Example: 198.4 Other parts of nervous system
Meninges **(cerebral) (spinal)**

:
Colons are used in the Tabular List after an incomplete term that needs one or more of the modifiers that follow to make it assignable to a given category.
Example: 021.1 Enteric tularemia
Tularemia:
    cryptogenic
    intestinal
    typhoidal

{ }
Braces are used to enclose a series of terms, each of which is modified by the statement appearing at the right of the brace
Example: 560.2 Volvulus
Knotting
Strangulation
Torsion   } of intestine, bowel, or colon
Twist

Boldface
Boldface type is used for all codes and titles in the Tabular List.

Italicized
Italicized type is used for all exclusion notes and to identify codes that should not be used for describing the primary diagnosis.

Includes
Instructional note that further defines or clarifies the content of the chapter, subchapter, category, subcategory, or subclassification.

Excludes
Terms following the word "Excludes" are not classified to the chapter, subchapter, category, subcategory, or specific subclassification code under which it is found. The instructional note also may provide the location of the excluded diagnosis. Excludes notes are not italicized.
Example: 461 Acute sinusitis
Includes   abscess
        empyema
        infection   } acute, of sinus (accessory) (nasal)
        inflammation
        suppuration
Excludes chronic or unspecified sinusitis
    (473.0-473.9)

*Some publishers use additional and/or other symbols.

Continued

Box 5-2 Official ICD-9-CM Code Book Conventions—cont'd

"And"	The word "and" should be interpreted to mean either "and" or "or" when it appears in a title.
"With"	The word "with" in the Alphabetic Index is sequenced immediately following the main term, not in alphabetic order.
"See" and "see also"	The "see" instruction following a main term in the index indicates that another term should be referenced. It is necessary to go to the main term referenced with the "see" note to locate the correct code.
	A "see also" instruction following a main term in the index instructs that there is another main term that may also be referenced that may provide additional index entries that may be useful. It is not necessary to follow the "see also" note when the original main term provides the necessary code.
Use additional code	This instruction signals the coder that an additional code should be used if the information is available to provide a more complete picture of that diagnosis.
	Example: 362.13 Changes in vascular appearance
	Vascular sheathing of retina
	Use additional code for any associated atherosclerosis (440.8)
Code first underlying disease	This instructional note is found under certain codes and is a sequencing rule.
	This rule applies to the manifestation convention and is found under the manifestation code.
	A manifestation code may never be used alone or as a primary diagnosis. The instructional note, the code, and its descriptor appear in italics in the Tabular List.
	Example: 590.81 Pyelitis or pyelonephritis in diseases classified elsewhere
	Code first underlying disease as: tuberculosis (016.0)
	Not all codes with a "Code first underlying disease" instructional note are part of the manifestation convention. The "Code first" note will appear, but the title of the code and the instructional note are not in italics. Report these codes alone or as the secondary diagnosis.
Code, if applicable any causal condition first	Instruction note that indicates this code may be assigned as a principal diagnosis when the causal condition is unknown or not applicable. If a causal condition is known, then the code for that condition should be sequenced as the principal or first-listed diagnosis.
	Example:590.0 Chronic pyelonephritis
	Chronic pyelitis
	Chronic pyonephrosis
	Code, if applicable, any causal condition first
Omit code	Instruction note found in the Alphabetic Index to diseases that indicates no code is to be assigned.
	Example: Metaplasia
	cervix—**omit code**
See Condition	Instruction note found in the Alphabetic Index to diseases that instructs the coder to refer to a main term for the condition.
	Example: Cervix—**see condition**
	Diffuse—**see condition**
Morphology codes	For each neoplastic disease listed in the index, a morphology code is given that identifies histologic type and behavior. The histology is identified by the first four digits and the behavior is identified by the digit following the slash.
	Example: Myelolipoma (**M8870/0**)—see Neoplasm, by site, benign

Symbols and Notations

•	A bullet at a code or line of text indicates the entry is new.
▲	A triangle in the Tabular List indicates the code title is revised. In the Alphabetic Index, the triangle indicates the code has changed.
►◄	When two triangle symbols meet at their points, they appear at the beginning and end of a section of new or revised text.
DEF:	This notation indicates a definition of disease or procedural term.
PDx:	This notation identifies a V code that can only be used as a primary diagnosis.
SDx:	This notation identifies a V code that can only be used as a secondary diagnosis. A V code without a symbol can be used as either a primary or secondary diagnosis.
♂♀	Age and sex symbols are used to detect inconsistencies between the patient's age and diagnosis.
	Examples:
	Newborn age: 0
	Pediatric age: 0 to 17
	Maternity age:12 to 55
	Adult age: 15 to 124
§	The section mark symbol preceding a code denotes the placement of a footnote at the bottom of the page that is applicable to all subdivisions in that code. This symbol is used only in the Tabular List of Diseases.
√	This symbol found only in the Alphabetic Index sections and the Table of Drugs and Chemicals indicates that an additional digit is required. Referring to the tabular section is essential to locate the appropriate additional digit.
④ ⑤ ✓4th ✓5th	Either of these symbols signals that a fourth or fifth digit is required for coding to indicate the highest level of specificity.

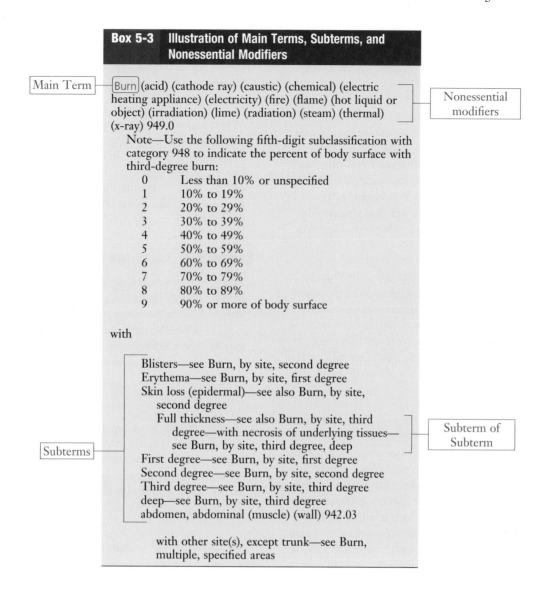

Box 5-3   Illustration of Main Terms, Subterms, and Nonessential Modifiers

Main Term → Burn (acid) (cathode ray) (caustic) (chemical) (electric heating appliance) (electricity) (fire) (flame) (hot liquid or object) (irradiation) (lime) (radiation) (steam) (thermal) (x-ray) 949.0 ← Nonessential modifiers

Note—Use the following fifth-digit subclassification with category 948 to indicate the percent of body surface with third-degree burn:

0	Less than 10% or unspecified
1	10% to 19%
2	20% to 29%
3	30% to 39%
4	40% to 49%
5	50% to 59%
6	60% to 69%
7	70% to 79%
8	80% to 89%
9	90% or more of body surface

with

Subterms →
Blisters—see Burn, by site, second degree
Erythema—see Burn, by site, first degree
Skin loss (epidermal)—see also Burn, by site, second degree
    Full thickness—see also Burn, by site, third degree—with necrosis of underlying tissues—see Burn, by site, third degree, deep ← Subterm of Subterm
First degree—see Burn, by site, first degree
Second degree—see Burn, by site, second degree
Third degree—see Burn, by site, third degree
deep—see Burn, by site, third degree
abdomen, abdominal (muscle) (wall) 942.03

with other site(s), except trunk—see Burn, multiple, specified areas

---

If the fourth or fifth digits are available for a particular three-digit category, then the use of a three-digit code is *NOT* optional unless the medical record does not provide information to select a fourth or fifth digit code. You may want to select a code book that has the categories marked and color coded so that it will not be easy to overlook fifth digits. The medical record should always be checked to see if there is sufficient information documented to select a more specific code. Near the end of this chapter (accompanying the section Rules for Coding, Diabetes Mellitus) is another example illustrating the use of fifth digits. When the fourth or fifth digit is missing, the code is not complete and technically is not a code but rather a category (Example 5-2). There are some valid three-digit codes (categories) but most have fourth digits (subcategories) and fifth digits (subclassifications). If the base code has a fourth or fifth digit, you must code up to that level.

Example 5-2   Fourth and Fifth Digits (Tabular List)

§645	Late pregnancy
[0, 1, 3]	Post-term pregnancy
	Pregnancy that has advanced beyond 42 weeks of gestation

Different symbols are shown by different publishers of ICD-9-CM to indicate when an additional digit is needed (i.e., the red dot [stop sign] or in this example the section mark (§) requires a fifth digit; valid digits are in [brackets] beneath each code. Use 0 as the fourth digit for this category.

When you are billing Medicare, you will find that some diagnostic codes are designated as invalid from year to year. If you work in a medical practice that sees Medicare patients, it is essential to access online the regional Medicare bulletins and read them, as well as attend

Medicare seminars periodically to keep abreast of these changes, or visit the CMS website.

Handy Hints in Diagnostic Coding

If your ICD-9-CM code books are not color-coded, mark manifestation (italicized) codes with a colored highlighter pen (e.g., 608.81 [italicized code]). This will remind you to **always code the underlying disease first.** Also, add tabs to main sections of Volume 1 (first page, V codes, E codes, Appendix E) and Volume 2 (sections I, II, and III). Refer to the end of this chapter for the step-by-step procedures for locating and selecting diagnostic codes.

Many times you locate a diagnostic code in Volume 2 only to find that the cross-referenced code is the same when verified in Volume 1. Indicate these codes in Volume 2 with a different colored highlighter pen to remind you that this code is correct as described in Volume 2, which saves the time you would spend checking Volume 1. But to be sure, always code from the tabular section.

Keep a list of diagnostic and *Current Procedural Terminology* (CPT) procedure codes commonly encountered by your office, making sure to include fourth and fifth digit specificity. Some insurance companies publish lists of codes specifying diagnostic codes that are acceptable for specific procedures. Consult payer guidelines by calling the insurance company or managed care plan to determine whether certain procedures are a covered benefit for certain diagnoses and if not, have the patient sign a waiver. Reference books that show codes that link between diagnostic and procedure codes are available. The American Medical Association (AMA) publishes a list of the most common diagnostic codes at the end of each of their mini-specialty code books. See the Appendix for information on how to obtain reference books that contain such data. Some medical practices develop an encounter form that is an all-encompassing billing document that is a reference page and acts as a shortcut to locating diagnostic codes for conditions commonly seen by a physician specialist.

These forms must be reviewed, updated, and changed on a regular basis (January 1 for procedure codes and in April and October for diagnostic codes).

V Codes—Supplementary Classification of Factors Influencing Health Status and Contact With Health Services

V codes are a supplementary classification of coding located in a separate section at the end of Volume 1, Tabular List. In Volume 2, the Alphabetic Index, the V codes are included in the major section Index of Diseases.

V codes may be used for the following four primary circumstances:

1. When a person who is not currently sick encounters health services for some specific purpose such as to act as a donor of an organ or tissue, receive a vaccination, discuss a problem that is not in itself a disease or injury, seek consultation about family planning, request sterilization, or obtain supervision of a normal pregnancy (Example 5-3).

Example 5-3   Supervision of First Pregnancy, Normal

Step 1. Find the heading **pregnancy** in Volume 2.

Step 2. Look for the subheading **supervision**.

Step 3. Look for the second subheading **normal** and a further subheading **first,** which gives you the code V22.0.

Step 4. Find **V22.0** in Volume 1. By Tabular List, you will see "**Supervision of Normal First Pregnancy.**"

---

2. When a person with a resolving disease or injury, such as a chronic, long-term condition that needs continuous care, seeks aftercare.
3. When a circumstance influences an individual's health status, but the illness is not current.
4. When it is necessary to indicate the birth status of a newborn.

These types of encounters are among the more common services for hospital outpatients and patients of private practitioners, health clinics, and others. Certain V codes may only appear as a primary code and others only as secondary codes.

Some key words in patient care that may indicate a V code might be necessary are *exposure, routine annual examination, admission, history of, encounter,* and *vaccination.* V codes also are used when some circumstance or problem is present that influences the person's health status but is not in itself a current illness or injury such as when the person is known to have an allergy to a specific drug. In this instance the V code cannot be used as a stand-alone code and should be used only as a supplementary code.

Additional code numbers are given for occupational health examinations and routine annual physical examinations; therefore select specific codes depending on the circumstances (Example 5-4).

Sometimes a patient receives a consultation for a pre-operative medical evaluation as an inpatient or outpatient (Example 5-5), and the majority of the results are

---

Example 5-4   Routine Annual Physical Examination

Step 1. Look up **examination,** and notice **annual** as a subterm and the code V70.0.

Step 2. Find **V70** in Volume 1, Tabular List, and the wording **"Routine general medical examination at a health facility."**

Example 5-5   Admission (Encounter) Code

A patient to have surgery for gallstones is sent to a cardiologist for evaluation of suspected cardiovascular disease.

Step 1. In Volume 2, look up **admission (encounter) (for) examination, preoperative, cardiovascular V72.81.** Verify it in Volume 1.

Step 2. Code the reason for the surgery—574.xx, cholelithiasis.

INDEX TO EXTERNAL CAUSES

Fall, falling (accidental) E888.9
  building E916
        burning E891.8
            private E890.8
  down
        escalator E880.0
        ladder E881.0
            in boat, ship, watercraft E833 ☑
        staircase E880.9
        stairs, steps – *see* Fall, from, stairs
  earth (with asphyxia or suffocation (by
        pressure) (*see also* Earth, falling) E913.3
  from off
        aircraft (at landing, take-off) (in-transit)
            (while alighting, boarding) E843 ☑
        resulting from accident to aircraft –
            see categories E840-E842 ☑
        animal (in sport or transport) E828 ☑
        animal-drawn vehicle E827 ☑
        balcony E882
        bed E884.4
        bicycle E826 ☑

FIGURE 5-1 E coding.

Example 5-6   E Codes

26720 Closed treatment of phalangeal shaft fracture, proximal phalanx, finger; without manipulation, each
816.02 Closed, fracture of one distal phalanx of hand
E880.1 Fall from sidewalk curb

NOTE: Code 26720 is a CPT code; CPT is discussed in Chapter 6.

---

negative for chronic or current illness. A good-health diagnosis code will trigger a rejection by the third-party payer unless it is mandated by the insurance company. From Volume 2, Section I, use an admission (encounter) code from the V72.X code series for "other specified examinations" instead of a treatment code. The term "admission (encounter)" is equivalent to *encounter for* and does not refer to an admission to the hospital.

When coding a healthy patient examination, V codes (V70 through V70.9) should be sequenced as primary diagnoses over all other diagnoses. Be cautious when using V codes as second or third diagnoses because Medicare might automatically reject the claim, and insurance companies that adopt Medicare policies may possibly do so, too.

E Codes—Index to External Causes of Injury and Poisoning

E codes are also a supplementary classification of coding in which you look for external causes of injury rather than disease. The code description refers to the circumstances that caused an injury rather than the nature of the injury. E codes are also used in coding adverse reactions to medications (Figure 5-1). In ICD-10-CM, E codes have a different title and the codes begin with different alpha letters.

E codes are listed in a separate section of Volume 1, Tabular List, after V codes. To look up E codes, use section III in Volume 2. The E codes are also in a separate section, Index to External Causes of Injury and Poisoning, which follows the regular Alphabetic Index. One

method of finding E codes is to use Appendix E: List of Three-Digit Categories found in the appendices of the code book.

The use of an E code after the primary or other acute secondary diagnosis explains the mechanism for the injury. For example, if a patient falls and fractures a finger, the fracture code is primary, and an E code following it helps explain how the accident or injury was incurred (Example 5-6). It can help speed the reimbursement process because a payer will see an acute injury code and know a third party is responsible for payment as in a workers' compensation injury or motor vehicle accident. E codes also play a role in gathering data such as in statistical reporting, credentialing, utilization review, and state injury prevention programs. On the negative side, however, many payers require chart notes to accompany E-code claims, which means generating a paper

Table 5-2	Table of Drugs and Chemicals					
	External Cause (E Code)					
SUBSTANCE	POISONING	ACCIDENT	THERAPEUTIC USE	SUICIDE ATTEMPT	ASSAULT	UNDETERMINED
Acetylsalicylic acid ...	965.1	E850.3	E935.3	E950.0	E962.0	E980.0

Example 5-7 Coding an Adverse Effect

An inpatient had an adverse effect (ventricular fibrillation) to the medication digoxin, which was prescribed by her physician and taken correctly.

Step 1. Refer to the Table of Drugs and Chemicals in Volume 2 and look up **digoxin.**

Step 2. Because this medication was for therapeutic use, locate the correct E code number under that column.

Step 3. The correct number is **E942.1.**

Step 4. Locate the main term **fibrillation** in the Index to Diseases.

Step 5. Find the subterm **ventricular**

Step 6. The correct code number is **427.41.**

Step 7. Verify the code number 427.41 in Volume I, Tabular Listing.

Sequencing: **427.41 Ventricular fibrillation (chief complaint)**
E942.1 Therapeutic use, Digoxin

NOTE: For outpatient billing, the E code would not be listed.

claim rather than sending it electronically. E codes often trigger a questionnaire to be sent to the beneficiary. This may lead to a delay in reimbursement. Although E codes do not generate revenue, it is recommended that they should be reported in addition to the appropriate procedural and diagnostic codes. This ensures that the most specific information possible is provided in regard to the patient's injury. E codes are billed by the initial entity seeing the patient. If the patient visits the physician's office after hospitalization for injuries sustained in a motor vehicle accident, the hospital assigns an E code and there is no requirement for repeating it for the office visit. An E code may never be sequenced as the primary diagnosis in the first position. When using E codes, be sure to list them last on the claim form. Instructions are included here for additional knowledge about the classification system.

The Table of Drugs and Chemicals found after the alphabetical index in Volume 2, Section II (Table 5-2), contains a classification of drugs and other chemical substances for identifying poisoning states and external causes of adverse effects. Read the introduction explanation at the beginning of the Table of Drugs and Chemicals.

Adverse effect is defined as an adverse or a pathologic reaction to a drug that occurs when appropriate doses are given to humans for prophylaxis (prevention of disease), diagnosis, and therapy (Example 5-7). When an adverse effect occurs (e.g., drug reaction, hypersensitivity, drug intolerance, or idiosyncratic reaction), a code is assigned to the diagnosis that classifies the specific reaction or symptom (e.g., dermatitis, syncope, tachycardia, or urticaria). You do not use a code from the 960 to 989 range but do code the specific reaction or symptom from use of the drug followed by a code from the E code column. The E code identifying the agent involved is taken solely from the Therapeutic Use column.

Poisoning is defined as a condition resulting from an intentional overdose of drugs or chemical substances or from the wrong drug or agent given or taken in error.

The following situations occur and are documented in the medical record to indicate poisoning:

● Taking the wrong medication
● Receiving the wrong medication
● Taking the wrong dose of the right medication
● Receiving the wrong dose of the right medication
● Ingesting a chemical substance not intended for human consumption
● Overdose of a chemical substance (drug)
● Prescription drug taken with alcohol
● Mixing prescription drugs and over-the-counter medications without the physician's advice or consent

Each of the substances listed in Table 5-2 is assigned a code according to the poisoning classification (960 through 989). These adverse effect codes are used when there is a state of poisoning, overdose, wrong substance given or taken, or intoxication. **Intoxication** is defined as an adverse effect rather than a poisoning when drugs such as digitalis and steroid agents are involved. However, whenever the term intoxication is used, the biller should clarify with the physician the circumstances surrounding the administration of the drug or chemical before assigning the appropriate code. This must be documented in the health record. If a diagnosis is stated as possible or suspected suicide attempt, then go to the column entitled "Undetermined" and not "Suicide Attempt."

Example 5-8 shows the steps for coding a case involving poisoning.

Example 5-8   Coding a Poisoning

Baby Kathy got into the kitchen cabinet and ingested liquid household ammonia.

Step 1.	Refer to the Table of Drugs and Chemicals in Volume 2 and look up **ammonia**
Step 2.	Find the subterm **liquid (household).**
Step 3.	Because this is a case of ingesting a chemical substance not intended for human use, locate the correct code number under the **Poisoning** column.
Step 4.	Write down the code number **983.2.**
Step 5.	Because this is an accident, locate the E code in the **Accident** column **(E861.4).**
Sequencing:	1.1 Poisoning code: 983.2 Poisoning, ammonia
	2.2 Manifestation(s): **Outcome of the poisoning (e.g., nausea and vomiting) would be coded in the second position if documented in the medical record.**
	3.3 E code from appropriate column, not Therapeutic Use: **E861.4 Poisoning, accidental, ammonia**

Example 5-9   No Precise Diagnosis

The patient has an enlarged liver and further diagnostic studies may or may not be done. Use code 789.1 for hepatomegaly.

Example 5-10   No Precise Diagnosis

The patient complains of painful urination and urinalysis is negative. Use code 788.1 for dysuria.

Example 5-11   Transient Sign and Symptom Code

The patient complains of **chest pain on deep inspiration.** On examination, the physician finds nothing abnormal and tells the patient to return in 1 week. When the patient returns, the pain has ceased. **Use code 786.52 for painful respiration.**

Example 5-12   Provisional Diagnosis

On examination, the physician documents abnormal percussion of the chest. The patient is sent for a chest x-ray and is asked to return for a recheck. The patient does not have the x-ray and fails to return. **Use code 786.7 for abnormal chest sounds.**

Example 5-13   Sign and Symptom Code Before Definite Diagnosis

A patient complains of nausea and vomiting and is referred to a gastroenterologist. **Use code 787.01 for nausea with vomiting.**

RULES FOR CODING

Signs, Symptoms, and Ill-Defined Conditions

Chapter 16 of the ICD-9-CM—Symptoms, Signs, and Ill-Defined Conditions (codes 780 to 799.9)—contains many but not all codes for symptoms. If the final diagnosis at the end of the encounter or at the time of discharge is qualified by any of the following terms (*apparent, likely, might, possible, probable, probably, questionable, rule out, suspected, or suspicion of*), do not code these conditions as if they existed or were established. Instead, document the condition to the highest degree of certainty for each encounter or visit (e.g., signs, symptoms, abnormal test results, or other reason for the visit) and code the chief complaint, sign, or symptom.

This is contrary to coding practices used by hospital health information management departments for coding the diagnoses of hospital inpatients. If one were to follow hospital coding guidelines and the patient was suspected of having a heart attack, this would be coded as a confirmed case of a myocardial infarction. The same holds true for "possible epilepsy." If the patient had a convulsion and epilepsy was the probable cause but had not been proved, code the convulsion.

The following are instances in which sign and symptom codes can be used:

- No precise diagnosis can be made (Examples 5-9 and 5-10).
- Signs or symptoms are transient, and a specific diagnosis was not made (Example 5-11).
- Provisional diagnosis for a patient who does not return for further care (Example 5-12).
- A patient is referred for treatment before a definite diagnosis is made (Example 5-13).

Sterilization

The code V25.2 is used only when the sterilization is performed for the major purpose of contraception rather than being an incidental result of the treatment of a disease. If the sterilization is purely elective, code V25.2 suffices as a single code for the diagnosis. If the sterilization is performed for contraceptive purposes during a current admission for obstetric delivery, sequence code V25.2 in the second position. If the sterilization is the end result of a hysterectomy performed because of injury or damage to the uterus during delivery, do not use code

Table 5-3	Coding for Neoplasms					
	Malignant					
	PRIMARY	**SECONDARY**	**CA IN SITU**	**BENIGN**	**UNCERTAIN BEHAVIOR**	**UNSPECIFIED**
neoplasm, neoplastic	199.1	199.1	234.9	229.9	238.9	239.9
abdomen, abdominal	195.2	198.89	234.8	229.8	238.8	239.8
Cavity	195.2	198.89	234.8	229.8	238.8	238.8
Organ	195.2	198.89	234.8	229.8	238.8	238.8
Viscera	195.2	198.89	234.8	229.8	238.8	239.8
Wall	173.5	198.2	232.5	216.5	238.2	239.2
connective tissue	171.5	198.89	—	215.5	238.1	239.2
abdominopelvic	195.8	198.89	234.8	229.8	238.8	239.8
accessory sinus—see						
Neoplasm, sinus						
acoustic nerve	192.0	198.4	—	225.1	237.9	239.7
acromion (process)	170.4	198.5	—	213.4	238.0	239.2
adenoid (pharynx) (tissue)	147.1	198.89	230.0	210.7	235.1	239.0
adipose tissue (see also Neoplasm,	171.9	198.89	—	215.9	238.1	239.2
connective tissue)						
adnexa (uterine)	183.9	198.82	233.3	221.8	236.3	239.5
adrenal (cortex) (gland) (medulla)	194.0	198.7	234.8	227.0	237.2	239.7
ala nasi (external)	173.3	198.2	232.3	216.3	238.2	239.2
alimentary canal or tract NEC	159.9	197.8	230.9	211.9	235.5	239.0

V25.2 but instead code the condition or procedure (i.e., hysterectomy and the diagnosis that precipitated the hysterectomy).

Neoplasms

A **neoplasm** is a spontaneous new growth of tissue forming an abnormal mass that is also known as a tumor. It may be benign or malignant. The main entry "Neoplasm" contains a table with the column headings Malignant, Benign, Uncertain Behavior, and Unspecified. The table is found in the alphabetic index under "Neoplasm" in Volume 2 (Table 5-3). First, check the index and if you are not able to locate the word (area that is in active treatment) you are searching for, then go to the table. Often, the index entry will produce the correct code and tell you what area of the table to look at. If you go to the table first, you may end up obtaining an incorrect code. Code numbers for neoplasms are given by anatomic site. For each site, there are six possible code numbers, indicating whether the neoplasm in question is malignant (primary, secondary, or carcinoma in situ), benign, of uncertain behavior, or of unspecified nature. The description of the neoplasm often indicates which of the six code numbers is appropriate (e.g., malignant melanoma of skin, benign fibroadenoma of breast, or carcinoma in situ of cervix uteri) (Example 5-14).

For a tumor that has not been diagnosed as benign or malignant by the pathologist, use the codes in the column labeled "Uncertain Behavior." If a tumor is suspected and not confirmed, use "mass." For example, a breast mass

---

Example 5-14 **Adenocarcinoma of the Breast With Metastases to the Pelvic Bone**

Step 1. Look up **adenocarcinoma** in Volume 2. Do not use the morphology code M8140/3. Notice it states, "see also Neoplasm, by site, malignant."

Step 2. Locate **neoplasm** in the table in Volume 2. At the top of the page notice the Malignant heading with the subheadings **Primary, Secondary,** and **Ca In Situ**. **Primary** means the first site of development of the malignancy. **Secondary** means metastasis from the primary site to a second site. **Ca In Situ** means cancer confined to the epithelium of the site of origin without invasion of the basement membrane tissue of the site.

Step 3. Find the site of the adenocarcinoma (in this case the breast), and look under the Malignant and Primary headings. Note that the code given is **174.9.**

Step 4. Next, find **bone** as a subterm in the Neoplasm Table and look for the subterm **pelvic.** Now look at the three columns under Malignant and using the Secondary column, find the **correct code number 198.5.** In listing these diagnoses on the insurance claim, you give the following: **174.9 and 198.5.**

---

would be coded 611.72. When coding a neoplasm, ask yourself the following questions:

- What is it now?
- Where did it start?
- What happened to it?

A **benign tumor** is one that does not have the properties of invasion and **metastasis** (e.g., spread or transfer of tumor cells from one organ to another site) and is usually surrounded by a fibrous capsule. Cysts and lesions are not neoplasms. A **malignant tumor** has the properties of invasion and metastasis. The term *carcinoma* refers to a cancerous or malignant tumor. Carcinoma **in situ** means cancer confined to the site of origin without invasion of neighboring tissues. A *primary malignancy* means the original neoplastic (malignant) site. A *secondary neoplasm* or malignancy is the site or location to which the original malignancy has spread or metastasized. If the diagnosis does not mention metastasis, then code the case as a primary neoplasm (Example 5-15). Lymphomas and leukemias are not classified using the primary and secondary terminology.

Example 5-15   Primary and Secondary Cancerous Tumors

Primary	189	Malignant neoplasm of kidney and other and unspecified urinary organs
	189.0	Kidney, except pelvis
		Kidney NOS
		Kidney parenchyma
Secondary	198	Secondary malignant cancerous neoplasm of other tumor specified sites
		Excludes lymph node metastasis (196.0 to 196.9)
	198.0	Kidney

The diagnostic statement "metastatic from" indicates primary stage carcinoma, whereas "metastatic to" indicates secondary stage carcinoma. If the diagnostic statement is "malignant neoplasm spread to," then code it as the primary site spread to the secondary site. The phrase "recurrent malignancy" is new and is coded as a primary neoplasm.

Anatomic sites marked with an asterisk (*) are always considered to be neoplasms of the skin.

In Appendix A of the Tabular List of Volume 1, there is a section titled "Morphology of Neoplasms," which gives M codes. These codes are not used for billing insurance claims by physicians' offices.

Circulatory System Conditions

Diseases of the circulatory system are difficult to code because of the variety and lack of specific terminology used by physicians in stating the diagnoses. Carefully read all inclusion, exclusion, and "use additional code" notations contained in the Tabular List of Volume 1.

Hypertension

The lay term "high blood pressure" is medically termed *hypertension*. Hypertension can cause various forms of heart and vascular disease, or it can accompany some heart conditions. In fact, there is a syndrome called *malignant hypertension* that has nothing to do with tumor formation. It is a condition of very high blood pressure with poor prognosis. A **syndrome** is another name for a symptom complex (a set of complex signs, symptoms, or other manifestations resulting from a common cause or appearing in combination, presenting a distinct clinical picture of a disease or inherited abnormality). Malignant hypertension is a symptom complex of markedly elevated blood pressure (diastolic pressure > 140 mm Hg) associated with papilledema. The term *malignant* here means "life threatening." *Benign hypertension* refers to high blood pressure that runs a relatively long and symptomless course. Only a physician can state whether the hypertension is malignant or benign. When in doubt, ask the physician.

When the diagnostic statement indicates a cause by stating "heart condition *due to* hypertension" or "hypertensive heart disease," use codes 402.0X through 402.9X. If the diagnostic statement reads "*with* hypertension" or "cardiomegaly *and* hypertension," you need two separate codes. Elevated blood pressure without mention of hypertension is coded 796.2. Secondary hypertension is coded 405.XX, and the cause of the hypertension should be coded when specified.

Myocardial Infarctions

A separate three-digit category (412) is provided for old myocardial infarction, healed myocardial infarction, or myocardial infarction diagnosed on electrocardiogram. Myocardial infarction of 8 weeks' duration or less (410.xx) is considered acute, if not specified otherwise. Symptoms of more than 8 weeks' duration are coded 414.8, other forms of chronic ischemic heart disease.

Chronic Rheumatic Heart Disease

When coding heart conditions, some conditions are presumed to be caused by rheumatic fever:

- Mitral valve of unspecified etiology 394.9
- Mitral valve insufficiency 394.1
- Mitral valve and aortic valve disorders of unspecified etiology 396.6
- Mitral stenosis 394.0

Aortic valve of unspecified etiology 424.1 is not presumed to be caused by rheumatic fever.

Arteriosclerotic Cardiovascular Disease and Arteriosclerotic Heart Disease

Use code 429.2 for a patient who has a diagnosis of arteriosclerotic cardiovascular disease (ASCVD). Code 440.9 excludes ASCVD because it is in conflict with the note given for 429.2. Code 429.2 is primary when the additional code 440.9 is necessary. However, a patient with arteriosclerotic heart disease (ASHD) is assigned code 414.0X. At code 429.2 in your copy of Volume 1, write in "see code 440" after "use additional code to identify, if desired, the presence of arteriosclerosis." To distinguish between ASCVD and ASHD, cardiovascular means pertaining to heart and blood vessels throughout the body, whereas ASHD means acute or chronic heart disability resulting from an insufficient supply of oxygenated blood to the heart.

Diabetes Mellitus

The two types of diabetes are type I and type II. The following are the clinical features important in the classification of diabetes (Table 5-4).

In type I diabetes, the patient's pancreas does not function and produce the necessary insulin. Thus this patient's body is dependent on insulin. In type II diabetes the patient's pancreas produces some insulin, but the insulin is ineffective in doing its job, which is removing sugar from the bloodstream. This diabetes may be controlled with diet, oral medication, or insulin.

Coding diabetes always requires five digits because of the types and complications that may accompany this disease. If the type is not documented, select the code for type II. This classification appears in ICD-9-CM, Volume 2, as the following:

"Fifth-digit subclassification with code 250 is not based on severity or age grouping of the case (Figure 5-2). It is a type grouping; use Table 5-5 as a guide."

Table 5-4	Features of Type I and Type II Diabetes
TYPE I DIABETES	**TYPE II DIABETES**
Insulin-dependent diabetes mellitus	Non–insulin-dependent diabetes mellitus
Patients must be treated with insulin	Patients may be treated with insulin
Insulin levels are very low	Insulin levels may be high, "normal," or low
Ketosis prone	Non-ketosis prone
Patients usually are lean	Patients usually are obese
Usually "juvenile onset" (peak onset at early puberty)	Usually "adult onset," although occasionally seen in children
Often little family history of diabetes mellitus	Often strong family history of diabetes mellitus

Always ask the physician for further clarification when a medical record contains the statement "discharged on insulin" with no further explanation of the type of diabetes. Do not assume that a patient taking insulin has insulin-dependent diabetes. If the patient routinely takes insulin, use diagnosis code V58.67, but not if the patient takes it temporarily to control blood sugar. If the patient receives an underdose because of pump failure, use code 996.57 as the primary code with the appropriate 250 series code. If the pump failure causes an insulin overdose, the second diagnosis code should be 962.3 (poisoning by insulins and antidiabetic agents) with the 250 series code.

When a diabetic patient has a complication, use a code from the 250 series with a corresponding code for each associated condition (Example 5-16).

Example 5-16	Complication Related to Diabetes
250.50	Diabetes with ophthalmic manifestations
366.41	Cataract related to diabetes

Do not use code 250.0X if the diabetes is stated with delivery of a child or as a complication of pregnancy. Use code 648.01.

Pregnancy, Delivery, or Abortion

The following main sections are included:

630 to 633 Ectopic and molar pregnancy
634 to 639 Other pregnancy with abortive outcome (*five-digit subclassifications must be used with categories 634 to 637*)
640 to 649 Complications mainly related to pregnancy (*five-digit subclassifications must be used*)
650 to 659 Normal delivery and other indications for care in pregnancy, labor, and delivery (*five-digit subclassifications must be used in categories 651-659*)
660 to 669 Complications occurring mainly in the course of labor and delivery (*five-digit subclassifications must be used*)
670 to 677 Complications of the puerperium (*five-digit subclassifications must be used for categories 670 to 676*)
678 to 679 *Other maternal and fetal complications*

The following guidelines are used:

1. Code 650 is used for a completely normal delivery. This means normal spontaneous delivery, cephalic (vertex) presentation of one live-born fetus, full-term gestation (with or without episiotomy), no manipulation necessary, and no laceration.
2. A code other than 650 should be used to provide greater detail about a complication of abortion, pregnancy, childbirth, or the puerperium when

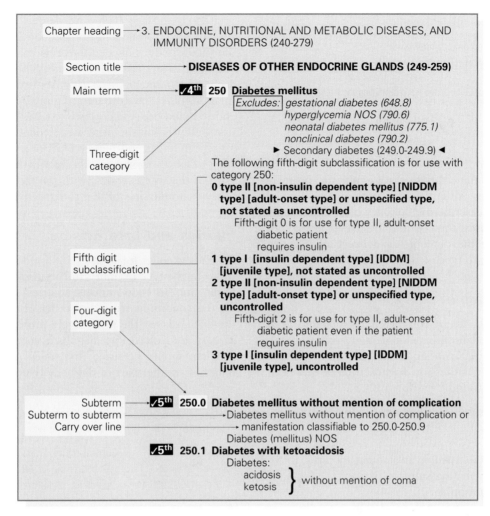

FIGURE 5-2 Classification of diabetes mellitus showing fifth-digit subclassification from *International Classification of Diseases, Ninth Revision, Clinical Modification* (ICD-9-CM), Volume 2.

Table 5-5	Type Grouping for Diabetes	
250.00 FOR NON–INSULIN-DEPENDENT DIABETES	**250.02 FOR NON–INSULIN-DEPENDENT DIABETES**
Adult onset	Adult onset
Type two, type II or unspecified	Type two, type II or unspecified
Stable or not stated as uncontrolled	Uncontrolled
Non-ketosis prone	
250.01 for insulin-dependent diabetes	**250.03 for insulin-dependent diabetes**
Juvenile onset	Juvenile onset
Type one, type I	Type one, type I
Stable or not stated as uncontrolled	Uncontrolled
Ketosis prone	

NOTE: Terms such as adult onset diabetes (AODM), insulin-dependent diabetes (IDDM), non–insulin-dependent diabetes (NIDDM), and maturity-onset diabetes are no longer used and the only differentiation is type I or type II.

information is available such as the presence of anemia, diabetes mellitus, or thyroid dysfunction (Example 5-17). Complication of the puerperium is a complication within 6 weeks after labor.

Example 5-17	Complications Related to Pregnancy	
648.01	250.00	Pregnancy (delivered) with diabetes mellitus
648.23	282.60	Pregnancy (antepartum) with sickle cell anemia

3. A V code is always required to report the outcome of delivery. In most instances an additional code is added to specify the patient's specific problem.

A multiple gestation (twins, triplets) is a complication of pregnancy and is considered high risk. When a patient

Example 5-18   Multiple Gestation

651.11	Triplet pregnancy (delivered)
675.02	Infection of nipple (postpartum)

NOTE: Code V27 series would be added when submitting the mother's bill.

delivers and experiences both antepartum and postpartum complications, different fifth digits may be applied on the codes to describe the episodes of care (Example 5-18). In such cases, there is also a need for using a V code to indicate the outcome of delivery of liveborn infants according to type of birth (V30 to V39).

Admitting Diagnoses

Some diagnostic codes are considered questionable when used as the first diagnosis on admission of a patient to the hospital (e.g., 278.00 obesity, 401.1 benign hypertension). The inpatient admission diagnosis may be expressed as one of the following:

1. One or more significant findings (symptoms or signs) representing patient distress or abnormal findings on examination.
2. A diagnosis established on an ambulatory care basis or previous hospital admission.
3. An injury or poisoning.
4. A reason or condition not classifiable as an illness or injury such as pregnancy in labor or follow-up inpatient diagnostic tests.

When a physician makes hospital visits, code the reason for the visit, which might not necessarily be the reason the patient was admitted to the hospital.

Reporting Same Diagnosis Code More Than Once

Each unique ICD-9-CM diagnosis code may be reported only once for an encounter. This applies to bilateral conditions or two different conditions classified to the same diagnosis code.

Burns

To be as specific as possible with coding burns, you need a code for each burn site and a single code to describe the total body surface area (TBSA) for all sites. The first code is for the exact site and degree of the burn (940 to 949). The second code found in category 948 describes the percentage of body surface area burned. The fourth digit indicates the total percentage of all burns—first, second, and third degree. A fifth digit is included in this category and is necessary to indicate how much of the total body surface had third-degree burns. Think of the body as a whole and not the body parts as a whole. The adult body is divided into regions: head, 9%; arms, 9% each; trunk, 18% front and 18% back; legs, 18% each; and perineum, 1% (Figure 5-3). Children's and infants' bodies have different regional percentages. Burn codes should be sequenced with the highest-degree burn first, followed by the other burn codes. However, when a first- and a second-degree burn of the same anatomic site (3-digit category) are listed, only the highest-degree burn of that site is coded, with the fifth digit indicating other anatomic sites of that category.

Injuries and Late Effects

Diagnostic codes for injuries are listed in the Alphabetic Index by the type of injury and are broken down by anatomic site. To code multiple injuries, list the diagnosis for the conditions treated in order of importance, with the diagnosis for the most severe problem listed first. If surgery is involved, the diagnostic code for the surgical problem should be listed first unless there is a severe injury of another part of the body (Example 5-19).

Example 5-19   Current Injury

824.8	**Current injury**: Fracture, left ankle
	OR
733.81 and 905.4	Late effect: Malunion fracture, left ankle

The most difficult part of assigning injury codes is to know what main terms to look for in the Alphabetic Index. Codes A 800 through 959 include fractures, dislocations, sprains, and other types of injury. Injuries are coded according to the general type of injury and broken down within each type by anatomic site. A list of common injury medical terms and the types of injuries included for each is shown in Table 5-6.

Use the following guides for coding injuries:

1. Decide whether a diagnosis represents a current injury or a late effect of an injury (Example 5-20).
2. Fractures are coded as closed if there is no indication of whether the fracture is open or closed.
3. The word "with" indicates involvement of both sites, and the word "and" indicates involvement of either one or two sites when multiple injury sites are given (Example 5-21).

Look up code 813 in your diagnostic code book and note that this code section relates to a fracture of the radius, ulna, or both.

FIGURE 5-3 A, The rules of nines estimation of total body surface area (TBSA) burned. **B,** The degrees of burn involving the layers of the skin: first-degree burns include the epidermis (redness), second-degree burns include the epidermis and dermis (blistering), third-degree burns include the first two layers and the subcutaneous tissues (full thickness), and deep-third burns involve all layers of the skin with resulting eschar (deep necrosis).

Table 5-6	Common Injury Medical Terms
MAIN TERM	**EXPLANATION**
Contusion	Bruise and hematoma without a fracture or open wound.
Crush	Crushing injury not complicated by concussion, fractures, injury to internal organs, or intracranial injury.
Dislocation	Displacement and subluxation. Dislocation may be open or closed. Closed dislocation may be complete, partial, simple, or uncomplicated. Open dislocation may be compound, infected, or with foreign body. A dislocation not indicated as closed or open is classified as closed.
Fracture	Fractures may be open or closed. A fracture not indicated as open or closed is classified as closed. An injury described as fracture dislocation is coded as a fracture. Open fractures may be described as compound, infected, missile, puncture, or with foreign body. Closed fractures may be described as comminuted, depressed, elevated, fissured, greenstick, impacted, linear, march, simple, slipped, epiphyseal, or spiral.
Injury, blood vessel	Described as arterial hematoma, avulsion, laceration, rupture, traumatic aneurysm, or traumatic fistula.
Injury, internal	Includes all injuries to internal organs such as the heart, lung, liver, kidney, and pelvic organs. Types of injuries to internal organs include laceration, tear, traumatic rupture, penetrating wounds, blunt trauma, crushing, blast injuries, or open wounds to internal organs with or without fracture in the same region.
Injury, intracranial	Includes concussion, cerebral laceration and contusion, or intracranial hemorrhage. These injuries may be open or closed. Intracranial injuries with skull fractures may be found under fracture.
Injury, superficial	Includes abrasion, insect bite (nonvenomous), blister, or scratch.
Sprain/strain	Injury to the joint capsule, ligament, muscle, or tendon described by the following terms: avulsion, hemarthrosis, laceration (closed), rupture, or tear. Open laceration of these structures should be coded as open wounds.
Wound, open	Includes open wounds not involving internal organs. Wounds may be to skin, muscle, or tendon, described as animal bite, avulsion, cut, laceration, puncture wound, or traumatic amputation. Open wounds may be complicated or uncomplicated. Complicated includes injuries with mention of delayed healing, delayed treatment, foreign body, or major infection.

Example 5-20   Injuries

Case: An intracranial injury, managed medically, and a fractured middle phalanx of the right hand, managed surgically,

854.00   Intracranial injury (first-listed primary diagnosis)
816.11   Fractured middle phalanx (secondary diagnosis)

Example 5-21   Multiple Injury Sites

806   Fracture of the vertebral column **with** spinal cord injury
813   Fracture of radius **and** ulna

Example 5-22   Late Effects

A. 905.4 *Malunion* (823.30) open **fracture**, right tibia
   905.4 Traumatic *arthritis* following (822.0) **fracture** of right knee;
   438.20 Hemiplegia following (432.9) **cerebrovascular thrombosis** 1 year previously
   906.7 *Scarring* caused by (943.33) third-degree **burn** of right arm
B. 905.2 Traumatic **arthropathy,** shoulder region 905.2 Traumatic **arthritis** of left shoulder due to old (812.10) **fracture** of left humerus followed by late effect of **fracture of upper extremities**

A **late effect** means "the residual effect (condition produced) after the acute phase of an illness or injury has terminated." An injury may have a late effect, which must be coded in a different fashion. An effect is considered to be late if the diagnosis reads "due to an old injury," "late," "due to" or "following" (previous illness or injury), or "due to an injury or illness that occurred 1 year or more before the current admission of encounter."

Example 5-22 illustrates late effects. Residuals are shown in italics, and the causes are shown in bold print. Code both the residual effect and the cause.

Use the following guides for coding late effects:

1. Refer to the main term "late—*see also* condition" in ICD-9-CM Volume 2 when coding a case with late effects.
2. Look for the condition.
3. Use two codes when late effects are involved for both the present condition and the initial condition. The late effect code is usually a secondary diagnosis code, with the primary diagnosis code listed as the current residual condition. In some cases the late effect is the sole reason for the office visit; in such cases the late effect code becomes the primary diagnosis.

Now that you have learned the basics of ICD-9-CM coding, the next step is to begin to learn the new system based on ICD-10.

ICD-10-CM DIAGNOSIS AND PROCEDURE CODES

Since 1950, the ICD-9-CM diagnosis system has been used. Although it has been updated, the system has outlived its usefulness because of advances in technology, discovery of new diseases, development of new procedures, the need to report more details for statistical purposes, and for global standardization with other countries. To satisfy this need, ICD-10 was published by the WHO in 1992. It was clinically modified (CM) by the National Center for Health Statistics (NCHS) before code adoption. The CM provides the specifics that the United States needs for collecting data on health status. This became known as the *International Classification of Diseases, Tenth Revision, Clinical Modification* (ICD-10-CM-diagnostic codes). Reasons for clinical modification are the removal of procedural codes, unique mortality codes, and "multiple" codes. Following that, *ICD-10 Procedure Coding System* (ICD-10-PCS-procedure codes) was developed in the mid-1990s by 3M Health Information Systems under contract with the CMS. This replaces Volume 3 of ICD-9-CM used in hospital billing but does not replace the CPT code book used in outpatient billing. The state entities that record vital statistics within the US adopted ICD-10 for reporting diagnosis and external causes on death certificates beginning in 1999. Both hospital and physician office insurance billers should be concerned with the new diagnosis codes, but only hospital billers need to concern themselves with the procedure codes. Beginning in 2005, this coding system has biannual updates on April 1 and October 1.

ICD-10-CM meets HIPAA criteria by providing specific information for outpatient and inpatient procedures, describing medical services using terminology in today's environment, expanding injury and disease codes and categories, and giving a precise, clear, clinical picture of the patient.

Reasons for development of ICD-10-CM and ICD-10-PCS are as follows:

1. ICD-9-CM was not expandable, comprehensive, or multiaxial (broken down into many subdivisions).
2. ICD-9-CM did not have standardized terminology and included diagnostic information.

ICD-10-CM Versus ICD-9-CM

ICD-10-CM differs from ICD-9-CM in the following ways:

1. Major changes in code book organization exist.
2. Many new categories and chapters have been added. For some chapters, the body or organ system is the axis of the classification. Other chapters are grouped together by the nature of the disease, disorder, injury, symptoms, signs, and abnormal findings. For some chapters, the body or organ system is the axis of the classification. Other chapters are grouped together by the nature of the disease, disorder, injury, symptoms, signs, and abnormal findings.
3. There is a replacement of the traditional numeric coding system with a six-digit and sometimes seven-digit alphanumeric scheme for ICD-10-CM (Figure 5-4). Obstetrics, injuries, and external causes of injuries may have seven-digit codes. Some codes include last-digit alpha characters "A," "B," "D," "G," "J," or "Q" to identify initial encounter, subsequent encounter, or sequelae. These are referred to as extensions and always occupy the final (seventh) character position in an extension code.
4. Old injury (800 to 999) codes have been changed to S and T codes. Currently, coding is done by type of injury, such as fractures, dislocations, and sprains/strains, but ICD-10 coding is by injury site (e.g., injuries to neck, injuries to thorax).
5. Explanatory notes and instructions for use have been greatly expanded and appear at the beginning of chapters or any of the subdivisions that follow. This is the same as in ICD-9-CM.

6. E codes in ICD-9-CM are in ICD-10-CM Chapter 20: External Causes of Morbidity and have developed into V, W, X, and Y Codes (V01 to Y98).
7. V codes in ICD-9-CM are now in Chapter 21: Factors Influencing Health Status and Contact With Health Services (Z00 to Z99).
8. The coding system allows for assignment of unique codes as new procedures are developed.
9. Combination diagnosis/symptom codes have been added. For example, poisoning/external cause codes have been combined.
10. Postoperative complication codes describe both the type and site of complication. A **complication** is a condition arising during the health care episode that modifies the course of the patient's illness or the medical care needed. The following several types of complications exist:
    a. *Misadventure,* an adverse event (accident) occurring during medical or surgical care that is caused by that treatment (e.g., accidental puncture or laceration of the ear during an ear procedure).
    b. *Early complication,* a condition that occurs within 29 days after a procedure but is not known at the time of the procedure.
    c. *Late complication,* a condition that occurs after 29 days following a procedure.
    d. *Sequela,* a current condition resulting from a previously occurring postoperative complication.
    e. *Transient postoperative condition,* a temporary state that exists during the postoperative period but is not regarded as a postoperative complication (e.g., headache, nausea, vomiting, confusion, hypertension, or electrolyte disturbances). Code as a complication when present at discharge, evident longer than normal, or if the physician documents the condition is a complication of the procedure.
11. An activity code category that describes activities in which a patient was engaged when he or she was injured (e.g., horseback riding Y93.013).
12. ICD-10-PCS is much more specific than the CPT coding system when making a comparison.

Format and Structure

As of the printing of this edition, all ICD-10-CM data and information for figures and examples have been obtained from the 2009 draft version. The general structure of ICD-10-CM is as follows:

Official Guidelines for Coding and Reporting

The Official Guidelines section contains definitions, standards, rules, general coding guidelines and 21 chapter specific guidelines. Whereas ICD-9-CM consists of 17 chapters and two supplemental classifications.

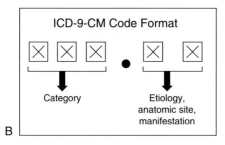

FIGURE 5-4 ICD-10-CM versus ICD-9-CM diagnostic code format. *(From Fordney MT: Fordney's medical insurance dictionary for billers and coders, St. Louis, 2010, Elsevier Science.)*

ICD-9-CM has one chapter for Diseases and Disorders of the Nervous System while ICD-10-CM has these conditions in three separate chapters. Disorders of the immune mechanism are included with diseases of the blood and blood forming organs. Immunity disorders in ICD-9-CM are with the endocrine, nutritional, and metabolic diseases. Some chapters are reordered (e.g., diseases of the skin and subcutaneous tissue [Chapter 12] and diseases of the musculoskeletal system and connective tissue [Chapter 13] follow the chapter for diseases of the digestive system). Next are chapters for diseases of the genitourinary system (Chapter 14), pregnancy, childbirth, and the puerperium (Chapter 15), certain conditions originating in the perinatal period (Chapter 16), and congenital malformations, deformations, and chromosomal abnormalities (Chapter 17).

Alphabetic Index to Diseases and Injuries

The Alphabetic Index contains the Tables of Drugs and Chemicals, Neoplasm Table, and Index to External Causes. It is formatted the same as the Index in the ICD-9-CM. Main code descriptor items are in alphabetic order, and indented subterms, applicable additional qualifiers, descriptors, or modifiers are beneath the main terms.

Tabular List of Diseases and Injuries

The Tabular List contains Chapters 1 through 21 and is composed of alphanumeric codes that represent diagnoses. The ICD-10-CM codes contain up to seven characters with a decimal point after the third character. This is shown as: digit #1 (alpha character), digits #2 to #3 (numeric character), and digits #4 to #7 (alpha or numeric character). The first three characters are placed to the left of the decimal point and indicate the category. The remaining digits to the right of the decimal point indicate the etiology, anatomic site, and severity. The sixth character can signify laterality, the intent of a drug poisoning (intentional self-harm, assault), "with" or "without" a given manifestation, the trimester of a pregnancy, the depth of a skin ulcer, or the nature of an injury. An "X" is used as a placeholder to save space for future code expansion and/or to meet the requirement of coding to the highest level of specificity (Figure 5-5).

ICD-10-CM Code Book Conventions

Quite a number of the conventions used in the ICD-9-CM system such as punctuation, symbols and terminology are used in ICD-10-CM (Box 5-4). However, exceptions not included in ICD-10-CM are the brace (}), lozenge (◇), and section mark (§). It is important to read the explanation for unfamiliar conventions such as how to use alpha extensions and the uppercase letters at the end of some codes that can identify encounter status or current condition.

Combination Code

A **combination code** is a situation in which a single code is used to classify two diagnoses or a diagnosis with an associated secondary process (manifestation) or a diagnosis with an associated complication. Identify a combination code by referring to subterm entries in the Alphabetic Index and by reading the inclusion and exclusion notes in the Tabular List. If the combination code does not specifically describe the manifestation or complication, then use a secondary code.

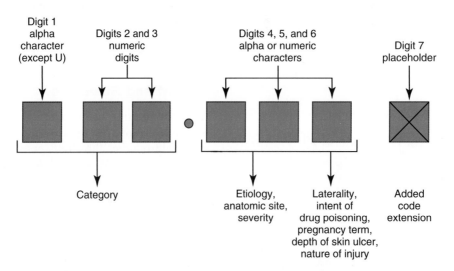

FIGURE 5-5 Explanation of the ICD-10-CM seven-digit positions.

Box 5-4	Official ICD-10-CM Code Book Conventions

Punctuation

[ ]   Brackets are used in the Tabular List to enclose synonyms, alternative wording, or explanatory phrases.
Example: J95.85 Mechanical complication of respirator **[ventilator]**

:   Colons are used in the Tabular List after an incomplete term, which needs one or more of the modifiers following the colon to make it assignable to a given category.
Example: L99 Other disorders of skin and subcutaneous tissue in diseases classified elsewhere
Code first underlying disease, such as:
amyloidosis (E85.-)

-   Dashes are used in both the ICD-10-CM Indexes and the Tabular List. The Indexes use the dash to show the level of indentation. A symbol (-) at the end of an index entry indicates an incomplete code so additional characters are needed. Locate the referenced category or subcategory elsewhere in the Tabular List, review the options, and assign the code.
Example:
Excludes2: cellulitis of fingers (L03.01-)

( )   Parentheses are used in the Tabular List to enclose supplementary words (nonessential modifiers) that may be present or absent in the statement of a disease/condition without affecting the code number to which it was assigned.
Example: N39.3 Stress incontinence **(female) (male)**

Abbreviations

NEC   Not Elsewhere Classifiable in the Tabular List under a code identifies it as an "other specified" code.
Example: A85 Other viral encephalitis, not elsewhere classified
           Includes: specified viral encephalomyelitis **NEC**

NOS   Not Otherwise Specified is equivalent to an unspecified code.
Example: Q66.8 Other congenital deformities of feet
        Congenital clubfoot **NOS**

And

and   This word represents and/or when used in a narrative statement.
Example: B35.0 Tinea barbae **and** tinea capitis

Code first/use additional code

Code first/Use additional code   Notes that certain conditions have both an underlying etiology and multiple body system manifestations due to the underlying etiology. Manifestation code titles have a phrase, "in diseases classified elsewhere." The underlying condition must be sequenced first followed by the manifestation.
Example:
E08 Diabetes mellitus due to underlying condition
Code first the underlying condition, such as:
Congenital rubella (P35.0)
Use additional code to identify any insulin use (Z79.4)

Code also

Code also   Note instructing that two codes may be needed to completely describe a condition dependent on the severity of the conditions and the reason for the encounter.
Example: S85 Injury of blood vessels at lower leg level
Code also any associated open wound (S81.-)

Includes

Includes   *Includes* appears under certain categories to add to the definition or give an example of the content of the category.
Example: S93 Dislocation and sprain of joints and ligaments at ankle, foot, and toe level
Includes: avulsion of joint or ligament of ankle, foot, and toe

Inclusion terms

Inclusion Terms   List of terms included under some codes such as conditions for which that code is to be used, synonyms, or various specified conditions assigned to 'other specified' codes.
Example: C46.1 Kaposi's sarcoma of soft tissue
        Kaposi's sarcoma of blood vessel
        Kaposi's sarcoma of connective tissue
        Kaposi's sarcoma of fascia
        Kaposi's sarcoma of ligament

Continued

Box 5-4   Official ICD-10-CM Code Book Conventions—cont'd

Excludes

Excludes1   An *Excludes1* note should never be used at the same time as the code above the Excludes1 note. It is used when two conditions cannot occur together such as a congenital form versus an acquired form of the same condition.
Example: E20 Hypoparathyroidism
Excludes1: Di George's syndrome (D82.1)

Excludes2   An *Excludes2* note indicates that the condition excluded is not part of the condition represented by the code but a patient may have both conditions at the same time. When an Excludes2 note appears under a code, use both the code and the excluded code together.
Example: I10 Essential (primary) hypertension
Excludes2: Essential (primary) hypertension involving vessels of brain (I60-I69)

See

See   Instruction that follows a main term in the Index indicating another term should be referenced. Go to the main term referenced with the "see" note to find the correct code.
Example: Postphlebitic syndrome—**see** Syndrome, postphlebitic

See also

See also   Instruction following a main term in the Index to indicate there is another main term that may also be referenced and may provide additional index entries that may be useful. It is not necessary to follow the "see also" note when the original main term gives the code.
Example: Preterm delivery (**see also** Pregnancy, complicated by, preterm labor) 060.10

With/without

with/without   When a condition may have two versions: *with* or *without* a specific sign, symptom, or manifestation, this is indicated by a change in one of the code characters. These words in the Alphabetic Index are sequenced following the main term, not in alphabetical order.
Example: Epilepsy, epileptic, epilepsia
    intractable G40.919
    with status epilepticus G40.911
    without status epilepticus G40.919

Examples

J44.0   Chronic obstructive pulmonary disease with acute lower respiratory infection
    Use additional code to identify the infection
G03   Meningitis due to other and unspecified causes
    Includes: arachnoiditis NOS
    Excludes1: meningomyelitis (G04.-)

Default Code

Default code is shown next to a main term in the Alphabetic Index and represents the condition that is commonly associated with the main term or is the unspecified code for the condition. For example, if the EHR documents appendicitis but does not list acute or chronic, then the default code should be assigned.

Example

Cracked tooth   K03.81

Morphology Codes

Morphology codes (M codes) are located in the Alphabetic Index the same as they were in ICD-9-CM, but do not confuse these with the codes in Chapter 13: Diseases of the Musculoskeletal System and Connective Tissue that also begin with the letter "M."

Example

Lymphosarcoma (diffuse) (M9592/3)

Neoplasm Codes

Neoplasm codes may begin with the letter "C" or "D."

Examples

C03 Malignant neoplasm of gum
D00.1 Carcinoma in situ of esophagus

Acute, Subacute, and Chronic Conditions

When the documentation mentions that a condition is both acute (subacute) and chronic and separate codes exist in the Alphabetic Index, both are coded with the acute (subacute) sequenced first followed by the code for the chronic condition.

Examples

Appendicitis (pneumococcal) (retrocecal) K37
    acute (catarrhal) (fulminating) (gangrenous)
        (obstructive) (retrocecal) (suppurative) K35.9
    subacute (adhesive) K36
    chronic (recurrent) K36

Bilateral Sites

The right side is always character 1 and the left side character 2. In those situations when a bilateral code is given, the bilateral character is always 3. If the side is not identified, an unspecified code is provided, which is either a character 0 or 9, depending on whether it is a fifth or sixth character.

Examples

S67.0 Crushing injury of thumb
    S67.00 Crushing injury of thumb of unspecified side
    S67.01 Crushing injury of right thumb
    S67.02 Crushing injury of left thumb

Other and Unspecified Codes

Codes titled "other" or "other specified" are for use when the information in the medical record gives detail for which a specific code does not exist. Alphabetic Index entries with NEC (not elsewhere classifiable) in the line designate "other" codes in the Tabular List. These Index entries represent specific disease entities for which no specific code exists so the term is included within an "other" code.

In ICD-10-CM a code with a fourth digit 9 or fifth digit 0 for diagnosis codes titled "unspecified" are used when the information in the medical record is insufficient to assign a more specific code. For those categories for which an unspecified code is not provided, the "other specified" code may represent both other and unspecified (Figure 5-6). Note: ICD-9-CM, four-digit subcategories .8 and .9 usually but not always are reserved for "other specified" and "unspecified" conditions, respectively. "Other specified" and "unspecified" subcategories are referred to as *residual subcategories*.

Residual subcategories are used for conditions that are specifically named in the medical record but not specifically listed under a code description. If there is a lack of details in the medical record and you cannot match to a specific subdivision, research the medical record for a qualifying statement in the physician's progress notes or history and physical examination report that will allow you to use a more specific diagnostic code (Figure 5-7).

Gender and Age Codes

Diagnostic codes must match the age and gender of the patient. If an adult female patient with breast cancer is seen (excluding carcinoma in situ and skin cancer of breast), a code from the ICD-10-CM Neoplasm Table must be used. In ICD-9-CM, codes 174.0 through 174.9 must be used. If a male with breast cancer is treated, an ICD-9-CM code from 175.0 through 175.9 must be chosen. Some codes apply only to newborns such as code P70.2 (ICD-10-CM) or 775.1 (ICD-9-CM) for neonatal diabetes mellitus.

Transition to ICD-10-CM

ICD-10-CM allows more code choices and requires greater documentation in the medical record. An experienced coder should develop a proactive, positive attitude toward accepting and learning the ICD-10-CM. A coder must have a higher level of clinical knowledge. It is wise to attend an anatomy and physiology course a year before the

	ICD-10-CM		ICD-9-CM	
M33.20	**Polymyositis**	710.4	**Polymyositis** ◄───────────────	Specified

M35.8	**Eosinophilia myalgia syndrome**	710.5	**Eosinophilia myalgia syndrome**
			    Toxic oil syndrome
			    Use additional E code to identify
			        drug if drug induced	

M35.8	**Other specified systemic
	involvement of connective tissue**
		710.8	**Other specified diffuse** ◄──────
			diseases of connective tissue
			    Multifocal fibrosclerosis (idiopathic)
			        NEC
			    Systemic fibrosclerosing syndrome
				Other specified

M35.9	**Systemic involvement of connective tissue, unspecified**	710.9	**Unspecified diffuse connective tissue** ◄── **disease** Collagen disease NOS	Unspecified

FIGURE 5-6 Example of specified, other specified, and unspecified disease conditions for ICD-9-CM and ICD-10-CM.

FIGURE 5-7 Insurance billing specialist looking up a patient's medical record file to verify documentation for a diagnostic code.

Example 5-23   Acute and Chronic Pelvic Inflammatory Disease (Female)

	ICD-10-CM	ICD-9-CM
Condition:	Disease	Disease
Subcategories:	Pelvis, Pelvic	Pelvis, Pelvic
Sub-subcategory:	Inflammatory (female) N73.9	Inflammatory
	Acute N73.0	Acute 614.3
	Chronic N73.1	Chronic 614.4

new system is adopted if you have not already done so. It is vital to attend training workshops that will be offered as the time approaches for mandatory use of ICD-10-CM. As of the publication of this textbook, the US House of Representatives legislation calls for an implementation date by October 1, 2013. To gain knowledge and proficiency, many hours of instruction may be necessary to learn the new system. Even after a person learns how to code, it takes a longer time to code under the new system.

The step-by-step procedure for the basic steps in selecting ICD-10-CM diagnostic codes is presented at the end of this chapter.

Publishers of ICD-10-CM may use different styles and formats, so it is important to study and compare the features of several books before making a decision to purchase. When choosing a book, the following questions should be asked: Is color coding being used for emphasis in locating items quickly? Are definitions or notes included to help one interpret and gain a better understanding of difficult medical terms and phrases? Are coding guidelines boxed for easy reference? Are icons or symbols used? All of these benefit the coder.

Selection of an ICD-9 Versus an ICD-10 Code

Now use a step-by-step approach to code acute and chronic pelvic inflammatory disease and refer to each volume, as shown in Example 5-23.

Identify possible codes from the Alphabetic Index, Volume 2. Then go to the Tabular List, Volume 1, to verify that the code number selected is in accord with the desired classification of the diagnosis. Look for important instructions that often appear. Check for exclusion notes, which refer to terms or conditions that are not included

within the code. These may further direct the coder to the correct ICD-9-CM code assignment (Figure 5-8, *A*).

An "excludes" note may appear listing diagnoses and additional codes to research to ensure that the correct code is assigned. As shown in Figure 5-8, *B*, this example appears on the insurance claim in ICD-10-CM as K30 and in ICD-9-CM keyed without the decimal as 5368. Heartburn is not coded because it is a symptom of dyspepsia and appears as an exclusion under dyspepsia.

Certain conditions are classified according to etiology (cause) of the disorder (Figure 5-9). In these cases, you should follow the instructions "Code first underlying disease. ..." Code the etiology in the first position. Code the disorder in the second position. Words to look for in the diagnostic statement include "acquired," "congenital," "associated with," "obstetric," "nonobstetric," "transmissible," "not transmissible," "traumatic," and "nontraumatic."

Special Points to Remember in the Tabular List

- Use two or more codes if necessary to completely describe a given diagnosis. Example: Arteriosclerotic cardiovascular *disease* I25.10 (ICD-10-CM) or 429.2 (ICD-9-CM) with congestive heart failure I50.9 (ICD-10-CM) or 428.0 (ICD-9-CM).
- Search for one code when two diagnoses or a diagnosis with an associated secondary process (manifestation) or complication is present. There are instances when two diagnoses are classified with a single code number called a *combination code*.
- Use category codes (three-digit codes) only if there are no subcategory codes (fourth-digit subdivisions).

Special Points to Remember in Volume 2

- Notice that appropriate sites or modifiers are listed in alphabetic order under the main terms, with further subterm listings as needed.

A   **The Patient's Diagnosis is Dyspepsia and Heartburn**

		ICD-10-CM	ICD-9-CM
Step 1.	Look for the code number—not the page number—in the tabular list.	K30	536.8
Step 2.	Notice that there is an exclusion note for heartburn indicating the code number.	R12	787.1
Step 3.	Be sure to check that code number in the tabular list.		

B   **Dyspepsia and other specified disorders of function of stomach**

ICD-10-CM   **ICD-9-CM**

K30 Dyspepsia
    Includes: indigestion
    Excludes1: heartburn (R12)
              nervous dyspepsia (F45.8)
              neurotic dyspepsia (F45.8)
              psychogenic dyspepsia (F45.8)

536.8 Dyspepsia and other specified disorders of function of stomach
    Achylia gastrica
    Hourglass contraction of stomach
    Hyperacidity
    Hyperchlorhydria
    Hypochlorhydria
    Indigestion
    Excludes: achlorhydria (536.0)
               heartburn (787.1)

FIGURE 5-8 A, Example of a disease to look up in the Tabular Lists of ICD-10-CM and ICD-9-CM. **B,** Illustration of coding showing exclusion notes from the Tabular Lists of ICD-10-CM and ICD-9-CM.

ICD-10-CM   **ICD-9-CM**
M07.60 Arthropathy associated   713.1 **Arthropathy associated**
    with gastrointestinal   **with gastrointestinal**
    conditions other than infections   **conditions other than infections**

Code first underlying disease as:
    regional enteritis   K50.90   555.0-555.9
    ulcerative colitis   K51.90   556

FIGURE 5-9 Coding by etiology for ICD-10-CM and ICD-9-CM.

Pancreatitis (annular) (apoplectic) (calcareous) ←—— **Nonessential**
    (edematous) (hemorrhagic) (malignant)   **modifiers**
    (recurrent) (subacute) (suppurative) K85.9

FIGURE 5-10 Coding with modifiers in parentheses.

    ➤ **Gamstorp's disease** (adynamia episodica hereditaria)
Eponyms   G72.3
    ➤ **Gandy-Nanta disease** (siderotic splenomegaly) D73.1

FIGURE 5-11 Coding diagnoses associated with an eponym.

- Examine all nonessential modifiers that appear in parentheses next to the main term. Check for nonessential modifiers that apply to any of the qualifying terms used in the statement of the diagnosis found in the patient's medical record (Figure 5-10).
- Notice that eponyms appear as both main term entries and modifiers under main terms such as "disease" or "syndrome" and "operation." As mentioned in Chapter 4 and shown in Example 4.2, an **eponym** is the name of a disease, structure, operation, or procedure, usually derived from the name of a place or a person who discovered or described it first.
- Look for sublisted terms in parentheses that are associated with the eponym (Figure 5-11).
- Locate closely related terms, code categories, and cross-referenced synonyms indicated by *see* and *see also* (Figure 5-12).

Inflammation, inflamed, inflammatory
(with exudation)-*continued*

spinal
    cord (*see also* Encephalitis) 323.9
    late effect—*see* category 326
    membrane—*see* Meningitis
    nerve—*see* Disorder, nerve

FIGURE 5-12 Cross-referencing synonyms, closely related terms, and code categories from the Alphabetic Index of *International Classification of Diseases, Ninth Revision, Clinical Modification* (ICD-9-CM), Volume 2.

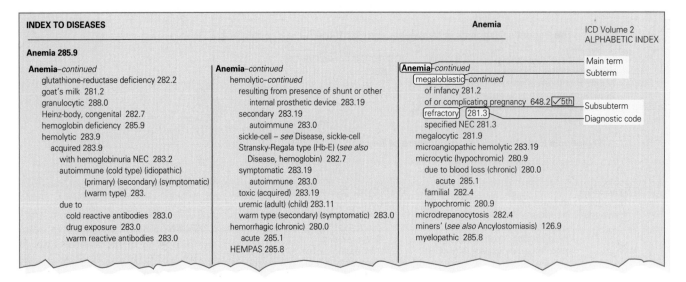

FIGURE 5-13 Excerpt from the Alphabetic Index of *International Classification of Diseases, 9th Revision, Clinical Modification* (ICD-9-CM), Volume 2.

PROCEDURE 5-1

Basic Steps in Selecting Diagnostic Codes From ICD-9-CM

OBJECTIVE: Accurately select and insert diagnostic codes for electronic transmission of an insurance claim

EQUIPMENT/SUPPLIES: Diagnostic code book (Volumes 1 and 2), medical dictionary, and pen or pencil

DIRECTIONS: Use a standard method and establish a routine for locating a code. Follow these recommended steps for coding the first diagnosis. There are no short-cuts. For each subsequent diagnosis in a patient's medical record, repeat these steps. Refer to Figure 5-13 as you go through Step 1.

DIAGNOSIS: Refractory megaloblastic anemia, with chronic alcoholic liver disease

1. Read the patient's medical record. Identify the main term or condition (not the anatomic site) in the Alphabetic Index, Volume 2 (anemia). To locate the main term, ask what is wrong with the patient.
2. Refer to any notes under the main term (none shown).
3. Read any notes or terms enclosed in parentheses after the main term (nonessential modifiers) (none shown).
4. Look for appropriate subterm (megaloblastic). *Do not* skip over any subterms indented under the main term.
5. Look for appropriate sub-subterm (refractory).

6. Follow any cross-reference instructions (none given).
7. Write down the code (281.3).
8. Verify the code number in the Tabular List, Volume 1 (Figure 5-14).
9. Read and be guided by any instructional terms in the Tabular List. In this example, there are none given.
10. Read complete description and then code to the highest specificity; that is, code to the highest number of digits (three, four, or five) in the classification (refractory megaloblastic anemia, 281.3). When a fourth or fifth digit is listed, its use is NOT optional. A three-digit code is considered a category unless no fourth or fifth digit appears after it. Fifth-digit codes appear either at the beginning of a chapter, section, or three-digit category, or within the four-digit subcategory. To facilitate locating those codes that require a fourth or fifth digit, some publishers may insert a symbol (e.g., *f*) in the code book. Do not arbitrarily use a zero as a filler character when listing a diagnostic code number. This may nullify the code or indicate a different disease. The code book includes decimal points, but these are not required for transmission of insurance claims.
11. Assign the code.

FIGURE 5-14 Excerpt from the Tabular List of *International Classification of Diseases, 9th Revision, Clinical Modification* (ICD-9-CM), Volume 1.

PROCEDURE 5-2

Basic Steps in Selecting Diagnostic Codes From ICD-10-CM

OBJECTIVE: Accurately choose and insert diagnostic codes for electronic transmission of an insurance claim

EQUIPMENT/SUPPLIES: ICD-10-CM diagnostic code book (download latest draft version from Internet), medical dictionary, and pen or pencil

DIRECTIONS: Use a standard method and establish a routine for locating a code. Follow these steps for coding the first diagnosis. For each subsequent diagnosis in a patient's medical record, repeat these steps.

1. Read the patient's medical record to find the main term. To identify the main term, ask what is wrong with the patient.

2. Next locate the main term (disease or condition), not the anatomic site, in Volume 3 of the Alphabetic Index. When reviewing the main terms, notice that ICD-10-CM has a higher level of specificity than ICD-9-CM. The Alphabetic Index is organized by main terms and has three sections:

   Section 1—Index to Diseases and Nature of Injury includes Neoplasm Table and Table of Drugs and Chemicals

   Section 2—Index to External Causes of Injury

   Section 3—Table of Drugs and Chemicals

3. Read any notes under the main term. Notice similar conventions as with ICD-9-CM such as "see," "see also," and notes that appear to define terms, provide directions, and give coding instructions. Follow any instructions. The alphanumeric structure of ICD-10-CM is also more specific than that of ICD-9-CM. Select and write down the code.

4. Next go to the Tabular List, review how it is organized for the subclassification, read and be guided by any instructional terms, and then verify that the selected code gives the highest level of specificity (up to seven alphanumeric characters). Possible errors may occur when using the Tabular List and when coding diseases or conditions that begin with categories "O" and "I." These can look like the numbers "zero" and "one" (e.g., I00 and O99 are correct and not 100 and 099). In these categories, special attention must be given. Do not confuse Morphology Codes (M codes) with the codes in Chapter 13, Diseases of the Musculoskeletal System and Connective Tissue that also begin with the letter "M."

5. Always read the specific chapter guidelines and refer to the general guidelines in the code book for certain diagnoses and/or conditions in the classification before choosing a code.

6. Assign the code.

KEY POINTS

This is a brief chapter review or summary of the key issues presented. To further enhance your knowledge of the technical subject matter, review the key terms and key abbreviations for this chapter by locating the meanings in the glossary at the end of this book that appear in a section before the index.

1. Accurate diagnostic coding can mean the financial success or failure of a medical practice.
2. Payment for outpatient services is related to procedure codes but must be supported and justified by the diagnosis.
3. Diagnostic coding was developed for the following reasons: (1) tracking of disease processes, (2) classification of causes of mortality, (3) medical research, and (4) evaluation of hospital service utilization.
4. When submitting insurance claims for patients seen in a physician's office or an outpatient hospital setting, the primary diagnosis, which is the main reason for the encounter, is listed first. For inpatient hospital coding, the principal diagnosis is the diagnosis obtained after study that prompted the hospitalization.
5. Always use ICD-9-CM Volume 2, the Alphabetic Index, and then go to Volume 1, the Tabular (numerical) List before assigning a diagnostic code. When selecting an ICD-10-CM code, do the same.

6. Always code to the highest degree of specificity. The more digits a code has, the more specific the description is.
7. Always code the underlying disease, the etiology or cause, first and subsequently list the secondary diagnosis.
8. V codes in ICD-9-CM are used when a person who is not currently sick encounters health services for some specific purpose such as to receive a vaccination. In ICD-10-CM these codes begin with the letter "Z."
9. E codes in ICD-9-CM are used for external causes of injury rather than the nature of the injury or disease and for coding adverse reactions to medications. In ICD-10-CM these codes begin with V, W, X, and Y.
10. Always follow coding conventions because they assist in the selection of correct codes for the diagnoses encountered. These conventions are rules or principles for determining a diagnostic code when using diagnostic code books such as each space, typefaces, indentations, punctuation marks, symbols, instructional notes, abbreviations, cross-reference notes, and specific usage of the words "and," "with," and "due to."

⊖volve INTERNET RESOURCES

For active links to the following resources, visit the Evolve website at
http://evolve.elsevier.com/fordney/handbook

● AHIMA diagnostic code guidelines for outpatient services and diagnostic coding and reporting requirements for physician billing.

● Code guidelines for the Centers for Medicare and Medicaid Services.
● Download the November 2010 final draft of ICD-10-PCS.

STUDENT ASSIGNMENT

✓ Study Chapter 5.
✓ Answer the fill-in-the-blank, multiple choice, and true/false review questions in the *Workbook* to reinforce theory learned in this chapter and to help prepare you for a future test.

✓ Complete the assignments in the *Workbook* to gain hands-on experience in diagnostic coding.
✓ Turn to the glossary at the end of this textbook for a further understanding of the key terms and key abbreviations used in this chapter.

KEY TERMS*

alternative billing codes
bilateral
bundled codes
comprehensive code
conversion factor
Current Procedural Terminology
customary fee
downcoding
fee schedule
global surgery policy

Healthcare Common Procedure
  Coding System
modifiers
never event
procedure code numbers
professional component
reasonable fee
relative value studies
relative value unit

resource-based relative value
  scale
surgical package
technical component
unbundling
upcoding
usual, customary, and
  reasonable

KEY ABBREVIATIONS*

ABCs
AHA
CF
CPT
DME
ECG

ED
E/M services
EMTALA
EOB
FTC
GAF

GPCIs
HCPCS
NCCI edits
PC
RVS
RVU

RBRVS
TC
UCR

*Definitions for the key terms and key abbreviations are located near the back of this textbook in the glossary.

CHAPTER 6

Procedural Coding

OBJECTIVES

After reading this chapter, you should be able to:

- Explain the purpose and importance of coding for professional services.
- Define terminology used in *Current Procedural Terminology* (CPT).
- Demonstrate an understanding of CPT code conventions.
- Describe various methods of payment by insurance companies and state and federal programs.
- Describe the process in which the Healthcare Common Procedure Coding System (HCPCS) and a Relative Value System (RVS) are used to create a fee schedule.

- Interpret the meaning of CPT code book symbols.
- Identify the complexity of Evaluation and Management (E/M) services codes.
- Compare a surgical package and a Medicare global package.
- Explain various types of code edits.
- Explain how to choose accurate procedure codes for descriptions of services and procedures documented in a patient's medical record.
- Explain correct usage of modifiers in procedure coding.

Service to Patients

Procedure codes must reflect the services rendered to the patient so that optimal payment is generated by an insurance plan based on selection of the correct code. Codes are chosen dependent on supporting documentation in the patient's medical record.

UNDERSTANDING THE IMPORTANCE OF PROCEDURAL CODING SKILLS

Now that you have learned some terminology and the basics of diagnostic coding, the next step is to learn how to code procedures.

Procedure coding is the transformation of written descriptions of procedures and professional services into numeric designations (code numbers). The physician rendering medical care either writes or dictates this information into the patient's health record. Then the insurance billing specialist reads through the pertinent information and verifies this with the procedure codes marked on the encounter form. Routine office visits and procedures usually are listed with codes and brief descriptions on the encounter form. These services are documented in the record and circled or checked off on the encounter form by the physician when they are performed during the patient's visit.

With the implementation of computer technology and stricter adherence to federal regulations, more emphasis is being placed on correct procedural coding. Coding must be correct if claims are to be paid promptly and optimally.

Performance objectives, testing and review material, and hands-on practical exercises for this chapter are available in these resources

 The Insurance Handbook Student Workbook   The Insurance Handbook Evolve Site

161

Every procedure or service must be assigned correct and complete code numbers. Because of the complexity of procedural coding, a working knowledge of medical terminology, including anatomy and physiology, is essential.

Procedure codes are a standardized method used to precisely describe the services provided by physicians and allied health care professionals. They allow claim forms to be optically scanned by insurance companies. The general acceptance of the codes by third-party payers and government agencies assures the physician who uses a standardized coding system that the services and procedures he or she performs can be objectively identified and priced. The American Hospital Association (AHA) and American Health Information Management Association (AHIMA) guidelines for outpatient services and procedure coding and reporting requirements for physician billing may be found by visiting the Evolve website listed in the Internet Resources at the end of this chapter. The website has active links to these associations. The AHA Central Office is the official clearinghouse for information on proper use of ICD-9-CM codes, Level I HCPCS codes (CPT-4 codes) for hospital providers, and certain Level II HCPCS codes for hospitals, physicians, and other health care professionals.

The primary coding system used in physicians' offices for professional services and procedures is *Current Procedural Terminology* **(CPT)***, published and updated annually by the American Medical Association (AMA). To obtain a current copy of CPT, visit the AMA's website listed in the Internet Resources at the end of this chapter. A relative value scale, called **relative value studies (RVS)**, is also used for services and procedures; it is the system used by Medicare called *resource-based relative value scale* (RBRVS). RVS and RBRVS provide unit values for CPT codes that can then be converted into dollars by use of geographic and conversion factors.

Some managed care plans develop a few internal codes for use by the plan only. Sometimes the codes are used for tracking; other times, they are used to provide reimbursement for a service not defined within CPT on the basis of their benefit structure and internal needs.

Current Procedural Terminology

The first edition of *Physicians' Current Procedural Terminology* appeared in 1966, and the book was subsequently revised in 1970, 1973, and 1977. Since 1984, *Current Procedural Terminology* (CPT), fourth edition, has been updated and revised annually. Code numbers are added

CODING COMPLIANCE PLAN

Because the government is more involved in health care, each medical practice should construct and maintain a policy and procedure manual in regard to coding guidelines for its medical practice so that it is in compliance with HIPAA. Establishing coding and billing policies and procedures helps physicians and their office staff address potential risk areas for fraud and abuse. A plan should include the medical practice's basic ethical philosophy, outline policies, detail coding procedures, and create an environment of confidentiality. Billers and coders should sign a statement annually indicating that they have read, understood, and agreed with the medical practice's standards of conduct (see Figure 2-5). The plan should provide coders with the framework for correct coding and indicate that health record documentation must support the codes billed. An internal audit should be done on a regular basis, and action should be taken to correct the offense if noncompliance is discovered. Such plans must have a compliance officer or a committee that oversees the audits, monitors compliance issues, and trains employees in compliance issues.

or deleted as new procedures are developed or existing procedures are modified. These changes are shown in each edition by the use of symbols, which are described and shown later in this chapter in Figure 6-4. The symbols with their meanings are located at the bottom of each page of code numbers in the CPT code book.

CPT uses a basic five-digit system for coding services rendered by physicians and two-digit add-on **modifiers** to indicate circumstances in which a procedure as performed differs in some way from that described in the code. **Procedure code numbers** represent diagnostic and therapeutic services on medical billing statements and insurance forms (Example 6-1).*

CPT emerged as the procedural coding of choice when the federal government developed the Health Care Financing Administration (HCFA) Common Procedure Coding System (HCPCS) (pronounced "hick-picks") for the Medicare Program. The HCFA changed its acronym to CMS (Centers for Medicare and Medicaid Services); therefore the HCPCS acronym is translated as **Healthcare Common Procedure Coding System (HCPCS)**. The Medicare HCPCS consists of the following two levels of coding:

---

*Available from Book and Pamphlet Fulfillment: OP-3416, American Medical Association, P.O. Box 10946, Chicago, IL 60610-0946, or visit CPT on the Internet at website www.amaassn.org/cpt.

---

*Examples shown in this chapter reflect wording pertinent to coding a specific procedure and may be missing complete chart entries, therefore there may be a gap of information for the reader.

Example 6-1 Current Procedural Terminology Procedure Code Numbers

A 45-year-old woman is seen for an initial office visit for evaluation of recurrent right shoulder pain. The patient's condition warranted a detailed history and physical examination (D HX & PX) with low complexity medical decision making (LCMDM). The patient complains of pain radiating down her right arm. A complete radiographic study of the right shoulder is obtained in the office and read by the physician. A corticosteroid solution is injected into the shoulder joint.

CPT Code	Description of Services
99203	Office visit, new patient **(E/M service)**
73030	Radiologic examination, shoulder, two views **(Diagnostic service)**
20610	Arthrocentesis inj.; major joint, shoulder **(Therapeutic service)**

- Level I: The AMA CPT codes and modifiers (national codes).
- Level II: CMS-designated codes and alpha modifiers (national codes). Table 6-1 lists the Level II HCPCS national code content and code ranges with details of each alphanumeric code category. Several companies annually publish Level II HCPCS code books. Content, numbers of the appendices, color-coded coverage instructions, notes, and unlisted procedures vary between the editions. Notes or special instructions may appear in or following subsections or headings or as part of the description in a heading or code. Unlisted procedures may use one of the following terms: *unlisted, not otherwise classified (NOC), unspecified, unclassified, other,* or *miscellaneous.* Examples of level II codes may be found in Table 2 of Appendix B of the *Workbook.*

Table 6-1 Level II HCPCS National Code Content

CODE CATEGORY	CONTENTS	CODE RANGES
Index	Alphabetically arranged.	
A codes	Transportation services, including ambulance (medical and surgical supplies, administrative, and miscellaneous and investigational services and supplies).	A0000-A9999
B codes	Enteral and parenteral therapy.	B4000-B9999
C codes	Outpatient prospective payment system (OPPS) services	C1000-C9999
D codes	Dental procedures (diagnostic, preventive, restorative, endodontic, periodontic, prosthodontic, prosthetic, orthodontic, and surgical). These codes have been removed from the official HCPCS list but remain available from and are maintained by the American Dental Association.	D0000-D9999
E codes	Durable medical equipment (canes, crutches, walkers, commodes, decubitus care, bath and toilet aids, hospital beds, oxygen and related respiratory equipment, monitoring equipment, pacemakers, patient lifts, safety equipment, restraints, traction equipment, fracture frames, wheelchairs, and artificial kidney machines).	E0100-E9999
G codes	Procedures and professional services (temporary) under review before inclusion in the CPT code book.	G0000-G9999
H codes	Alcohol and drug abuse treatment services.	H0001-H9999
J codes	Drugs administered other than oral method (chemotherapy drugs, immunosuppressive drugs, inhalation solutions, and miscellaneous drugs and solutions).	J0100-J9999
K codes	Temporary codes (durable medical equipment and drugs). When these codes are approved for permanent inclusion in HCPCS, they become A, E, or J codes.	K0000-K9999
L codes	Orthotic procedures and devices (prosthetic devices, scoliosis equipment, orthopedic shoes, and prosthetic implants).	L0100-L4999
M codes	Medical services (office services, cellular therapy, prolotherapy, intragastric hypothermia, IV chelation therapy, and fabric wrapping of an abdominal aneurysm).	M0000-M0301
P codes	Pathology and laboratory services.	P0000-P9999
Q codes	Miscellaneous temporary codes.	Q0000-Q9999
R codes	Diagnostic radiology services codes.	R0000-R9999
S codes	Temporary national codes (non-Medicare) replaced many of the Level III (local) codes, which have been phased out.	S0009-S9999
T codes	National T codes established for state Medicaid agencies and not valid for Medicare.	T1000-T9999
V codes	Vision, hearing, and speech-language pathology services.	V0000-V2999
Appendix 1	Table of Drugs. (Drugs listed by their generic names with amount, route of administration, and code number. Brand names are listed with reference to the generic drug name.)	
Appendix 2	Modifiers.	
Appendix 3	Abbreviations and Acronyms.	
Appendix 4	Pub 100 References (lists revisions to the CMS Manual).	
Appendix 5	New, changed, deleted, and reinstated HCPCS codes.	
Appendix 6	Place of service and type of service.	

Additional contents in some HCPCS code books are place of service and type of service codes for professional claims.
CMS, Centers for Medicare and Medicaid Services; *CPT, Current Procedural Terminology; HCPCS,* Healthcare Common Procedure Coding System; *IV,* intravenous.

You may discover that one case can be coded in two coding levels. The CPT code should be used when both a CPT and Level II code have the same description. The Level II code should be used if the descriptions are not identical (e.g., if the CPT code narrative is generic and the HCPCS Level II code is specific).

The guideline for selecting a code that most accurately identifies the service is as follows:

- *Level I HCPCS CPT code* describes physician or provider service (PPS)
- *Level II HCPCS national code* describes ambulance, medical and surgical supplies, enteral and parenteral therapy, outpatient PPS, dental procedures, durable medical equipment, procedures/professional services, alcohol and drug abuse treatment services, drugs administered other than oral method, orthotic procedures, prosthetic procedures, other medical services, pathology and laboratory services, casting and splinting supplies, diagnostic radiology services, temporary non-Medicare codes, T codes for state Medicaid agencies, and vision and hearing services

Some private insurance companies have begun to accept Level II HCPCS codes. It is wise to check the payer's provider manual or telephone the third-party payer before sending in claims for medications and durable medical equipment. The HCPCS is updated each January 1 with periodic updates made throughout the year as needed. (See Chapter 12 for additional information on coding for Medicare cases.) In some states the TRICARE and Medicaid programs accept HCPCS codes. Most commercial insurance companies have adopted the Level I (CPT) and Level II (HCPCS) code systems.

A step-by-step procedure is presented at the end of this chapter on how to use a HCPCS code book for billing purposes.

Under HIPAA, providers and medical facilities are responsible for using ICD-9-CM diagnostic codes to document why patients are seen and CPT-4 and HCPCS for what is done to patients during their encounter. They are also responsible for implementing the updated codes in a timely manner, using the HIPAA-mandated transaction code set codes, and deleting old or obsolete codes.

Alternative Billing Codes

Alternative billing codes (ABCs) were created and distributed by Alternative Links and approved for a pilot study. They are five-character alphabetic symbols with appended two-character practitioner modifiers that represent the practitioner type. These codes represent more than 4000 integrative health care products and services (Example 6-2). Integrative health care is care that incorporates the best approaches from conventional and complementary and alternative medicine.

The following areas of health care are represented by the ABC codes and are within specialty areas:

Acupuncturist	Massage therapy
Ayurvedic medicine	Mental health care
Body work	Midwifery
Botanical medicine	Minority health care
Chiropractic	Naturopathic medicine
Clinical nutrition	Oriental medicine
Conventional nursing	Osteopathic medicine
Holistic dentists and	Physical medicine
physicians	Somatic educational
Homeopathy	Spiritual and prayer-
Indigenous medicine	based healing

Example 6-2   ABC Code With Modifier

The following descriptions illustrate the coding hierarchy of ABC codes with modifiers.
CODE: CEBAM-1G High-risk pregnancy identification, Antepartum, Midwifery, Practice specialties

Section	Subsection	Heading	Code	Practitioner modifier
C	E	B	AM	-1G
↓	↓	↓	↓	↓
Practice Specialties	Midwifery	Prenatal	Intervention Management	Certified Nurse Midwife

CODE: BFBAJ-1H Weight management

Section	Subsection	Heading	Code	Practitioner modifier
B	F	B	AJ	-1H
↓	↓	↓	↓	↓
Multispecialty	Nutrition Services	Management	Interventions Weight Management, group, each 15 min	Nurse Practitioner

As of October 16, 2006, Alternative Link discontinued its pilot study. Covered entities under HIPAA may not use the codes in HIPAA transactions but may use them for non-HIPAA transactions, for research, management, and manual or paper-based commerce. Alternative Links continually refines the code set and has modeled the structure of the code set and fee schedule after systems that are already part of the transaction and code set regulations of HIPAA to ease their anticipated assimilation. This company established a relative value unit scale similar to the reimbursement process of the Medicare physician fee schedule. It includes a conversion factor that is annually updated. For electronic commerce, which is a federally regulated use of code sets under HIPAA, ABC codes may be used by any of more than 10,000 entities that secured rights to use the codes under section 45CFR162.940 of the Code of Federal Regulations and their contractual trading partners. Some coded procedures require additional certification or training, and those codes may be used if a practitioner can supply the documentation.

ABC codes may become mandatory. Sandia Health System in New Mexico has been paying ABC-coded claims since 1999. Numerous payers are in the process of implementing the ABC codes for payment. For current information on this subject, to order code resources, or to file a petition for the rights to use the codes, visit the Evolve website listed in the Internet Resources at the end of this chapter for an active link to Alternative Links.

METHODS OF PAYMENT

Private insurance companies, as well as federal and state programs, adopt different methods for establishing payment rates for outpatient services: (1) fee schedules; (2) usual, customary, and reasonable (UCR); and (3) relative value scales or schedules. Additional methods of payment for inpatient hospital claims are discussed in Chapter 17.

Fee Schedule

A **fee schedule** is simply a listing of accepted charges or established allowances for specific medical procedures. A medical practice can have more than one fee schedule unless specific state laws restrict this practice. Charges refer to the regular rates established by the provider for services rendered to both Medicare beneficiaries and to other paying patients. Charges should be related consistently to the cost of the services and uniformly applied to all patients whether inpatient or outpatient. The following situations can occur:

1. Providers *participating* in the Medicare program would typically be paid by the fiscal agent an amount from a fee schedule for Medicare patients.

2. Providers *not participating* in the Medicare program would be paid by the fiscal agent an amount based on limiting charges for each service set by the Medicare program.
3. Providers having a contractual arrangement with a managed care plan (e.g., health maintenance organization, individual practice association, preferred provider organization) would be paid on the basis of the fee schedule written into the negotiated contract.
4. Providers rendering services to those who have sustained industrial injuries use a separate workers' compensation fee schedule (see Chapter 15).

Section 1128(b) of the Social Security Act states that a physician may risk exclusion or suspension from the Medicare program if his or her Medicare charges are "substantially in excess of such individual's or entity's usual charges." An exception is charges negotiated for managed care contracts that are not considered the physician's usual charges. In those cases, it is possible that Medicare patients may be charged more than managed care patients. By implementing multiple fee schedules, a provider may risk charging federal or state health programs a fee that might be construed as more than the provider's "usual" charge for a given service. This could potentially result in a violation of the Social Security Act and managed care agreements.

To prevent a possible violation of Section 1128(b) of the Social Security Act, the provider should assign one fee for each procedure code when establishing a fee schedule. This fee should be billed to all third-party payers and to self-pay patients. The provider can establish fees on the basis of the amount that the payer reimburses, which is based on the contract with the insurance plan. By establishing one fee for each procedure instead of multiple fees for each procedure, the provider helps establish the usual and customary fee for his or her geographic area. By monitoring payments, it is possible to observe when third-party payers raise their allowable rates, which cannot be done if sending a claim on the basis of the payer's allowable. It is equally important to monitor third-party payer adjustments to determine how much revenue is lost because of poor contracts and to monitor employee theft.

The fees should be above the maximums paid by the third-party payers to whom the practice generally bills. Your physician employer may wish to evaluate the fee schedules annually to decide whether fees should be raised for certain procedures or services.

Because mistakes can be costly in terms of lost revenue and possible violations, one fee schedule for all patients, with provisions for financial hardship cases, is usually the safest course for health care providers. The physician may want to evaluate the fee schedule in use to annually increase fees caused by cost-of-living and cost-of-supply increases. Such a process is discussed later in the section on Developing a Fee Schedule Using Relative Value Studies Conversion Factors.

Usual, Customary, and Reasonable

Usual, customary, and reasonable (UCR) is a complex system in which three fees are considered in calculating payment. UCR is used mostly in reference to fee-for-service reimbursement. Figure 6-1 illustrates how a surgeon's payment is determined under this method. The usual fee is the fee that a physician usually charges (submitted fee) for a given service to a private patient. A fee is a **customary fee** if it is in the range of usual fees charged by providers of similar training and experience in a geographic area (e.g., the history of charges for a given service). The **reasonable fee** is the fee that meets the aforementioned criteria or is, in the opinion of the medical review committee, justifiable considering the special circumstances of the case. Reimbursement is based on the lower of the two fees (usual and customary)

and determines the approved or allowed amount. In a UCR system, payment can be extremely low for a rarely performed but highly complex procedure because there may be no history of billed charges from other physicians on which to base payment. Many private health insurance plans use this method and pay a physician's full charge if it does not exceed UCR charges. Depending on the policies of each insurance company, the UCR system is periodically updated. UCR is a method chosen by third-party payers and not the provider. If the physician has a UCR that is significantly lower than those of other practices in his or her area, document this and ask the third-party payer for a review and possible adjustment. Increasing numbers of plans are beginning to discontinue the UCR system and are adopting the Medicare RBRVS method for physician reimbursement. A description of this system is found under Relative Value Studies, which follows.

To be considered *customary* for Medicare reimbursement, a provider's charges for like services must be imposed on most patients regardless of the type of patient treated or the party responsible for payment of such services. Customary charges are those uniform charges

---

PARTICIPATING SURGEON
UCR CALCULATION

Four Example Cases

Surgeon's bill	Usual fee	compared to	Customary fee		Payment
1) $400	$350	————→	$350——→	declared reasonable (extenuating circumstances)	$400
2) $400	$350	————→	$350——→	declared customary (no unusual circumstances)	$350
3) $375	$350	————→	$400——→	declared customary (does not exceed customary level)	$375
4) $350	$350	————→	$400——→	declared customary (falls within customary range)	$350

Usual Fee– usual submitted fee for a given service to patient.

Customary Fee– in the range of usual fees charged by providers of similar training and experience in a geographical area (i.e., the history of charges for a given service).

Reasonable Fee– meets the aforementioned criteria or is, in the opinion of the medical review committee, justifiable considering the special circumstances of the case.

Payment– based on the lower of usual and customary fees.

FIGURE 6-1 Usual, customary, and reasonable calculation for four participating surgeons' cases.

listed in a provider's established charge schedule that is in effect and applied consistently to most patients and recognized for Medicare program reimbursement.

Relative Value Studies

In 1956 the California Medical Association Committee on Fees published the first edition of the *California Relative Value Studies* (CRVS).

CRVS was subsequently revised and published in 1957, 1960, 1964, 1969, and 1974. RVS, referred to as either relative value studies or scale, is a coded listing of procedure codes with unit values that indicate the relative value of the various services performed, taking into account the time, skill, and overhead cost necessary for each service (Example 6-3).

Example 6-3   Relative Value Scale

Procedure

Code	Description	Units
10060	Incision & drainage of cyst	**0.8**

Using a hypothetical figure of $153/unit, this procedure is valued at $122.40.

Math: $153.00 × 0.8 = $122.40

Units in RVS are based on the median charges of all physicians during the time period in which the RVS was published. A **conversion factor** is used to translate the abstract units in the scale to dollar fees for each service.

The RVS is a sophisticated system for coding and billing of professional services. After the successful use of the California RVS, many state and medical specialty associations adopted the CRVS method. In 1975 the Federal Trade Commission (FTC) challenged the legality of using the RVS as a fee schedule, stating it could be interpreted as a form of price fixing in violation of antitrust laws. Since that time, many medical societies and medical specialty associations issued new publications that omitted unit values for the procedures listed but retained the procedure code portion of RVS.

Some states passed legislation mandating the use of RVS codes for procedures and the unit values as the schedule of fees for workers' compensation claims. In these states the conversion factor to be used in applying the units is also stated in the law. The third-party payer pays a specific dollar amount for each unit listed for each procedure in the RVS code book.

An insurer or other third party could devise an RVS on the basis of its own data. This type of RVS would not be created by physicians in an effort to regulate fees and,

therefore, would be acceptable on the basis of FTC guidelines. An example is *Ingenix Relative Values for Physicians* (RVP) (refer to the Appendix for information on where to obtain this book). Additionally, a national RVS developed under a government contract may be acceptable and would not be in violation of antitrust laws.

Resource-Based Relative Value Scale

The **resource-based relative value scale (RBRVS)** is an RVS developed for CMS by William Hsiao and associates of the Harvard School of Public Health. Centers for Medicaid and Medicare Services used it to devise the Medicare fee schedule that was phased in from 1992 through 1996. This approach to fees was developed to redistribute Medicare dollars more equitably among physicians and to control escalating fees that were out of control using the UCR system. This became the basis for physicians' payments nationwide for a 5-year phase-in that began on January 1, 1992. This system consists of a fee schedule based on relative values. The formula for obtaining relative value units is somewhat complex and involves a bit of mathematics in computing three components: a **relative value unit (RVU)** for the service, a geographic adjustment factor (GAF), and a monetary conversion factor (CF).

Relative Value Unit Formula

RVU × GAF × CF = Medicare $ per service

RVUs are based on the physician work RVU, the practice expense RVU, and the malpractice insurance RVU. To bring the fees in line for the region where the physician practices and to adjust for regional overhead and malpractice costs, each of the RVUs is adjusted for each Medicare local fiscal agent by geographic practice cost indices (GPCIs), pronounced "gypsies."

A CF is used to convert a geographically adjusted relative value into a payment amount. This CF is updated to a new amount each year. Figure 6-2 provides an example of calculating payment for one procedure code.

HCPCS/CPT CODE	WORK RVUs	PRACTICE EXPENSE RVUs	MALPRACTICE RVUs	
91000 RVUs	1.04	0.70	0.06	
GPCI*	×1.028	×1.258	×1.370	= Total adjusted
	1.07	0.88	0.08	RVUs, 2.03

For 2011, the conversion factor for nonsurgical care is
$35.98 × 2.03 = Allowed amount $68.98

*The geographical practice cost indices (GPCI) for the medical practice whose location in the example is Oakland, California.

FIGURE 6-2 Formula used to calculate the fee for a specific procedure using the resource-based relative value scale system.

A	B	C	D	E	F	G	H
Table 6-2	**RBRVS Crosswalk**						
CODE	CODE DESCRIPTION	RBRVS/RVU	CONVERSION FACTOR	FEE	CONTRACT CONVERSION FACTOR	CONTRACT FEE	% CONTRACT PAYMENT
99212	Office Visit	0.68	72.06	$49	64.71	$44.00	90%

RBRVS, Resource-based relative value scale; *RVU*, relative value unit.

The figures to work out this formula in the chart for each service are published annually in the *Federal Register*.

RVUs help when determining cost accounting because they take into account the practice expense, malpractice expense, work effort, and cost of living. They are also helpful when negotiating the best contract available with managed care plans; therefore office managers or individuals assisting physicians should know and understand RBRVS data. A crosswalk is an effective way to see how the practice may be affected by an RBRVS contract (Table 6-2). To develop one, make several columns using spreadsheet software. In column A, list common procedure codes used by the practice; column B, the code description; and column C, the RBRVS RVUs. Leave column D blank to insert a conversion factor. In column E, put in the present fee-for-service rate (rounded-out figure). Divide the fee in column E by column C to get the conversion factor. Leave a blank for column F to insert a conversion factor for the contract. List the managed care contract payment in column G. Divide column G by column C to get the conversion factor for column F. Then divide the plan's contract fee by the physician's fee for column H to work out the percentage being paid at the contract rate.

Medicare Fee Schedule

Beginning in 1996, each local Medicare administrative contractor (MAC) annually sent each physician a Medicare fee schedule for his or her area or region number listing three columns of figures: participating amount, nonparticipating amount, and limiting charge for each procedure code number. Currently, fee schedules may be accessed online at your local MAC's website. To see an example of this, refer to the Mock Fee Schedule shown in Appendix A of the *Workbook*.

Developing a Fee Schedule Using Relative Value Studies Conversion Factors

A physician's fees can be adjusted if they are too high or low, but doing this can present a problem. It is legal to use an RVS guide for setting, realigning, or evaluating fees as long as the physician does not enter into any price-fixing agreements. Updating or establishing a fee schedule can be accomplished in a number of ways ranging from easy to difficult. They are as follows:

1. Use the RBRVS fee profile sent to each physician's practice in the latter part of each year. This lists the codes most frequently used by the practice with their allowable charges and limiting charge amounts for the coming year. This is used for billing patients under the Medicare program. However, it can help you update the office fee schedule but you must make sure the charges are above the allowances on that schedule and above the allowances of the majority of the other third-party payers to whom the medical practice generally sends insurance claims.

2. Obtain the *Federal Register* with the printed relative values for most of the CPT code numbers and geographic cost indices for the region of service. Using a simple formula, calculate the actual Medicare reimbursement for the procedures the physician most frequently performs, making up a set of separate conversion factors for the Evaluation and Management (E/M), Anesthesia, Surgery, Radiology, Pathology, and Medicine sections. A fee schedule can be either updated or established from the calculations. Take into consideration that the fees should be above the maximums paid by the third-party payers to whom the practice generally bills. This procedure is detailed at the end of this chapter to assist you in gaining experience and skill if choosing to use this method.

3. A more time-consuming method is to review the medical practice's patient mix, that is, those patients with Medicare, the Blue Plans, Medicaid, managed care, private pay, workers' compensation, TRICARE, CHAMPVA, and so on. This may involve a detailed chart review of a large representative sampling of patients seen in the medical practice. Next, review the current fee schedule and current reimbursement amounts for the most commonly billed codes and the payments generated from each insurance plan in the study. A new fee schedule can be created from these data. See Appendix A for information on how to obtain the code books mentioned in this chapter.

FORMAT AND CONTENT OF THE CPT CODE BOOK

The following explains content and procedures for the 2009 edition of the CPT published by the American Medical Association. CPT code books published by other companies may contain differences, such as the Index, may appear at the beginning and not the end of the book. CPT codes have three categories: I, II, and III. This code book is a systematic listing of five-digit code numbers with no decimals. CPT I is divided into six code sections with categories and subcategories. The CPT content is as follows:

Category I Codes	(99201 to 99607)
Evaluation and Management (E/M)	99201 to 99499
Anesthesia	00100 to 01999
Surgery	10021 to 69990
Radiology, Nuclear Medicine, and Diagnostic Ultrasound	70010 to 79999
Pathology and Laboratory	80047 to 89398
Medicine	90281 to 99607
Category II Codes	0001F to 7025F
Category III Codes	0016T to 0207T

Appendix A Modifiers
Appendix B Summary of Additions, Deletions, and Revisions
Appendix C Clinical Examples
Appendix D Summary of CPT Add-on Codes
Appendix E Summary of CPT Codes Exempt from Modifier 51
Appendix F Summary of CPT Codes Exempt from Modifier 63
Appendix G Summary of CPT Codes That Include Moderate (Conscious) Sedation
Appendix H Alphabetic Index of Performance Measures by Clinical Condition or Topic
Appendix I Genetic Testing Code Modifiers
Appendix J Electrodiagnostic Medicine Listing of Sensory, Motor, and Mixed Nerves
Appendix K Product Pending FDA Approval
Appendix L Vascular Families
Appendix M Deleted CPT Codes
Appendix N Summary of Resequenced CPT Codes
Index

Each main section is divided into categories and subcategories according to anatomic body systems, procedure, condition, description, and specialty. Figure 6-3, A, illustrates the format of the Index, which is where you go to locate the CPT section, and Figure 6-3, B, illustrates the format of the CPT section.

Read through the clinical examples presented in Appendix C of the CPT. These examples will help you become familiarized with some common case scenarios that might occur for the codes that appear in the E/M section of the CPT.

When on the job, you might want to make your CPT into a reference manual by customizing it. This can help you find codes, modifiers, and rules, making your job easier. Break apart the manual into as many sections as needed on the basis of specialty, three-hole punch it, and place it into a binder. You may want to add indexes with tabs to the frequently used sections. You can also add coding edits, Medicare updates, and notes at any place in the binder. Color code any codes to which you usually add modifiers or that should not be used until you have reviewed certain data. For example, use red to highlight codes, descriptions, or entire sections, to alert you or anyone using the reference to codes that are often denied. Use yellow to highlight a code that needs to be checked before using it in combination with other codes. Use a symbol (e.g., * or ?) to identify services not covered under certain conditions. Appendix A of the CPT code book is a comprehensive list of the modifiers, so you might want to add any insurance plan bulletins pertinent to modifiers that affect the specialty you bill for in this section of the binder. Customizing the CPT code book with a reference like this can save time and reduce coding errors.

Category I, II, and III Codes

To improve the existing CPT-4 code system, a CPT-5 Project was implemented, which is a revision of CPT-4 and includes two new code sets: category II codes, intended for performance measurement, and category III codes, intended for new and emerging technology. Existing CPT codes are considered category I.

Category II codes describe clinical components that may be typically included in E/M services or clinical services and do not have a relative value associated with them. They also describe results from clinical laboratory

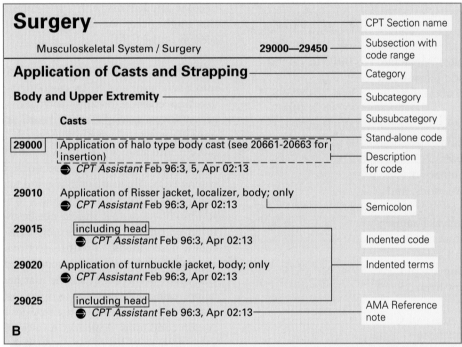

FIGURE 6-3 **A,** CPT format illustrating conventions of the index and a section. **B,** CPT format illustrating conventions of the index and a section.

or radiology tests and other procedures, identified processes intended to address patient safety practices, or services reflecting compliance with state or federal laws.

Beginning with the CPT 2005 edition, Category II codes appear in a separate section located immediately after the Medicine section. They also have an alphanumeric identifier with a letter in the last field (e.g., 0502F Subsequent prenatal care visit) to distinguish them from category I codes. Two modifiers are used to indicate that a service specified by a performance measure was considered but, because of either medical or patient circumstance(s) documented in the medical record, the service was not provided. The modifiers are 1P, 2P, 3P, and 8P.

Use of these codes is optional for correct coding.

Category III codes are a temporary set of tracking codes used to code emerging technologies that do not yet have any procedure code assignment in category I. They are intended to expedite data collection and assessment of new services and procedures to substantiate widespread use and clinical effectiveness. A category III code may become a category I code. When it is deleted from category III and adopted as category I code, the CPT book provides clear indication of this change by inserting a cross reference in place of the former category III code; for example, ▶(0024T has been deleted. To report use 93799)◀. The AMA website posts updates to this category in July and January every year.

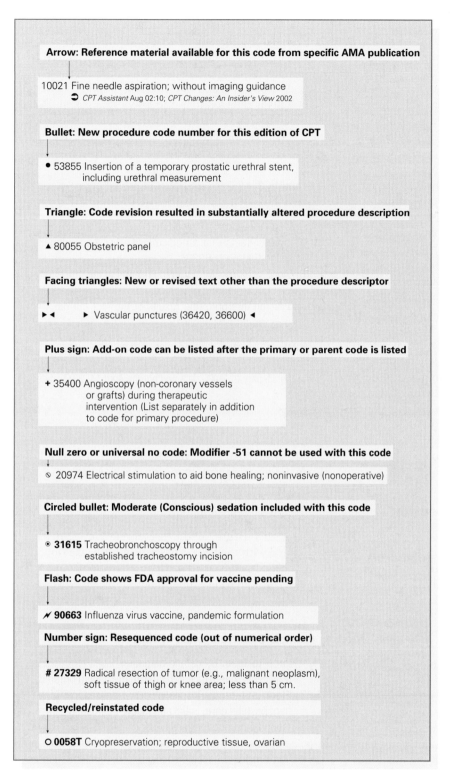

Arrow: Reference material available for this code from specific AMA publication

10021 Fine needle aspiration; without imaging guidance
⮑ *CPT Assistant* Aug 02:10; *CPT Changes: An Insider's View* 2002

Bullet: New procedure code number for this edition of CPT

• 53855 Insertion of a temporary prostatic urethral stent, including urethral measurement

Triangle: Code revision resulted in substantially altered procedure description

▲ 80055 Obstetric panel

Facing triangles: New or revised text other than the procedure descriptor

►◄   ► Vascular punctures (36420, 36600) ◄

Plus sign: Add-on code can be listed after the primary or parent code is listed

+ 35400 Angioscopy (non-coronary vessels or grafts) during therapeutic intervention (List separately in addition to code for primary procedure)

Null zero or universal no code: Modifier -51 cannot be used with this code

⊘ 20974 Electrical stimulation to aid bone healing; noninvasive (nonoperative)

Circled bullet: Moderate (Conscious) sedation included with this code

⊙ **31615** Tracheobronchoscopy through established tracheostomy incision

Flash: Code shows FDA approval for vaccine pending

⚡ **90663** Influenza virus vaccine, pandemic formulation

Number sign: Resequenced code (out of numerical order)

27329 Radical resection of tumor (e.g., malignant neoplasm), soft tissue of thigh or knee area; less than 5 cm.

Recycled/reinstated code

○ **0058T** Cryopreservation; reproductive tissue, ovarian

FIGURE 6-4 Symbols that appear in the 2011 *Current Procedural Terminology* (CPT) code book and a brief explanation of what they tell the coder. These symbols and their meanings appear at the bottom of each page of codes in the CPT code book.

Code Book Symbols

With each new issuance of CPT, deletions and new codes and description changes are added. Become familiar with the new codes and any description changes or deleted codes for codes that may exist on your medical practice's fee schedule. Figure 6-4 shows how to identify new codes and description changes by following the symbols that are used. The symbols ⮑ and ⮒ placed below many codes throughout the code book indicate that the AMA has published reference material on that particular code. The reference citation is also provided. When using a new code, marked with a bullet (•), it may take as long as 6 months before a third-party payer has a mandatory value assignment; therefore reimbursements are received in varying amounts during that time. An exception is in the Medicare program, which has a value assignment published annually in the fall in the *Federal Register*. For revised codes or revised text, marked with a triangle (▲) or (▶ ◀), highlight what is new or deleted. This saves time in trying to figure out what was changed and prevents using these codes incorrectly. Appendix B in the CPT code book provides a summary of code additions, deletions, and revisions. Add-on codes, shown with a plus sign (+), means the code can be listed after the primary or parent code has been listed. Modifier -51 exempt codes, shown with a symbol (⊘), means the modifier cannot be used with this code. More explanation about the add-on codes and modifier -51 appears at the end of this chapter. The symbol ⊙ is used to identify codes that include moderate (conscious) sedation, and Appendix G in the CPT code book provides a complete list of these codes. The symbol ⊁ is used to identify codes for vaccines that are pending Food and Drug Administration (FDA) approval. A complete list of these appears in Appendix K in the CPT code book. Resequenced codes that are not placed numerically are identified with the # symbol, and a reference placed numerically (e.g., "Code is out of numerical sequence. See ...") is a navigational alert to direct the user to the location of the out-of-sequenced code. A list appears in Appendix N. All of these symbols are located at the bottom of each page of codes in the CPT code book.

Evaluation and Management Section

The insurance billing specialist must become familiar with the terminology in the procedure code book to use it efficiently. Basic procedural code terminology is reviewed in Chapter 4 to give you a good foundation to begin coding. By now you should know the difference between a new and an established patient, a consultation and a referral, and concurrent care versus continuity of care. This section familiarizes you with specific coding policies in relation to some of the terminology you have learned thus far.

The E/M section is divided into office visits, hospital visits, and consultations, and these codes describe physician's services involving the E/M of a patient's problem. Two subcategories of office visits exist: new patient and established patient. Hospital visits also have two subcategories: initial and subsequent. Each subcategory has levels of E/M services identified by specific codes. This classification is based on the nature of the physician's work such as type of service, place of service, and the patient's status.

In Chapter 4, you learned the CPT definitions for new patient and established patient. However, Medicare's revised definition of new patient is "Patient who has not received any professional services (i.e., E/M service or other face-to-face service [e.g., surgical procedure]) from the physician or physician group practice (same physician/same specialty) within the previous 3 years" (Example 6-4). This is referred to as the *3-year rule*. The CPT has a decision tree in the E/M services guidelines section for new versus established patients to help the provider.

Example 6-4 **Determination of a Medicare New Patient**

On January 2, 20XX, Jason Emerson, new patient, is seen by Dr. Practon for an office visit. The service is billed using E/M code 99204.

On April 14, 20XX, Mr. Emerson returns to the office for an electrocardiogram, in-office laboratory test, and Dr. Practon interprets the results of the test but does not perform an E/M service.

NOTE: In this case, the time interval to determine whether the patient is considered a new patient or established patient reverts to the January 2, 20XX, date and not the April 14, 20XX, date.

The format for the levels of E/M service is as follows: First, under new patient or established patient a code number is listed. Second, the place and/or type of service is listed. Third, the content of the service is defined (e.g., comprehensive history and comprehensive examination). Fourth, the nature of the presenting problem usually associated with the level is described. Fifth, the time typically needed to give the service is stated (Example 6-5). You are allowed to use time to determine an E/M service

---

Example 6-5 **Categories of Time**

1. **Face-to-face:** Office and outpatient visits
   (Physician meets face to face with the patient or family.)
2. **Floor/unit time:** Hospital observation services, inpatient hospital care, initial and follow-up hospital consultations, and nursing facility services
   (Physician is present on the patient's hospital floor or unit providing bedside services to the patient such as time with patient, time working on patient's chart, discussing patient's care with nurses.)
3. **Non-face-to-face time:** Inpatient hospital pre-encounter and post-encounter time, obtaining records and test results, talking with other health care providers, arranging for additional services
   (Physician does work related to the patient before or after face-to-face time or floor/unit time.)

level when counseling and/or coordinating care takes up more than 50% of the visit. Refer to Table 6-4, which appears later in this chapter and shows a summary of the E/M codes with these five components.

There are seven elements when selecting an E/M code to bill and providers consider the following in this order:

1. History
2. Examination
3. Medical decision making
4. Nature of presenting problem
5. Counseling
6. Coordination of care
7. Time

Hospital Inpatient Services

In the E/M section of the code book, the hospital inpatient service codes range from 99221 to 99239. If a patient is seen in the emergency department and is subsequently admitted to the hospital, it is billed as initial hospital care when done on the same date as the admission. The physician includes the services related to the admission that he or she provided in the other sites of hospital service departments, as well as in the inpatient setting.

Consultation

As learned in Chapter 4, a consultation includes services rendered by a physician whose opinion or advice is requested by another physician or agency in the evaluation or treatment of a patient's illness or a suspected problem. A referral is the transfer of the total or specific care of a patient from one physician to another for known problems.

Some insurance policies pay for only one consultation per patient per year and often require a written report to be generated.

A consulting physician must submit a written report containing his or her findings and opinions to the requesting physician. Codes for consultations are as follows:

- Office or other outpatient consultations (new or established patient): 99241 through 99245 (Example 6-6).
- Inpatient consultations (new or established patient): 99251 through 99255 (Example 6-7).

In the office setting, use the appropriate initial consultation code for the initial encounter and if a follow-up visit is required for additional diagnostic testing or examination, then use the appropriate established patient code. In a hospital setting, use the appropriate inpatient hospital consultation code and if a follow-up is required for additional services, then use subsequent hospital care codes.

Example 6-6 Outpatient Consultation

A 20-year-old female is seen for an office consultation for cystitis. She complains of burning on urination and urinary frequency. The patient's records from the referring physician were reviewed. Urine culture confirmed a urinary tract infection which was reported to her primary care physician for treatment. Obtained problem focused history and examination with straightforward medical decision making.

| 99241 | Office consultation |
| 87086 | Urine culture, bacterial |

Example 6-7 Inpatient Consultation

A 50-year-old male is seen for an initial inpatient consultation with a status post left hip fracture and a history of well-controlled type II diabetes mellitus. Consultation is requested for surgical clearance. Reviewed medical data on the unit. Obtained a detailed history and performed a detailed examination with low complexity medical decision making. Discussed diagnosis and treatment options with patient and completed medical record documentation. Will give ongoing consultation to referring physician.

| 99253 | Inpatient consultation |

Effective January 1, 2010, the Center for Medicare and Medicaid Services (CMS) issued a policy that eliminated the use of all consultation codes (ranges 99241 through 99245 and 99251 through 99255 for inpatient and office/outpatient settings and for various places of service except for telehealth consultation (HCPCS G-codes). CMS says to use the initial hospital care codes 99221 through 99223 when billing a consultation on a hospital inpatient. The attending physician must append HCPCS Level II modifier AI (A-eye) *principal physician of record* to the code. If a transfer of care, codes 99201 through 99205 and 99211 through 99215 may be used. Note: Continue to bill consultation codes to non-Medicare payers.

As learned in Chapter 4, remember the four Rs: There must be a *requesting* physician, and the consultant must *render* an opinion and send a *report*. The requesting physician must document the *reason* on the medical record.

Critical Care

According to CPT guidelines, critical care is the direct delivery of medical care by a physician for a critically ill or injured patient. A critical illness or injury acutely impairs one or more vital organ systems and makes an imminent or life-threatening deterioration in the patient's condition highly probable. Critical care involves highly complex decision making to assess, manipulate, and support vital system functions to treat single or multiple vital organ system failure or prevent further life-threatening deterioration of the patient's condition. Examples of vital organ system failure include, but are not limited to, central nervous system failure; circulatory failure; shock; and renal, hepatic, metabolic, or respiratory failure.

Although critical care typically requires interpretation of multiple physiologic parameters or application of advanced technologies, critical care may be provided in life-threatening situations when these elements are not present. Critical care may be provided on multiple days, even if no changes are made in the treatment rendered to the patient, as long as the patient's condition continues to require the level of physician attention described in the preceding paragraph.

Providing medical care to a critically ill, injured, or postoperative patient qualifies as a critical care service only if both the illness or injury and the treatment being provided meet the preceding requirements. Critical care is usually, but not always, given in a critical care area such as the coronary care unit, intensive care unit, pediatric intensive care unit, respiratory care unit, or emergency care facility. It could occur in the patient's room or in the emergency department.

Inpatient critical care services provided to neonates and infants 29 days through 24 months of age are reported with pediatric critical care codes 99468 through 99476. The pediatric critical care codes are reported as long as the infant or young child qualifies for critical care services during the hospital stay. Inpatient critical care services provided to neonates (28 days of age or younger) are reported with the neonatal critical care codes 99468 and 99469. The neonatal critical care codes are reported as long as the neonate qualifies for critical care services through the twenty-eighth postnatal day. The reporting of the pediatric and neonatal critical care services is not based on time or the type of unit (e.g., pediatric or neonatal critical care unit) nor is it dependent on the type of provider delivering the care. For additional instructions on reporting these services, see the section on Inpatient Neonatal and Pediatric Critical Care in the Evaluation and Management section of CPT.

Services for a patient who is not critically ill but is in a critical care or intensive care unit are reported by use of other appropriate in-hospital E/M codes.

Critical care and other E/M services may be provided to the same patient on the same date by the same physician.

The following services are included in critical care codes used to report critical care when performed during the critical period by the physician providing critical care: the interpretation of cardiac output measurements (93561, 93562), chest radiographs (71010, 71015, 71020), pulse oximetry (94760, 94761, 94762), blood gases and information data stored in computers (e.g., electrocardiograms, blood pressures, hematologic data [99090]), gastric intubation (43752, 91105), temporary transcutaneous pacing (92953), ventilator management (94002 through 94004, 94660, 94662), and vascular access procedures (36000, 36400, 36405, 36406, 36410, 36415, 36591, 36600). These services are not coded in addition to the critical care codes.

Any services performed in excess of those listed earlier should be reported separately. Many third-party payers attempt to downcode claims by stating the procedure is included with critical care. If denied, these claims should be appealed by attaching supporting documentation such as a copy of the critical care guidelines. The payer may tell you the codes are inclusive or that they are not a covered benefit.

Codes 99289 through 99290 should be reported for the physician's attendance during the transport of critically ill or injured pediatric patients younger than 24 months of age to or from a facility or hospital.

Critical care codes 99291 and 99292 are used to report the total duration of time spent by a physician providing critical care services to a critically ill or injured patient, even if the time spent by the physician on that date is not continuous. For any given period of time spent providing critical care services, the physician must devote his or her full attention to the patient and therefore cannot provide services to any other patient during the same period of time.

Time spent with the individual patient must be recorded in the patient's record. Time spent engaged in work directly related to the individual patient's care, whether that time was spent at the immediate bedside or elsewhere on the floor or unit even if not continuous, is reported as critical care. For example, time spent on the unit or at the nursing station on the floor reviewing test results or imaging studies, discussing the critically ill patient's care with other medical staff, or documenting critical care services in the medical record is reported as critical care, even though it does not occur at the bedside. Also, when the patient is unable or clinically incompetent to participate in discussions, time spent on the floor or unit with family members or surrogate decision makers obtaining a medical history, reviewing the patient's condition or prognosis, or discussing treatment or limitations of treatment may be reported as critical care, as long as the conversation bears directly on the management of the patient.

Time spent in activities that occur outside of the unit or off the floor (e.g., telephone calls, whether taken at home, in the office, or elsewhere in the hospital) may not be reported as critical care because the physician is not immediately available to the patient.

Time spent in activities that do not directly contribute to the treatment of the patient may not be reported as critical care, even if they are performed in the critical care unit (e.g., participation in administrative meetings or telephone calls to discuss other patients). Time spent performing separately reportable procedures or services should not be included in the time reported as critical care time.

Code 99291 is used to report the first 30 to 74 minutes of critical care on a given date. It should be used only once per date even if the time spent by the physician is not continuous on that date. Critical care of less than 30 minutes total duration on a given date should be reported with the appropriate E/M code.

Code 99292 is used to report additional blocks of time, of up to 30 minutes each, beyond the first 74 minutes. This code has a plus sign (+) and is an "add-on" code. It is never used alone.

Pediatric and Neonatal Critical Care

According to CPT guidelines, the codes 99468 through 99476 are used to report inpatient services provided by a physician directing the care of a critically ill neonate or infant. The same definitions for critical care services apply for the adult, child, and neonate.

The initial day neonatal critical care code (99468) can be used, in addition to codes 99360 Physician standby service, 99464 Attendance, or 99465 Newborn resuscitation as appropriate, when the physician is present for the delivery and newborn resuscitation is necessary. Other procedures performed as a necessary part of the resuscitation (e.g., endotracheal intubation) are also reported separately when performed as part of the preadmission delivery room care. They must be performed as a necessary component of the resuscitation and not done for convenience.

Codes 99468 and 99469 are used to report services provided by a physician directing the care of a critically ill neonate through the first 28 days of life. These codes describe care for the date of admission (99468) and subsequent days (99469) and should be reported only once per day per patient. Once the neonate is no longer

considered critically ill, the Intensive Low Birth Weight Services codes for those with present body weight of less than 1500 grams (99478, 99479, and 99480) or the codes for Subsequent Hospital Care (99231 through 99233) for those with present body weight more than 5000 grams should be used.

Codes 99471 and 99472 are used to report services provided by a physician directing the care of a critically ill infant or young child from 29 days of postnatal age up through 24 months of age. These codes represent care for the date of admission (99471) and subsequent days (99472) and should be reported by a single physician only once per day per patient in a given setting. The critically ill or injured child older than 2 years of age when admitted to an intensive care unit is reported with hourly critical care service codes (99291 and 99292). When an infant is no longer considered critically ill but continues to require intensive care, the Intensive Low Birth Weight Services code 99478 should be used to report services for infants with a body weight of less than 1500 grams. When the body weight of those infants exceeds 1500 grams, the Subsequent Intensive Care 99479 and 99480 codes should be used.

The pediatric and neonatal critical care codes include those procedures previously listed for the hourly critical care codes (99291 and 99292). In addition, the following procedures also are included in the bundled (global) pediatric and neonatal critical care service codes (99469 to 99471):

- Umbilical venous (36510) and umbilical arterial (36660) catheters
- Central (36555) or peripheral vessel catheterization (36000)
- Other arterial catheters (36140, 36620)
- Oral or nasogastric tube placement (43752)
- Endotracheal intubation (31500)
- Lumbar puncture (62270)
- Suprapubic bladder aspiration (51100)
- Bladder catheterization (51701, 51702)
- Initiation and management of mechanical ventilation (94002 through 94004) or continuous positive airway pressure (94660)
- Surfactant administration (94610)
- Vascular access procedures (36400, 36405, 36406)
- Transfusion of blood components (36430 and 36440)
- Vascular punctures oral (36420 and 36600)
- Invasive or noninvasive electronic monitoring of vital signs
- Bedside pulmonary function testing (94375)
- Monitoring or interpretation of blood gases for oxygen saturation (94760 through 94762)

Any services performed that are not listed in the preceding should be reported separately.

Emergency Care

Codes 99281 through 99285 describe various levels of emergency care provided in an emergency department. An *emergency department* (ED) is defined as an organized hospital-based facility for the provision of unscheduled episodic services to patients who present for immediate medical attention. However, some facilities must use the ED to accommodate after-hours patients, overflow clinic patients, or administer minor procedures in the absence of a clinic. When a patient is seen in the ED for a scheduled procedure, he or she must have a valid order for services. The patient should be registered as a clinic patient because his or her visit is not deemed an emergency. Medical necessity rules apply and the hospital should screen the procedure and diagnosis. As learned in Chapter 4, medical necessity is services provided that are consistent with the diagnosis. This type of patient falls under the regulations of the Emergency Medical Treatment and Active Labor Act (EMTALA). The facility may either perform an EMTALA screening for the patient or have the patient sign a document indicating he or she is not in the ED for emergency services. In these cases, there is a charge for the scheduled service provided but it is usually inappropriate to charge an E/M visit in addition to the procedure charge.

Code 99288 is used when advanced life support is necessary during emergency care and the physician is located in a hospital emergency or critical care department and is in two-way voice communication with ambulance or rescue personnel outside the hospital.

If office services are provided on an emergency basis, code 99058 (office services provided on an emergency basis—found in the Medicine Section) may be used when billing private insurance cases. CPT codes 99281 through 99285 should not to be used to report emergency care provided in an office setting. Medicare does not pay for code 99058, and other third-party payers also may deny this code. When a physician spends several hours attending to a patient, coding for prolonged services (99354 through 99357), in addition to an E/M service office visit, might be indicated.

If a patient comes into the office requiring emergency care for a wound trauma, you might bill for the office visit, suturing of the laceration, and the surgical tray. Most third-party payers only pay for suturing. Typically, the payer will state that the office visit is included or bundled (codes grouped together that are related to a procedure) into the suture procedure. The payer will also typically state that surgical trays/supplies are included or bundled into the suture procedure. If you view the CMS National Correct Coding Initiative (NCCI) edits, you can see which codes are normally considered part of another procedure.

Example 6-8 Office Emergency	
Incorrect Coding	
99212	Office visit, level 2, established patient
12005	Simple repair of scalp laceration, 12.6 cm
99070	Surgical tray (itemized)
Correct Coding	
99212	Office visit, level 2, established patient
99058	Office services provided on an emergency basis
12005	Simple repair of scalp laceration, 12.6 cm

If the NCCI edits do not show the codes as being inclusive, you should appeal the third-party payer's decision or bill the patient if allowed by federal or state law. This topic is explained in more detail later in the section on Coding Guidelines for Code Edits. To obtain further information about the NCCI edits, refer to the Internet Resources at the end of this chapter and go to the Evolve website, which has an active link to this initiative. However, if documentation supports coding the claim for office services provided on an emergency basis (99058), most payers will reimburse for the office visit in addition to the repair (Example 6-8). For example, if a patient has an extensive open wound of the arm, a bill should be submitted only for the wound repair. If a patient has an extensive wound of the arm with abrasions of the shoulder, contusions of the ribs, and a sprained finger, then a bill should be submitted for the wound repair and an E/M code. The wound diagnosis would be associated to the wound repair, and the diagnosis for the injuries would support the E/M visit. Make sure the appropriate modifiers are appended to the CPT codes on the claim. For example, modifier -25 is used to report a significant and separate procedure that was performed in addition to an E/M. A -25 modifier should be appended to the E/M in the previous example, but the documentation in the chart must support the reasons for the codes.

Miscellaneous service codes 99050 through 99058 can be used depending on the hour at which the patient is seen as an emergency either in the physician's office or if taken to the emergency room of a hospital (24-hour facility). Most payers, including Medicare, do not pay for these codes. Some payers might pay for these codes and require documentation from the provider to support the code. Other codes under Miscellaneous Services in the Medicine Section may be applicable for a patient receiving emergency care, so these should be scrutinized carefully.

Preventive Medicine

Counseling. Preventive medicine is composed of services provided to prevent the occurrence of illness, injury, and disease such as vaccine immunizations, antiseptic measures, regular exercise, routine physical examinations, and screening programs for detection of signs of disorders. Sometimes one aspect of preventive medicine is counseling, which is a discussion between the physician and a patient, family, or both concerning the diagnosis, recommended studies or tests, treatment options, risks, and benefits of treatment, treatment options, patient and family education, and so on.

Codes 99381 through 99397 include counseling that is provided at the time of the initial or periodic comprehensive preventive medicine examination. Codes 99401 through 99412 should be used for reporting counseling given at an encounter separate from the preventive medicine examination.

Sometimes a Medicare patient may have an annual checkup but while having the examination he or she tells the physician of experiencing pain. The physician provides both the preventive and problem-focused services at the same time. You may bill Medicare only for covered screenings or services (e.g., problem-focused E/M, Pap smear, colon/rectal cancer screening, or prostate cancer screening) and must properly "carve out" the rest of the noncovered and/or preventive services (codes 99381 through 99397) to bill to the patient. Carve out refers to medical services not included as benefits. This term may also be seen in managed care billing and is further discussed in Chapter 11. For preventive medicine when

billing a Medicare case, an Advance Beneficiary Notice is not required.

Categories and Subcategories

The E/M section of CPT has categories and subcategories that have from three to five levels for reporting purposes. These levels are based on key components, contributory factors, and face-to-face time with the patient or family. To begin the coding process, the provider of service must identify the category (e.g., office, hospital inpatient or outpatient, or consultation) and then select the subcategory (e.g., new patient or established patient). The description should be read thoroughly to note the key components (e.g., history, examination, and medical decision making), and the contributory factors (e.g., counseling, coordination of care, and nature of the presenting problem) and face-to-face time of the service should be noted. Review the sample in Figure 6-5 illustrating an E/M code for a new patient seen in the office or in an outpatient or ambulatory setting.

Because key components are clinical in nature, the physician must document these factors in the patient's record. In a case in which counseling and coordination of care dominate (more than 50%) the face-to-face physician-patient encounter, then time is considered the key component to qualify for a particular level of E/M services. Tables 6-3 and 6-4 give a concise view of the components for each code number.

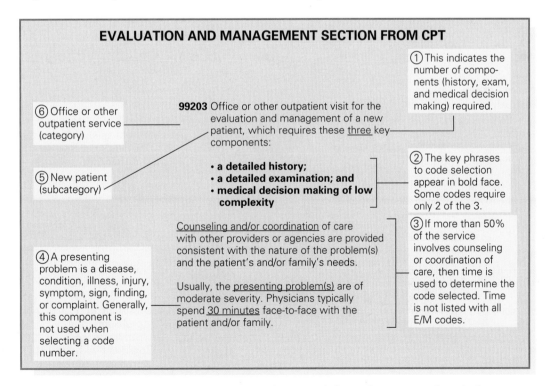

FIGURE 6-5 Evaluation and Management code 99203 defining the main words and phrases. This code is used for a new patient seen in the office or in an outpatient or ambulatory setting.

Table 6-3	**Selection of Evaluation and Management Codes**					
CODE	HISTORY	EXAMINATION	MEDICAL DECISION MAKING	PROBLEM SEVERITY	COORDINATION OF CARE AND COUNSELING	TIME SPENT (AVG)
Office or Other Outpatient Services (Includes Hospital Observation Area)						
New Patient*						
99201	Problem focused	Problem focused	Straightforward	Minor or self-limited	Consistent with problem(s) and patient's needs	10 min face to face
99202	Expanded problem focused	Expanded problem focused	Straightforward	Low to moderate	Consistent with problem(s) and patient's needs	20 min face to face
99203	Detailed	Detailed	Low complexity	Moderate	Consistent with problem(s) and patient's needs	30 min face to face
99204	Comprehensive	Comprehensive	Moderate complexity	Moderate to high	Consistent with problem(s) and patient's needs	45 min face to face
99205	Comprehensive	Comprehensive	High complexity	Moderate to high	Consistent with problem(s) and patient's needs	60 min face to face
Established Patient*†						
99211	—	—	Physician supervision, but presence not required	Minimal	Consistent with problem(s) and patient's needs	5 min face to face
99212	Problem focused	Problem focused	Straightforward	Minor or self-limited	Consistent with problem(s) and patient's needs	10 min face to face
99213	Expanded problem focused	Expanded problem	Low complexity	Low to moderate	Consistent with problem(s) and patient's needs	15 min face to face
99214	Detailed	Detailed	Moderate complexity	Moderate to high	Consistent with problem(s) and patient's needs	25 min face to face
99215	Comprehensive	Comprehensive	High complexity	Moderate to high	Consistent with problem(s) and patient's needs	40 min face to face
Hospital Observation Services						
99217	—	—	—	—	—	—
99218	Detailed or comprehensive	Detailed or comprehensive	Straightforward or low complexity	Low	Consistent with problem(s) and patient's needs	—
99219	Comprehensive	Comprehensive	Moderate complexity	Moderate	Consistent with problem(s) and patient's needs	—
99220	Comprehensive	Comprehensive	High complexity	High		—
Hospital Inpatient Services						
Initial Care‡						
99221	Detailed or comprehensive	Detailed or comprehensive	Straightforward or low complexity	Low	Consistent with problem(s) and patient's needs	30 min unit/ floor
99222	Comprehensive	Comprehensive	Moderate complexity	Moderate	Consistent with problem(s) and patient's needs	50 min unit/ floor
99223	Comprehensive	Comprehensive	High complexity	High	Consistent with problem(s) and patient's needs	70 min unit/ floor

Table 6-3	Selection of Evaluation and Management Codes—cont'd					
CODE	HISTORY	EXAMINATION	MEDICAL DECISION MAKING	PROBLEM SEVERITY	COORDINATION OF CARE AND COUNSELING	TIME SPENT (AVG)
Subsequent Care‡§						
99231	Problem focused interval	Problem focused	Straightforward or low complexity	Stable, recovering or improving	Consistent with problem(s) and patient's needs	15 min unit/floor
99232	Expanded problem focused interval	Expanded problem focused	Moderate complexity	Inadequate response to treatment; minor complication	Consistent with problem(s) and patient's needs	25 min unit/floor
99233	Detailed interval	Detailed	High complexity	Unstable significant new problem(s) or complication(s)	Consistent with problem(s) and patient's needs	35 min unit/floor
99234	Detailed or comprehensive	Detailed or comprehensive	Straightforward or low complexity	Low	Consistent with problem(s) and patient's needs	—
99235	Comprehensive	Comprehensive	Moderate	Moderate	Consistent with problem(s) and patient's needs	—
99236	Comprehensive	Comprehensive		High	Consistent with problem(s) and patient's needs	—
99238	Hospital discharge day management					30 min or less
99239	Hospital discharge day management					more than 30 min

CPT codes, descriptions, and material are from *Current Procedural Terminology, CPT 2011, Standard Edition*, 2010, American Medical Association. All Rights Reserved.

*Key component: For new patients for initial office and other outpatient services, all three components (history, physical examination, and medical decision making) are required in selecting the correct code. For established patients, at least two of these three components are required. Although average time spent is shown in the table, it is NOT a factor when billing but is shown to assist physicians in selecting the most appropriate level of evaluation and management service.

†Includes follow-up, periodic reevaluation, and management of new problems.

‡Key components: For initial care, all three components (history, physical examination, and medical decision making) are required in selecting the correct code. For subsequent care, at least two of these three components are required.

§All subsequent levels of service include a review of the medical record, diagnostic studies, and changes in the patient's status such as history, physical condition, and response to treatment since the last assessment.

Many physicians refer to the E/M codes as level 5 for the most complex to level 1 as the lowest, least complex. These levels coincide with the fifth or last digit of the CPT code, for example, 99205. It is common to hear a physician say "Ted Brown was seen for a level 5 today." This terminology may appear on encounter forms with five-digit CPT code numbers and be referred to as levels 1 through 5 (Example 6-9).

Alternatively, this terminology may be seen abbreviated as L-1, L-2, and so on, but this usage is not preferred because it can be confused with the nomenclature for the sections of the lumbar vertebrae. The level also may be written out as level one, level two, and so on, depending on the complexity of the case. A breakdown of the E/M levels with code numbers is shown in Table 6-5.

In some cases, it is necessary to use a two-digit modifier to give a more accurate description of the services rendered. This is used in addition to the procedure code. Refer to the comprehensive list of modifiers at the end of this chapter for more information.

Surgery Section

Coding From an Operative Report

It is best to obtain a copy of the patient's operative report from the hospital when coding surgery. A photocopy can be used so that you can make notes right on the document. When reviewing the report, use a ruler or highlighter pen. Use the ruler to read the report line by line. Highlight words that could indicate that the procedure

Table 6-4   Selection Criteria for Consultations

E/M CODE	HISTORY*	EXAMINATION	MEDICAL DECISION MAKING*	PROBLEM SEVERITY	COORDINATION OF CARE AND COUNSELING	TIMES (AVG)
Office or Other Outpatient						
99241	Problem focused	Problem focused	Straightforward	Minor or self-limited	Consistent with problem(s) and patient's needs	15 min face to face
99242	Expanded problem focused	Expanded problem focused	Straightforward	Low	Consistent with problem(s) and patient's needs	30 min face to face
99243	Detailed	Detailed	Low complexity	Moderate	Consistent with problem(s) and patient's needs	40 min face to face
99244	Comprehensive	Comprehensive	Moderate complexity	Moderate to high	Consistent with problem(s) and patient's needs	60 min face to face
99245	Comprehensive	Comprehensive	High complexity	Moderate to high	Consistent with problem(s) and patient's needs	80 min face to face
Initial Inpatient†						
99251	Problem focused	Problem focused	Straightforward	Minor or self-limited	Consistent with problem(s) and patient's needs	20 min unit/ floor
99252	Expanded problem focused	Expanded problem focused	Straightforward	Low	Consistent with problem(s) and patient's needs	40 min unit/ floor
99253	Detailed	Detailed	Low complexity	Moderate	Consistent with problem(s) and patient's needs	55 min unit floor
99254	Comprehensive	Comprehensive	Moderate complexity	Moderate to high	Consistent with problem(s) and patient's needs	80 min unit/ floor
99255	Comprehensive	Comprehensive	High complexity	Moderate to high	Consistent with problem(s) and patient's needs	110 min unit/ floor

CPT codes, descriptions, and material are taken from *Current Procedural Terminology, CPT 2007, Standard Edition*, 2006, American Medical Association. All Rights Reserved.
*Key component: For office and initial inpatient consultations, all three components (history, physical examination, and medical decision making) are required for selecting the correct code.
†These codes also are used for residents of nursing facilities.

Example 6-9   Current Procedural Terminology Code Digit Analysis

performed may be altered by specific circumstances and to remind you that a code modifier may be necessary. Look up any unfamiliar terms using a medical dictionary or anatomic reference book and write the definition in the margin.

Assign the code for the postoperative diagnosis shown at the beginning of the operative report. Also search for additional diagnoses in the body of the report that you can add as secondary diagnostic codes to support medical necessity, especially if the case is complex.

If the complex surgical procedure is not accurately described in the procedure code nomenclature, include an operative report and list "Attachment" in Block 19 of the insurance claim form so that the claims adjuster clearly understands the case and maximum payment is generated.

Code numbers that describe a part of the body treated render higher reimbursement, depending on their location (e.g., suturing of a facial laceration pays a higher rate than suturing of an arm laceration).

Code only the procedures that actually were documented in the report. Check to make sure they were neither a part of the main procedure nor bundled by NCCI edits, which is discussed later in this chapter.

Remember the rule: not documented, not done.

Do not code using only the name of the procedure as it is given in the heading of the operative report. Read the report thoroughly before coding to see whether additional procedures were performed and whether they were

Table 6-5 | Levels With Code Numbers

	Office Visits		Consultations	
	NEW	ESTABLISHED	OFFICE	HOSPITAL
Level 1	99201	99211	99241	99251
Level 2	99202	99212	99242	99252
Level 3	99203	99213	99243	99253
Level 4	99204	99214	99244	99254
Level 5	99205	99215	99245	99255

Example 6.10 | Integral Code

Partial and complete, which means the partial procedure is included in the complete procedure.
56620   Vulvectomy simple; partial
56625   complete
Partial and total, which means the partial procedure is included in the total procedure.
58940   Oophorectomy, partial or total, unilateral or bilateral
Unilateral and bilateral, which means the unilateral procedure is included in the bilateral procedure.
58900   Biopsy of ovary, unilateral or bilateral
Single and multiple, which means the single procedure is included in the multiple procedure.
49321   Laparoscopy, surgical, with biopsy (single or multiple)

part of the main procedure, performed independently, or were unrelated. If the surgical position is noted, this can help you identify the right approach code. You can also consult a good medical dictionary with illustrations of the various surgical positions. All codes include approach and closure except some skull base surgery codes. Information on how to code multiple procedures that are not inherent in a major procedure may be found at the end of this chapter under modifier -51.

Check to see how many surgeons were involved in the operative procedure and their roles (assistant surgeon, co-surgeon, or team surgeon).

Reread the report to make certain that all procedural and diagnostic codes have been identified. Compare the content with the codes you are using. You cannot code circumstances that the physician relays to you verbally. Be sure the words "extensive complications" are in the report if there are such complications.

Look for unusual details such as special instruments used, unusually long or complex procedures, rare approach techniques, reoperation, or extensive scarring encountered. These conditions may need one or more modifiers appended to the code.

Surgical code descriptions may define a correct coding relationship wherein one code is part of another based on the language used in the description (Example 6-10). An

explanation of how to read a description for standalone codes and indented codes can be found in Procedure 6.3: Choose Correct Procedural Codes for Professional Services at the end of this chapter.

Confirm that the report findings agree with the procedure codes on the claim.

Surgical Package for Non-Medicare Cases

Surgical package is a phrase commonly encountered when billing. Generally, a surgical procedure includes the following:

- The operation.
- Local infiltration; topical anesthesia or metacarpal, metatarsal, or digital block.
- After the decision for surgery is billed, the surgical package includes one related E/M encounter on the date immediately before or on the date of procedure (including history and physical). Also, see the later section on -57 Decision for Surgery.
- Immediate postoperative care, including dictating operative notes and talking with the family and other physicians.
- Writing orders.
- Evaluating the patient in the postanesthesia recovery area.
- Typical postoperative follow-up care (hospital visits, discharge, or follow-up office visits).

This is referred to as a "surgical package" for operative procedures, and one fee covers the entire set of services (Figure 6-6, *A*). The majority of surgical procedures, including fracture care, are handled in this manner. Typical postoperative follow-up care includes only care that is usually a part of the surgical service. Complications, exacerbations, recurrence, or the presence of other diseases or injuries that require additional services should be separately reported. The global period under CPT is not specifically stated, so from a CPT perspective, the global surgical period extends from no more than one day before the day of the procedure to as long as is necessary for typical postoperative follow-up care to be completed. In essence, the postoperative period is open-ended. Medicare defines the postoperative global periods of 0, 10, 30, or 90 days, and most third-party insurance companies apply the same criteria.

Visits not related to the original surgery and complications of the surgery (infection of the wound) are billable using modifier -24. Preoperative services, such as consultations, office visits, and initial hospital care, are often billed separately. An appropriate five-digit E/M code should be selected for these type services. Payment of these services depends on third-party payment policy and the documentation—some are paid separately; some are not.

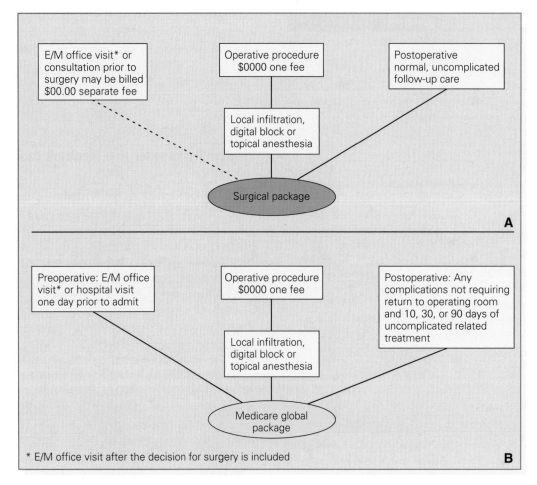

FIGURE 6-6 A, Surgical package concept. **B,** Medicare global package.

Insurance policies and managed care plans vary in what is included in the surgical package fee. Most follow Medicare guidelines; some do not. Plans may include all visits several weeks before surgery, or they may include only visits that occur 1 day before the surgery. When a decision is made for surgery, a commonly asked question is whether a charge may be made for the consultation or office visit and admission if done on the same day. In most cases the admission should be billed listing initial hospital care codes 99221 through 99223. However, the guidelines are different for surgeons. For example, surgical package rules apply if a patient is referred by his or her primary care physician for consultation by a surgeon and the surgeon recommends that the patient receive immediate transfer of care and admission for surgery. The consultation that resulted in the decision for surgery may be billed by adding modifier -57 (decision for surgery) to the consultation procedure code number. The surgeon may not charge for an admission because all E/M services provided within 24 hours of surgery are included in (bundled) the surgical fee. Most third-party reimbursement systems will not pay medical and surgical services to the same physician on the same date of service.

Medicare Global Package

Medicare has a **global surgery policy** for major operations that is similar to the surgical package concept. The Medicare global fee is a single fee for all necessary services normally furnished by the surgeon before, during, and after the procedure. This became effective January 1, 1992 (see Figure 6-6, *B*). As previously mentioned, CMS issued a policy that eliminated the use of all consultation codes (ranges 99241 through 99245 and 99251 through 99255 for inpatient and office/outpatient settings. Included in the global surgery package are the following:

● Preoperative visits (1 day before or day of surgery)
● Intraoperative services that are a usual and necessary part of the surgical procedure
● Complications after surgery that do not require additional trips to the operating room (medical and surgical services)
● Postoperative visits, including hospital visits, discharge, and office visits, for variable postoperative periods: 0, 10, 30, or 90 days

- Writing orders
- Evaluating the patient in the recovery area
- Normal postoperative pain management

Procedures shown in the *Federal Register* may show one of the three-digit or three-alpha codes in the global period column. These codes are not used on the claim form. They give information related to billing rules and regulations that indicate whether a global time period is part of a CPT code. This is particularly important when a patient comes in for a visit after surgery and helps in deciding if the visit can be billed or is included in the surgical fee. These codes appear as follows:

000 No global period.
010 For minor procedure with expected normal follow-up in a 10-day period.
090 For major surgery with a one-day preoperative period and a 90-day postoperative period included in the fee.

MMM No global period. This is a service furnished in uncomplicated maternity cases, which includes prenatal care, delivery, and postnatal care.

XXX No global period. Visits, procedures, and follow-up services may be charged separately.

YYY The global period will be determined by the local Medicare fiscal agent because the code is for an unlisted procedure.

ZZZ The code is part of another service and falls within that service's global period.

Services provided for a Medicare patient not included in the global surgery package that may be billed are the following:

- Initial evaluation (regardless of when it occurs). Also, see the later section on -57 Decision for Surgery.
- Postoperative visits unrelated to the diagnosis for which the surgical procedure was performed (modifier -24 applies).
- Treatment necessary to stabilize a seriously ill patient before surgery.
- Diagnostic tests and procedures.
- Related procedure for postoperative complications that requires a return trip to the operating room (modifier -78 applies).
- Immunosuppressive therapy after transplant surgery.

Never Event

Effective January 15, 2009, Medicare will not cover certain surgical never events and some insurance

Understanding which services are included, what constitutes the global surgical period, and how to code related or unrelated services in the global surgical package for Medicare patients is critical in ensuring correct payment and meeting compliance guidelines.

companies have stopped payment to hospitals for never events A **never event** is an occurrence related to a surgical procedure that is performed on the wrong side, wrong site, wrong body part, or wrong person; retention of a foreign object in a patient after a procedure; patient death or disability associated with the use of contaminated drugs, devices, or biologics provided by the health care facility; patient death or serious disability associated with a medication error; stage 3 or 4 pressure ulcers acquired after admission to the health care facility; and patient death or disability associated with a fall while being cared for at the health care facility. Such occurrences should never happen in a medical practice and are usually preventable. Medicare will not cover hospitalization and other services related to these non-covered procedures. After discharge, reasonable and necessary services are covered whether they are or are not related to the surgical error.

Transfer to Another Facility

If a Medicare patient is discharged from one hospital facility and admitted to a different hospital or facility on the same day, a provider may get paid for both, depending on the circumstances of the case. A low-level admission code (e.g., 99221) is used for the second hospital admission. A higher-level admission code may be used when the patient goes from a regular room status to a type of specialized hospital. Two separate revised CMS-1500 claim forms, one for the discharge and another for the admission, must be used because two different locations of service (hospital names) must appear on the claim forms.

Follow-up (Postoperative) Days

The number of follow-up (postoperative) days that are included in the surgical package varies. The CPT code book does not specify how many days should be given, so an additional reference manual is necessary. Most states use an RVS for workers' compensation cases, which lists the follow-up days allowed for most surgical procedures. Another source that lists surgical follow-up days for Medicare services is published in the *Federal Register* at the end of each year. Locate Appendix B (the Medicare Fee

Schedule). Follow-up days are listed as a global fee period in the ninth column. Obtain the RVS used in your state or a copy of the *Federal Register* for this information.

Medicare lists a 30- or 90-day global period for all major procedures and 10 days for minor procedures. Some commercial third-party payers have a 45-day global period for all or some major procedures. A few commercial third-party payers treat major procedures like minor procedures in the surgical package by allowing 10 follow-up days instead of 90. But most third-party insurance companies follow Medicare guidelines and adhere to the 10-, 30-, and 90-day global periods. To obtain specific payer information, send the insurance company a list of the most common surgical procedures and ask for the surgical package rules and the number of global days that apply to each code. If this information is not available, it is wise to bill the private payer for the preoperative and all postoperative visits. When this information is received, a table should be created that shows global days on a payer-by-payer and procedure-by-procedure basis. On the chart of each patient scheduled for surgery, the type of surgery and how many days the insurance policy allows should be indicated. A bill should be submitted for all visits after the surgical package period expires.

For office visits by the physician during the postoperative period, use CPT code number 99024 on the patient's financial account to indicate "No Charge." This code is located in the Medicine Section under Special Services and Reports; Miscellaneous Services. It has no value, is unbundled with other codes, and is used for tracking purposes. Code number 99024 on itemized billing statements lets the patient know how many office visits after surgery have been provided at no charge. There is no Medicare guideline for this code. It is not necessary to list this code when completing an insurance claim unless the third-party payer has specific instructions requesting that it be shown. If the patient has to be seen beyond the normal postoperative period, the reason must be documented in the patient's medical record and an applicable procedure code and fee for this service should be indicated on the claim form. A bill may be submitted for the office visit if the patient returns to the provider for treatment of an unrelated illness or injury during the postoperative (global) period. The diagnosis codes should support the reason for the visit. If the provider did not perform the surgery but is performing the postoperative care, the provider can charge for the visits but must use the appropriate modifier (-55) to explain the charge.

Repair of Lacerations

If multiple lacerations are repaired with the same technique and are in the same anatomic category, the insurance billing specialist should add up the total length of all the lacerations and report one code to obtain maximum reimbursement. Anatomic categories are the scalp, neck, axillae, external genitalia, trunk, extremities (hands or feet), face, ears, eyelids, nose, lips, or mucous membranes. If the patient had three repairs and each was listed with a different code, the second and third codes are downcoded (coded down one level) by the third-party payer so that a smaller payment is generated. If a patient has lacerations on both sides of the face, the lengths of all the lacerations should be combined because the anatomic region is the same, and a claim should be submitted for the total length. No modifier is used, and the right and left side of the face are not billed separately (Example 6-11).

Example 6-11   Repair of Multiple Lacerations

Three lacerations of the face totaling 8.2 cm
Incorrect Coding
12011   Repair 2.5-cm laceration of face
12013   Repair 2.7-cm laceration of face
12013   Repair 3-cm laceration of face
Correct Coding
12015   Repair 8.2-cm laceration of face

Multiple Lesions

The descriptions for the surgical codes that relate to accessory structures (e.g., scalp, arms, or legs) and lesions found in the integumentary system (pertaining to the skin) can cause confusion. Code descriptions, including indentations, should be read completely with attention paid to terms such as complex, complicated, extensive, and multiple (lesions). Lesion excision code selection is based on the lesion's clinical diameter plus margin before excision and the character of the lesion-benign or malignant. Measurements should be taken before excision because a specimen subject to pathology may shrink. Do not refer to a pathology report because the diameter of the mass may be measured after shrinkage or fragmentation of the specimen. Example 6-12 is a guide to obtain maximum reimbursement for paring of seven corns.

Example 6-12   Paring of Seven Corns

Incorrect Coding
11055   Paring; single lesion
11056-51   Two to four lesions
11057-51   More than four lesions
        or
11055 ×7   Paring; single lesion (×seven corns)
Correct Coding
11057   Paring; more than four lesions (seven corns)

If possible, delay submission of the insurance claim for removal of a lesion or lesions until the pathology report is received. Usually, a malignant lesion is reimbursed at a higher rate because of the more detailed nature of the procedure.

Supplies

When billing for office surgery and supplies used, checklists for the items used on the sterile tray (Figure 6-7, *A*) and for determining complete and incomplete records (see Figure 6-7, *B*) should be used. These items can only be charged for if the surgery required the use of additional items not normally used for this type of surgery.

MINOR OPERATING ROOM INSTRUMENT TRAY SUPPLY CHECKLIST

1 Adson Brown tissue forceps
1 Adson tissue forceps with teeth
1 long tissue forceps
2 mosquito clamps
1 Peck Joseph dissecting scissors
1 Kahn dissecting scissors
1 Reynolds dissecting scissors
1 Stratte needle holder
1 Webster needle holder
4 small piercing towel clips
2 double-skin hooks
2 single-skin hooks
1 knife handle
1 #15 blade
10 4 x 4s
2 cotton-tipped applicators
1 small basin
3 sterile towels (drapes)
1 Bovie pencil
Sutures:_____ _____ _____
Dressings: ½-inch Steri-strips

A

OFFICE SURGERY MEDICAL RECORD CHECKLIST

Patient information sheet
H and P or progress note
Consent form
Diagnostic studies
Pathology report(s)
Anesthesia record
Circulating nurse's note
Doctor's orders
Discharge note
Operative report
Signature/operative report

B

FIGURE 6-7 A, Checklist to document supplies used when billing for office surgery. This list can be kept with the patient's medical record. **B,** Checklist for identifying complete and incomplete medical records used for a patient receiving office surgery. As each item or document is completed, it is checked off so that the person reviewing the chart can see at a glance what needs to be finalized.

Medicare pays for trays with some procedure codes but not for others.

Incident-to Services

According to federal Medicare billing guidelines, physicians can bill for services provided by allied health professionals who are members of their practice, such as physician assistants, therapists, nurses, and nurse practitioners, as long as the services relate to the professional services that the physician provides and direct supervision occurs. Examples for using E/M code 99211 (established patient office visit) not requiring the presence of a physician might include:

- Rechecking a patient for conjunctivitis
- Checking blood pressure for a patient who is being treated for high blood pressure
- Checking a wound beyond the global period
- Reading a tuberculin test result
- Recheck for issuing a return-to-work certificate

The physician must be present in the office suite; thus being available by telephone does not count as direct supervision of the allied health professional. It is important that documentation includes the date of service, reason for the visit, medical necessity, patient encounter information, and signature of the practitioner. To verify that there was a supervising physician, add a place for the physician to countersign that he or she was available and directly supervised the visit.

Prolonged Services, Detention, or Standby

Code numbers 99354 through 99359 should be used to indicate prolonged services with direct face-to-face patient contact; for example, the physician has spent time beyond the usual amount allotted for the service (e.g., 30 to 60 minutes). There are specific codes for services with face-to-face contact and without face-to-face contact. Prolonged service that is less than 30 minutes should not be billed using these codes because the time is included in the E/M code. Time should be documented in the health record to justify use of these codes. Reimbursement for prolonged attendance in the hospital is higher than payment for many other types of care, and reimbursement for critical care is even higher.

Physician standby services over the first 30 minutes are billed using code 99360. Some insurance programs or plans (e.g., Medicare) do not pay for physician standby services, so be sure to check before billing to see whether the commercial payer will pay. The charge for this type of service is based on what the physician believes is the value of an hour of his or her time. An example of this might be when a pediatrician is on standby during a high-risk cesarean section performed on a pregnant woman.

Unlisted Procedures

When an unusual service is rendered, an unlisted code (Example 6-13) should be used rather than guessing or using an incorrect code. Supporting documentation (letter and copy of operative report) should be sent explaining the service.

Example 6-13 Unlisted Procedure Code

31599 Unlisted procedure, larynx

Since the development of category III codes, it is important to double check that section of the CPT code book to verify whether a code exists before using an unlisted code. Unlisted codes may or may not end in -99 and are found at the end of each section or subsection. A comprehensive listing of unlisted codes is found at the beginning of each section. Some MACs do not pay for any of the special -99 adjunct or unlisted codes. The following are guidelines for submitting a claim with an unlisted code to obtain maximum payment:

- Always send or transmit supporting documentation with the claim to clearly identify the procedure performed and the medical necessity. If detailed documentation cannot be electronically submitted or faxed to the third-party payer, send a paper claim with supporting documentation in a large envelope so that it is not folded. Do not use paper clips, staples, or tape to affix the attachments to the claim. Mark each attachment with the patient's name, insurance identification number, date of service, page number of the attachment, and total number of pages submitted (e.g., page 2 of 3). This helps the claim's processor match the documentation to the claim in case they are separated. Do not use a highlighter to point out the pertinent operative note sections because it may not show up when payers scan the claim. Instead, underline, star, or bracket the applicable sections for quick identification.
- File claims with unlisted procedure codes in a separate "tickler" file or in an electronic tracking system. Follow up the status of the claim if there is no response within 1 month.

Coding Guidelines for Code Edits

In 1996 the Medicare program implemented the NCCI. This initiative involves a code editing system consistent with Medicare policies to eliminate inappropriate reporting of CPT codes. *Code editing* is a computer software function that performs online checking of codes on an insurance claim to detect unbundling, splitting of codes, and other types of improper code submissions. Some

coders refer to this process as *code screening*. NCCI edits are updated quarterly. Updated information may be obtained by referring to the Internet Resources at the end of this chapter and visiting the Evolve website, which has an active link to this initiative. Such software is used by private payers, federal programs, and state Medicaid programs. Some code pairs in the NCCI edits are followed by a 0 and others by a 1. If the superscript 0 appears with a code pair, it means Medicare never allows a modifier to be used with the codes, so the code pair could never be reported together. The superscript 1 means that you may use a modifier under certain circumstances with appropriate documentation to get both codes reimbursed.

Because every medical practice has billing problems and questions unique to its specialty that arise because of denial or reduction in payment of claims, the billing specialist must become a detective and discover how to obtain maximum reimbursements in the appropriate specialty. The best way is to telephone the third-party payer inquiring about new coding options and by noting improvements in reimbursement. Coding takes expertise. It is an art not an exact science. The following explanations of various ways of coding claims assist in obtaining maximum reimbursement for each service rendered and avoiding denials, lowered reimbursement, and possible audit.

Comprehensive and Component Edits

A **comprehensive code** means a single code that describes or covers two or more component codes that are bundled together as one unit. A component code is a lesser procedure and is considered part of the major procedure. Each component code represents a portion of the service described in the comprehensive code and should be used only if a portion of the comprehensive service was performed (Example 6-14).

Example 6-14 Comprehensive and Component Codes

Comprehensive code	93015	Cardiovascular stress test
Component codes	93016, 93017, 93018	
93015		Cardiovascular stress test using maximal or submaximal treadmill or bicycle exercise, continuous electrocardiographic monitoring, or pharmacologic stress; with physician supervision, with interpretation and report
93016		physician supervision only, without interpretation and report
93017		tracing only, without interpretation and report
93018		interpretation and report only

Under the Medicare program, NCCI component code edits involve procedures that meet any of the following criteria:

1. Code combinations that are specified as "separate procedures" by CPT
2. Codes that are included as part of a more extensive procedure
3. Code combinations that are restricted by the guidelines outlined in CPT
4. Component codes that are used incorrectly with the comprehensive code

If any one of these restricted code combinations is billed, Medicare allows payment for only the procedure with the highest relative value (Example 6-15).

Example 6-15   Separate Procedure

Separate procedure example: Inguinal hernia repair with lesion excised from spermatic cord

Comprehensive code: 49505 Repair initial hernia age 5 years or older; reducible

Component code: 55520 Excision of lesion of spermatic cord (separate procedure)

For example, when performing an inguinal hernia repair, the surgeon makes an incision in the groin and dissects tissue to expose the hernia sac, internal oblique muscle, and spermatic cord. If a lesion is excised from the spermatic cord, it is considered a component of the comprehensive hernia repair procedure and is not separately billable. Medicare will deny code 55520 (lesion excision) as a component of procedure code 49505 (hernia repair) when performed during the same operative session.

Mutually Exclusive Code Denials

Mutually exclusive code edits relate to procedures that meet any of the following criteria:

1. Code combinations that are restricted by the guidelines outlined in CPT
2. Procedures that represent two methods of performing the same service
3. Procedures that cannot reasonably be done during the same session
4. Procedures that represent medically impossible or improbable code combinations

In Example 6-16, if one were to submit both codes 47605 and 47563, both of the procedures noted in the example are different methods of accomplishing the same result (removal of the gallbladder with cholangiography). They represent a duplication of efforts and an overlap of services, therefore Medicare would deny code 47563 (laparoscopy) as mutually exclusive to code 47605 (the excision).

Example 6-16   Mutually Exclusive

47605   **Excision,** cholecystectomy; with cholangiography
47563   **Laparoscopy,** surgical; cholecystectomy with cholangiography
NOTE: Different methods of accomplishing same procedure.

Bundled Codes

For insurance claim purposes, **bundled codes** means to group related codes together. To completely understand bundled codes, one must have a thorough knowledge of the service or procedure that is being provided or use an unbundling book as a reference guide.

Example 6-17 illustrates one type of bundling found in the CPT code book. Because code 19271 (excision of chest wall tumor without mediastinal lymphadenectomy) does not include mediastinal lymphadenectomy and code 19272 (with mediastinal lymphadenectomy) does include it, reporting both codes together would be a contradiction in the actual performance of the services at the same session. Hence when mediastinal lymphadenectomy is part of the procedure, submit code 19272 because code 19271 is bundled with it.

Example 6-17   Bundled Code

| **Component code** | 19271 | Excision of chest wall tumor involving ribs, with plastic reconstruction; without mediastinal lymphadenectomy |
| **Comprehensive code** | 19272 | with mediastinal lymphadenectomy |

In the Medicare program, a number of services may be affected because CMS considers the services bundled. Because many commercial third-party payers may follow Medicare guidelines, an understanding of this bundling concept is necessary. When dealing with private insurance, an explanation of benefits (EOB) document may print out with a statement "Benefits have been combined," which means the same thing as bundling.

For example, when listing a sterile tray for an in-office surgical procedure, the tray is bundled with the procedure unless additional supplies are necessary in addition to those usually used. CPT code 99070 (supplies and materials) is not reimbursed by Medicare; however, HCPCS level II alphanumeric codes may be used in such cases. The cost of some services and supplies are bundled into E/M codes (e.g., telephone services, reading of test results). However, Medicare pays for slings, splints, rib belts, cast supplies, Hexcelite and light casts, pneumatic

---

Example 6-18   Unbundled Code

Incorrect Coding

43235   Upper gastrointestinal (GI) endoscopy

43600   Biopsy of stomach

Correct Coding

43239   Upper GI endoscopy with biopsy of stomach

Example 6-19   Unbundling (Comprehensive Code)

Unbundled Claim

58150   Total abdominal hysterectomy (corpus and cervix) with removal of tubes and with removal of ovary ($1200)

58700   Salpingectomy ($650)

58940   Oophorectomy ($685)

Total Charge: $2535

Claim Coded Correctly

58150   Comprehensive code for all three services

Total Charge: $1200

Example 6-20   Unbundling (Bilateral)

Incorrect Coding

77055-RT   Right mammography

77055-LT   Left mammography

Correct Coding

77056   Mammography, bilateral

Example 6-21   Bundling (Surgical Approach)

Incorrect Coding

49000   Exploratory laparotomy

44150   Colectomy, total, abdominal

Correct Coding

44150   Colectomy, total, abdominal (correct because it includes exploration of the surgical field)

---

ankle-control splints, and prosthetics, but a supplier (provider) number is necessary to bill for take-home surgical supplies and durable medical equipment (DME). Medicare claims for supplies and DME go to one of four regional DME fiscal agents. These may be found by visiting the Evolve website listed in Internet Resources at the end of this chapter for an active link to the DME regional contacts. A reference book published by Ingenix has a comprehensive list of the codes that CMS considers bundled for the Medicare program. (See the Appendix for further information.)

When appealing a claim, a great deal of time may be spent on paperwork only to discover that the code is bundled and denial is imminent. When in doubt about whether services are combined or not, contact the third-party payer and ask.

Unbundling

Unbundling is coding and billing numerous CPT codes to identify procedures that usually are described by a single code. It is also known as *exploding*, or *a la carte*, medicine.

Some practices do this unwittingly, but it is considered fraud if it is done intentionally to gain increased reimbursement. Unbundling can lead to downward payment adjustments and possible audit of claims.

Types of unbundling are as follow:

- Fragmenting one service into component parts and coding each component part as if it were a separate service (Example 6-18)
- Reporting separate codes for related services when one comprehensive code includes all related services (Example 6-19)
- Coding **bilateral** (both sides of the body) procedures as two codes when one code is proper (Example 6-20)
- Separating a surgical approach from a major surgical service that includes the same approach (Example 6-21)

Insurers use special software designed to detect unbundling. To avoid this problem, always use a current CPT code book. The use of outdated codes often inadvertently

results in unbundling. A new technology or technique may have its own code when it is developed but may be bundled with another code as it becomes commonplace. If the practice uses a billing service, request in writing that its computer system include no unbundling programming.

Always submit current CPT codes because if outdated codes are used, it could red flag a provider with Medicare as being in noncompliance.

Downcoding

Downcoding occurs when the coding system used on a claim submitted to a third-party payer does not match the coding system used by the company receiving the claim. The computer system converts the code submitted to the closest code in use, which is usually down one level from the submitted code. Therefore the payment that is generated is usually less. In many states, it is illegal for an insurance company to downcode a claim. Insurance commissioners have published bulletins warning payers to cease this claims adjudication practice. When a payer receives a claim, the payer is allowed to pay or deny the claim. If additional information is necessary to adjudicate the claim, it should be requested from the patient or provider. The payer is limited by the number of days it has to review the claim. At completion of the review, the payer must pay or deny the claim.

Make sure that the documentation from the provider supports the code that is being submitted to prevent downcoding.

Use current CPT manuals. Review all Medicare updates for changes to HCPCS codes. Always monitor reimbursements and look for downcoding so that you become knowledgeable about which codes are affected (Example 6-22).

Example 6-22   Downcoding

Incorrect Coding
20010   Incision of abscess with suction irrigation
(**NOTE:** 20010 has been deleted from CPT and would result in downcoding.)
Correct Coding
20005   Incision of abscess, deep or complicated

Downcoding also occurs when a claims examiner converts the CPT code submitted to a code in the RVS being used by the payer. This can occur in workers' compensation claims. When there is a choice between two or three somewhat similar codes, the claims examiner chooses the lowest paying code. Any time the code that was submitted is changed, appeal the change immediately.

Downcoding also may occur when a claims examiner compares the code used with the written description of the procedure included in an attached document. If the two do not match, the payer will reimburse according to the lowest paying code that fits the description given (Example 6-23). In this example the word "bone" is a clue to go to the musculoskeletal section of the code book and not the integumentary section. See Chapter 9 for additional information and solutions to downcoding.

Example 6-23   Downcoding

Document states: Excision of bone tumor from anterior tibial shaft.
    Pathology report states: Tibia bone tumor; benign
Incorrect Coding
11400   Excision of benign lesion including margins except skin tag, trunk, arms or legs; excised diameter 0.5 cm or less
Correct Coding
27635   Excision of bone tumor of tibia, benign

Upcoding

The term **upcoding** is used to describe deliberate manipulation of CPT codes for increased payment. This practice can be spotted by Medicare fiscal agents and third-party payers using prepayment and postpayment screens or "stop alerts," which are built into most computer coding software programs. An example of intentional upcoding might be a physician who selects one level of service code for all visits with the theory that the costs even out, such as always using code 99213. This opens the door to audits and in the end may cost the practice money. Upcoding may occur unintentionally if the coder is ill informed or does not keep current. Join a free list service (listserv) to keep current, make national coding contacts, and post questions to others who may know the answer to a current coding or billing dilemma; for example, if you wish to join a free listserv visit the Evolve website listed in the Internet Resources at the end of this chapter. It has an active link to Listserv.

Code Monitoring

Monitoring of CPT codes is done to maximize reimbursement from all third-party payers. First, determine which codes are used most often in the physician's practice. Many computer programs can generate a list of codes, ranking them according to frequency of use. If the practice does not have a computer, take a sampling of the charge slips to determine the prevalent codes. Once the high-volume codes are known, focus on coding strategies for the best possible reimbursement (Figure 6-8). Monitor every Remittance Advice/Explanation of Benefits that comes in directly or via patients. Every private insurance, Medicare, Medicaid, and TRICARE payment received should be checked for accuracy to see whether it is consistently the same or if coding changes have occurred. Incorrect payments should be investigated and appealed. Examine all payments made for codes that do not match those submitted. Be sure to appeal every payment that is less than half of what the physician bills. An example of

CODE/PAYMENT TRACKING LOG					Date: 1-XX
CPT CODE	Practice fee	Medicare date and amount paid	Medicaid date and amount paid	TRICARE date and amount paid	Blue Shield date and amount paid
99201	$00.00	11-XX $00.00	8-XX $00.00	7-XX $00.00	4-XX $00.00
99202	$00.00	12-XX $00.00	9-XX $00.00	10-XX $00.00	6-XX $00.00
99211	$00.00	12-XX $00.00			11-XX $00.00
99212	$00.00				12-XX $00.00
99221	$00.00				
99231	$00.00				
99232	$00.00				
99241	$00.00				

FIGURE 6-8 Example of a code/payment tracking log.

a code and payment tracking log to help monitor payments received is shown in Figure 6-8.

HELPFUL HINTS IN CODING

Office Visits

When an established patient is seen for an office visit and a clinical medical assistant incidentally takes the patient's blood pressure per the physician's standing order, the physician includes that service with the appropriate level of E/M code number (e.g., 99213 or 99214). If the clinical medical assistant takes the blood pressure and the patient is not seen by the physician but the physician reviews the results, the appropriate E/M code number is 99211 (presence of physician not necessary). If more than one office visit is necessary per day, the requirements for use of modifiers -25 and -59 should be read before submitting a claim to determine whether one of them may be applicable.

Some insurance policies allow only two moderate- or high-complexity office visits per patient per year. Therefore contact the insurance company either online or by telephone to validate whether the patient is insured and also to learn if there are any limitations. A physician's practice should have a system in place to track this.

Drugs and Injections

When submitting claims for Medicare, Medicaid, and some private insurance carriers, insert the name, amount of dosage, strength, and how it was administered for the Not Otherwise Classified (NOC) drug in Block 19 on the CMS-1500 claim form. This information must be documented in the patient's health record. If a drug is experimental or expensive, you need to attach a copy of the invoice. CPT codes for immunization administration for vaccines are 90465 through 90474 and for therapeutic or diagnostic are 96372 to 96379. Separate codes are used to identify the product being administered, either immune globulin codes 90281 through 90399, vaccine/toxoid codes 90476 through 90749, or when billing a Medicare case, Level II HCPCS national alphanumeric codes A0000 or J0000. In Medicaid cases, it is permissible to bill for injectable medications. Separate codes are available for combination vaccines. See CPT codes 95004 through 95199 for allergy testing and codes 95115 through 95199 for allergen immunotherapy. If an anesthetic agent is being used, determine whether it is diagnostic, therapeutic, or prophylactic for pain. Medicare bills for immunosuppressive therapy are submitted to durable medical equipment fiscal agents, regional carriers (private companies) that contract with Medicare to process and pay insurance claims for medical equipment. *Immunosuppressive therapy* is treatment by administering an agent that significantly interferes with the ability of the body's immune system to respond to antigenic stimulation by inhibiting cellular and humoral immunity, such as preparing someone for a bone marrow transplant or to prevent rejection of donor tissue.

Some providers give mass immunizations to Medicare patients. A simplified process called *roster billing* was created that allows a provider to submit a vaccine roster with the CMS-1500 (08-05) claim form. The roster must include the Medicare patients' identification numbers, names, addresses, dates of birth, genders, and signatures when they received vaccinations for influenza and pneumococcal vaccines covered by Medicare. Paper or electronic claims may be submitted with the roster. Medicare annual Part B deductible and coinsurance amounts do not apply to these vaccines. HCPCS codes G0008, G0009, and G0010 are used with the appropriate vaccine product code and a V code from ICD-9-CM indicating the need for the immunization. For e-prescribing, a bonus is given to providers who electronically prescribe drugs. As of 2010, HCPCS code G8553 should be used for reporting.

Adjunct Codes

Adjunct codes are referred to in the Medicine Section of the CPT as Special Services, Procedures and Reports and fall under the category of Miscellaneous Services. They are important to consider when billing because these codes provide the reporting physician with a means of identifying special services and reports that are provided in addition to the basic services provided. The circumstances that are covered under these codes (99000 through 99091) include handling of laboratory specimens, telephone calls, seeing patients after hours, office emergency services, supplies and materials, special reports, travel, and educational services rendered to patients. Explain the circumstances on an attached document to justify the use of these codes when submitting an insurance claim. Some insurance companies pay for these services, but others do not.

Basic Life or Disability Evaluation Services

Use code 99450 when reporting examinations done on patients for the purpose of trying to obtain life or disability insurance. Codes 99455 and 99456 may be used for work-related or medical disability examinations. Additional information about life or health insurance examinations is given in Chapter 7.

CODE MODIFIERS

The use of a CPT code's two-digit add-on modifier permits the physician to indicate circumstances in which a procedure as performed differs in some way from that described by its usual five-digit code (Example 6-24). It may be necessary when using a modifier to include an operative, pathology, x-ray, or special report to justify its use to a third-party payer. For each modifier listed in Table 6-6, there is a statement as to when it is appropriate to include a report. A modifier can indicate the following:

- A service or procedure has either a professional or technical component.
- A service or procedure was performed by more than one physician or in more than one location.
- A service or procedure has been increased or reduced.
- A service or procedure was provided more than once.
- Only part of a service was performed.

Example 6-24   How to Report Modifier on Claim Form

Add a two-digit modifier to the five-digit code number
Single line item:
       12345-**22** *OR* **1234522**

- An adjunctive service was performed.
- A bilateral procedure was performed.
- Unusual events occurred.

Correct Use of Common CPT Modifiers

A choice of any modifier that fits the situation that is being coded may be used except when the modifier definition restricts the use of specific codes; for example, modifier -51, Multiple Procedures, states that -51 is to be appended for "multiple procedures, other than Evaluation and Management Services . . ." Discussion of the most commonly used modifiers follows.

-22 Increased Procedural Services

Modifier -22 is used when the service provided is substantially greater than that typically required for the listed procedure. If you add modifier -22, the documentation in the health record, such as operative reports and/or chart note, must support the substantial additional work. Encourage your physician to use appropriate descriptions in the report, and call these words to his or her attention. The reasons for use of this modifier are that the work encompasses increased intensity, time, technical difficulty of procedure, severity of the patient's condition, and physical and mental effort needed. This modifier may not be used with E/M services. Most third-party payers send an insurance claim to medical review before payment is made if modifier -22, indicating unusual services, appears on the claim. Because payments may be delayed, be cautious when using this modifier. An operative report should be submitted with the claim. If the third-party payer routinely denies the claim with modifier -22, an appeal for review should be made. See Chapter 9 for details on the Medicare redetermination (appeal) process.

-25 Significant, Separately Identifiable Evaluation and Management Service

For information on the modifier -25 (significant, separately identifiable E/M service by the same physician on the same day of the procedure or other service), see the explanation of modifier -57.

-26 Professional Component

Certain procedures are a combination of a **professional component (PC)** and a **technical component (TC)** and are considered a global service. Usually these involve radiology and pathology procedures. The professional (physician) component refers to a portion of a test or procedure that the physician does, such as interpreting an electrocardiogram (ECG), reading an x-ray film, or

Text continued on page 202.

Table 6-6	CPT Modifier Codes							
MODIFIER	EXPLANATION	**USE IN MAIN TEXT SECTIONS**						
		E/M	ANESTHESIA	SURGERY	RADIOLOGY	PATHOLOGY	MEDICINE	TYPE
-22	**Increased Procedural Service:** When the work required to provide a service is substantially greater than typically required, it may be identified by adding modifier -22 to the usual procedure code. Documentation must support the substantial additional work and the reason for the additional work (i.e., increased intensity, time, technical difficulty of procedure, severity of patient's condition, physical and mental effort required). Note: This modifier should not be appended to an E/M service.	Ø	Y	Y	Y	Y	Y	
-23	**Unusual Anesthesia:** Occasionally a procedure that usually requires either no anesthesia or local anesthesia must be done under general anesthesia because of unusual circumstances. This circumstance may be reported by adding the modifier -23 to the procedure code of the basic service.† **Examples:** A proctoscopy might require no anesthesia. A skin biopsy or excision of a subcutaneous tumor might require local anesthesia. If general anesthesia is necessary, append the procedure code with -23.	Ø	Y	Y	N	N	Ø	ANES
-24	**Unrelated E/M Service by the Same Physician During a Postoperative Period:** The physician may need to indicate that an evaluation and management service was performed during a postoperative period for a reason(s) unrelated to the original procedure. This circumstance may be reported by adding the modifier -24 to the appropriate level of E/M service.† **Example:** A patient seen for a postoperative visit after an appendectomy complains of a lump on the leg. The physician takes a history and examines the site, and a biopsy is scheduled. The E/M code 99024 is used for the postsurgery examination and the modifier -24 is added for unrelated service rendered during a postoperative period. **Medicare Payment Rule:** No effect on payment: however, failure to use this modifier when appropriate may result in denial of the E/M service. CMS memo FQA-541 reads "a documented, separately identifiable related service is to be paid for. We would define 'related' as being caused or prompted by the same symptoms or conditions." Make sure to document that the E/M service was related to the procedure.	Y	Ø	Ø	Ø	Ø	Ø	GP E/M

Modified with permission from the American Medical Association, Chicago.
ANES, Modifier related to anesthesia; *BUN*, modifier related to bundling or CCI; *CPT*, *Current Procedural Terminology*; *E/M*, Evaluation and Management only modifier; *GP*, global package modifier; *LAB*, modifier related to laboratory service; *N*, not usually used with the codes in that section of CPT; *Y*, yes commonly used with the codes in that section of CPT; *#*, modifier related to number of surgeons; *Ø*, never used with the codes in that section of CPT.
*This modifier may affect reimbursement by third-party payer.
†This modifier may affect reimbursement, depending on the payer.

Table 6-6	CPT Modifier Codes—cont'd							
MODIFIER	EXPLANATION	**USE IN MAIN TEXT SECTIONS**						
		E/M	ANESTHESIA	SURGERY	RADIOLOGY	PATHOLOGY	MEDICINE	TYPE
-25	**Significant, Separately Identifiable E/M Service by the Same Physician on the Same Day of the Procedure or Other Service:** It may be necessary to indicate that on the day a procedure or service identified by a CPT code was performed, the patient's condition required a significant, separately identifiable E/M service above and beyond the other service provided or beyond the usual preoperative and postoperative care associated with the procedure that was performed. A significant, separately identifiable E/M service is defined or substantiated by documentation that satisfies the relevant criteria for the respective E/M service to be reported (see CPT Evaluation and Management Services Guidelines for instructions on determining level of E/M service). The E/M service may be prompted by the symptom or condition for which the procedure and/or service was provided. As such, different diagnoses are not required for reporting of the E/M services on the same date. This circumstance may be reported by adding modifier -25 to the appropriate level of E/M service. **Note:** This modifier is not used to report an E/M service that resulted in a decision to perform surgery. See modifier -57. For significant, separately identifiable non-E/M services, see modifier -59. **Example:** A patient is seen for a diabetic follow-up and the physician discovers a suspicious mole on the patient's neck (0.4 cm), which is removed. The physician makes a minor adjustment of the oral diabetes medication. This case illustrates a significant E/M service provided on the same day as a procedure, so -25 is added to the E/M code. Code 11420 is used for removal of the benign lesion. **Note:** This modifier is not used to report an E/M service that resulted in a decision to perform surgery. See modifier -57.† **Medicare Payment Rule:** No effect on payment; however, failure to use this modifier when appropriate may result in denial of the E/M service.	Y	Ø	Ø	Ø	Ø	Ø	BUN GP E/M
-26	**Professional Component:** Certain procedures are a combination of a professional physician component and a technical component. When the professional (physician) component is reported separately, the service may be identified by adding the modifier -26 to the usual procedure number.* **Note:** The professional component comprises only the professional services performed by the physician during radiologic, laboratory, and other diagnostic procedures. These services include a portion of a test or procedure that the physician does, such as interpretation of the results. The technical component includes personnel, materials including usual contrast media and drugs, film or xerograph, space, equipment, and other facilities but excludes the cost of radioisotopes. When billing for the technical component, use the usual five-digit procedure number with modifier -TC. **Example:** 70450-26 Computerized axial tomography, head or brain; without contrast material. *The modifier -26 indicates the physician interpreted this test only.* 70450-TC Computerized axial tomography, head or brain; without contrast material. *The modifier indicates the facility is billing only for the use of the equipment.*	N	N	Y	Y	Y	Y	BUN

*This modifier may affect reimbursement by third-party payer.
†This modifier may affect reimbursement, depending on the payer.

Continued

| Table 6-6 | CPT Modifier Codes—cont'd | | | | | | | |

MODIFIER#	EXPLANATION	E/M	ANESTHESIA	SURGERY	RADIOLOGY	PATHOLOGY	MEDICINE	TYPE
-27	**Multiple Outpatient Hospital E/M Encounters on the Same Date:** For hospital outpatient reporting purposes, utilization of hospital resources related to separate and distinct E/M encounters performed in multiple outpatient hospital settings on the same date may be reported by adding the modifier -27 to each appropriate level outpatient and/or emergency department E/M code(s). This modifier provides a means of reporting circumstances involving evaluation and management services provided by physician(s) in more than one (multiple) outpatient hospital settings (e.g., hospital emergency department, clinic). Do not use this modifier for physician reporting emergency department, or preventative medicine service codes. **Example:** Patient is seen in a hospital outpatient clinic. The patient falls in the treatment room and receives a cut on the right arm. The patient is taken to the emergency department for two stitches and a dressing. **Medicare Payment Rule:** Do not use modifier -27 for Medicare outpatients. Continue to use the -G0 (G-zero) modifier that CMS established to cover multiple procedures, same patient, same day.	Y	N	N	N	N	Y	E/M
-32	**Mandated Services:** Services related to mandated consultation and/or related services (e.g. third-party payer, governmental, legislative, or regulatory requirement) may be identified by adding the modifier -32 to the basic procedure.‡ **Example:** A patient is referred to the physician by an insurance company for an unbiased opinion regarding permanent disability after a year of treatment following an accident. Add modifier -32 to the E/M code because the second opinion is mandated by the insurance company. **Medicare Payment Rule:** No effect on payment.	Y	Y	Y	Y	Y	Y	
-47	**Anesthesia by Surgeon:** Regional or general anesthesia provided by the surgeon may be reported by adding the modifier -47 to the basic service (this does not include local anesthesia† **Note:** Modifier -47 would not be used for anesthesia procedures 00100 through 01999. **Example:** A gastroenterologist performs an endoscopy for removal of esophageal polyps using the snare technique. The physician sedates the patient with Versed to perform the procedure. 43217 Esophagoscopy with removal of polyps by snare technique 43217-47 Administered Versed **Medicare Payment Rule:** Medicare will not reimburse the surgeon to administer anesthesia (any type).	Ø	Ø	Y	Ø	Ø	Ø	ANES
-50	**Bilateral Procedure:** Unless otherwise identified in the listings, bilateral procedures that are performed at the same session should be identified by adding modifier -50 to the appropriate 5-digit code. **Note:** It is important to read each surgical description carefully to look for the word "bilateral." A bilateral modifier on a unilateral procedure code indicates that the procedure was performed on both sides of a paired organ during the same operative session. **Example A:** 71060 Bronchography, bilateral (would be listed with no modifier) **Example B:** 19305 Mastectomy, radical 19305-50 Mastectomy, radical; bilateral **Medicare Payment Rule:** Payment is based on 150% (200% for x-rays) of the fee schedule amount.	N	N	Y	N	N	N	

†This modifier may affect reimbursement, depending on the payer.
‡Modifier is informational in nature. Do not ask for an adjustment in reimbursement. Monitor reimbursement when using this modifier.
#**Modifier -33 Preventive Service:** When the primary purpose of the service is the delivery of an evidence-based service in accordance with a US Preventive Services Task Force A or B rating in effect and other preventive services identified in preventive services mandates (legislative or regulatory), the service may be identified by appending modifier 33, Preventive Service to the service. For separately reported services specifically identified as preventive, the modifier should not be used. **This modifier allows a provider to identify a service as preventive under the Patient Protection and Affordable Care Act and indicates cost sharing does not apply.**

Table 6-6	CPT Modifier Codes—cont'd							
MODIFIER	**EXPLANATION**	USE IN MAIN TEXT SECTIONS						
		E/M	ANESTHESIA	SURGERY	RADIOLOGY	PATHOLOGY	MEDICINE	TYPE
-51	**Multiple Procedures:** When multiple procedures, other than E/M services, physical medicine and rehabilitation services, or provision of supplies (e.g., vaccines) are performed at the same session by the same provider, the primary procedure or service(s) may be identified by appending modifier -51 to the additional procedure or service code(s). **Note:** This modifier should not be appended to designated "add-on" codes (see Appendix D of CPT). Always list the procedure of highest dollar value first. **Example:** Patient had herniated disk in lower back with stabilization of the area where the disk was removed. 63030 Lumbar laminectomy with disk removal 22612-51 Arthrodesis (modifier used after the lesser of the two procedures) **Medicare Payment Rules:** Standard multiple surgery policy—100% of the fee schedule amount is allowed for the highest valued procedure, 50% for the second through fifth procedures, and "by report" for subsequent procedures.	N	Y	Y	Y	Ø	Y	
-52	**Reduced Services:** Under certain circumstances a service or procedure is partially reduced or eliminated at the physician's election. Under these circumstances the service provided can be identified by its usual procedure number and the addition of the modifier -52 signifying that the service is reduced. This provides a means of reporting reduced services without disturbing the identification of the basic service.§ **Note:** This means there will be no effect on the physician's fee profile in the computer data. It is not necessary to attach a report to the claim when using this modifier because it indicates a reduced fee. When a physician performs a procedure but does not charge for the service, such as a postoperative follow-up visit that is included in a global service, remember to use code 99024. Some physicians prefer to bill the insurance carrier the full amount and accept what the carrier pays as payment in full. In such cases, a modifier would not be used. **Example:** A patient is not able to participate or cooperate in a minimal psychiatric interview (90801) and the physician decides to attempt this at a later date. Modify the code with -52. **Medicare Payment Rule:** Payment is based on the extent of the procedure or service performed. Submit documentation with the claim.	Y	N	Y	Y	Y	Y	
-53	**Discontinued Procedure:** Under certain circumstances, the physician may elect to terminate a surgical or diagnostic procedure. Due to extenuating circumstances or those that threaten the well-being of the patient, it may be necessary to indicate that a surgical or diagnostic procedure was started but discontinued. This circumstance may be reported by adding the modifier "-53" to the code for the discontinued procedure. **Note:** This modifier is not used to report the elective cancellation of a procedure before the patient's anesthesia induction and/or surgical preparation in the operating suite. For outpatient hospital/ambulatory surgery center (ACS), see modifiers -73 and -74. **Example:** The physician is beginning a cholecystectomy on a patient. An earthquake of great magnitude occurs and the electricity is shut off. The backup generator comes on and electricity is restored; however, because of the disarray in the operative suite, the physician decides to discontinue the surgery. Code 47562 is used with -53 appended to it. **Medicare Payment Rule:** The carrier will determine the amount of payment "by report." Submit documentation with the claim identifying the extent of the procedure performed and the extenuating circumstances.	Ø	Y	Y	Y	Y	Y	

§This modifier affects reimbursement but not the physician's fee profile.

Continued

Table 6-6	CPT Modifier Codes—cont'd							
MODIFIER	**EXPLANATION**		**USE IN MAIN TEXT SECTIONS**					
		E/M	ANESTHESIA	SURGERY	RADIOLOGY	PATHOLOGY	MEDICINE	TYPE
-54	**Surgical Care Only:** When one physician performs a surgical procedure and another provides preoperative and/or postoperative management, surgical services may be identified by adding the modifier -54 to the usual procedure number.* **Note:** Because many surgical procedures encompass a "package" concept that includes normal uncomplicated follow-up care, the surgeon will be paid a reduced fee when using this modifier. **Example:** A patient presents in the emergency department with severe abdominal pain. Dr. A, the on-call surgeon, examines the patient and performs an emergency appendectomy. Dr. A is leaving on vacation the next morning, so he calls his friend and colleague Dr. B. He asks him to visit the patient in the hospital the following day and take over the postoperative care. Dr. A bills using the appendectomy procedure code 44950 and modifies it with -54. **Medicare Payment Rule:** Payment is limited to the amount allotted for intraoperative services only.	N	N	Y	N	N	N	GP
-55	**Postoperative Management Only:** When one physician performs the postoperative management and another physician performs the surgical procedure, the postoperative component may be identified by adding the modifier -55 to the usual procedure number. **Note:** The fee to list would be approximately 30% of the surgeon's fee. **Example:** The Dunmires are relocating to Memphis, TN, when Mrs. Dunmire discovers a lump on her arm. She visits her family physician, Dr. A, who tells her it needs to be excised. She wants her physician (Dr. A) to do the surgery and Dr. A agrees if she promises to arrange for a physician in Memphis to follow up postoperatively. She makes arrangements with Dr. B in Memphis. Dr. B bills using the correct excision code that he obtained from Dr. A and modifies it with -55. **Medicare Payment Rule:** Payment will be limited to the amount allotted for postoperative services only. Payment to more than one physician for split surgical care of a patient will not exceed the amount paid for the total global surgical package.	N	N	Y	N	N	Y	GP
-56	**Preoperative Management Only:** When one physician performs the preoperative care and evaluation and another physician performs the surgical procedure, the preoperative component may be identified by adding the modifier -56 to the usual procedure number.† **Example:** Dr. A sees Mrs. Jones and determines she needs to have a lung biopsy. He admits her to the hospital and Dr. A becomes ill. Dr. B is called in and performs the surgery. Dr. A bills for the preoperative care using the surgical code he obtained from Dr. B and modifies it with -56. **Medicare Payment Rule:** Payment for this component is included in the allowable for the surgery. If another physician performed the surgery, use an appropriate E/M code to bill for the preoperative service.	N	N	Y	N	N	Y	GP
-57	**Decision for Surgery:** An E/M service that resulted in the initial decision to perform the surgery may be identified by adding the modifier -57 to the appropriate level of E/M service.‡ **Example:** A trauma patient is seen in the emergency department by an orthopedic surgeon for a consultation to determine whether surgery on a fractured femur is necessary. The surgeon subsequently performs surgery 24 hours later in order to provide time for the patient to clear his intestinal contents. The surgeon bills the E/M consultation code and adds the -57 modifier. By adding this modifier, the third-party payer is informed that the consultation is not part of the global surgical procedure. Medicare will pay if it is for major surgery that requires a 90-day postoperative follow-up but not for a minor surgical procedure (0- to 10-day postoperative follow-up). **Medicare Payment Rule:** Payment will be made for the E/M service in addition to the global surgery payment.	Y	N	N	N	N	Y	GP E/M

| Table 6-6 | CPT Modifier Codes—cont'd |

MODIFIER	EXPLANATION	E/M	ANESTHESIA	SURGERY	RADIOLOGY	PATHOLOGY	MEDICINE	TYPE
-58	**Staged or Related Procedure or Service by the Same Physician During the Postoperative Period:** It may be necessary to indicate that the performance of a procedure or service during the postoperative period was (a) planned or anticipated (staged), (b) more extensive than the original procedure, or (c) for therapy after a surgical procedure. This circumstance may be reported by adding the modifier -58 to the staged or related procedure.‡ **Note:** For treatment of a problem that requires a return to the operating or procedure room (e.g., unanticipated clinical condition) see modifier -78. **Example:** A patient has breast cancer and a surgeon performs a mastectomy. During the postoperative global period, the surgeon inserts a permanent prosthesis. The -58 modifier is added to the code for inserting the prosthesis, indicating that this service was planned at the time of the initial operation. If the modifier is not used, the insurance carrier may reject the claim because surgery occurred during the surgery's global period.	N	N	Y	Y	N	Y	GP BUN
-59	**Distinct Procedural Service:** Under certain circumstances, it may be necessary to indicate that a procedure or service was distinct or independent from other non-E/M services performed on the same day. Modifier -59 is used to identify procedures/services, other than E/M services, that are not normally reported together but are appropriate under the circumstances. Documentation must support a different session, different procedure or surgery, different site or organ system, separate incision/excision, separate lesion, or separate injury (or area of injury in extensive injuries) not ordinarily encountered or performed on the same day by the same individual. However, when another already established modifier is appropriate, it should be used rather than modifier -59. Modifier -59 should only be used if no more descriptive modifier is available and the use of modifier -59 best explains the circumstances. **Note:** Modifier -59 should not be appended to an E/M service. To report a separate and distinct E/M service with a non-E/M service performed on the same date, see modifier -25. **Example:** A patient is seen at a physician's office in the morning and the doctor orders a single view (71010) chest x-ray because the patient is complaining of a cough and chest congestion. The physician treats the patient for pneumonia. Later that same day, the patient is seen in the physician's office complaining of chest pain. The physician again orders a chest x-ray, but this time a two-view x-ray (71020). Ordinarily, the single-view chest x-ray will be denied as a component of the two-view chest x-ray. However, because they were obtained at separate encounters, addition of the -59 modifier will indicate that these services are not combination components and should be paid for separately. **Medicare Payment Rule:** No effect on payment amount; however, failure to use modifier when appropriate may result in denial of payment for the services.	N	Y	Y	Y	Y	Y	BUN
-62	**Two Surgeons:** When two surgeons work together as primary surgeons performing distinct parts of a single reportable procedure, each surgeon should report his or her distinct operative work using the same procedure code and adding the modifier -62. If additional procedures (including add-on procedures) are performed during the same surgical session, separate codes may be reported without the modifier -62. **Note:** If the co-surgeon acts as an assist in the performance of additional procedure(s) during the same surgical session, those services may be reported using separate procedure code(s) with modifier -80 or -81. **Example:** A procedure for scoliosis is performed by a thoracic surgeon who does the anterior approach and an orthopedic surgeon who does the posterior approach and repair. **Medicare Payment Rule:** Medicare allows 125% of the approved fee schedule amount for the -62 modifier if reported by both surgeons. That total fee is divided in half and dispersed to each surgeon at 62.5% of the approved amount.	Ø	Ø	Y	Y	Ø	N	#

Continued

Table 6-6	CPT Modifier Codes—cont'd							
		USE IN MAIN TEXT SECTIONS						
MODIFIER	EXPLANATION	E/M	ANESTHESIA	SURGERY	RADIOLOGY	PATHOLOGY	MEDICINE	TYPE
-63	**Procedure Performed on Infants less than 4 kg:** Procedures performed on neonates and infants up to a present body weight of 4 kg may involve significantly increased complexity and physician work commonly associated with these patients. This circumstance may be reported by adding the modifier -63 to the procedure number. **Note:** Unless otherwise designated, this modifier may only be appended to procedures/services listed in the 20000-69999 code series. Modifier -63 should not be appended to any codes listed in the E/M services, Anesthesia, Radiology, Pathology/Laboratory, or Medicine sections.	N	N	Y	Y	N	Y	
-66	**Surgical Team:** Under some circumstances, highly complex procedures (requiring the concomitant services of several physicians, often of different specialties, plus other highly skilled, specially trained personnel and various types of complex equipment) are carried out under the "surgical team" concept. Such circumstances may be identified by each participating physician with the addition of the modifier -66 to the basic procedure number used for reporting services.* **Example:** A kidney transplant, requiring use of a vascular surgeon, urologist, and nephrologist, with the assistance of anesthesiologist and pathologist, or open heart surgery using perfusion personnel, three cardiologists, and an anesthesiologist. **Medicare Payment Rule:** Carrier medical staff will determine the payment amounts for team surgeries on a report basis. Submit supporting documentation with the claim.	Ø	Ø	Y	Y	Ø	N	#
-73	**Discontinued Outpatient Hospital/Ambulatory Surgery Center (ASC) Procedure Before the Administration of Anesthesia:** Because of extenuating circumstances or those that threaten the well-being of the patient, the physician may cancel a surgical or diagnostic procedure subsequent to the patient's surgical preparation (including sedation when provided, and being taken to the room where the procedure is to be performed), but prior to the administration of anesthesia (local, regional block[s], or general). Under these circumstances, the intended service that is prepared for but canceled can be reported by its usual procedure number and the addition of modifier -73. **Note:** The elective cancellation of a service before the administration of anesthesia and/or surgical preparation of the patient should not be reported. For physician reporting of a discontinued procedure, see modifier -53.	N	N	Y	N	N	N	
-74	**Discontinued Outpatient Hospital/Ambulatory Surgery Center (ASC) Procedure After Administration of Anesthesia:** Because of extenuating circumstances or those that threaten the well-being of the patient, the physician may terminate a surgical or diagnostic procedure after the administration of anesthesia (local, regional block[s], or general) or after the procedure was started (incision made, intubation started, or scope inserted). Under these circumstances, the procedure started but terminated can be reported by its usual procedure number and the addition of modifier -74. **Note:** The elective cancellation of a service before the administration of anesthesia and/or surgical preparation of the patient should not be reported. For physician reporting of a discontinued procedure, see modifier -53.	N	N	Y	N	N	N	

Table 6-6	CPT Modifier Codes—cont'd								
MODIFIER	**EXPLANATION**				**USE IN MAIN TEXT SECTIONS**				
		E/M	**ANESTHESIA**	**SURGERY**	**RADIOLOGY**	**PATHOLOGY**	**MEDICINE**	**TYPE**	
-76	**Repeat Procedure or Service by Same Physician or Other Qualified Health Care Professional:** It may be necessary to indicate that a procedure or service was repeated by the same physician or other qualified health care professional subsequent to the original procedure or service. This circumstance may be reported by adding modifier -76 to the repeated procedure or service. **Note:** This modifier should not be appended to an E/M service. **Example:** A patient is seen by his family physician in the morning for his regular appointment. At that time, his doctor orders an ECG (93000). The patient calls in to his doctor's office in the afternoon to state that he is having some odd chest pain. The physician may request that the patient return to the office for another ECG (93000). The second ECG should be billed with a -76 modifier. **Medicare Payment Rule:** Failure to use this modifier when appropriate (and to submit supporting documentation) may result in denial of the subsequent procedure.	N	N	Y	Y	N	Y	GP	
-77	**Repeat Procedure or Service by Another Physician or Other Qualified Health Care Professional:** It may be necessary to indicate that a basic procedure or service was repeated by another physician or other qualified health care professional subsequent to the original procedure or service. This circumstance may be reported by adding modifier -77 to the repeated procedure or service. **Note:** This modifier should not be appended to an E/M service. **Example:** A femoral–popliteal bypass graft (35556) is performed in the morning and in the afternoon it becomes clotted. The original surgeon is not available, and a different surgeon performs the repeat operation later in the day. The original surgeon reports 35556. The second surgeon reports 35556-77. **Medicare Payment Rule:** Failure to use this modifier when appropriate (and to submit supporting documentation) may result in denial of the subsequent surgery.	N	N	Y	Y	N	Y	GP	
-78	**Unplanned Return to the Operating/Procedure Room by the Same Physician or Other Qualified Health Care Professional Following Initial Procedure for a Related Procedure During the Postoperative Period:** It may be necessary to indicate that another procedure was performed during the postoperative period of the initial procedure (unplanned procedure following initial procedure). When the procedure is related to the first, and requires the use of the operating or procedure room, it may be reported by adding the modifier -78 to the related procedure. (For repeat procedures, see modifier -76.)† **Example:** A patient has an open reduction with fixation of a fracture of the elbow. While still hospitalized, the patient develops an infection and is returned to surgery for removal of the pin because it appears to be the cause of an allergic reaction. The original procedure would be billed for the open treatment of the fracture. The pin removal would be billed with modifier -78 because it is a related procedure. **Medicare Payment Rule:** Medicare will pay the full value of the intraoperative portion of a given procedure. Documentation should be submitted with the claim to describe the clinical circumstances.	N	N	Y	Y	N	Y	GP	

Continued

Table 6-6	CPT Modifier Codes—cont'd								
MODIFIER	**EXPLANATION**					**USE IN MAIN TEXT SECTIONS**			
		E/M	ANESTHESIA	SURGERY	RADIOLOGY	PATHOLOGY	MEDICINE		TYPE
-79	**Unrelated Procedure or Service by the Same Physician During the Postoperative Period:** The physician may need to indicate that the performance of a procedure or service during the postoperative period was unrelated to the original procedure. This circumstance may be reported by using the modifier -79. (For repeat procedures on the same day, see -76).† **Example:** A patient in the hospital has colon resection surgery and is discharged home. After 7 days, the patient develops acute renal failure, is hospitalized, does not recover renal function, and hemodialysis is ordered. A nephrologist inserts a cannula for the dialysis. When billing for the nephrologist, the code for hemodialysis is shown with a -79 modifier indicating that this is unrelated to the initial surgery. If modifier -79 is not used, the insurance carrier may not realize the service is not related to the initial surgery and may reject the claim. **Medicare Payment Rule:** No effect on payment; however, failure to use this modifier when appropriate may result in denial of the subsequent surgery. Specific diagnostic codes will substantiate the medical necessity of the unrelated procedure. Documentation may be required to describe the clinical circumstances. A new global period begins for any procedure modified by -79.	N	N	Y	Y	N	Y		GP
-80	**Assistant Surgeon:** Surgical assistant services may be identified by adding the modifier -80 to the usual procedure number(s).* **Note:** Some insurance policies do not include payment for assistant surgeons, such as for 1-day surgery, but do pay for major or complex surgical assistance. In some instances, prior approval may be indicated owing to the patient's physiologic condition. Medicare will not pay assistant surgeons for operations that are not life threatening. Therefore Medigap insurance will not pay on this service because the service is not allowable. Assisting surgeons usually charge 16% to 30% of the primary surgeon's fee. **Example:** The primary surgeon performs a right ureterectomy submitting code 50650-RT. The assistant surgeon would bill using the primary surgeon's code with modifier -80 (50650-80). **Medicare Payment Rule:** Payment is based on the billed amount or 16% of the global surgical fee, whichever is lower, for procedures approved for assistant-at-surgery. Medicare will deny payment for an assistant-at-surgery for surgical procedures in which a physician is used as an assistant in less than 5% of the cases nationally.	Ø	N	Y	Y	N	N		#
-81	**Minimum Assistant Surgeon:** Minimum surgical assistant services are identified by adding the modifier -81 to the usual procedure number. **Note:** Payment is made to physicians but not registered nurses or technicians who assist during surgery.* **Example:** A primary surgeon plans to perform a surgical procedure but during the operation circumstances arise that require the services of an assistant surgeon for a relatively short period. In this scenario, the second surgeon provides minimal assistance and may report using the procedure code with the -81 modifier appended.	Ø	N	Y	N	N	N		#
-82	**Assistant Surgeon:** (When qualified resident surgeon is not available.) The unavailability of a qualified resident surgeon is a prerequisite for use of modifier -82 appended to the usual procedure code number(s).* **Note:** This modifier is usually used for services rendered at a teaching hospital. **Example:** A resident surgeon is scheduled to assist with an anorectal myomectomy (45108). Surgery is delayed due to the previous surgery, the shift rotation changes, and the resident is not available. A nonresident assists with the surgery and reports the procedure, appending it with modifier -82 (45108-82).	Ø	N	Y	N	N	N		#

Table 6-6	CPT Modifier Codes—cont'd								
MODIFIER	**EXPLANATION**			**USE IN MAIN TEXT SECTIONS**					
		E/M	ANESTHESIA	SURGERY	RADIOLOGY	PATHOLOGY	MEDICINE	TYPE	
-90	**Reference (Outside) Laboratory:** When laboratory procedures are performed by a party other than the treating or reporting physician, the procedure may be identified by adding the modifier -90 to the usual procedure number.† **Note:** Use this modifier when the physician bills the patient for the laboratory work and the laboratory is not doing its own billing. **Example:** Dr. Input examines the patient, performs venipuncture, and sends the specimen to an outside laboratory for a liver panel. The physician has an arrangement with the laboratory to bill for the test, and, in turn, he bills the patient. Dr. Input bills for the examination (E/M code), venipuncture (36415 or for Medicare 0001), and acute hepatitis panel (80074), using modifier -90 (80074-90) to append to the hepatitis panel code.	N	N	Y	Y	Y	Y	LAB	
-91	**Repeat Clinical Diagnostic Laboratory Test:** In the course of treatment of the patient, it may be necessary to repeat the same laboratory test on the same day to obtain subsequent (multiple) test results. Under these circumstances, the laboratory test performed can be identified by its usual procedure number and the addition of modifier -91. **Note:** This modifier may not be used when tests are rerun to confirm initial results, due to testing problems with specimens or equipment, or for any other reason when a normal, one-time, reportable result is all that is required. This modifier may not be used when other code(s) describe a series of test results (e.g., glucose tolerance tests, evocative/suppression testing). This modifier may only be used for laboratory test(s) performed more than once on the same day on the same patient. **Example:** A patient is scheduled for a nonobstetric dilation and curettage for dysfunctional uterine bleeding. When the patient arrives at the office, a routine hematocrit is obtained. During the procedure, the patient bleeds excessively. After the procedure, the physician orders a second hematocrit to check the patient for anemia due to blood loss. The first hematocrit is billed using CPT code 85013. The second hematocrit is billed using the same code appended with modifier -91 (85013-91).	N	N	Y	Y	Y	Y	LAB	
-92	**Alternative Laboratory Platform Testing:** When laboratory testing is being performed using a kit or transportable instrument that wholly or in part consists of a single-use, disposable, analytic chamber, the service may be identified by adding modifier -92 to the usual laboratory procedure code (HIV testing 86701-86703). The test does not require permanent dedicated space; hence by its design it may be hand carried or transported to the vicinity of the patient for immediate testing at that site, although location of the testing is not in itself determinative of the use of this modifier.	N	N	Y	Y	Y	Y	LAB	
-99	**Multiple Modifiers:** Under certain circumstances, two or more modifiers may be necessary to delineate a service completely. In such situations modifier -99 should be added to the basic procedure, and other applicable modifiers may be listed as part of the description of the service.‡ **Example:** An assistant surgeon helps repair an enterocele where unusual circumstances appear because of extensive hemorrhaging. 57270-99 Repair of enterocele -22 Extensive hemorrhaging (unusual service) -80 Assistant surgeon **Medicare Payment Rule:** No effect on payment; however, the individual modifier payment policies apply including any inherent effect they may have on payment.	N	N	Y	Y	N	Y		

making an observation and determination using a microscope. The technical component refers to the use of the equipment, the supplies, and the operator who performs the test or procedure such as ECG machine and technician, radiography machine and technician, and microscope and technician. The technical component is billed by the entity that owns the equipment. Do not modify procedures that are either 100% technical or 100% professional or when the physician performs both the professional and technical components. Modifier -26 represents the professional component only. Use of this modifier alerts the insurance company to expect a separate claim from another provider or facility for the TC.

In Example 6-25, the physician is performing only one of two services—he or she is interpreting the results of bilateral hip x-ray films.

Example 6-25   Professional/Technical Components

73520-26	**Professional component** only for a radiograph of both hips. Use to bill physician's fee for interpretation of X-ray film.	$
73520-TC or 73525	**Technical component** only for a radiograph of both hips. Use to bill facility fee that owns equipment and employs technician. Modifier –TC is at carrier's discretion.	$
73520	**Global service:** Radiologic examination, hips, bilateral. Minimum of two views of each hip. Use to bill complete fee when physician owns equipment, employs technician, and interprets x-ray film.	$

The facility where the patient had the x-ray film taken bills only for the technical component by either using 73525 or 73520 with modifier -TC. If the physician owns the equipment and reads the x-ray film, there is no need to modify the x-ray code (73520) because both the professional and technical components were done in the office. Modifier -TC is assigned at the carrier's discretion.

-51 Multiple Procedures

Multiple procedures are when more than one surgical service and/or related surgical service is performed on the same day or at the same surgical session by the same physician. In such cases, first report the primary service or procedure, which can be determined easily by highest dollar value. Identify all additional services or procedures by appending codes with modifier -51 (Example 6-26).

The operative report should clearly state which procedures were done through separate incisions and which were done through the same incision. There are many

---

Example 6-26   Multiple Procedure Modifier -51

Excision of 2.0-cm benign lesion on the nose and at the same session a biopsy of the skin and subcutaneous tissue of the forearm.

Code	RVU	Description of Services
11442	$	Excision, other benign lesion including margins, face, ears, eyelids, nose, lips, mucous membrane; excised diameter 1.1 to 2.0 cm
11100-**51**		Biopsy of skin, subcutaneous tissue, or mucous membrane (including simple closure), unless otherwise listed; single lesion **(second; multiple procedure)**

---

circumstances when multiple procedures are performed. Modifier -51 may be used to identify the following:

- Multiple surgical procedures performed at the same session by the same provider
- Multiple related surgical procedures performed at the same session by the same provider
- Surgical procedures performed in combination at the same session, whether through the same or another incision or involving the same or different anatomy
- A combination of medical and surgical procedures performed at the same session by the same provider

Usually payment by third-party payers for the primary code is 100% of the allowable charge, second code 50%, third code 25%, fourth and remaining codes 10%. However, under NCCI guidelines, Medicare pays 100% of the allowable charge for the primary code and 50% for two to five secondary procedures and does not require the assignment of modifier -51. Some computer systems can determine code order and automatically make the code adjustment for you. Many carriers no longer require modifier -51 because they process claims electronically and the software program recognizes when multiple procedures are performed and automatically makes the reduction in payment. Contact insurance carriers and ask which method is preferred when reporting multiple surgical procedures. Then note this for each payer's policy to refer to for future billings. Always bill the full amount and let the third-party payer make the payment adjustments for percentage considerations. For all third-party payers, it is recommended that you monitor the Remittance Advice/Explanation of Benefits to ensure correct payment. A decision flow chart is provided for reference to help simplify the modifier decision process (Figure 6-9). As you read through the remainder of this chapter, follow the steps by answering the questions in Figure 6-9, *A*, as they apply to your billing scenario and refer to Figure 6-9, *B*, for key information and descriptions.

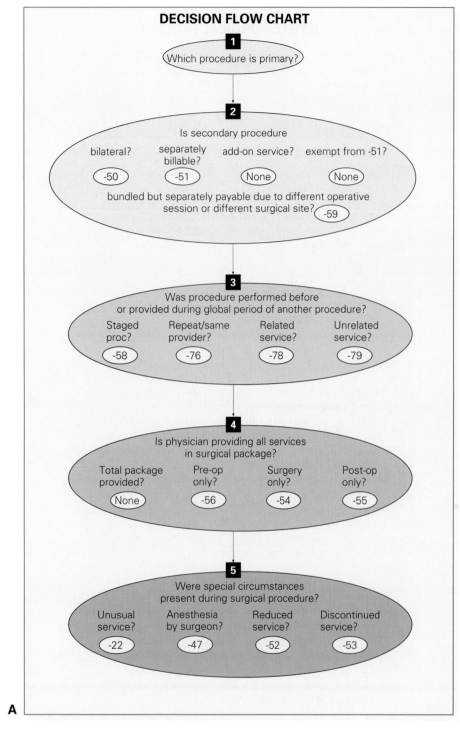

FIGURE 6-9 A, Decision flow chart for surgical procedures. **B,** Guidelines and description of modifiers for multiple surgical procedures. *Continued*

MULTIPLE SURGICAL PROCEDURES

Multiple services must be related to:
• Same patient
• Same provider
• Same date of service

• List all procedures in order of reimbursement, highest to lowest
• Most comprehensive service brings greatest reimbursement
  and is considered primary
• Check all procedures to make sure there is no unbundling, i.e.,
  using two codes when one code describes procedure
• Decision making expands at this point. Follow numbered
  question to determine correct modifier usage

-50 bilateral procedure, not described by code
-51 not bundled, separately billable
-59 ordinarily bundled, separately payable due to special circumstance

• The term "primary procedure" can also refer to the first procedure
  initiating a global surgical period
-58 Current service was planned prospectively at time of first service
-76 Physician repeats procedure subsequent to original procedure
-78 Return to operating room for subsequent procedure, complication
    relating to original procedure
-79 Unrelated procedure performed during global period of previous surgery

4

• Surgical package means one fee covers the whole package,
  surgical procedure and postoperative care

5

-22 An extremely difficult procedure due to altered anatomy or unusual
    circumstances (add 10% to 30% reimbursement)
-47 When the surgeon administers regional or general anesthesia
-52 Procedure/service reduced or eliminated at the discretion
    of the physician
-53 Procedure is discontinued due to extenuating circumstances
    or because of threat to the patient

B

FIGURE 6-9 cont'd.

If multiple procedures are done as in-office procedures or services and one is using E/M codes, it may be possible to bill a higher-level E/M visit because the -51 modifier is not used with E/M services. Do not use the -51 modifier with add-on codes designated with a "+" (see Appendix D in CPT) or codes listed as exempt to modifier -51 (see Appendix E in CPT). Add-on codes are codes that cannot stand alone. When billing with add-on codes, you must first list another code referred to as the "parent code" to give a full description for service billed (Example 6-27).

When making a decision about when to use an add-on code, look for a clue phrase that indicates additional

Example 6-27   Add-on Code

| Parent code | 11000 | Biopsy of skin … single lesion each separate/additional lesion (list separately in addition to code for primary procedure) |
| Add-on code | +11101 | |

Example 6-28   Decision for Surgery

A new patient is seen in the office complaining of a great deal of pain. Cholangiography is done and reveals blocked bile ducts. The patient is scheduled for surgery the next day.

| 8-1-20XX | 99204-**57** | New patient office visit | $00.00 |
| 8-2-20XX | 47600 | Cholecystectomy | $000.00 |

procedures such as "each additional," "list in addition to," and "second lesion."

-52 Reduced Services

Use of the modifier -52 indicates that under certain circumstances a service or procedure is partially reduced or eliminated at the physician's discretion. It is wise to provide an explanation of why the service was reduced. A cover letter or a copy of the operative report should not accompany these claims because usually they are not sent to medical review and attached documents may impede processing. Never use this modifier if the fee is reduced because of a patient's inability to pay.

-57 Decision for Surgery

The modifier -57 is used strictly to report an E/M service that resulted in the initial decision to perform a major surgical procedure within 24 hours of the office visit (e.g., those with a 90-day follow-up period); see Examples 6-28 and 6-29. A -57 modifier may be used for inpatient or outpatient consultations, inpatient hospital visits, and new or established patient visits that occur the day of or the day before surgery. Do not attach modifier -57 to a hospital visit code for the day before surgery or the day of surgery when a decision for a major surgical procedure was made a week before surgery. Think of -57 as telling the insurance company that the office visit is not part of the global fee.

-25 Significant Separately Identifiable Evaluation and Management Service

In some cases, you may be confused whether to assign modifier -25 or -57. Modifier -25 is defined as "significant, separately identifiable evaluation and management

Example 6-29   Decision for Surgery

A new patient comes to the office after sustaining a fall while in-line skating. She is in distress, complaining of right wrist pain and swelling of the joint. The injury is evaluated **(1)** with an x-ray film. **(2)** It is determined that the patient has a Smith fracture and manipulation is performed. A long-arm cast is applied **(3)** using fiberglass (Hexcelite) material **(4)**.

(1)	99203-**57**	Initial office evaluation (detailed) **with decision for surgery**
(2)	73100-RT	Radiologic examination, right wrist, anteroposterior (AP) and lateral (lat) views
(3)	25605	Closed treatment of distal radial fracture (e.g., Colles or Smith type), with manipulation
(4)	99070	Supplies: Casting material (third-party payer) Medicine Section code or Supplies: Hexcelite material (Medicare fiscal agent)
	A4590	HCPCS Level II code

The patient returns in 4 weeks for follow-up care **(1)**. The wrist is radiographed again **(2)**, the long-arm cast is removed **(3)**, and a short-arm cast is applied **(4)** using plaster material **(5)**.

(1)	No code	Follow-up care included in global fee
(2)	73100-RT	Radiologic examination, right wrist, AP and lat views
(3)	No code	Cast removal included in original fracture care (25605)
(4)	29075-**58**	Application, plaster, elbow to finger (short arm) **staged procedure**
(5)	99070	Supplies: Casting material (third-party payer) Medicine Section code or Supplies: Plaster material (Medicare fiscal agent)
	A4580	HCPCS Level II code

service by same physician on the same day of the procedure or other service." The industry standard is to use -25 when a diagnostic procedure or minor procedure is involved (e.g., those with a 0- to 10-day follow-up period). Typically, E/M services that are modified with -25 are office visits performed on the day of a minor procedure for an established patient. However, the confusion results because the CPT code book states, "This modifier is not used to report an E/M service that resulted in a decision to perform surgery. See modifier -57."

Consult Figure 6-10 when making the decision about which modifier to use for a surgical procedure that is performed within 24 hours of an office visit.

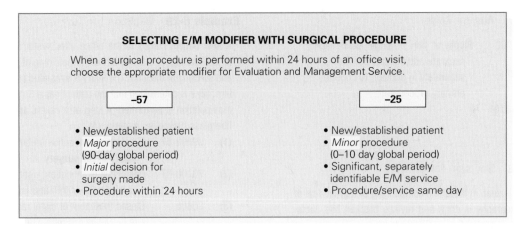

FIGURE 6-10 Two selections, with criteria to evaluate, when choosing the appropriate code or modifier for evaluation and management (E/M) services when a surgical procedure is performed within 24 hours of an office visit.

In Medicare cases, the CMS has published in the NCCI the specific codes for modifier -25 use after October 2000. Refer to the bulletin or newsletter pertinent to this update.

-58 Staged or Related Procedure

The modifier -58 is used to indicate that the performance of a procedure or service during the postoperative period was as follows:

- Planned (staged) at the time of the original procedure
- More extensive than the original procedure
- For therapy after a surgical procedure

Such circumstances should be reported by adding modifier -58 to the staged or related procedure. The use of this modifier requires accurate documentation of events leading up to the initial surgery and any subsequent surgery. It is only possible to modify procedures if the coder has all of the relevant facts and circumstances. In Example 6-27, the fracture is considered surgery because it is in the surgery section of the CPT book. All fracture codes have 90-day postoperative periods.

-62, -66, -80, -81, -82 More Than One Surgeon

If more than one surgeon is involved, clarify for whom you are billing by using the appropriate two-digit modifier as follows:

-62, Co-surgeon: Two surgeons work together as primary surgeons performing distinct parts of a procedure. Each physician reports his or her distinct operative work by adding this modifier.

-66, Team surgery: A group of surgeons work together. Each participating physician adds this modifier to the basic procedure number for the service.

Example 6-30   Assistant at Surgery

Closure of intestinal cutaneous fistula		
Operating surgeon bills	44640	**No modifier**
Assistant surgeon bills	44640-**80**	**With modifier**

-80, Assistant at surgery: Used when the surgery is not performed in a teaching hospital.

-81, Minimum assistant surgeon.

-82, Assistant surgeon: Used for surgeries performed in a teaching hospital when a qualified resident surgeon is not available to act as assistant at surgery.

The assistant physician adds one of these modifiers to the usual procedure number (see Examples 6-30 and 6-31).

Modifier -80 (assistant at surgery) is commonly used when billing for a physician who assists the primary physician in performing a surgical procedure (Example 6-30).

The assisting doctor is paid a reduced fee of 16% to 30% of the allowed fee the primary surgeon receives for performing the surgery on the basis of the patient's contract. The assisting physician uses the same surgical code as the primary surgeon and adds the -80 modifier to it. The fee indicating a reduced percentage typically is listed as the fee on the claim form. However, some third-party payers may prefer having the full fee listed and making the reduction themselves. Under some insurance contracts, there may be some surgical procedures that restrict payment for an assistant surgeon.

-99 Multiple Modifiers

If a procedure requires more than one modifier code, use the two-digit modifier -99 after the usual five-digit CPT code number, all typed on one line; then list each modifier on a separate line (Example 6-31). Some insurance companies require -99 with a separate note in Block 19 of the CMS-1500 claim form or in the freeform area of electronic submissions, indicating which two or more modifiers are being used.

Example 6-31   Multiple Modifiers

A physician sees a patient who is grossly obese. The operative report documents that a bilateral sliding-type inguinal herniorrhaphy was performed, and the procedure took 2 hours 15 minutes.

49525-**99**   Bilateral repair sliding inguinal hernia requiring 2 hours 15 minutes

-**50**

-**22**

HCPCS

Besides CPT modifiers, HCPCS Level II modifiers are used by Medicare and may be used by some commercial payers. HCPCS Level II modifiers may be two alpha digits (Example 6-32), two alphanumeric characters (Figure 6-11), or a single alpha digit used for reporting

ambulance services or results of positron emission tomography scans. A brief list of these modifiers is found in Appendix A of the CPT code book. Modifiers also appear on the inside cover of the CPT code book. A comprehensive list may be found in an HCPCS national Level II code book. HCPCS reference books may be obtained from resources listed in Appendix A.

Use the two-digit HCPCS modifiers whenever they are necessary. HCPCS modifiers further describe the services provided and can increase or decrease the physician's fee. If not used properly, they can drastically affect the physician's fee profile by reducing future payments to the physician.

Comprehensive List of Modifier Codes

Now that you have learned about some basic modifiers, read through the comprehensive list shown in Table 6-6 to gain information on additional modifiers and their use illustrated by clinical examples.

Example 6-32   HCPCS Modifiers

When taking x-ray films of both feet, the billing portion of the insurance claim appears as follows:

05/06/XX   73620 **RT**   Radiologic examination, foot—right
05/06/XX   73620 **LT**   Radiologic examination, foot—left

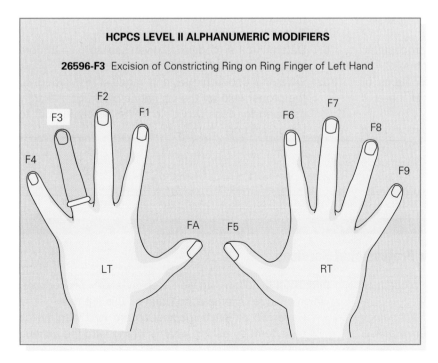

HCPCS LEVEL II ALPHANUMERIC MODIFIERS

26596-F3 Excision of Constricting Ring on Ring Finger of Left Hand

FIGURE 6-11 HCPCS Level II alpha modifiers (*LT* and *RT* used to identify left and right hands) and alphanumeric modifiers (*FA* through *F9*) used to identify digits (fingers) of left and right hands.

PROCEDURE 6-1

Determine Conversion Factors

OBJECTIVE: To determine the conversion factors for several procedure codes

EQUIPMENT/SUPPLIES: *Current Procedural Terminology* (CPT) code book, geographic practice cost indices and relative value unit (RVU) pages from the Federal Register, calculator, and pen or pencil

DIRECTIONS: Follow these step-by-step procedures, which include rationales, to practice this job skill.

1. Choose 10 or more procedure codes commonly used in the medical practice and in the same section (E/M, Anesthesia, Surgery, Radiology, Pathology, or Medicine) and list the code numbers, at least 60 code numbers.

2. Use the relative value unit formula: RVU × GAF × CF = Medicare $ per service, and the geographic practice cost indices and RVU pages from the Federal Register. From the 60 or more codes you have assembled, locate the first procedure code from the RVUs page of the Federal Register.

3. For the work amount, obtain the dollar amount from the Work RVUs and multiply that by the GPCI of the locality name of where the medical practice is located.

4. For the overhead amount, obtain the dollar amount from the Practice expense RVUs and multiply that by the figure in the GPCI practice expense column.

5. For the malpractice amount, obtain the dollar amount from the Malpractice RVUs and multiply that by the figure in the GPCI malpractice column.

6. Take the three results and add them together to obtain the total adjusted RVUs.

7. Use the current year Medicare conversion factor amount and multiply that by the total adjusted RVUs amount to get the allowed amount for the procedure code.

8. Repeat steps 2 through 7 for all additional procedure codes commonly used by the medical practice for each section of the CPT code book.

9. Look at all of the dollar figures that you have determined for all of the procedure codes selected. For each section of the CPT code book, they should fall within the same general range. If they do not, reevaluate those fees that are too high or low and readjust them depending on the service descriptions and market competition comparisons.

PROCEDURE 6-2

Locate Correct Level II HCPCS Codes for Professional Services

OBJECTIVE: Accurately locate and select Level II HCPCS codes for professional services

EQUIPMENT/SUPPLIES: HCPCS code book, medical dictionary, and pen or pencil

DIRECTIONS: Follow these step-by-step procedures, which include rationales, to practice this job skill.

1. Read the patient's medical record for items or services that might be covered under Level II HCPCS codes.

2. Go to the index that is arranged alphabetically and locate the name of the supply, drug, or service. This will direct you to the proper code. Never code from the index.

3. Turn to the code number in the section and verify that it is the proper code for the item or service the provider supplied to the patient.

4. Select the code.

5. Determine if a modifier is necessary to give a more accurate description of the service or item.

6. Enter the code number and modifier (if needed) to the proper field on the insurance claim form exactly as given for each service or item. Be careful not to transpose code numbers.

PROCEDURE 6-3

Choose Correct Procedural Codes for Professional Services

OBJECTIVE: Accurately locate and select procedural codes for professional services

EQUIPMENT/SUPPLIES: *Current Procedural Terminology* (CPT) code book, medical dictionary, and pen or pencil.

DIRECTIONS: Follow these step-by-step procedures, which include rationales, to practice this job skill.

1. Read the patient's medical record and identify the main term by asking what is wrong with the patient.

PROCEDURE 6-3—cont'd

Choose Correct Procedural Codes for Professional Services

2. Always read the Introduction section at the beginning of the code book, which may change annually with each edition.
3. Use the index at the back of the book to locate a specific item by generalized code numbers, not by page numbers. Never code from the index. Listings may be looked up according to names of procedures or services, organs, conditions, synonyms, eponyms, and abbreviations; for example, some primary entries might be as follows:
   a. Procedure or service
      Example: Anastomosis; Endoscopy; Splint
   b. Organ or other anatomic site
      Example: Salivary Gland; Tibia; Colon
   c. Condition
      Example: Abscess; Entropion; Tetralogy of Fallot
   d. Synonyms, eponyms, and abbreviations
      Example: EEG; Bricker operation; Clagett procedure
      If the procedure performed is not listed, check for the organ involved. If the procedure or organ is difficult to find, look up the condition. Key words, such as synonyms or eponyms, and abbreviations, will help you find the appropriate code.
4. Locate the code number in the code section for the code range given in the index.
5. Turn to the beginning of the section for the code range given in the index and read the Guidelines at the beginning of the section. This gives general information and instructions on coding certain procedures within the section, defines commonly used terms, explains classifications within the section, and gives instructions specific to the section.
6. Turn to the correct section, subsection, category, or subcategory, and read through the narrative description to locate the most appropriate code to apply to the patient's procedure. Look at the size of the title to find out the area you are in. Some code books have color-coded titles, making this determination easier. In the surgery section, each subsection is further divided into categories based on anatomic site. Within each category are subcategories listed by type of procedure (e.g., excision, repair, destruction, graft) or condition (burn, fracture). Read the notes and special subsection information throughout the section.
7. Notice punctuation and indenting. Descriptions for stand-alone codes begin at the left margin and have a full description. No matter how many indented codes are listed, always go back to the stand-alone code to begin reading the description. A semicolon (;) separates common portions from subordinate designations; subterms are indented (Figure 6-12). Any terminology after the semicolon has a dependent status, as do the subsequent indented entries. In Figure 6-12, the procedure code number 11044 should read as follows: Debridement; skin, subcutaneous tissue, muscle, and bone. Figure 6-13 shows an insurance claim for a patient who has had six corns pared.
8. When trying to locate an E/M code, identify the place or type of service rendered. Then identify whether the patient is new or established and locate the category or subcategory. Review any guidelines or instructions pertaining to the category or subcategory. Read the descriptors of the levels of E/M service. Identify the requirements necessary for code assignment. Make sure the components necessary were performed by the physician and documented in the chart for the assigned E/M code. Commercial templates are available to aid in E/M code selection and help tremendously when verifying a code that has been selected by the physician.
9. For a code that has been assigned, note the following:
   • Parentheses ( ) further define the code and tell where other services are located (Figure 6-14).
   • Measurements throughout the code book are based on the metric system (Figure 6-15).
   • All anesthesia services are reported by use of the five-digit anesthesia code plus a physical status modifier. The use of other modifiers to explain a procedure further is optional. Example: Patient is a healthy 23-year-old Caucasian woman. Anesthesia is given for a vaginal delivery. The procedure code with modifier is 01960-P1.
   • The Surgery section is the largest segment of the code book. It has many subsections and subheadings. You must be able to break down a procedure and identify various terms that will direct you to

11040	Debridement; skin, partial thickness
11041	skin, full thickness
11042	skin, and subcutaneous tissue
11043	skin, subcutaneous tissue, and muscle
11044	skin, subcutaneous tissue, muscle, and bone

FIGURE 6-12 Use of a semicolon.

Continued

PROCEDURE 6-3—cont'd

Choose Correct Procedural Codes for Professional Services

CODING FOR MULTIPLE LESIONS

Paring or Cutting

11055   Paring or cutting of benign hyperkeratotic lesion (e.g., corn or callus); single lesion

11056   two to four lesions

11057   more than four lesions

A

24. A. DATE(S) OF SERVICE						B. PLACE OF SERVICE	C. EMG	D. PROCEDURES, SERVICES, OR SUPPLIES (Explain Unusual Circumstances)		E. DIAGNOSIS POINTER	F. $ CHARGES		G. DAYS OR UNITS	H. EPSDT Family Plan	I. ID. QUAL.	J. RENDERING PROVIDER ID. #
From			To					CPT/HCPCS	MODIFIER							
MM	DD	YY	MM	DD	YY											
05	11	2001				11		99203		1	00	00	1		NPI	4627889700
05	11	2001				11		11057		1	00	00	1		NPI	4627889700
															NPI	
															NPI	
															NPI	
															NPI	

B

FIGURE 6-13 A, Procedure codes from the Surgery Section of *Current Procedural Terminology*. **B,** Blocks 24A through 24J of the revised CMS-1500 (08-05) insurance claim form showing placement of the code on Line 2.

BIOPSY

Defining further ─────────→ 11100   Biopsy of skin, subcutaneous tissue and/or mucous membrane (including simple closure), unless otherwise listed (separate procedure); single lesion

11101   each separate/additional lesion

Location of other services ──────→ (For biopsy of conjunctiva, see 68100; eyelid, see 67810)

FIGURE 6-14 Use of parentheses in the Surgery Section of *Current Procedural Terminology*.

13150   Repair, complex, eyelids, nose, ears, and/or lips; 1.0 cm or less (See also 40650–40654, 67961–67975)

13151   1.1 cm to 2.5 cm

13152   2.6 cm to 7.5 cm

FIGURE 6-15 Metric measurements from the Surgery Section of *Current Procedural Terminology*.

PROCEDURE 6-3—cont'd

Choose Correct Procedural Codes for Professional Services

the correct code. Blocks 24A through 24J of the revised CMS-1500 (08-05) insurance claim form show placement of the code on Line 2 (Example 6-33).

10. Determine if one or more modifiers are necessary to give a more accurate description of the services

rendered or the circumstances in which they were performed.

11. Enter the five-digit code number and modifier to the proper field on the insurance claim form exactly as given for each procedure or service rendered. Be careful not to transpose code numbers.

Example 6.33   Blocks 24A Through 24J of the CMS-1500 Claim Form

Closed Manipulative Treatment of a Clavicular Fracture

Section:	Surgery, Musculoskeletal System
Anatomic subheading:	Shoulder
Condition:	Fracture or Dislocation
Code:	23505

Thus when completing an insurance claim form for closed manipulative treatment, clavicular fracture, the billing portion appears as follows (Figure 6-16):

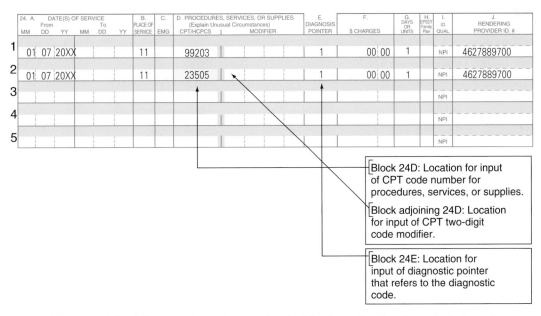

Block 24D: Location for input of CPT code number for procedures, services, or supplies.

Block adjoining 24D: Location for input of CPT two-digit code modifier.

Block 24E: Location for input of diagnostic pointer that refers to the diagnostic code.

FIGURE 6-16 The billing portion of a completed claim form for closed manipulation of a clavicular fracture.

KEY POINTS

This is a brief chapter review or summary of the key issues presented. To further enhance your knowledge of the technical subject matter, review the key terms and key abbreviations for this chapter by locating the meanings in the glossary at the end of this book before the index.

1. CPT codes are a standardized five-digit numeric method used to precisely describe each service and procedure provided by physicians and allied health care professionals.

2. Medicare's Healthcare Common Procedure Coding System (HCPCS) has two levels: Level I—the American Medical Association's CPT codes and modifiers and Level II—Centers for Medicare and Medicaid Services (CMS) designated codes and alpha modifiers. HCPCS national codes are used to bill for ambulance, medical and surgical supplies, durable medical equipment, drugs administered other than oral method, and so on.

3. Alternative billing codes (ABCs) are five-character alphabetic symbols with appended two-character practitioner modifiers that represent the practitioner type. ABC codes are used to bill for integrative health care such as alternative medicine.

4. A fee schedule is a listing in an insurance policy of procedure code numbers with charges or pre-established allowances for specific medical services and procedures. The Medicare fee schedule is annually published and shows the maximum dollar amounts Medicare will allow for each service rendered for a beneficiary.

5. The various methods of payment by insurance companies and state and federal programs are (1) fee schedules; (2) usual, customary, and reasonable (UCR); and (3) relative value studies or scale (RVS).

6. Each year when a new CPT code book is published, become familiar with code deletions, new codes, description changes, and observe the symbols and their interpretation in relation to the codes.

7. In CPT coding, a surgical package is a term used to describe a surgical procedure code that includes the operation, local infiltration, digital block, or topical anesthesia, and normal, uncomplicated postoperative care all included in one fee. Under Medicare, a global surgery policy (GSP) relates to surgical procedures in which preoperative and postoperative visits (24 hours before [major] and day of [minor]), usual intraoperative services, and complications not requiring an additional trip to the operating room are included in one fee.

8. Code edits are performed on submitted insurance claims to detect unbundling, splitting of codes, and other types of improper code submissions.

9. Make sure that the documentation from the provider supports the code submitted to prevent downcoding by the third-party payer.

10. Use two-digit add-on CPT modifiers to indicate circumstances in which a procedure as performed differs in some way from that described by its usual five-digit code.

11. In final summary, the seven steps to accurate coding are:
    a. Read the patient's encounter form completely and any notes made by the health care provider.
    b. Highlight words important to the selection of diagnostic and procedural codes.
    c. Ask the provider to clarify any inconsistent or missing information and code only from actual documentation. Do not assume or guess.
    d. Code each confirmed diagnosis and accompanying signs or symptoms using the highest level of specificity.
    e. Code each medical service, procedure, and treatment provided in the documentation.
    f. Verify medical necessity by associating each procedure code to the diagnostic code.
    g. Recheck the codes selected by rereading the code descriptions and match them with the provider's notes to confirm the codes assigned.

evolve INTERNET RESOURCES

For active links to the following resources, visit the Evolve website at
http://evolve.elsevier.com/fordney/handbook

- AHIMA and AHA diagnostic code guidelines for outpatient services and diagnostic coding and reporting requirements for physician billing
- Alternative links for Alternative Billing Codes (ABCs) for current information on this subject, to order code resources, or to file a petition for the rights to use the codes
- Changes in HCPCS Level II
- *Current Procedural Terminology* (CPT) code books are available from Book and Pamphlet Fulfillment:

OP-3416, American Medical Association, P.O. Box 10946, Chicago, IL 60610-0946, or visit the website: http://www.ama-assn.org/cpt.
- *Federal Register* at website: www.archives.gov/federal_register/index.html.
- Listserv, if you wish to join a free listserv.
- Medicare
- Medicare durable medical equipment regional contractors (DMERC)
- Medicare National Correct Coding Initiative (NCCI) Edits

STUDENT ASSIGNMENT

✓ Study Chapter 6.
✓ Answer the fill-in-the-blank, multiple choice, and true/false review questions in the *Workbook* to reinforce the theory learned in this chapter and help prepare you for a future test.
✓ Complete the assignments in the *Workbook* to assist you in hands-on practical experience in procedural coding and learning medical abbreviations.

✓ Assignments related to the resource-based relative value scale (RBRVS) because of the complexity of that subject are presented later in the course when studying the chapter about Medicare.
✓ Turn to the glossary at the end of this textbook for a further understanding of the key terms and key abbreviations used in this chapter.

KEY TERMS*

clean claim
deleted claim
dirty claim
durable medical equipment
  number
electronic claim
employer identification number
facility provider number

group National Provider
  Identifier
Health Insurance Claim Form
  (CMS-1500 [08-05])
incomplete claim
intelligent character recognition
invalid claim
National Provider Identifier

optical character recognition
"other" claims
paper claim
pending claim
physically clean claim
rejected claim
Social Security number
state license number

KEY ABBREVIATIONS*

CMS-1500	FDA	MSP	PAYERID
DME	HHA	NA, N/A	PRO
DNA	ICR	NOC	SOF
EIN	IDE	NPI	SSN
EMG	LMP	OCNA key	TMA
EPSDT	MG	OCR	

---

*Definitions for the key terms and key abbreviations are located near the back of this textbook in the glossary.

CHAPTER 7

The Paper Claim CMS-1500 (08-05)

OBJECTIVES

After reading this chapter, you should be able to:

- Discuss the history of the Health Insurance Claim Form (CMS-1500 [08-05]).
- State when the CMS-1500 (08-05) claim form may or may not be used.
- Define two types of claims submission.
- Explain the difference between clean, pending, rejected, incomplete, and invalid claims.
- Abstract from the patient record relevant information for completing the CMS-1500 (08-05) insurance claim form.
- Describe basic guidelines for submitting insurance claims.

- Describe reasons why claims are rejected.
- Explain procedures that will minimize the number of insurance forms returned because of improper completion.
- Identify techniques required for optically scanned insurance claims.
- Demonstrate the ability to complete the CMS-1500 (08-05) claim form accurately for federal, state, and private payer insurance contracts using current basic guidelines.

HISTORY

In 1958 the Health Insurance Association of America (HIAA) and the American Medical Association (AMA) attempted to standardize the insurance claim form by jointly developing the Standard Form. It was not universally accepted by all third-party payers, and as the types of coverage became more variable, new claim forms were instituted that required more information than the original Standard Form. The form eventually became known as *COMB-1*, or *Attending Physician's Statement*. In 1968 the HIAA*decided to revamp the

form so that it would be more adaptable to electronic data processing.

In April 1975 the AMA approved a "universal claim form," called the Health Insurance Claim Form, referred to as the *HCFA-1500*, which was an abbreviation for the *Health Care Financing Administration*. In July 2001 the HCFA became the Centers for Medicare and Medicaid Services (CMS); thus the form became known as CMS-1500. CMS adopted the form because of the need for a standard format and to expedite claims processing. The CMS-1500 claim form answered the needs of many health insurers processing claims manually. The National Association of Blue Shield Plans Board of Directors adopted a motion supporting the concept of a uniform national claim form.

---

*In 2003 the HIAA, Group Health Association of America (GHAA), and the American Managed Care and Review Association (AMCRA) merged with American Association of Health Plans (AAHP) and created what is now known as *America's Health Insurance Plans* (AHIP).

Performance objectives, testing and review material, and hands-on practical exercises for this chapter are available in these resources

 The Insurance Handbook Student Workbook   The Insurance Handbook Evolve Site

In 1990 the CMS-1500 (12-90) was revised and printed in red ink, which allowed claims to be optically scanned by the insurance carriers. Beginning on May 1, 1992, all services for Medicare patients from physicians and suppliers, except for ambulance services, had to be billed on the scannable CMS-1500 (12-90) form.

The revised form was adopted by TRICARE Management Activity (TMA), formerly known as the *Office of Civilian Health and Medical Programs of the Uniformed Services* (OCHAMPUS). It also received the approval of the AMA Council on Medical Services. The HIAA endorsed and recommended that their members (private insurance companies) accept the form. In some states the Medicaid program and industrial (workers' compensation) cases use this form to process claims. After October 16, 2003, the Health Insurance Portability and Accountability Act (HIPAA) required that claims be transmitted electronically in the HIPAA format by providers who are not small providers (institutional organizations with fewer than 25 full-time employees or physicians with fewer than 10 full-time employees).

In 2005, it became necessary to change the CMS-1500 (12-90) so that it could accommodate the reporting of the National Provider Identifier (NPI) for providers; this form is presently referred to as *CMS-1500 (08-05)*.

Widespread use of the CMS-1500 (08-05) has saved time and simplified processing of claims for both physicians and carriers because it has eliminated the need to complete the many various insurance forms brought into the office by patients. Another way of billing that may be accepted by insurance companies is to complete the CMS-1500 (08-05) and attach it to the patient's encounter form. The patient's and employer's portions of the private insurance form should be complete and accurate, and the patient should sign the assignment of benefits, if applicable. Both forms are sent directly to the insurance carrier. If the patient is insured by two companies (dual coverage or duplication of coverage), assignment for both insurance carriers should be obtained. Most offices use a standard assignment of benefits form, which becomes part of the patient's health record. The primary carrier should be determined, and the claim submitted to that carrier first. After the primary insurance carrier has paid out, a claim should be submitted to the secondary carrier with a copy of the payment check voucher (or patient's explanation of benefits [EOB] document) attached.

Insurance carriers with various computer programs and equipment that optically scan claims may have instructions on completion of the form that vary by locality and program. Local representatives of insurance carriers should always be contacted to find out whether the form is acceptable before any claims are submitted. A

photocopy is not acceptable if the form is processed by the insurance carrier through scanning equipment because the statements on the back of the form are critical to the block-by-block data on the claim form side. Quantities of the CMS-1500 (08-05) can be purchased from many medical office supply companies or from the AMA by calling toll free to 800-621-8335. In many cases the computerized practice management system will produce the CMS-1500 (08-05) claim form, but an original claim form is required for submission. Also, the CMS-1500 (08-05) claim form may be downloaded from the CMS website but may not be used for submission of claims (see Internet Resources at the end of this chapter). The Evolve website has an active link to the National Uniform Claim Committee.

In this chapter, instructions for completing a paper claim using optical character recognition (OCR) format are emphasized. HIPAA allows small providers with fewer than 10 full-time employees to continue to send paper claims. Medicare advised that the purchased red ink versions of the CMS-1500 (08-05) claim form cannot be duplicated by computer printer; therefore, if the Medicare carrier uses OCR scanning technology, the claims must be originals and not photocopies or they will not be processed. This chapter focuses on the paper claim, and Chapter 8 explains the intricacies of transmitting electronic claims as mandated by HIPAA.

TYPES OF SUBMITTED CLAIMS

A **paper claim** is one that is submitted on paper including optically scanned claims that are converted to electronic form by insurance companies. Paper claims may be typed or generated via computer.

An **electronic claim** is one that is submitted to the insurance carrier via dial-up modem (telephone line or computer modem), direct data entry, or over the Internet by way of digital subscriber line (DSL) or file transfer protocol (FTP). Electronic claims are digital files that are not printed on paper claim forms when submitted to the payer.

 COMPLIANCE ISSUES RELATED TO INSURANCE CLAIM FORMS

HIPAA federal laws affect insurance claim submission. The provider rendering the service or procedure must be properly identified with the correct provider number. Claims must only show services rendered that have been properly documented and are medically necessary without evidence of fraud or abuse issues. HIPAA mandates use of electronic standards for automated transfer

COMPLIANCE ISSUES RELATED TO INSURANCE CLAIM FORMS—cont'd

of certain health care data among health care payers, plans, and providers. The National Provider Identifier (NPI) system for health care providers became effective May 27, 2007, in connection with the electronic transactions identified in HIPAA. Refer to Chapters 2 and 8 for a complete discussion about health care providers that are required to submit claims electronically.

Claim Status

Paper or electronic claims can be designated as clean, rejected, or pending (suspended).

A **clean claim** means that the claim was submitted within the program or policy time limit and contains all necessary information so that it can be processed and paid promptly. A **physically clean claim** is one that has no staples or highlighted areas and on which the bar code area has not been deformed.

A **rejected claim** means that the claim has not been processed or cannot be processed for various reasons (e.g., the patient is not identified in the payer system, the provider of services is not active in the third-party payer records, or the claim was not submitted in a timely manner). A rejected claim is one that requires investigation and needs further clarification and possibly answers to some questions. Such a claim should be resubmitted after proper corrections are made.

A **pending claim** is an insurance claim that is held in suspense for review or other reason by the third-party payer. These claims may be cleared for payment or denied.

Medicare Claim Status

In the Medicare program, besides the phrase "clean claims," specific terms such as *incomplete*, *rejected*, and *dirty* are used to describe various claim-processing situations. These terms may or may not be used by other insurance programs. The Omnibus Budget Reconciliation Act (OBRA) requires Medicare administrative contractors to pay the Prompt Payment Interest Rate on all clean claims not paid timely. The government updates the interest rate January 1 and July 1 each year on the Treasury's Financial Management Service page.

A *clean claim* means the following:

1. The claim has no deficiencies and passes all electronic edits.
2. The carrier does not need to investigate outside of the carrier's operation before paying the claim.
3. The claim is investigated on a postpayment basis, meaning a claim is not delayed before payment and may be paid. After investigation, payments may be considered "not due" and a refund may be requested from the provider.
4. The claim is subject to medical review with attached information or forwarded simultaneously with electronic medical claim (EMC) records.

Further information on the many methods to ensure clean claims is given in the next chapter.

Medicare claims not considered "clean" claims, which require investigation or development on a prepayment basis (developed for Medicare Secondary Payer information), are known as **"other" claims**.

Participating provider electronic submissions are processed within approximately 14 days of receipt. Participating provider paper submissions and nonparticipating provider claims are not processed until at least 27 days after receipt.

An **incomplete claim** is any Medicare claim missing required information. It is identified to the provider so that it can be resubmitted as a new claim.

An **invalid claim** is any Medicare claim that contains complete, necessary information but is illogical or incorrect (e.g., listing an incorrect provider number for a referring physician). An invalid claim is identified to the provider and may be resubmitted.

A **dirty claim** is a claim submitted with errors, one requiring manual processing for resolving problems, or one rejected for payment. Pending or suspense claims are placed in this category because something is holding the claim back from payment, perhaps review or some other problem.

A **deleted claim** is a claim canceled, deleted, or voided by a Medicare fiscal intermediary for the following reasons: CMS-1500 (08-05) or current CMS-1450 is not used, itemized charges are not provided, more than six line items are submitted on the CMS-1500 (08-05) claim form, patient's address is missing, internal clerical error was made, Certificate of Medical Necessity (CMN) was not with the Part B claim or was incomplete or invalid, and name of the store is not on the receipt that includes the price of the item.

ABSTRACTING FROM MEDICAL RECORDS

Abstraction of technical information from patient records may be requested for three situations: (1) to complete insurance claim forms, (2) when sending a letter to justify a health insurance claim after professional services are rendered, or (3) when a patient applies for life, mortgage, or health insurance. Abstracting to complete insurance claims is discussed later in this chapter.

Cover Letter Accompanying Insurance Claims

A letter accompanying insurance claims should include the patient's name, subscriber's name if different, subscriber identification number, date and type of service, total amount of the claim, a short history, and a clear but concise explanation of the medical necessity, difficulty or complexity, or unusual circumstance (e.g., emergency). The letter and insurance claim should be sent to the attention of the claims supervisor so that it may be directed to the appropriate person for processing.

Life or Health Insurance Applications

When a patient applies for insurance, the insurance company may request information from the patient's private physician, require a physical examination, or both.

On some application forms, the release of medical information signed by the patient may appear as a separate sheet or as a perforated attachment to a multiple-paged form. In the latter, page 1 is completed by the insurance agent when interviewing the client, page 2 is filled in by the prospective insured, and page 3 is completed by the physician at the time of the physical examination of the prospective insured. Sometimes a form is sent to the client's attending physician along with a check requesting medical information. The amount of the check may vary, depending on how much information is requested. If the check is not included, the physician should request a fee on the basis of the length of the report before sending in the completed report form. The fee is required before completion of the form or payment may not be received. Examples of pages 2 and 3 of a life insurance application form may be found on the Evolve website.

Be extremely accurate when abstracting medical information from the patient's record. Figure 7-1 is a chart note identifying important abstracting components. Abbreviations on the chart must be understood, and only the requested information should be provided. If the form has questions about high blood pressure, kidney infection, or heart problems, the patient could be prohibited from obtaining life, health, or mortgage insurance if the answers are derogatory. Part of HIPAA laws (Insurance Portability, Part I) provides guidance on circumstances when an individual can be excluded from health insurance benefits coverage. Be sure to check with the insurance company for more information. Because this part of HIPAA is more involved than would apply in the role of a billing specialist, this topic is not discussed in depth here.

If a patient tests positive for human immunodeficiency virus (HIV), legal counsel may be necessary because some state laws allow information on HIV infection and acquired immunodeficiency syndrome (AIDS) to be given only to the patient or to the patient's spouse. In some states, it is illegal to require a blood test for HIV antibodies, a urinalysis for HIV, or an HIV antigen test as a condition of coverage. It also may be illegal to question applicants about HIV status or prior symptoms of and treatment for AIDS or other forms of immune deficiency. Sometimes, private group plans allow medical coverage for people testing positive for HIV or an AIDS-related illness through a state major risk medical insurance program. However, the waiting period may exceed 1 year if the maximum enrollment number has been reached. A separate release of information statement is necessary before any information can be released regarding an HIV/AIDS patient.

In some situations, it is preferable to submit a narrative report dictated by the physician instead of completing the form, which has numerous check-off columns and no space for comments. It may be necessary to attach a copy of an operative, pathology, laboratory, or radiology report and an electrocardiogram (ECG) tracing.

A "Please Read" note should be placed on the insurance questionnaire to have the physician check it over thoroughly before signing it and to make sure that the information is accurate and properly stated.

An insurance company may ask a copy service to come to your office to photocopy the patient's record. Usually this is done at the convenience of the office staff, and an appointment should be made. The insurance company should be reminded that an authorization form signed by the patient is necessary to release medical information. An appropriate fee for this service is charged and quoted at the time of the telephone request. The physician should review the records in advance to ensure that they are in proper order.

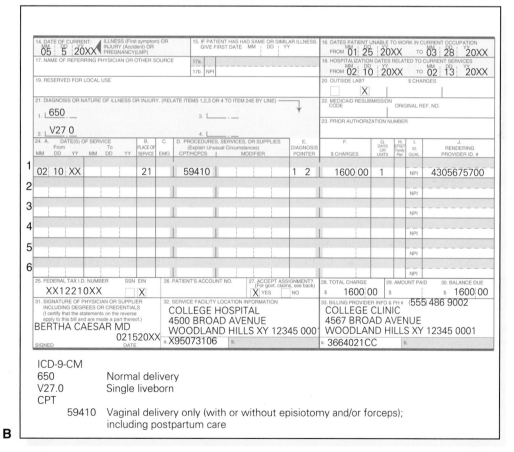

FIGURE 7-1 A, Example of a chart note illustrating important information to read through and abstract for insurance claim completion. **B,** The location of the abstracted information placed in the blocks on a CMS-1500 (08-05) insurance claim form in OCR format.

HEALTH INSURANCE CLAIM FORM (CMS-1500 [08-05])

Basic Guidelines for Submitting a Claim

The **Health Insurance Claim form (CMS-1500 [08-05])**, often known simply as the CMS-1500 claim form, is the form required when submitting Medicare claims and is accepted by nearly all state Medicaid programs and private third-party payers, as well as by TRICARE and workers' compensation.

A claim form should be completed and submitted as required by payer rules on behalf of a patient who is covered by third-party insurance. If coverage is in question, the insurance carrier should be contacted about eligibility status. An official rejection from the insurance company is the best answer to present to the patient in this situation. The patient may be unaware of the status of his or her health care policy coverage and current deductible status. It is recommended that you submit an insurance claim and get paid for services rendered if there is coverage rather than have the patient receive payment from his or her insurance company.

 In this chapter, icons are used as they are shown in previous chapters. The paper CMS-1500 (08-05) icon identifies physicians' offices that are paper based, meaning they do not file electronic claims. The computer icon is used to indicate physicians' offices that operate in an electronic environment.

Individual Insurance

When a patient brings in a form from a private insurance plan that is not a CMS-1500 (08-05) claim form, he or she should sign it. This occurs less frequently today than in the past. In addition, the patient should sign the CMS-1500 (08-05) claim form in Block 13 (Assignment of Benefits). If you have a signed assignment of benefits form in the patient's health record, you can state "signature on file" on the CMS-1500 (08-05) claim form. The patient's portion of the private insurance form should be checked to ensure that it is complete and accurate. The forms should then be mailed together to the insurance carrier. Some companies allow staples and some do not. It is not recommended to let patients direct their own forms to insurance companies or employers. Patients have been known to lose forms or alter data on documents before mailing, forget to send them, or mail them to an incorrect address.

Group Insurance

When a patient has group insurance through an employer, be sure all the information about the employer is complete and correct. If the employer's section is complete, both the CMS-1500 (08-05) and the group insurance forms should be sent directly to the insurance carrier after the physician's portion is completed.

Secondary Insurance

When two insurance policies are involved (sometimes called *dual coverage* or *duplication of coverage*), one is considered primary and the other secondary (Example 7-1). For billing purposes, generally the primary policy is the policy held by the patient when the patient and his or her spouse are both covered by employer-paid insurance. The patient's signature should always be acquired for assignment of benefits for both insurance companies. In regard to children, refer to the section explaining the birthday law and divorced parents in Chapter 3.

Example 7-1   Primary/Secondary Insurance Plans

A husband and wife have insurance through their employers and both have added the spouse to their plans for secondary coverage. If the wife is seen for treatment, the insurance plan to which she is the subscriber is the primary carrier for her.

After payment is made by the primary plan, a claim is submitted with a copy of the explanation of benefits from the primary carrier to the secondary carrier.

Completion of Insurance Claim Forms

The recommendation is to answer all required (R) and conditionally required (C) questions on the form whether the form is optically scanned or not. If any questions are unanswerable, do not use DNA (Does Not Apply), NA, or N/A (Not Applicable), but leave the space blank.

Diagnosis

In Block 21, diagnosis field of the CMS-1500 (08-05) claim form, all accurate diagnostic codes that affect the patient's condition should be inserted, with the primary diagnosis code listed first followed by any secondary diagnosis codes. Electronic claims have the ability to hold a maximum of eight diagnoses codes allowed by the ANSI 837P 4010A1 claim format. However, to allow twelve diagnostic codes, this will become the electronic ASC X12 837 version 5010 to be implemented on January 1, 2012. Check with your regional Medicare administrative contractor to learn the procedure for conveying more than four diagnostic codes when submitting paper claims. A diagnosis should never be submitted without supporting documentation in the medical record. The diagnosis must agree with the medical necessity of the treatment and services rendered. If there is no formal diagnosis at the conclusion of an encounter, the code(s) for the patient's symptom(s) should be submitted.

It is best to list only one illness or injury and its treatment per form, unless there are concurrent conditions to avoid confusing services with multiple medical conditions.

Service Dates

Dates of service must be entered with no spaces using a 6-digit or 8-digit format; for example, January 2, 20XX, should appear as either 0102XX or 010220XX. However, if you choose to enter 8-digit dates for Blocks 11b, 14, 16, 18, 19, or 24A, the dates must be consistent for all blocks; the same rule applies if you choose 6-digit dates. Blocks 12 and 31 are exempt from this rule. Do not use ditto marks (") to indicate repetition of dates for services performed on subsequent lines. Charges for services rendered in different years on the same claim form should not be submitted. Sometimes such practices can be affected by deductible and eligibility factors, thereby delaying reimbursement.

Consecutive Dates

Some carriers allow medical services or hospital or office visits to be grouped if each visit is consecutive, occurs in the same month, uses the same procedure code, or results in the same fee. The total fee for the procedures should be listed in Block 24F, and the number of times the procedure was performed or service supplied should be listed in Block 24G as illustrated in the graphic at the bottom of this page (Example: $55.56 × 5 =$277.80). However, private insurance carriers should be contacted because some carriers require a single fee listed in Block 24F rather than the total fee for the procedures. If there is a difference in the procedure code or fee for several visits listed on the claim, each separately coded hospital or office visit must be itemized and each procedure or service code and charge entered on a separate line.

No Charge

Insurance claims should not be submitted for services that have no charge, such as global or surgical package postoperative visit, unless the patient requests that it be

sent. These services should appear documented in the patient's health and financial records.

Physicians' Identification Numbers

Insurance companies and federal and state programs require certain identification numbers on claim forms to be submitted from health care providers and facilities who provide and bill for services to patients. This can be confusing to the beginner, as well as to someone experienced in insurance billing procedures, because there are so many different numbers.

- *State license number.* To practice within a state, each physician must obtain a physician's **state license number.** Sometimes this number is requested on forms and is used as a provider number.
- *Employer identification number.* In a medical group or solo practice, each physician must have his or her own federal tax identification number, known as an **employer identification number (EIN)** or tax identification number (TIN). This is issued by the Internal Revenue Service for income tax purposes.

25. FEDERAL TAX I.D. NUMBER	SSN EIN
74 10640XX	☐ ☒

- *Social security number.* In addition, each physician has a **Social Security number (SSN)** for other personal use and may have one or more EINs for financial reasons. These are not typically used on the claim form unless the provider does not have an EIN, in which case the Social Security number may be required.

25. FEDERAL TAX I.D. NUMBER	SSN EIN
082 XX 1707	☒ ☐

Provider Numbers. Claims may require several NPI numbers: one for the referring physician, one for the ordering physician, and one for the performing physician (billing entity). It is possible that the ordering physician and performing physician are the same. On rare occasions, the number may be the same for all three, but more frequently different numbers are required, depending on the circumstances of the case. For placement of the NPI number on the CMS-1500 (08-05) claim form, refer to the block-by-block instructions for Blocks 17a and 24J. Keep in mind what role the physicians and their numbers represent in relationship to the provider listed in Block 33. The following examples of blocks from the CMS-1500 (08-05) insurance claim form show where these

24. A. DATE(S) OF SERVICE						B. PLACE OF SERVICE	C. EMG	D. PROCEDURES, SERVICES, OR SUPPLIES (Explain Unusual Circumstances)		E. DIAGNOSIS POINTER	F. $ CHARGES	G. DAYS OR UNITS	H. EPSDT Family Plan	I. ID. QUAL.	J. RENDERING PROVIDER ID. #
From MM DD YY			To MM DD YY					CPT/HCPCS	MODIFIER						
1	10 04 XX		10 08 XX			21		99232		1	277 80	5			32783127XX
2													NPI		

numbers are commonly placed. Insurance billing manuals from major insurers give specific directions.

When a non-physician practitioner (NPP) bills incident-to a physician in the same group, but that physician is out of the office on a day the NPP sees the patient, another physician in the same group can provide direct supervision to meet the incident-to requirements. Incident-to services are discussed in Chapter 6. When the ordering and supervising doctors are different individuals, the ordering doctor's name goes in Block 17 and his or her NPI goes in Block 17a. The NPI of the supervising doctor goes in Block 24J and the supervising physician signs the form in Block 31. The group's NPI goes in Block 33.

To assist with claims completion, a reference list of provider numbers should be compiled for all ordering physicians and physicians who frequently refer patients. For Medicare claims, physicians' provider numbers can be obtained by calling their offices, contacting the Medicare carrier, or searching the NPI Registry on the Internet. For license numbers, search the state licensing board on the Internet. Refer to Appendix A for all physician provider numbers when completing *Workbook* assignments.

- *Provider identification number (PIN).* With the implementation of the NPI for compliance by May 23, 2007, PINs are no longer used.
- *Unique provider identification number (UPIN).* With the implementation of the National Provider Identifier on May 23, 2007, UPINs are no longer used.
- *Group National Provider Identifier (group NPI).* The **group NPI** is used instead of the individual NPI for the performing provider who is a member of a group practice that submits claims to insurance companies under the group name.

33. BILLING PROVIDER INFO & PH #   (555)486 9002
COLLEGE CLINIC
4567 BROAD AVENUE
WOODLAND HILLS XY 12345 0001
a.   3664021CC   b.

- *National Provider Identifier.* The **National Provider Identifier (NPI)** is a lifetime 10-digit number that will replace all other numbers assigned by various health plans. It will be recognized by state (Medicaid), federal (Medicare, TRICARE, and CHAMPVA), and private programs. Most providers required to submit standard electronic transactions under HIPAA applied for an NPI from the National Provider System beginning May 23, 2005. Each provider began using the NPI on May 23, 2007, except for small health plans whose compliance date is May 23, 2008. A health care provider will be assigned only one NPI, which is retained for a lifetime even if he or she moves to another state.

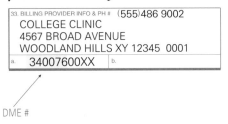

NPI root
check digit
locator code

- *Durable medical equipment number.* Medicare providers who charge patients a fee for supplies and equipment such as crutches, urinary catheters, ostomy supplies, surgical dressings, and so forth must bill Medicare using a **durable medical equipment (DME) number.** These claims are not sent to the regional fiscal intermediary but to another specific location.

33. BILLING PROVIDER INFO & PH #   (555)486 9002
COLLEGE CLINIC
4567 BROAD AVENUE
WOODLAND HILLS XY 12345 0001
a.   34007600XX   b.

DME #

- *Facility provider number.* Each facility (e.g., hospital, laboratory, radiology office, skilled nursing facility) is issued a **facility provider number** to be used by the performing physician to report services done at the location.

32. SERVICE FACILITY LOCATION INFORMATION
COLLEGE HOSPITAL
4500 BROAD AVENUE
WOODLAND HILLS XY 12345
a. X9507310XX   b.

- *Taxonomy code.* Some payers may either assign a provider identifier or prefer the taxonomy code to be inserted on CMS-1500 claim forms. Depending on issues of each case, provider taxonomy codes may or may not be required on the form. When needed, the blocks affected are Blocks 17a, 19, 24I, 24J, 32b, or 33b.

A FINAL NOTE

AN NPI NUMBER PAYS BECAUSE IT'S UNIVERSAL!

Physician's Signature

The physician should sign the insurance claim form above or under the typed or preprinted physician's name. A stamped signature is allowed in some instances and discussed later in this chapter. A removable indicator "Sign Here" tag may be used to help the physician locate where to sign the claim.

In the computerized office environment, the practice management system will generate a paper CMS-1500 (08-05) form. The participating contract with the third-party payer (including Medicare, Medicaid, and the Blue Plans) that is signed by the physician allows the physician's name to be printed in the signature block as it would normally be signed. This is an acceptable method for the provider's signature.

Insurance Biller's Initials

If more than one person is assigned to complete insurance paper claims, then the insurance biller should place his or her initials in the bottom left or top right corner of the claim form. Placement of this reference should be consistent. The following are three good reasons to adopt this habit:

- To identify who in the office is responsible for the insurance form
- To decrease errors
- To avoid being accused of someone else's error, especially if another biller submitted a fraudulent claim

Proofread

Ideally, every paper claim should be proofread for transposition of numbers (group, policy, physician's ID, procedure, and diagnostic codes), misspelled name, missing date of birth, blanks, and attachments. Larger, more complex claims require special attention because they involve greater sums of money and may be more difficult to complete. Check to make sure the bill is for the right patient by checking the address and date of birth to verify the correct individual. Review the encounter form to charge for the correct tests and number of tests so the patient is not charged more than once for the same service. Review the bill for the correct amount of time (e.g., a patient seen for 16 minutes should show a billing for one 15-minute session). Check for any overcoding such as do not bill for a longer office visit that included paperwork time when only actual face-to-face time should have been charged. Double check to see if there are charges for items that can be included in the cost of something else because unbundled charges are not allowed. Proofreading data prevents denials and time-consuming questions coming up later.

Supporting Documentation

Occasionally, claims need supporting documents to further explain services billed and to obtain maximum reimbursement.

On any submitted supplemental document, the patient's name, subscriber's name (if different from that of the patient), date of service, and insurance identification number should be included in case the document becomes separated from the claim during processing. This same information should be placed on each page of the document, front and back if two-sided.

If a medication is expensive or experimental, a copy of the invoice received from the supply house or pharmacy should be sent.

When a procedure is complicated, a copy of all pertinent reports (operative, radiology, laboratory, pathology, and discharge summary) should be included.

For a treatment not listed in the procedure code book, a special detailed report should be sent that gives the nature, extent, and need for the services along with the time, effort, supplies, and equipment required. The correct code number should be used for unlisted services or procedures, which may or may not always end in "99" (Example 7-2).

Example 7-2   Unlisted Procedure

95199 Unlisted Allergy Testing Procedure

Office Pending File

As mentioned in Chapter 3, the office copy of the insurance form should be filed in a separate alpha (tickler) file for insurance claim copies or in the back of the patient's medical chart, unless the computer system maintains files. The tickler file should be reviewed for follow-up every 30 days.

 The practice management system will keep an accurate record of all patients and activity on their accounts.

COMMON REASONS WHY CLAIM FORMS ARE DELAYED OR REJECTED

It is wise to be aware of common billing errors and how to correct them for quicker claim settlements and to reduce the number of appeals. This may help avoid additional administrative burdens such as telephone calls, resubmission of claims, and appeal letters. Also see Chapter 9 for information on solutions to denied or delayed claims, as well as prevention measures. Table 7-1 contains some reasons why claims are rejected or delayed and suggested solutions when completing the CMS-1500 (08-05) insurance claim form blocks.

Table 7-1   The Paper Claim: Problem Solving

BLOCK NUMBER	PROBLEM	SOLUTION
1	When submitting a paper claim, wrong block is checked (i.e., claim submitted to the secondary insurer instead of the primary insurer).	Obtain data from the patient during the first office visit as to which company is the primary insurer, depending on illness, injury, or accident. Submit the claim to the primary carrier and then send in a claim with a copy of the primary carrier's explanation of benefits (EOB) to the secondary carrier.
1 to 13	Information missing on patient portion of the claim form.	Obtain a complete patient registration form from which information can be extracted. Educate patients on data requirements at the time of the first visit to the physician's office if patients are filling out their portion. Be sure to ask if there have been any changes on subsequent office visits.
1a	Patient's insurance number is incorrect or transposed (especially in Medicare and Medicaid cases).	Proofread numbers carefully from source documents. Always photocopy front and back sides of insurance identification cards.
2	Patient's name and insured's name are entered as the same when the patient is a dependent. A common error is the patient listed as insured when he or she is not the insured (e.g., spouse or child). Block 4 is used for listing the insured's name.	Verify the insured party and check for Sr., Jr., and correct birth date.
3	Incorrect gender identification, resulting in a diagnosis or procedure code that is inconsistent with patient's gender.	Proofread claim before mailing and review patient's medical record to locate gender, especially if the patient's first name could be male or female.
9a through 9d	Incomplete entry for other insurance coverage.	Accurately abstract data from the patient's registration form and input to the computer database. Telephone the patient if information is incomplete.
10	Failure to indicate whether patient's condition is related to employment or an "other" type of accident.	Review patient's medical history to find out details of injury or illness and proofread claim before mailing. Telephone the employer to see if permission was given to treat the patient as a workers' compensation case.
14	Date of injury, date of last menstrual period (LMP), or dates of onset of illness are omitted. This information is important for determining whether accident benefits apply, patient is eligible for maternity benefits, or there was a preexisting condition.	Do not list unless dates are clearly documented in the patient's medical record. Read the patient's medical history and call the patient to obtain the date of accident or LMP. Compose an addendum to the record, if necessary. Always proofread a paper claim before mailing in case data are missing.
17 through 17a	Incorrect or missing name or NPI of referring physician on claim for consultation or other services requiring this information.	Check the patient registration form and the chart note for reference to the referring physician. Develop a list of NPI numbers for all physicians in the area.
19	Attachments (e.g., prescription, operative report, manufacturer's invoice) or Medicaid verification (e.g., labels, identification numbers) are missing.	Submit all information required for pricing or coverage on an 8.5- × 11-inch paper with the patient's name, subscriber name (if other than patient), and insurance identification number on each attachment (enclosure). Type the word "ATTACHMENT" in Block 19 or 10d. Never staple or clip documentation to a claim.
21	The diagnostic code is missing, incomplete, invalid, or not in standard nomenclature (e.g., missing fourth or fifth digit); it includes a written description or does not correspond to the treatment (procedure code) rendered by the physician.	Update encounter forms twice a year (October 1 and January 1). Verify and submit correct diagnostic codes by referring to an updated diagnostic code book and reviewing the patient record. Check with the physician if the diagnosis code listed does not go with the procedure code shown.
24A	Omitted, incorrect, overlapping, or duplicate dates of service.	Verify against the encounter form or medical record that all dates of service are listed and accurate and appear on individual lines on paper claims. Date spans for multiple services must be adequate for the number and types of services provided. Each month should be on a separate line and each year should be on a separate claim.

Table 7-1	The Paper Claim: Problem Solving—cont'd	
BLOCK NUMBER	**PROBLEM**	**SOLUTION**
24B	Missing or incorrect place of service code. If a physician sees a patient in a skilled nursing facility (SNF) that is in the same building as a domicile rest home or a hospice, it is possible to incorrectly document the SNF as the site for each patient.	Verify the place of service from the encounter form or medical record and list the correct code for place of service and submitted procedure.
24D	Procedure codes are incorrect, invalid, or missing.	Verify the coding system used by the third-party payer and submit correct procedure code(s) by referring to a current procedure code book. For Medicare patients and certain private insurance plans, check the HCPCS manual for CMS national and local procedure codes.
24D	Incorrect or missing modifier(s).	Verify usage of modifiers by referring to a current procedure code book and HCPCS manual. Submit valid modifiers with the correct procedure codes (Chapter 6).
24F	Omitted or incorrect amount billed.	Be certain the fee column is filled in. Check the amounts charged with the appropriate fee schedule.
24G	Reasons for multiple visits made in 1 day are not stated on an attachment sheet.	Depending on insurance guidelines, submit documentation explaining reason for multiple visits. Use appropriate modifiers or upcode evaluation and management services to include all visits.
24G	Incorrect quantity billed.	Verify charge amounts. Make sure that the number of units listed is equal to the date span when more than one date of service is billed (e.g., hospital visits).
24J	Provider's identification number is missing.	Verify and insert the required provider's number in this block.
24A through 24J, Line 6	More than six lines entered on a paper claim.	Insert service date and corresponding procedure on lines one to six only. Complete an additional paper claim if more services should be billed.
28	Total amounts do not equal itemized charges.	Total charges for each claim and verify amounts with patient account. If number of units listed in 24G is more than 1, multiply the units by the fee listed in 24F and add to all other charges listed.
31	Physician's signature is missing.	Have the physician or physician's representative sign the claim using a removable indicator "Sign Here" tag to indicate the correct location or key in "SOF" or "signature on file."
32	Information is not centered in block as required when submitting a paper claim.	Enter data centered in block.
33	Provider's address, PIN, or group number are missing.	Obtain provider's data from a list that contains all physicians' professional information.

ADDITIONAL CLAIM SUBMISSION ERRORS

PROBLEM: Carolyn, the insurance biller, telephoned the insurance company and discovered there was no record of the claim at the third-party payer.

SOLUTION: Always keep copies of paper claims or electronic transmission receipts. Send claims with large dollar amounts by certified mail, return receipt requested. Another option is to request that the customer service representative search the insurance carrier's imaging file for the period beginning on the date of service forward until the date you are calling. Sometimes the claim was received and scanned but was never crossed over to the processing unit.

PROBLEM: Claire is in a hurry and submits a claim form that is illegible.

SOLUTION: Never handwrite a claim form. Check printer ink, toner, or typewriter ribbon and replace when necessary.

PROBLEM: Untimely or lack of response to claim development letters.

SOLUTION: Pay close attention to the due date shown in the letter, and reply to development letters (third-party payer's request for additional information) as soon as possible. Send a copy of the claim with the letter and appropriate medical documentation listing the claim control number, if assigned.

PROBLEM: Duplicate claim or duplicate service.

SOLUTION: For an electronically transmitted claim, check the Medicare Interactive Voice Recognition system for claim status and rebill only the denied detail or line item, not the entire claim. Verify the claim was transmitted with correct data.

PROBLEM: Phillip reviews the Medicare remittance advice and discovers a noncovered service that is deemed not a medical necessity.

SOLUTION: For Medicare claims, check the local coverage determination policies and national coverage determination policies for diagnosis requirements or for private claims, the insurance policy for the service. Verify that the diagnosis billed indicates necessity for the medical procedure or service.

PROBLEM: Noncovered service because a routine screening procedure is performed in conjunction with a routine examination.

SOLUTION: Determine if it is a diagnostic or preventive service and if the code is correct. Use the GY modifier when submitting a statutory excluded service for payment by the secondary insurance carrier.

PROBLEM: Payment adjusted because the care may be covered by another insurance plan per coordination of benefits.

SOLUTION: Annually check all Medicare patients' coverage. Verify eligibility on the Medicare Interactive Voice Recognition system before transmitting the claim.

PROBLEM: Noncovered charge.

SOLUTION: Claim must be transmitted electronically and only providers granted a waiver may submit paper claims.

PROBLEM: Payment adjusted because the medical service is not paid separately because it is a global surgery or a National Correct Coding Initiative (NCCI) denial.

SOLUTION: Determine the global period for the surgical procedure. Use a modifier to report an unrelated or exception service within a global period. Check the NCCI edits to see if the code selected has been deleted or is a bundled service.

PROBLEM: Irene submits a claim with missing/incomplete/invalid information on where the medical services were performed.

SOLUTION: Include the ZIP code of where the service was performed.

PROBLEM: In reviewing a Medicare remittance advice document, Anne notices it indicates that Mrs. Bentley's medical expenses were incurred before insurance coverage.

SOLUTION: Annually verify all Medicare patients' coverage. Review the patient's Medicare card for entitlement and effective dates. Verify eligibility on the Medicare Interactive Voice Recognition system before transmitting the claim. Verify the claim is submitted with the correct Medicare number including the Alpha suffix.

OPTICAL SCANNING FORMAT GUIDELINES

Optical Character Recognition

Optical character recognition (OCR), also less commonly referred to as **intelligent character recognition (ICR)** or *image copy recognition (ICR)*, devices (scanners) are being used across the nation in processing insurance claims because of their speed and efficiency. A scanner can transfer printed or typed text and bar codes to the insurance company's computer memory. Scanners read at such a fast speed that they reduce data entry cost and decrease processing time.

More control is gained over data input by using OCR. It improves accuracy, thus reducing coding errors because the claim is entered exactly as coded by the insurance biller.

Do's and Don'ts for Optical Character Recognition

The CMS-1500 (08-05) form was developed so that insurance carriers could process claims efficiently by OCR. Keying a form for OCR scanning requires different techniques than preparing one for standard claims submission. Because the majority of insurance carriers accept the OCR format, it is suggested that it be routinely used. Basic do's and don'ts for completing claims using OCR format follow:

Do: Use original claim forms printed in red ink; photocopies and forms generated from ink jet or laser printers cannot be scanned.

Don't: Handwrite information on the document. Handwriting is only accepted for signatures. Handwritten claims require manual processing.

2 nd request

			PICA	
FECA BLK LUNG *(SSN)*	OTHER *(ID)*	1a. INSURED'S I.D. NUMBER	*(FOR PROGRAM IN ITEM 1)*	
		111704521	A482	

Do: Align the printer correctly so that characters appear exactly in the proper fields. Enter all information within designated fields.

Don't: Allow characters to touch lines.

Correct

Incorrect

Don't: Use broken characters (dot matrix), script, slant, minifont, or italicized fonts or expanded, compressed, or bold print. Use fonts that have the same width for each character (proportional).

Do: Enter all information in upper case (CAPITAL) letters. Keep characters within the borders of each field. Use 10 pitch Pica or Arial or 10-, 11-, or 12-point type.

Correct

> 2. PATIENT'S NAME (Last Name, First Name, Middle Initial)
> DOE JANE E

Incorrect

> 2. PATIENT'S NAME (Last Name, First Name, Middle Initial)
> Doe, Jane E.

Don't: Strike over any errors when correcting or crowd preprinted numbers; OCR equipment does not read corrected characters on top of correction tape or correction fluid.

Correct

> 3. PATIENT'S BIRTH DATE   SEX
> MM | DD | YY
> 01 | 06 | 1946   M [X]   F [ ]

Incorrect

> 3. PATIENT'S BIRTH DATE   SEX
> MM | DD | YY
> 01 | 06 | 1946   M [X]   F [ ]

Do: Indicate a deletion for a delete field and go to the next line to insert the data if an optically scanned form has a delete field. Lines, marks, or characters entered in a delete field cause deletion of the entire line.

Do: Complete a new form for additional services if the case has more than six lines of service.

Correct

> 6 04:07 XX   11   99214

> 24. A. DATE(S) OF SERVICE   B. C. D. PROCEDURES, SERVICES, OR SUPPLIES
> From   To   PLACE OF   (Explain Unusual Circumstances)
> MM DD YY MM DD YY SERVICE EMG CPT/HCPCS   MODIFIER
> 1 04:10 XX   21   30520

Incorrect

> 6 040720XX   11   99214
>   041020XX   21   30520

Don't: Use highlighter pens or colored ink on claims because OCR equipment will not recognize these.

Do: Use alpha or numeric symbols.

Don't: Use symbols (#, -, /), periods (.), ditto marks ("), parentheses, or commas (,).

Correct

> 25. FEDERAL TAX I.D. NUMBER   SSN EIN
> 123 XX 6789   [X] [ ]

Incorrect

> 25. FEDERAL TAX I.D. NUMBER   SSN EIN
> 123-XX-6789   [X] [ ]

Don't: Use decimals in Block 21 or dollar signs ($) in the money column.

Correct   **Incorrect**

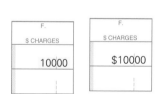

Don't: Use narrative descriptions of procedures, modifiers, or diagnoses; code numbers are sufficient.

Correct

> D. PROCEDURES, SERVICES, OR SUPPLIES
> (Explain Unusual Circumstances)
> CPT/HCPCS   MODIFIER
> 42820

Incorrect

Don't: Use N/A or DNA when information is not applicable. Leave the space blank.

Correct

17. NAME OF REFERRING PHYSICIAN OR OTHER SOURCE

Incorrect

17. NAME OF REFERRING PHYSICIAN OR OTHER SOURCE
DNA

Do: Enter comments in Block 19 (e.g., ATTACHMENT) for primary EOB submitted with claim to secondary insurance company.

Correct

19. RESERVED FOR LOCAL USE
ATTACHMENT

Incorrect

Don't: Use paper clips, cellophane tape, stickers, rubber stamps, or staples.

Do: Enter 6-digit or 8-digit date formats: 0601XX or 060120XX or 06 01 20XX, depending on the block instructions.

Correct

24. A. DATE(S) OF SERVICE
From / To
MM DD YY MM DD YY
1 03 03 XX
2

Correct

24. A. DATE(S) OF SERVICE
From / To
MM DD YY MM DD YY
1 030320XX
2

Do: Keep signature within signature block. Use of rubber stamps is discouraged; however, they may be used if they are accepted by insurance carrier and produce complete, clean images, without smudges or missing letters.

Correct

reference initials

Incorrect

31. SIGNATURE OF PHYSICIAN OR SUPPLIER INCLUDING DEGREES OR CREDENTIALS
(I certify that the statements on the reverse apply to this bill and are made a part thereof.)
CONCHA ANTRUM MD
030320XX
SIGNED   DATE

Concha Antrum MD
reference initials

Don't: Overtrim or undertrim forms when bursting (taking apart multipage computer printouts). Use care in separating forms and discard any forms with tears or holes.

Don't: Fold or spindle forms when mailing because they will not feed into OCR equipment properly if creased or torn.

Do: Enter information via computer keyboard. Use clean equipment and quality ink-jet or laser printers, if possible, not dot matrix.

PROCEDURE 7-1

Instructions for the Health Insurance Claim Form (CMS-1500 [08-05])

The Health Insurance Claim Form is divided into two major sections: patient information and physician information. The Patient and Insured (Subscriber) Information section is the upper portion of the claim form and contains 13 blocks numbered 1 through 13 (11 data elements and 2 signature blocks). The Physician or Supplier Information section is the lower portion of the claim form and consists of 20 blocks numbered 14 through 33 (19 data elements and 1 signature block). Some of the blocks are subdivided, with the subdivisions labeled a, b, c, d, and so forth. More than 100 places are available to enter specific information.

The instructions are straightforward and contain all pertinent information needed to complete a claim (see Figures 7-3 through 7-12, pp. 278 through 287). Much information on specific coverage guidelines, program policies, and practice specialties could not be included here.

A brief description of each block and of its applicability to the requirements of private insurance payers, Medicaid, Medicare, TRICARE, CHAMPVA, and workers' compensation is presented. Because guidelines vary at the state and local levels for completing the CMS-1500 (08-05) claim form for the aforementioned insurance plans, consult your local intermediary or private carriers.

Question: Do the HIPAA transactions and code sets standards apply to paper claims and other nonelectronic transactions?

Answer: No. The HIPAA transactions and code sets standards only apply to electronic transactions conducted by covered entities. Other entities such as employers or casualty insurance plans may decide to use them voluntarily but are not required to do so.

For paper transactions, health plans are free to set their own data requirements. Other federal or state laws may require plans or providers to use specific code sets for certain paper transactions. All covered health plans and providers must, however, be able to use the HIPAA standards for electronic transactions. Health plans may choose to require that paper claims include the same data elements, codes, and identifiers that are required by the HIPAA regulations for electronic transactions.

Block numbers match those on the Health Insurance Claim Form. Blocks marked with **R** (Required) or **C** (Conditionally Required) will cause your claim to be rejected if they are missing, invalid, or incomplete. However, there are many other blocks on the claim form that must be properly completed or your claim will be delayed or denied. Italicized sections refer students to guidelines in completing the Workbook assignments when there are optional ways of completing a block. However, whenever a Block number is mentioned in these block-by-block instructions, the related concept and information required also applies to equivalent fields for electronically transmitted claims discussed in Chapter 8, Table 8-5, and Table 8-6. Icon meanings are as follows:

All Payers: All payer guidelines including all private insurance companies and all federal and state programs.

All Private Payers: All private insurance companies.

CHAMPVA: Civilian Health and Medical Program of the Department of Veterans' Affairs.

Medicaid: State Medicaid programs.

Medicare: Federal Medicare programs, Medicare/Medicaid, Medicare/Medigap, and Medicare Secondary Payer (MSP).

TRICARE: TRICARE Standard (formerly CHAMPUS), TRICARE Prime, TRICARE Extra.

Workers' Compensation: State workers' compensation programs.

Top of Form

Do not enter the name and address of third-party payer in the top right corner of the insurance form.

Some carriers prefer this area of the claim to be left blank because identifying data are printed during the initial processing stage.

If a commercial payer requires this section of the form completed, use a four-line address. If the third line of the address is not used, leave the line blank and enter the city, state, and zip code on the fourth line.

PICA							PICA

1a. INSURED'S I.D. NUMBER 111704521 (For Program in Item 1) A482

2. PATIENT'S NAME: FOREHAND HARRY N
3. PATIENT'S BIRTH DATE 01 06 1946 M X
4. INSURED'S NAME: SAME

Block 1

Required

PICA								PICA

1. MEDICARE	MEDICAID	TRICARE CHAMPUS	CHAMPVA	GROUP HEALTH PLAN	FECA BLK LUNG	OTHER	1a. INSURED'S I.D. NUMBER	(For Program in Item 1)
(Medicare #)	(Medicaid #)	(Sponsor's SSN)	(Member ID#) X	(SSN or ID)	(SSN)	(ID)	111704521	A482

2. PATIENT'S NAME (Last Name, First Name, Middle Initial)	3. PATIENT'S BIRTH DATE MM DD YY	SEX	4. INSURED'S NAME (Last Name, First Name, Middle Initial)
FOREHAND HARRY N	01 06 1946	M X F	SAME

 All Private Payers: Check the name of the insurance plan or type of insurance for where you are sending the form to and do not check the secondary coverage.
Individual Health Plan: Check "Other" for an individual who is covered under an individual policy.
Group Health Plan: Check this box for those covered under any group contract insurance (e.g., insurance obtained through employment) and for patients who receive services paid by managed care programs (e.g., HMOs, PPOs, IPAs). Some Blue Plans prefer that "Other" be checked even if the patient has a group plan. If in doubt, check with the insurance carriers for their preference.
→ *When completing the **Workbook** assignments, if the insured is employed, assume the insurance is through the employer and is "group" insurance; otherwise, assume it is an individual policy and enter "Other."*

 Medicaid: Check for person receiving Medicaid benefits.

 Medicare: Check for patient who receives Medicare benefits.
Medicare/Medicaid: Check "Medicare" and "Medicaid" if the patient is covered under Medicare and Medicaid programs. Some reference manuals state that when there is secondary insurance, check the insurance plan on the claim form for the one you are sending that form to and insert the secondary insurance information in the correct location on the form.
Medicare/Medigap: Check "Medicare" and, if the patient has group or individual or Medigap coverage, check "Group" or "Other," depending on the health plan. Some reference manuals state that when there is secondary insurance, check the insurance plan on the claim form for the one you are sending that form to and insert the secondary insurance information in the correct location on the form.
→ *When completing the **Workbook** assignments, if the insured is employed, assume the insurance is through the employer and is "group" insurance; otherwise, assume it is an individual policy and enter "Other."*
MSP: Check "Group" or "Other" (depending on health plan) and "Medicare" when a Medicare patient has insurance primary to Medicare coverage. Some reference manuals state that when there is secondary insurance, check the insurance plan on the claim form for the one you are sending that form to and insert the secondary insurance information in the correct location on the form.

 TRICARE: Check "TRICARE/CHAMPUS" for individual receiving TRICARE benefits.

 CHAMPVA: Check "TRICARE/CHAMPVA" for individual receiving CHAMPVA benefits.

 Workers' Compensation: Check "Other" for all workers' compensation claims except FECA Black Lung. Check "FECA Black Lung" for patients who receive black lung benefits under the Federal Employee Compensation Act.

Block 1a

Required

	PICA							PICA		
1. MEDICARE	MEDICAID	TRICARE CHAMPUS	CHAMPVA	GROUP HEALTH PLAN	FECA BLK LUNG	OTHER	1a. INSURED'S I.D. NUMBER		(For Program in Item 1)	
(Medicare #)	(Medicaid #)	(Sponsor's SSN)	(Member ID#) X	(SSN or ID)	(SSN)	(ID)	111704521		A482	
2. PATIENT'S NAME (Last Name, First Name, Middle Initial)			3. PATIENT'S BIRTH DATE MM DD YY		SEX		4. INSURED'S NAME (Last Name, First Name, Middle Initial)			
FOREHAND HARRY N			01 06 1946	M X	F		SAME			

 All Private Payers: Enter the patient's policy (identification or certificate) number in the left portion of the block and the group number, if applicable, in the right portion of the block as it appears on the insurance card, without punctuation.

 Medicaid: Enter the Medicaid number in the left portion of the block. Do not enter dashes or other special characters in this block.

 Medicare: Enter the patient's Medicare Health Insurance Claim number (HICN) from the patient's Medicare card in the left portion of this block, regardless of whether Medicare is the primary or secondary payer.
Medicare/Medicaid: Enter the patient's Medicare number in the left portion of this block.
Medicare/Medigap: Enter the patient's Medicare number in the left portion of this block.
MSP: Enter the patient's Medicare number in the left portion of this block. Refer to Block 11 for primary insurance.

 TRICARE: First enter the sponsor's SSN in the left portion of this block. Then, if the patient is a NATO (North Atlantic Treaty Organization) beneficiary, add "NATO" or, if the sponsor is a security agent, add "SECURITY." Do not provide the patient's SSN unless the patient and sponsor are the same.

 CHAMPVA: Enter the Veterans' Affairs file number (omit prefix or suffix) or sponsor's SSN in the left portion of this block. Do not use any other former service numbers.

 Workers' Compensation: Enter the claim number. If none is assigned, enter the employer's policy number or patient's SSN.

Block 2

Required

	PICA							PICA		
1. MEDICARE	MEDICAID	TRICARE CHAMPUS	CHAMPVA	GROUP HEALTH PLAN	FECA BLK LUNG	OTHER	1a. INSURED'S I.D. NUMBER		(For Program in Item 1)	
(Medicare #)	(Medicaid #)	(Sponsor's SSN)	(Member ID#) X	(SSN or ID)	(SSN)	(ID)	111704521		A482	
2. PATIENT'S NAME (Last Name, First Name, Middle Initial)			3. PATIENT'S BIRTH DATE MM DD YY		SEX		4. INSURED'S NAME (Last Name, First Name, Middle Initial)			
FOREHAND HARRY N			01 06 1946	M X	F		SAME			

Example 7-3   Surname Format

Hyphenated name: Smith-White = SMITH-WHITE

Prefixed name: MacIverson = MACIVERSON

Seniority name with numeric suffix: John R. Ellis, III = ELLIS III JOHN R

All Payers: Enter the last name, first name, and middle initial of the patient—in that order—as shown on the patient's identification card, even if it is misspelled. Do not use nicknames or abbreviations. Do not use commas. A hyphen may be used if a name is hyphenated (Example 7-3).

Block 3

Required

PICA							PICA
1. MEDICARE	MEDICAID	TRICARE CHAMPUS	CHAMPVA	GROUP HEALTH PLAN	FECA BLK LUNG	OTHER	1a. INSURED'S I.D. NUMBER (For Program in Item 1)
(Medicare #)	(Medicaid #)	(Sponsor's SSN)	(Member ID#) X	(SSN or ID)	(SSN)	(ID)	111704521 A482
2. PATIENT'S NAME (Last Name, First Name, Middle Initial)			3. PATIENT'S BIRTH DATE SEX				4. INSURED'S NAME (Last Name, First Name, Middle Initial)
FOREHAND HARRY N			MM 01 DD 06 YY 1946 M X F				SAME

All Payers: Enter the patient's birth date using eight digits (01272000). The patient's age must be as follows to correlate with the diagnosis in Block 21:
- Birth: Newborn diagnosis
- Birth to 17 years: Pediatric diagnosis
- 12 to 55 years: Maternity diagnosis
- 15 to 124 years: Adult diagnosis

Check the appropriate box for the patient's sex. If left blank, gender block defaults to "female."

Block 4

Conditionally Required

PICA							PICA
1. MEDICARE	MEDICAID	TRICARE CHAMPUS	CHAMPVA	GROUP HEALTH PLAN	FECA BLK LUNG	OTHER	1a. INSURED'S I.D. NUMBER (For Program in Item 1)
(Medicare #)	(Medicaid #)	(Sponsor's SSN)	(Member ID#) X	(SSN or ID)	(SSN)	(ID)	111704521 A482
2. PATIENT'S NAME (Last Name, First Name, Middle Initial)			3. PATIENT'S BIRTH DATE SEX				4. INSURED'S NAME (Last Name, First Name, Middle Initial)
FOREHAND HARRY N			MM 01 DD 06 YY 1946 M X F				SAME

All Private Payers: Enter "SAME" when the insured is also the patient. If the insured is not the patient, enter the name of the insured (last name first).

Medicaid: Refer to Medicare guidelines.

Medicare: Leave blank if Medicare is primary and if the insured is also the patient. Enter the insured's name, if different from the patient's.
Medicare/Medicaid: Refer to Medicare guidelines.
Medicare/Medigap: Refer to Medicare guidelines.
MSP: Enter the name of the insured (last name first), which is the subscriber to the primary insurance coverage.

TRICARE: Enter the sponsor's last name, first name, and middle initial, not a nickname or abbreviation. Enter "SAME" if the sponsor and patient are the same.

CHAMPVA: Enter the veteran's name, last name first.

Workers' Compensation: Enter the employer's name. If the employer is a large corporation, enter the name of the insured corporation in Block 4 and the local employer in Block 11b (e.g., Saunders is the insured corporation [4] and Elsevier is the employer and would be listed in Block 11b).

Block 5

Required

5. PATIENT'S ADDRESS (No., Street)		6. PATIENT RELATIONSHIP TO INSURED		7. INSURED'S ADDRESS (No., Street)	
1456 MAIN STREET		Self [X] Spouse [ ] Child [ ] Other [ ]			
CITY WOODLAND HILLS	STATE XY	8. PATIENT STATUS		CITY	STATE
		Single [ ] Married [X] Other [ ]			
ZIP CODE 12345 0000	TELEPHONE (Include Area Code) (555) 490 9876	Employed [X] Full-Time Student [ ] Part-Time Student [ ]		ZIP CODE	TELEPHONE (INCLUDE AREA CODE) ( )

All Private Payers: Enter the patient's mailing address and residential telephone number.

Medicaid: Enter the patient's mailing address and residential telephone number.

Medicare: Enter the patient's mailing address and residential telephone number. On the first line, enter the street address; on the second line, the city and two-character state code (e.g., AZ = Arizona); on the third line, the ZIP code and residential telephone number. Punctuation is not necessary (e.g., ST LOUIS, no period after ST).
Medicare/Medicaid: Enter the patient's mailing address and residential telephone number.
Medicare/Medigap: Enter the patient's mailing address and residential telephone number.
MSP: Enter the patient's mailing address and residential telephone number.

TRICARE: Enter the patient's mailing address and residential telephone number. Do not enter a post office box number; provide the actual place of residence. If a rural address, the address must contain the route and box number. An APO/FPO address should not be used unless that person is residing overseas.

CHAMPVA: Enter the patient's mailing address and residential telephone number. Do not enter a post office box number; provide the actual place of residence. If a rural address, the address must contain the route and box number. An APO/FPO address should not be used unless that person is residing overseas.

Workers' Compensation: Enter the patient's mailing address and residential telephone number.

Block 6

Conditionally Required

5. PATIENT'S ADDRESS (No., Street)		6. PATIENT RELATIONSHIP TO INSURED	7. INSURED'S ADDRESS (No., Street)	
1456 MAIN STREET		Self [X] Spouse [ ] Child [ ] Other [ ]		
CITY	STATE	8. PATIENT STATUS	CITY	STATE
WOODLAND HILLS	XY	Single [ ] Married [X] Other [ ]		
ZIP CODE TELEPHONE (Include Area Code)		Employed [X] Full-Time [ ] Part-Time [ ]	ZIP CODE TELEPHONE (INCLUDE AREA CODE)	
12345 0000 (555) 490 9876		Student Student	( )	

All Private Payers: Check the patient's relationship to the insured. If the patient is an unmarried "domestic partner," check "Other."

Medicaid: Leave blank. Check appropriate box only if there is third-party coverage.

Medicare: Indicate relationship to insured when Block 4 is completed; otherwise, leave blank.
Medicare/Medicaid: Refer to Medicare guidelines.
Medicare/Medigap: Refer to Medicare guidelines.
MSP: Indicate patient's relationship to insured.

TRICARE: Check the patient's relationship to the sponsor. If the patient is the sponsor, check "Self" (e.g., retiree). If the patient is a child or stepchild, check the box for child. If "Other" is checked, indicate how the patient is related to the sponsor in Block 19 or on an attachment (e.g., former spouse).

CHAMPVA: Indicate the patient's relationship to the sponsor. If the patient is the sponsor, check "Self." If the patient is a child or stepchild, check the box for child. If "Other" is checked, indicate how the patient is related to the sponsor (e.g., former spouse) in Block 19 or on an attachment.

Workers' Compensation: Check "Other."

Block 7

Conditionally Required

5. PATIENT'S ADDRESS (No., Street) 1456 MAIN STREET		6. PATIENT RELATIONSHIP TO INSURED Self [X] Spouse [ ] Child [ ] Other [ ]	7. INSURED'S ADDRESS (No., Street)	
CITY WOODLAND HILLS	STATE XY	8. PATIENT STATUS Single [ ] Married [X] Other [ ]	CITY	STATE
ZIP CODE 12345 0000	TELEPHONE (Include Area Code) (555) 490 9876	Employed [X] Full-Time Student [ ] Part-Time Student [ ]	ZIP CODE	TELEPHONE (INCLUDE AREA CODE) ( )

All Private Payers: Leave blank if Block 4 indicates "same." Enter "SAME" if Block 4 is completed and the address is identical to that listed in Block 5. Enter address if different from that listed in Block 5.

Medicaid: Refer to Medicare guidelines.

Medicare: Leave blank if Block 4 is blank. Enter "SAME" if Block 4 is completed and the address is identical to that listed in Block 5. Enter address if different from that listed in Block 5. Complete this block only when Blocks 4, 6, and 11 are completed.
Medicare/Medicaid: Refer to Medicare guidelines.
Medicare/Medigap: Refer to Medicare guidelines.
MSP: Complete only when Block 4 is completed. If insured is other than the patient, list insured's address and if the address is the same as in Block 5, enter "SAME."

TRICARE: Enter "SAME" if address is the same as that of the patient listed in Block 5. Enter the sponsor's address (e.g., an APO/FPO address or active duty sponsor's duty station or the retiree's mailing address) if different from the patient's address.

CHAMPVA: Enter "SAME" if address is the same as that of the patient. Enter the sponsor's address if different from the patient's address.

Workers' Compensation: Enter the employer's address.

Block 8

Required/Conditionally Required

5. PATIENT'S ADDRESS (No., Street) 1456 MAIN STREET		6. PATIENT RELATIONSHIP TO INSURED Self [X] Spouse [ ] Child [ ] Other [ ]	7. INSURED'S ADDRESS (No., Street)	
CITY WOODLAND HILLS	STATE XY	8. PATIENT STATUS Single [ ] Married [X] Other [ ]	CITY	STATE
ZIP CODE 12345 0000	TELEPHONE (Include Area Code) (555) 490 9876	Employed [X] Full-Time Student [ ] Part-Time Student [ ]	ZIP CODE	TELEPHONE (INCLUDE AREA CODE) ( )

All Private Payers: Check the appropriate box for the patient's marital status and whether employed or a student. Check "Single" if widowed or divorced. The "Other" box should be checked when a patient is covered under his or her children's health insurance plan or for a domestic partner. For individuals between the ages of 19 and 23, some insurance carriers require documentation from the school verifying full-time student status. This may be obtained as a signed letter from the school or by using a special form supplied by the insurance carrier.

 Medicaid: Leave blank.

 Medicare: Check the appropriate box or boxes for the patient's marital status and whether employed or a student (e.g., a beneficiary may be employed, a student, and married). Check "Single" if widowed or divorced. In some locales, this block is not required by Medicare.
   Medicare/Medicaid: Check appropriate box for the patient's marital status and whether employed or a student. Check "Single" if widowed or divorced.
   Medicare/Medigap: Check appropriate box for the patient's marital status and whether employed or a student. Check "Single" if widowed or divorced.
   MSP: Check appropriate box for the patient's marital status and whether employed or a student. Check "Single" if widowed or divorced.

 TRICARE: Check the appropriate box for the patient's marital status and whether employed or a student.

 CHAMPVA: Check the appropriate box for the patient's marital status and whether employed or a student.

 Workers' Compensation: Check "Employed." Some workers' compensation carriers may have requirements for marital status; otherwise, leave blank.
   → *When completing the **Workbook** assignments, leave marital status blank.*

Block 9

Conditionally Required

9. OTHER INSURED'S NAME (Last Name, First Name, Middle Initial)	10. IS PATIENT'S CONDITION RELATED TO:	11. INSURED'S POLICY GROUP OR FECA NUMBER
a. OTHER INSURED'S POLICY OR GROUP NUMBER	a. EMPLOYMENT? (CURRENT OR PREVIOUS) ☐ YES ☒ NO	a. INSURED'S DATE OF BIRTH MM DD YY SEX M ☐ F ☐
b. OTHER INSURED'S DATE OF BIRTH MM DD YY M ☐ F ☐	b. AUTO ACCIDENT? PLACE (State) ☐ YES ☒ NO	b. EMPLOYER'S NAME OR SCHOOL NAME
c. EMPLOYER'S NAME OR SCHOOL NAME	c. OTHER ACCIDENT? ☐ YES ☒ NO	c. INSURANCE PLAN NAME OR PROGRAM NAME
d. INSURANCE PLAN NAME OR PROGRAM NAME	10d. RESERVED FOR LOCAL USE	d. IS THERE ANOTHER HEALTH BENEFIT PLAN? ☐ YES ☒ NO *If yes,* return to and complete item 9 a-d.

All Private Payers: For submission to primary insurance, leave blank. For submission to secondary insurance, enter patient's full name in last name, first name, and middle initial order.

Medicaid: If Medicaid is the primary insurance, leave blank. If Medicaid is the secondary insurance, enter patient's full name in last name, first name, and middle initial order.

Medicare: For primary insurance, leave blank. Do not list Medicare supplemental coverage (private, not Medigap) on the primary Medicare claim. Beneficiaries are responsible for filing a supplemental claim if the private insurer does not contract with Medicare to send claim information electronically.
Medicare/Medicaid: Enter Medicaid patient's full name in last name, first name, and middle initial order.
Medicare/Medigap: Enter the last name, first name, and middle initial of the Medigap enrollee if it differs from that in Block 2; otherwise, enter "SAME." Only Medicare-participating physicians and suppliers should complete Block 9 and its subdivisions, and only when the beneficiary wishes to assign his or her benefits under a Medigap policy to the participating physician or supplier. If no Medigap benefits are assigned, leave blank.
MSP: Leave blank.

TRICARE: For primary insurance, leave blank. For secondary insurance held by someone other than the patient, enter the name of the insured. Blocks 11a through d should be used to report other health insurance held by the patient.

CHAMPVA: For primary insurance, leave blank. For secondary insurance held by someone other than the patient, enter the name of the insured. Blocks 11a through d should be used to report other health insurance held by the patient.

Workers' Compensation: Leave blank. If case is pending and not yet declared as workers' compensation, insert other insurance.

Block 9a

Conditionally Required

All Private Payers: Enter the policy and/or group number of the other (secondary) insured's insurance coverage.

Medicaid: Leave blank.

Medicare: Refer to appropriate secondary coverage guidelines.

Medicare/Medicaid: Enter Medicaid number here or in Block 10d. Some states may have different guidelines, so check with your local fiscal intermediary if in doubt.

→ *When completing the **Workbook** assignments, enter the Medicaid policy number in Block 10d.*

Medicare/Medigap: Enter the policy or group number of the Medigap enrollee preceded by the word "MEDIGAP," "MG," or "MGAP." In addition to Medicare/Medigap, if a patient has a third insurance (e.g., employer-supplemental), all information for the third insurance should be submitted on an attachment.

→ *When completing the **Workbook** assignments, enter the word "MEDIGAP."*

MSP: Leave blank.

TRICARE: Enter the policy or group number of the other (secondary) insured's insurance policy.

CHAMPVA: Enter the policy or group number of the other (secondary) insured's insurance policy.

Workers' Compensation: Leave blank.

Block 9b

Conditionally Required

All Private Payers: Enter the other insured's date of birth and gender.

Medicaid: Leave blank.

Medicare: Refer to appropriate secondary coverage guidelines.

Medicare/Medicaid: Enter the Medicaid enrollee's birth date, using eight digits (e.g., 030620XX), and gender. If this information is the same as the patient's, leave blank.

Medicare/Medigap: Enter the Medigap enrollee's birth date, using eight digits (e.g., 030620XX), and gender. If this information is the same as the patient's, leave blank.

MSP: Leave blank.

TRICARE: For secondary coverage held by someone other than the patient, enter the other insured's date of birth and check the appropriate box for gender.

CHAMPVA: For secondary coverage held by someone other than the patient, enter the other insured's date of birth and check the appropriate box for gender.

Workers' Compensation: Leave blank.

Block 9c

Conditionally Required

 All Private Payers: For secondary coverage, enter employer's name, if applicable.

 Medicaid: Leave blank.

 Medicare: Refer to appropriate secondary coverage guidelines.
Medicare/Medicaid: Leave blank.
Medicare/Medigap: Enter the Medigap insurer's claims processing address. Ignore "Employer's name or school name." Abbreviate the street address to fit in this block by deleting the city and using the two-letter state postal code and ZIP code. For example, 1234 Wren Drive, Any City, Pennsylvania 19106 would be typed "1234 WREN DR PA 19106."Note: If a carrier-assigned payer identification (PAYERID) number that is sometimes called "Other Carrier Name and Address" or OCNA key for a Medigap insurer appears in Block 9d, then Block 9c may be left blank.
MSP: Leave blank.

 TRICARE: For secondary coverage held by someone other than the patient, enter the name of the other insured's employer or name of school.

 CHAMPVA: For secondary coverage held by someone other than the patient, enter the name of the other insured's employer or name of school.

 Workers' Compensation: Leave blank.

Block 9d

Conditionally Required

 All Private Payers: Enter name of secondary insurance plan or program.

Medicaid: Leave blank.

Medicare: Refer to appropriate secondary coverage guidelines.
Medicare/Medicaid: Leave blank.
Medicare/Medigap: Enter the Medigap insurer's nine-digit alphanumeric PAYERID number if known (often called the "Other Carrier Name and Address," or OCNA key), and Block 9c may be left blank. If not known, enter the name of the Medigap enrollee's third-party payer. If you are a participating provider, all of the information in Blocks 9 through 9d must be complete and correct or the Medicare carrier cannot electronically forward the claim information to the Medigap insurer. For multiple insurance information, enter "ATTACHMENT" in Block 10d and provide information on an attached sheet.
MSP: Leave blank.

TRICARE: For secondary coverage held by someone other than the patient, insert the name of the insured's other health insurance program. On an attached sheet, provide a complete mailing address for all other insurance information and enter the word "ATTACHMENT" in Block 10d. If the patient is covered by a health maintenance organization (HMO), attach a copy of the brochure showing that the service is not covered by the HMO.

CHAMPVA: For secondary coverage held by someone other than the patient, insert the name of the insured's other health insurance program. On an attached sheet, provide a complete mailing address for all other insurance information and enter the word "ATTACHMENT" in Block 10d. If the patient is covered by an HMO, attach a copy of the brochure showing that the service is not covered by the HMO.

Workers' Compensation: Leave blank.

Block 10a

Required

9. OTHER INSURED'S NAME (Last Name, First Name, Middle Initial)	10. IS PATIENT'S CONDITION RELATED TO:	11. INSURED'S POLICY GROUP OR FECA NUMBER
a. OTHER INSURED'S POLICY OR GROUP NUMBER	a. EMPLOYMENT? (CURRENT OR PREVIOUS) ☐ YES ☒ NO	a. INSURED'S DATE OF BIRTH MM DD YY SEX M ☐ F ☐
b. OTHER INSURED'S DATE OF BIRTH MM DD YY SEX M ☐ F ☐	b. AUTO ACCIDENT? PLACE (State) ☐ YES ☒ NO	b. EMPLOYER'S NAME OR SCHOOL NAME
c. EMPLOYER'S NAME OR SCHOOL NAME	c. OTHER ACCIDENT? ☐ YES ☒ NO	c. INSURANCE PLAN NAME OR PROGRAM NAME
d. INSURANCE PLAN NAME OR PROGRAM NAME	10d. RESERVED FOR LOCAL USE	d. IS THERE ANOTHER HEALTH BENEFIT PLAN? ☐ YES ☒ NO *If yes*, return to and complete item 9 a-d.

All Payers: Check "Yes" or "No" to indicate whether the patient's diagnosis described in Block 21 is the result of an accident or injury that occurred on the job or an industrial illness.

Block 10b

Required

 All Private Payers: A "Yes" checked in Block 10b indicates a third-party liability case; file the claim with the other liability insurance or automobile insurance carrier. List the abbreviation of the state in which the accident took place (e.g., CA for California).

 Medicaid: Check appropriate box.

 Medicare: Check "No." If "Yes," bill the liability insurance as primary insurance and Medicare as secondary insurance.
Medicare/Medicaid: Refer to Medicare guidelines.
Medicare/Medigap: Refer to Medicare guidelines.
MSP: Refer to Medicare guidelines.

 TRICARE: Check "Yes" or "No" to indicate whether another accident (not work related or automobile) applies to one or more of the services described in Block 24. If so, provide information concerning potential third-party liability. If a third party is involved in the accident, the beneficiary must complete Form DD 2527 (Statement of Personal Injury—Possible Third-Party Liability) and attach it to the claim.

 CHAMPVA: Check "Yes" or "No" to indicate whether automobile liability applies to one or more of the services described in Block 24. If "Yes," provide information concerning potential third-party liability.

 Workers' Compensation: Check "Yes" to indicate an automobile accident that occurred while the patient was on the job.

Block 10c

Required

 All Private Payers: Check "Yes" or "No" to indicate whether the patient's condition is related to an accident other than automobile or employment. Verify primary insurance.

 Medicaid: Check if applicable.

Medicare: Check "Yes" or "No" to indicate whether the patient's condition is related to an accident other than automobile or employment. Verify primary insurance.
Medicare/Medicaid: Refer to Medicare guidelines.
Medicare/Medigap: Refer to Medicare guidelines.
MSP: Refer to Medicare guidelines.

TRICARE: Check "Yes" or "No" to indicate whether automobile liability applies to one or more of the services described in Block 24. If "Yes," provide information concerning potential third-party liability. If a third party is involved in the accident, the beneficiary must complete Form DD 2527 (Statement of Personal Injury—Possible Third-Party Liability) and attach it to the claim.

CHAMPVA: Refer to TRICARE guidelines.

Workers' Compensation: Check "No."

Block 10d

Conditionally Required

All Private Payers: Leave blank. However, if required to provide a subset of Condition Codes to indicate such things as employment status, same day transfer, or a pregnancy indicator (e.g., AA = Abortion performed due to rape), enter code in this field.

Medicaid: Generally, this block is used exclusively for Medicaid as a secondary payer. Enter the patient's Medicaid (MCD) number preceded by "MCD." Note, however, that this guideline is under discussion, so carriers may not yet notify providers of a usage change for this block. Some carriers state that if more than one type of other insurance applies to the claim, the identifiers for each type should be shown, for example:
Medicare/Medigap and Medicaid coverage = MG/MCD
Medicare/Medigap and Employer-Supp coverage = MG/SP
Medicaid and Employer-Supp coverage = MCD/SP
Primary (MSP) and Medicaid Secondary coverage = MSP/MCD
Two primary insurance plans = 2MSP
→ *When completing the **Workbook** assignments, enter the patient's Medicaid number preceded by "MCD."*

Medicare: Leave blank.
Medicare/Medicaid: Enter the patient's Medicaid (MCD) number preceded by "MCD."
Medicare/Medigap: Leave blank.
MSP: Leave blank.

TRICARE: Generally, leave blank unless regional fiscal intermediary gives special guidelines. However, if Block 11d is checked "Yes," then the mailing address of the insurance carrier must be attached to the claim form, and in this block enter "ATTACHMENT."
→ *When completing the **Workbook** assignments, leave blank.*

CHAMPVA: Generally, leave blank unless regional fiscal intermediary gives special guidelines. If Block 11d is checked "Yes," the mailing address of the insurance carrier must be attached to the claim form, and in this block enter "ATTACHMENT."
→ *When completing the **Workbook** assignments, leave blank.*

Workers' Compensation: Leave blank.

Block 11

Required

9. OTHER INSURED'S NAME (Last Name, First Name, Middle Initial)	10. IS PATIENT'S CONDITION RELATED TO:	11. INSURED'S POLICY GROUP OR FECA NUMBER
a. OTHER INSURED'S POLICY OR GROUP NUMBER	a. EMPLOYMENT? (CURRENT OR PREVIOUS) ☐ YES ☒ NO	a. INSURED'S DATE OF BIRTH MM DD YY M ☐ SEX F ☐
b. OTHER INSURED'S DATE OF BIRTH MM DD YY M ☐ SEX F ☐	b. AUTO ACCIDENT? PLACE (State) ☐ YES ☒ NO	b. EMPLOYER'S NAME OR SCHOOL NAME
c. EMPLOYER'S NAME OR SCHOOL NAME	c. OTHER ACCIDENT? ☐ YES ☒ NO	c. INSURANCE PLAN NAME OR PROGRAM NAME
d. INSURANCE PLAN NAME OR PROGRAM NAME	10d. RESERVED FOR LOCAL USE	d. IS THERE ANOTHER HEALTH BENEFIT PLAN? ☐ YES ☒ NO *If yes*, return to and complete item 9 a-d.

All Private Payers: Leave blank. If (private) secondary insurance, see Blocks 9 through 9d.

Medicaid: Generally, leave blank. Enter a rejection code if the patient has other third-party insurance coverage and the claim was rejected.

Medicare: If other insurance is not primary to Medicare, enter "NONE" and go to Block 12. Block 11 must be completed. By completing this block, the physician/supplier acknowledges having made a good faith effort to determine whether Medicare is the primary or secondary payer.
Medicare/Medicaid: Refer to Medicare guidelines.
Medicare/Medigap: Refer to Medicare guidelines.
MSP: When insurance is primary to Medicare, enter the insured's policy or group number, or both, and complete Blocks 11a through 11c.

TRICARE: Leave blank.

CHAMPVA: Enter the three-digit number of the VA station that issued the identification card.

 Workers' Compensation: Leave blank.

Block 11a

Conditionally Required

 All Private Payers: Leave blank.

 Medicaid: Leave blank.

 Medicare: Leave blank.
Medicare/Medicaid: Leave blank.
Medicare/Medigap: Leave blank.
MSP: Enter the insured's eight-digit date of birth (061220XX) and gender if different from that listed in Block 3; otherwise, leave blank.

 TRICARE: Enter sponsor's date of birth and gender, if different from that listed in Block 3; otherwise, leave blank.

 CHAMPVA: Enter sponsor's date of birth and gender, if different from that listed in Block 3.

 Workers' Compensation: Leave blank.

Block 11b

Conditionally Required

 All Private Payers: When submitting to secondary insurance, enter the name of the employer, school, or organization if primary policy is a group plan; otherwise, leave blank.

 Medicaid: Leave blank.

Medicare: Leave blank.
Medicare/Medicaid: Leave blank.
Medicare/Medigap: Leave blank.
MSP: Enter the employer's name of primary insurance. Also use this block to indicate a change in the insured's insurance status (e.g., "RETIRED" and the six-digit or eight-digit retirement date). Submit paper claims with a copy of the primary payer's Remittance Advice (RA) document to be considered for Medicare Secondary Payer benefits. Instances when Medicare may be secondary include the following:

1. Group health plan coverage
   a. Working aged
   b. Disability (large group health plan)
   c. End-stage renal disease
2. No fault, other liability, or both
   a. Automobile
   b. Homeowner
   c. Commercial
3. Work-related illness, injury, or both
   a. Workers' compensation
   b. Black lung
   c. Veterans' benefits

TRICARE: Indicate sponsor's branch of service, using abbreviations (e.g., United States Navy = USN).

CHAMPVA: Indicate sponsor's branch of service, using abbreviations (e.g., United States Army = USA).

Workers' Compensation: If a large corporation's name is listed in Block 4, enter the name of the patient's local employer; otherwise, leave this block blank.

Block 11c

Conditionally Required

All Private Payers: When submitting to secondary insurance, enter the name of the primary insurance plan; otherwise, leave this block blank.

Medicaid: Leave blank.

Medicare: Must be completed. If there is no insurance primary to Medicare, enter "NONE."
Medicare/Medicaid: Leave blank.
Medicare/Medigap: Leave blank.
MSP: Enter the nine-digit PAYERID number or complete name of the insurance plan or program that is primary to Medicare. If the primary payer's EOB does not contain the claims processing address, record the primary payer's claim processing address and telephone number directly on the EOB.

TRICARE: Enter "TRICARE."

CHAMPVA: Indicate name of the secondary coverage held by the patient, if applicable; otherwise, leave this block blank.

Workers' Compensation: Leave blank.

Block 11d

Conditionally Required

All Private Payers: Check "Yes" or "No" to indicate if there is another health plan. If "Yes," Blocks 9a through 9d must be completed.

Medicaid: Leave blank.

Medicare: Generally, leave blank; some regions require "Yes" or "No" to be checked, so verify this requirement with your local fiscal intermediary.
*When completing the **Workbook** assignments, leave blank.*
Medicare/Medicaid: Refer to guidelines for Medicare.
Medicare/Medigap: Refer to guidelines for Medicare.
MSP: Leave blank.

TRICARE: Check "Yes" or "No" to indicate if there is another health plan. If "Yes," Blocks 9a through 9d must be completed.

CHAMPVA: Check "Yes" or "No" to indicate if there is another health plan. If "Yes," Blocks 9a through 9d must be completed.

Workers' Compensation: Leave blank.

Block 12

Required

READ BACK OF FORM BEFORE COMPLETING & SIGNING THIS FORM. 12. PATIENT'S OR AUTHORIZED PERSON'S SIGNATURE I authorize the release of any medical or other information necessary to process this claim. I also request payment of government benefits either to myself or to the party who accepts assignment below. SIGNED _Harry N. Forehand_ DATE _March 3, 20XX_	13. INSURED'S OR AUTHORIZED PERSON'S SIGNATURE I authorize payment of medical benefits to the undersigned physician or supplier for services described below. SIGNED _Harry N. Forehand_

or

READ BACK OF FORM BEFORE COMPLETING & SIGNING THIS FORM. 12. PATIENT'S OR AUTHORIZED PERSON'S SIGNATURE I authorize the release of any medical or other information necessary to process this claim. I also request payment of government benefits either to myself or to the party who accepts assignment below. SIGNED ___SIGNATURE ON FILE___ DATE ___	13. INSURED'S OR AUTHORIZED PERSON'S SIGNATURE I authorize payment of medical benefits to the undersigned physician or supplier for services described below. SIGNED ___SIGNATURE ON FILE___

All Private Payers: Medical office policy varies for obtaining the patient's signature for release of medical information, but know this is *not* a HIPAA compliance requirement. For offices that prefer the patient's signature in this block, a signature here authorizes the release of medical information for claims processing. Have the patient or authorized representative sign and date this block. If the patient has signed a consent form, "Signature on File" can be entered here. Some third-party payers accept the acronym "SOF." The consent form must be current, possibly may be lifetime, and must be in the medical practice's office files for the patient. Many offices routinely annually renew consent forms. When the patient's representative signs, that person's relationship to the patient must be indicated. If the signature is indicated by a mark (X), a witness must sign his or her name and enter the address next to the mark. If a patient is seen in the hospital and never comes to the doctor's office, the signature forms obtained by the hospital cover the physician.

➡ *When completing the Workbook assignments, enter "Signature on File," not "SOF," in this block.*

Medicaid: Leave blank.

Medicare: A signature here authorizes payment of benefits to the physician (if the physician accepts assignment). Have the patient or authorized representative sign and date this block. If the patient has signed a consent form, "Signature on File" can be typed here. The form must be current, may be lifetime, and must be in the physician's file. When the patient's representative signs, that person's relationship to the patient must be indicated. If the signature is by mark (X), a witness must sign his or her name and enter the address next to the mark. Enter either a six-digit date, eight-digit date, or an alphanumeric date unless the signature is on file.

➡ *When completing the **Workbook** assignments, enter "Signature on File," not "SOF," in this block.*
Medicare/Medicaid: Refer to Medicare guidelines.
Medicare/Medigap: Refer to Medicare guidelines.
MSP: Guidelines for this block are the same as for Medicare.

TRICARE: A signature here authorizes payment of benefits to the physician (if the physician accepts assignment). Have the patient or the authorized representative sign and date this block. If the patient has signed a consent form, "Signature on File" or "SOF" can be typed here. The form must be current, may be lifetime, and must be in the physician's file. When the patient's representative signs, that person's relationship to the patient must be indicated. If the signature is by mark (X), a witness must sign his or her name and enter the address next to the mark.

➡ *When completing the **Workbook** assignments, enter "Signature on File," not "SOF," in this block.*

CHAMPVA: Refer to TRICARE guidelines.

 Workers' Compensation: No signature is required.

Block 13

Conditionally Required

READ BACK OF FORM BEFORE COMPLETING & SIGNING THIS FORM.	13. INSURED'S OR AUTHORIZED PERSON'S SIGNATURE I authorize
12. PATIENT'S OR AUTHORIZED PERSON'S SIGNATURE I authorize the release of any medical or other information necessary to process this claim. I also request payment of government benefits either to myself or to the party who accepts assignment below.	payment of medical benefits to the undersigned physician or supplier for services described below.
SIGNED *Harry N. Forehand* DATE *March 3, 20XX*	SIGNED *Harry N. Forehand*

or

READ BACK OF FORM BEFORE COMPLETING & SIGNING THIS FORM.	13. INSURED'S OR AUTHORIZED PERSON'S SIGNATURE I authorize
12. PATIENT'S OR AUTHORIZED PERSON'S SIGNATURE I authorize the release of any medical or other information necessary to process this claim. I also request payment of government benefits either to myself or to the party who accepts assignment below.	payment of medical benefits to the undersigned physician or supplier for services described below.
SIGNED SIGNATURE ON FILE DATE	SIGNED SIGNATURE ON FILE

 All Private Payers: Patient's signature is necessary when benefits are assigned. "SOF" may be listed if the patient's signature is on file.
→ *When completing the **Workbook** assignments, enter "Signature on File," not "SOF," in this block.*

 Medicaid: Leave blank.

 Medicare: Leave blank.
Medicare/Medicaid: Leave blank.
Medicare/Medigap: For participating provider, a signature here authorizes payment of "mandated" Medigap benefits when required Medigap information is included in Blocks 9 through 9d. List the signature of the patient or authorized representative, or list "Signature on File" if the signature is on file as a separate Medigap authorization.
→ *When completing the **Workbook** assignments, enter "Signature on File" in this block.*
MSP: The signature of the patient or authorized representative should appear in this block, or list "Signature on File" if the signature is on file for benefits assigned from the primary carrier.
→ *When completing the **Workbook** assignments, enter "Signature on File" in this block.*

 TRICARE: Leave blank.

CHAMPVA: Leave blank.

 Workers' Compensation: Leave blank. All payment goes directly to the physician.

Block 14

Conditionally Required

14. DATE OF CURRENT: MM / DD / YY ◄ ILLNESS (First symptom) OR INJURY (Accident) OR PREGNANCY(LMP)	15. IF PATIENT HAS HAD SAME OR SIMILAR ILLNESS. GIVE FIRST DATE MM / DD / YY	16. DATES PATIENT UNABLE TO WORK IN CURRENT OCCUPATION MM / DD / YY MM / DD / YY FROM TO
03 / 01 / 20XX		
17. NAME OF REFERRING PHYSICIAN OR OTHER SOURCE PERRY CARDI MD	17a. 17b. NPI 67805027XX	18. HOSPITALIZATION DATES RELATED TO CURRENT SERVICES MM / DD / YY MM / DD / YY FROM TO
19. RESERVED FOR LOCAL USE		20. OUTSIDE LAB? $ CHARGES ☐ YES ☒ NO

 All Private Payers: Enter the eight-digit date that the patient's first symptoms occurred from the current illness, if stated in the medical record; date of injury or accident; or for pregnancy, first day of LMP. For chiropractic treatment, enter the eight-digit date that treatment began.

 Medicaid: Leave blank.

 Medicare: Enter either a six-digit or eight-digit date that the patient's first symptoms occurred from the current illness, if stated in the medical record; date of injury or accident; or for pregnancy, first day of LMP. For chiropractic treatment, enter either a six-digit or eight-digit date that treatment began and enter a six-digit or eight-digit date in Block 19.
Medicare/Medicaid: Refer to Medicare guidelines.
Medicare/Medigap: Refer to Medicare guidelines.
MSP: Refer to Medicare guidelines.

 TRICARE: Enter the eight-digit date the patient's first symptoms occurred from the current illness, if stated in the medical record; date of injury or accident; or for pregnancy, first day of LMP. For chiropractic treatment, enter the eight-digit date that treatment began.

 CHAMPVA: Refer to TRICARE guidelines.

 Workers' Compensation: Enter first date of injury, accident, or industrial illness; it should coincide with the date specified in the Doctor's First Report of Injury.

Block 15

Conditionally Required

14. DATE OF CURRENT: ◀ ILLNESS (First symptom) OR INJURY (Accident) OR PREGNANCY(LMP) MM · DD · YY 03 · 01 · 20XX	15. IF PATIENT HAS HAD SAME OR SIMILAR ILLNESS. GIVE FIRST DATE MM · DD · YY	16. DATES PATIENT UNABLE TO WORK IN CURRENT OCCUPATION MM · DD · YY MM · DD · YY FROM TO
17. NAME OF REFERRING PHYSICIAN OR OTHER SOURCE PERRY CARDI MD	17a. 17b. NPI 67805027XX	18. HOSPITALIZATION DATES RELATED TO CURRENT SERVICES MM · DD · YY MM · DD · YY FROM TO
19. RESERVED FOR LOCAL USE		20. OUTSIDE LAB? $ CHARGES ☐ YES ☒ NO

 All Private Payers: Enter the eight-digit date when the patient had the same or similar illness, if applicable, and document in the medical record.

 Medicaid: Leave blank.

 Medicare: Leave blank.
Medicare/Medicaid: Leave blank.
Medicare/Medigap: Leave blank.
MSP: Leave blank.

 TRICARE: Enter the eight-digit date when the patient had the same or similar illness, if applicable, and document in the medical record.

 CHAMPVA: Refer to TRICARE guidelines.

 Workers' Compensation: Enter the eight-digit date, if appropriate, and document in the medical record.

Block 16

Conditionally Required

14. DATE OF CURRENT: ◀ ILLNESS (First symptom) OR INJURY (Accident) OR PREGNANCY(LMP) MM · DD · YY 03 · 01 · 20XX	15. IF PATIENT HAS HAD SAME OR SIMILAR ILLNESS. GIVE FIRST DATE MM · DD · YY	16. DATES PATIENT UNABLE TO WORK IN CURRENT OCCUPATION MM · DD · YY MM · DD · YY FROM TO
17. NAME OF REFERRING PHYSICIAN OR OTHER SOURCE PERRY CARDI MD	17a. 17b. NPI 67805027XX	18. HOSPITALIZATION DATES RELATED TO CURRENT SERVICES MM · DD · YY MM · DD · YY FROM TO
19. RESERVED FOR LOCAL USE		20. OUTSIDE LAB? $ CHARGES ☐ YES ☒ NO

All Private Payers: Enter the eight-digit dates the patient is employed but cannot work in his or her current occupation. *From:* Enter first full day the patient was unable to perform job duties. *To:* Enter last day the patient was disabled before returning to work.

Medicaid: Leave blank.

Medicare: Enter either six-digit or eight-digit dates the patient is employed but cannot work in his or her current occupation. *From:* Enter first full day the patient was unable to perform job duties. *To:* Enter last day the patient was disabled before returning to work.
Medicare/Medicaid: Refer to Medicare guidelines.
Medicare/Medigap: Refer to Medicare guidelines.
MSP: Refer to Medicare guidelines.

TRICARE: Refer to Medicare guidelines.

CHAMPVA: Refer to Medicare guidelines.

Workers' Compensation: May be completed but is not mandatory and must be verified with documentation in Doctor's First Report of Injury. *From:* Enter first full day the patient was unable to perform job duties. *To:* Enter last day the patient was disabled before returning to work.
→ *When completing the* **Workbook** *assignments, enter information when documented in the medical record.*

Block 17

Conditionally Required

14. DATE OF CURRENT: ILLNESS (First symptom) OR INJURY (Accident) OR PREGNANCY(LMP) MM DD YY 03 01 20XX		15. IF PATIENT HAS HAD SAME OR SIMILAR ILLNESS. GIVE FIRST DATE MM DD YY	16. DATES PATIENT UNABLE TO WORK IN CURRENT OCCUPATION MM DD YY MM DD YY FROM TO
17. NAME OF REFERRING PHYSICIAN OR OTHER SOURCE PERRY CARDI MD	17a. 17b. NPI 67805027XX		18. HOSPITALIZATION DATES RELATED TO CURRENT SERVICES MM DD YY MM DD YY FROM TO
19. RESERVED FOR LOCAL USE			20. OUTSIDE LAB? $ CHARGES ☐ YES ☒ NO

All Private Payers: Enter complete name and degree of referring physician, when applicable. Do not list other referrals (i.e., family or friends).

Medicaid: Enter the complete name and degree of the referring physician, when applicable. Do not list other referrals (i.e., family or friends).

Medicare: Enter the name and degree of the referring or ordering physician on all claims for Medicare-covered services and items resulting from a physician's order or referral. Use a separate claim form for each referring or ordering physician.

Surgeon: A surgeon must complete this block. When the patient has not been referred, enter the surgeon's name. On an assistant surgeon's claim, enter the primary surgeon's name.

Referring physician: A physician who requests a service for the beneficiary for which payment may be made under the Medicare program. When a physician extender (e.g., nurse practitioner) refers a patient for a consultative service, enter the name of the physician supervising the physician extender.

Ordering physician: A physician who orders a consultation or nonphysician services for the patient such as diagnostic radiology, laboratory, or pathology tests; pharmaceutical services; durable medical equipment (DME); parenteral and enteral nutrition; or immunosuppressive drugs.

When the ordering physician is also the performing physician (e.g., the physician who actually performs the in-office laboratory tests), the performing physician's name and assigned UPIN/NPI number must appear in Block 17 and taxonomy code in Block 17a.

When a patient is referred to a physician who also orders and performs a diagnostic service, a separate claim form is necessary for the diagnostic service.

Enter the original referring physician's name and NPI in Blocks 17 and 17a of the first claim form.

Enter the ordering (performing) physician's name and NPI in Blocks 17 and 17a of the second claim form.

Medicare/Medicaid: Refer to Medicare guidelines.

Medicare/Medigap: Refer to Medicare guidelines.

MSP: Refer to Medicare guidelines.

TRICARE: Enter the name, degree, and address of the referring provider. This is required for all consultation claims. If the patient was referred from a Military Treatment Facility (MTF), enter the name of the MTF and attach DD Form 2161 or SF 513, "Referral for Civilian Medical Care."

CHAMPVA: Refer to TRICARE guidelines.

Workers' Compensation: Indicate name and degree of referring provider.

Block 17a

14. DATE OF CURRENT: ILLNESS (First symptom) OR INJURY (Accident) OR PREGNANCY(LMP)		15. IF PATIENT HAS HAD SAME OR SIMILAR ILLNESS. GIVE FIRST DATE MM DD YY	16. DATES PATIENT UNABLE TO WORK IN CURRENT OCCUPATION MM DD YY FROM ___ TO ___ MM DD YY
MM DD YY 03 01 20XX			
17. NAME OF REFERRING PHYSICIAN OR OTHER SOURCE	17a.		18. HOSPITALIZATION DATES RELATED TO CURRENT SERVICES MM DD YY FROM ___ TO ___ MM DD YY
PERRY CARDI MD	17b. NPI 67805027XX		
19. RESERVED FOR LOCAL USE			20. OUTSIDE LAB? ☐ YES ☒ NO $ CHARGES

All Private Payers: Block 17a may be used for either a taxonomy code, state license number, Blue Shield provider, Medicare provider, Medicaid provider, or Social Security number, depending on the guidelines of the payer, and Block 17b is for the NPI of the referring provider.

Block 17b

Required

 All Payers: Effective May 23, 2007, an NPI MUST be reported when a service was ordered or referred by a physician.

Block 18

Conditionally Required

14. DATE OF CURRENT: ◄ ILLNESS (First symptom) OR INJURY (Accident) OR PREGNANCY(LMP) MM DD YY 03 01 20XX	15. IF PATIENT HAS HAD SAME OR SIMILAR ILLNESS. GIVE FIRST DATE MM DD YY	16. DATES PATIENT UNABLE TO WORK IN CURRENT OCCUPATION MM DD YY MM DD YY FROM TO
17. NAME OF REFERRING PHYSICIAN OR OTHER SOURCE PERRY CARDI MD	17a. 17b. NPI 67805027XX	18. HOSPITALIZATION DATES RELATED TO CURRENT SERVICES MM DD YY MM DD YY FROM TO
19. RESERVED FOR LOCAL USE		20. OUTSIDE LAB? $ CHARGES ☐ YES [X] NO

 All Payers: Complete this block when a medical service is furnished as a result of, or subsequent to, a related (inpatient) hospitalization, skilled nursing facility, or nursing home visit. Do not complete for outpatient hospital services, ambulatory surgery, or emergency department services. Enter either six-digit or eight-digit admitting and discharge dates. If the patient is still hospitalized at the time of the billing, enter eight zeros in the "TO" field.

Block 19

Conditionally Required

14. DATE OF CURRENT: ◄ ILLNESS (First symptom) OR INJURY (Accident) OR PREGNANCY(LMP) MM DD YY 03 01 20XX	15. IF PATIENT HAS HAD SAME OR SIMILAR ILLNESS. GIVE FIRST DATE MM DD YY	16. DATES PATIENT UNABLE TO WORK IN CURRENT OCCUPATION MM DD YY MM DD YY FROM TO
17. NAME OF REFERRING PHYSICIAN OR OTHER SOURCE PERRY CARDI MD	17a. 17b. NPI 67805027XX	18. HOSPITALIZATION DATES RELATED TO CURRENT SERVICES MM DD YY MM DD YY FROM TO
19. RESERVED FOR LOCAL USE		20. OUTSIDE LAB? $ CHARGES ☐ YES [X] NO

 All Private Payers: This block may be completed in a number of different ways depending on commercial carrier guidelines. Some common uses are:

- Enter the word "ATTACHMENT" when an operative report, discharge summary, invoice, or other attachment is included.
- Enter an explanation about unusual services or unlisted services.
- Enter the drug name and dosage when submitting a claim for Not Otherwise Classified (NOC) drugs. Enter the word "ATTACHMENT" and attach the invoice.
- Describe the supply when the code 99070 is used.
- Enter the x-ray date for chiropractic treatment.
- Do not bill with attachments smaller than 8½ inches by 11 inches.
- Enter the phrase "faxed documentation" when a report included is faxed.
- NUCC-approved ID qualifiers and numbers (as shown in Field 17a).

Medicaid: Check with the regional fiscal intermediary, who may have special guidelines for entries in this block.

→ *When completing the **Workbook** assignments, refer to private payer guidelines.*

Medicare: Although the block is labeled "Reserved for Local Use," CMS guidelines state it may be completed in a number of different ways depending on the circumstances of the services provided to the patient. This block can only contain up to three conditions per claim. Some common uses are:

- Enter the attending physician's NPI and taxonomy code. Enter either the six-digit or eight-digit date of the patient's latest visit for claims submitted by a physical or occupational therapist, psychotherapist, chiropractor, or podiatrist.
- Enter all applicable modifiers when modifier 99 (multiple modifiers) is entered in item 24D. For each line item containing a 99 modifier, list as follows: 1= (mod). This means all modifiers applicable to line item number 1.
- Enter the drug's name and dosage when submitting a claim for Not Otherwise Classified (NOC) drugs. Enter the word "ATTACHMENT" and include a copy of the invoice.
- Describe the procedure for unlisted procedures. Enter a concise description of the unlisted procedure code or if there is not sufficient room in this block, send an attachment.
- Enter "Homebound" when an independent laboratory renders an electrocardiogram or collects a specimen from a patient who is homebound or institutionalized.
- Enter the statement "Patient refuses to assign benefits" when a Medicare beneficiary refuses to assign benefits to a participating provider. No payment to the physician will be made on the claim in this case.
- Enter "Testing for hearing aid" when submitting a claim to obtain an intentional denial from Medicare as the primary payer for hearing aid testing and a secondary payer is involved.
- Enter the specific dental surgery for which a dental examination is being performed.
- Enter the name and dosage when billing for low osmolar contrast material for which there is no Level II HCPCS code.
- Enter either a six-digit or eight-digit assumed and relinquished date of care for each provider when providers share postoperative care for global surgery claims.
- Enter the statement "Attending physician, not hospice employee" when a physician gives service to a hospice patient but the hospice in which the patient resides does not employ the physician.
- Enter the NPI of the physician who is performing a purchased interpretation of a diagnostic test.

Medicare/Medicaid: Refer to Medicare guidelines.
Medicare/Medigap: Refer to Medicare guidelines.
MSP: Refer to Medicare guidelines.

TRICARE: Generally, this block is reserved for local use (e.g., to indicate referral number or enter x-ray date for chiropractic treatment).

CHAMPVA: Refer to TRICARE guidelines.

Workers' Compensation: Leave blank.

Block 20

Conditionally Required

14. DATE OF CURRENT: ◀ ILLNESS (First symptom) OR MM | DD | YY ◀ INJURY (Accident) OR 03 | 01 | 20XX PREGNANCY(LMP)	15. IF PATIENT HAS HAD SAME OR SIMILAR ILLNESS. GIVE FIRST DATE MM | DD | YY	16. DATES PATIENT UNABLE TO WORK IN CURRENT OCCUPATION MM | DD | YY MM | DD | YY FROM TO
17. NAME OF REFERRING PHYSICIAN OR OTHER SOURCE PERRY CARDI MD	17a. 17b. NPI 67805027XX	18. HOSPITALIZATION DATES RELATED TO CURRENT SERVICES MM | DD | YY MM | DD | YY FROM TO
19. RESERVED FOR LOCAL USE		20. OUTSIDE LAB? $ CHARGES ☐ YES ☒ NO

 All Private Payers: Enter "Yes" or "No" when billing diagnostic laboratory tests. "No" means the tests were performed by the billing physician/laboratory. "Yes" means that the laboratory test was performed outside of the physician's office and that the physician is billing for the laboratory services. If "Yes," enter purchase price of the test in the "Charges" portion of this block and complete Block 32.

 Medicaid: Check "No"; outside laboratories must bill directly.

 Medicare: Enter "Yes" or "No" when billing diagnostic laboratory tests. "No" means the tests were performed by the billing physician or laboratory. "Yes" means that the laboratory test was performed outside of the physician's office and that the physician is billing for the laboratory services. If "Yes," enter purchase price of the test in the "Charges" portion of this block and complete Block 32. Clinical laboratory services must be billed to Medicare on an assigned basis. When billing for multiple purchased diagnostic tests, each test must be submitted on a separate claim form.
Medicare/Medicaid: Refer to Medicare guidelines.
Medicare/Medigap: Refer to Medicare guidelines.
MSP: Refer to Medicare guidelines.

 TRICARE: Refer to Medicare guidelines.

 CHAMPVA: Refer to Medicare guidelines.

 Workers' Compensation: Refer to Private Payer guidelines.

Block 21

Required/Conditionally Required

21. DIAGNOSIS OR NATURE OF ILLNESS OR INJURY. (RELATE ITEMS 1,2,3 OR 4 TO ITEM 24E BY LINE)		22. MEDICAID RESUBMISSION CODE	ORIGINAL REF. NO.
1. ∟ 382 . 00 3. ∟___ . ___		23. PRIOR AUTHORIZATION NUMBER	
2. ∟___ . ___ 4. ∟___ . ___			

24. A. DATE(S) OF SERVICE		B. PLACE OF SERVICE	C. EMG	D. PROCEDURES, SERVICES, OR SUPPLIES (Explain Unusual Circumstances)		E. DIAGNOSIS POINTER	F. $ CHARGES	G. DAYS OR UNITS	H. EPSDT Family Plan	I. ID. QUAL.	J. RENDERING PROVIDER ID. #
From	To			CPT/HCPCS	MODIFIER						
MM DD YY	MM DD YY										
1										NPI	

 All Payers: On paper claims, enter up to four diagnostic codes in priority order, with the primary diagnosis in the first position. However, because Medicare administrative contractors (MACs) may accept and process up to a maximum of eight diagnoses, check with your regional Medicare administrative contractor to learn the procedure for submitting more than four codes. Electronic claims hold a maximum of eight diagnostic codes. Codes must be carried out to their highest degree of specificity. Do not use decimal points or add any code narratives. Code only the conditions or problems that the physician is actively treating and that relate directly to the services billed. All narrative diagnoses for nonphysician specialties must be submitted on an attachment. Claims submitted by ambulance suppliers are not required to complete this block.

Block 22

Conditionally Required

21. DIAGNOSIS OR NATURE OF ILLNESS OR INJURY. (RELATE ITEMS 1,2,3 OR 4 TO ITEM 24E BY LINE)		22. MEDICAID RESUBMISSION CODE	ORIGINAL REF. NO.
1. ∟ 382 . 00 3. ∟___ . ___		23. PRIOR AUTHORIZATION NUMBER	
2. ∟___ . ___ 4. ∟___ . ___			

24. A. DATE(S) OF SERVICE		B. PLACE OF SERVICE	C. EMG	D. PROCEDURES, SERVICES, OR SUPPLIES (Explain Unusual Circumstances)		E. DIAGNOSIS POINTER	F. $ CHARGES	G. DAYS OR UNITS	H. EPSDT Family Plan	I. ID. QUAL.	J. RENDERING PROVIDER ID. #
From	To			CPT/HCPCS	MODIFIER						
MM DD YY	MM DD YY										
1										NPI	

 All Private Payers: Leave blank.

 Medicaid: Complete for resubmission.

 Medicare: Leave blank.
Medicare/Medicaid: Refer to Medicaid guidelines.
Medicare/Medigap: Leave blank.
MSP: Leave blank.

TRICARE: Leave blank.

 CHAMPVA: Leave blank.

 Workers' Compensation: Leave blank.

Block 23

Conditionally Required

 All Private Payers: Enter the professional or peer review organization (PRO) 10-digit prior authorization number.

 Medicaid: Enter the Professional (Peer) Review Organization (PRO) 10-digit prior authorization or precertification number for procedures requiring PRO prior approval. If billing for an investigational device, enter the Investigational Device Exemption (IDE) number.

 Medicare: Although this block is labeled "Prior Authorization Number," CMS guidelines state it may be completed in a number of different ways depending on the circumstances of the services provided to the patient. Some common uses are:
- Enter the Quality Improvement Organization (QIO) 10-digit prior authorization or precertification number for procedures requiring QIO prior approval.
- Enter the Investigational Device Exemption (IDE) number if billing for an investigational device.
- Enter the 10-digit Clinical Laboratory Improvement Amendments (CLIA) federal certification number when billing for laboratory services billed by a physician office laboratory.
- Enter the NPI number of the hospice or home health agency (HHA) when billing for care plan oversight services (G0181 or G0182).
- Post Market Approval (PMA) number should be placed in this block when applicable.
- Enter the NPI number of the skilled nursing facility (SNF) when a physician provides services to an SNF patient and the services were given to the SNF patient outside of the SNF.

NOTE: Block 23 can contain only one condition. Additional conditions must be reported on separate claim forms. When reporting multiple page claims, only the diagnoses listed on the first page may be used on subsequent pages.

Medicare/Medicaid: Refer to Medicare guidelines.

Medicare/Medigap: Refer to Medicare guidelines.

MSP: Refer to Medicare guidelines.

TRICARE: Enter the professional (peer) review organization (pro) 10-digit prior authorization or precertification number for procedures requiring pro approval. If billing for an investigational device, enter the investigational device exemption (ide) number. Attach a copy of the authorization.

 CHAMPVA: Refer to TRICARE guidelines.

 Workers' Compensation: Leave blank.

Blocks 24A through 24J may not contain more than six detail lines. If the case requires more than six detail lines, put the additional information on a separate claim form, treat it as an independent claim, and total all charges on each claim. Claims cannot be "continued" from one to another. Do not list a procedure on the claim form for which there is no charge. The CMS-1500 (08-05) claim form six service lines have been divided horizontally for submission of both the NPI and legacy identifier during the NPI transition and for submission of supplemental information to support the billed service. The top portion in each of the six service lines is shaded and is the location for reporting supplemental information. Use the unshaded portion for all service entries. Do not treat this feature as allowing 12 service lines of billing.

Block 24A

Required

24. A. DATE(S) OF SERVICE From MM DD YY / To MM DD YY	B. PLACE OF SERVICE	C. EMG	D. PROCEDURES, SERVICES, OR SUPPLIES (Explain Unusual Circumstances) CPT/HCPCS | MODIFIER	E. DIAGNOSIS POINTER	F. $ CHARGES	G. DAYS OR UNITS	H. EPSDT Family Plan	I. ID. QUAL.	J. RENDERING PROVIDER ID. #
1 03 03 XX	11		99203	1	70 92	1		NPI	12458977XX
2								NPI	
3								NPI	
4								NPI	
5								NPI	
6								NPI	

25. FEDERAL TAX I.D. NUMBER	SSN EIN	26. PATIENT'S ACCOUNT NO.	27. ACCEPT ASSIGNMENT? (For govt. claims, see back)	28. TOTAL CHARGE	29. AMOUNT PAID	30. BALANCE DUE
XX12210XX	X	010	X YES NO	$ 70 92	$	$ 70 92

24. A. DATE(S) OF SERVICE From MM DD YY / To MM DD YY	B. PLACE OF SERVICE	C. EMG	D. PROCEDURES, SERVICES, OR SUPPLIES (Explain Unusual Circumstances) CPT/HCPCS | MODIFIER	E. DIAGNOSIS POINTER	F. $ CHARGES	G. DAYS OR UNITS	H. EPSDT Family Plan	I. ID. QUAL.	J. RENDERING PROVIDER ID. #
1 11 30 XX	21		99231	1	37 74	1		NPI	32783127XX
2 12 01 XX 12 03 XX	21		99231	1	37 74	3		NPI	32783127XX
3								NPI	
4								NPI	
5								NPI	
6								NPI	

25. FEDERAL TAX I.D. NUMBER	SSN EIN	26. PATIENT'S ACCOUNT NO.	27. ACCEPT ASSIGNMENT? (For govt. claims, see back)	28. TOTAL CHARGE	29. AMOUNT PAID	30. BALANCE DUE
XX12210XX	X	102	X YES NO	$ 150 96	$	$ 150 96

All Private Payers: Enter the month, day, and year (eight digits with no spaces) for each procedure, service, or supply reported in Block 24D. Make sure the dates shown are no earlier than the date of the current illness if listed in Block 14. If the "From" and "To" dates are the same, enter only the "From" date. Enter the "To" date when reporting a consecutive range of dates for the same procedure code. Use a separate line for each month. Some third-party payers may use different date formats (e.g., December 4, 20XX = 20XX1204).

 Medicaid: Enter an eight-digit "From" date (month, day, and year with no spaces) for each service or supply. Leave "To" date blank. No date ranging is allowed for consecutive dates.

 Medicare: Enter the month, day, and year (six or eight digits with no spaces) for each procedure, service, or supply reported in Block 24D. Make sure the dates shown are no earlier than the date of the current illness if listed in Block 14. If the "From" and "To" dates are the same, enter only the "From" date. Enter the "To" date when reporting a consecutive range of dates for the same procedure code. Use a separate line for each month except when reporting weekly radiation therapy, durable medical equipment, or oxygen rental.
Medicare/Medicaid: Refer to Medicare guidelines.
Medicare/Medigap: Refer to Medicare guidelines.
MSP: Refer to Medicare guidelines.

 TRICARE: Enter the month, day, and year (eight digits with no spaces) for each procedure, service, or supply reported in Block 24D. Make sure the dates shown are no earlier than the date of the current illness if listed in Block 14. If the "From" and "To" dates are the same, enter only the "From" date. Enter the "To" date when reporting a consecutive range of dates for the same procedure code. Use a separate line for each month.

 CHAMPVA: Refer to TRICARE guidelines.

 Workers' Compensation: Enter the month, day, and year (eight digits with no spaces) for each procedure, service, or supply reported in Block 24D. Date ranging is not the preferred format for consecutive dates.

Block 24B

Required

24. A. DATE(S) OF SERVICE						B. PLACE OF SERVICE	C. EMG	D. PROCEDURES, SERVICES, OR SUPPLIES (Explain Unusual Circumstances)		E. DIAGNOSIS POINTER	F. $ CHARGES	G. DAYS OR UNITS	H. EPSDT Family Plan	I. ID. QUAL.	J. RENDERING PROVIDER ID. #
From MM	DD	YY	To MM	DD	YY			CPT/HCPCS	MODIFIER						
1 03	03	XX				11		99203		1	70 92	1		NPI	12458977XX
2														NPI	
3														NPI	
4														NPI	
5														NPI	
6														NPI	

25. FEDERAL TAX I.D. NUMBER	SSN EIN	26. PATIENT'S ACCOUNT NO.	27. ACCEPT ASSIGNMENT? (For govt. claims, see back)	28. TOTAL CHARGE	29. AMOUNT PAID	30. BALANCE DUE
XX12210XX	☐ ☒	010	☒ YES ☐ NO	$ 70 92	$	$ 70 92

All Payers: Enter the appropriate "Place of Service" code shown in Figure 7-2. Identify by location where the service was performed or an item was used. Use the inpatient hospital code only when a service is provided to a patient admitted to the hospital for an overnight stay. Enter the name, address, and provider number of the hospital in Block 32.

Medical practices that have multiple offices must show the address of where the service was rendered in Block 32.

Block 24C

24. A. DATE(S) OF SERVICE						B. PLACE OF SERVICE	C. EMG	D. PROCEDURES, SERVICES, OR SUPPLIES (Explain Unusual Circumstances)		E. DIAGNOSIS POINTER	F. $ CHARGES	G. DAYS OR UNITS	H. EPSDT Family Plan	I. ID. QUAL.	J. RENDERING PROVIDER ID. #
From MM	DD	YY	To MM	DD	YY			CPT/HCPCS	MODIFIER						
1 03	03	XX				11		99203		1	70 92	1		NPI	12458977XX
2														NPI	
3														NPI	
4														NPI	
5														NPI	
6														NPI	

25. FEDERAL TAX I.D. NUMBER	SSN EIN	26. PATIENT'S ACCOUNT NO.	27. ACCEPT ASSIGNMENT? (For govt. claims, see back)	28. TOTAL CHARGE	29. AMOUNT PAID	30. BALANCE DUE
XX12210XX	☐ ☒	010	☒ YES ☐ NO	$ 70 92	$	$ 70 92

All Private Payers: Leave blank.

Medicaid: EMG stands for the word "emergency" and means that the service was rendered in hospital emergency department. Enter "Y" for "Yes" if emergency care is provided in an emergency department or leave blank if "No" in the bottom, unshaded area of the block.

BLOCK 24B
PLACE OF SERVICE CODES

01 Pharmacy
02 Unassigned
03 School
04 Homeless shelter
05 Indian health service free-standing facility
06 Indian health service provider-based facility
07 Tribal 638 free-standing facility
08 Tribal 638 provider-based facility
09 Prison/correctional facility
10 Unassigned
11 Doctor's office
12 Patient's home
13 Assisted living facility
14 Group home
15 Mobile unit
16 Temporary lodging
17-19 Unassigned
20 Urgent care facility
21 Inpatient hospital
22 Outpatient hospital or urgent care center
23 Emergency department—hospital
24 Ambulatory surgical center
25 Birthing center
26 Military treatment facility/uniformed service treatment facility
27-30 Unassigned
31 Skilled nursing facility (swing bed visits)
32 Nursing facility (intermediate/long-term care facilities)
33 Custodial care facility (domiciliary or rest home services)
34 Hospice (domiciliary or rest home services)
35-40 Unassigned
41 Ambulance—land
42 Ambulance—air or water
43-48 Unassigned
49 Independent clinic
50 Federally qualified health center
51 Inpatient psychiatric facility
52 Psychiatric facility—partial hospitalization
53 Community mental health care (outpatient, twenty-four-hours-a-day services, admission screening, consultation, and educational services)
54 Intermediate care facility/mentally retarded
55 Residential substance abuse treatment facility
56 Psychiatric residential treatment center
57 Non-residential substance abuse treatment facility
58-59 Unassigned
60 Mass immunization center
61 Comprehensive inpatient rehabilitation facility
62 Comprehensive outpatient rehabilitation facility
63-64 Unassigned
65 End-stage renal disease treatment facility
66-70 Unassigned
71 State or local public health clinic
72 Rural health clinic
73-80 Unassigned
81 Independent laboratory
82-98 Unassigned
99 Other place of service not identified above

FIGURE 7-2 Block 24B Place of Service codes.

Medicare: Leave blank.
Medicare/Medicaid: Leave blank.
Medicare/Medigap: Leave blank.
MSP: Leave blank.

TRICARE: Leave blank.

CHAMPVA: Leave blank.

Workers' Compensation: Leave blank.

Block 24D

Required

24. A. DATE(S) OF SERVICE From MM DD YY	To MM DD YY	B. PLACE OF SERVICE	C. EMG	D. PROCEDURES, SERVICES, OR SUPPLIES (Explain Unusual Circumstances) CPT/HCPCS	MODIFIER	E. DIAGNOSIS POINTER	F. $ CHARGES	G. DAYS OR UNITS	H. EPSDT Family Plan	I. ID. QUAL.	J. RENDERING PROVIDER ID. #
1 03 03 XX		11		99203		1	70 92	1		NPI	12458977XX
2										NPI	
3										NPI	
4										NPI	
5										NPI	
6										NPI	

25. FEDERAL TAX I.D. NUMBER SSN EIN	26. PATIENT'S ACCOUNT NO.	27. ACCEPT ASSIGNMENT? (For govt. claims, see back)	28. TOTAL CHARGE	29. AMOUNT PAID	30. BALANCE DUE
XX12210XX ☐ ☒	010	☒ YES ☐ NO	$ 70 92	$	$ 70 92

All Private Payers: Enter the appropriate CPT/HCPCS code for each procedure, service, or supply and applicable modifier without a hyphen. Note that the CMS-1500 (08-05) allows for four modifiers. During the transition period of CMS-1500 (12-90) to CMS-1500 (08-05), some third-party payers may still accept use of multiple modifier -99 in Block 24D with the modifiers listed in Block 19.

Medicaid: Enter the appropriate CPT/HCPCS code for each procedure, service, or supply and applicable modifier without a hyphen. Note that the CMS-1500 (08-05) allows for four modifiers.

Medicare: Enter CPT/HCPCS code and applicable modifiers without a hyphen for procedures, services, and supplies without a narrative description. When procedure codes do not require modifiers, leave modifier area blank—do not enter "00" or any other combination. Note that the CMS-1500 (08-05) allows for four modifiers. For multiple surgical procedures, list the procedure with the highest fee first. For unlisted procedure codes, include a narrative description in Block 19 (e.g., 99499, "Unlisted Evaluation and Management Service"). If information does not fit in Block 19, include an attachment. When entering an unlisted surgery code, submit the operative notes with the claim as an attachment.
Medicare/Medicaid: Refer to Medicare guidelines.
Medicare/Medigap: Refer to Medicare guidelines.
MSP: Refer to Medicare guidelines.

TRICARE: Enter the appropriate CPT/HCPCS code for each procedure, service, or supply and applicable modifier without a hyphen. Note that the CMS-1500 (08-05) allows for four modifiers. When Not Otherwise Classified (NOC) codes are submitted (e.g., supplies and injections), provide a narrative of the service in Block 19 or on an attachment.

CHAMPVA: Refer to TRICARE guidelines.

Workers' Compensation: Enter appropriate RVS codes and applicable modifiers (without a hyphen) used in your state or region. Note that the CMS-1500 (08-05) allows for four modifiers.
⟶ *When completing the **Workbook** assignments, use appropriate CPT codes.*

Block 24E

Required/Conditionally Required

21. DIAGNOSIS OR NATURE OF ILLNESS OR INJURY. (RELATE ITEMS 1,2,3 OR 4 TO ITEM 24E BY LINE)		22. MEDICAID RESUBMISSION CODE / ORIGINAL REF. NO.
1. ⌊ 382 . 00 ◄	3. ⌊___ . ___	
2. ⌊___ . ___	4. ⌊___ . ___	23. PRIOR AUTHORIZATION NUMBER

24. A. DATE(S) OF SERVICE From / To — MM DD YY MM DD YY	B. PLACE OF SERVICE	C. EMG	D. PROCEDURES, SERVICES, OR SUPPLIES (Explain Unusual Circumstances) CPT/HCPCS / MODIFIER	E. DIAGNOSIS POINTER	F. $ CHARGES	G. DAYS OR UNITS	H. EPSDT Family Plan	I. ID. QUAL.	J. RENDERING PROVIDER ID. #
1 03 03 XX	11		99203	1	70 92	1			12458977XX
2								NPI	
3								NPI	
4								NPI	
5								NPI	
6								NPI	

25. FEDERAL TAX I.D. NUMBER	SSN EIN	26. PATIENT'S ACCOUNT NO.	27. ACCEPT ASSIGNMENT? (For govt. claims, see back)	28. TOTAL CHARGE	29. AMOUNT PAID	30. BALANCE DUE
XX12210XX	☐ ☒X	010	☒X YES ☐ NO	$ 70 92	$	$ 70 92

All Private Payers: Enter all of the diagnosis code reference "pointer" numbers (1, 2, 3, 4) per line item that apply to the CPT code. This links the diagnostic code(s) listed in Block 24E to Block 21. When multiple services are performed, enter the corresponding diagnostic reference number for each service (e.g., 1, 2, 3, 4). DO NOT USE ACTUAL ICD-9-CM CODES IN THIS BLOCK.
→ *When completing **Workbook** assignments, more than one diagnosis reference "pointer" number per line item is allowed.*

 Medicaid: Refer to Medicare guidelines. In some states, completion may not be required.

 Medicare: Enter only one diagnosis code reference "pointer" number per line item linking the diagnostic codes listed in Block 21. When multiple services are performed, enter the corresponding diagnostic reference number for each service (e.g., 1, 2, 3, 4). DO NOT USE ACTUAL ICD-9-CM CODES IN THIS BLOCK.
Medicare/Medicaid: Refer to Medicare guidelines.
Medicare/Medigap: Refer to Medicare guidelines.
MSP: Refer to Medicare guidelines.

 TRICARE: Enter the diagnosis reference number (e.g., indicating up to four ICD-9-CM codes) as shown in Block 21 to relate the date of service and the procedures performed to the appropriate diagnosis. If multiple procedures are performed, enter the diagnosis code reference number for each service.

 CHAMPVA: Refer to TRICARE guidelines.

 Workers' Compensation: Enter all appropriate diagnosis code reference "pointer" numbers from Block 21 to relate appropriate diagnosis to date of service and procedures performed. A maximum of four diagnosis pointers may be referenced. Place commas between multiple diagnosis reference pointers on the same line.

Block 24F

Required

All Private Payers: Enter the fee for each listed service from the appropriate fee schedule. DO NOT ENTER DOLLAR SIGNS OR DECIMAL POINTS. ALWAYS INCLUDE CENTS. If the same service is performed on consecutive days, list the fee for the procedure in this block times the number of units it was performed as shown in Block 24G.

*When completing the **Workbook** assignments for private, Medicaid, TRICARE, and workers' compensation cases, use the Mock Fee. For Medicare participating provider cases, use the Participating Provider Fee. For nonparticipating provider cases, use the Limiting Charge.*

Block 24G

Required

24. A. DATE(S) OF SERVICE		B. PLACE OF SERVICE	C. EMG	D. PROCEDURES, SERVICES, OR SUPPLIES (Explain Unusual Circumstances) CPT/HCPCS | MODIFIER	E. DIAGNOSIS POINTER	F. $ CHARGES	G. DAYS OR UNITS	H. EPSDT Family Plan	I. ID. QUAL.	J. RENDERING PROVIDER ID. #
From MM DD YY	To MM DD YY									
1 03 03 XX		11		99203	1	70 92	1		NPI	12458977XX
2									NPI	
3									NPI	
4									NPI	
5									NPI	
6									NPI	

25. FEDERAL TAX I.D. NUMBER	SSN EIN	26. PATIENT'S ACCOUNT NO.	27. ACCEPT ASSIGNMENT? (For govt. claims, see back)	28. TOTAL CHARGE	29. AMOUNT PAID	30. BALANCE DUE
XX12210XX	[X]	010	[X] YES [ ] NO	$ 70 92	$	$ 70 92

All Private Payers: Enter the number of days or units that apply to each line of service. This block is important for calculating multiple visits, anesthesia minutes, or oxygen volume.

Medicaid: Each service must be listed on separate lines (no date ranging). Indicate that each service was performed one time by listing "1" in this block. List number of visits in 1 day.

Medicare: Enter the number of days or units that apply to each line of service. This block is important for calculating multiple visits, number of miles, units of supplies including drugs, anesthesia minutes, or oxygen volume. For anesthesia, show the elapsed time (minutes) in Block 24G. Convert hours into minutes and enter the total minutes for the procedure. See the Medicare Manual for rounding out figures when billing gas and liquid oxygen units.
Medicare/Medicaid: Refer to Medicare guidelines.
Medicare/Medigap: Refer to Medicare guidelines.
MSP: Refer to Medicare guidelines.

TRICARE: Refer to Medicare guidelines.

CHAMPVA: Refer to Medicare guidelines.

 Workers' Compensation: Refer to Medicare guidelines.

Block 24H

Conditionally Required

24. A. DATE(S) OF SERVICE	B.	C.	D. PROCEDURES, SERVICES, OR SUPPLIES	E.	F.	G.	H.	I.	J.
From / To	PLACE OF SERVICE	EMG	CPT/HCPCS | MODIFIER	DIAGNOSIS POINTER	$ CHARGES	DAYS OR UNITS	EPSDT Family Plan	ID. QUAL.	RENDERING PROVIDER ID. #
1 03 03 XX	11		99203	1	70 92	1		NPI	12458977XX
2								NPI	
3								NPI	
4								NPI	
5								NPI	
6								NPI	

25. FEDERAL TAX I.D. NUMBER SSN EIN	26. PATIENT'S ACCOUNT NO.	27. ACCEPT ASSIGNMENT?	28. TOTAL CHARGE	29. AMOUNT PAID	30. BALANCE DUE
XX12210XX ☐ ☒	010	☒ YES ☐ NO	$ 70 92	$	$ 70 92

 All Private Payers: Leave blank.

 Medicaid: EPSDT means early, periodic, screening, diagnosis, and treatment, and refers to a Medicaid service program for children 12 years of age or younger. Enter "E" for EPSDT services or "F" for family planning services, if applicable.

 Medicare: Leave blank.
Medicare/Medicaid: Leave blank.
Medicare/Medigap: Leave blank.
MSP: Leave blank.

 TRICARE: Leave blank.

 CHAMPVA: Leave blank.

Workers' Compensation: Leave blank.

Block 24I

Conditionally Required

24. A. DATE(S) OF SERVICE		B. PLACE OF SERVICE	C. EMG	D. PROCEDURES, SERVICES, OR SUPPLIES (Explain Unusual Circumstances)		E. DIAGNOSIS POINTER	F. $ CHARGES	G. DAYS OR UNITS	H. EPSDT Family Plan	I. ID. QUAL.	J. RENDERING PROVIDER ID. #
From MM DD YY	To MM DD YY			CPT/HCPCS	MODIFIER						
1 03 03 XX		11		99203		1	70 92	1		NPI	12458977XX
2										NPI	
3										NPI	
4										NPI	
5										NPI	
6										NPI	

25. FEDERAL TAX I.D. NUMBER	SSN EIN	26. PATIENT'S ACCOUNT NO.	27. ACCEPT ASSIGNMENT? (For govt. claims, see back)	28. TOTAL CHARGE	29. AMOUNT PAID	30. BALANCE DUE
XX12210XX	☐ ☒	010	☒ YES ☐ NO	$ 70 92	$	$ 70 92

 All Private Payers: If the provider does not have an NPI number, enter the ID qualifier "1C" in the shaded portion of the block. The qualifier indicates the non-NPI number being reported. NUCC-approved ID qualifiers and numbers (as shown in Block 17a) may be reported.

 Medicaid: Refer to Medicare guidelines.

 Medicare: If the provider does not have an NPI number, enter the ID qualifier "1C" in the shaded portion of the block. The qualifier indicates the non-NPI number being reported.
Medicare/Medicaid: Refer to Medicare guidelines.
Medicare/Medigap: Refer to Medicare guidelines.
MSP: Refer to Medicare guidelines.

 TRICARE: Refer to Medicare guidelines.

 CHAMPVA: Refer to Medicare guidelines.

 Workers' Compensation: Refer to Medicare guidelines.

Block 24J

Required

24. A. DATE(S) OF SERVICE						B. PLACE OF SERVICE	C. EMG	D. PROCEDURES, SERVICES, OR SUPPLIES (Explain Unusual Circumstances) CPT/HCPCS | MODIFIER		E. DIAGNOSIS POINTER	F. $ CHARGES		G. DAYS OR UNITS	H. EPSDT Family Plan	I. ID. QUAL.	J. RENDERING PROVIDER ID. #
From MM	DD	YY	To MM	DD	YY											
1 03	03	XX				11		99203		1	70	92	1		NPI	12458977XX
2															NPI	
3															NPI	
4															NPI	
5															NPI	
6															NPI	

25. FEDERAL TAX I.D. NUMBER	SSN EIN	26. PATIENT'S ACCOUNT NO.	27. ACCEPT ASSIGNMENT? (For govt. claims, see back)	28. TOTAL CHARGE	29. AMOUNT PAID	30. BALANCE DUE
XX12210XX	☐ ☒X	010	☒X YES ☐ NO	$ 70 92	$	$ 70 92

 All Private Payers: In the upper portion, enter the provider's taxonomy code. Enter the rendering provider's NPI number in the lower portion. NUCC-approved ID qualifiers and numbers (as shown in Block 17a) may be reported.

 Medicaid: In the upper portion, enter the provider's taxonomy code. Enter the rendering provider's NPI number in the lower portion.

 Medicare: In the upper portion, enter the provider's taxonomy code. Enter the rendering provider's NPI number in the lower portion when billing for a group. In the case of a service provided incident-to the service of a physician or NPP, when the person who ordered the service is not supervising, enter the NPI of the supervisor. When billing for a solo provider, leave blank.

Medicare/Medicaid: In the upper portion, enter the provider's taxonomy code. Enter the rendering provider's NPI number in the lower portion when billing for a group.

Medicare/Medigap: In the upper portion, enter the provider's taxonomy code. Enter the rendering provider's NPI number in the lower portion when billing for a group.

MSP: In the upper portion, enter the provider's taxonomy code. Enter the rendering provider's NPI number in the lower portion when billing for a group.

 TRICARE: In the upper portion, enter the provider's taxonomy code. Enter the rendering provider's NPI number in the lower portion when billing for a group.

 CHAMPVA: In the upper portion, enter the provider's taxonomy code. Enter the rendering provider's NPI number in the lower portion when billing for a group.

 Workers' Compensation: In the upper portion, enter the provider's taxonomy code. Enter the rendering provider's NPI number in the lower portion when billing for a group.

Block 25

Required

25. FEDERAL TAX I.D. NUMBER SSN EIN	26. PATIENT'S ACCOUNT NO.	27. ACCEPT ASSIGNMENT? (For govt. claims, see back)	28. TOTAL CHARGE	29. AMOUNT PAID	30. BALANCE DUE
XX12210XX [X]	010	[X] YES ☐ NO	$ 70 92	$	$ 70 92

31. SIGNATURE OF PHYSICIAN OR SUPPLIER INCLUDING DEGREES OR CREDENTIALS (I certify that the statements on the reverse apply to this bill and are made a part thereof.)
CONCHA ANTRUM MD 030320XX

SIGNED *Concha Antrum MD* DATE

32. SERVICE FACILITY LOCATION INFORMATION

a.   b.

33. BILLING PROVIDER INFO & PH # (555) 486 9002
COLLEGE CLINIC
4567 BROAD AVENUE
WOODLAND HILLS XY 12345 0001

a. 3664021CC   b.

reference initials

All Payers: Enter the physician or supplier's federal tax ID. This number may be the EIN or SSN. A provider who is an independent contractor must insert his or her federal tax ID. If physicians in a group are employees and the claim is being reported as a group, enter the group's federal tax ID. Check the corresponding box.
- A Medicaid case may or may not require a physician's tax ID number, depending on individual state guidelines.
- In a Medicare/Medigap case, the physician's federal tax ID number is not necessary for Medigap because the Medicare contractor will retrieve the tax ID information from his or her internal provider file.

➔ *When completing the **Workbook** assignments, enter the group's federal tax ID number and check the appropriate box except in Medicare/Medigap cases.*

Block 26

Conditionally Required

25. FEDERAL TAX I.D. NUMBER SSN EIN	26. PATIENT'S ACCOUNT NO.	27. ACCEPT ASSIGNMENT? (For govt. claims, see back)	28. TOTAL CHARGE	29. AMOUNT PAID	30. BALANCE DUE
XX12210XX [X]	010	[X] YES ☐ NO	$ 70 92	$	$ 70 92

31. SIGNATURE OF PHYSICIAN OR SUPPLIER INCLUDING DEGREES OR CREDENTIALS (I certify that the statements on the reverse apply to this bill and are made a part thereof.)
CONCHA ANTRUM MD 030320XX

SIGNED *Concha Antrum MD* DATE

32. SERVICE FACILITY LOCATION INFORMATION

a.   b.

33. BILLING PROVIDER INFO & PH # (555) 486 9002
COLLEGE CLINIC
4567 BROAD AVENUE
WOODLAND HILLS XY 12345 0001

a. 3664021CC   b.

reference initials

All Payers: Enter the patient's account number assigned by the physician's accounting system. Do not use dashes or slashes. When Medicare is billed electronically, this block must be completed.
➔ *When completing the **Workbook** assignments, list the patient account number when provided.*

Block 27

Required

25. FEDERAL TAX I.D. NUMBER SSN EIN	26. PATIENT'S ACCOUNT NO.	27. ACCEPT ASSIGNMENT? (For govt. claims, see back)	28. TOTAL CHARGE	29. AMOUNT PAID	30. BALANCE DUE
XX12210XX [X]	010	[X] YES ☐ NO	$ 70 92	$	$ 70 92

31. SIGNATURE OF PHYSICIAN OR SUPPLIER INCLUDING DEGREES OR CREDENTIALS (I certify that the statements on the reverse apply to this bill and are made a part thereof.)
CONCHA ANTRUM MD 030320XX

SIGNED *Concha Antrum MD* DATE

32. SERVICE FACILITY LOCATION INFORMATION

a.   b.

33. BILLING PROVIDER INFO & PH # (555) 486 9002
COLLEGE CLINIC
4567 BROAD AVENUE
WOODLAND HILLS XY 12345 0001

a. 3664021CC   b.

reference initials

All Private Payers: Check "Yes" or "No" to indicate whether the physician accepts assignment of benefits. If "Yes," then the physician agrees to accept the amount allowed by the third party. You may need to bill the patient for any copayment or deductible amount.
↪ *When completing the* ***Workbook*** *assignments, check "Yes."*

Medicaid: Check "Yes."

Medicare: Check "Yes" or "No" to indicate whether the physician accepts assignment of benefits. If "Yes," then the physician agrees to accept the allowed amount paid by the third party plus any copayment or deductible as payment in full. If this field is left blank, "No" is assumed, and a participating physician's claim will be denied. The following provider or supplier must file claims on an assignment basis:

- Clinical diagnostic laboratory services performed in physician's office.
- Physicians wishing to accept assignment on clinical laboratory services but not other services should submit two separate claims, one "assigned" for laboratory and one "nonassigned" for other services. Submit all charges on a nonassigned claim, as indicated in Block 27, and write "I accept assignment for the clinical laboratory tests" at the bottom of Block 24.
- Participating physician or supplier services.
- Physician's services to Medicare/Medicaid patients.
- Services of physician assistants, nurse practitioners, clinical nurse specialists, nurse midwives, certified registered nurse anesthetists, clinical psychologists, and clinical social workers.
- Ambulatory surgical center services.
- Home dialysis supplies and equipment paid under Method II (monthly capitation payment).

↪ *When completing the* ***Workbook*** *assignments, check "Yes."*
Medicare/Medicaid: Check "Yes."
Medicare/Medigap: Check "Yes."
MSP: Check "Yes" or "No" to indicate whether the physician accepts assignment of benefits for primary insurance and Medicare.
↪ *When completing the* ***Workbook*** *assignments, check "Yes."*

TRICARE: Refer to Medicare guidelines. However, participation in TRICARE may be made on a case-by-case basis.

CHAMPVA: Refer to Medicare guidelines.

Workers' Compensation: Leave blank.

Block 28

Required

25. FEDERAL TAX I.D. NUMBER SSN EIN	26. PATIENT'S ACCOUNT NO.	27. ACCEPT ASSIGNMENT? (For govt. claims, see back)	28. TOTAL CHARGE	29. AMOUNT PAID	30. BALANCE DUE
XX12210XX ☐ X	010	X YES ☐ NO	$ 70 92	$	$ 70 92
31. SIGNATURE OF PHYSICIAN OR SUPPLIER INCLUDING DEGREES OR CREDENTIALS (I certify that the statements on the reverse apply to this bill and are made a part thereof.) CONCHA ANTRUM MD 030320XX SIGNED *Concha Antrum MD* DATE	32. SERVICE FACILITY LOCATION INFORMATION a. b.		33. BILLING PROVIDER INFO & PH # (555)486 9002 COLLEGE CLINIC 4567 BROAD AVENUE WOODLAND HILLS XY 12345 0001 a. 3664021CC b.		

reference initials

 All Payers: Enter total charges for services listed in Block 24F. Do not enter dollar signs or decimal points. Always include cents.

Block 29

Conditionally Required

25. FEDERAL TAX I.D. NUMBER SSN EIN	26. PATIENT'S ACCOUNT NO.	27. ACCEPT ASSIGNMENT? (For govt. claims, see back)	28. TOTAL CHARGE	29. AMOUNT PAID	30. BALANCE DUE
XX12210XX ☐ X	010	X YES ☐ NO	$ 70 92	$	$ 70 92
31. SIGNATURE OF PHYSICIAN OR SUPPLIER INCLUDING DEGREES OR CREDENTIALS (I certify that the statements on the reverse apply to this bill and are made a part thereof.) CONCHA ANTRUM MD 030320XX SIGNED *Concha Antrum MD* DATE	32. SERVICE FACILITY LOCATION INFORMATION a. b.		33. BILLING PROVIDER INFO & PH # (555)486 9002 COLLEGE CLINIC 4567 BROAD AVENUE WOODLAND HILLS XY 12345 0001 a. 3664021CC b.		

reference initials

 All Private Payers: Enter only the amount paid for the charges listed on the claim.

 Medicaid: Enter only the payment on claim by a third-party payer, excluding Medicare.

 Medicare: Enter only the amount paid for the charges listed on the claim.
Medicare/Medicaid: Refer to Medicare guidelines.
Medicare/Medigap: Enter only the amount paid for the charges listed on the claim.
MSP: Enter only the amount paid for the charges listed on the claim. It is mandatory to enter amount paid by primary carrier and attach an explanation of benefits document when billing Medicare.

 TRICARE: Enter only amount paid by other carrier for the charges listed on the claim. If the amount includes payment by any other health insurance, the other health insurance explanation of benefits, work sheet, or denial showing the amounts paid must be attached to the claim. Payment from the beneficiary should not be included.

CHAMPVA: Refer to TRICARE guidelines.

Workers' Compensation: Leave blank.

Block 30

Conditionally Required

25. FEDERAL TAX I.D. NUMBER SSN EIN	26. PATIENT'S ACCOUNT NO.	27. ACCEPT ASSIGNMENT? (For govt. claims, see back)	28. TOTAL CHARGE	29. AMOUNT PAID	30. BALANCE DUE
XX12210XX ☐ ☒	010	☒ YES ☐ NO	$ 70 92	$	$ 71 92

| 31. SIGNATURE OF PHYSICIAN OR SUPPLIER INCLUDING DEGREES OR CREDENTIALS (I certify that the statements on the reverse apply to this bill and are made a part thereof.) CONCHA ANTRUM MD 030320XX SIGNED *Concha Antrum MD* DATE | 32. SERVICE FACILITY LOCATION INFORMATION a.   b. | 33. BILLING PROVIDER INFO & PH # (555)486 9002 COLLEGE CLINIC 4567 BROAD AVENUE WOODLAND HILLS XY 12345 0001 a. 3664021CC   b. |

reference initials

All Private Payers: Enter balance due on claim (Block 28 less Block 29).

Medicaid: Leave blank or enter balance due on claim depending on individual state guidelines.
→ *When completing the **Workbook** assignments, enter the balance due.*

Medicare: Leave blank.
Medicare/Medicaid: Leave blank.
Medicare/Medigap: Leave blank.
MSP: Leave blank.

TRICARE: Enter balance due on claim (Block 28 less Block 29).

CHAMPVA: Enter balance due on claim (Block 28 less Block 29).

Workers' Compensation: Enter balance due on claim (Block 28 less Block 29).

Block 31

Required

25. FEDERAL TAX I.D. NUMBER	SSN EIN	26. PATIENT'S ACCOUNT NO.	27. ACCEPT ASSIGNMENT? (For govt. claims, see back)	28. TOTAL CHARGE	29. AMOUNT PAID	30. BALANCE DUE
XX12210XX	X	010	X YES NO	$ 70 92	$	$ 70 92

| 31. SIGNATURE OF PHYSICIAN OR SUPPLIER
INCLUDING DEGREES OR CREDENTIALS
(I certify that the reverse statements on the reverse
apply to this bill and are made a part thereof.)
CONCHA ANTRUM MD 030320XX

SIGNED *Concha Antrum MD* DATE | 32. SERVICE FACILITY LOCATION INFORMATION

a.   b. | 33. BILLING PROVIDER INFO & PH # (555) 486 9002
COLLEGE CLINIC
4567 BROAD AVENUE
WOODLAND HILLS XY 12345 0001
a. 3664021CC   b. |

reference initials

All Payers: Type the provider's name and show the signature of the physician or the physician's representative above or below the name. Enter either six-digit, eight-digit, or alphanumeric date that the form was prepared. Use of a stamped signature is discouraged but some insurance carriers may accept it. However, the stamp must be completely inside the block. Do not type the name of the association or corporation.

In the case of a service that is provided incident to the service of a physician or NPP, when the ordering physician or non-physician practitioner is directly supervising the service, the signature of the ordering physician or NPP shall be entered in Block 31. When the ordering physician or NPP is not supervising the service, enter the signature of the physician or NPP providing the direct supervision in Block 31.

In a computerized office environment, the participating contract with the third-party payer including Medicare, Medicaid, and the Blue Plans signed by the physician allows the physician's name to be printed in the signature block as it would normally be signed.

NOTE: The claim can be processed if a physician, supplier, or authorized person's signature is missing but the signature is on file; an authorization is attached to the claim; or the signature block has "Signature on File" or a computer-generated signature.

Block 32

Required

25. FEDERAL TAX I.D. NUMBER	SSN EIN	26. PATIENT'S ACCOUNT NO.	27. ACCEPT ASSIGNMENT? (For govt. claims, see back)	28. TOTAL CHARGE	29. AMOUNT PAID	30. BALANCE DUE
XX12210XX	X	010	X YES NO	$ 70 92	$	$ 70 92

| 31. SIGNATURE OF PHYSICIAN OR SUPPLIER
INCLUDING DEGREES OR CREDENTIALS
(I certify that the statements on the reverse
apply to this bill and are made a part thereof.)
CONCHA ANTRUM MD 030320XX

SIGNED *Concha Antrum MD* DATE | 32. SERVICE FACILITY LOCATION INFORMATION

a.   b. | 33. BILLING PROVIDER INFO & PH # (555) 486 9002
COLLEGE CLINIC
4567 BROAD AVENUE
WOODLAND HILLS XY 12345 0001
a. 3664021CC   b. |

reference initials

All Payers: Enter the physical location (name, address, and ZIP code) of the facility if the services were furnished in a hospital, clinic, laboratory, or facility other than the patient's home or physician's office. The name, address, and ZIP code of the physical location for all services other than those furnished in place of service home 12 must be indicated in this block or the claim will be rejected. Only one name, address, and ZIP code may be entered in the block. If additional entries are necessary, separate claim forms should be submitted.

Block 32a

Conditionally Required

All Payers: If a service facility is inserted in Block 32, insert the NPI.

Block 32b

Conditionally Required

All Payers: Used for taxonomy code. NUCC-approved ID qualifiers and numbers (as shown in Block 17a) may be reported. For purchased diagnostic tests, insert the supplier's PIN. For certified mammography screening centers, insert the 6-digit FDA-approved certification number. For durable medical orthotic and prosthetic claims, insert the PIN of the location where the order was accepted if the name and address is not in Block 32.

Block 33

Required

25. FEDERAL TAX I.D. NUMBER	SSN EIN	26. PATIENT'S ACCOUNT NO.	27. ACCEPT ASSIGNMENT? (For govt. claims, see back)	28. TOTAL CHARGE	29. AMOUNT PAID	30. BALANCE DUE
XX12210XX	☐ ☒	010	☒ YES ☐ NO	$ 70 92	$	$ 70 92
31. SIGNATURE OF PHYSICIAN OR SUPPLIER INCLUDING DEGREES OR CREDENTIALS (I certify that the statements on the reverse apply to this bill and are made a part thereof.) CONCHA ANTRUM MD 030320XX SIGNED *Concha Antrum MD* DATE		32. SERVICE FACILITY LOCATION INFORMATION a.　　　　　　　b.		33. BILLING PROVIDER INFO & PH #　(555)486 9002 COLLEGE CLINIC 4567 BROAD AVENUE WOODLAND HILLS XY 12345 0001 a. 3664021CC　　　b.		

reference initials

All Payers: Enter the provider of service/supplier's billing name, address, ZIP code, and telephone number. Enter the NPI for the performing provider of service/supplier who is not a member of a group practice. Enter the group NPI for the performing provider of service/supplier who is a member of a group practice. Suppliers billing the durable medical equipment regional carrier/contractor (DMERC) use the National Supplier Clearinghouse (NSC) number in this block.

Block 33a

Required

All Payers: Enter the NPI of the billing provider or group.

Block 33b

Required

 All Payers: Block 33b is reserved for a taxonomy code when a case requires it. NUCC-approved ID qualifiers and numbers (as shown in Block 17a) may be reported.

Bottom of Form Enter insurance billing specialist's initials in lower left corner of the insurance claim form.

Insurance Program Templates

The following pages show completed CMS-1500 (08-05) insurance claim forms and templates for the most common insurance programs encountered in a medical practice. Screened areas on each form do not apply to the insurance program example shown and should be left blank. Add a tab at the page margin for ease in flipping to this reference section when completing *Workbook* assignments. The following examples illustrate entries for basic cases:

Figure 7-3 Private payer.
Figure 7-4 Back of CMS-1500 (08-05) insurance claim form.
Figure 7-5 Medicaid.
Figure 7-6 Medicare.
Figure 7-7 Medicaid/Medicare—a crossover claim.

Figure 7-8 Medicare/Medigap—a crossover claim.
Figure 7-9 MSP—other insurance primary and Medicare secondary.
Figure 7-10 TRICARE—Standard.
Figure 7-11 CHAMPVA.
Figure 7-12 Workers' compensation.

KEY POINTS

This is a brief chapter review or summary of the key issues presented. To further enhance your knowledge of the technical subject matter, review the key terms and key abbreviations for this chapter by locating the meanings in the glossary at the end of this book that appear in a section before the index.

1. There are two types of claims submitted to insurance companies for payment: *paper claims* and *electronic claims*.
2. A *clean claim* is one that was submitted to the third-party payer within the time limit and had the necessary information for processing and was paid promptly. Under the Medicare program, a clean claim is one that has passed all electronic edits and is routed for payment.
3. Other types of claims are called *dirty* when a claim is submitted with errors, *incomplete* when missing required information, *invalid* when illogical or incorrect, *pending* when a claim is held in suspense for review, *rejected* when the claim needs investigation and answers to some questions, or *deleted* when the Medicare fiscal intermediary cancels, deletes, or voids a claim.
4. When two insurance policies are involved (*dual coverage* or *duplication of coverage*), one is considered primary and the other secondary. First an insurance claim is submitted to the primary plan, and after payment the secondary carrier is billed with a copy of the explanation of benefits from the primary carrier.
5. A diagnosis should never be submitted on an insurance claim without supporting documentation in the medical record.
6. Every insurance claim should be proofread for completeness and accuracy of content before it is submitted to the insurance carrier.
7. Be aware of common billing errors and learn how to correct them for quicker claim settlements and to reduce the number of appeals.
8. HIPAA transactions and code sets standards only apply to electronic transactions conducted by covered entities.
9. Copies of submitted insurance claim forms should be filed in a tickler file and reviewed for follow-up every 30 days unless the computer system maintains the files.
10. Be sure the correct NPI is shown on the claim for the physician rendering the medical service to the patient.

evolve INTERNET RESOURCES

For active links to the following resources, visit the Evolve website at **http://evolve.elsevier.com/fordney/handbook**

- CMS-1500 (08-05) claim form instruction manual and access to the form
- HIPAA regulations and guidance
- Standard Code Set (rules and information for electronic claim submission)
- Centers for Medicare and Medicaid Services

STUDENT ASSIGNMENT

✓ Study Chapter 7.

✓ Answer the fill-in-the-blank, multiple choice, and true/false questions in the *Workbook* to reinforce the theory learned in this chapter and to help prepare you for a future test.

✓ Complete the assignments in the *Workbook* to give you hands-on experience in abstracting information from case histories and financial accounting record cards, as well as completing insurance claim forms.

✓ Study the claim sample in the *Workbook* and try to locate as many errors as possible on the basis of the instructions you have been given in this chapter.

✓ Turn to the glossary at the end of this textbook for a further understanding of the key terms and key abbreviations used in this chapter.

PRIVATE PAYER
No secondary coverage

1. MEDICARE	MEDICAID	TRICARE CHAMPUS	CHAMPVA	GROUP HEALTH PLAN	FECA BLK LUNG	OTHER	1a. INSURED'S I.D. NUMBER	(For Program in Item 1)
(Medicare #)	(Medicaid #)	(Sponsor's SSN)	(Member ID#) X	(SSN or ID)	(SSN)	(ID)	111704521	A482

2. PATIENT'S NAME (Last Name, First Name, Middle Initial)	3. PATIENT'S BIRTH DATE	SEX	4. INSURED'S NAME (Last Name, First Name, Middle Initial)
FOREHAND HARRY N	01 06 1946 M X F		SAME

5. PATIENT'S ADDRESS (No., Street)
1456 MAIN STREET

6. PATIENT RELATIONSHIP TO INSURED
Self X Spouse Child Other

7. INSURED'S ADDRESS (No., Street)

CITY	STATE	8. PATIENT STATUS	CITY	STATE
WOODLAND HILLS	XY	Single Married X Other		

ZIP CODE	TELEPHONE (Include Area Code)		ZIP CODE	TELEPHONE (INCLUDE AREA CODE)
12345 0000	(555) 490 9876	Employed X Full-Time Student Part-Time Student		( )

9. OTHER INSURED'S NAME (Last Name, First Name, Middle Initial)

10. IS PATIENT'S CONDITION RELATED TO:

11. INSURED'S POLICY GROUP OR FECA NUMBER

a. OTHER INSURED'S POLICY OR GROUP NUMBER

a. EMPLOYMENT? (CURRENT OR PREVIOUS)
YES X NO

a. INSURED'S DATE OF BIRTH   MM DD YY   SEX   M   F

b. OTHER INSURED'S DATE OF BIRTH   MM DD YY   SEX   M   F

b. AUTO ACCIDENT?   PLACE (State)
YES X NO

b. EMPLOYER'S NAME OR SCHOOL NAME

c. EMPLOYER'S NAME OR SCHOOL NAME

c. OTHER ACCIDENT?
YES X NO

c. INSURANCE PLAN NAME OR PROGRAM NAME

d. INSURANCE PLAN NAME OR PROGRAM NAME

10d. RESERVED FOR LOCAL USE

d. IS THERE ANOTHER HEALTH BENEFIT PLAN?
YES X NO   If yes, return to and complete item 9 a-d.

READ BACK OF FORM BEFORE COMPLETING & SIGNING THIS FORM.
12. PATIENT'S OR AUTHORIZED PERSON'S SIGNATURE I authorize the release of any medical or other information necessary to process this claim. I also request payment of government benefits either to myself or to the party who accepts assignment below.

SIGNED *Harry N. Forehand*   DATE *March 3, 20XX*

13. INSURED'S OR AUTHORIZED PERSON'S SIGNATURE I authorize payment of medical benefits to the undersigned physician or supplier for services described below.

SIGNED *Harry N. Forehand*

14. DATE OF CURRENT: ILLNESS (First symptom) OR INJURY (Accident) OR PREGNANCY(LMP) MM DD YY 03 01 20XX	15. IF PATIENT HAS HAD SAME OR SIMILAR ILLNESS. GIVE FIRST DATE MM DD YY	16. DATES PATIENT UNABLE TO WORK IN CURRENT OCCUPATION MM DD YY FROM TO MM DD YY

17. NAME OF REFERRING PHYSICIAN OR OTHER SOURCE
PERRY CARDI MD

17a.
17b. NPI 67805027XX

18. HOSPITALIZATION DATES RELATED TO CURRENT SERVICES   MM DD YY   FROM   TO   MM DD YY

19. RESERVED FOR LOCAL USE

20. OUTSIDE LAB? $ CHARGES
YES X NO

21. DIAGNOSIS OR NATURE OF ILLNESS OR INJURY. (RELATE ITEMS 1,2,3 OR 4 TO ITEM 24E BY LINE)
1. 38200
2.
3.
4.

22. MEDICAID RESUBMISSION CODE   ORIGINAL REF. NO.

23. PRIOR AUTHORIZATION NUMBER

24. A. DATE(S) OF SERVICE			B. PLACE OF SERVICE	C. EMG	D. PROCEDURES, SERVICES, OR SUPPLIES (Explain Unusual Circumstances) CPT/HCPCS MODIFIER	E. DIAGNOSIS POINTER	F. $ CHARGES	G. DAYS OR UNITS	H. EPSDT Family Plan	I. ID. QUAL.	J. RENDERING PROVIDER ID. #
From MM DD YY	To MM DD YY										
03 03 20XX			11		99203	1	71 00	1		NPI	1245897700
										NPI	
										NPI	
										NPI	
										NPI	
										NPI	

25. FEDERAL TAX I.D. NUMBER SSN EIN	26. PATIENT'S ACCOUNT NO.	27. ACCEPT ASSIGNMENT? (For govt. claims, see back)	28. TOTAL CHARGE	29. AMOUNT PAID	30. BALANCE DUE
XX12210XX X	010	X YES NO	$ 71 00	$	$ 71 00

31. SIGNATURE OF PHYSICIAN OR SUPPLIER INCLUDING DEGREES OR CREDENTIALS (I certify that the statements on the reverse apply to this bill and are made a part thereof.)
CONCHA ANTRUM MD 030320XX
SIGNED *Concha Antrum MD* DATE

32. SERVICE FACILITY LOCATION INFORMATION
a.   b.

33. BILLING PROVIDER INFO & PH # (555) 486 9002
COLLEGE CLINIC
4567 BROAD AVENUE
WOODLAND HILLS XY 12345 0001
a. 3664021CC   b.

reference initials

FIGURE 7-3 Front side of the scannable Health Insurance Claim Form approved by the American Medical Association's Council on Medical Service. This form is also known as the CMS-1500 (08-05) and is shown illustrating completion to a private third-party payer with no secondary coverage. Third-party payer, state, and local guidelines vary and may not always follow the visual guide presented here. Screened blocks should not be completed for this type of case.

BECAUSE THIS FORM IS USED BY VARIOUS GOVERNMENT AND PRIVATE HEALTH PROGRAMS, SEE SEPARATE INSTRUCTIONS ISSUED BY APPLICABLE PROGRAMS.

NOTICE: Any person who knowingly files a statement of claim containing any misrepresentation or any false, incomplete or misleading information may be guilty of a criminal act punishable under law and may be subject to civil penalties.

REFERS TO GOVERNMENT PROGRAMS ONLY

MEDICARE AND TRICARE PAYMENT: A patient's signature requests that payment be made and authorizes release of any information necessary to process the claim and certifies that the information provided in Blocks 1 through 12 is true, accurate and complete. In the case of a Medicare claim, the patient's signature authorizes any entity to release to Medicare medical and nonmedical information, including employment status, and whether the person has employer group health insurance, liability, no-fault, worker's compensation or other insurance which is responsible to pay for the services for which the Medicare claim is made. See 42 CFR 411.24(a). If item 9 is completed, the patient's signature authorizes release of the information to the health plan or agency shown. In Medicare assigned or TRICARE participation cases, the physician agrees to accept the charge determination of the Medicare carrier or TRICARE fiscal intermediary as the full charge determination of the Medicare carrier or TRICARE fiscal intermediary if this is less than the charge submitted. TRICARE is not a health insurance program but makes payment for health benefits provided through certain affiliations with the Uniformed Services. Information on the patient's sponsor should be provided in those items captioned in "Insured", i.e., items 1a, 4, 6, 7, 9, and 11.

BLACK LUNG AND FECA CLAIMS

The provider agrees to accept the amount paid by the Government as payment in full. See Black Lung and FECA instructions regarding required procedure and diagnosis coding systems.

SIGNATURE OF PHYSICIAN OR SUPPLIER (MEDICARE, TRICARE, FECA AND BLACK LUNG)

I certify that the services shown on this form were medically indicated and necessary for the health of the patient and were personally furnished by me or were furnished incident to my professional service by my employee under my immediate supervision, except as otherwise expressly permitted by Medicare or TRICARE regulations.

For services to be considered as "incident" to a physician's professional service, 1) they must be rendered under the physician's immediate personal supervision by his/her employee, 2) they must be an integral, although incidental part of a covered physician's service, 3) they must be of kinds commonly furnished in physician's offices, and 4) the services of nonphysicians must be included on the physician's bills.

For TRICARE claims, I further certify that I (or any employee) who rendered services am not an active duty member of the Uniformed Services or a civilian employee of the United States Government or a contract employee of the United States Government, either civilian or military (refer to 5 USC 5536). For Black-Lung claims, I further certify that the services performed were for a Black Lung-related disorder.

No Part B Medicare benefits may be paid unless this form is received as required by existing law and regulations (42 CFR 424.32).

NOTICE: Any one who misrepresents or falsifies essential information to receive payment from Federal funds requested by this form may upon conviction be subject to fine and imprisonment under applicable Federal laws.

NOTICE TO PATIENT ABOUT THE COLLECTION AND USE OF MEDICARE, TRICARE, FECA, AND BLACK LUNG INFORMATION
(PRIVACY ACT STATEMENT)

We are authorized by CMS, TRICARE and OWCP to ask you for information needed in the administration of the Medicare, TRICARE, FECA, and Black Lung programs. Authority to collect information is in section 205(a), 1862, 1872 and 1874 of the Social Security Act as amended, 42 CFR411.24(a) and 424.5(a) (6), and 44 USC 3101; CFR 101 et seq and 10 USC 1079 and 1086; 5 USC 8101 et seq; and 30 USC 901 et seq; 38 USC 613; E.O. 9397.

The information we obtain to complete claims under these programs is used to identify you and to determine your eligibility. It is also used to decide if the services and supplies you received are covered by these programs and to insure that proper payment is made.

The information may also be given to other providers of services, carriers, intermediaries, medical review boards, health plans, and other organizations or Federal agencies, for the effective administration of Federal provisions that require other third parties payers to pay primary to Federal program, and as otherwise necessary to administer these programs. For example, it may be necessary to disclose information about the benefits you have used to a hospital or doctor. Additional disclosures are made through routine uses for information contained in systems of records.

FOR MEDICARE CLAIMS: See the notice modifying system No. 09-70-0501, titled 'Carrier Medicare Claims Record,' published in the Federal Register, Vol. 55 No. 177, page 37549, Wed., Sept. 12, 1990, or as updated and republished.

FOR OWCP CLAIMS: Department of Labor, Privacy Act of 1974, "Republication of Notice of Systems of Records," Federal Register, Vol. 55 No. 40, Wed., Feb. 28, 1990, See ESA-5, ESA-6, ESA-12, ESA-13, ESA-30, or as updated and republished.

FOR TRICARE CLAIMS: PRINCIPAL PURPOSE(S): To evaluate eligibility for medical care provided by civilian sources and to issue payment upon establishment of eligibility and determination that the services/supplies received are authorized by law.

ROUTINE USE(S): Information from claims and related documents may be given to the Dept. of Veterans Affairs, the Dept. of Health and Human Services and/or the Dept. of Transportation consistent with their statutory administrative responsibilities under TRICARE/CHAMPVA; to the Dept. of Justice for representation of the Secretary of Defense in civil actions; to the Internal Revenue Service, private collection agencies, and consumer reporting agencies in connection with recoupment claims; and to Congressional Offices in response to inquiries made at the request of the person to whom a record pertains. Appropriate disclosures may be made to other federal, state, local, foreign government agencies, private business entities, and individual providers of care, on matters relating to entitlement, claims adjudication, fraud, program abuse, utilization review, quality assurance, peer review, program integrity, third-party liability, coordination of benefits, and civil and criminal litigation related to the operation of TRICARE.

DISCLOSURES: Voluntary; however, failure to provide information will result in delay in payment or may result in denial of claim. With the one exception discussed below, there are no penalties under these programs for refusing to supply information. However, failure to furnish information regarding the medical services rendered or the amount charged would prevent payment of claims under these programs. Failure to furnish any other information, such as name or claim number, would delay payment of the claim. Failure to provide medical information under FECA could be deemed an obstruction.

It is mandatory that you tell us if you know that another party is responsible for paying for your treatment. Section 1128B of the Social Security Act and 31 USC 3801-3812 provide penalties for withholding this information.

You should be aware that P.L. 100-503, the "Computer Matching and Privacy Protection Act of 1988," permits the government to verify information by way of computer matches.

MEDICAID PAYMENTS (PROVIDER CERTIFICATION)

I hereby agree to keep such records as are necessary to disclose fully the extent of services provided to individuals under the State's Title XIX plan and to furnish information regarding any payments claimed for providing such services as the State Agency or Dept. of Health and Humans Services may request.

I further agree to accept, as payment in full, the amount paid by the Medicaid program for those claims submitted for payment under that program, with the exception of authorized deductible, coinsurance, co-payment or similar cost-sharing charge.

SIGNATURE OF PHYSICIAN (OR SUPPLIER): I certify that the services listed above were medically indicated and necessary to the health of this patient and were personally furnished by me or my employee under my personal direction.

NOTICE: This is to certify that the foregoing information is true, accurate and complete. I understand that payment and satisfaction of this claim will be
          from Federal and State funds, and that any false claims, statements, or documents, or concealment of a material fact, may be prosecuted under applicable Federal or State laws.

Public reporting burden for this collection of information is estimated to average 15 minutes per response, including time for reviewing instructions, searching existing date sources, gathering and maintaining data needed, and completing and reviewing the collection of information. Send comments regarding this burden estimate or any other aspect of this collection of information, including suggestions for reducing the burden, to CMS, Office of Financial Management, P.O. Box 26684, Baltimore, MD 21207; and to the Office of Management and Budget, Paperwork Reduction Project (OMB-0938-0008), Washington, D.C. 20503.

FIGURE 7-4 Back side of the CMS-1500 (08-05) Health Insurance Claim Form approved by the American Medical Association's Council on Medical Service.

MEDICAID
No secondary coverage

1. MEDICARE	MEDICAID	TRICARE CHAMPUS	CHAMPVA	GROUP HEALTH PLAN	FECA BLK LUNG	OTHER	1a. INSURED'S I.D. NUMBER (For Program in Item 1)
☐ (Medicare #)	X (Medicaid #)	☐ (Sponsor's SSN)	☐ (Member ID#)	☐ (SSN or ID)	☐ (SSN)	☐ (ID)	276835090

2. PATIENT'S NAME (Last Name, First Name, Middle Initial) ABRAMSON ADAM	3. PATIENT'S BIRTH DATE MM 02 DD 12 YY 1995 SEX M X F ☐
	4. INSURED'S NAME (Last Name, First Name, Middle Initial)

5. PATIENT'S ADDRESS (No., Street) 760 FINCH STREET	6. PATIENT RELATIONSHIP TO INSURED Self ☐ Spouse ☐ Child ☐ Other ☐
	7. INSURED'S ADDRESS (No., Street)

CITY WOODLAND HILLS	STATE XY	8. PATIENT STATUS Single ☐ Married ☐ Other ☐

CITY		STATE

ZIP CODE 12345 TELEPHONE (Include Area Code) (555) 482 6789	Employed ☐ Full-Time Student ☐ Part-Time Student ☐
	ZIP CODE TELEPHONE (INCLUDE AREA CODE) ( )

9. OTHER INSURED'S NAME (Last Name, First Name, Middle Initial)	10. IS PATIENT'S CONDITION RELATED TO:
	11. INSURED'S POLICY GROUP OR FECA NUMBER
a. OTHER INSURED'S POLICY OR GROUP NUMBER	a. EMPLOYMENT? (CURRENT OR PREVIOUS) ☐ YES X NO
	a. INSURED'S DATE OF BIRTH MM DD YY SEX M ☐ F ☐
b. OTHER INSURED'S DATE OF BIRTH MM DD YY SEX M ☐ F ☐	b. AUTO ACCIDENT? PLACE (State) ☐ YES X NO ☐
	b. EMPLOYER'S NAME OR SCHOOL NAME
c. EMPLOYER'S NAME OR SCHOOL NAME	c. OTHER ACCIDENT? X YES ☐ NO
	c. INSURANCE PLAN NAME OR PROGRAM NAME
d. INSURANCE PLAN NAME OR PROGRAM NAME	10d. RESERVED FOR LOCAL USE
	d. IS THERE ANOTHER HEALTH BENEFIT PLAN? ☐ YES ☐ NO If yes, return to and complete item 9 a-d.

READ BACK OF FORM BEFORE COMPLETING & SIGNING THIS FORM.

12. PATIENT'S OR AUTHORIZED PERSON'S SIGNATURE I authorize the release of any medical or other information necessary to process this claim. I also request payment of government benefits either to myself or to the party who accepts assignment below. SIGNED _____ DATE _____	13. INSURED'S OR AUTHORIZED PERSON'S SIGNATURE I authorize payment of medical benefits to the undersigned physician or supplier for services described below. SIGNED _____

14. DATE OF CURRENT: MM DD YY ◄ ILLNESS (First symptom) OR INJURY (Accident) OR PREGNANCY(LMP)	15. IF PATIENT HAS HAD SAME OR SIMILAR ILLNESS. GIVE FIRST DATE MM DD YY
	16. DATES PATIENT UNABLE TO WORK IN CURRENT OCCUPATION FROM MM DD YY TO MM DD YY
17. NAME OF REFERRING PHYSICIAN OR OTHER SOURCE 17a. 17b. NPI	18. HOSPITALIZATION DATES RELATED TO CURRENT SERVICES FROM MM DD YY TO MM DD YY
19. RESERVED FOR LOCAL USE	20. OUTSIDE LAB? ☐ YES X NO $ CHARGES

21. DIAGNOSIS OR NATURE OF ILLNESS OR INJURY. (RELATE ITEMS 1,2,3 OR 4 TO ITEM 24E BY LINE) 1. 931 . __ 3. __ . __ 2. __ . __ 4. __ . __	22. MEDICAID RESUBMISSION CODE ORIGINAL REF. NO.
	23. PRIOR AUTHORIZATION NUMBER

A. DATE(S) OF SERVICE From MM DD YY	To MM DD YY	B. PLACE OF SERVICE	C. EMG	D. PROCEDURES, SERVICES, OR SUPPLIES (Explain Unusual Circumstances) CPT/HCPCS	MODIFIER	E. DIAGNOSIS POINTER	F. $ CHARGES	G. DAYS OR UNITS	H. EPSDT Family Plan	I. ID. QUAL.	J. RENDERING PROVIDER ID. #
1 07 14 XX		23	Y	99282		1	37 00	1		NPI	37640017XX
2 07 04 XX		23	Y	69200		1	49 00	1		NPI	37640017XX
3										NPI	
4										NPI	
5										NPI	
6										NPI	

25. FEDERAL TAX I.D. NUMBER XX12210XX SSN ☐ EIN X	26. PATIENT'S ACCOUNT NO. 030	27. ACCEPT ASSIGNMENT? (For govt. claims, see back) X YES ☐ NO	28. TOTAL CHARGE $ 86 00	29. AMOUNT PAID $	30. BALANCE DUE $ 86 00

31. SIGNATURE OF PHYSICIAN OR SUPPLIER INCLUDING DEGREES OR CREDENTIALS (I certify that the statements on the reverse apply to this bill and are made a part thereof.) PEDRO ATRICS MD 071420XX SIGNED Pedro Atrics MD DATE	32. SERVICE FACILITY LOCATION INFORMATION COLLEGE HOSPITAL 4500 BROAD AVENUE WOODLAND HILLS XY 12345 0001 a. HSC 43700F b.	33. BILLING PROVIDER INFO & PH # (555) 486 9002 COLLEGE CLINIC 4567 BROAD AVENUE WOODLAND HILLS XY 12345 0001 a. 3664021CC b.

reference initials

FIGURE 7-5 A Medicaid case with no secondary coverage emphasizing basic elements and screened blocks that do not require completion.

FIGURE 7-6 Example of a completed CMS-1500 (08-05) Health Insurance Claim Form for a basic Medicare case with no other insurance coverage. The physician has accepted assignment. Screened blocks should not be completed for a Medicare case with no other insurance.

MEDICARE/MEDICAID
(primary) (secondary)
Crossover claim

1. MEDICARE [X] (Medicare #) MEDICAID [X] (Medicaid #) TRICARE CHAMPUS (Sponsor's SSN) CHAMPVA (Member ID#) GROUP HEALTH PLAN (SSN or ID) FECA BLK LUNG (SSN) OTHER (ID)	1a. INSURED'S I.D. NUMBER (For Program in Item 1) 660 XX 2715A
2. PATIENT'S NAME (Last Name, First Name, Middle Initial) JOHNSON KATHRYN	3. PATIENT'S BIRTH DATE MM 09 DD 07 YY 1937 SEX M [ ] F [X]	4. INSURED'S NAME (Last Name, First Name, Middle Initial)
5. PATIENT'S ADDRESS (No., Street) 218 VEGA DRIVE	6. PATIENT RELATIONSHIP TO INSURED Self [ ] Spouse [ ] Child [ ] Other [ ]	7. INSURED'S ADDRESS (No., Street)
CITY WOODLAND HILLS STATE XY	8. PATIENT STATUS Single [ ] Married [X] Other [ ]	CITY STATE
ZIP CODE 12345 TELEPHONE (Include Area Code) (555) 482 9112	Employed [ ] Full-Time Student [ ] Part-Time Student [ ]	ZIP CODE TELEPHONE (INCLUDE AREA CODE) ( )
9. OTHER INSURED'S NAME (Last Name, First Name, Middle Initial)	10. IS PATIENT'S CONDITION RELATED TO:	11. INSURED'S POLICY GROUP OR FECA NUMBER NONE
a. OTHER INSURED'S POLICY OR GROUP NUMBER	a. EMPLOYMENT? (CURRENT OR PREVIOUS) YES [ ] NO [X]	a. INSURED'S DATE OF BIRTH MM DD YY SEX M [ ] F [ ]
b. OTHER INSURED'S DATE OF BIRTH MM DD YY SEX M [ ] F [ ]	b. AUTO ACCIDENT? PLACE (State) YES [ ] NO [X]	b. EMPLOYER'S NAME OR SCHOOL NAME
c. EMPLOYER'S NAME OR SCHOOL NAME	c. OTHER ACCIDENT? YES [ ] NO [X]	c. INSURANCE PLAN NAME OR PROGRAM NAME
d. INSURANCE PLAN NAME OR PROGRAM NAME	10d. RESERVED FOR LOCAL USE MCD016745289	d. IS THERE ANOTHER HEALTH BENEFIT PLAN? YES [ ] NO [ ] If yes, return to and complete item 9 a-d.

READ BACK OF FORM BEFORE COMPLETING & SIGNING THIS FORM.

12. PATIENT'S OR AUTHORIZED PERSON'S SIGNATURE I authorize the release of any medical or other information necessary to process this claim. I also request payment of government benefits either to myself or to the party who accepts assignment below.

SIGNED *Kathryn Johnson* DATE 10/1/XX

13. INSURED'S OR AUTHORIZED PERSON'S SIGNATURE I authorize payment of medical benefits to the undersigned physician or supplier for services described below.

SIGNED

14. DATE OF CURRENT: ILLNESS (First symptom) OR INJURY (Accident) OR PREGNANCY(LMP) MM DD YY	15. IF PATIENT HAS HAD SAME OR SIMILAR ILLNESS. GIVE FIRST DATE MM DD YY	16. DATES PATIENT UNABLE TO WORK IN CURRENT OCCUPATION FROM MM DD YY TO MM DD YY
17. NAME OF REFERRING PHYSICIAN OR OTHER SOURCE BRADY COCCIDIOIDES MD	17a. 17b. NPI 64211067XX	18. HOSPITALIZATION DATES RELATED TO CURRENT SERVICES FROM MM DD YY TO MM DD YY
19. RESERVED FOR LOCAL USE		20. OUTSIDE LAB? YES [ ] NO [X] $ CHARGES
21. DIAGNOSIS OR NATURE OF ILLNESS OR INJURY. (RELATE ITEMS 1,2,3 OR 4 TO ITEM 24E BY LINE) 1. 172.7 3. 2. 4.		22. MEDICAID RESUBMISSION CODE ORIGINAL REF. NO.
		23. PRIOR AUTHORIZATION NUMBER 7680560012

24. A. DATE(S) OF SERVICE From MM DD YY To MM DD YY	B. PLACE OF SERVICE	C. EMG	D. PROCEDURES, SERVICES, OR SUPPLIES (Explain Unusual Circumstances) CPT/HCPCS MODIFIER	E. DIAGNOSIS POINTER	F. $ CHARGES	G. DAYS OR UNITS	H. EPSDT Family Plan	I. ID. QUAL.	J. RENDERING PROVIDER ID. #
1 10 01 XX	24		11600	1	195 00	1		NPI	50307117XX
2								NPI	
3								NPI	
4								NPI	
5								NPI	
6								NPI	

25. FEDERAL TAX I.D. NUMBER SSN [ ] EIN [X] XX12210XX	26. PATIENT'S ACCOUNT NO. 050	27. ACCEPT ASSIGNMENT? (For govt. claims, see back) [X] YES [ ] NO	28. TOTAL CHARGE $ 195 00	29. AMOUNT PAID $	30. BALANCE DUE $
31. SIGNATURE OF PHYSICIAN OR SUPPLIER INCLUDING DEGREES OR CREDENTIALS (I certify that the statements on the reverse apply to this bill and are made a part thereof.) COSMO GRAFF MD 100320XX SIGNED *Cosmo Graff, MD* DATE	32. SERVICE FACILITY LOCATION INFORMATION WOODLAND HILLS AMBULATORY CENTER 1229 CENTER STREET WOODLAND HILLS XY 12345 0001 a. X950513700 b.	33. BILLING PROVIDER INFO & PH # (555)486 9002 COLLEGE CLINIC 4567 BROAD AVENUE WOODLAND HILLS XY 12345 0001 a. 3664021CC b.

reference initials

FIGURE 7-7 Example of a Medicare/Medicaid crossover claim. The CMS-1500 (08-05) claim form is sent to Medicare (primary payer) and then processed automatically by Medicaid (secondary payer). Screened blocks should not be completed for this type of case.

MEDICARE/MEDIGAP
(primary) (secondary)
Crossover claim

1. MEDICARE MEDICAID TRICARE CHAMPUS CHAMPVA GROUP HEALTH PLAN FECA BLK LUNG OTHER	1a. INSURED'S I.D. NUMBER (For Program in Item 1)
X (Medicare #) ☐ (Medicaid #) ☐ (Sponsor's SSN) ☐ (Member ID#) X (SSN or ID) ☐ (SSN) ☐ (ID)	419 XX 7272A

2. PATIENT'S NAME (Last Name, First Name, Middle Initial)	3. PATIENT'S BIRTH DATE MM 08 DD 29 YY 1917 SEX M [X] F ☐	4. INSURED'S NAME (Last Name, First Name, Middle Initial)
BARNES AGUSTA E		

5. PATIENT'S ADDRESS (No., Street)	6. PATIENT RELATIONSHIP TO INSURED	7. INSURED'S ADDRESS (No., Street)
356 ENCINA AVENUE	Self ☐ Spouse ☐ Child ☐ Other ☐	

CITY WOODLAND HILLS	STATE XY	8. PATIENT STATUS Single [X] Married ☐ Other ☐	CITY	STATE

ZIP CODE 12345 0000	TELEPHONE (Include Area Code) (555) 467 2646	Employed ☐ Full-Time Student ☐ Part-Time Student ☐	ZIP CODE	TELEPHONE (INCLUDE AREA CODE) ( )

9. OTHER INSURED'S NAME (Last Name, First Name, Middle Initial) SAME	10. IS PATIENT'S CONDITION RELATED TO:	11. INSURED'S POLICY GROUP OR FECA NUMBER NONE
a. OTHER INSURED'S POLICY OR GROUP NUMBER MEDIGAP 419167272	a. EMPLOYMENT? (CURRENT OR PREVIOUS) YES ☐ X NO	a. INSURED'S DATE OF BIRTH MM DD YY SEX M ☐ F ☐
b. OTHER INSURED'S DATE OF BIRTH MM DD YY SEX M ☐ F ☐	b. AUTO ACCIDENT? PLACE (State) YES ☐ X NO	b. EMPLOYER'S NAME OR SCHOOL NAME
c. EMPLOYER'S NAME OR SCHOOL NAME	c. OTHER ACCIDENT? YES ☐ X NO	c. INSURANCE PLAN NAME OR PROGRAM NAME
d. INSURANCE PLAN NAME OR PROGRAM NAME CALFCA002	10d. RESERVED FOR LOCAL USE	d. IS THERE ANOTHER HEALTH BENEFIT PLAN? YES ☐ NO ☐ If yes, return to and complete item 9 a-d.

READ BACK OF FORM BEFORE COMPLETING & SIGNING THIS FORM.

12. PATIENT'S OR AUTHORIZED PERSON'S SIGNATURE I authorize the release of any medical or other information necessary to process this claim. I also request payment of government benefits either to myself or to the party who accepts assignment below. SIGNED *Agusta E. Barnes* DATE *11/21/XX*	13. INSURED'S OR AUTHORIZED PERSON'S SIGNATURE I authorize payment of medical benefits to the undersigned physician or supplier for services described below. SIGNED *Agusta E. Barnes*

14. DATE OF CURRENT: ILLNESS (First symptom) OR INJURY (Accident) OR PREGNANCY(LMP) MM DD YY	15. IF PATIENT HAS HAD SAME OR SIMILAR ILLNESS. GIVE FIRST DATE MM DD YY	16. DATES PATIENT UNABLE TO WORK IN CURRENT OCCUPATION FROM MM DD YY TO MM DD YY

17. NAME OF REFERRING PHYSICIAN OR OTHER SOURCE GASTON INPUT MD	17a. 17b. NPI 32783127XX	18. HOSPITALIZATION DATES RELATED TO CURRENT SERVICES FROM MM DD YY TO MM DD YY

19. RESERVED FOR LOCAL USE	20. OUTSIDE LAB? $ CHARGES YES ☐ X NO

21. DIAGNOSIS OR NATURE OF ILLNESS OR INJURY. (RELATE ITEMS 1,2,3 OR 4 TO ITEM 24E BY LINE) 1. 78659 3.	22. MEDICAID RESUBMISSION CODE ORIGINAL REF. NO.
2. 4.	23. PRIOR AUTHORIZATION NUMBER

24. A. DATE(S) OF SERVICE From MM DD YY To MM DD YY	B. PLACE OF SERVICE	C. EMG	D. PROCEDURES, SERVICES, OR SUPPLIES (Explain Unusual Circumstances) CPT/HCPCS MODIFIER	E. DIAGNOSIS POINTER	F. $ CHARGES	G. DAYS OR UNITS	H. EPSDT Family Plan	I. ID. QUAL.	J. RENDERING PROVIDER ID. #
1 11 21 XX	11		93350	1	183 00	1		NPI	67805027XX
2 11 21 XX	11		93017	1	68 00	1		NPI	67805027XX
3								NPI	
4								NPI	
5								NPI	
6								NPI	

25. FEDERAL TAX I.D. NUMBER SSN EIN ☐	26. PATIENT'S ACCOUNT NO. 060	27. ACCEPT ASSIGNMENT? (For govt. claims, see back) X YES ☐ NO	28. TOTAL CHARGE $ 251 00	29. AMOUNT PAID $	30. BALANCE DUE $

31. SIGNATURE OF PHYSICIAN OR SUPPLIER INCLUDING DEGREES OR CREDENTIALS (I certify that the statements on the reverse apply to this bill and are made a part thereof.) PERRY CARDI MD SIGNED *Perry Cardi, MD* DATE 112220XX	32. SERVICE FACILITY LOCATION INFORMATION a. b.	33. BILLING PROVIDER INFO & PH # (555)486 9002 COLLEGE CLINIC 4567 BROAD AVENUE WOODLAND HILLS XY 12345 0001 a. 3664021CC b.

reference initials

FIGURE 7-8 Example of a completed CMS-1500 (08-05) Health Insurance Claim Form for a Medicare (primary) and Medigap (secondary) crossover claim. Shaded blocks should not be completed for this type of case.

OTHER INSURANCE/MEDICARE-MSP
(primary)   (secondary)

1. MEDICARE	MEDICAID	TRICARE CHAMPUS	CHAMPVA	GROUP HEALTH PLAN	FECA BLK LUNG	OTHER	1a. INSURED'S I.D. NUMBER	(For Program in Item 1)
[X] (Medicare #)	[ ] (Medicaid #)	[ ] (Sponsor's SSN)	[ ] (Member ID#)	[X] (SSN or ID)	[ ] (SSN)	[ ] (ID)	609 XX 5523A	

2. PATIENT'S NAME (Last Name, First Name, Middle Initial)	3. PATIENT'S BIRTH DATE	SEX	4. INSURED'S NAME (Last Name, First Name, Middle Initial)
BLAIR GWENDOLYN	09 01 1931 M [ ]	F [X]	BLAIR GWENDOLYN

5. PATIENT'S ADDRESS (No., Street)	6. PATIENT RELATIONSHIP TO INSURED	7. INSURED'S ADDRESS (No., Street)
416 RICHMOND STREET	Self [X] Spouse [ ] Child [ ] Other [ ]	SAME

CITY	STATE	8. PATIENT STATUS	CITY	STATE
WOODLAND HILLS	XY	Single [ ] Married [X] Other [ ]		

ZIP CODE	TELEPHONE (Include Area Code)		ZIP CODE	TELEPHONE (INCLUDE AREA CODE)
12345 0000	(555) 459 1519	Employed [X] Full-Time Student [ ] Part-Time Student [ ]		( )

9. OTHER INSURED'S NAME (Last Name, First Name, Middle Initial)	10. IS PATIENT'S CONDITION RELATED TO:	11. INSURED'S POLICY GROUP OR FECA NUMBER
		7845931Q

a. OTHER INSURED'S POLICY OR GROUP NUMBER	a. EMPLOYMENT? (CURRENT OR PREVIOUS)	a. INSURED'S DATE OF BIRTH	SEX
	YES [ ] NO [X]	MM DD YY M [ ]	F [ ]

b. OTHER INSURED'S DATE OF BIRTH	SEX	b. AUTO ACCIDENT? PLACE (State)	b. EMPLOYER'S NAME OR SCHOOL NAME
MM DD YY M [ ] F [ ]		YES [ ] NO [X]	CITY LIBRARY

c. EMPLOYER'S NAME OR SCHOOL NAME	c. OTHER ACCIDENT?	c. INSURANCE PLAN NAME OR PROGRAM NAME
	YES [ ] NO [X]	ABC INSURANCE COMPANY

d. INSURANCE PLAN NAME OR PROGRAM NAME	10d. RESERVED FOR LOCAL USE	d. IS THERE ANOTHER HEALTH BENEFIT PLAN?
		YES [ ] NO [ ] *If yes*, return to and complete item 9 a-d.

READ BACK OF FORM BEFORE COMPLETING & SIGNING THIS FORM.

12. PATIENT'S OR AUTHORIZED PERSON'S SIGNATURE I authorize the release of any medical or other information necessary to process this claim. I also request payment of government benefits either to myself or to the party who accepts assignment below.	13. INSURED'S OR AUTHORIZED PERSON'S SIGNATURE I authorize payment of medical benefits to the undersigned physician or supplier for services described below.
SIGNED SIGNATURE ON FILE DATE	SIGNED SIGNATURE ON FILE

14. DATE OF CURRENT: ILLNESS (First symptom) OR INJURY (Accident) OR PREGNANCY(LMP) MM DD YY	15. IF PATIENT HAS HAD SAME OR SIMILAR ILLNESS. GIVE FIRST DATE MM DD YY	16. DATES PATIENT UNABLE TO WORK IN CURRENT OCCUPATION MM DD YY MM DD YY FROM TO

17. NAME OF REFERRING PHYSICIAN OR OTHER SOURCE	17a.	18. HOSPITALIZATION DATES RELATED TO CURRENT SERVICES MM DD YY MM DD YY
GERALD PRACTON MD	17b. NPI 46278897XX	FROM TO

19. RESERVED FOR LOCAL USE	20. OUTSIDE LAB? $ CHARGES
	YES [ ] NO [X]

21. DIAGNOSIS OR NATURE OF ILLNESS OR INJURY. (RELATE ITEMS 1,2,3 OR 4 TO ITEM 24E BY LINE)	22. MEDICAID RESUBMISSION CODE ORIGINAL REF. NO.
1. 110 1 3. ___ . ___	
2. ___ . ___ 4. ___ . ___	23. PRIOR AUTHORIZATION NUMBER

24. A. DATE(S) OF SERVICE From — To MM DD YY MM DD YY	B. PLACE OF SERVICE	C. EMG	D. PROCEDURES, SERVICES, OR SUPPLIES (Explain Unusual Circumstances) CPT/HCPCS MODIFIER	E. DIAGNOSIS POINTER	F. $ CHARGES	G. DAYS OR UNITS	H. EPSDT Family Plan	I. ID. QUAL.	J. RENDERING PROVIDER ID. #
1	03 15 XX	11		99243 25	1	103 00	1		NPI	54022287XX
2	03 15 XX	11		11750	1	193 00	1		NPI	54022287XX
3									NPI	
4									NPI	
5									NPI	
6									NPI	

25. FEDERAL TAX I.D. NUMBER SSN EIN	26. PATIENT'S ACCOUNT NO.	27. ACCEPT ASSIGNMENT? (For govt. claims, see back)	28. TOTAL CHARGE	29. AMOUNT PAID	30. BALANCE DUE
XX12210XX [X]	070	[X] YES [ ] NO	$ 296 00	$ 100 00	$

31. SIGNATURE OF PHYSICIAN OR SUPPLIER INCLUDING DEGREES OR CREDENTIALS (I certify that the statements on the reverse apply to this bill and are made a part thereof.)	32. SERVICE FACILITY LOCATION INFORMATION	33. BILLING PROVIDER INFO & PH # (555)486 9002
NICK PEDRO DPM 031620XX		COLLEGE CLINIC
SIGNED *Nick Pedro, DPM* DATE	a. b.	4567 BROAD AVENUE
	a. 3664021CC b.	WOODLAND HILLS XY 12345 0001

reference initials

FIGURE 7-9 Template for a case in which another insurance carrier is the primary payer and Medicare is the secondary payer (MSP).

TRICARE
No secondary coverage

1. MEDICARE (Medicare #) ☐ MEDICAID (Medicaid #) ☐ TRICARE CHAMPUS (Sponsor's SSN) ☒ CHAMPVA (Member ID#) ☐ GROUP HEALTH PLAN (SSN or ID) ☐ FECA BLK LUNG (SSN) ☐ OTHER (ID) ☐	1a. INSURED'S I.D. NUMBER (For Program in Item 1) 581147211
2. PATIENT'S NAME (Last Name, First Name, Middle Initial) SMITH SUSAN J	3. PATIENT'S BIRTH DATE 03 16 1976 SEX M ☐ F ☒	4. INSURED'S NAME (Last Name, First Name, Middle Initial) SMITH WILLIAM D
5. PATIENT'S ADDRESS (No., Street) 420 MAPLE STREET	6. PATIENT RELATIONSHIP TO INSURED Self ☐ Spouse ☒ Child ☐ Other ☐	7. INSURED'S ADDRESS (No., Street) SAME
CITY WOODLAND HILLS STATE XY	8. PATIENT STATUS Single ☐ Married ☒ Other ☐	CITY STATE
ZIP CODE 12345 0000 TELEPHONE (Include Area Code) (555) 789 9898	Employed ☐ Full-Time Student ☐ Part-Time Student ☐	ZIP CODE TELEPHONE (INCLUDE AREA CODE) ( )
9. OTHER INSURED'S NAME (Last Name, First Name, Middle Initial)	10. IS PATIENT'S CONDITION RELATED TO:	11. INSURED'S POLICY GROUP OR FECA NUMBER
a. OTHER INSURED'S POLICY OR GROUP NUMBER	a. EMPLOYMENT? (CURRENT OR PREVIOUS) YES ☐ NO ☒	a. INSURED'S DATE OF BIRTH 06 12 1974 SEX M ☒ F ☐
b. OTHER INSURED'S DATE OF BIRTH MM DD YY SEX M ☐ F ☐	b. AUTO ACCIDENT? PLACE (State) YES ☐ NO ☒	b. EMPLOYER'S NAME OR SCHOOL NAME USN
c. EMPLOYER'S NAME OR SCHOOL NAME	c. OTHER ACCIDENT? YES ☐ NO ☒	c. INSURANCE PLAN NAME OR PROGRAM NAME TRICARE/CHAMPUS
d. INSURANCE PLAN NAME OR PROGRAM NAME	10d. RESERVED FOR LOCAL USE	d. IS THERE ANOTHER HEALTH BENEFIT PLAN? YES ☐ NO ☒ If yes, return to and complete item 9 a-d.
READ BACK OF FORM BEFORE COMPLETING & SIGNING THIS FORM. 12. PATIENT'S OR AUTHORIZED PERSON'S SIGNATURE I authorize the release of any medical or other information necessary to process this claim. I also request payment of government benefits either to myself or to the party who accepts assignment below. SIGNED SIGNATURE ON FILE DATE	13. INSURED'S OR AUTHORIZED PERSON'S SIGNATURE I authorize payment of medical benefits to the undersigned physician or supplier for services described below. SIGNED

14. DATE OF CURRENT: ILLNESS (First symptom) OR INJURY (Accident) OR PREGNANCY(LMP) 10 28 20XX	15. IF PATIENT HAS HAD SAME OR SIMILAR ILLNESS. GIVE FIRST DATE MM DD YY	16. DATES PATIENT UNABLE TO WORK IN CURRENT OCCUPATION FROM 07 21 20XX TO 09 17 20XX
17. NAME OF REFERRING PHYSICIAN OR OTHER SOURCE ADAM LANGERHANS MD	17a. 17b. NPI 47680657XX	18. HOSPITALIZATION DATES RELATED TO CURRENT SERVICES FROM 08 06 20XX TO 08 08 20XX
19. RESERVED FOR LOCAL USE		20. OUTSIDE LAB? YES ☐ NO ☒ $ CHARGES
21. DIAGNOSIS OR NATURE OF ILLNESS OR INJURY. (RELATE ITEMS 1,2,3 OR 4 TO ITEM 24E BY LINE) 1. 650 3. 2. 4.		22. MEDICAID RESUBMISSION CODE ORIGINAL REF. NO. 23. PRIOR AUTHORIZATION NUMBER

24. A. DATE(S) OF SERVICE From / To MM DD YY	B. PLACE OF SERVICE	C. EMG	D. PROCEDURES, SERVICES, OR SUPPLIES CPT/HCPCS MODIFIER	E. DIAGNOSIS POINTER	F. $ CHARGES	G. DAYS OR UNITS	H. EPSDT	I. ID. QUAL.	J. RENDERING PROVIDER ID. #
1 08 06 XX	21		59400	1	1864 00	1		NPI	43056757XX
2								NPI	
3								NPI	
4								NPI	
5								NPI	
6								NPI	

25. FEDERAL TAX I.D. NUMBER SSN EIN XX12210XX ☒	26. PATIENT'S ACCOUNT NO. 080	27. ACCEPT ASSIGNMENT? YES ☒ NO ☐	28. TOTAL CHARGE $ 1864 00	29. AMOUNT PAID $	30. BALANCE DUE $ 1864 00
31. SIGNATURE OF PHYSICIAN OR SUPPLIER INCLUDING DEGREES OR CREDENTIALS (I certify that the statements on the reverse apply to this bill and are made a part thereof.) BERTHA CAESAR MD 081020XX SIGNED *Bertha Caesar, MD* DATE	32. SERVICE FACILITY LOCATION INFORMATION COLLEGE HOSPITAL 4500 BROAD AVENUE WOODLAND HILLS XY 12345 0001 a. X950731067 b.		33. BILLING PROVIDER INFO & PH # (555)486 9002 COLLEGE CLINIC 4567 BROAD AVENUE WOODLAND HILLS XY 12345 0001 a. 3664021CC b.		

reference initials

FIGURE 7-10 Example of a completed CMS-1500 (08-05) claim form, used when billing for professional services rendered in a TRICARE Standard case. Screened blocks should not be completed for this type of case.

CHAMPVA
No secondary coverage

1. MEDICARE ☐ (Medicare #) MEDICAID ☐ (Medicaid #) TRICARE CHAMPUS ☐ (Sponsor's SSN) CHAMPVA ☒ (Member ID#) GROUP HEALTH PLAN ☐ (SSN or ID) FECA BLK LUNG ☐ (SSN) OTHER ☐ (ID)	**1a.** INSURED'S I.D. NUMBER (For Program in Item 1) 560 XX 4444
2. PATIENT'S NAME (Last Name, First Name, Middle Initial) DEXTER BRUCE R	**3.** PATIENT'S BIRTH DATE MM 03 DD 13 YY 1934 SEX M ☒ F ☐	**4.** INSURED'S NAME (Last Name, First Name, Middle Initial) DEXTER BRUCE R
5. PATIENT'S ADDRESS (No., Street) 226 IRWIN ROAD	**6.** PATIENT RELATIONSHIP TO INSURED Self ☒ Spouse ☐ Child ☐ Other ☐	**7.** INSURED'S ADDRESS (No., Street) SAME
CITY WOODLAND HILLS STATE XY	**8.** PATIENT STATUS Single ☒ Married ☐ Other ☐	CITY STATE
ZIP CODE 12345 0000 TELEPHONE (Include Area Code) (555) 497 1338	Employed ☐ Full-Time Student ☐ Part-Time Student ☐	ZIP CODE TELEPHONE (INCLUDE AREA CODE) ( )
9. OTHER INSURED'S NAME (Last Name, First Name, Middle Initial)	**10.** IS PATIENT'S CONDITION RELATED TO:	**11.** INSURED'S POLICY GROUP OR FECA NUMBER 023
a. OTHER INSURED'S POLICY OR GROUP NUMBER	**a.** EMPLOYMENT? (CURRENT OR PREVIOUS) YES ☒ NO ☐	**a.** INSURED'S DATE OF BIRTH MM DD YY SEX M ☐ F ☐
b. OTHER INSURED'S DATE OF BIRTH MM DD YY SEX M ☐ F ☐	**b.** AUTO ACCIDENT? PLACE (State) YES ☐ NO ☒	**b.** EMPLOYER'S NAME OR SCHOOL NAME USAF
c. EMPLOYER'S NAME OR SCHOOL NAME	**c.** OTHER ACCIDENT? YES ☐ NO ☒	**c.** INSURANCE PLAN NAME OR PROGRAM NAME
d. INSURANCE PLAN NAME OR PROGRAM NAME	**10d.** RESERVED FOR LOCAL USE	**d.** IS THERE ANOTHER HEALTH BENEFIT PLAN? YES ☐ NO ☒ *If yes*, return to and complete item 9 a-d.

READ BACK OF FORM BEFORE COMPLETING & SIGNING THIS FORM.

12. PATIENT'S OR AUTHORIZED PERSON'S SIGNATURE I authorize the release of any medical or other information necessary to process this claim. I also request payment of government benefits either to myself or to the party who accepts assignment below.

SIGNED SIGNATURE ON FILE   DATE

13. INSURED'S OR AUTHORIZED PERSON'S SIGNATURE I authorize payment of medical benefits to the undersigned physician or supplier for services described below.

SIGNED

14. DATE OF CURRENT: MM DD YY ILLNESS (First symptom) OR INJURY (Accident) OR PREGNANCY(LMP)	**15.** IF PATIENT HAS HAD SAME OR SIMILAR ILLNESS. GIVE FIRST DATE MM DD YY	**16.** DATES PATIENT UNABLE TO WORK IN CURRENT OCCUPATION MM DD YY FROM TO MM DD YY
17. NAME OF REFERRING PHYSICIAN OR OTHER SOURCE GERALD PRACTON MD	**17a.** **17b.** NPI 46278897XX	**18.** HOSPITALIZATION DATES RELATED TO CURRENT SERVICES MM DD YY FROM 07 29 20XX TO 07 31 20XX
19. RESERVED FOR LOCAL USE		**20.** OUTSIDE LAB? $ CHARGES YES ☐ NO ☒
21. DIAGNOSIS OR NATURE OF ILLNESS OR INJURY. (RELATE ITEMS 1,2,3 OR 4 TO ITEM 24E BY LINE) 1. 600 .0 3. ___.___ 2. ___.___ 4. ___.___		**22.** MEDICAID RESUBMISSION CODE ORIGINAL REF. NO. **23.** PRIOR AUTHORIZATION NUMBER

24. A. DATE(S) OF SERVICE From MM DD YY	To MM DD YY	B. PLACE OF SERVICE	C. EMG	D. PROCEDURES, SERVICES, OR SUPPLIES (Explain Unusual Circumstances) CPT/HCPCS MODIFIER	E. DIAGNOSIS POINTER	F. $ CHARGES	G. DAYS OR UNITS	H. EPSDT Family Plan	I. ID. QUAL.	J. RENDERING PROVIDER ID. #
1 07 29 XX		21		52601	1	1193 00	1		NPI	25678831XX
2									NPI	
3									NPI	
4									NPI	
5									NPI	
6									NPI	

25. FEDERAL TAX I.D. NUMBER SSN ☐ EIN ☒ XX12210XX	**26.** PATIENT'S ACCOUNT NO. 090	**27.** ACCEPT ASSIGNMENT? (For govt. claims, see back) YES ☒ NO ☐	**28.** TOTAL CHARGE $ 1193 00 **29.** AMOUNT PAID $ **30.** BALANCE DUE $ 1193 00
31. SIGNATURE OF PHYSICIAN OR SUPPLIER INCLUDING DEGREES OR CREDENTIALS (I certify that the statements on the reverse apply to this bill and are made a part thereof.) GENE ULIBARRI MD 073020XX SIGNED *Gene Ulibarri MD* DATE	**32.** SERVICE FACILITY LOCATION INFORMATION COLLEGE HOSPITAL 4500 BROAD AVENUE WOODLAND HILLS XY 12345 0001 **a.** X950731067 **b.**		**33.** BILLING PROVIDER INFO & PH # (555)486 9002 COLLEGE CLINIC 4567 BROAD AVENUE WOODLAND HILLS XY 12345 0001 **a.** 3664021CC **b.**

reference initials

FIGURE 7-11 An example of a completed CMS-1500 (08-05) Health Insurance Claim Form for a CHAMPVA case with no secondary coverage. Screened blocks should not be completed for this type of case.

WORKERS' COMPENSATION

1. MEDICARE (Medicare #) **MEDICAID** (Medicaid #) **TRICARE CHAMPUS** (Sponsor's SSN) **CHAMPVA** (Member ID#) **GROUP HEALTH PLAN** (SSN or ID) **FECA BLK LUNG** (SSN) **OTHER** [X] (ID)	**1a. INSURED'S I.D. NUMBER** (For Program in Item 1) 667289

2. PATIENT'S NAME (Last Name, First Name, Middle Initial) BARTON PETER A	**3. PATIENT'S BIRTH DATE** MM 11 DD 14 YY 1976 **SEX** M [X] F	**4. INSURED'S NAME** (Last Name, First Name, Middle Initial) D F CONSTRUCTION
5. PATIENT'S ADDRESS (No., Street) 14890 DAISY AVENUE	**6. PATIENT RELATIONSHIP TO INSURED** Self [ ] Spouse [ ] Child [ ] Other [X]	**7. INSURED'S ADDRESS** (No., Street) 1212 HARDROCK PLACE
CITY WOODLAND HILLS **STATE** XY	**8. PATIENT STATUS** Single [ ] Married [ ] Other [ ]	**CITY** WOODLAND HILLS **STATE** XY
ZIP CODE 12345 0000 **TELEPHONE** (Include Area Code) (555) 427 7698	Employed [X] Full-Time Student [ ] Part-Time Student [ ]	**ZIP CODE** 12345 0000 **TELEPHONE** (INCLUDE AREA CODE) (555) 427 8200

9. OTHER INSURED'S NAME (Last Name, First Name, Middle Initial)	**10. IS PATIENT'S CONDITION RELATED TO:**	**11. INSURED'S POLICY GROUP OR FECA NUMBER**
a. OTHER INSURED'S POLICY OR GROUP NUMBER	**a. EMPLOYMENT?** (CURRENT OR PREVIOUS) [X] YES [ ] NO	**a. INSURED'S DATE OF BIRTH** MM DD YY **SEX** M [ ] F [ ]
b. OTHER INSURED'S DATE OF BIRTH MM DD YY **SEX** M [ ] F [ ]	**b. AUTO ACCIDENT?** PLACE (State) [ ] YES [X] NO	**b. EMPLOYER'S NAME OR SCHOOL NAME**
c. EMPLOYER'S NAME OR SCHOOL NAME	**c. OTHER ACCIDENT?** [ ] YES [X] NO	**c. INSURANCE PLAN NAME OR PROGRAM NAME**
d. INSURANCE PLAN NAME OR PROGRAM NAME	**10d. RESERVED FOR LOCAL USE**	**d. IS THERE ANOTHER HEALTH BENEFIT PLAN?** [ ] YES [ ] NO *If yes*, return to and complete item 9 a-d.

READ BACK OF FORM BEFORE COMPLETING & SIGNING THIS FORM.

12. PATIENT'S OR AUTHORIZED PERSON'S SIGNATURE I authorize the release of any medical or other information necessary to process this claim. I also request payment of government benefits either to myself or to the party who accepts assignment below. SIGNED _____ DATE _____	**13. INSURED'S OR AUTHORIZED PERSON'S SIGNATURE** I authorize payment of medical benefits to the undersigned physician or supplier for services described below. SIGNED _____

14. DATE OF CURRENT: MM 01 DD 04 YY 20XX ◄ ILLNESS (First symptom) OR INJURY (Accident) OR PREGNANCY(LMP)	**15. IF PATIENT HAS HAD SAME OR SIMILAR ILLNESS.** GIVE FIRST DATE MM DD YY	**16. DATES PATIENT UNABLE TO WORK IN CURRENT OCCUPATION** FROM MM 01 DD 04 YY 20XX TO MM 03 DD 27 YY 20XX
17. NAME OF REFERRING PHYSICIAN OR OTHER SOURCE	17a. 17b. NPI	**18. HOSPITALIZATION DATES RELATED TO CURRENT SERVICES** FROM MM DD YY TO MM DD YY
19. RESERVED FOR LOCAL USE		**20. OUTSIDE LAB?** [ ] YES [ ] NO $ CHARGES

21. DIAGNOSIS OR NATURE OF ILLNESS OR INJURY. (RELATE ITEMS 1,2,3 OR 4 TO ITEM 24E BY LINE) 1. 71831 3. _____ 2. _____ 4. _____	**22. MEDICAID RESUBMISSION** CODE _____ ORIGINAL REF. NO. _____ **23. PRIOR AUTHORIZATION NUMBER**

24. A. DATE(S) OF SERVICE From MM DD YY — To MM DD YY	B. PLACE OF SERVICE	C. EMG	D. PROCEDURES, SERVICES, OR SUPPLIES (Explain Unusual Circumstances) CPT/HCPCS	MODIFIER	E. DIAGNOSIS POINTER	F. $ CHARGES	G. DAYS OR UNITS	H. EPSDT Family Plan	I. ID. QUAL.	J. RENDERING PROVIDER ID. #
1 02 27 XX	11		29055		1	150 00	1		NPI	12678547XX
2									NPI	
3									NPI	
4									NPI	
5									NPI	
6									NPI	

25. FEDERAL TAX I.D. NUMBER XX12210XX SSN [ ] EIN [X]	**26. PATIENT'S ACCOUNT NO.** 100	**27. ACCEPT ASSIGNMENT?** (For govt. claims, see back) [ ] YES [ ] NO	**28. TOTAL CHARGE** $ 150 00	**29. AMOUNT PAID** $	**30. BALANCE DUE** $ 150 00

31. SIGNATURE OF PHYSICIAN OR SUPPLIER INCLUDING DEGREES OR CREDENTIALS (I certify that the statements on the reverse apply to this bill and are made a part thereof.) RAYMOND SKELTON MD 022820XX SIGNED *Raymond Skelton, MD* DATE	**32. SERVICE FACILITY LOCATION INFORMATION** a. b.	**33. BILLING PROVIDER INFO & PH #** (555) 486 9002 COLLEGE CLINIC 4567 BROAD AVENUE WOODLAND HILLS XY 12345 0001 a. 3664021CC b.

reference initials

FIGURE 7-12 An example of a completed CMS-1500 (08-05) Health Insurance Claim Form for a workers' compensation case. Screened blocks should not be completed for this type of case.

KEY TERMS*

Accredited Standards
   Committee X12
Accredited Standards
   Committee X12 Version 5010
application service provider
back up
batch
business associate agreement
cable modem
clearinghouse

code sets
covered entity
data elements
digital subscriber line
direct data entry
electronic data interchange
electronic funds transfer
electronic remittance advice
encoder
encryption

HIPAA Transaction and Code
   Set Rule
National Standard Format
password
real time
standard transactions
T-1
taxonomy codes
trading partner agreement

KEY ABBREVIATIONS*

ANSI	DSL	ePHI	PMS
ASC X12	EDI	ERA	TCS rule
ASET	EFT	HHS	UPS
ASP	EHR	IRS	
ATM	EMC	MTS	
DDE	EOMB	NSF	

*Definitions for the key terms and key abbreviations are located near the back of this textbook in the glossary.

Electronic Data Interchange: Transactions and Security

OBJECTIVES

After reading this chapter, you should be able to:

- Summarize advantages of electronic claim submission.
- Identify the transactions and code sets to use for insurance claims transmission.
- State which insurance claim data elements are required or situational for the 837P standard transaction format.
- Describe necessary components when adopting a practice management system.
- Describe the use of patient encounter forms and scannable encounter forms in electronic claim submission.
- Name some methods of interactive computer transactions for transmitting insurance claims.

- Explain the difference between carrier-direct and clearinghouse electronically transmitted insurance claims.
- List computer transmission problems that can occur.
- List HIPAA administrative safeguards for electronic protected health information.
- State technical and physical safeguards used to secure privacy of electronic mail, Internet, and instant messaging.
- Explain the handling of data storage and data disposal for good electronic records management.

ELECTRONIC DATA INTERCHANGE

Electronic data interchange (EDI) is the exchange of data in a standardized format through computer systems (e.g., health insurance claims). This is a process by which understandable data are sent back and forth via computer linkages between entities that function alternatively as sender and receiver. Technology and the use of EDI has made the processing of transactions more efficient and reduced administrative overhead costs in other industries. Electronic transmissions are sent encrypted so that they cannot be opened and read if intercepted (received) by the wrong individual. **Encryption** is used to assign a code to represent data and is done for security purposes. This

"secret code" makes data unintelligible to unauthorized parties. In encrypted (encoded) versions, the data look like gibberish to unauthorized users and must be decoded to use or read. In electronically secure environments, the sending computer system encrypts/encodes the data being sent and the receiving computer decodes the data to make them understandable. Therefore both computers must speak the same "language." Standardizing transaction and code sets is required to use EDI effectively, so the industry has witnessed the implementation of standard formats, procedures, and data content through Health Insurance Portability and Accountability Act (HIPAA) regulations.

Performance objectives, testing and review material, and hands-on practical exercises for this chapter are available in these resources

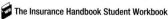 The Insurance Handbook Student Workbook   The Insurance Handbook Evolve Site

ELECTRONIC CLAIMS

An electronic claim, like a paper claim, is constructed from data that are used in the reimbursement process (the life cycle of a claim is discussed in Chapter 3). However, the method for submitting an electronic claim is by means of EDI rather than the United States (US) Postal Service ("snail mail") or paper fax transmission.

In the 1960s and early 1970s, large hospitals began submitting electronic claims for payment to third-party payers. Today, most health care providers submit electronic claims for reimbursement. As the Medicare program expanded, thereby increasing the number of covered individuals, the Centers for Medicaid and Medicare Services (CMS) began to emphasize electronic claims submission to reduce the number of paper claims and administrative costs. This system of transmission was practical only for hospitals and large medical practices because some carriers required 25 or more claims per batch. A **batch** is a group of claims for different patients sent at the same time from one facility.

ADVANTAGES OF ELECTRONIC CLAIM SUBMISSION

Nearly all insurance companies are required under HIPAA to participate in the electronic claim processing standards. Unlike paper claims, electronic transactions require no signature or stamp, no search for a third-party payer's address, no postage fees or trips to the post office, and no storage of claim forms in a file cabinet. Electronic transactions build an audit trail, a chronologic record of submitted data that can be traced to the source to determine the place of origin. Generally, cash flow is improved and less time is spent processing claims, thereby freeing staff for other duties. Information goes from one computer to another, which reduces overhead by decreasing labor costs and human error. After electronic submission of claims, payment can be received in 2 weeks or less. In comparison, when claims are completed manually and sent by mail, payment may take 4 to 6 weeks on average. With EDI, the audit trail offers a proof of receipt and is generated by the carrier, thus eliminating the potential for insurance payers to make the excuse that the claim was never received and therefore not processed.

Another important advantage of electronic claims submission is the online error-edit process that may be incorporated into the software in the physician's office, clearinghouse, or insurance company. This feature alerts the person processing the claim to any errors immediately so that a correction can be made before transmission of the claim. Information about problem claims can be telecommunicated immediately, allowing quicker submission of corrected or additional data.

Both paper and electronic claims begin with gathering data before, during, and after the service is rendered. You have learned that the information you need to obtain is crucial when submitting a paper claim for payment; therefore accurate information is key to successful electronic claim submission and timely reimbursement.

CLEARINGHOUSES

For a seamless business process, a **clearinghouse** is an entity that receives the electronic transmission of claims (EDI) from the health care provider's office and translates it into a standard format prescribed in HIPAA regulations. This HIPAA standard is readable by the processing parties (insurance payers) to complete the reimbursement cycle. The clearinghouse's duties include separating the claims by carrier, performing software edits on each claim to check for errors, and transmitting claims electronically to the correct insurance payer (Figure 8-1).

After receiving the claims transmission, a typical clearinghouse process works as follows:

- Claims are checked electronically (scrubbed) for missing or incorrect information using an elaborate editing process. Claims that do not meet all required data for further processing are rejected and not forwarded to the payer.
- Claims that are rejected during the editing process are electronically sent back to the health care provider along with a report that lists needed corrections.
- Groups of batches of claims that pass all edits are then sent to each separate insurance payer. Several claims can be submitted to various insurance payers in a single-batch electronic transmission.
- Once corrections are made, the claims can be resubmitted for processing and go through the same previous edits to ensure the correct data are present.

Some medical practices have carrier direct links to the insurance companies and do not use the services of a clearinghouse.

CMS has a Medicare Transaction System (MTS) for Part A (hospital services) and Part B (outpatient medical services) claims processing. This system replaces the numerous software programs formerly used by Medicare's claims processing contractors with a national electronic standard program. The system called *electronic medical claims* (EMC) is used for nearly all Medicare transactions, including claims submission, payment, direct deposit, online eligibility verification, coordination of benefits, and claims status.

Using a clearinghouse offers the following several advantages:

Thank You for being a member

20%off

your entire purchase in-store or online*

NOW THROUGH SATURDAY, AUGUST 3RD

20% off your entire purchase*

P2220000980692UCFEM

This is a one-time use coupon valid either in-store or online.

For online purchases use coupon code:

2A1YZ2UCFEM

ULTA
B E A U T Y ®

1135 Arbor Drive,
Romeoville, IL 60446

Member Number

2 810050 744650

A4
May Padayao
Apt. 3
4444 Hamilton Ave.
San Jose, CA 95130-1475

The Breast Cancer Research Foundation.

PRSRT-STD
US Postage
Paid
ULTA

Postmaster, please deliver between
Wed. July 24th - Fri. July 26th

LW25-13 **A**

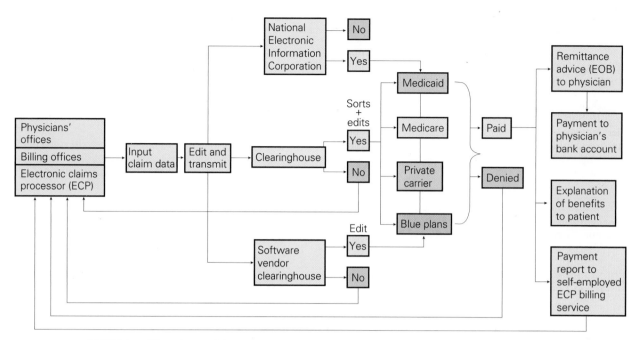

FIGURE 8-1 Flow sheet of electronic transmission systems showing path for claim payment via the National Electronic Information Corporation (NEIC), clearinghouse, and independent software vendor. This system also indicates when payment is made to physician and depicts locations where claims may not pass an edit or are denied.

- Translation of various formats to the HIPAA-compliant standard format
- Reduction in time of claims preparation
- Cost-effective method through loss prevention
- Fewer claim rejections
- Fewer delays in processing and quicker response time
- More accurate coding with claims edits
- Consistent reimbursement

TRANSACTION AND CODE SET REGULATIONS: STREAMLINING ELECTRONIC DATA INTERCHANGE

The **HIPAA Transaction and Code Set (TCS) Rule** was developed to introduce efficiencies into the health care system. The objectives are to achieve a higher quality of care and to reduce administrative costs by streamlining the processing of routine administrative and financial transactions. The US Department of Health and Human Services (HHS) has estimated that by implementing TCS, almost $30 billion over 10 years would be saved.

TCS regulation required the implementation of specific standards for transactions and code sets by October 16, 2003. The intent of TCS requirements is to achieve a single standard.

For example, in the pre-HIPAA environment, when submitting claims for payment, health care providers had been doing business with insurance payers who required the use of their own version of local code sets (e.g., state Medicaid programs) or identifiers and paper forms. More than 400 versions of a **National Standard Format (NSF)** exist to submit a claim for payment. Health care providers' offices benefit from less paperwork, and standardizing data results in more accurate information and a more efficient organization.

HIPAA standardization actions are similar to using a bank's automatic teller machine (ATM) or the grocery store's self-checkout. A magnetic strip on a bank card or the bar code on a grocery item can be swiped across a scanning device, allowing customers to process a transaction more quickly than with traditional methods. As these methods are adapted, there are benefits to both the end user and the business providing the technology (Table 8-1).

As learned in Chapter 2, HIPAA governs how a covered entity may handle health information. Whether a provider transmits health information in electronic form in connection with a transaction covered by HIPAA will determine whether a provider is considered a covered entity (Figure 8-2). Under HIPAA, the following circumstances would likely make the provider a **covered entity:**

- If the provider submits electronic transactions to any payer.
- Large providers: If the provider submits paper claims to Medicare and has 10 or more employees,

Table 8-1	Recognized Benefits of TCS and EDI	
BENEFIT	**RESULT**
More reliable and timely processing—quicker reimbursement from payer	Fast eligibility evaluation; reduced time in claim life cycle; industry averages for claim turnarounds are 9-15 days for electronic versus 30-45 days for paper claims, improving cash flow.
Improved accuracy of data	Decreases processing time, increases data quality, and leads to better reporting.
Easier and more efficient access to information	Improves patient support.
Better tracking of transactions	Assists tracking of transactions (i.e., when sent and received), allowing for monitoring (e.g., prompt payments).
Reduction of data entry/manual labor	Electronic transactions assist automated processes (e.g., automatic payment posting).
Reduction in office expenses	Lowers office supplies, postage, and telephone expenses.

Data from HIPAAdocs Corporation, Columbia, MD.
EDI, Electronic data interchange; *TCS,* transaction and code set.

FIGURE 8-2 Decision flow chart of who is subject to the HIPAA Transaction and Code Set (TCS) rule.

the provider is required to convert to electronic transactions (no later than October 16, 2003). Therefore HIPAA compliance is required.

A provider is not considered a covered entity under HIPAA in the following circumstances:

- Small providers: If the provider has fewer than 10 employees and submits claims only on paper to Medicare (not electronic). The provider may continue to submit on paper and therefore is not required to comply with HIPAA guidelines (i.e., not required to submit electronically).
- If the provider only submitted paper claims until and after April 14, 2003 and does not send claims to Medicare, the provider is not required to comply with sending electronic claims.

According to CMS, "Providers who are not small providers (institutional organizations with fewer than 25 full-time employees or physicians with fewer than 10 full-time employees) must send all claims electronically in the HIPAA format."

Transaction and Code Set Standards

TCS standards have been adopted for health care transactions. HIPAA **standard transactions** are the electronic files in which medical data are compiled to produce a specific format to be used throughout the health care industry.

In general, **code sets** are the allowable set of codes that anyone could use to enter into a specific space (field) on a form. All health care organizations using electronic transactions have to use and accept (either directly or through a clearinghouse) the code set systems required under HIPAA that document specific health care data elements, including medical diagnoses and procedures, drugs, physician services, and medical suppliers. These codes have already been in common use throughout the industry and should have helped ease the transition to the new transaction requirements. What has been a standard in the health care industry and recognized by most payers has now been *mandated* under HIPAA.

HIPAA standard codes are used in conjunction with the standard electronic transactions. It is necessary that the health care industry recognize a standard that eliminates ambiguity when processing transactions. In turn, this will ultimately improve the quality of data and result in improved decision-making and reporting in administrative and clinical processes.

Medical code sets are **data elements** used uniformly to document why patients are seen (diagnosis, ICD-9-CM) and what is done to them during their encounter (procedure, CPT-4 and HCPCS). Each covered entity organization is responsible for implementing the updated codes in a timely manner, using the new HIPAA-mandated TCS codes, and deleting old or obsolete ones (Table 8-2). Because of this, medical practices may opt to subscribe to coding software or data files that have frequent updates and include new, updated, and deleted codes. Deleted codes become obsolete but are not removed because they have been used when billing past accounts.

Data Requirements

Your role as an insurance billing specialist will likely require you to understand which data elements are required to construct an HIPAA standard transaction in comparison with those essential for a paper CMS-1500 (08-05) form or the old electronic NSF.

The office's practice management software system produces the required HIPAA standard electronic formats. If the software is not capable of producing such formats, the continued use of clearinghouses eliminates much of the confusion by translating into the HIPAA standard format. You will be trained on the practice management software system on where to insert or input additionally captured data that have not been collected on the CMS-1500 (08-05) form or electronic NSF.

When a patient comes into your office and is treated, his or her confidential health information is collected and put into the computerized practice management system. The services rendered are assigned a standard code from the HIPAA-required *code sets* (e.g., CPT), and the diagnosis is selected from another code set (e.g., ICD-9-CM)—much the same as pre-HIPAA.

When claims are generated for electronic submission, all data collected are compiled and constructed into a HIPAA *standard transaction*. This EDI is recognized across the health care sector in computer systems maintained by providers, clearinghouses, and insurance payers. The harmony among the covered entities results in a more efficient claim life cycle.

Table 8-2	HIPAA Medical Code Sets and Elements	
STANDARD CODE SETS	**MEDICAL DATA ELEMENTS**
International Classification of Diseases, Ninth Edition, Clinical Modification (ICD-9-CM), volumes 1 and 2 ICD-9-CM replaces *Diagnostic and Statistical Manual of Mental Disorders*, fourth edition (DSM-IV)	Diseases Injuries Impairments Other health-related problems and their manifestations Causes of injury, disease, impairment, or other health-related problems
ICD-9-CM, volume 3	Procedures or other actions taken for diseases, injuries, and impairments on hospital inpatients reported by hospitals, including prevention, diagnosis, treatment, and management
Current Procedural Terminology, fourth edition (CPT-4)	Physician services Physical and occupational therapy services Radiologic procedures Clinical laboratory tests Other medical diagnostic procedures Hearing and vision services Transportation services (e.g., helicopter, ambulance) Other services
Code on Dental Procedures and Nomenclature (*Current Dental Terminology*) National Drug Codes (NDC) for Retail Pharmacy transactions *International Classification of Diseases, Tenth Edition, Clinical Modification* (ICD-10-CM) (diagnosis) *International Classification of Diseases, Tenth Edition, Procedural Coding System* (to replace ICD-9-CM, volume 3 Procedural Coding System)	Dental services Pharmaceuticals Biologics Implementation date October 2013

Required and Situational

In addition to the major code sets (ICD-9 and CPT/HCPCS), several *supporting code sets* encompass both medical and nonmedical data (Table 8-3). When constructing a claim, the supporting code sets are made up of "Required" and "Situational" data elements, similar to those on the CMS-1500 (08-05) paper form. These supporting code sets are embedded in the data elements identified by the HIPAA standard electronic formats. You will not need to know all of these specific codes, but it will be helpful to know they do exist, especially if you are active in the claims processing procedures. When reviewing reports from the clearinghouse or the insurance payer, you may have to correct claims that were rejected for not having correct data elements.

Required refers to data elements that must be used to be in compliance with a HIPAA standard transaction. Conversely, *situational* means that the item depends on the data content or context (Example 8-1). For the required and situational status of data elements when electronically transmitting 837P claims, refer to the extreme right column of Table 8-5.

Example 8-1 Situational Data

Baby's birth weight when an infant is delivered.
Last menstrual period (LMP) when a woman is pregnant.

Determining the required and situational data elements not currently collected for the CMS-1500 (08-05) claim or NSF electronic format can be complex; you will learn this process when you are in the office performing claims processing duties. As an insurance billing specialist, you are directly involved in the claims processing procedures and need to know the most important items to look for related to HIPAA requirements and situational data to successfully construct a compliant and payable insurance claim.

In addition to other data elements required under HIPAA TCS, examples include the following:

● *Taxonomy codes.* Taxonomy is defined as the science of classification; thus these are numeric and alpha provider specialty codes, which are assigned and which classify each health care provider. Common **taxonomy codes** include "general practice 208D0000X," "family practice 207Q00000X," and "nurse practitioner 363L00000X." Beginning January 2, 2007, CMS required providers submitting claims for their primary facility to include a taxonomy code. This code allows crosswalking to the Online Survey Certification and Reporting (OSCAR) System. Taxonomy codes are necessary because some institutional providers may not choose to apply for a unique national provider number for each of its subparts (e.g., psychiatric unit or rehabilitation unit).

Table 8-3	HIPAA Transaction Functions and Formats	
STANDARD TRANSACTION FUNCTION		**INDUSTRY FORMAT NAME**
Official Title: Health Care Eligibility Benefit Inquiry and Response **Purpose:** Eligibility verification/response When obtaining issues regarding benefits and coverage, this standard is used from a health care provider to a health plan or between two health plans. The 270 is the "inquiry for eligibility verification." The 271 is the "response."		ASC X12N 270/271
Official Title: Health Care Claim Status Request and Response **Purpose:** Health claim status inquiry/response The 276 is the "inquiry" to determine the status of a claim. The 277 is the "response."		ASC X12N 276/277
Official Title: Health Care Services Review—Request for Review and Response **Purpose:** Referral certification and authorization for patient health care services		ASC X12N 278
Official Title: Payroll Deducted and Other Group Premium Payment for Insurance Products **Purpose:** Health plan premium payments including payroll deductions		ASC X12N 820
Official Title: Benefit Enrollment and Maintenance **Purpose:** Transmission of subscriber enrollment information to a health plan to establish coverage or terminate the policy		ASC X12N 834
Official Title: Payment and Remittance Advice **Purpose:** Transmission indicating the explanation of benefits or remittance advice from a health plan payer to the health care provider. This may also be data sent from a health plan directly to the provider's financial institution (bank) and may include payment and information about the processing of the claim.		ASC X12N 835
Official Title: Health Care Claim or Equivalent Encounter **Purpose:** To obtain payment for the transmitted health services encounter information. The 837P (Professional) replaces the paper CMS-1500 form and the electronic national standard format (NSF). The 837I (Institutional) replaces the paper UB-04 often used in hospitals. The 837D (Dental) is used for dentistry. Additionally, the Coordination of Benefits for claims and payment will be transmitted through the 837 format.		ASC X12N 837 Includes: 837P—Health Care Claim, Professional 837I—Health Care Claim, Institutional 837D—Health Care Claim, Dental
Proposed Official Title: First Report of Illness, Injury or Incident **Potential Purpose:** This standard will be used to report information on a claim pertaining to factors such as date of onset of illness or date of accident.		PROPOSED ASC X12N 148
Proposed Official Title: Health Claims Attachment **Potential Purpose:** Transmit additional information to claim. This means no more photocopied attachments stapled to paper claims or additional information mailed after the claim is initially received.		PROPOSED ASC X12 275 and HL7

- *Patient account number.* To be assigned to every claim.
- *Relationship to patient.* Expanded to 25 different relationships including indicators such as "grandson," "adopted child," "mother," and "life partner."
- *Facility code value.* Facility-related element that identifies the place of service, with at least 29 to choose from including "office," "ambulance air or water," and "end-stage renal disease treatment facility."
- *Patient signature source code.* Indicates how the patient or subscriber signatures were obtained for authorization and how signatures are retained by the provider. Codes include letters such as "B" for "signed signature authorization form or forms for both CMS-1500 (08-05) claim form block 12 and block 13 are on file" and "P" for "signature generated by provider because the patient was not physically present for services."

TRANSITION FROM PAPER CMS-1500 (08-05) TO ELECTRONIC STANDARD HIPAA 837P

The American National Standards Institute (ANSI) formed the **Accredited Standards Committee X12 (ASC X12),** which developed the US standards body for the cross-industry development, maintenance, and publication of electronic data exchange standards. In regard to the health care industry, processing administrative functions can be costly and involve many paper forms and communications via telephone, fax, and postal services. Also, the security and privacy of an individual's health information may be jeopardized. So, to address the burden of these high overhead costs, the uniform adoption of HIPAA standards has brought forth electronic formats to complete the following health care–related transactions:

Box 8-1   HIPAA Supporting Code Sets

Adjustment reason code	Entity identifier code	Provider organization code
Agency qualifier code	Exception code	Product/service procedure code
Ambulatory patient group code	Functional status code	Prognosis code
Amount qualifier code	Facility type code	Provider code
Attachment report type code	Hierarchical child code	Provider specialty certification code
Attachment transmission code	Hierarchical level code	Provider specialty code
Claim adjustment group code	Hierarchical structure code	Record format code
Claim filing indicator code	Immunization status code	Reject reason code
Claim frequency code	Immunization type code	Related-causes code
Claim payment remark code	Individual relationship code	Service type code
Claim submission reason code	Information release code	Ship/delivery or calendar pattern code
Code list qualifier code	Insurance type code	Ship/delivery pattern time code
Condition codes	Measurement reference ID code	Student status code
Contact function code	Medicare assignment code	Supporting document response code
Contract code	Nature of condition code	Surgical procedure code
Contract type code	Nonvisit code	Transaction set identifier code
Credit/debit flag code	Note reference code	Transaction set purpose code
Currency code	Nutrient administration method code	Unit or basis measurement code
Disability type code	Nutrient administration technique code	Version identification code
Discipline type code	Place of service code	X-ray availability indicator code
Employment status code	Policy compliance code	

- Obtain authorization to refer to a specialist
- Submit a claim for reimbursement
- Request and respond to additional information needed to process a claim
- Health care claims or equivalent encounter information
- Health care payment and remittance advice
- Coordination of benefits
- Health care claim status
- Enrollment and disenrollment in a health plan
- Eligibility for a health insurance plan
- Health plan premium payments
- Referral certification and authorization
- First report of injury
- Health claims attachments
- Other transactions HHS may prescribe by regulation

Each of these standard transactions is identified by a three-digit number preceded by "ASC X12N." The transactions, however, are referred to in the office simply by the three-digit number (e.g., 837 or 837P [professional]). The 837P replaces the paper CMS-1500 (08-05) form and more than 400 versions of the electronic National Standard Format (NSF). HIPAA also provides standards for the complete cycle of administrative transactions and electronic standard formats. Use Box 8-1 to become better acquainted with these HIPAA-supporting code sets.

Levels of Information for 837P Standard Transaction Format

Because the 837P is an electronic claims transmittal format, data collected to construct and submit a claim are grouped by levels. It is important for claims processing staff to know the language when following up on claims. You do not need to know exactly how these are grouped. However, if the clearinghouse or payer states that you have an invalid item at the "high level," you will need to understand that it could be incomplete or erroneous information pertaining to the provider, subscriber, or payer (Table 8-4).

A "friendlier" way to understand this new stream-of-data format is to address a "crosswalk" between the legacy CMS-1500 (08-05) and the 837P (Table 8-5; note that dates on HIPAA transactions will be in the 8-digit format YYYYMMDD [20090806]). Refer to a paper CMS-1500 (08-05) Health Insurance Claim Form template as shown in Chapter 7. Use Table 8-6 and compare the block number on the CMS-1500 (08-05) paper claim with the data element number in the 837 electronic format.

Accredited Standards Committee X12 (ASC X12) Version 5010

From time to time the software for transmission of insurance claims data must be upgraded due to the continual changes to policies and regulations for payment of claims. Because of the implementation of ICD-10-CM/PCS in 2013, the X12 HIPAA transaction standards have been upgraded to a version known as **ASC X12 Version 5010.** On January 1, 2012, providers, payers, and clearinghouses must be using the new standards exclusively. This version allows providers and payers to transmit either ICD-9 or ICD-10 data. There are many system improvements such as returning claims to the provider that need corrections sooner, assignment of claim numbers closer

Table 8-4 | Data Grouping in 837P Standard Transaction Format

LEVEL	INFORMATION
High-level information: Applies to the entire claim and reflects data pertaining to the billing provider, subscriber, and patient.	Billing/pay to provider information Subscriber/patient information Payer information
Claim-level information: Applies to the entire claim and all service lines and is applicable to most claims.	Claim information
Specialty claim–level information: Applies to specific claim types.	Specialty
Service line–level information: Applies to specific procedure or service that is rendered and is applicable to most claims.	Service line information
Specialty service line–level information: Applies to specific claim types. Required data are only required for the specific claim type.	Specialty service line information
Other information	Coordination of benefits (COB) Repriced claim/line Credit/debit information Clearinghouse/Value added network (VAN) tracking

Table 8-5 | Comparison of CMS-1500 and 837 v5010

CMS-1500 BLOCK #	CMS-1500 BLOCK DESCRIPTION	ANSI 837 v5010 LOOP, SEGMENT, ELEMENT	STATUS
1	Government program	Identification code qualifier	R
1a	Insured ID number	Loop 2010BZ, NM1/IL, 09	R
2	Patient last name	2010BA, NM1/IL, 03	R
2	Patient first name	2010BA, NM1/IL, 04	R
3	Patient date of birth	2010BA, DMG, 02	R
3	Patient sex	2010BA, DMG, 03	R
4	Insured last name	2330A, NM1/IL, 03	S
4	Insured first name	2330A, NM1/IL, 04	S
5	Patient street address	2010BA, N3, 01	R
5	Patient city	2010BA, N4, 01	R
5	Patient state	2010BA, N4, 02	R
5	Patient ZIP code	2010BA, N4, 03	R
5	Patient telephone number	Not used in 837 v5010	
6	Patient relationship to insured, self, spouse	2000B, SBR, 02	S
7	Insured's address	Not used—Use only if insured is different than patient	S
7	City		S
7	State		S
7	ZIP code		S
7	Telephone	Not used in 837 v5010	
8	Patient status single, married	Not used in 837 v5010	
8	Other	Not used in 837 v5010	
8	Employed	Not used in 837 v5010	
8	Full-time student	Not used in 837 v5010	
8	Part-time student	Not used in 837 v5010	
9	Other insured last name	2330A, NM1/IL, 03	S
9	Other insured first name	2330A, NM1/IL, 04	S
9	Other insured middle initial	2330A, NM1/IL, 05	S
9a	Other insured policy or group number	2330A, NM1/IL, 09	S
9b	Other insured date of birth and sex	Not available in format	S
9c	Employer's name or school name	2330B, NM1/PR, 03	S
9d	Insurance plan name or program name	2330B, NM1/PR, 09	S
10	Is patient's condition related to:	2300, CLM, 11	S
10a	Employment (current or previous)	2300, CLM, 11	S
10b	Auto accident	2300, CLM, 11	S
10b	Place (state)	2300, CLM, 11	S
10c	Other accident	2300, CLM, 11	S
11	Insured's policy group or FECA number	No direct match for blocks 11-11d of the CMS-1500 claim form to the ANSI 837 v5010 format.	S

Continued

Table 8-5   Comparison of CMS-1500 and 837 v5010—cont'd

CMS-1500 BLOCK #	CMS-1500 BLOCK DESCRIPTION	ANSI 837 v5010 LOOP, SEGMENT, ELEMENT	STATUS
11a	Insured's date of birth	See note in 11.	S
11a	Sex	See note in 11.	S
11b	Employer's name or school name	See note in 11.	S
11c	Insurance plan name or program name	See note in 11.	S
11d	Is there another health benefit plan?	See note in 11.	S
12	Patient's or authorized person's signature (and date)	2300, CLM, 10 (Patient signature source code)	R
13	Insured's or authorized person's release of information signature	2300, CLM, 09	S
14	Date of current: illness, injury, pregnancy (LMP)	2300, DTP/439, 03	S
14	Initial treatment date	2300 or 2400, DTP/454, 03	S
15	If patient has had same or similar illness, give first date	Not used	S
16	Dates patient unable to work in current occupation	2300, DTP/360/361/or 314, 03	S
17	Onset of current illness or injury	2300 or 2400, DTP/431, 03	S
17	Last name of referring physician or other source	2310A or 2420F, NM1/DN, 03	S
17	First name of referring physician	2310A or 2420F, NM1/DN, 04	S
17	Ordering provider last name	2420E, NM1/DK, 03	S
17	Ordering provider first name	2420E, NM1/DK, 04	S
17a	Ordering provider ID number	Not used	S
17a	Referring provider secondary identifier	Not used	S
17b	Ordering provider NPI	2420E, NM1/DK, 09	S
17b	Referring provider NPI	2310A or 2420F, NM1/DN, 09	S
18	Hospitalization dates related to current services: from / to		S
19	Ordering provider primary Identifier (SSN or EIN)	Not available in format	S
19	Referring provider primary identifier (SSN or EIN)	Not used	S
19	Narrative	2300 or 2400, NTE, 02	S
19	Date last seen and X-ray	2300 or 2400, DTP/304, 03	S
19	Supervising NPI	2310D or 2420D, NMI/DQ, 09	S
19	Anesthesia minutes	2400, SV1, 04 (03=MJ)	S
19	Homebound indicator	2300, CRC/75, 03	S
19	Hospice employed provider indicator	2400, CRC/70, 02	S
19	Assumed & relinquished care dates	2300, DTP/90 or 91, 03	S
20	Outside lab? Purchased service $ charges	2400, PS1, 02	S
21	Diagnosis or nature of illness or injury, 1	2300, HI, 01-2	S
21	Diagnosis 2	2300, HI, 02-2	S
21	Diagnosis 3	2300, HI, 03-2	S
21	Diagnosis 4	2300, HI, 04-2	S
21	Diagnosis 5	2300, HI, 05-2	S
21	Diagnosis 6	2300, HI, 06-2	S
21	Diagnosis 7	2300, HI, 07-2	S
21	Diagnosis 8	2300, HI, 08-2	S
21	Diagnosis 9	2300, HI, 09-2	S
21	Diagnosis 10	2300, HI, 10-2	S
21	Diagnosis 11	2300, HI, 11-2	S
21	Diagnosis 12	2300, HI, 12-2	S
22	Medicaid resubmission code	Not used in 837 v5010	
22	Original reference number	Not used in 837 v5010	
23	CLIA number	2300 or 2400, REF/X4, 02	S
23	Prior authorization number	2300 or 2400, REF/G1, 02	S
23	Investigational device exemption number	2300, REF/LX, 02	S
23	Care plan oversight services: HHA or hospice NPI	2300/REF/1J/02	S
24a	Dates of service: *from* mm dd yy	2400, DTP/472, 03	R
24a	*to* mm dd yy	2400, DTP/472, 03	R
24b	Place of service	2300, CLM, 05 or 2400, SV1, 05	S
24c	Type of service	Not required in 837 v5010	

Table 8-5 Comparison of CMS-1500 and 837 v5010—cont'd

CMS-1500 BLOCK #	CMS-1500 BLOCK DESCRIPTION	ANSI 837 v5010 LOOP, SEGMENT, ELEMENT	STATUS
24d	CPT/HCPCS procedure code and modifier for services or supplies	2400, SV/1, 01-2	R
24e	Diagnosis pointer	2400, SV1, 07-1	S
24f	$ Charges	2400, SV1, 02	R
24g	Days or units of service	2400, SV1, 04 (03=UN)	R
24g	Anesthesia minutes	2400, SV1, 04 (03=MJ)	R
24h	EPSDT family plan	Not required by Medicare.	
24i	Emg (emergency indicator)	Not used	
24j	COB	Not required for Medicare.	
24j	Rendering provider legacy number (shaded area)	Not used	
24j	NPI of rendering provider (unshaded area)	2310B or 2420A, NM1/82, 09 (08=XX)	
25	Federal tax ID number provider SSN or EIN#	2010AA, REF, 02 (REF01=EI or SY)	R
26	Patient's account no.	2300, CLM, 01	R
27	Accept assignment	2300, CLM, 07	R
28	Total charge	2300, CLM, 02	R
29	Amount paid	2300, AMT/F5, 02	S
30	Balance due	Not required for Medicare.	
31	Signature of provider (and date)	2300, CLM, 06	R
32	Name of facility where services were rendered	2310C, NM1/77, 03	S
32	Place of service address	2310C, N3, 01	S
32	Place of service city	2310C, N4, 01	S
32	Place of service state	2310C, N4, 02	S
32	Place of service ZIP code	2310C, N4, 03	S
32	Laboratory ID	2400, PS1, 01	R
32	Mammography certification no.	2300 or 2400, REF/EW, 02	R
32a	Facility NPI number	2310C, NMI/77, 09	R
32b	Facility qualifier and legacy no.	Not used	
33	Organization name	2010AA, NM1/85, 03	R
33	Provider's last name	2010AA, NM1/85, 03	R
33	Provider's first name	2010AA, NM1/85, 04	R
33	Address	2010AA, N3, 01	R
33	City	2010AA, N4, 01	R
33	State	2010AA, N4, 02	R
33	ZIP code	2010AA, N4, 03	R
33	Billing provider NPI	2010AA/NM1/85/09 (08=XX)	R
33	Billing provider legacy number or PIN	No longer used, effective 5/23/08	

to the time received by the payer, and more consistency of claims editing and error handling.

CLAIMS ATTACHMENTS STANDARDS

The proposed Claims Attachments Standards rule (as of September 2010) is intended to develop an electronic standard for claims attachments as required by HIPAA. Currently, practice management and claims software include a data field that allows you to indicate that a paper claims attachment is included with the claim. An electronic standard transaction for claims attachment would be used to transmit clinical data, in addition to those data contained in the claims standard, to help establish medical necessity for coverage and eliminate the need for the paper attachment.

Standard Unique Identifiers
Standard Unique Employer Identifier

The employer identification number (EIN) is assigned by the Internal Revenue Service (IRS) and is used to identify employers for tax purposes. HIPAA requires that the EIN be used to identify employers rather than inputting the actual name of the company when submitting claims. The date to comply was July 30, 2004. Employers will use their EINs to identify themselves in transactions involving premium payments to health plans on behalf of their employees or to identify themselves or other employers as the source or receiver of information about eligibility. Employers also will use EINs to identify themselves in transactions when enrolling or disenrolling employees in a health plan.

Table 8-6 Medicare Requirements When Submitting Paper and Electronic Claims

BLOCK NUMBER	PAPER CLAIMS	ELECTRONIC CLAIMS
Mandatory Information		
1.	Check mark for insurance plan	
1a.	Insured's ID number	Insured's ID number
2.	Patient's name	Patient's last name and first name
3.	Patient's birth date	
5.	Patient's address	
10a.	Patient's employment	
10b.	Check if auto accident	
10c.	Check for other type of accident	
11.	Insured's policy group number	Group number/source of payment
12.	Patient's signature source	Patient's signature source/release of information indicator
17b.	NPI of referring/ordering provider	Referring/ordering provider's NPI, referring provider's NPI
24A.	Dates of service	Service from/through dates
24B.	Place of service	Place of service
24D.	CPT/HCPCS codes and modifiers	HCPCS procedure codes
24F.	$ Charges	Line charges
24G.	Days of units of service	Units of service
24J.	Rendering provider's NPI	Rendering provider's NPI
25.	Federal tax ID number	
27.	Accept assignment?	
28.	Total charge	
31.	Provider's signature indicator	Provider's signature indicator
32.	Facility name and address	Facility/laboratory name and/or facility/laboratory NPI
33.	Provider's billing name and address	Provider's last and first names
		Payer organization, name
		Provider's Medicare number (batch level)
		Provider's pay-to address 1
		Provider's pay-to city
		Provider's pay-to state
		Provider's pay-to ZIP code
		Provider's pay-to telephone number
33a.	Billing provider's NPI	Billing provider's NPI
Conditional Requirements		
4.	Insured's name	Insured's last and first names
6.	Patient's relationship to insured	Patient's relationship to insured
7.	Insured's address	Insured's address—line 1. Insured's city, state, ZIP code, and telephone number
9c.	Employer's or school name	Insured's employer name
9d.	Insurance plan or program name	Group name
10d.	Leave blank unless third-party payer requires specific data	
11a. through 11d.	Other third-party payer insurance coverage	
13.	Assigned benefits	
14.	Date of current illness and so on	Accident/symptom date
15.	Date of same or similar illness	
16.	Dates patient unable to work	
17.	Name of referring/ordering provider	Referring/ordering provider's last name
18.	Dates of hospitalization	
19.	Reserved for local use	Dates last seen, supervising provider's NPI, date of last x-ray
20.	Outside lab	Laboratory indicator, laboratory charges, purchased service indicator, purchased service charge
21.	Diagnosis	Diagnosis 1, 2, 3, 4
22.	Medicaid resubmission	
23.	Prior authorization number	
24D.	HCPCS modifier 1, 2, 3, 4	
24H.	Medicaid EPSDT program	
26.	Patient's account number	
29.	Amount paid on the claim	
30.	Balance due	

CPT, Current Procedural Terminology; EPSDT, early and periodic screening diagnosis and treatment program; *HCPCS,* Healthcare Common Procedure Coding System; *NPI,* National Provider Identifier.

Standard Unique Health Care Provider Identifier

Health insurance plans have been assigning an identifying number to each provider with whom they conduct business. Providers have many different identifier numbers when submitting claims to several different payers. HIPAA requires that a National Provider Identifier (NPI) be assigned to each provider to be used in transactions with all health plans. The NPI is all numeric and is 10 characters in length; it was required by May 23, 2007. In April 2005, CMS announced that Fox Systems, Inc, received and processed NPI applications. Fox operates a help desk for providing more information (visit www.foxsys.com).

According to CMS, NPI is a lasting identifier that would not change on the basis of changes in a health care provider's name, address, ownership or membership in health plans, or Healthcare Provider Taxonomy classification (taxonomy identifies the specialty). If an NPI is used for fraudulent purposes, an investigation will take place and a different NPI may be assigned.

Standard Unique Health Plan Identifier

The Standard Unique Health Plan Identifier rule is under development and like the NPI, will assign a standard identifier to identify health plans that process and pay certain electronic health care transactions. As of September, 2010, a Notice of Proposed Rule-Making has not been published in the *Federal Register*. The American Medical Association has encouraged a final rule to create an implementation date of October 1, 2012. Check for updates at www.cms.hhs.gov.

Standard Unique Patient Identifier

The intention to create a standard for a uniform patient identifier prompted protest among public interest groups who saw a universal identifier as a civil liberties threat. Therefore the issue of a universal patient identifier is "on hold."

PRACTICE MANAGEMENT SYSTEM

The most important function of a practice management system (PMS) is accounts receivable. Many offices use features, such as scheduling, electronic health record (EHR), and word processing, to run an efficient office. However, the goal of maximum value can be attained if the PMS is able to prepare, send, receive, and process HIPAA standard electronic transactions. For older PMS versions, a clearinghouse converts old formats into the HIPAA standard transactions. Keep in mind that HIPAA does not apply to the format of stored data within the PMS databases. Computer systems are free to use any

data format when storing data because HIPAA standards apply only to the format in which data are transmitted.

If your practice is in the market for a new PMS, it is important to find a vendor that understands HIPAA thoroughly—including the privacy and security rules. A PMS can help with the administrative burdens such as tracking the receipt of the Notice of Privacy Practices (NPP), noting a patient's treatment consent or authorization, and mapping disclosures. A HIPAA-ready PMS may allow the following:

- Setting security access to patient files in the software
- Indicating date of receipt and signature of NPP
- Inserting date of patient's authorization
- Maintaining files of practice's authorization and notification forms
- Tracking requests for amendments, request for restrictions on use and disclosure of protected health information (PHI), and indication of whether the physician agreed to the request or denied the request
- Tracking expiration dates

When assessing the PMS's functionality in accounts receivable management, consider the ability to perform the following:

- Set up all practice providers as individuals to bill using correct and appropriate identifiers for each and every health care provider.
- Key in all patient demographics and insurance information.
- Electronic claim batch submission either direct to payer or through clearinghouse. Note that some PMS vendors sell an "add-on" module to go directly to some carriers such as Medicare, Medicaid, and Blue Cross Blue Shield.

BUILDING THE CLAIM

Encounter or Multipurpose Billing Forms

As mentioned in Chapter 3, an *encounter form* (also known as *charge slip, multipurpose billing form, patient service slip, routing form, super bill,* or *transaction slip*) is a document used to record information about the service rendered to a patient. The style and format of the billing form varies because it is customized to meet the needs of each health care office. For easy reference in selecting levels of service and diagnosis, many billing forms include preprinted procedural and diagnostic codes. The list of codes printed on the form is specific to the medical practice's specialty. This aids the health care provider in determining the correct level of evaluation and management (E/M) service, ensures each component is addressed in the physician's dictation, and expedites data entry of professional services. The provider circles the codes, and the insurance billing specialist takes that information and enters it into the computer system. Billing forms cannot be used in place of documentation in the patient record and may not withstand an external audit. Remember that the encounter form's procedure and diagnostic code sections should be updated and reprinted with correct descriptions because changes, additions, and deletions occur that may affect the medical practice (October 1 for changes in diagnostic codes and January 1 for changes in procedural codes).

Scannable Encounter Form

Some encounter forms are designed so that they may be scanned to input charges and diagnoses into the patient's computerized account. Time is saved and fewer errors occur because no keystrokes are involved (Figure 8-3).

Keying Insurance Data for Claim Transmission

Manual claim completion is accomplished by obtaining patient and insurance data, looking up a diagnosis and procedure in an index, referring to medical and financial records, and following block-by-block guidelines for the CMS-1500 (08-05) insurance claim form. Much of this source information is found on an encounter form that is used to post charges and payments. Additionally, scanning or copying the front and back of the patient's insurance card and driver's license can assist when obtaining information for a claim or following up on a delinquent account.

When one is operating computer software, the encounter form also may be used to obtain patient information (Figure 8-4). A prompt (question field) appears on the screen, and the data are keyed in reply to the prompt. Reusable data are entered initially in a file and identified by a number. Each treating physician, referring physician, patient, and third-party payer has an assigned computer code number. Notice in Figures 8-4, 8-5, and 8-6 that a patient, John Bordon, is input as an account number BORJO000; Blue Cross Blue Shield insurance is BLU01; and Dr. J.D. Mallard is keyed in as JM. This information is stored in the database and is the same as that necessary for completing a claim manually. It is automatically retrieved by the system when a computer code number is keyed in and used to generate a computerized claim or electronic claim. Because there are computer code numbers and prompts for each item, there is less chance for error or omitting mandatory information. The program checks to see that data are complete and in proper format. It is important to understand how your particular management system works.

Some entries are made using a "macro." This technique involves a series of menu selections, keystrokes, or commands that have been recorded into memory and assigned a name or key combination. When the macro name is keyed in, the steps or characters in the macro are executed from beginning to end, saving time and key strokes. However, when using a macro, template, or other automated billing system, be sure the provider accurately individualizes each record to reflect what occurred during the visit. The practice of cutting and pasting diagnosis and treatment language from one record to another can generate a false claim.

Some general do's and don'ts guidelines for keying in data and billing electronic claims follow.

Do: Use the patient account numbers to differentiate between patients with similar names.

Do: Use correct numeric locations of service code, current valid CPT, or HCPCS procedure codes.

Do: Print an insurance billing worksheet or perform a front-end edit (online error checking) to look for and correct all errors before the claim is transmitted to the third-party payer.

Do: Request electronic-error reports from the third-party payer to make corrections to the system.

Do: Obtain and cross-check the electronic status report against all claims transmitted.

Don't: Use special characters (dashes, spaces, or commas).

Don't: Bill codes using modifier -22 electronically unless the carrier receives documents (called attachments) to justify more payment.

After input is complete, the information is stored in memory and a claim may be transmitted individually or in batches. Batched claims can be divided according to insurance type or date(s) of service and are ideally sent during low-volume times.

Because the health care provider is responsible for submitting an accurate bill, the insurance billing specialist inputs the codes and the third-party payer's claims examiners will not recode. Medicare is forbidden to recode a claim. This eliminates transposition of numbers or missing or added digits on transmitted claims. However, if a patient's records are requested after a prepayment audit, a third-party payer may determine that a different code is required for the case. During the edit and error process, software code editors identify invalid codes, age conflicts, gender conflicts, procedural and diagnostic code conflicts, and other data before issuing payment. If certain information is submitted incorrectly (e.g., patient's name or insurance identification number

CFR

PAT 4140.0

( ) 985-6575 01/22/1936 F63	**DOCTOR:** 2 FRANK CHI, M.D.
PRI: (Y) BLUE SHIELD ENVOY	ROOM:
201-XX-9969	APPTLOC:
SEC:	APPTCD:

DOCTOR: 2 FRANK CHI, M.D.
ROOM:
APPTLOC:
APPTCD:
REASON: OX, F/U visit
LAST DX: 000.0 No diagnosis applicable
SSN/STA: 201-XX-9969, 1 Active
OVERLAY: 1 INTERNAL MEDICINE

APPT DATE: 05/27/XX
APPT TIME: 2:30 PM
APPT LEN: 10 min.
DEPT/LOC: 0, n/a
DSET/PRT: 1, 12
ACCT BAL: 75.00
PAT DUE: 0.00
VOUCHER: 7887

NEW PT OFFICE VISITS
①②③④Ⓟ/Ⓛ 99203 NP LEVEL THREE
①②③④Ⓟ/Ⓛ 99204 NP LEVEL FOUR
①②③④Ⓟ/Ⓛ 99205 NP LEVEL FIVE
EST PT OFFICE VISIT
①②③④Ⓟ/Ⓛ 99211 EST PT LEVEL ONE
①②③④Ⓟ/Ⓛ 99212 EST PT LEVEL TWO
①②③④Ⓟ/Ⓛ 99213 EST PT LEVEL THREE
①②③④Ⓟ/Ⓛ 99214 EST PT LEVEL FOUR
①②③④Ⓟ/Ⓛ 99215 EST PT LEVEL FIVE
①②③④Ⓟ/Ⓛ 00003 GLOBAL VISIT

OTHER PROCEDURES
①②③④Ⓟ/Ⓛ 99000 COLL & PREP/PAP TEST
①②③④Ⓟ/Ⓛ 93000 EKG WITH INTERPRETATION
①②③④Ⓟ/Ⓛ 82270 HEMOCCULT
①②③④Ⓟ/Ⓛ 81000 URINALYSIS

INJECTIONS
①②③④Ⓟ/Ⓛ ~FLU FLU INJ/ADMIN/MCR
①②③④Ⓟ/Ⓛ ~9065 FLU INJ/NON MCR
①②③④Ⓟ/Ⓛ ~PNEU PNEUMO/ADMIN/MCR
①②③④Ⓟ/Ⓛ ~9073 PNEUMO INJ NON MCR

UNLISTED PROCEDURES
_____

STOP FOR VERIFICATION
BREASTS
①②③④Ⓟ/Ⓛ 610.2 FIBROADENOSIS, BREAST
①②③④Ⓟ/Ⓛ 611.72 LUMP OR MASS IN BREAST

CARDIOVASCULAR
①②③④Ⓟ/Ⓛ 441.4 ABDOM AORTIC ANEURYSM
①②③④Ⓟ/Ⓛ 411.1 ANGINA
①②③④Ⓟ/Ⓛ 424.1 AORTIC VALVE DISORDER
①②③④Ⓟ/Ⓛ 427.31 ATRIAL FIBRILLATION
①②③④Ⓟ/Ⓛ 427.32 ATRIAL FLUTTER
①②③④Ⓟ/Ⓛ 427.61 ATRIAL PREMATURE BEATS
①②③④Ⓟ/Ⓛ 426.11 ATRIOVENT BLOCK-1ST DE
①②③④Ⓟ/Ⓛ 785.2 CARDIAC MURMURS NEC
①②③④Ⓟ/Ⓛ 429.3 CARDIOMEGALY
①②③④Ⓟ/Ⓛ 428.0 CONGESTIVE HEART FAILU
①②③④Ⓟ/Ⓛ 425.1 HYPERTR OBSTR CARDIOMY
①②③④Ⓟ/Ⓛ 414.01 ISCHEMIC CHR HEART DIS
①②③④Ⓟ/Ⓛ 426.2 LEFT BB HEMIBLOCK
①②③④Ⓟ/Ⓛ 424.0 MITRAL VALVE DISORDER
①②③④Ⓟ/Ⓛ 785.1 PALPITATIONS
①②③④Ⓟ/Ⓛ 427.0 PAROX ATRIAL TACHYCARD
①②③④Ⓟ/Ⓛ 427.1 PAROX VENTRIC TACHYCAR

CHEST
①②③④Ⓟ/Ⓛ 466.0 BRONCHITIS, ACUTE
①②③④Ⓟ/Ⓛ 491.0 BRONCHITIS, CHRONIC
①②③④Ⓟ/Ⓛ 493.20 CH OB ASTH W/O STAT AS
①②③④Ⓟ/Ⓛ 493.00 EXT ASTHMA W/O STAT AS

①②③④Ⓟ/Ⓛ 491.21 OBS CHR BRNC W ACT EXA
①②③④Ⓟ/Ⓛ 491.20 OBS CHR BRNC W/O ACT E

ENDOCRINE
①②③④Ⓟ/Ⓛ 250.61 DMI NEURO CMP CONTROLL
①②③④Ⓟ/Ⓛ 250.01 DMI WO CMP CONTROLLED
①②③④Ⓟ/Ⓛ 250.03 DMI UNCONTROLLED
①②③④Ⓟ/Ⓛ 250.60 DMII NEURO CMP CONTROL
①②③④Ⓟ/Ⓛ 250.00 DMII WO CMP CONTROLLED
①②③④Ⓟ/Ⓛ 250.02 DMII UNCONTROLLED
①②③④Ⓟ/Ⓛ 272.0 HYPERCHOLESTEROLEMIA
①②③④Ⓟ/Ⓛ 272.1 HYPERGLYCERIDEMIA
①②③④Ⓟ/Ⓛ 245.2 HYPOTHYROIDISM
①②③④Ⓟ/Ⓛ 278.01 MORBID OBESITY
①②③④Ⓟ/Ⓛ 241.0 THYROID NODULE

EXTREMITIES
①②③④Ⓟ/Ⓛ 782.3 EDEMA
①②③④Ⓟ/Ⓛ 440.22 LOWER EXT EMBOLISM
①②③④Ⓟ/Ⓛ 451.0 PHLEBITIS-LEG
①②③④Ⓟ/Ⓛ 440.21 PVD W/CLAUDICATION
①②③④Ⓟ/Ⓛ 454.9 VARICOSE VEIN OF LEG

GI
①②③④Ⓟ/Ⓛ 789.06 ABDMNAL PAIN EPIGASTRI
①②③④Ⓟ/Ⓛ 789.02 ABDMNAL PAIN LFT UP QU
①②③④Ⓟ/Ⓛ 789.04 ABDMNAL PAIN LT LWR QU
①②③④Ⓟ/Ⓛ 789.05 ABDMNAL PAIN PERIUMBIL
①②③④Ⓟ/Ⓛ 789.03 ABDMNAL PAIN RT LWR QU
①②③④Ⓟ/Ⓛ 789.01 ABDMNAL PAIN RT UPR QU
①②③④Ⓟ/Ⓛ 578.1 BLOOD IN STOOL
①②③④Ⓟ/Ⓛ 575.12 CHOLECYSTITIS, ACUTE
①②③④Ⓟ/Ⓛ 564.0 CONSTIPATION
①②③④Ⓟ/Ⓛ 787.91 DIARRHEA
①②③④Ⓟ/Ⓛ 562.11 DIVERTICULITIS
①②③④Ⓟ/Ⓛ 562.10 DIVERTICULOSIS
①②③④Ⓟ/Ⓛ 574.20 GALLSTONE(S), CHRONIC
①②③④Ⓟ/Ⓛ 535.00 GASTRITIS
①②③④Ⓟ/Ⓛ 530.81 GERD
①②③④Ⓟ/Ⓛ 455.3 HEMORRHOID, EXT W/O COM
①②③④Ⓟ/Ⓛ 455.0 HEMORRHOID, INT W/O COM
①②③④Ⓟ/Ⓛ 564.1 IRRITABLE COLON
①②③④Ⓟ/Ⓛ 787.01 NAUSEA WITH VOMITING
①②③④Ⓟ/Ⓛ 569.3 RECTAL & ANAL HEMORRHA
①②③④Ⓟ/Ⓛ 530.11 REFLUX ESOPHAGITIS
①②③④Ⓟ/Ⓛ V76.41 SCREEN COLORECTAL

GU
①②③④Ⓟ/Ⓛ 601.0 ACUTE PROSTATITIS
①②③④Ⓟ/Ⓛ 600 BPH
①②③④Ⓟ/Ⓛ 592.0 CALCULUS OF KIDNEY
①②③④Ⓟ/Ⓛ 592.1 CALCULUS OF URETER
①②③④Ⓟ/Ⓛ 595.0 CYSTITIS, ACUTE
①②③④Ⓟ/Ⓛ 595.1 CYSTITIS, CHRONIC
①②③④Ⓟ/Ⓛ 599.7 HEMATURIA
①②③④Ⓟ/Ⓛ 607.84 IMPOTENCE, ORGANIC ORI
①②③④Ⓟ/Ⓛ 791.0 PROTEINURIA

HEENT
①②③④Ⓟ/Ⓛ 380.4 CERUMEN, IMPACTED
①②③④Ⓟ/Ⓛ 372.02 CONJUNCTIVITIS
①②③④Ⓟ/Ⓛ 784.7 EPISTAXIS
①②③④Ⓟ/Ⓛ 784.0 HEADACHE
①②③④Ⓟ/Ⓛ 464.0 LARYNGITIS/TRACHEITI
①②③④Ⓟ/Ⓛ 465.0 LARYNGOPHARYNGITIS, A
①②③④Ⓟ/Ⓛ 780.4 LIGHT-HEADEDNESS
①②③④Ⓟ/Ⓛ 346.00 MIGRAINE
①②③④Ⓟ/Ⓛ 460 NASOPHARYNGITIS, ACUT
①②③④Ⓟ/Ⓛ 381.01 OTITIS MEDIA
①②③④Ⓟ/Ⓛ 462 PHARYNGITIS, ACUTE
①②③④Ⓟ/Ⓛ 477.0 RHINITIS ALLERGIC
①②③④Ⓟ/Ⓛ 461.0 SINUSITIS, ACUTE
①②③④Ⓟ/Ⓛ 780.2 SYNCOPE/VERTIGO

HEMATOLOGIC
①②③④Ⓟ/Ⓛ 280.0 CHR BLOOD LOSS ANEMI
①②③④Ⓟ/Ⓛ 280.1 IRON DEF ANEMIA DIET
①②③④Ⓟ/Ⓛ 281.0 PERNICIOUS ANEMIA

HYPERTENSION
①②③④Ⓟ/Ⓛ 404.12 BEN HY HT/REN/CHF
①②③④Ⓟ/Ⓛ 403.10 BEN HTN REN W/O REN
①②③④Ⓟ/Ⓛ 403.11 BEN HYP WITH REN FAI
①②③④Ⓟ/Ⓛ 401.1 BENIGN HYPERTENSION
①②③④Ⓟ/Ⓛ 401.0 MALIGNANT HYPERTENSI
①②③④Ⓟ/Ⓛ 458.0 ORTHOSTATIC HYPOTENS

NEURO
①②③④Ⓟ/Ⓛ 345.10 GEN CNV EPIL W/O INT
①②③④Ⓟ/Ⓛ 435.3 TIA
①②③④Ⓟ/Ⓛ 433.10 CAROTID STENOSIS
①②③④Ⓟ/Ⓛ 437.0 CEREBRAL ATHEREOSCLER

OB GYN
①②③④Ⓟ/Ⓛ 112.1 CANDIDAL VULVOVAGINI
①②③④Ⓟ/Ⓛ 627.2 MENOPAUSAL SYMPTOMS
①②③④Ⓟ/Ⓛ V76.2 SCREEN MAL NEOP-CERV

RHEUMATOLOGIC
①②③④Ⓟ/Ⓛ 723.1 CERVICAL PAIN
①②③④Ⓟ/Ⓛ 274.0 GOUT
①②③④Ⓟ/Ⓛ 724.2 LUMBAGO/BACK PAIN
①②③④Ⓟ/Ⓛ 729.5 PAIN IN LIMB
①②③④Ⓟ/Ⓛ 724.1 PAIN IN THORACIC SPI
①②③④Ⓟ/Ⓛ 714.0 RHEUMATOID ARTHRITIS
①②③④Ⓟ/Ⓛ 724.3 SCIATICA
①②③④Ⓟ/Ⓛ 710.0 SYST LUPUS ERYTHEMAT

MISC
①②③④Ⓟ/Ⓛ 780.6 FEVER UNKN ORGIN
①②③④Ⓟ/Ⓛ 054.9 HERPES SIMPLEX NOS
①②③④Ⓟ/Ⓛ 786.05 SHORTNESS OF BREATH

UNLISTED DIAGNOSIS
①②③④Ⓟ/Ⓛ STOP FOR VERIFICATION

---

①②③④Ⓟ/Ⓛ **REFERRALS**
①②③④Ⓟ/Ⓛ
①②③④Ⓟ/Ⓛ
①②③④Ⓟ/Ⓛ
①②③④Ⓟ/Ⓛ

①②③④Ⓟ/Ⓛ **LOCATIONS**
①②③④Ⓟ/Ⓛ
①②③④Ⓟ/Ⓛ
①②③④Ⓟ/Ⓛ
①②③④Ⓟ/Ⓛ

①②③④Ⓟ/Ⓛ **DOCTORS**
①②③④Ⓟ/Ⓛ
①②③④Ⓟ/Ⓛ F. CHI, MD
①②③④Ⓟ/Ⓛ A. SWERD, MD
①②③④Ⓟ/Ⓛ J. STEVEN, MD

①②③④Ⓟ/Ⓛ **NEXT VISIT**
①②③④Ⓟ/Ⓛ _____ DAYS
①②③④Ⓟ/Ⓛ _1_ WEEKS
①②③④Ⓟ/Ⓛ _____ MONTHS
①②③④Ⓟ/Ⓛ

FIGURE 8-3 Scannable encounter form. Primary service or procedure is marked (with a No. 2 pencil) in the Number 1 location and linked to the primary diagnosis, which also is marked in the Number 1 location. The secondary procedures are marked in the Number 2 location, as is the secondary diagnosis. The primary linkage for all services and procedures is connected to the physician performing the service and the location in which it took place. Because there are five levels for both new and established patient office visits, an encounter form should include all levels. If information is missing, such as is shown in this example, an audit could be triggered because it appears to construe that this medical practice never bills any service lower than a Level 3, indicating fraud to an auditor. (Form template from Pearson NCS, Inc, Bloomington, MN. Form data are fictitious and not a part of the template.)

FIGURE 8-4 Medisoft screen of an open patient account with patient data fields. (Screenshots used by permission of MCKESSON Corporation. All Rights Reserved. MCKESSON Corporation 2008.)

is incorrect, a diagnosis code is missing a fourth or fifth digit, or a provider's identification number is omitted), the claim is rejected and must be resubmitted with correct data. Incorrect coding may be keying errors, or it may be a deliberate attempt to obtain fraudulent payment. The edit check allows immediate feedback about the status of an electronically transmitted claim.

Medicare requires certain information when submitting paper and electronic claims for some blocks of the CMS-1500 (08-05) claim form. Carriers may return claims if this information is omitted. A list of mandatory information and conditional requirements is shown in Table 8-6.

The physician may revise coding on the health record and on the claim to reflect the services more accurately up until the time at which the claim is transmitted for payment.

Encoder

An **encoder** is add-on software to practice management systems that can greatly reduce the time it takes to build

or review a claim before batching. This may or may not improve overall coding accuracy. The billing specialist or other user is prompted with a series of questions or choices leading to or affecting a specific code assignment by displaying code-specific edits. Using an encoder can enhance a medical practice's compliance program when it comes to accuracy in its billing procedures. Used as an audit tool, the encoder can also be helpful in performance improvement by identifying problem areas in the billing process.

However, there are instances when an encoder does not accurately assign codes; therefore one must never be completely dependent on code-assist software. For example, if a patient has three thorns incised and extracted (removed), the CPT code 10120 "incision and removal of foreign body, subcutaneous tissue; simple (integumentary system)" might be generated by the encoder. But if internally audited, the case may warrant CPT code 27372 "removal of foreign body, deep, thigh region in knee area (musculoskeletal system)." Thus one learns that not all procedures involving the skin are found in the integumentary system and, if deeper skin layers are affected, a code may be found in another system. A *grouper* is

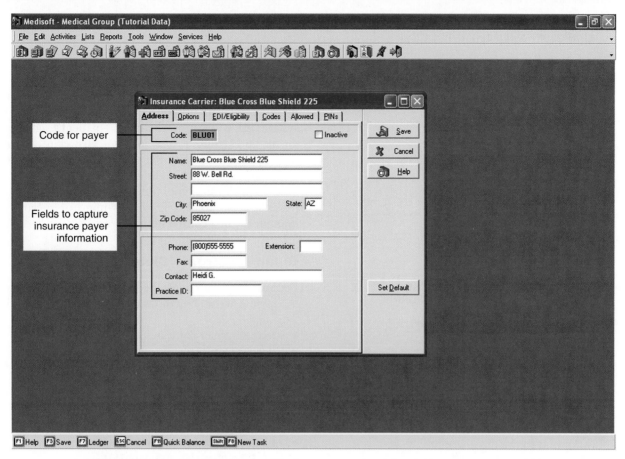

FIGURE 8-5 Medisoft screen of a payer file showing completed data fields. Notice that the Code for the Payer is "BLU01." (Screenshots used by permission of MCKESSON Corporation. All Rights Reserved. MCKESSON Corporation 2008.)

FIGURE 8-6 Medisoft screen of the provider file of Dr. J. D. Mallard. Note that he is identified in the PMS as "JM," so all information keyed into the PMS under "JM" is assigned as Dr. Mallard being the responsible physician. (Screenshots used by permission of MCKESSON Corporation. All Rights Reserved. MCKESSON Corporation 2008.)

PATIENT'S MEDICARE ELECTRONIC SIGNATURE MONTHLY AUTHORIZATION FORM

I authorize any holder of medical or other information about me to release to the Social Security Administration and Centers for Medicare and Medicaid Services or its intermediaries or carriers any information needed for this or a related Medicare claim. I permit a copy of this authorization to be used in place of the original, and request payment of medical insurance benefits either to myself or to the party who accepts assignment.

_____   _____
Signature of Patient   Date

A

PATIENT'S MEDICARE ELECTRONIC SIGNATURE ONE-TIME AUTHORIZATION FORM

I request that payment of authorized Medicare benefits be made either to me or on my behalf to _____ for services furnished me by that physician or supplier. I permit a copy of this authorization to be used in place of the original and authorize any holder of medical information about me to release to the Centers for Medicare and Medicaid Services or its agents any information needed to determine these benefits or the benefits payable for related services.

_____   _____
Signature of Patient   Date

B

FIGURE 8-7 Examples of patients' Medicare electronic signature authorization forms. **A,** Monthly form. **B,** One-time form.

software designed for use in a network that serves a group of users working on a related project that allows access to the same data.

The final considerations in building a claim are the signature requirements for both the patient and the physician or provider of service.

Signature Requirements

Physician. The physician's signature on the agreement or contract with the third-party payer is a substitute for his or her signature on the claim form.

Patient. For assignment of benefits, each patient's signature must be obtained and retained in the office records because there are no handwritten signatures on electronic claims (Figure 8-7). Office policy varies on obtaining the patient's signature for release of medical information. A clause on the patient registration form or an authorization and assignment release document may be designed specifically for obtaining signatures for transmitting electronic claims and acceptance of financial responsibility by the patient. The CMS-1500 (08-05)

Health Insurance Claim form also may be used for this purpose, and the patient should sign in Block 12 or 13 for a specific date of service. Most practice management systems ask a question whether the patient's signature is on file and require a "yes" or "no" answer to complete the required field when the claim is submitted. When a physician sees a patient in the hospital who has never been to the office, the authorizations obtained by the hospital apply to that provider's filing of a claim, for example, as in a consultation process.

Clean Electronic Claims Submission

Because dirty claims cost medical practices, the following is a review of some methods used to ensure clean claims.

● Claim scrubber software (prebill/edit processing)
● Encoder software
● Electronic clearinghouse
● Single and batch claims review

PUTTING HIPAA STANDARD TRANSACTIONS TO WORK

Interactive Transactions

Interactive transaction is back-and-forth communication between two computer systems. One requests information and the other provides information during what is referred to as online **real time.** Real time allows for instant information. An inquiry is made and an answer received within seconds. It can involve eligibility verification, deductible status, claim inquiries, status of claims, and other insurance claim data. Other information also may be accessed such as limiting charges, fee schedules, allowables, procedure codes, and postoperative days for specific procedures. Many insurance companies such as Medicare fiscal intermediaries provide access to information on assigned pending and paid claims. Additional information that may be determined includes whether the individual has other coverage and which third-party payer should be billed as primary. In addition, some third-party payers deposit payments into the physician's bank account automatically via **electronic funds transfer (EFT).** EFT is a paperless computerized system that enables funds to be debited, credited, or transferred and eliminates the need for personal handling of checks. A deposit-only bank account, sometimes called *zero-balance account* (ZBA), provides protection against cyber thieves (identity or other theft). This account has blocks and filters so that it only accepts deposits. However, if the health plan's EFT agreement allows it to recoup overpayments from the provider's bank account, this restriction would have to be removed.

ELECTRONIC REMITTANCE ADVICE

An online transaction about the status of a claim is called an **electronic remittance advice (ERA).** This gives information on charges paid or denied. If the medical practice elects to set the software system to automatically post the information to patients' accounts, then data entry is not required. The computer tests the claims computer data against various guidelines or parameters known as screens. If the services billed on the claim exceed the screens, the claim is denied, returned to the physician for more information, or sent for review. If a claim is denied or rejected, the billing specialist receives a printout stating the reason. The missing, miscoded, or incomplete information should be added or corrected and the claim resubmitted; this process is more efficient than remaining on a telephone on hold or resubmitting a claim via standard mail.

A Medicare ERA, formerly known as *explanation of Medicare benefits* (EOMB or EOB), is based on the American National Standards Institute (ANSI) Accredited Standards Committee X12 (ASC X12) Health Care Claim Payment/Advice (835), or "ANSI 835" (Figure 8-8). *A* subcommittee, X12N, has developed standards for a variety of electronic transactions between third-party payers and health care providers.

The use of ANSI 835 Version 4010 generates an electronic Medicare remittance advice instead of the paper RA. To improve cash flow, ANSI 835 also allows EFT of Medicare payments to the physician's bank account, which is called *direct deposit.*

DRIVING THE DATA

Basic procedures for transmission of a claim electronically are as follows:

1. Set up the database.
2. Enter data.
3. Batch or compile a group of claims.
4. Connect the computerized database with the clearinghouse or direct to the payer.
5. Transmit the claims.
6. Review the clearinghouse reports.

METHODS FOR SENDING CLAIMS

The methods for getting claims submitted to either the payer or the clearinghouse vary according to the office system in place. Methods can include the following:

1. Data transmission via cable modem, DSL, T-1
   a. **Cable modem.** A modem used to connect a computer to a cable television system that offers online services.
   b. **Digital subscriber line (DSL).** A high-speed connection through a telephone line jack and usually a means of accessing the Internet.
   c. **T-1.** A T-carrier channel that can transmit voice or data channels quickly.
2. Data directly keyed into payer system: DDE via dial-up modem or Internet
   a. **Direct data entry (DDE).** Keying claim information directly into the payer system by accessing over modem dial-up or DSL. This is a technology to directly enter the information into the payer system via the access whether it is dial-up or DSL.
3. Practice management system (PMS)—in-house shared systems or application service provider (ASP)
   a. **Application service provider (ASP).** "Renting" a PMS available over the Internet. All data are housed on the server of the ASP, but the accounts are managed by the health care provider's staff. Claims are batched and submitted similarly as though the software is stored on the desktop at the provider's office.

COMPUTER CLAIMS SYSTEMS

Payer or Carrier-Direct

For a better understanding of how insurance claims are transmitted, know the types of systems and how they work (e.g., payer or carrier-direct and clearinghouse).

Fiscal agents for Medicaid, Medicare, TRICARE, and many private third-party payers use the carrier-direct system. With this system, the data are transmitted electronically directly into the payer's system. This eliminates the need for a clearinghouse.

It is necessary to have a signed agreement with each carrier with whom the physician wishes to submit electronic claims.

Once enrollment is complete, a submitter number may be assigned. Submitters must send a test file to the insurance carrier to ensure accurate file format, completeness, and validity. Any problems discovered during the test period must be corrected and a new test submitted for review before final approval. Test submissions may be a cross section of claim type data (from previously adjudicated claims) that might be expected in a production environment. The test file must consist of a minimum number of claims, dependent on the requirements of the insurance carrier, for each claim type to be billed. The test procedure must be completed for each claim type. A new test must be submitted when software is upgraded or the submission method changes. Test claims are not processed for payment. It is only after receiving written

No. 1 ABC INSURANCE COMPANY	5780 MAIN STREET			XY	12345		TEL # 5557639836	
No. 2 Prov #	No. 3 Prov Name		No. 4 Part B	No. 5	Paid Date:	No. 6 Remit #	Page:	

Field	Prov Name / Detail	NACHG / COST	HICHG / COVDY	TOB / NCOVDY	RC (No. 20)	REM (No. 21)	DRG	No. 5	Paid Date:	No. 6 Remit #	Page:
PATIENT NAME No. 7	PATIENT CNTRL NUMBER No. 12				RC No. 20	REM No. 21	DRG # No. 22	DRG OUT AMT No. 27	COINSURANCE No. 30	PAT REFUND No. 34	CONTRACT ADJ No. 38
HIC NUMBER No. 8	ICN NUMBER No. 13				RC No. 20	REM No. 21	OUTCD Nos. 23	CAPCD 24	COVD CHGS No. 31	ESRD NET ADJ No. 35	PER DIEM RTE No. 39
FROM DT–THRU DT Nos. 9 10		NACHG Nos. 14	HICHG 15	TOB 16	RC No. 20	REM No. 21	PROF COMP No. 25	MSP PAYMT No. 28	NCOVD CHGS No. 32	INTEREST No. 36	PROC CD AMT No. 40
CLM STATUS No. 11		COST Nos. 17	COVDY 18	NCOVDY 19	RC No. 20	REM No. 21	DRG AMT No. 26	DEDUCTIBLES No. 29	DENIED CHGS No. 33	PRE PAY ADJ No. 37	NET REIMB No. 41
SUBTOTAL FISCAL YEAR		Nos. 17	18	19			No. 25 No. 26	No. 27 No. 28 No. 29	No. 30 No. 31 No. 32 No. 33	No. 34 No. 35 No. 36 No. 37	No. 38 No. 39 No. 40 No. 41
SUBTOTAL PART B		Nos. 17	18	19			No. 25 No. 26	No. 27 No. 28 No. 29	No. 30 No. 31 No. 32 No. 33	No. 34 No. 35 No. 36 No. 37	No. 38 No. 39 No. 40 No. 41

FIGURE 8-8 A, Example of a computer-generated Medicare Part B Remittance Advice document received by a provider from the payer or fiscal intermediary.

A

Medicare Remittance Advice

No. 1   The payer name, address, city, state, ZIP code, and telephone number
No. 2   Medicare provider number
No. 3   Provider name
No. 4   Claim type (Part A and Part B claims are listed on separate pages of the remittance advice)
No. 5   Date the claim was paid
No. 6   Sequential remittance advice assigned code and page number
No. 7   Beneficiary's last name, first initial, and middle initial
No. 8   Beneficiary's Health Insurance Claim Number (HICN)
No. 9   Statement covers from date (MMDDCCYY)
No. 10   Statement covers through date (MMDDCCYY)
No. 11   Claim Status Code:
         1—Paid as primary
         2—Paid as secondary
         3—Paid as tertiary
         4—Denied
         5—Pended
         10—Received, but not in process

         19—Paid as primary and crossed over
         20—Paid as secondary and crossed over
         21—Paid as tertiary and crossed over
         22—Reversal of previous payment
         23—Not our claim and crossed over
No. 12   Patient control number
No. 13   Internal control number
No. 14   Patient name change (74 = change in patient name and QC = No change in patient name)
No. 15   HIC number change (C = Change in HIC number and N = No change in HIC number)
No. 16   Type of bill (three digit code)
No. 17   *Cost report days
No. 18   *Covered days
No. 19   *Noncovered days
No. 20   Reason codes (up to 4 occurrences—see ANSI code list)

No. 21   Remark codes. These codes are used to return claim-specific information to the provider. Only ANSI codes are used.
No. 22   *Diagnosis Related Group (DRG) number
No. 23   *Outlier code 70 = Code is present if a cost outlier is paid
No. 24   *Capital code 22 is present if capital is present
No. 25   *Professional fees billed but not payable by the FI
No. 26   *PPS-DRG operating amount (DSH+OLD+CAP+HSP+FSP)
No. 27   *PPS-DRG outlier amount
No. 28   MSP primary payer amount
No. 29   Deductible amounts (Cash deductible and/or blood deductible)
No. 30   Coinsurance amounts (including LTR days)
No. 31   Covered charges
No. 32   Noncovered charges
No. 33   Denied charges
No. 34   Patient refund amounts
No. 35   ESRD Network reduction
No. 36   Interest paid to provider and/or beneficiary for claim. The amount paid by Medicare when there is a delay in processing a clean claim
No. 37   Presumptive payment adjustment–forced balancing amount (standard paper remittance only)
No. 38   Contractual adjustment (amount used to balance claim charges to payment amount). Amount calculated as follows:
         Minus the sum of all value codes for MSP
         Minus claim noncovered charges
         Minus Gramm-Rudman reduction
         Minus ESRD Network reduction
         Minus claim denied charges
         Minus the value code amount for professional component
         Minus blood deductible
         Minus cash deductible
         Minus coinsurance amount
         Minus net provider reimbursement amount
         Minus patient refund amount
         *Do not subtract if satisfied by MSP payment
No. 39   Per diem rate
No. 40   Fee schedule amount payable amount
No. 41   Reimbursement amount paid to the provider for this claim

FIGURE 8-8, cont'd B, Explanation of the Medicare Remittance Advice. (From a handout, "How to Read a Remittance Advice [RA]," supplied by TrailBlazer Health Enterprises, LLC, Dallas, Medicare contractor.)

B

notification from the insurance carrier that claims may be transmitted electronically.

Clearinghouses

Clearinghouses may charge a flat fee per claim or a monthly charge. Some clearinghouses offer to file claims free of charge to the provider, but they recoup the expense from the payer. Most often, a vendor agreement of sorts will be in place between the clearinghouse and the provider submitting the claims. These contracts may be a **business associate agreement,** a **trading partner agreement,** or other contract.

TRANSMISSION REPORTS

Whether claims are submitted carrier-direct or through a clearinghouse, reports are generated and accessible to track each function of the claims process. Examples are as follows:

- *Send and receive files reports* show that a file is received by the clearinghouse and/or payer and also notifies the billing specialist when a file has been sent to the provider's account for review (Figure 8-9).
- *Batch claim report billed summary* lists each patient's name, total charges for medical services, batch number, billing number, name of insurance company billed, and chronologically the date the claim was transmitted (Figure 8-10).
- *Scrubber report* indicates the total number of claims, charges, and dollar amounts that were received by the clearinghouse and scrubbed for claim submitted to Massachusetts Insurance Plan (Figure 8-11). The billing specialist reviews the scrubber report for each insurance payer when claims have been transmitted through the clearinghouse.
- *Transaction transmission summary* shows how many claims were originally received by the clearinghouse and/or payer and how many claims were rejected automatically [not included for further processing] (Figure 8-12).
- *Rejection analysis report* identifies the most common reasons claims are rejected and indicates what claims were not included for processing (Figure 8-13). Corrections must be made by the billing specialist and the claims need to be refiled.
- *Electronic inquiry* or *claims status review* lists files received from the provider's office and indicates the progress of the claim. For example, if a claim is sent to a clearinghouse and forwarded to a payer, then the clearinghouse can indicate the status is confirmed received by the payer.

Electronic Processing Problems

Some problems can occur in electronic claims submission. Usually a status report of claims is received electronically from the third-party payer. It consists of an acknowledgment report and indicates assigned and unassigned claims, crossed over and not crossed over claims, claims accepted with errors, and rejected claims (see Figure 8-13). Data transmission problems arise periodically because of hardware or software problems.

Most billing software bundles claims into a batch, and they are all transmitted together. If one claim in the batch contains an error (e.g., missing patient name or missing diagnosis code), the third-party payer may reject the entire batch and return all claims to the provider. Some batches contain errors that occur in every transaction in the batch. These are called *syntax errors*. Syntax errors are inaccuracies that violate the HIPAA standard transaction format such as incorrect sequence of patient information or incorrect batch header. Such errors make it difficult for the third-party payer's software to read the transactions in a batch. There are other errors in which only one transaction in the batch has a syntax error or one of the batch's transactions has a data content error. In these instances, it would be inappropriate for a third-party payer to reject the entire batch. Usually the payer returns any noncompliant claims and processes the remaining claims in the batch. To avoid these types of rejections, it is important to use software that will separate out noncompliant transactions so that those can be removed from the batch and fixed before submission.

Billing and Account Management Schedule

Maintaining a schedule will help with EDI transmissions, which will enable a better cash flow. Table 8-7 suggests guidelines and procedures to tailor to the needs of your billing office.

Administrative Simplification Enforcement Tool

To address issues of noncompliance in regard to TCS, the federal government has implemented the use of an electronic tool to assist health care providers, payers, clearinghouses, and others to submit complaints regarding the HIPAA TCS rule. This online tool, the *Administrative Simplification Enforcement Tool,* or *ASET,* enables individuals or organizations to file a complaint online against an entity "whose actions impact the ability of a transaction to be accepted and/or efficiently processed."

The Security Rule: Administrative, Physical, and Technical Safeguards

Security measures encompass all the administrative, physical, and technical safeguards in an information system. The Security Rule addresses only electronic PHI

```
                        Raw 837
                        =========

              Electronic Technologies, Inc.
              ===========================


ISA*00* *00*
*ZZ*1234*ZZ*VB6786786*041110*0310*U*00401*123456789*0*P*:~GS*HC*12
34*VB6786786*20041110*0310*123456789*X*004010X098A1~ST*837*0001~B
HT*0019*00*1*20041110*0310*CH~REF*87*004010X098A1~NM1*41*2*GERI
ATRIC ASSOCIATES LLC*****46*1234~PER*IC*JIM
JONES*TE*8005551212~NM1*40*2*MASSACHUSETTS INS
PLAN*****46*XYZ1~HL*1**20*1~NM1*85*2*ALABAMA MEDICAL
ASSOC*****24*54-5555555~N3*PO BOX
123456~N4*BOSTON*MA*12345~REF*1D*123456789~HL*2*1*22*0~SBR*P*1
8******MC~NM1*IL*1*JONES*DEBRA*K***MI*123456789123~N3*11
JEFFERS POND
ROAD~N4*BOSTON*MA*12345~DMG*D8*19640812*F~NM1*PR*2*VMAP
FHSC FA*****PI*DMAS~N3*PO BOX
123~N4*BOSTON*MA*12345~CLM*123456*150***11::1*Y*A*Y*Y*B~REF*X
4*1242522DD~HI*BK:6110~NM1*DN*1*JACKSON*DONALD~REF*1D*12345
6789~NM1*82*1*ROWLAND*DAVID****24*54-
5555555~PRV*PE*ZZ*207ZP0102X~REF*1D*123456789~NM1*77*2*NORTH
OFFICE*****24*54-5555555~N3*123 LIPPLE
AVENUE~N4*BOSTON*MA*12345~LX*1~SV1*HC:88305:26*150*UN*1***1~
DTP*472*D8*20041028~REF*6R*11265594~
               .
               .
               .
               .
SE*160*0001~GE*1*123456789~IEA*1*123456789~
```
A

```
                  Human-Readable 837
                  ==================
              Electronic Technologies, Inc.
              =========================


=====================================            =====================================
INTERCHANGE HEADER - Production File             Account Number:                 123456
=====================================            Claim Amount:                   $150
Authorization: none        Password: none        Facility:                       Office
SubmitterID: 1234          ReceiverID: VB6786786  This Claim is                   ORIGINAL
Date: 11.10.2004           Time: 0310             Provider Signature:             On File Assignment Code: Assigned
Run #: 003                 Control #: 123456789   Assignment of Benefits Indicator:  Y
Request Acknowledgement: No Sub-element Separator: :   Release of Information:     Yes, Provider Has a Signed Statement
                                                 Permitting Release of Medical Billing
FUNCTIONAL GROUP HEADER - HC                     Data Related to a Claim
=====================================            CLIA Number:                    1242522DD
Submitter ID: 1234         ReceiverID: VB6786786  Principal Diagnosis Code:       6110
Date: 11.10.2004           Time: 0310 Control #: 123456789
ANSI X10 Version: 004010X098A1                   Referring Prov. - Person
                                                 ---------------
TRANSACTION SET HEADER- 837                      JACKSON, DONALD
=====================================            MA Provider Number: 123456789
Control #: 0001
Structure Code: 0019       Purpose Code: 00       Rendering Prov. - Person
Reference ID: 1            Type: CH               ---------------
Date: 11.10.2004           Time: 0310             ROWLAND, DAVID  (Employer ID Number,54-5555555)
Functional Category: 004010X098A1                Provider Taxonomy Code: 207ZP0102X
                                                 MA Provider Number: 123456789
Submitter - Non-Person
---------                                         Service Location - Non-Person
GERIATRIC ASSOCIATES LLC (Electronic Transmitter ID #,1234)   ---------------
Contact: JIM JONES                               NORTH OFFICE (Employer ID Number,54-5555555)
Phone Number: 800.555.1212                       123 LIPPLE AVENUE
                                                 BOSTON, MA 12345
Receiver - Non-Person
---------                                         Service Line # 1
MASSACHUSETTS INS PLAN (Electronic Transmitter ID #,XYZ1)   ---------------
                                                 Service Code:                   88305
BATCH #1                                         Modifier:                       26
=====================================            Amount:                         $150 Measurement: Unit Quantity: 1
                                                 Diagnosis Pointer:              1
Billing Provider - Non-Person                    Date of Service:                20041028
---------------                                   Prov. Control #:                11265594
ALABAMA MEDICAL ASSOC (Employer ID Number,54-5555555)
PO BOX 123456                                    PATIENT #2
BOSTON, MA 12345                                 =====================================
Provider Number: 123456789                                    .
                                                             .
PATIENT #1                                                   .
=====================================                         .
Primary Insurance                                            .
---------------                                   TRANSACTION SET TRAILER
Patient Relationship: Self                       =====================================
                                                 Included Segments: 160
Subscriber - Person                              Control #: 0001
---------
JONES, DEBRA K (Member ID Number,123456789123)   FUNCTIONAL GROUP TRAILER
11 JEFFERS POND ROAD                             =====================================
BOSTON, MA  12345                                Transaction Sets Included: 1
                                                 Group Control #: 123456789
Date of Birth: 19640812 Gender Code: F
                                                 INTERCHANGE TRAILER
Payer - Non-Person                               =====================================
-----                                             Included Functional Groups: 1
VMAP FHSC FA (Payer ID Number,DMAS)              Control #: 123456789
PO BOX 123
BOSTON, MA 12345
```
B

FIGURE 8-9 A, Raw 837 clearinghouse transmission report. If you print the 837 electronic claims transmission file, it looks similar to **A;** however, the report becomes readable after it comes back from the clearinghouse showing the patients' claims that were submitted. **B,** Readable 837 clearinghouse transmission report. (Reports supplied by Electronic Technologies, Inc, Delmar, NY.)

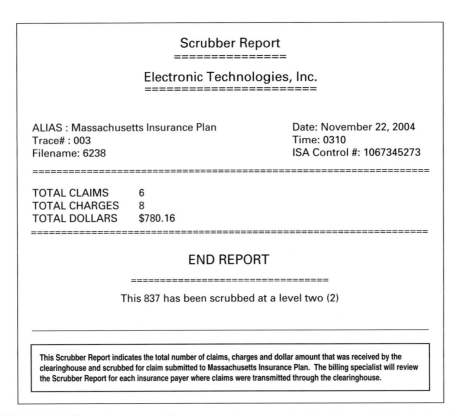

BATCH CLAIM REPORT Billed Summary

Patient code	Total charges	Batch #	Billing #	Insurance co. billed	Date sent
BORTOLUSSI	465.00	2	1005	ABCI000001	05/25/2005
BLACKWOOD	16.07	3	1006	TRICARE	05/25/2005
HELMS	33.25	4	1007	MDCR	05/25/2005
JAMESON	41.07	5	1008	ROYAL	05/25/2005
KELSEY	66.23	8	1010	XYZI000001	06/09/2005
	621.62				

FIGURE 8-10 Batch Claim Report billed summary by chronologic date.

Scrubber Report
===============

Electronic Technologies, Inc.
========================

ALIAS : Massachusetts Insurance Plan   Date: November 22, 2004
Trace# : 003   Time: 0310
Filename: 6238   ISA Control #: 1067345273

===

TOTAL CLAIMS   6
TOTAL CHARGES   8
TOTAL DOLLARS $780.16

===

END REPORT

=================================
This 837 has been scrubbed at a level two (2)

This Scrubber Report indicates the total number of claims, charges and dollar amount that was received by the clearinghouse and scrubbed for claim submitted to Massachusetts Insurance Plan. The billing specialist will review the Scrubber Report for each insurance payer where claims were transmitted through the clearinghouse.

FIGURE 8-11 Clearinghouse scrubber report. (Report supplied by Electronic Technologies, Inc, Delmar, NY.)

(ePHI), but the concept of protecting PHI that will become ePHI puts emphasis on security for the entire office. The Security Rule is divided into the following three main sections:

- Administrative safeguards
- Technical safeguards
- Physical safeguards

Administrative safeguards prevent unauthorized use or disclosure of PHI through administrative actions that manage the selection, development, implementation, and maintenance of security measures to protect ePHI. These management controls guard data integrity, confidentiality, and availability and include the following:

- Information access controls authorize each employee's physical access to PHI. This is management of password and access for separate employees that restricts their access to records in accordance with their responsibility in the health care organization. For example, usually the health information records clerk who has authorization to retrieve health records will not have access to billing records located on the computer.
- Internal audits allow the ability to review who has had access to PHI to ensure that there is no intentional or accidental inappropriate access, in both the practice management software system and the paper records or charges.

FIGURE 8-12 Clearinghouse 997 report that shows which 837 claim files were accepted and rejected. (Report supplied by Electronic Technologies, Inc, Delmar, NY.)

- Risk analysis and management is a process that assesses the privacy and security risks of various safeguards and the cost in losses if those safeguards are not in place. Each organization must evaluate their vulnerabilities and the associated risks and decide how to lessen those risks. Reasonable safeguards must be implemented to protect against known risks.
- Termination procedures should be formally documented in the office policies and procedures (P&P) manual and include terminating an employee's access to PHI. Other procedures would include changing office security pass codes, deleting user access to computer systems, deleting terminated employees' e-mail accounts, and collecting any access cards or keys.

Technical safeguards are technologic controls in place to protect and control access to information on computers in the health care organization and include the following:

- Access controls consist of user-based access (system set up to place limitations on access to data tailored to each staff member) and role-based access (limitations created for each job category [e.g., receptionist, administrative medical assistant, clinical medical assistant, bookkeeper, or insurance billing specialist]).

- Audit controls keep track of log-ins to the computer system, administrative activity, and changes to data. This includes changing passwords, deleting user accounts, or creating new user accounts.
- Automatic logoffs prevent unauthorized users from accessing a computer when it is left unattended. The computer system or software program should automatically log off after a predetermined period of inactivity. Your office's practice management software may have this useful feature; if not, the feature may be temporarily mimicked using a screen saver and password.
- Each user should have a unique identifier or "username" and an unshared, undisclosed **password** to log into any computer with access to PHI. Identifying each unique user allows the functions of auditing and access controls to be implemented. Other authentication techniques involve more sophisticated devices such as a magnetic card or fingerprints. Most likely you will be dealing with a password in your office. Passwords for all users should be changed on a regular basis and should never be common names or words.

Physical safeguards also prevent unauthorized access to PHI. These physical measures and P&P protect a covered entity's electronic information systems and related

```
             ALIAS: Massachusetts Insurance Plan 997 Report
        ==========================================
                 CLAIMS 997 ACKNOWLEDGMENT FILE


Trace#: 941                              ID: 114120941
SUBMISSION DATE: 11.22.2004             997 DATE: 11.23.2004
TIME SUBMITTED: 0112                     997 TIME: 111346
===============        =========================================
```

ERROR CODE	PATIENT ACCT #	LINE# / CHARGE#
251:NM1:9	628263478	2893

DESCRIPTION: Payer Name
Segment Has Data Element Errors
DETAIL: Subscriber Identifier - (Mandatory data element missing)
SUBMITTED:

ERROR CODE	PATIENT ACCT #	LINE# / CHARGE#
251:NM1:10	123456	5454545

DESCRIPTION: Payer Name
Segment Has Data Element Errors
DETAIL: (Invalid character in data element)
SUBMITTED:

ERROR CODE	PATIENT ACCT #	LINE# / CHARGE#
251:NM1:8	4515485	3157654

DESCRIPTION: Payer Name
Segment Has Data Element Errors
DETAIL: Identification Qualifier (Conditional required data element missing)
SUBMITTED:

This transaction was :	Rejected
Rejection Reason :	One or More Segments in Error
This Functional Group was :	Rejected
Transaction Sets Included :	1
Transaction Sets Received :	1
Transaction Sets Accepted :	0

FIGURE 8-13 Clearinghouse 997 report showing the claims acknowledgment file. This report shows error codes and details the types of errors made. It also shows patient account numbers and names of the payers. (Report supplied by Electronic Technologies, Inc, Delmar, NY.)

Table 8-7	Daily, Weekly, and End-of-Month Guidelines and Protocols	
DAILY	**WEEKLY**	**END OF MONTH**
Post charges in practice management system.	Batch, scrub, edit, and transmit claims (daily or weekly).	Run month-end aging reports.
Post payments in practice management system.	Analyze previous week's rejected and resubmitted claims.	Review all claim rejection reports (clearinghouse and payer), making sure all problems are resolved and claims accepted.
Batch, scrub, edit, and transmit claims (daily or weekly); retrieve transmission reports.	Note any problematic claims and resolve outstanding files.	Update practice management system with payer information, such as EIN, and NPI.
Run day sheet.	Research unpaid claims.	Run patient statements in office or through clearinghouse.
Review clearinghouse/payer transmission confirmation reports.	Make follow-up calls to resolve reasons for rejections, such as incorrect NPI, missing patient ID, incomplete data elements, and wrong format.	
Audit claims batched and transmitted with confirmation reports.		
Correct rejections and resubmit claims.		

EIN, Employer identification number; *NPI*, National Provider Identifier.

COMPUTER CONFIDENTIALITY

Confidentiality Statement

Most information in patients' medical records and physicians' financial records is considered confidential and sensitive. Employees who have access to such computer data should have integrity and be well chosen because they have a high degree of responsibility and accountability. It is wise to have those handling sensitive computer documents sign an annual confidentiality statement, as recommended by the Alliance of Claims Assistance Professionals (Figure 8-14). This way the statement can be updated when an individual's responsibilities increase or decrease. The statement should contain the following:

- Written or oral disclosure of information pertaining to patients is prohibited.
- Disclosure of information without consent of the patient results in serious penalty (e.g., immediate dismissal).

An additional example of an employee confidentiality agreement that may be used by an employer when hiring an insurance biller is shown in Figure 2-5.

Prevention Measures

Employees can take a number of preventive measures to maintain computer security:

YOUR COMPANY NAME
ADDRESS
PHONE/FAX

CONFIDENTIALITY STATEMENT

I, _____ , understand and acknowledge that as a
  (Type in individual's name)
principle/employee of _____(company name)_____ my position
as ___(job title)_____ requires that I access and use computer equipment and
software applications owned or leased by____(company name)_____ .
I understand that my position as a principle/employee of this company obligates me to abide by
the purchase, lease or rental agreements applicable to this equipment and software.

I understand and acknowledge that my position may require that I handle information regarding
the physicians and medical suppliers who are clients of ___(company name)_____ .
I understand and acknowledge that such client information, including financial data, fees,
corporate structure, etc., is privileged and confidential and that I am not at liberty to divulge or
discuss such information with unauthorized individuals within this company or to anyone outside
this company.

I understand and acknowledge that my duties may require me to access and/or process specific
patient data for individuals under the care of____(company name)_____ client
physicians and/or medical suppliers. I understand and acknowledge that all patient's data is
protected under federal privacy legislation and that discussion or release of this information in any
form without the patient's express permission is prohibited by federal law and subject to
prosecution and civil monetary penalties for any violation.

I further understand that violations of this confidentiality agreement will result in termination of
employment with____(company name)_____ .

My signature below is to verify my understanding and acceptance of the above data
confidentiality requirements and to signify my explicit agreement to abide by these requirements.

_____   _____
        Signature   Date

_____   _____
        Type Name   Title

FIGURE 8-14 Example of a confidentiality statement for an employee using computer equipment and software. (From National Association of Claims Assistance Professionals, Inc, Downers Grove, IL.)

COMPUTER CONFIDENTIALITY—cont'd

1. Obtain a software program that stores files in coded form.
2. Never leave disks or tapes unguarded on desks or anywhere else in sight.
3. Use a privacy filter over the computer monitor so that data may be read only when one is directly in front of the computer.
4. Log off the computer terminal before leaving a workstation, especially if working in a LAN (local area network) environment, which is used in most hospitals, clinics, or large offices.
5. Check and double-check the credentials of any consultant hired.
6. Read the manuals for the equipment, especially the sections entitled "Security Controls," and follow all directions.
7. Store confidential data on disks rather than only to the computer's hard drive. Disks should be stored in a locked, secure location, preferably one that is fireproof and away from magnetic fields.
8. Make sure the computer system has a firewall installed and proper antivirus/antispyware software. This can keep amateurs, but not professional hackers, from accessing an electronic system. Hackers can access digital copiers, laser printers, fax machines, and other electronic equipment with internal memories. Some offices leave modems on for transmitting and receiving data during low-cost, low-volume hours.
9. Develop passwords for each user and access codes to protect the data. A password is a combination of letters, numbers, or symbols that an individual is assigned to access the system. Passwords should be changed at regular intervals and never written down. A good password is composed of more than five characters and is case sensitive. Case sensitive means that the password must be entered exactly as stored using upper- or lower-case characters. Delete obsolete passwords from the system. Change any passwords known by an employee who is fired or resigns. Individuals with their own passwords allow the employer to distinguish work done by each employee. If errors or problems occur, focus may then be directed toward correcting the individual user.
10. Send only an account number (not the patient's name) when e-mailing a colleague with specific questions (e.g., about coding).

buildings and equipment from natural and environmental hazards and unauthorized intrusion. Appropriate and reasonable physical safeguards should include the following:

- Media and equipment controls are documented in the office P&P manual regarding the management of the PHI. Typical safeguard policies include how the office handles the retention, removal, and disposal of paper records, as well as recycling computers and destroying obsolete data disks or software programs containing PHI.
- Physical access controls limit unauthorized access to areas in which equipment and medical charts are stored. Locks on doors are the most common type of control.
- Secure workstation locations minimize the possibility of unauthorized viewing of PHI. This includes making sure that password-protected screen savers are in use on computers when unattended and that desk drawers are locked. **TIP:** Adjust the timing of your computer's screen saver to a lower time setting if you find yourself frequently called away from your desk. Most screen savers can be activated after 1 to 60 minutes of inactivity. This practice protects open documents.

HIPAA: APPLICATION TO THE PRACTICE SETTING

Because HIPAA affects all areas of the health care office, from the reception area to the provider, every staff member must be educated about HIPAA and trained in the P&P pertinent to the organization. This is in addition to being trained on job responsibilities.

Reasonable safeguards are measurable solutions based on accepted standards that are implemented and periodically monitored to demonstrate that the office is in compliance. Reasonable efforts must be made to limit the use or disclosure of PHI. If you are the receptionist and you close the privacy glass between your desk and the reception room area when you are making a call to a patient, this is a reasonable safeguard to prevent others in the waiting room from overhearing.

Incidental uses and disclosures are permissible under HIPAA only when reasonable safeguards or precautions have been implemented to prevent misuse or inappropriate disclosure of PHI. When incidental uses and disclosures result from failure to apply reasonable safeguards or adhere to the minimum necessary standard, the Privacy

Rule has been violated. If you are in the reception area and you close the privacy glass when having a confidential conversation and are still overheard by an individual in the waiting room, this would be "incidental." You have applied a reasonable safeguard to prevent this from happening.

RECORDS MANAGEMENT

Data Storage

A paperless office requires an organized and efficient system for keeping files that have been saved to the hard drive protected against accidental destruction. Keep financial records on computer disks or tapes and store them in an area that does not have temperature extremes or magnetic fields.

When data are keyboarded, it is wise to **back up** (save data) frequently, preferably daily. Automated backup is possible, and the computer regularly initiates the process. Most financial software programs display a screen prompt instructing the operator to back up before quitting the program. If there is no automated backup, always back up files at the end of the day or several times a week so that information is not lost during a power outage (e.g., surge, spike, blackout, brownout, lightning strike), computer breakdown, or head crash. Head crash occurs when the read-write head on a disk drive strikes the surface of the disk, causing damage at the point of impact.

About once a week, a verification process should be done that compares the original records with the copies. This can take 20% to 30% longer than ordinary backup, but if a comparison is not made, there is no way to ensure that the data have been backed up. Store backup copies away from the office in case of fire, flood, or theft.

Maintain a notebook (log) of the documents on computer disks or CDs with an index located at the front of the book. The log enables one to keep track of files and should list when the files were backed up last so that they can be located quickly. Be sure another employee knows where this notebook is kept and is familiar with how to track down files through this system. Note the code for accessing these documents and date revisions when updating old documents. Do not put anything related to personal health information in this log (e.g., 31403.DOC, Mrs. Private Patient Positive HIV Report).

Data Disposal

Another HIPAA security rule is the establishment of policies and procedures for final disposal of electronic protected health information (ePHI) and the hardware or electronic media on which it is stored. It is easy to recover ePHI off of hard drives, CD-ROMs, and other media storage devices if they are not properly erased or destroyed. Simply deleting files or formatting drives is not sufficient to keep ePHI from being accessed. Some acceptable methods are as follows:

- Reformat and overwrite the disk media several times to sanitize the hard drive.
- Reinitialize the storage space of the computer hardware, if possible.
- Break, incinerate, crush, or destroy the storage device.
- Shred audiotapes, microfilm, or microfiche.

Electronic Power Protection

Plug equipment into power surge suppressors or, better yet, receptacles with an uninterruptible power supply (UPS) to prevent computer and data file damage. In addition, the entire office should be protected by a surge suppressor installed near the electric circuit breaker panel. This device is called an *all-office* or *whole-office surge suppressor*.

Selection of an Office Computer System

A medical practice wishing to use an in-office computer or an individual wishing to set up his or her own business should consider the following:

1. What is the cost of the basic equipment and will it be purchased or leased?
2. What accessories will be necessary and what are their costs?
3. How much space will be necessary for the equipment and accessories for the office or home office business?
4. What type of electrical installation should be done to handle electronic transmission of data?
5. Should a computer fax or modem be obtained or should there be a separate fax line installed?
6. How much electrical energy will be used and how much additional cost will be necessary?
7. If the computer is on a time-sharing system with other users, how much will the telephone line cost when communicating online or directly to the computer?
8. What are the hardware maintenance costs and who will do the repair work?
9. What initial software will be necessary and will it be compatible with the operating system?
10. What is the estimated cost of software upgrades and will upgrades require an expanded operating system?
11. What are the software maintenance costs and who will provide technical support?
12. Should a document scanner be obtained?

13. What forms will be used as output from the computer? Also consider their size, design, acquisition, storage, waste, and cost.

14. What other supplies will be necessary and what will their costs be?

15. How many people on the staff will operate the computer? Will recruitment be necessary? Who will train employees? How much training time is necessary?

16. Will there be financing when the equipment is purchased and, if so, what type?

17. Will there be insurance and a warranty on the system?

18. How much will the consulting costs be?

19. What is the backup support and response time when there is a system crash (software or hardware)? Who will respond to software problems and who will respond to hardware problems?

20. How much time will it take to convert the current accounting system to the computerized system, and who will be doing the conversion?

Major mistakes made by practice administrators and physicians when selecting an office computer system are as follows:

- Practice software process is not structured.
- Specific needs and requirements are not fully addressed.
- Consultant selected for advice is biased.
- Primary users omitted from decision purchasing process.
- Buying more than is required by the practice.
- Allowing vendors to dictate the purchasing process.
- Senior management team finalizes the choice of systems in the process rather than giving end users more input.
- Equating the vendor representative with the product.
- Refusing to use the Request for Proposal concept.

KEY POINTS

This is a brief chapter review or summary of the key issues presented. To further enhance your knowledge of the technical subject matter, review the key terms and key abbreviations for this chapter by locating the meanings in the glossary at the end of this book that appear in a section before the index.

1. The American National Standards Institute (ANSI) formed the Accredited Standards Committee X12 (ASC X12), which developed the US standards body for the cross-industry development, maintenance, and publication of electronic data exchange standards.

2. Through HIPAA regulations, standardized transaction and code sets have been implemented to use electronic data interchange effectively.

3. A clearinghouse receives the electronic transmission of claims from the health care provider's office and translates it into a standard format prescribed in HIPAA regulations.

4. Under HIPAA rules, a provider who sends Medicare claims is considered a covered entity that has 10 or more employees and must transmit claims electronically. Those medical practices with fewer than 10 employees are not considered a covered entity and are not required to submit Medicare claims electronically.

5. Practice management software is used to input data, which helps generate a variety of documents including the 837P (professional) in electronic National Standard Format (NSF), formerly the CMS-1500 (08-05) paper form.

6. When constructing an insurance claim, the supporting code sets are made up of "required" and "situational" data elements identified by the HIPAA standard electronic formats.

7. Ten-character alphanumeric provider specialty taxonomy codes are assigned and classify each health care provider. These codes are used when transmitting electronic insurance claims.

8. Employers use their employer identification numbers (EINs) to identify themselves in transactions involving premium payments to health plans on behalf of their employees or to identify themselves to other employers as the source or receiver of information about eligibility. Employers use EINs to identify themselves in transactions when enrolling or disenrolling employees in health plans.

9. HIPAA requires that a National Provider Identifier (NPI), a 10-character numeric identifier, be assigned to each provider to be used in transactions with all health plans.

10. An encoder is helpful because it can reduce the time it takes to build or review a claim and help improve coding accuracy before batching and transmitting to a third-party payer.

11. An electronic remittance advice (ERA) is the equivalent of a paper summarized statement called

an *explanation of benefits*, which gives the status of insurance claims with payment details for one or more beneficiaries. It is referred to as *ANSI 835* or *Health Care Claim Payment/Advice (835)*.

12. Several methods are available for getting claims submitted to either the payer or clearinghouse such as cable modem, digital subscriber line (DSL), T-1, direct data entry (DDE), and application service provider (ASP).

13. The HIPAA Security Rule addresses only electronic protected health information (ePHI) and is divided into three sections: administrative safeguards, technical safeguards, and physical safeguards.

14. Computer confidentiality and security measures must be followed at all times to prevent unauthorized disclosure of electronic protected health information.

15. Back up data frequently to prevent loss of files and information.

⊖volve INTERNET RESOURCES

For active links to the following resources, visit the Evolve website at
http://evolve.elsevier.com/fordney/handbook

- Administrative Simplification Enforcement Tool (ASET)
- American Academy of Professional Coders
- American Health Information Management Association's Clinical Coding Forum
- American Medical Association
- Association for Electronic Health Care Transactions (AFEHCT)
- Blue Cross Blue Shield Association
- Centers for Medicaid and Medicare Services

- *Federal Register*
- Healthcare Information and Management Systems Society
- Joint Healthcare Information Technology Alliance (JHITA)
- North Carolina Healthcare Information and Communications Alliance, Inc. (NCHICA)
- Office of Inspector General
- State Insurance Commissioners
- TRICARE
- TRICARE Support Office
- Workers' Compensation–related links
- Workgroup for Electronic Data Interchange (WEDI)

STUDENT ASSIGNMENT

✓ Study Chapter 8.
✓ Answer the fill-in-the-blank, multiple choice, and true/false review questions in the *Workbook* to reinforce the theory learned in this chapter and to help prepare for a future test.

✓ Complete the assignments in the *Workbook* to edit and correct insurance claims that have been transmitted and rejected with errors.
✓ Turn to the glossary at the end of this textbook for a further understanding of the key terms and key abbreviations used in this chapter.

KEY TERMS*

appeal
delinquent claim
denied paper or electronic
    claim
explanation of benefits
inquiry

lost claim
overpayment
peer review
rebill (resubmit)
rejected claim
remittance advice

review
suspended claim
suspense
tracer

KEY ABBREVIATIONS*

ALJ	EOB	HIPAA	NPI
CMS	ERISA	HMO	RA
DAB	FTC	HO	

Receiving Payments and Insurance Problem Solving

OBJECTIVES

After reading this chapter, you should be able to:

- Identify three health insurance payment policy provisions.
- Interpret and post a patient's explanation of benefits document.
- Indicate time limits for receiving payment for manually versus electronically submitted claims.
- Name three claim management techniques.
- Identify purposes of an insurance company payment history reference file.
- Explain reasons for claim inquiries.
- Define terminology pertinent to problem paper and electronic claims.
- State solutions for denied and rejected paper and electronic claims.

- Identify reasons for rebilling a claim.
- Describe situations for filing appeals.
- Name Medicare's five levels in the redetermination (appeal) process.
- Determine which forms to use for the Medicare review and redetermination process.
- Name three levels of review under the TRICARE appeal process.
- List four objectives of state insurance commissioners.
- Mention seven problems to submit to insurance commissioners.

Service to Patients

To reduce insurance problems and obtain correct maximum payments, it is vital to extend service to patients by doing the following:

- Assist patients with in-office registration procedures so that complete and accurate personal and financial data are obtained initially and during follow-up visits to help diminish denied claims.
- Verify the patient's insurance coverage. If a patient does not have active coverage and services are going to be provided, it is important to communicate that he or she is responsible for all charges.
- Implement an appeals process to help settle any improper claim denials by notifying the patient with a telephone call

that an appeal letter was sent to the third-party payer. This informs the patient that the practice is investigating and explains why the claim was appealed.
- Telephone or send a letter to the patient telling him or her of the third-party payer's final decision. Give a clear explanation to the patient of the remittance advice (RA) or explanation of benefits (EOB) when questions are asked because these documents can lead to confusion or misunderstandings.
- Prepare a letter or form for the patient's signature if the patient has a complaint about a third-party payer and send it to the local insurance commissioner explaining the problem and asking for help in resolving it.

Performance objectives, testing and review material, and hands-on practical exercises for this chapter are available in these resources

 The Insurance Handbook Student Workbook   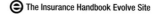 The Insurance Handbook Evolve Site

FOLLOW-UP AFTER CLAIM SUBMISSION

For an overall picture of where and when insurance claim problems occur after submission, all aspects of the insurance picture must be studied from beginning to end. This chapter begins with the provisions for payment in the insurance contract and explains how this affects the timeliness for payment. Then the text demonstrates how to interpret the document that accompanies the payment and how to manage and organize financial records. To improve cash flow, numerous problems that can occur are presented and some solutions are offered. Finally, the review and appeal processes are discussed for various programs.

With the development of proficient skills and experience in following up on claims, one can become a valuable asset to his or her employer and bring in revenue that might otherwise be lost to the business.

CLAIM POLICY PROVISIONS

Insured

Each health insurance policy has provisions relating to insurance claims. There may be a provision that the claimant has an obligation to notify the insurance company of a loss (injury, illness, or accident) within a certain period of time or the insurer has the right to deny benefits for the loss.

In some policies, if the insured is in disagreement with the insurer for settlement of a claim, a suit must begin within 3 years after the claim is submitted. Another provision states that an insured person cannot bring legal action against an insurance company until 60 days after a claim is submitted.

Payment Time Limits

The health insurance policy also has a provision about the insurance company's obligation to pay benefits promptly when a claim is submitted. However, time limits vary in this provision from one third-party payer to another. Specific time limits will be stated either in the insurance contract or the payer's manual outlining claims filing rules. It is reasonable to expect payment within 4 to 12 weeks if claims are submitted on paper or in as little as 7 days when transmitted electronically. If a payment problem develops and the insurance company is slow or ignores, denies, or exceeds time limits to pay a claim, then it is prudent to contact the insurance company. In the letter, the contracted time limit should be stated, the reason the claim has not been paid should be asked, and a copy should be retained for the physician's files. If the problem persists and there is no favorable response, the state insurance commissioner should be contacted to see whether he or she can take action to improve the situation. A copy of the correspondence should also be mailed. Many state insurance commissioners have broad powers to regulate the insurance companies within their state; others have no powers at all. If the carrier is a self-insured plan, a Medicaid or Medicare health maintenance organization (HMO), or an Employee Retirement Income Security Act (ERISA)-based plan, the insurance commissioner will not be able to assist with carrier issues. Claims may be submitted to the insurance company repeatedly with none of them ever being recorded. The one claim that will make it to the insurance company is the one that arrives after the self-determined timely filing deadline. If the provider has no contract with the carrier, the provider is not obligated to the carrier's deadline. Their denial should be appealed and payment demanded.

Managed care plans usually process claims on a daily basis, but some plans release payments quarterly. Some plans withhold a percentage that is reserved in a pool and distributed at the end of the fiscal year. In some states, managed care plans do not come under the jurisdiction of the state insurance commissioner. Read through the contract and if the responsible entity is still unable to find out who the responsible entity is, then check with your state medical society. Because managed care plans vary considerably in payment policies and administrative procedures, Chapter 10 details follow-up procedures and problem-solving techniques.

EXPLANATION OF BENEFITS

An **explanation of benefits (EOB)** may also be referred to as a **remittance advice (RA),** *check voucher*, or *payment voucher*. It is a document issued stating the status of the claim, that is, whether it is paid, adjusted, suspended (pending), rejected, or denied. A **suspended claim** is one that is processed by a third-party payer but is held in an indeterminate (pending) state about payment either because of an error or the need for additional information from the provider of service or the patient. The EOB also states the allowed and disallowed amounts by the third-party payer. The allowed amount is the maximum dollar value the insurance company assigns to each procedure and service on which payment is based. Insurance companies pay different percentages (e.g., 80%) of the allowed amount or flat rate on the basis of the service depending on the type of contract. If benefits have been assigned, the health care provider receives a copy of the EOB/RA along with a payment check. If benefits have not been assigned, payment goes to the patient and the provider's office personnel should bill the patient.

Components of an EOB

At first glance the form may seem difficult to understand. Unfortunately, there is no standard format for EOBs from one carrier to the next, but information contained in each one is usually the same. If one line at a time is read, the description and calculations for each patient may be understood easily. The EOB breaks down how payment was determined and contains the following information in categories or columns:

1. Insurance company's name and address
2. Provider of services
3. Dates of services
4. Service or procedure code numbers
5. Amounts billed by the providers
6. Reduction or denial codes. Comment codes (reason, remarks, or notes) indicating reasons payments were denied or payment reduced, asking for more information to determine coverage and benefits, or stating amounts of adjustment because of payments by other insurance companies (coordination of benefits)
7. Claim control number
8. Subscriber's and patient's name and policy numbers
9. Analysis of patient's total payment responsibility (amount not covered, copayment amount, deductible, coinsurance, other insurance payment, and patient's total responsibility)
10. Copayment amount(s) due from the patient
11. Deductible amounts subtracted from billed amounts
12. Total amount paid by the insurance carrier

Figure 9-1 illustrates an EOB for a private third-party payer and identifies each component mentioned in the preceding list.

Interpretation of an EOB

Reading and interpreting an EOB may be a bit overwhelming initially, so take time to read the document carefully. If several patients' claims are submitted to a third-party payer, the EOB may reflect the status of all of those claims and one check voucher may be issued. If the provider has signed a contract agreeing to discount fees with a number of third-party payers and managed care plans, payment amounts may vary along with the percentage of the fee that is adjusted off of the account. In addition, if more than one provider is in the medical practice and the practice is submitting claims using one group tax identification number, more than one physician's patients' claims may appear on a single EOB. The explanation of benefits shown in Figure 9-1 should be read line by line to interpret the meanings under each category or column, and the numbered explanations should be referred to when necessary. A helpful way to separate patients and their corresponding payments is to use a highlighter or ruler to underline the entire row across the EOB. This helps reduce errors when posting payments.

Posting an EOB

When an EOB is received in the physician's office, the claim(s) should be pulled or the patient's computerized account should be referenced, and every payment against the applicable insurance contract should be checked to establish whether the amount paid is correct. Refer to Chapter 3 and see Figure 3-14 that illustrates a patient's financial accounting record that shows posting of professional service descriptions, fees, payments, adjustments, and running balance due.

If services are reimbursed but you cannot totally understand what appears on an EOB, a telephone call to the payer usually clarifies and resolves the problem so that posting can be completed.

 Claims paid with no errors are put into a file designated for closed claims. An EOB for a single payment may be stapled to the claim form and then filed with the closed claims according to the date the payment was posted. EOBs that have many patients' payments listed may be filed in an EOB file. Some offices prefer to make copies of each multiple EOB, highlight the appropriate patient account, and attach the copy to the individual claim or file it in each patient's financial record.

 After posting payments and adjustments to applicable patient accounts, the paper EOB/RA should be filed in a designated area clearly marked in a folder. Some offices may group these remittances by payer, by month received, or by some other method. If your office receives electronic EOBs/RAs and you print them out, file accordingly. Some practice management systems allow for paper EOBs to be scanned into the software and some do automatic posting of payment by downloading electronic files that work in sync with the format of the remittances.

Additional information and examples of documents may be found in the following chapters: Chapter 11 explains a Statement of Remittance for managed care systems. Chapters 8 and 12 explain both a Medicare electronic RA and a hard copy RA, formerly known as *Explanation of Medicare Benefits* (EOMB). Chapter 14 shows a Summary Payment Voucher for the TRICARE program.

CLAIM MANAGEMENT TECHNIQUES

Insurance Claims Register

As discussed in Chapter 3, completed paper claims are logged into an insurance claims register. After logging in to a register, place a copy

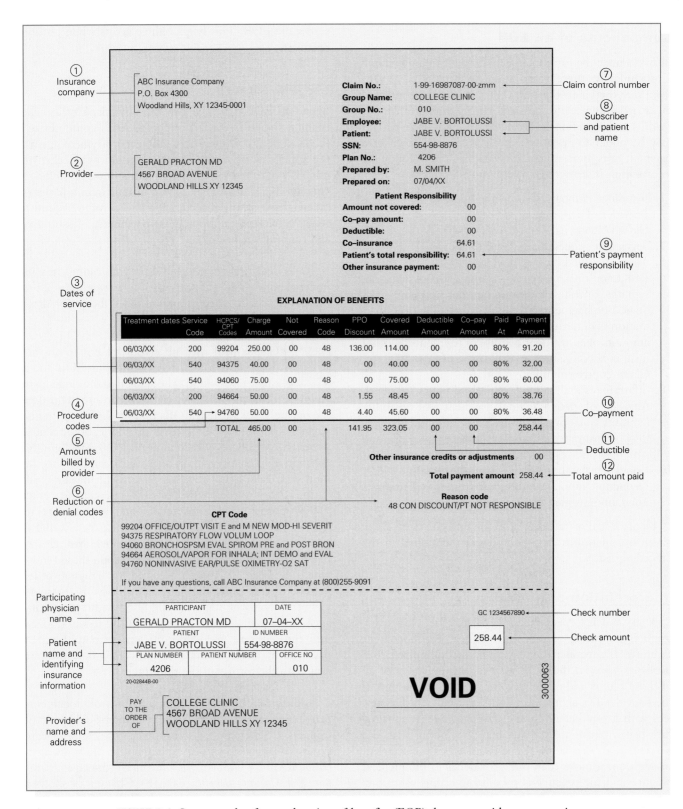

FIGURE 9-1 One example of an explanation of benefits (EOB) document with accompanying check that the provider received from a private third-party payer. These payment voucher documents vary among insurance companies.

of all insurance claims in a pending file labeled for each month of service so that the unpaid claims can be retrieved for timely follow-up. Or, place a copy of the insurance claim in an alphabetic file by insurance company name. This method permits an inquiry on multiple outstanding claims in one letter to the third-party payer each month rather than many letters covering individual claims. Place the insurance claims register in a loose-leaf notebook indexed according to the various insurance companies. When referring to a claims register, delinquent claims can be quickly located by simply looking through the book under the Date Claim Paid column. If that column is blank, check the Date Claim Submitted column and follow up as needed.

When a payment is received, pull all copies of claims that correspond with the payments and attach the EOB/RA. Post the payment received and the contracted adjustment to the patient's financial accounting record and to the day sheet or the computerized financial record. File the EOB/RA and deposit the payment check in the physician's bank account. Use a check mark or draw a line through the pertinent information in the claim register but do not obscure data. When all claims on the page have been paid, draw a diagonal line across the page. Some medical practices prefer to date stamp and insert "complete" in the upper right corner of the sheet. Pages may be retained for future reference.

 A log like this also could be developed and updated with little effort if using a spreadsheet software program, which would allow statistical data to be retrieved quickly and easily.

Most medical software programs offer practice management reports that can be used to track insurance payments (see Figure 3-18).

Some claims are aged according to date submitted, allowing easy reference for timely follow-up. Other offices age by date of service, which is when charges are initiated.

Tickler File

An alternative manual method used to track pending or resubmitted insurance claims is a "tickler file." This file is also called a *suspense* or *follow-up file*. A type of tickler file is also used to remind patients of upcoming or missed appointments. Tickler files also can be set up in computer systems that prompt the insurance billing specialist to telephone or send inquiries about unpaid insurance claims.

To create a manual reminder system, divide active claims by month and file them in chronologic order by date of service. Subdivisions also can be made by patient name or in numeric order by account number. Maintain the active file (unpaid claims) for the calendar year and put inactive resolved claims (older than 1 year) in storage that is accessible.

To incorporate this manual system into the billing process, start by printing two completed CMS-1500 (08-05) claim forms or copy completed claim forms. Send the original to the payer and file the copy in the tickler file by date of service. After receiving the payment check and EOB/RA, pull all claims noted on the EOB/RA from the tickler file. Post the payment to the patient's account (financial accounting record) and day sheet or financial record in the computer system. Compare the charges made on each claim to the payments listed on the EOB/RA. If it is a managed care plan, refer to the insurance contract made with the provider, if necessary. If a patient has received many services and the claim was submitted on several forms, determine whether services on all forms were processed for payment. After performing this reconciliation process, attach a copy of the EOB/RA to the claim and put it in a paid file. Each claim should be referenced with the date of payment posted to the patient's account.

Delinquent claims remaining in the tickler file and exceeding the contract time limits should be traced. Complete the insurance claim tracer form shown in Figure 9-2. If a claim has been denied because of a billing error, send a letter to the appeals division of the insurance company as shown in Figure 9-3. Attach a copy of the tracer or letter to the claim and refile it in the tickler file. It is recommended to send a copy of correspondence marked "For your information" to the patient. Follow-up procedures for claim inquiries are discussed next.

Aging Reports

 Each month a report should be run that will indicate which claims are outstanding. The report can be selected to be aged as "current," "30 days," "60 days," "90 days," "120 days," and so on. After running the report, proper follow-up should be made by inquiry as to why a claim has not yet been paid. The insurance billing specialist can write notes on the aging report documenting calls to the payer or adjustment made. For example, a note indicating that the claim is to be corrected and rebilled would be helpful.

After investigating each outstanding item on the aging report, the documentation should be retained properly for future reference. If the office protocol allows notes to be placed directly in the practice management system under the pertinent patient account, then follow the office procedure.

COLLEGE CLINIC
4567 Broad Avenue
Woodland Hills, XY 12345-0001
Telephone (555) 486-9002
Fax (555) 487-8976

INSURANCE CLAIM TRACER

INSURANCE COMPANY NAME American Insurance   DATE: 09/14/XX   .

ADDRESS P.O. Box 5300, New York, New York 12000   .

Patient name: Marcella Austin

Date of birth: May 25, 1970

Employer: TC Corporation

Insured: Marcella Austin

Policy/certificate No.   9635 402-A

Group name/No.   B0105

Date of initial claim submission: 08/02/XX

Date(s) of service: 07/02/XX to 07/10/XX

Total charges submitted: $536.24

An inordinate amount of time has passed since submission of our original claim. We have not received a request for additional information and still await payment of this assigned claim. Please review the attached duplicate and process for payment within 7 days.

DETAILS OF INQUIRY

Please check the claim status and return this letter to our office. Thank you.

- ☐ No record of claim.
- ☐ Claim received and payment is in process.
- ☐ Claim is in suspense (comment please).
- ☐ Claim is in review (comment please).
- ☐ Additional information needed (comment please).
- ☐ Applied to deductible. Amount: $_____
- ☐ Patient not eligible for benefits.
- ☐ Determination issued to beneficiary.
- ☐ Claim paid. Date: _____ Amount: $_____ To whom: _____
- ☐ Claim denied (comment please).

Comments: _____
_____

Thank you for your assistance in this important matter. Please contact the insurance specialist named below if you have any questions regarding this claim.

Insurance Specialist: Katelyn Chang   (555) 486-9002 Ext. 236   .

Treating Physician: Gene Ulibarri, MD   State license number C1480XX   .

Provider Number: 256788831XX   Provider's IRS number 77-86531XX .

FIGURE 9-2 One example of an insurance claim tracer showing how a form may be set up to follow up on a delinquent claim.

ABC MEDICAL GROUP, INC.

123 Main Street
Woodland Hills, XY 12345-0239
Tel. 555/487-4900
Fax. No. 555/486-4834

September 12, 20XX

Ms. Jane Hatfield
Appeals Division
XYZ Managed Care Plan
100 South H Street
Anytown, XY 12345-0001

Dear Ms. Hatfield:

Re: Claim number: A0958
       Patient: Carolyn B. Little
       Dates of service: August 2–10, 20XX

Recently I received a denied claim from your office (see enclosure). A review of the contract I have with your managed care plan shows that these services should have been approved and paid according to your fee schedule.

Enclosed is a photocopy of my chart notes for the professional services rendered to the patient on these dates. I have seen Ms. Little five times in the last nine days and each service was medically necessary by the specific complaints expressed by the patient.

On examination, I found the complaints by the patient were valid.

If after review of this claim you still feel reimbursement is not appropriate, please forward this request to the Peer Review Committee for a final determination.

If you need additional information, please telephone, fax, or write my office.

Sincerely,

John Doe, MD

mtf
Enclosures

FIGURE 9-3 A letter signed by the physician asking for a review about a claim submitted and denied by a managed care plan.

Because time is of the essence, it is wise to be aggressive on claims that are outstanding for more than 60 days, especially when there are issues concerning timely filing.

Insurance Company Payment History

Manually obtaining information on the payment history of insurance companies can be done by making a file of 3- × 5-inch index cards or 8½- × 11-inch three-hole-punched sheets in a loose-leaf binder listing the insurance companies or managed care plans that send claim payments directly to the physician. Every time a payment is received, pull out the card or the loose-leaf sheet for that company and update the information. The following information is necessary for tracking:

- Insurance company name and regional office addresses
- Claims filing procedures
- Payment policies (provisions) for each plan
- Time limits to submit claims
- Time limit for receiving payments
- Dollar amount paid for each procedure code number
- Allowable charges for each procedure code number
- Names of patients covered and their policy and group numbers

If the patients' names and group policy numbers are listed, this file is helpful when discussing with the patient what the insurance company may be expected to pay for certain services. Remember that group numbers may change annually as benefits increase or decrease, so keep the policy numbers current.

 Using the practice management system's monthly reporting capabilities is useful when tracking the payment history of insurance companies. This is an easy method to discover which companies pay slowly or pay less on certain services, and it provides excellent reports for tax purposes or to understand trends in the financial operations of the health care office.

An insurance company payment history system can help avoid potential problems and pinpoint requirements that must be met to help secure additional payment on a reduced or denied claim.

CLAIM INQUIRIES

An **inquiry,** most often referred to as a follow-up or **tracer,** is a written request made to an insurance company to either locate the status of an insurance claim (i.e., claim in review, claim never received, or clarification about something related to the member's health plan), inquire about payment determination shown on the EOB/RA, or ask about general information such as deductible or entitlement. As mentioned, claim status can be accessed electronically or telephonically by digital response systems, thus speeding up response time. Claim status also may be accessed with a telephone call or by mail. The following are reasons for making inquiries:

- There was no response to a submitted claim within 45 days.
- Payment was not received within the time limit for the plan or program.
- Payment is received, but the amount is incorrect.
- Payment is received, but the amount allowed and the patient's responsibility is not defined.
- Payment received was for a patient not seen by the provider. It is possible to receive a payment check made out to a payee's name that is different from the patient's name. Making a call may quickly clarify for whom the payment is being made.

In addition to nonpayment or reduced payment, there are other reasons for inquiries to an insurance company, including the following:

- EOB/RA shows that a professional or diagnostic code was changed from what was submitted.
- EOB/RA shows that the service was disallowed when it was a benefit.

- The claim should be revised and resubmitted. Check to see whether the procedure codes were correct and that the services listed were described fully enough to justify the maximum allowable benefits. If services were coded correctly and a particular service was disallowed, be sure to meet the requirements of your office in documenting this situation. You may need to talk to your supervisor to better understand how to handle this particular issue.
- There is an error on the EOB/RA.
- The check received was made out to the wrong physician.

Inquire about the claim if any of these situations occurs. If the inquiry is submitted in writing, some programs require special forms to be completed with a copy of the claim attached. Figure 9-3 is an example of a letter used when asking for a review about a denied claim that was submitted to a managed care plan. If a claim must be reviewed after payment has been rendered, send in the letter as shown in Figure 9-4. To establish efficient secretarial procedures when calling, document the name of the person spoken to, date and time of call, department or extension of the person, and an outline of the conversation.

PROBLEM PAPER AND ELECTRONIC CLAIMS

Types of Problems

Many types of problem claims (e.g., delinquent, in suspense [pending], lost, rejected, denied, downcoded, partial payment, payment lost in the mail, payment paid to patient, and overpayment) exist. Table 9-1 has a complete list of the types of problems and their descriptions.

To keep accounting accurate and up to date, these problems require some type of follow-up action. The claim status may be indicated on an EOB; however, sometimes a claim is submitted and no status is reported. As mentioned, sending a claim inquiry form (tracer) is often the quickest way of determining the status of a claim (see Figure 9-2).

To prevent repeated claims errors, if the office manager understands and has a good overview of the insurance claims process, he or she should identify the source of the errors within the medical office. Often a claim may be denied because of an error that occurred when collecting registration information at the front desk or when posting charges to the account. Other errors occur because of wrong procedure or diagnostic codes, incorrect provider numbers, and a variety of situations mentioned in prior chapters. Many claims are denied for wrong gender and

COLLEGE CLINIC
4567 Broad Avenue
Woodland Hills, XY
12345-0001
Telephone 555/486-9002
Fax (555) 487-8976

Committee on Physician's Services

Re: Underpayment	
Identification No.:	M18876782
Patient:	Peaches Melba
Type of Service:	Plastic & Reconstructive Surgery
Date of Service:	1 - 3 - XX
Amount Paid:	$ 75.00
My Fees:	$ 180.00

Dear Sirs:

Herewith a request for a committee review of the above-named case, since I consider the allowance paid very low having in mind the location, the extent, the type, and the necessary surgical procedure performed: The skin graft, one inch in diameter, included the lateral third of eyebrow and was full thickness to preserve hair follicles.

Operative report for the surgery has been sent to you with the claim.

Considering these points I hope that you will authorize additional payment in order to bring the total fee to within reasonable and customary charges.

Sincerely,

Cosmo Graff, M.D.

Cosmo Graff, M.D.

mf
enclosure

FIGURE 9-4 A letter signed by the physician appealing a fee reduction. This letter lists important data and is sent to the third-party payer after payment has been received that the physician believes should be increased.

wrong year of birth. The more unusual or foreign-sounding a name is, the more denials occur on the basis of gender. Be aware that some names (e.g., Alex, Cameron) could be either male or female.

The individual handling the front desk must collect insurance information accurately and update patient demographic information routinely (e.g., insurance identification number and address). The person posting to accounts must be certain to post to the correct account and see that supplemental insurers are billed after the primary insurance company has paid. Identified errors should be brought to the attention of the responsible individuals to improve accuracy of outgoing claims and avoid future problems.

Delinquent, Pending, or Suspense

The following are specific claim problems and possible solutions.

PROBLEM: The term **delinquent claim** means payment is overdue from a nonpayer. The nonpayer can be an insurance company, managed care plan, or intermediary for the Medicaid, Medicare, or TRICARE programs. Sometimes nonpayment is caused by a claim in **review** or in **suspense** because of an error or the need for additional information. The carrier may be investigating a claim because of preexisting conditions or possibly because the patient may have a work-related injury. If a service is not covered, sometimes there is no response; however, a follow-up should be initiated to further investigate.

PAPER CLAIM SOLUTION: Use claim management techniques (e.g., insurance claims register, tickler file, or insurance company payment history) to keep on top of delinquent claims so that follow-up can be accomplished in a timely manner. If the office handles a large volume of claims, divide the unpaid claims into four groups, one for each of the three largest insurers and the fourth for all others. Work on one group each week so that the work

Table 9-1	**Insurance Claim Adjudication Problems**
TYPE	**DESCRIPTION**
Delinquent claims	Payment overdue from nonpayer
Denied claims	Lack of insurance coverage (canceled, service provided before effective insurance, or lapsed beyond renewal date)
	Selected diagnoses not covered
	• Frequency limitations or restrictions per benefit period
	• Procedure performed by ineligible specialty provider (e.g., podiatrist would not be paid for neurosurgery)
	• Bundled with other services
	• Payable only in certain locations (e.g., outpatient only)
	• Prior approval needed and not obtained
	• Service or procedure not justified by diagnosis
	• Missing or incorrect place of service code
	Insurance policy issue (preexisting condition or preauthorization required under plan)
	Experimental procedure not reimbursable
	Incorrect code for service rendered
	Code selected from incorrect system (CPT code instead of HCPCS Level II national code)
	Unbundled codes when one code should have been submitted
	Unspecified diagnostic code reported
Downcoded claims	Computer software selects procedure code at lower level than medical service requires
Lost claims	Claim not received by third-party payer
Overpayment	Third-party payer pays more than the bill or the allowed amount
	Third-party payer pays more than one's fee or contract rate
	• Third-party payer sends provider payment intended for patient
	• Provider receives duplicate payments from two or more insurance companies or from the patient and one or more third-party payers
	• Provider receives payment for someone who is not the provider's patient
Payment errors	Third-party payer sends provider payment intended for patient
	Patient paid by third-party payer when provider should have been paid
Pending (suspense) claims	Claim has an error
	Additional information required
	Claim review needed by third-party payer (complex procedure, high reimbursement, utilization management)
Rejected (soft denial) claims	Claim contains technical error (missing or incorrect information, numbers transposed, invalid diagnostic or procedural code numbers, duplicate charges, duplicate dates of service, and so on)
	Third-party payer instructions not followed
Two-party check	Check written to both the provider and the hospital
Underpayment	Third-party payment at less than negotiated contract rate

is spread out over the 4 weeks in the month. Write a follow-up letter to the insurance company asking for payment and enclose a copy of the original claim form or complete the insurance company's claim tracer form or create one as shown in Figure 9-2. If the insurance contract does not bar the provider from billing members for noncovered services and the plan has not responded, send the plan a letter with a copy to the member. In the letter, say that you assume the nonresponse means the service is not covered, so you will bill the member directly.

ELECTRONIC CLAIM SOLUTION: In-house editing includes trying to resolve the issue as to why the claim is still not paid. Look for evidence of the claim being submitted, which should be identified in the practice management system. If the claim was submitted and confirmed received, then it is wise to look at how the claim was billed (e.g., CPT and ICD-9-CM codes). If this information is correct and the dates are correct on the claim, then contact the payer to find out what other information is

holding up the claim or why the claim was denied. If the claim was not successful in being received by the clearinghouse and there is no clear-cut reason on reports or investigating the claim data showing exactly what information was amiss, then perhaps there was a problem with the format. Contacting the clearinghouse gives you more insight as to why the claim was not successfully received or rejected. The insurance billing specialist can contact the payer immediately after finding out that the claim is delinquent or the payer can be contacted after initial steps of investigation take place such as the in-house editing and contacting the clearinghouse.

Lost Claims

PROBLEM: When an insurance claim is received by the insurance company, the claim is date stamped usually within 24 hours, assigned a claim number, and logged into the payer system. However, if there is a backlog of claims, it may take several days to be logged into the system. If one calls to find out the status of the claim during that time, one may be told it has not been received or it may be considered a **lost claim.**

PAPER CLAIM SOLUTION: Ask if there is a backlog of claims to resolve the situation. This indicates that the claim probably has not been logged into the system. Always verify that the patient is insured by the insurance company and is covered for the basic benefits claimed. If it is determined to be lost, then submit a copy of the original claim referencing it "copy of the original claim submitted on (date)." Before sending it, verify the correct mailing address (e.g., post office box number, ZIP code). There are several ways to track the claim if there have been various problems with the same insurance company. Send it by certified mail with return receipt or fax the claim and ask for a confirmation. Another method available to show proof that a special communication was sent by a deadline is to obtain and complete a Certificate of Mailing form from the post office. The form is initialed and postmarked at the post office and returned to the insurance biller for office file records. Because the post office does not keep a record of the mailing, this certificate costs less than certified mail. If there is verifiable information of a lost claim, call or write to the provider relations department or member services and explain the problem. If a managed care plan, possibly check the time limit in the contract with the payer in question. Some contracts have a clause that specifies any claims not paid within a certain number of days (e.g., 30 days) after receipt will be paid at an increased rate or in full. If there is a possibility that claims have been mishandled, gather documentation and send a letter to the state insurance commission with a letter to the third-party payer about the action taken.

ELECTRONIC CLAIM SOLUTION: Always retain the electronic response or confirmation from the carrier saying it received the specific claim. Keep all clearinghouse reports that confirm received transmission and relay information back regarding claim status. Practice management software programs show the date of every claim submitted. Tamper-proof data recorded by the computer may be used as a legal form of proof that the claim was submitted to the third-party payer. Unfortunately this does not "prove" the payer received the claim, so some payers do not always accept this. Send a printed copy of the electronic proof of timely filing to the third-party payer. Or you may send a letter with the proof of filing, a copy of the claim, and a copy of the denial if you received one for exceeding the timely filing limit.

Rejected Claims

Chapter 7 discusses some common reasons why paper claims are rejected or delayed. A **rejected claim,** also called *soft denial,* is a submitted claim that does not follow specific third-party payer instructions or contains a technical error. Such claims may be disapproved or discarded by the system and returned to the biller. Technical errors consist of missing or incorrect information and are found through computer edits, screening processes for benefit provisions, and proofreading. Medicare-mandated prepayment screens are discussed in Chapter 12.

PROBLEM: Paper or electronic claim rejections may occur due to one or more of the following:

- Transposed numbers
- Missing required Health Insurance Portability and Accountability Act (HIPAA) transaction code sets
- Missing subscriber date of birth
- Missing, invalid, or incorrect procedure codes and modifiers
- Missing or invalid place of service
- Mismatch of place of service to type of service
- Missing referring physician when billing tests
- Missing or invalid provider number when the patient was referred
- Incorrect, invalid, nonspecific, or missing diagnostic code numbers
- Incorrect dates of service
- Incorrect year of service
- Incorrect number of days in the month (e.g., February)
- Code description does not match services rendered
- Duplicate dates of service
- Duplicate charges

PAPER CLAIM SOLUTION: If a claim is rejected and returned, add the missing or incomplete information and resubmit a corrected claim for regular claims processing. Never send a corrected claim for review or appeal because this type of claim should always be resubmitted.

ELECTRONIC CLAIM SOLUTION: Likely, an electronic claim will not make it in a batch to be transmitted to the payer if a series of computer edits have been performed before batching (grouping claims together). The system will flag this particular claim as needing edits and will not batch it in with the rest. Correct the data in the appropriate fields and rebatch the claim.

If the claim does go through to the payer and is reported as being rejected, review the rejection reason code and correct the field. Then, rebatch the claim and submit again.

PROBLEM: A claim is submitted for several services. One service is rejected for incomplete information but the other services are paid.

PAPER CLAIM SOLUTION: Complete a new CMS-1500 (08-05) claim form, including all information and resubmit for the rejected services only. Note in Block 19 that it is a resubmission.

ELECTRONIC CLAIM SOLUTION: As with a paper claim, add the required information and retransmit only the claim that was rejected, not all the claims that were originally batched and transmitted. Because this was rejected, it will likely be in the payer system for processing.

PROBLEM: Third-party payer requests further information or information about another insurance carrier.

PAPER CLAIM SOLUTION: Verify primary and secondary insurance information with the patient, obtain signed patient release of information form that follows HIPAA guidelines, and call or mail the information to the insurance company. Identify the subscriber, subscriber number, and date of service on all correspondence.

ELECTRONIC CLAIM SOLUTION: As with a paper claim, verify all insurance information and provide accurate payer information in all applicable fields and resubmit.

PROBLEM: Resubmitted claim is returned a second time.

PAPER CLAIM SOLUTION: Review the EOB/RA statement to determine whether there is a denial code or narrative explanation. Examine the claim for missing, incomplete, or incorrect information and, if found, correct it. Evaluate the claim to determine whether it is a candidate for the appeal process. Determine whether a specific appeal form must be submitted. Submit chart notes, a detailed summary, or a copy of the operative or pathology report, as applicable, to clearly identify the procedure or service. Enclose a cover letter with the resubmitted data. The letter must specifically say what course of action is being requested (i.e., review) and it must have the name and signature of the person requesting the review.

ELECTRONIC CLAIM SOLUTION: Verify all data required for processing the claim at the payer end. Determine whether an appeal process is warranted and follow steps as outlined by the payer.

Denied Claims

A **denied paper or electronic claim** is one that may be denied because of benefits coverage policy issues or program issues. It stands to reason that insurance companies save money when a claim is denied, and only a small percentage of individuals pursue appeals. State laws require insurance companies to notify the insured of a denial and state why the claim was denied. It is possible that payment can be received even after a claim has been denied in whole or in part.

When a claim is denied and the responsible party is the patient, then transfer the balance to the patient's financial account record. However, an exception is a Medicare patient who must have signed an Advance Beneficiary Notice acknowledging the service will not be paid by Medicare and that he or she is responsible for the fee.

If the patient has not been contacted by the insurance company, notify the patient by telephone or mail as soon as possible to keep him or her informed. Always retain the correspondence from the insurance company so that it can be quickly retrieved in case a patient inquires and has additional questions. The recourse to a denied claim is to appeal and request a review in writing. The appeals process varies among third-party payers. A Medicare claim may be redetermined (appealed) by requesting a review in writing, and federal laws require that an explanation be given for each denied service. In Medicare Part B redetermination cases, carriers have been instructed to pay an appealed claim if the cost of the hearing process is more than the amount of the claim.

Some reasons why paper or electronic claims are not paid because of denial include the following:

- Selected diagnoses not covered
- Frequency limitations or restrictions per benefit period
- Procedure performed by ineligible specialty provider (e.g., podiatrist would not be paid for neurosurgery)
- Bundled with other services
- Payable only in certain locations (e.g., outpatient only)
- Prior approval needed and not obtained
- Service or procedure not justified by diagnosis
- Missing or incorrect place of service code

Because denials usually involved policy coverage issues, electronic claims may be denied for the same reasons as a paper claim.

In either case of paper or electronic claim denial, simply changing information on the claim and resubmitting will not resolve the problem. Additional examples with suggested solutions are as follows:

PROBLEM: Service was not a policy or program benefit (e.g., routine physical examination, routine tests, routine foot care, routine dental care, cosmetic surgery, custodial care, eye or hearing examinations for glasses or hearing aids, and some immunizations). Plastic surgery is considered a general exclusion in many insurance policies.

PAPER AND ELECTRONIC CLAIM SOLUTION: Send the patient a statement with a notation of the response from the insurance company. Before providing services, always verify coverage for routine physical examinations or tests and services that are in question as to whether they will be paid by the insurance policy. Discuss this with the patient before service is provided and advise of the likelihood of no coverage. It may be appropriate to request payment at the time of service. Before service is given in a Medicare case, have the patient sign an Advance Beneficiary Notice of Noncoverage (see Figure 12-9).

PROBLEM: Treatment is given for a preexisting condition. (Currently some policies do not include this exclusion.)

PAPER AND ELECTRONIC CLAIM SOLUTION: When a patient is referred, ask the referring physician to forward information on all preexisting conditions that may be relevant to the surgery or procedure to be performed. Under HIPAA policies, physicians may treat patients, seek payment, and conduct routine health care operations without having to obtain a patient's written consent. Request verification of insurance coverage from the insurer for the surgery or procedure with regard to preexisting conditions. Request authorization for the surgical procedure or diagnostic tests. If authorization is denied, have the physician discuss other treatment or payment options with the patient. If the physician believes that the patient's condition is not preexisting, send an appeal to the insurance company. Otherwise, bill the patient, noting the insurance company's response on the statement.

PROBLEM: Insurance coverage is canceled before service.

PAPER AND ELECTRONIC CLAIM SOLUTION: Send the patient a statement with notation of the insurance determination on the bill.

PROBLEM: Insurance coverage lapsed before service is rendered.

PAPER AND ELECTRONIC CLAIM SOLUTION: Send the patient a statement with notation of the response from the insurance company on the bill.

PROBLEM: Service is provided before coverage is in effect.

PAPER AND ELECTRONIC CLAIM SOLUTION: Send the patient a statement with notation of the response from the insurance company on the bill.

PROBLEM: Insurance company indicates provided service was not medically necessary.

PAPER AND ELECTRONIC CLAIM SOLUTION: Determine under what circumstances the third-party payer considers the service to be medically necessary. The problem may be that the diagnostic code does not properly support the procedural codes being reported. It is vital that the physician's documentation be specific enough to support the necessity of the services provided. If the physician believes the patient's condition supported the medical necessity for the service, send an appeal for review to the insurance company, explaining in detail the reasons why. Keep a list of codes that have been denied for medical necessity and what further determinations were made in the insurance company payment history. Check the insurance contract to determine whether the patient may be billed. Consider asking patients to sign an Advance Beneficiary Notice or Waiver of Liability form before treatment. Beware that you do not have every patient sign such documents because then such documents would be considered a blanket waiver. Bill the patient if payment may be denied.

PROBLEM: Service was for an injury that is considered as payable or covered under workers' compensation. Create a workers' compensation information sheet asking the employee and employer to fill out separate sections with space for the following: explanation of the injury, insurance information, adjuster's name and telephone number, and claim or case number.

PAPER AND ELECTRONIC CLAIM SOLUTION: Locate the carrier for the industrial injury, request permission to treat, and send the carrier a report of the case with a bill. Notify the patient's health insurance carrier monthly about the status of the case.

PROBLEM: Service was not precertified for a surgery, hospitalization, or diagnostic procedure.

PAPER AND ELECTRONIC CLAIM SOLUTION: Telephone the insurance company and ask whether precertification was necessary for the service or if any sanctions were imposed. The office may want to institute a policy that all surgical procedures and durable medical equipment/supplies be called in to insurance companies before rendering the service. Document the contact name, date, and time of the call. If there were problems or difficulties about the case leading to the reason that precertification was not obtained, write a letter of appeal noting the history. Insurance payers can change their policies on certain procedure codes throughout the year.

PROBLEM: Patient or employer did not pay premium.

PAPER AND ELECTRONIC CLAIM SOLUTION: Verify insurance coverage before treatment begins, especially for procedures and surgery. Change patient's account to "cash" if insurance is not in force and discuss this with the patient.

PROBLEM: Service or procedure is experimental.

PAPER AND ELECTRONIC CLAIM SOLUTION: Verify whether the procedure is approved by the insurance company before the procedure is done.

PROBLEM: Deductible was not met.

PAPER AND ELECTRONIC CLAIM SOLUTION: Ask the patient when he or she arrives at the office about the status of the deductible. Or telephone the payer to find out this information, which often may be obtained from an automated system. Collect the deductible from the patient if it has not been paid. Consider holding the claim if several services are performed during the same time period and the patient paid the deductible at another office but the deductible has not been recorded by the insurance company.

PROBLEM: Services are considered cosmetic.

PAPER AND ELECTRONIC CLAIM SOLUTION: Appeal the claim if the problem was treated because of a medical condition, not for cosmetic reasons. Otherwise, collect from the patient before services are provided.

PROBLEM: Claim duplicates an existing claim.

PAPER AND ELECTRONIC CLAIM SOLUTION: Verify the services or charges have not been previously submitted and processed. Double billing may occur to medical practices with more than one location. All facilities should have the same software or programs that can communicate with each other. Update software system and write a check to the third-party payer if overpayment has occurred.

PROBLEM: Claim is missing a modifier or has an incomplete or invalid modifier.

PAPER AND ELECTRONIC CLAIM SOLUTION: Become familiar with the modifier descriptions and their appropriate use, and verify that the payer recognizes them.

Measures to Prevent Denied Claims. Prevention measures to avoid denied claims are as follows:

1. Be proactive and verify insurance coverage at the first visit—this saves time and surprises for everyone. Make sure demographic information is current at each visit.
2. Include progress notes and orders for tests for extended hospital services.
3. Submit a letter from the prescribing physician documenting necessity when ambulance transportation is used.
4. Clarify the type of service (e.g., primary surgical services versus assist-at-surgery services).
5. Use modifiers to further describe and identify the exact service rendered.
6. Keep abreast of the latest policies for all contracted payers, as well as the federal programs by going to the Centers for Medicare and Medicaid Services (CMS) website to read currently posted Medicare Transmittals (formerly called Program Memorandums). For example, know the Medicare Local Coverage Determinations (LCDs) and National Coverage Determinations (NCDs) that state which conditions and services are covered and limitations on coverage. Read news releases from the Blue Plans, Medicaid, TRICARE, workers' compensation insurance companies, and managed care plans.
7. Obtain current provider manuals for all contracted managed care payers, as well as the Blue Plans, Medicaid, Medicare, and TRICARE for quick reference. When bulletins or pages are received from these programs during the year, keep the manuals up to date by inserting the current material.

Downcoding

Lowered reimbursement is the result of downcoding. As mentioned in Chapter 6, downcoding occurs in the following problems.

PROBLEM: There is insufficient diagnostic information on a claim.

PAPER CLAIM SOLUTION: Be sure each procedure listed on the paper claim form is linked to an appropriate diagnosis. Refer to the health record if necessary. A code link book is an excellent resource and is available from Ingenix (see the Appendix).

PROBLEM: Unspecified diagnoses are listed on the claim form. Routine use of too many nonspecific diagnostic codes (ICD-9-CM codes that have number "9" as the fourth or fifth digit) result in denials, especially if extensive or specific surgery is involved.

PAPER CLAIM SOLUTION: Make sure the physician dictates specific diagnoses and does not circle nonspecific diagnoses on an encounter form. Always code to the highest level of specificity. Refer to the patient's health record when necessary.

Payment Paid to Patient

PROBLEM: Sometimes an insurance payment may be sent in error to the patient after an assignment of benefits has been signed and sent in with the insurance claim. In some cases a clause may be in the insurance policy that payment may be made only to the insured. In another instance, this might happen when a patient uses the services of a provider who is outside of his or her preferred provider organization.

PAPER AND ELECTRONIC CLAIM SOLUTION: Call the insurance company to verify whether the payment was made and to whom. If the provider has a participating agreement, then the insurance company is obligated to pay the provider and must proceed by correcting the error. If the account is substantially overdue, ask for a copy of the endorsed check or EOB/RA statement that indicates where payment was sent. If the carrier refuses, ask for help from the supervisor of the provider or customer relations department. The following are two different courses of action to take after this has been verified:

1. Call the patient explaining that the insurance company sent payment to the patient in error and ask when full payment can be expected. Document the commitment in the patient's financial record. If the patient cannot be reached by telephone, send a letter by certified mail to the patient. Document each effort that went into collection of the payment from the patient and the patient's responses. Then discuss with the physician

whether he or she wishes to discharge the patient from the practice.

2. Send a letter to the insurance company, including a copy of the claim with EOB/RA indicating payment was made to the patient and a copy of the assignment of benefits. Demand payment from the insurance company, stating the need to honor the assignment and the signed participation agreement. The insurance company must recover the payment from the patient. If a dead-end is reached after pursuing reimbursement from the insurance company, then file a complaint with the state insurance commissioner. After receiving the physician's complaint, the commissioner will write to the insurance company and request a review of the claim. If the insurance company admits that there is an assignment of benefits and that it inadvertently paid the patient, the insurance company must pay the physician within 2 to 3 weeks and honor the assignment even before it recovers its money from the patient. The insurance company then files for payment from the patient.

Two-Party Check

PROBLEM: A received check is made out to both the physician and the hospital and only part of the sum is the physician's payment. This might occur when the provider is contracted with the hospital.

SOLUTION: If you do not receive an EOB containing the breakdown of both party's payments, then call the insurance company and ask how much should be retained by the physician. Request the allocation be sent in writing. Ask whose tax identification number will be used on the 1099 form for reporting income to the Internal Revenue Service. The hospital's income should not be reflected on the physician's 1099 form. To avoid another problem like this, inquire why the insurance company paid in this manner. Sometimes a participating agreement may exist that the physician did not know about.

Underpayment

It is important that the insurance biller perform random checks and monitor large claim payments made during the first 3 months of a new contract to ensure the third-party payer's system has the contract loaded into the software correctly. Track the charge, allowable, deductible, and paid amount to determine whether the amounts are correct (Figure 9-5).

PROBLEM: Underpaid claims.

SOLUTION: Print the incorrectly paid claims and give them to the third-party payer's contract negotiator to be resolved. Ask them to readjudicate the claims on the basis of the correct contract, but make sure they are not processed and returned as duplicate claims. Use codes or notations on the claims to indicate they are updated.

Overpayment

An **overpayment** is a sum of money paid by the third-party payer or patient to the provider of service that is more than the bill or more than the allowed amount. Overpayments may be discovered immediately, called to one's attention by the patient or third-party payer, or not discovered for several months or years. The Office of Inspector General strongly advises to return overpayment promptly. Not doing so can lead to severe fines and implicate fraudulent activity.

Some states have laws or court decisions barring or restricting managed care plans and other insurers from recovering mistaken payments from providers. Some states bar insurers from collecting any mistaken payment from an innocent provider. Some states will not let insurers recover if the provider "changed its position" in reliance on the payment (i.e., the provider spent the money to pay its bills). First, determine whether an overpayment exists by reviewing the available financial documents on the case in question. Then decide how to handle the

Method for Calculating Over- and Underpayments						
Third-party payer: _____						
Patient name	Procedure/ service	Claims paid date	Provider charge	Allowed amount	Amount paid	Overpayment (+) Underpayment (−)
May Ito	Colonoscopy	5/2/20XX	$1500	$900	$2000	$1100+

FIGURE 9-5 Audit method used for calculating overpayments and underpayments. Subtract the allowed amount, which is the insurance contract's fee schedule amount minus any patient copayment or deductible from the amount paid. Any positive (+) number is an overpayment and any negative (−) number is an underpayment.

overpayment. Be sure to get the physician's attorney's advice on the extent to which you can challenge a plan's demand for repayment on the basis of state law or court decisions.

It is wise to develop an overpayment policy and procedure for each type of insurer, program, or managed care plan and for every type of overpayment situation that may occur.

PROBLEM: Overpayment scenarios that may occur are as follows:

- Receiving more than one's fee from a third-party payer
- Receiving more than the contract rate from a managed care plan
- Receiving payments that should have been paid to the patient
- Receiving duplicate payments from two or more insurance companies or from the patient and one or more third-party payers
- Receiving payment made for someone who is not the provider's patient

SOLUTION: When an overpayment occurs, post the activity to the appropriate patient account with additional notation that it was received in error and a refund was made. Creation of an account specifically for overpayments is advisable to track all funds in this category. In any type of overpayment situation, cash the third-party payer's check and make out a refund check payable to the originator of the overpayment. Keep a copy of the third-party payer check before it is deposited. The refund check should always be sent to the attention of a specific person at the insurance company. In case of an audit, this establishes documentation showing the problem has been resolved. Usually insurance companies process a credit of the overpayment amount to the next check voucher.

Refund checks should be given top priority and written as soon as reasonably possible. Make sure the office policy is clearly stated and adhered to in all cases. If the patient pays and a third-party pays and the overpayment must be refunded to the patient, always write a check—never refund in cash. Send the patient a letter with a check to explain the overpayment. If the patient pays by credit card, wait until the charges have cleared to draft a check or preferably process a credit card refund to the credit card company.

If the patient cannot be located to return the money, send a check by registered mail to the patient's last known address. When it comes back marked "undeliverable," retain the document as legal proof that an honest effort was made to return the overpayment. The money should be listed as taxable income and put in the bank.

Commercial Carriers

 PROBLEM: Usually an overpayment mistake made by a commercial carrier is the insurer's problem.

SOLUTION: First call and notify the patient; then proceed cautiously before refunding money by doing the following:

- Investigate the refund request by sending a letter to the insurance payer disputing the recoupment. Include documentation as proof (e.g., operative report, health record, or bundling guidelines).
- Obtain documentation from the insurance payer to prove why the refund is legitimate.
- The general rule is to not pay old recoupments dating back more than 4 or 5 years.
- If two or more third-party payers send duplicate payments, write a letter to each explaining the situation and let them straighten it out. Then send a refund to the correct third-party payer to the attention of a specific person after receiving a letter explaining to whom the money should be sent.

Managed Care Plan

 PROBLEM: An overpayment from a managed care plan is discovered.

SOLUTION: Review the payer's policy about overpayments and be sure it is clearly documented in the provider's contract. Address this issue if it is not defined by the payer. Follow your office protocol for documenting overpayments.

Medicare

 PROBLEM: An overpayment is made from Medicare, Medicaid, or a Blue Plan.

SOLUTION: Check the billing and health records to determine whether the provider made any mistakes. The physician has 30 days from the date of the letter to mail a refund back to the address in the letter. However, if an error has been made by the insurance company, send a letter with documentation to appeal and prove the provider's case. Medicare, Medicaid, and the Blue Plans usually process a credit of the overpayment on the next payment voucher.

PROBLEM: An overpayment is made by a Medicare patient.

SOLUTION: For assigned claims, if Medicare sends a letter to the physician, respond with a letter and overpayment check to the patient within 15 days. For nonassigned claims, if Medicare sends a letter to the physician, a refund check must be made within 15 days or the physician may be subject to civil monetary penalties and sanctions.

REBILLING

If a claim has not been paid, do not automatically **rebill (resubmit)** the third-party payer without researching the reason why it is still outstanding. Simply rebilling claims can be considered duplicate claims, and the insurance company may audit the physician's practice for trying to collect duplicate payment unless you mark it "Possible duplicate." Instead, follow up on the claim as indicated in the previous section. If it is discovered that an error has been made in billing a case, then send in a corrected claim or use a claim correction form (Figure 9-6) if the third-party payer will accept it. This form was developed by a special committee convened by the American Association of Health Plans, the Healthcare Financial Management Association, and the Specialty Society Coalition, which included representatives of the American Academy of Family Physicians, the American College of Obstetricians and Gynecologists, and the American Academy of Dermatology. Medical practices may adapt it or photocopy it for use.

Generally, if a bill has not been paid, the provider's office personnel have a strategy to automatically rebill the claim or the patient every 30 days. Bill patients on a monthly basis, even when insurance payment is expected so that they understand what has been submitted and what is pending. The statement should clearly identify the claim that has been submitted and what action is expected from the patient. If collection becomes a problem, action can be referenced to the date of service if the patient has been billed consistently. See Chapter 10 for the wording of notations on statements and in the collection process.

In December 2004 the CMS implemented a process that allows providers to resubmit corrected claims that have been rejected for minor errors or omissions rather than appealing those claims. For example, claims with missing or incorrect provider numbers, incorrect modifiers, or claims with keying errors (incorrect date or place of service) can be rebilled.

REVIEW AND APPEAL PROCESS

An **appeal** is a request for payment by asking for a review of an insurance claim that has been inadequately or incorrectly paid or denied by an insurance company. In the Medicare program, appeals are referred to as *redeterminations.* Usually there is a time limit for appealing a claim. Always check every private third-party payer, Medicare, TRICARE, managed care, and workers' compensation

payment against the appropriate fee schedule or customary profile to determine whether the benefits were allowed correctly. To find out this information, read the payment voucher document or refer to provider manuals for the various programs.

An appeal on a claim should be based not only on billing guidelines but also on state and federal insurance laws and regulations.

There may be a discrepancy in the way the physician or physician's staff and insurance company interpret a coding guideline. The decision to appeal a claim should be based on several factors. The provider should determine that there is sufficient information to back up his or her claim, and the amount of money in question should be sufficient in the physician's opinion. Ultimately the decision to appeal rests in the physician's hands, not the insurance billing specialist's. It takes a team effort to appeal a claim successfully. To proceed, make a telephone call to the insurance company. It may save time and money, and an expert who is able to solve the problem may be reached. The following are basic guidelines:

- Assemble all documents needed (e.g., patient's medical record, copy of the insurance claim form, and EOB/RA).
- Remain courteous at all times.
- Obtain the name and extension number of the insurance claims representative or adjuster and keep this with the telephone records. After developing rapport, one may wish to call on him or her in the future for help. Ask for any toll-free numbers that the company may have, and keep these for future reference.
- Listen carefully. Jot down the date and take notes of how to solve the problem. This may be of help if another problem of the same type occurs.

An appeal is filed in the following circumstances:

- Payment is denied and the reason for denial is not known.
- Payment is received, but the amount is incorrect. Verify that initially the correct amount was billed. Perhaps there was an excessive reduction in the allowed payment.
- The physician disagrees with the decision by the third-party payer about a preexisting condition.
- Unusual circumstances warranted medical treatments that are not reflected in payment.
- Precertification was not obtained within contract provisions because of extenuating circumstances, and the claim was denied.
- Inadequate payment was received for a complicated procedure.
- "Not medically necessary" is stated as the reason for denial and the physician disagrees.

Claim Correction Form

Physician offices are encouraged to submit claims electronically. This form should be used in situations where the provider cannot submit corrected claims electronically or where electronic submissions would not adequately address the issue.

Submitted To:

Plan/Payer Name:_____ Date Submitted:_____

Plan/Payer Address: _____

City:_____ State _____ Zip_____

Telephone: (____)_____ Fax: (____)_____ E-mail:_____

Patient Name: _____ D.O.B.:_____
                    First   M.I.   Last

Subscriber Name: _____ Date of Service: _____

Policy #:_____ Group #: _____ Original Claim #:_____

Submitted From:

Provider Name: _____ TIN or ID#: _____

Contact: _____ Telephone: (____)_____ Ext._____

Fax:(____)_____ E-mail _____

THE FOLLOWING WAS CORRECTED ON THIS CLAIM:

❏ The patient's policy/group number was incorrect. The correct number(s) are shown above.

❏ The correct CPT code is _____ instead of _____

❏ Wrong date of service was filed. The correct date is _____

❏ Visits were denied based on the diagnosis given. Proper diagnosis code is_____ instead of _____

❏ Visit: ❏ Procedure: denied as over carrier's utilization limits. Please see attached letter to justify extensions of these limits.

❏ Carrier indicated that the patient is covered by another plan that is Primary. This is incorrect. Patient indicates you are Primary.

❏ The secondary carrier is: _____ ❏ There is no secondary carrier.

❏ The procedure was denied as medically not necessary. Documentation to support the medical necessity of this service is attached.

❏ Our clerk: ❏ Carrier's clerk: failed to enter correct number of times (units) procedure was performed. Correct units are as follows:

D.O.S.: _____ Code: _____ Units: _____ Charge Total $: _____

❏ Multiple Surgical Procedures:

  ❏ Carrier failed to approve any procedure at 100%.   ❏ Carrier approved incorrect procedure at 100%.

  Carrier should have approved code _____ @ ❏ 100% or ❏ 50% instead of _____

  Carrier should have approved code _____ @ ❏ 100% or ❏ 50% instead of _____

  Carrier should have approved code _____ @ ❏ 100% or ❏ 50% instead of _____

❏ Modifiers should be attached to code(s)

Code	Code		Code	Code
❏ -50 ____ ____		❏ -51 ____ ____		
❏ -58 ____ ____		❏ -59 ____ ____		
❏ -79 ____ ____		❏ -GA ____ ____		
❏ __ ____ ____		❏ ____ ____		

❏ The following E/M visit was denied as included in the global surgical fee. In fact, the service was a significant separately identifiable service provided above and beyond the procedure and submitted with appropriate E/M modifier. Please reconsider with attached documentation:

  Code: _____ with modifier(s); ❏ -24 ❏ -25   Charge $ _____

❏ UPIN information for code _____ was omitted. Physician Name: _____ UPIN: _____

❏ Plan specific provider I.D. omitted. The I.D. # is_____

❏ CLIA number was omitted. The CLIA number is_____

❏ The place of service was incorrect. The place of service should be _____

❏ The service was rendered at the physician's physical location listed in Box 32 of the claim form.

❏ Failed to attach EOB from Primary carrier. The EOB is attached to this form.

❏ Failed to enter correct information on indicated line of claim form.

  Line #:_____ Correct Information: _____

❏ Other reason for claim correction: _____

❏ Comment: _____

June 2003

FIGURE 9-6 One example of a claim correction form that may be adapted or photocopied for use by medical practices that was developed by a special committee convened by the American Association of Health Plans, the Healthcare Financial Management Association, and the Specialty Society Coalition, June 2003. These data may not always apply to all third-party insurers because each has its own procedures.

FILING AN APPEAL

Refer to the end of this chapter for carrying out the procedure when filing an appeal that is not a Medicare case.

If the appeal is won but copies of the same documents must be submitted each time this issue arises, ask the third-party payer how future claims with the same issue may be handled. Keep track of this information in a file.

Appeals must be in writing, but some programs require completion of special forms. Always send a copy of the original claim, EOB/RA, and any other documents to justify the appeal.

It is always important to keep track of the status after inquiry or appeal until payment for the case is resolved. Use the insurance claims register mentioned in Chapter 3 or a separate active file labeled "Appeals Pending."

If an appeal is not successful, the physician may want to proceed to the next step, which is a peer review. A **peer review** is an evaluation done by a group of unbiased practicing physicians to judge the effectiveness and efficiency of professional care rendered. This group determines the medical necessity and subsequent payment for the case in question. Some insurance companies send a claim for peer review routinely for certain procedures that have been done for particular diagnoses.

Additional information on tracing delinquent claims, appealing or reviewing a claim, or submitting a claim for a deceased patient can be found in the chapters on Medicaid, Medicare, TRICARE, and workers' compensation.

Medicare Review and Redetermination Process

A physician or beneficiary has the right to appeal a claim after payment or denial. The Medicare program has five levels of redetermination and special guidelines to follow:

Level 1: Redetermination (telephone, letter, or CMS-20027 Form)
Level 2: Reconsideration (Hearing officer [HO] hearing)
Level 3: Administrative law judge (ALJ) hearing
Level 4: Medicare Appeals Council (MAC)
Level 5: Federal District Court

Telephone Review

Most Medicare carriers have a telephone appeals phone (TAP) service, which may save you from filing a formal paper "Post Payment Review." When requesting a telephone appeal, gather information such as the beneficiary's name, date of birth, Medicare health insurance claim number, name and address of provider of service, telephone and group tax identification number, date of initial determination, date of service for which the initial determination was issued, and which items are at issue in the appeal (progress notes, operative report).

Table 9-2 illustrates the Medicare Part B appeals process. Because Medicare guidelines frequently change, refer to the website; see Internet Resources at the end of this chapter.

Redetermination (Level 1)

On October 1, 2004, the redetermination step became effective. If the claim was denied because of a simple error made by the insurance biller, such as omission of the National Provider Identifier (NPI) of the referring physician or failure to code a diagnosis, then complete a CMS-20027 form and resubmit a corrected claim (Figure 9-7). Include only the denied services and indicate in Block 19 "resubmission, corrected claim." In the event the third-party payer made an error—for example, a procedure code was different from what was submitted or the date of service was entered incorrectly from the paper claim into the payer's computer—then resubmit the claim with an attachment explaining the error. If response to the resubmission indicates that the claim has been "processed" previously, then go to the next appeal level.

A notice must be mailed by the Medicare intermediary within 60 days of receipt of a request from a beneficiary or provider. It must include reasons for the decision, a summary of clinical or scientific evidence used in making the redetermination, a description of how to obtain additional information, a notification of the right to appeal, and instructions on how to appeal the decision to the next level. If requested, the Medicare intermediary must provide information about the policy, manual, or regulation used in making the redetermination decision. The decision must be written in language the beneficiary can understand.

Reconsideration (Level 2)

The physician may ask for a review when a claim is assigned. The request must be within 6 months from the date of the original determination shown on the RA. Figure 9-8 shows Form CMS-20033, which may be used in requesting a reconsideration of Medicare Part B claims. However, some carriers have developed their own request forms. Contact the carrier to find out the necessary form to use. Review the RA for the denial code or narrative stating why the claim has been denied. Check the claim for accuracy of diagnostic, procedural, or Healthcare

Table 9-2	Medicare Part B Redetermination Process				
LEVEL		TIME LIMIT FOR REQUEST	AMOUNT IN CONTROVERSY	JURISDICTION	FORM
1	Redetermination (telephone, letter, or CMS-20027 form)	120 days from initial claim determination	None	Medicare carrier/ Medicare Administrative Contractor (MAC)	CMS-2007 or CMS-20027 form (possibly fax) CMS-1500 (08-05) corrected claim resubmitted
2	Reconsideration (hearing officer [HO] hearing)	180 days from receipt of Medicare Redetermination Notice	None	Carrier/Qualified Independent Contractor (QIC)	CMS-20033
3	Administrative law judge (ALJ) hearing	60 days from receipt of the HO determination	$130 or more (2010)	Carrier/Social Security Bureau of Hearings and Appeals	CMS-5011A/B
4	Medicare Appeals Council	60 days from receipt of hearing decision	None	Federal District Court	HA-520
5	Federal District Court	60 days from receipt of the departmental appeal board's (DAB) decision	At least $1220 (2010)		

Common Procedure Coding System (HCPCS) codes or missing modifiers, as well as any other item that might be incorrect or missing.

Attach the following with the reconsideration request:

1. Copy of the original insurance claim
2. Copy of the RA showing the denial
3. Photocopy of other documents, such as operative or pathology report or detailed summary about the procedure, with appropriate words highlighted to help the reviewer
4. In the reconsideration form, explain the procedure indicating justification for the services and the reason the provider should receive more reimbursement.

Mail the documents by certified mail with return receipt requested and retain copies of all documents sent to the carrier in the provider's pending file.

If a claim is unassigned, the beneficiary (patient) can pursue the review or appoint the physician as an authorized representative. The patient completes form SSA-1696-U4 (Figure 9-9) and obtains the physician's acceptance signature. Decisions on unassigned claims are sent to the patient.

Send all requests to the review department. Most insurance companies have an address or post office box for review of requests that is different from initial claim submissions, so be sure to send it to a correct current address. A review is usually completed by the third-party payer within 30 to 45 days. Make a follow-up inquiry if no response is received in that time frame.

If certain procedures are consistently denied, ask the carrier what information is necessary to process the claim. If the provider is not satisfied with the results of the review, move to the next level.

Administrative Law Judge Hearing (Level 3)

A request for a hearing before an ALJ may be made if the amount still in question is $130 or more (usually in combined claims). The request must be made within 60 days of receiving the reconsideration officer's decision (Figure 9-10). It may take 18 months to receive an ALJ assignment. Proof that the claim represents an unusual case and warrants special consideration may lead to a successful conclusion. However, the decision might be reversed, allow partial adjustment of the carrier's payment, or deny payment. If the final judgment is not satisfactory, then proceed to the next level.

Medicare Appeals Council (Level 4)

The MAC is part of the Office of Hearings and Appeals of the Social Security Administration. A request must be made within 60 days of the ALJ decision; if there is a question that the final judgment was not made in accordance with the law, the council by its own election may review the ALJ decision. If the council denies a review, the provider may file a civil action for a federal district court hearing.

Federal District Court (Level 5)

The amount in controversy must be at least $1220, and an attorney must be hired to represent the provider and manage the case. The case may be filed where the

Text continued on page 346.

DEPARTMENT OF HEALTH AND HUMAN SERVICES
CENTERS FOR MEDICARE & MEDICAID SERVICES

MEDICARE REDETERMINATION REQUEST FORM

1. Beneficiary's Name: ___Carolyn N. Harvey___

2. Medicare Number: ___072-XX-1461___

3. Description of Item or Service in Question: ___office visit (99215)___

4. Date the Service or Item was Received: ___07-24-20XX___

5. I do not agree with the determination of my claim. MY REASONS ARE:
___Established patient is 60 years old and has diabetic nephropathy with increasing edema and dyspnea.___

6. Date of the initial determination notice ___09-02-20XX___
(If you received your initial determination notice more than 120 days ago, include your reason for not making this request earlier.)

7. Additional Information Medicare Should Consider: ___Comprehensive history and comprehensive examination was performed because patient had not been seen for a year. Her case had to be discussed with a cardiologist because of possibility of congestive heart failure condition.___

8. Requester's Name: ___Gerald Practon, MD___

9. Requester's Relationship to the Beneficiary: ___attending physician___

10. Requester's Address: ___4567 Broad Avenue___
___Woodland Hills, XY 12345___

11. Requester's Telephone Number: ___555-486-9002___

12. Requester's Signature: _____

13. Date Signed: ___10-04-20XX___

14. ☒ I have evidence to submit. (Attach such evidence to this form.)
❑ I do not have evidence to submit.

NOTICE: Anyone who misrepresents or falsifies essential information requested by this form may upon conviction be subject to fine or imprisonment under Federal Law.

Form CMS-20027 (05/05) EF 05/2005

FIGURE 9-7 Medicare Redetermination Request Form, CMS-20027, which can be used by the Medicare beneficiary or physician when requesting a redetermination of a submitted claim.

DEPARTMENT OF HEALTH AND HUMAN SERVICES
CENTERS FOR MEDICARE & MEDICAID SERVICES

MEDICARE RECONSIDERATION REQUEST FORM

1. Beneficiary's Name: _Jose F. Perez_

2. Medicare Number: _032-XX-6619_

3. Description of Item or Service in Question: _electrocardiographic monitoring, 24 hrs (93224)_

4. Date the Service or Item was Received: _01-21-20XX_

5. I do not agree with the determination of my claim. MY REASONS ARE:
Patient had heart palpitations, tachycardia, and light headedness (near syncopal episode).
Although patient had a previous Holter monitor within the 60 months time limitation, it
did not provide any clinical evidence of disease. Patient underwent recent monitoring after
experiencing additional symptoms that were more severe than the initial.

6. Date of the redetermination notice _03-24-20XX_
(If you received your redetermination notice more than 180 days ago, include your reason for not making this request earlier.)

_____

_____

_____

7. Additional Information Medicare Should Consider: _____

_____

_____

_____

8. Requester's Name: _Gerald Practon, MD_

9. Requester's Relationship to the Beneficiary: _attending physician_

10. Requester's Address: _4567 Broad Avenue_
Woodland Hills, XY 12345

11. Requester's Telephone Number: _555-486-9002_

12. Requester's Signature: _____

13. Date Signed: _06-05-20XX_

14. ☒ I have evidence to submit. (Attach such evidence to this form.)
☐ I do not have evidence to submit.

15. Name of the Medicare Contractor that Made the Redetermination: _Nancy W. Owens_

NOTICE: Anyone who misrepresents or falsifies essential information requested by this form may upon conviction be subject to fine or imprisonment under Federal Law.

Form CMS-20033 (05/05) EF 05/2005

FIGURE 9-8 Medicare Reconsideration Request Form, CMS-20033, which can be used in requesting a reconsideration of Medicare Part B claims.

**DEPARTMENT OF
HEALTH AND HUMAN SERVICES
CENTERS FOR MEDICARE & MEDICAID SERVICES**

NAME (Print of Type)
Carol T. Usner

H.I. CLAIM NUMBER
432-XX-9821

WAGE EARNER (if different)

SOCIAL SECURITY NUMBER

Section I   **APPOINTMENT OF REPRESENTATIVE**

I appoint this individual Gene Ulibarri, MD 4567 Broad Ave., Woodland Hills, XY 12345
(Print or type name and address of individual you want to represent you)

to act as my representative in connection with my claim or asserted right under Titles XI, or XVIII of the Social Security Act. I authorize this individual to make or give any request or notice; to present or to elicit evidence; to obtain information; and to receive any notice in connection with my claim wholly in my stead.

SIGNATURE (Beneficiary)
Carol T. Usner

ADDRESS
530 Hutch Street, Woodland Hills, XY 12345

TELEPHONE NUMBER
(555) 386-0122
(Area Code)

DATE
August 3, 20XX

Section II   **ACCEPTANCE OF APPOINTMENT**

I, Gene Ulibarri, MD , hereby accept the above appointment. I certify that I have not been suspended or prohibited from practice before the Social Security Administration; that I am not, as a current or former officer or employee of the United States, disqualified from acting as the claimant's representative; and that I will not charge or receive any fee for the representation unless it has been authorized in accordance with the laws and regulations referred to on the reverse side hereof. In the event that I decide not to charge or collect a fee for the repesentation, I will notify the Social Security Administration. (Completion of Section III satisfies this requirement.)

I am a/an medical doctor
(Attorney, union representative, relative, law student, etc.)

SIGNATURE (Representative)

ADDRESS
4567 Broad Ave., Woodland Hills, XY 12345

TELEPHONE NUMBER
(555)-486-9002
(Area code)

DATE
August 3, 20XX

Section III (Optional)   **WAIVER OF FEE OR DIRECT PAYMENT**
(Note to Representative: You may use this portion of the form to waive a fee or to waive direct payment of the fee from withheld past-due benefits.)

I waive my right to charge and collect a fee for representing _____
_____ before the Social Security Administraion or the Centers for Medicare & Medicaid Services.

SIGNATURE

DATE

(See important information on reverse)
Form SSA-1696-U4 (3-88)

A

FIGURE 9-9 A, Form SSA-1696-U4 completed by a Medicare patient appointing the physician as his or her authorized representative.   *Continued*

HOW TO COMPLETE THIS FORM

Print or type your full name and your Social Security Number.

Section I—APPOINTMENT OF REPRESENTATIVE

You may appoint as your representative an attorney or any other qualified individual. You may appoint more than one person, but see "The Fee You Owe The Representative(s)." You may NOT appoint as your representative an organization, the law firm, a group, etc. For example, if you go to a law firm or legal aid group for help with your claim, you may appoint any attorney or other qualified individual from that firm or group, but NOT the firm or group itself.

Check the block(s) for the program in which you have a claim. Title II, check if your claim concerns disability or retirement benefits, etc. Title XVI, check if the claim concerns Supplemental Security Income (SSI) payments. Title IV FMSHS (Federal Mine Safety and Health Act), check if the claim is for black lung benefits. Title XVIII, check only in connection with a proceeding before the Social Security Administration involving entitlement to medicare coverage or enrollment in the supplementary medical insurance plan (SMIP). More than one block may be checked.

Section II—ACCEPTANCE OF APPOINTMENT

The individual whom you appoint in Section I above completes this part. Completion of this section is desirable in all cases, but it is mandatory only if the appointed individual is not an attorney.

Section III—WAIVER OF FEE

This section may be completed by your representative if he/she will not charge any fee for services performed in this claim. If you had appointed a co-counsel (second representative) in Section I and he/she will also not charge you a fee, then the co-counsel should also sign this section or give a separate waiver statement.

GENERAL INFORMATION

1. When you have representative:

   We will deal directly with your representative on all matters that affect your claim. Occasionally, with the permission of your representative, we may deal directly with you on the specific issues. We will rely on your representative to keep you informed on the status of your claim, but you may contact us directly for any information about your claim.

2. The authority of your representative:

   Your representative has the authority to act totally on your behalf. This means he/she can (1) obtain

information about your claim the same as you; (2) submit evidence; (3) make statements about facts and provisions of the law; and (4) make any request (including a fee request). It is important, therefore, that you are represented by a qualified individual.

3. When will the representative stop:

   We will stop recognizing or dealing with your representative when (1) you tell us that he/she is no longer your representative; (2) your representative does any one of the following; (a) submits a fee petition, or (b) tells us that he/she is withdrawing from the claim, or (c) he/she violates any of our rules and regulations, and a hearing is held before an administrative law judge (designated as hearing officer) who orders your representative disqualified or suspended as representative of any Social Security claimant.

4. The fee you owe the representative(s):

   Every representative you appoint has a right to petition for a fee. To charge you a fee, a representative must first file a fee petition with us. Irrespective of your fee agreement, you never owe more than the fee we have authorized in a written notice to you and representative(s). (Out-of-pocket expenses are not included). If your claim went to court, you may owe an additional fee for your representative's service before the court.

5. How we determine the fee:

   We use the criteria on the back of the fee petition (Form SSA 1560-U4), a copy of which your representative must send you.

6. Review of the fee authorization:

   If you or your representative disagrees with the fee authorization, either of you may request a review. Instructions for filing this review are on the fee authorization notice.

7. Payment of fees:

   If past-due benefits are payable in your claim, we generally withhold 25 percent of the past-due benefits toward possible attorney fees. If no past-due benefits are payable or this is an SSI claim, then payment of the fee we have authorized is your responsibility.

8. Penalty for charging an unauthorized fee:

   If your representative wants to charge and collect from you a fee that is greater than what we had authorized, then he/she is in violation of the law and regulations. Promptly report this to your nearest Social Security office.

Form SSA-1696-U4 (3-88)

B

FIGURE 9-9, cont'd B, Form SSA-1696-U4 completed by a Medicare patient appointing the physician as his or her authorized representative.

DEPARTMENT OF HEALTH AND HUMAN SERVICES
OFFICE OF MEDICARE HEARINGS AND APPEALS

REQUEST FOR MEDICARE HEARING BY AN ADMINISTRATIVE LAW JUDGE
Effective July 1, 2005. For use by party to a reconsideration/fair hearing determination issued by a Fiscal Intermediary (FI), Carrier, or Quality Improvement Organization (QIO)
(Amount in controversy must be $100 or more.)

❏ **Part A**
☑ **Part B**

Send copies of this completed form to:
Original—The FI, Carrier, or QIO that issued the Reconsideration/Fair Hearing Notice
Copy—Appellant

Appellant *(The party appealing the reconsideration determination)*
Gaston Input, MD

Beneficiary *(Leave blank if same as the appellant.)* Deborah P. Sawyer	Provider or Supplier *(Leave blank if same as the appellant.)*
Address 1065 Evans Road	Address
City Woodland Hills / State XY / Zip Code 12345	City / State / Zip Code
Area Code/Telephone Number (555) 742-1821 / E-mail Address dpsawyer@gmail.net	Area Code/Telephone Number / E-mail Address
Health Insurance (Medicare) Claim Number 481-XX-6491	Document control number assigned by the FI, Carrier, or QIO 320-486-9002
FI, Carrier, or QIO that made the reconsideration/fair hearing determination Medicare Blue Cross/Blue Shield of North Dakota	Dates of Service From 02/03/20XX To 06/03/20XX

I DISAGREE WITH THE DETERMINATION MADE ON MY APPEAL BECAUSE:
Complications arose during surgical procedure requiring additional procedures to be performed. See attached chart notes and medical reports.

You have a right to be represented at the hearing. If you are not represented but would like to be, your Office of Medicare Hearings and Appeals Field Office will give you a list of legal referral and service organizations. *(If you are represented and have not already done so, complete form CMS-1696.)*

Check Only One Statement:	❏ I **wish** to have a hearing. ☑ I **do not wish** to have a hearing and I request that a decision be made on the basis of the evidence in my case. *(Complete form HHS-723, "Waiver of Right to an ALJ Hearing.")*	Check Only One Statement:	☑ I **have** additional evidence to submit. ❏ I **have no** additional evidence to submit.

The appellant should complete No. 1 and the representative, if any, should complete No. 2. If a representative is not present to sign, print his or her name in No. 2. Where applicable, check to indicate if appellant will accompany the representative at the hearing. ❏Yes ❏ No

1.(Appellant's Signature) *Gaston Input, MD*	Date 10/11/20XX	2.(Representative's Signature/Name)	Date
Address 4567 Broad Avenue		Address	❏ Attorney ❏ Non-Attorney
City Woodland Hills / State XY / Zip Code 12345		City / State / Zip Code	
Area Code/Telephone Number (555) 486-9002 / E-mail Address Inputclinic@cmail.net		Area Code/Telephone Number / E-mail Address	

Answer the following questions that apply:
A) Does request involve multiple claims? ❏ Yes ☑ No
(If yes, a list of all the claims must be attached.)
B) Does request involve multiple beneficiaries? ❏ Yes ☑ No
(If yes, a list of beneficiaries, their HICNs and the dates of the applicable reconsideration determinations must be attached.)
C) Did the beneficiary assign his or her appeal rights to you as the provider/supplier? ☑ Yes ❏ No
(If yes, you must complete and attach form CMS-20031. Failure to do so will prevent approval of the assignment.)
D) If there was no assignment, are you a physician being held liable pursuant to 1842(I)(1)(A) ❏ Yes ☑ No
of the Social Security Act?

CMS-5011A/B U2 (08/05) EF 08/2005 ATTACH A COPY OF THE RECONSIDERATION/FAIR HEARING DETERMINATION
(IF AVAILABLE) TO THIS COPY.

FIGURE 9-10 Request for Medicare Hearing by an Administrative Law Judge CMS-5011A/B.

physician's business is located. Contact the local medical society for suggestions of names of attorneys experienced at this level of the appeals process.

CMS Regional Offices

One final suggestion (and this can be done with steps for a hearing or a review) is to write or telephone the medical director at one of the CMS regional offices. Sometimes a regional officer intercedes or takes steps to correct problems or inequities. CMS regional offices may be located by accessing the Medicare website; see Internet Resources at the end of this chapter for an active link from the Evolve website.

Medigap

Insurance companies that sell Medigap policies must be certified before being allowed to sell in each state. The certification can be lifted from any insurer that does not honor its contract agreements. Only the state insurance commissioner can exert pressure on Medigap insurance companies. If payment is slow in coming or is not received from a Medigap insurer, first try the paper or electronic claim solutions for delinquent claims mentioned previously in this chapter. As a last resort, tell the insurer, "If I do not receive payment, I will have no alternative but to contact the state insurance commissioner."

Document complete follow-up information on each Medigap insurer (firm name, address, telephone number, and policy numbers) of every patient seen.

TRICARE Review and Appeal Process

A provider who treats a TRICARE patient but is out of network is not able to obtain information from TRICARE. Contact the patient for their assistance. Also, out-of-network providers who wish to treat an obstetric case may need a nonavailability request form completed and processed before a patient can receive care. There must be a reason the patient cannot go to a providing facility and TRICARE determines whether it will approve the request. Otherwise, claims will be denied.

Before appealing a TRICARE claim, if the patient wishes the provider to appeal, then the patient must complete an Appointment of Appeal Representative form as shown in Figure 9-11. After that is completed, an inquiry should be sent to verify claim status and attempt to resolve the problem. Figure 9-12 shows an example of a form that may be used for inquiring about a TRICARE Standard claim. TRICARE appeals procedures applicable to the routine processing of TRICARE Standard claims are described here. However, TRICARE managed

care contracts have been adopted throughout the United States and the appeals procedures that TRICARE contractors use in these areas may vary. For information on how to file reviews and appeals for those contracts, ask the contracting insurance company for instructions and forms.

The following three levels for review under TRICARE Standard appeal procedures exist:

1. Reconsideration (conducted by the claims processor or other TRICARE contractor responsible for the decision in a particular case). This is a formal written request by the appealing party to resolve a disputed statement of fact. To file an appeal, see Procedure 9-2 at the end of this chapter.
2. Formal review (conducted by TRICARE headquarters)
3. Hearing administered by TRICARE headquarters but conducted by an independent hearing officer

Reconsideration

Participating providers may appeal certain decisions made by TRICARE and request reconsideration. Providers who do not participate may not appeal, but TRICARE Standard patients and parents or guardians of patients younger than 18 years of age who seek care from non-participating providers may file appeals. Providers who do not participate may not receive any information about a particular claim without the signed authorization of the patient or the patient's parent or guardian.

Matters that can be appealed include the following:

1. Medical necessity disagreements (inappropriate care, level of care, investigational procedures)
2. Factual determinations (hospice care, foreign claims, provider sanction cases)
   a. Denials or partial denials of requests for preauthorization for certain services or supplies
   b. Coverage issues—notification that TRICARE will not pay for services before or after a certain date

Matters that cannot be appealed include the following:

1. Denial of services received from a provider not authorized to provide care under TRICARE
2. A specific exclusion of law or regulation
3. Allowable charges for particular services
4. Issues relating to the establishment and application of diagnosis-related groups
5. Decisions by the claims processor to ask for additional information on a particular case
6. A determination of a person's eligibility as a TRICARE beneficiary

Appointment of Appeal Representative

I, _____ , appoint
(Print/Type name of person giving consent)

_____
(Print/Type name and address of Representative)

to act as my representative in connection with my appeal under 32 CFR 199.10, Appeal and hearing procedures. To avoid the possibility of conflict of interest, I understand that an office or employee of the United States, to include an employee or member of a Uniformed Service, an employee of a Uniformed Service legal office, an MTF provider or a Health Benefits Advisor, is not eligible to serve as a representative. An exception to this is made when an employee of the United States or member of a Uniformed Service is representing an immediate family member.

I authorize the TRICARE Management Activity and Wisconsin Physicians Service (WPS)/TRICARE to release to said representative information related to my medical treatment, and if necessary, photocopies of any medical records which may be required for adjudication on my claim for TRICARE benefits.

I understand that the representative shall have the same authority as the party to the appeal and notice given to the representative shall constitute notice to the party.

This consent will expire upon the issuance of the final agency decision regarding my appeal; however, I reserve the right to withdraw this authorization at any time to the extent that TMA and WPS have not already taken action in reliance on it.

_____   _____
(Signature of Person Giving Consent)   (Date)

_____
(Sponsor Number)

TRICARE will not condition treatment, payment, enrollment, or eligibility for benefits on this authorization.

The potential exists for information disclosed pursuant to this authorization to be subject to redisclosure by the recipient and no longer protected by the Privacy Act and HIPAA Privacy Rule.

Prohibition on Redisclosure:
This information has been disclosed to you from records whose confidentiality is protected by Federal Law. Federal Regulations (42 CFR Part 2) prohibit you from making any further disclosure of this information except with specific written consent of the person to whom it pertains. A general authorization for the release of medical or other information, if held by another party, is NOT sufficient for this purpose. Federal regulations state that any person who violates any provision of this law shall be fined not more than $500 in the case of a first offense and not more than $5000 in the case of each subsequent offense.

FIGURE 9-11 Appointment of appeal representative.

The TRICARE department that handles appeals collects and organizes all information necessary to review the case effectively. Usually a determination decision is made within 60 days from receipt of the appeal. Disagreements about the amount allowed for a particular claim may be reviewed by the claims processor to determine whether it was calculated correctly. However, an individual cannot appeal the amount that the TRICARE contractor determines to be the allowable charge for a certain medical service.

Requests must be sent to the claims processor of the state in which services were provided and must be postmarked within 90 days of the date the provider receives the Summary Payment Voucher (formerly referred to as an EOB). Include photocopies of the claim, Summary Payment Voucher, and other supporting documents with the request form or letter. The claim identification number assigned by the claims processor should be included in any inquiry concerning payment of the claim. If TRICARE denies the initial request, then the other two levels of review, formal review and hearing, may be pursued.

Formal Review

A formal review must be done within 60 days from the date on the reconsideration decision notice. Include photocopies of the notice, as well as any other information or documents to support why there is a disagreement in the TRICARE decision. The case is reviewed again, and a formal review decision is issued. The formal review decision is final if the amount in dispute is less than $300.

TRICARE CLAIM INQUIRY

Date: _____

TO: TRICARE
           Address of fiscal intermediary
           City, State, Zip Code

FROM: Provider's name   Telephone number
           Address   Fax number
           City, State, Zip Code

RE: Sponsor's Social Security Number _____

      Sponsor's Name _____

      Patient's Name _____

      Patient's Mailing Address:

      _____
      Street   City   State   Zip Code

      Dates of service claim: _____

      Total charges billed on claim: _____

      Claim number that appears on TRICARE Explanation of Benefits
      (leave blank if the claim has not been paid and information is not available)

      _____

A. _____   I have submitted a claim, but have not received any payment
                or other notification from you.

B. _____   I have received notification or payment concerning the claim,
                but feel it may have been processed incorrectly.

C. _____   Deductible Status. Please confirm that individual and family
                deductibles have been applied correctly.

D. _____   Coverage for this patient is under

                _____ TRICARE   _____ CHAMPVA

E. _____   Additional information or explanation that will assist
                reviewing or processing the claim is attached to this letter or
                written in this area.

FIGURE 9-12 A TRICARE Standard claim inquiry form that may be completed to obtain a quick reply. Mail to the TRICARE fiscal intermediary for your region.

Hearing

An independent hearing may be pursued if the amount in dispute is $300 or more. The request must be postmarked or received within 60 days from the date of the formal review decision. A hearing is conducted by an independent hearing officer at a location convenient to both the requesting party and the government.

STATE INSURANCE COMMISSIONER

Commission Objectives

The insurance industry is protected by a special exemption from the Federal Trade Commission (FTC) under the McCarran Act (named for the late Senator Pat McCarran of Nevada). Under the exemption, the FTC cannot attack unfair or deceptive practices if there is any state law about such practices. The regulations vary widely from state to state, and by no means are all 50 states equally strict. If a complaint arises about an insurance policy, medical claim, or insurance agent or broker, the insurance department of the state of residence or the state where the insurance company's corporate office is headquartered should be contacted. Sometimes this department is referred to as the *insurance commission of the state*. State insurance departments usually have various objectives, including the following:

- To make certain that the financial strength of insurance companies is not unduly diminished
- To monitor the activities of insurance companies to make sure the interests of the policyholders are protected
- To verify that all contracts are carried out in good faith
- To make sure that all organizations authorized to transact insurance including agents and brokers are in compliance with the insurance laws of that state
- To release information on how many complaints have been filed against a specific insurance company in a year
- To help explain correspondence related to insurance company bankruptcies and other financial difficulties
- To assist if a company funds its own insurance plan
- To help resolve insurance conflicts

The insurance commissioner can hold a hearing to determine whether licensed insurers, agents, or brokers are in compliance with the insurance laws of the state, but the commissioner does not have the authority vested in a court of law to order an insurance company to make payment on a specific claim.

The insurance commissioner reviews the policy to determine whether the denial of a claim by the insurance company was based on legal provisions of the insurance contract and advises the patient if there is an infraction of the law. If there is an infraction, the patient should consult an attorney to determine whether the claim should be submitted to a court of law.

Types of Problems

Problems that should be submitted to the insurance commissioner are as follows:

1. Improper denial of a claim or settlement for an amount less than that indicated by the policy, after proper appeal has been made
2. Delay in settlement of a claim, after proper appeal has been made
3. Illegal cancellation or termination of an insurance policy
4. Misrepresentation by an insurance agent or broker
5. Misappropriation of premiums paid to an insurance agent or broker
6. Problems about insurance premium rates
7. Two companies that cannot determine which is primary

COMMISSION INQUIRIES

An insurance billing specialist may not be in a position to know the particulars about a case and should never assume or accuse unless he or she is certain or has concrete evidence. Remember, "Jump to conclusions, suffer contusions."

Requests to the insurance commissioner must be submitted in writing. An example of an insurance complaint form showing pertinent necessary information when making a request for assistance from the state insurance commissioner is shown in Figure 9-13. Refer to the Internet Resources at the end of this chapter for an active link at the Evolve website to contact your state insurance commissioner to determine whether a specific form is required and available. In some states the insurance commissioner requires that the complaint come from the patient even if an assignment of benefits form has been signed. In such a case, a letter or form should be prepared for the patient to sign and then submit. Depending on the circumstances of the case, one may wish to send copies to the state medical association or an attorney. Mail may be sent certified, return receipt requested. The request should contain the following information:

1. The inquiring person's (patient) or policyholder's name because the commissioner's responsibility is to the patient (the consumer), not the physician
2. The policyholder's address
3. The policyholder's telephone number

INSURANCE COMPLAINT FORM

To: State Insurance Commissioner
Address
City, State, ZIP code

1. → Your Name _____Grace T. O'Neal_____   _____XYZ Insurance Company_____ ← **8.**
                                                            (Agent or Company Complaint Against)

2. → Address _____4572 Southport St._____   Policy No. _____531 OK 492_____ ← **9.**

                      _____Woodland Hills, XY 12345_____   Date of Loss: _____10-11-20XX_____ ← **10.**

3. → Day Telephone No. _____555-421-0733_____   Claim or File No. _____

4. → Insured: _____Grace T. O'Neal_____

Is this the only complaint you have filed with the insurance commissioner concerning this matter?
Yes ____X____   No _____

5. → Have you taken up this problem with an official of the company, agent, or broker: If yes, give name, address, and title.   Yes ____X____   No _____

_____John Knave, Insurance Agent_____

_____

The following is a brief statement of what the agent or company has done, or failed to do:

6. → Insurance payment has been denied by insurance company as a noncovered service, but policy covers professional procedure performed.

7. → *Grace T. O'Neal*   _____12-15-20XX_____ ← **11.**
       Signature of Patient   Date

Attach a copy of the insurance policy, related documents, correspondence, etc.

FIGURE 9-13 Insurance complaint form signed by the patient, showing pertinent necessary information when stating a complaint and making a request for assistance from the state insurance commissioner.

4. The insured's name
5. Name, address, and title of the insurance agent or official of the insurance company
6. A statement of the complaint including, if possible, a copy of the policy, medical bills, unpaid medical insurance claim, canceled checks, and any correspondence from the company pertaining to the claim
7. The patient's signature
8. The name and address of the insurance company, agent, or broker, or name and address of the finance company if the premium was financed
9. The policy or claim number
10. The date of loss
11. The date the patient signed the complaint form

If an insurance company is continually a slow payer, a method to speed up payments is to include a note to the carrier that reads, "Unless this claim is paid or denied within 30 days, a formal written complaint will be filed with the state insurance commissioner."

Another method is to send a letter to the insurance commissioner with a copy notation inserted at the end to the insurance company. It might read, "The attached claim has been submitted to the XYZ Insurance Company. It has not been paid or denied. Please accept this letter as a formal written complaint against the XYZ Insurance Company."

Insurance companies are rated according to the number of complaints received about them, so they do not want the insurance commissioner to be alerted to any problems. Some states have information available to the public on how many claims have been submitted against a company if this information is necessary. Refer to the Internet Resources at the end of this chapter to contact the state insurance commissioner in your state for assistance or information about state laws.

PROCEDURE 9-1

Trace an Unpaid Insurance Claim

OBJECTIVE: To complete an insurance claim tracer and attach to this document a photocopy of the claim submitted

EQUIPMENT/SUPPLIES: Typewriter or computer, insurance claims register (tracing or log file), insurance Claim Tracer Form, a previously submitted insurance claim form, and pen or pencil

DIRECTIONS: Follow these basic step-by-step procedures, which include rationales, to learn this skill and practice it by completing the *Workbook* assignment.

1. Review the insurance claims register (tracing or log file) to learn and verify which claims are overdue for payment and have not been paid by the third-party payers.

2. Obtain a copy of the previously submitted insurance claim that has not been paid.
3. Abstract data from the insurance claim and insert it on the insurance claim tracer form.
4. Make a photocopy of the unpaid insurance claim form.
5. Have the physician, office manager, or insurance biller sign the form.
6. Post an entry to either the patient's accounting financial record or insurance claims register (tracing or log file) indicating a tracer was submitted to the third-party payer.

PROCEDURE 9-2

File an Appeal

OBJECTIVE: To compose, format, key, proofread, and print a letter of appeal and attach to this document photocopies of information to substantiate reimbursement requested

EQUIPMENT/SUPPLIES: Typewriter or computer, printer, letterhead paper, envelope, attachments (if necessary), thesaurus, English dictionary, medical dictionary, and pen or pencil

DIRECTIONS: Follow these basic step-by-step procedures, which include rationales, to learn this skill and practice it by completing the *Workbook* assignment.

1. Refer to Figure 9-14 and to the end of Chapter 4 and follow the procedure to compose, format, key, proofread, and print a letter.
2. Include the beneficiary's name, health insurance claim number, date of initial determination, dates of service in question, items or services in question, name and address of the provider, and signature of appellant.
3. Compose a letter with an introduction that stresses the medical practice's qualifications, the physician's commitment to complying with regulations and providing appropriate services, and the importance of the practice to the payer's panel of physicians or specialists.

4. Provide a detailed account of the necessity of the treatment given and its relationship to the patient's problems and chief complaint. You might cross reference the medical record and emphasize parts of it that the reviewer may have missed.
5. Explain the reason why the provider does not agree with the claim denial listed on the EOB/RA.
6. Abstract excerpts from the coding resource book and attach a photocopy of the article or pertinent information showing the name of the article, coding resource, and date of publication.
7. Send copies of similar cases with increased reimbursement from the same insurance company, if available from the insurance company payment history file.
8. Call the insurance company and speak to the individual responsible for appeals, explaining what the resubmission is trying to accomplish. Direct the correspondence to this person.
9. Retain copies of all data sent for the physician's files.
10. Use a method that confirms the payer received the letter, such as a certified return receipt or signature using Federal Express or Airborne Express services.

PHYSICIAN'S LETTERHEAD

January 2, 20XX

Committee on Physician's Services
Medicare
Street address of fiscal intermediary
City, State, ZIP Code

Dear Madam or Sir:

Re: Underpayment

Identification No.:	1910-2192283-101
Patient:	Mrs. Sarah C. Nile
Type of Service:	Exploratory laparotomy
Date of Service:	December 1, 20XX
Amount Paid:	$000.00
My Fees:	$0000.00

Herewith a request for a committee review of the above-named case, since I consider the allowance paid very low having in mind the patient's condition prior to surgery, the location, the extent, the type, and the necessary surgical procedure performed.

Enclosed are photocopies of the history and physical showing the grave status of the patient prior to surgery, operative report, pathology report, and discharge summary. The Medicare Remittance Advice and the Medicare CMS-1500 claim originally submitted are also enclosed.

Considering these points, I hope that you will authorize additional payment in order to bring the total fee to a more reasonable amount.

Sincerely,
Hugh R. Aged, MD
Hugh R. Aged, MD
NPI# 73542109XX

mf

FIGURE 9-14 A cover letter signed by the physician appealing a claim.

KEY POINTS

This is a brief chapter review or summary of the key issues presented. To further enhance your knowledge of the technical subject matter, review the key terms and key abbreviations for this chapter by locating the meanings in the glossary at the end of this book that appear in a section before the index.

1. Payment from a third-party payer after submission of a paper claim should occur within 4 to 12 weeks and for an electronic claim within 7 days. When a payment problem develops and the insurance company is slow, ignores, denies, or exceeds time limits, then contact the third-party payer.

2. An explanation of benefits or electronic remittance advice should be read and interpreted line by line, checked to establish whether the amount paid is correct, and amounts posted to each patient's financial account.

3. Routine periodic checks of the insurance claims electronic tracking report or insurance paper claims register (log) or tickler file should be done to manually follow up on delinquent claims.

4. The individual handling the front desk must collect insurance information accurately and update patient demographic information routinely to avoid future collection problems.

5. To avoid denied claims and assist in solving claim problems, keep abreast of the latest policies for all contracted payers, as well as the federal programs.

6. A decision to appeal a claim should be based on whether there is ample information to back up the claim and if there is a substantial amount of money in question.

7. The levels of a Medicare appeal are (1) redetermination by telephone, letter, or form; (2) reconsideration by a hearing officer; (3) hearing by an administrative law judge; (4) review by the Medicare Appeals Council; and (5) judicial review in the Federal District Court.

8. The levels of a TRICARE appeal are (1) reconsideration by a claims processor, (2) formal review conducted by TRICARE headquarters, and (3) a hearing conducted by an independent hearing officer.

9. To complain about a problem with an insurance contract or claim involving a private third-party payer or a Medigap supplemental plan, the state insurance commission must be contacted.

10. Always file the appropriate form or write a letter to begin the appeal process for resolving an insurance problem or complaint.

evolve INTERNET RESOURCES

For active links to the following resources, visit the Evolve website at
http://evolve.elsevier.com/fordney/handbook

- Medicare forms may be downloaded and printed and regional offices may be located at the Medicare website.
- A bimonthly newsletter that links to regulatory information online and a subscription repository of appeal letters and comments that assists the health care community in sharing successful appeal information is located at the Appeal Solutions website (http://www.appealsolutions.com)
- State insurance commissioners may be found at the National Association of Insurance Commissioners website.

STUDENT ASSIGNMENT

✓ Study Chapter 9.
✓ Answer the fill-in-the-blank, multiple choice, and true/false review questions in the *Workbook* to reinforce the theory learned in this chapter and to help prepare you for a future test.
✓ Complete the assignments in the *Workbook* to fill in a form for tracing a delinquent claim, locate errors on a returned claim, and complete a form to appeal a Medicare case.
✓ Turn to the glossary at the end of this textbook for a further understanding of the key terms and key abbreviations used in this chapter.

KEY TERMS*

accounts receivable
age analysis
*American Medical Association
   (AMA) Code of Ethics*
automatic stay
balance
bankruptcy
bonding
cash flow
Code of Medical Ethics
collateral
collection ratio
credit
credit card

creditor
cycle billing
debit card
debt
debtor
discount
dun messages
embezzlement
estate administrator
estate executor
fee schedule
financial accounting record
garnishment
insurance balance billing

itemized statement
lien
manual billing
netback
no charge
nonexempt assets
professional courtesy
reimbursement
secured debt
skip
statute of limitations
unsecured debt
write-off

KEY ABBREVIATIONS*

A/R
ATM
CMS
e-check
ERISA

FACT
FCBA
FCRA
FDCPA
FEHBA

FTC
HMO
N/A
NC
NSF

TILA
W2

---

*Definitions for the key terms and key abbreviations are located near the back of this textbook in the glossary.

Office and Insurance Collection Strategies

After reading this chapter, you should be able to:

- Define credit and collection key words terminology and abbreviations.
- Define accounts receivable and explain how it is handled.
- Recite types of fee adjustments available to patients.
- Name payment options available to patients.
- Define aging analysis.
- List the names of the federal credit laws applicable to a physician office setting.

- Perform oral and written communication collection techniques.
- State the role of a billing service, collection agency, and credit bureau in the collection process.
- Explain the purpose of small claims court in the collection process.
- Name basic actions in tracing a debtor who has moved and left no forwarding address.

Service to Patients

Explain fees and answer questions at initial encounter or during registration, or both, to establish the patient's responsibility for the service to be rendered. Offer payment options to the patient who is experiencing financial problems. If you can make the financial aspect of the medical service go smoothly, you can ease a patient's troubles. Patients rely on the insurance biller for timely, accurate reporting of services. This helps avoid making patients pay for your mistakes and adding expense and causing delays in payment.

CASH FLOW CYCLE

The practice of medicine is both a profession and a business. Although the physician decides what type of medicine he or she will practice, it is often the practice manager or administrator who is responsible for the business portion of the practice. It is extremely important for the physician and insurance specialist to work together to

provide all patients the best possible medical care and ensure that the physician is paid fairly for services rendered.

Today this process has become increasingly complex. Physician office and billing practices have evolved from the barter system of days past, and since the Great Depression, the availability of credit and credit cards has become a common feature of the financial marketplace. The word **credit** comes from the Latin word *credere*, which means "to believe" or "to trust." This trust is in an individual's business integrity and his or her financial ability to meet obligations when they become due. For many, the idea of credit has changed and may simply mean to put off paying today what one can pay tomorrow.

A large percentage of **reimbursement** to physicians' offices is generated from third-party payers (private insurance, government plans, managed care contracts,

Performance objectives, testing and review material, and hands-on practical exercises for this chapter are available in these resources

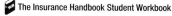 The Insurance Handbook Student Workbook   The Insurance Handbook Evolve Site

355

and workers' compensation). The physician, the practice administrator responsible for financial affairs, and the patient must understand these insurance contracts, which list the following:

- Reimbursement provisions
- Medical services not covered
- Portion of the bill the patient is responsible for
- Process for reimbursing the office

Figure 10-1 is a flow chart and overview of a medical practice's billing procedures that illustrates the sequence from beginning to end.

ACCOUNTS RECEIVABLE

Accounts receivable (A/R) include the unpaid balances due from patients and third-party payers for services that have been rendered. Each medical practice has a policy about handling A/R. The effectiveness of this policy and its enforcement are reflected in the practice's cash flow. The **cash flow** is the ongoing availability of actual cash in the medical practice. When charges are collected at the time of service, the A/R is zero. In an ideal situation, all outstanding balances are paid within 60 days; however, this is not possible for the following reasons:

1. Health care expenses have increased and exceed the expenses the patient pays for everyday living.
2. The public seems to have an attitude that it is a right, rather than a privilege, to receive the best possible health care. Therefore care of the indigent becomes an unreimbursable expense in the medical office.
3. Legal proceedings often delay the payment of medical expenses.
4. Third-party payers do not pay claims in a timely manner, resulting in further delays in the collection of patient copayments.

FIGURE 10-1 Medical office flow chart showing a medical practice's billing procedures from the patient's appointment to producing practice management reports.

5. Managed care plans seek discounted rates for members obtaining medical services.

By monitoring the A/R, the insurance billing specialist is able to evaluate the effectiveness of the collection process. Later in this chapter, A/R ratio formulas are presented in the section on A/R and age analysis.

The best way to keep the A/R down is to verify insurance benefits before sending claims, collect copayments and deductibles at the time of service, obtain authorizations for noncontracted health maintenance organization (HMO) patients, and monitor the A/R weekly. Set up the computer system so that it flags the self-pay patients. This reminds the receptionist to ask for a copayment, deductible, or noncovered fee. Electronic claims that have not been paid within 30 days and paper claims unpaid within 45 days of submission may have problems that can range from the carrier asking for additional information from the patient to the patient not being one of the carrier's insured.

The **collection ratio** is the relationship of the amount of money owed to a physician and the amount of money collected on the physician's A/R. A collection rate of 100% is obviously desirable, although unrealistic, and should always be sought as a goal for the person managing collections in the physician's office. To calculate the collection rate for a 1-month period, divide the amount of monies collected during the current month by the total amount of the A/R.

PATIENT EDUCATION

Information should be provided about office fees and payment policies during the initial contact with the patient. This decreases the number of billing statements sent and increases collections. Never allow a patient to believe that he or she is not responsible for the bill. Discuss copayment requirements (see Chapter 3) with patients who are enrolled in managed care plans, and convey the office policy of collecting this amount when registering the patient for the office visit. A new patient information pamphlet or brochure and confirmation letter (Figure 10-2) may be sent to welcome the new patient to the practice. This letter informs the patient about the practice, clearly outlines payment expectations, provides collection policies and procedures in printed form, establishes a contact person, invites questions, and confirms all specific details discussed.

Patient Registration Form

There is no substitution for good information-gathering techniques at the time of initial patient registration because this assists later in billing and collection. Always obtain complete and accurate demographic and identifying information from the patient on the first visit and confirm the accuracy of that information on each subsequent visit. Chapter 3 describes what data should be obtained from the patient; Figure 3-6 is an example of a patient registration information form, also called a *patient information sheet*. For commercial insurance plans, have the guarantor agree in writing to pay for all medical treatment. By obtaining the guarantor's signature, he or she is then bound by contract to pay the bill.

Learn as much as possible about the patient before any services are provided. This is when the patient is likely to be the most cooperative. Information provided on the patient information sheet will prove critical to any billing and collection efforts. The patient should be instructed to answer all questions and indicate any spaces on the form that do not apply by marking **N/A** (not applicable). Review of the completed patient information sheet ensures that all blanks have been addressed and accurate information has been collected. It also alerts office staff of an account that may be a future problem. Items often overlooked are the street address, when a post office box is given; an apartment or mobile home park number; a cell phone number; and a business telephone number with department and extension. These help trace a patient who has moved. If a patient refuses to divulge any information, invoking privacy laws, it should be policy to require payment for services at the time care is rendered. A potential nonpaying patient may be recognized at this time. Some indications to look for follow:

- Incomplete information on the registration form
- Multiple changes of residence
- Questionable employment record
- No telephone numbers (business, cell, or home)
- Post office box listed with no street address
- Motel address
- Incomplete insurance information or no insurance coverage
- No referral information or authorization from a primary care physician for patients enrolled in a managed care plan

Employers are changing health plans with increasing frequency and patients are more transient than ever, so update this form each time the patient is seen or every 6 months. This can be done by printing out a data sheet or having the patient review a copy of his or her registration form and inserting changes or corrections with a red pen.

FEES

Fee Schedule

Most medical practices operate with a set of fees that must be applied to all patients in the practice uniformly. As discussed in Chapter 6, a **fee schedule** is a listing of

COLLEGE CLINIC
4567 Broad Avenue
Woodland Hills, XY 12345-0001
Tel. (555) 486-9002
FAX (555) 487-8976

February 3, 20XX

Mrs. Mary M. McLean
4919 Dolphin Way
Woodland Hills, XY 12345-0001

Dear Mrs. McLean:

Thank you for making an appointment with Dr. Ulibarri and entrusting us with your personal health care. Your appointment has been scheduled on _____ (date) at ___o'clock (time). Please arrive 15 minutes early and bring the completed patient registration and history form.

The fee for your physical examination is approximately $_____ (charge). If laboratory tests, an electrocardiogram, or any procedures are necessary, there will be additional charges. For patients covered by insurance, our office policy requires a payment of 20% of all charges at the time of service. Please expect to pay this on the day of your visit. For your convenience, we accept cash, checks, and credit cards (Visa, American Express, and MasterCard).

Enclosed is a brochure with information regarding our medical practice and a map on the back for your convenience. We look forward to your visit. Please call me at (555) 486-9002 if you have any questions.

Sincerely,

Fran Staple, CMA
Office Manager

Enc: brochure, patient registration, history form

1. State with which doctor the patient has the appointment.

2. Confirm the date and time.

3. State the approximate fee for services ahead of time.

4. Alert the patient that additional charges may be added for additional services.

5. Offer payment options.

6. Enclose patient brochure, patient registration, and history form.

7. Establish a contact person and invite questions.

FIGURE 10-2 New patient confirmation letter emphasizing information to incorporate when writing to a new patient.

accepted charges or established allowances for specific medical procedures. Always quote fees and state policies about the collection of fees to the patient at the initial visit. Under federal regulations, a list of the most common services the physician offers, including procedure code numbers with a description of each service and its price, must be available to all patients. A sign must be posted in the office advising patients of this.

Occasionally, a physician assigns a fee for a service that is not on the fee schedule and not reimbursed by insurance such as completion of an insurance form, a long-distance telephone consultation, a narrative medical report for an insurance company, or interest assessed on a delinquent account. It is advisable to inform patients before billing for any such services to preserve the patient-physician relationship. If such charges are imposed or the fee schedule is increased at a later date, a notice should be placed in the reception room and communicated to patients via their monthly billing

statements. This information should be included in the medical practice's information brochure that is given to patients.

Missed Appointments

As of June 2007 the Centers for Medicare and Medicaid Services (CMS) allows a no-show fee billed to patients as long as the medical practice does the following:

- Establishes a written office policy on missed appointments that emphasizes it is a missed business opportunity and not the cost of the service itself.
- Informs all patients of what will happen for a missed appointment if there is no cancellation. For example, on the patient's second no-show occurrence, there is a $45 charge. A fee of $35 to $50 is the range most providers use.
- Applies the missed appointment policy to all patients.
- Bills all patients for missed appointments.

Fee Adjustments
Discounted Fees

A physician may choose to discount his or her fees for various reasons, but it is ill-advised and may be illegal in some circumstances. A **discount** is a reduction of the normal fee based on a specific amount of money or a percentage of the charge. When a physician offers a discount, it must apply to the total bill, not just the portion that is paid by the patient (copayment or coinsurance amount). By following this rule, the physician is giving a discount to the patient and the insurance company, but the same discount must be given to each member of the insurance plan. This practice could reduce the physician's profile with the insurance company and trigger a reduction in the physician's allowable reimbursement schedule; therefore the physician should consider the outcome of discounting fees. All discounts must be electronically posted to the patient's **financial accounting record**, and any financial reasons or special circumstances should be documented in the patient's medical record. This ensures complete record keeping and safeguards any questions that may be asked during a financial audit.

Cash Discounts

Cash discounts may be offered (5% to 20%) to patients who pay the entire fee, in cash, at the time of service (Figure 10-3). If a cash discount system is offered, this policy should be posted in the office and every active patient sent notification. Research your state laws because some states do not allow cash discounts, and check the medical practice's insurance contracts to determine whether they are affected. Also, refer to your office's compliance protocol to be sure any such discounts do not implicate fraud.

Financial Hardship

Financial hardship cases are the most difficult for the physician to determine. The insurance billing specialist should never assume anything about a patient's financial status, nor judge a patient's ability to pay by his or her appearance. The Department of Health and Human Services published a 2007 guideline on poverty income (Figure 10-4), which is used to determine eligibility for uncompensated services under the Hill-Burton, Community Services Block Grant, and Head Start programs. Physicians may choose to follow these guidelines to direct patients to government-sponsored programs, obtain public assistance, and determine who is eligible for a hardship waiver. A hardship waiver can vary from 25% to 100% of the bill. Various financial forms are available to obtain this information; a copy of the patient's wage and tax statement (W2) or income tax return should be examined to make a reliable decision. The patient also should sign a written explanation to verify true financial hardship. This helps in the collection process and allows the physician to accept the insurance as payment in full, in certain circumstances, without being suspected of insurance fraud. The reason for a fee reduction must be documented in the patient's medical record.

Be careful about giving a discount because it can be construed as discriminatory if not given to other patients consistently. To avoid problems, develop a written policy about what qualifies a patient for a financial hardship discount.

Write-Off or Courtesy Adjustment

A **write-off** or *courtesy adjustment* (preferred term) is an asset or **debt** that has been determined to be uncollectable and is taken off (subtracted/credited) the accounting books. It is considered lost income but may not be claimed as a loss for tax purposes. The insurance specialist should obtain financial information on all patients who request a write-off. Office policies about adjustments and all discounts should be in writing, and all staff members should be informed. The physician must approve the portion of the charge to be credited to the financial record before the debt is forgiven. A write-off is possible in three circumstances. The first is as stated in the preceding discussion, when the patient has proved a financial hardship. The second is when it will cost more to bill the balance than what is owed. For example, the balance may be $1.05. It will cost the practice more to collect this than what is worth. This type of write-off is known as a *small*

The Office of the Inspector General issued guidance to providers that they are free to use whatever policy they want on charity care, discounts, write-offs, and collections, as long as it is done consistently and the reasons for granting these are documented, for example, in the medical practice's compliance manual. Make sure that these deviations from standard collection procedures are not tied to or conditioned on referrals or use of the provider's services. Be sure office policy states the minimum effort in collection of debts such as one or more letters or telephone calls. The provider that uses minimum collection efforts can waive the obligations of patients in financial need in accordance with office policy and try to collect more aggressively from other patients who are not financially needy.

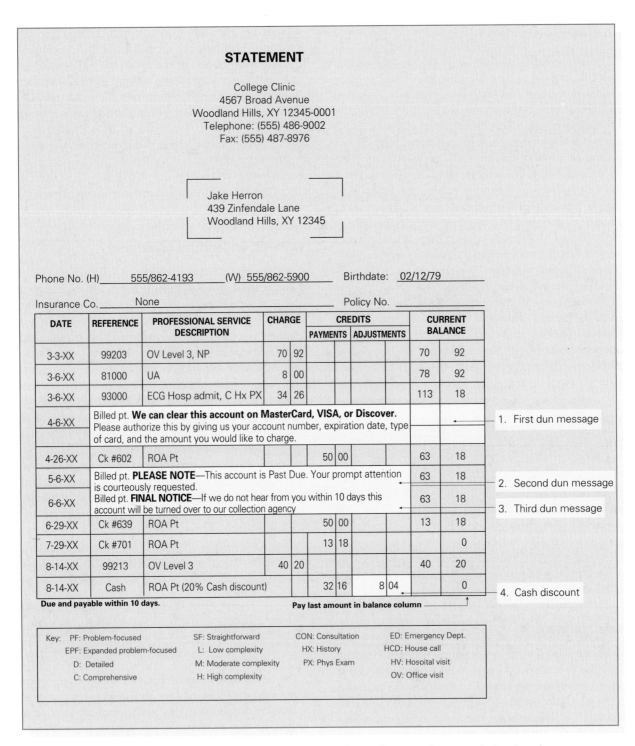

STATEMENT

College Clinic
4567 Broad Avenue
Woodland Hills, XY 12345-0001
Telephone: (555) 486-9002
Fax: (555) 487-8976

Jake Herron
439 Zinfendale Lane
Woodland Hills, XY 12345

Phone No. (H) ____555/862-4193____ (W) _555/862-5900___   Birthdate: __02/12/79__

Insurance Co. _____None_____   Policy No. _____

DATE	REFERENCE	PROFESSIONAL SERVICE DESCRIPTION	CHARGE		CREDITS		CURRENT BALANCE	
					PAYMENTS	ADJUSTMENTS		
3-3-XX	99203	OV Level 3, NP	70	92			70	92
3-6-XX	81000	UA	8	00			78	92
3-6-XX	93000	ECG Hosp admit, C Hx PX	34	26			113	18
4-6-XX	Billed pt. **We can clear this account on MasterCard, VISA, or Discover.** Please authorize this by giving us your account number, expiration date, type of card, and the amount you would like to charge.							
4-26-XX	Ck #602	ROA Pt			50	00		63	18
5-6-XX	Billed pt. **PLEASE NOTE**—This account is Past Due. Your prompt attention is courteously requested.						63	18
6-6-XX	Billed pt. **FINAL NOTICE**—If we do not hear from you within 10 days this account will be turned over to our collection agency						63	18
6-29-XX	Ck #639	ROA Pt			50	00		13	18
7-29-XX	Ck #701	ROA Pt			13	18		0	
8-14-XX	99213	OV Level 3	40	20			40	20
8-14-XX	Cash	ROA Pt (20% Cash discount)			32	16	8	04	0	

1. First dun message
2. Second dun message
3. Third dun message
4. Cash discount

Due and payable within 10 days.   **Pay last amount in balance column**

Key:	PF: Problem-focused	SF: Straightforward	CON: Consultation	ED: Emergency Dept.
	EPF: Expanded problem-focused	L: Low complexity	HX: History	HCD: House call
	D: Detailed	M: Moderate complexity	PX: Phys Exam	HV: Hospital visit
	C: Comprehensive	H: High complexity		OV: Office visit

FIGURE 10-3 Electronic hard copy of a patient's financial accounting record showing dun messages, posted payments, and cash discount.

balance write-off. The last situation is when the provider has made a good faith effort to collect the balance with no success. In this case the balance is written off and the account may or may not be sent to a professional collection agency depending on whether the agency accepts balances less than, for example, $35 for collection.

Professional Courtesy

Professional courtesy is a concept attributed to Hippocrates, but the foundations actually are derived from Thomas Percival's *Code of Medical Ethics,* written in 1803. The *American Medical Association (AMA) Code of Ethics,* formulated and adopted in 1847, closely

2010 GUIDELINES ON POVERTY INCOME

Size of family unit	48 contiguous states and D.C.	Alaska	Hawaii
1	$10,830	$13,530	$12,460
2	$14,570	$18,210	$16,760
3	$18,310	$22,890	$21,060
4	$22,050	$27,570	$25,360
5	$25,790	$32,250	$29,660
6	$29,530	$36,930	$33,960
7	$33,279	$41,610	$38,260
8	$37,010	$46,290	$42,560
For each additional person add:	$ 3,740	$ 4,500	$ 4,140

FIGURE 10-4 Department of Health and Human Services 2010 guidelines on poverty income, published in the *Federal Register* 73:15, January 23, 2008, pp. 3971-3972. Congress kept the 2009 guidelines in place for 2010.

mirrored Percival's code. The practice of professional courtesy served to build bonds between physicians and reduce the incentive for physicians to treat their own families. Most physicians agree that one of the greatest honors and privileges in the practice of medicine is to be asked to care for a physician and his or her family members. The practice of professional courtesy often was extended to others in the health care profession and members of the clergy. Most hospitals and many surgeons have given up the practice of free care today because most physicians now have insurance coverage for medical expenses.

Professional courtesy means either a discount or exemption from charges that may be given to certain people at the discretion of the physician rendering the service.

An interim rule from the CMS, effective July 24, 2004, identifies proper ways to offer professional courtesy:

1. The professional courtesy is offered to all physicians on the entity's bona fide medical staff or in the entity's local community or service area without regard to volume or value of referrals or other business generated between the parties.
2. The health care items and services provided are of a type routinely provided by the entity.
3. The entity's professional courtesy policy is written and approved in advance by the entity's governing body.
4. The professional courtesy is not offered to a physician (or immediate family member) who is a federal health care program beneficiary unless there has been a good faith showing of financial need.
5. If the professional courtesy involves any whole or partial reduction of any coinsurance obligation, the insurer is informed in writing of the reduction.

6. The arrangement does not violate the Anti-Kickback statute (section 1128b[b] of the act), or any federal or state law or regulation governing billing or claims submission.

Physicians must examine their policies on professional courtesy to ensure that they do not violate the contractual terms in private or managed care insurance policies or Medicare/Medicaid laws and regulations. If the treating physician does not bill the physician-patient for services rendered, the third-party payer is relieved of its contractual obligation. If the treating physician waives the deductible and copayment, the physician may be accused of not treating others with the same insurance coverage in an equal manner. Although there may be some situations in which it is defensible to not charge for services to health care professionals, the physician should ensure that this professional courtesy is not linked to patients who have been referred to the practice. Laws prohibit any inducement or kickbacks from physicians (or others) that could influence the decision of a physician (or other) to refer patients or that may affect a patient's decision to seek care.

Professional courtesy may violate fraud and abuse laws depending on how the recipients of the professional courtesy are selected and how the courtesy is extended. If selection depends on referral of individuals, then it may implicate the Anti-Kickback statute. An insurance claim submitted as a result of such a professional courtesy may also be affected by the False Claims Act.

Copayment Waiver

Waiving copayments is another way physicians have reduced the cost of medical care for patients in the past. In doing so, the physician accepts the insurance payment only. In most situations, both private insurers and the federal government ban waiving the copayment, therefore it is not recommended. Waiving copayments could violate the contract between the patient and third-party payer. If the physician has contracted with a third-party payer, waiving copayment may be a violation of the physician and managed care contract. Some insurance companies look at this as a means of recouping its losses by undergoing litigation against the provider or demanding the return of all payments made to the provider.

No Charge

No charge (NC) means waiving the entire fee for professional care. This is permitted as long as it is not part of a fraudulent scheme and is offered to all patients. All NC visits must be fully documented in the clinical portion of the patient's medical record and the financial record. As a way of trying to satisfy a patient's deductible, a physician or insurance specialist cannot assess a fee for services for which the insurance company or third-party payer does not cover.

Another instance when "NC" occurs on a patient's account is when follow-up visits are posted after a patient undergoes surgery considered under a surgical package or Medicare global fee structure. When posting such charges in a computer system, Current Procedural Terminology (CPT) procedure code 99024 (postoperative follow-up visit included in global fee) may be used.

Reduced Fee

Precautions should be taken before reducing the fee of a patient who dies. The doctor's sympathy in this case could be misinterpreted and result in a malpractice suit. A fee reduction should never be based on a poor result in the treatment of a patient.

If a patient disputes a fee and the physician agrees to settle for a reduced fee, the agreement should be in writing with a definite time limit for payment and the words "without prejudice" inserted. By doing this, the physician protects the right to collect the original sum if the patient fails to pay the reduced fee. The physician and patient should sign the agreement, and each should receive a copy.

Because the patient's financial history is personal, in-the-office conversations about fees must be private so that other individuals cannot overhear. The patient should be made to feel comfortable so that he or she feels free to discuss any financial problems. Be firm. Use tact. Always use a courteous but businesslike approach when discussing financial matters.

Communicating Fees

People have a difficult time asking each other for money and talking about financial obligations. Financial arrangements should be discussed up front and in great detail before any services are provided (Figure 10-5). Many medical practices create their own collection problems by not being clear about how and when they expect to be paid. If patients are not told that payment is due at the time of service, most assume they can pay at a later time. Patients are unaware of additional absorbed services given to patients during an office visit. Figure 10-6 presents a detailed description of some of those tasks that may be pointed out to patients so that they have a better understanding of the time expended by the provider and staff. Following are some guidelines to help communicate effectively about money:

1. Be courteous at all times but express a firm, businesslike approach that will not offend the patient.
2. Never badger or intimidate a patient into paying; merely state the payment policy and educate the patient.

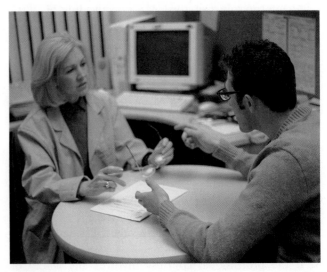

FIGURE 10-5 Insurance billing specialist discussing fees with the patient.

ABSORBED MEDICAL SERVICES

✔ Create and maintain patient's permanent medical records.

✔ Order, review/interpret, document/file, and telephone laboratory test results to the patient.

✔ Order x-rays, review/interpret, compare with previous studies if abnormal, consult with radiologist, document/file, and telephone results to the patient.

✔ Write and send consultation reports/letters to referring or consulting physicians and other providers.

✔ Telephone consultations with physicians.

✔ Complete family medical leave forms, disability forms, waivers for handicapped plates, waivers of insurance premiums, automotive forms, life insurance premium forms, travel insurance forms, and school, camp, or athletic participation forms.

✔ E-mail responses to patients.

✔ Write letters of referral to specialists.

✔ Create patient education materials.

✔ Conduct medical research pertinent to the patient's case.

✔ Write prescriptions and communicate with pharmacies about patients' prescriptions.

✔ Transmit (or complete) patients' insurance claim forms and complete insurance application forms.

✔ Conduct utilization review negotiations with hospitals and insurance companies.

✔ Review and maintain documentation for patients' hospital medical records.

✔ Write medical orders for hospitalized patients and orders for those in nursing facilities.

✔ Write letters to obtain medical services, instruments, or equipment for patients.

✔ Arrange for hospital admissions and follow-up consultations with nurses and other physicians.

FIGURE 10-6 Details of additional absorbed services the provider and staff give to patients during an office visit or depending on the complexity of a medical problem.

3. Inform the patient of the fee and any deductible and balance due in a clear manner.
4. Verify the patient's copayment listed on his or her insurance card and collect this amount before the patient's office visit.
5. Make it easier for the patient to pay rather than leave without making payment.
6. Do not give the patient an option by asking if he or she would like to pay now or have a bill sent.
7. Motivate the patient to pay by appealing to his or her honesty, integrity, and pride.

The following are examples of communicating in a positive manner and letting the patient know exactly what is expected:

● "The office visit is $62, Mrs. Smith. Would you like to pay by cash, check, credit card, or debit card?"
● "Your copayment for today's visit is $20, Mr. Jones, and you can pay by cash, check, credit, or debit card."
● "Your insurance policy shows a $100 deductible that is your responsibility and currently has not been met, Miss Rodriguez. You must pay the full fee today, which is $75."
● "Mrs. Merryweather, I must collect $4.77 today for your vitamin B$_{12}$ injection. The injection is not covered by your insurance policy."
● "We look forward to seeing you on Tuesday, March 3, at 10 AM, Mr. Gillespie. The consultation fee will be approximately $150, and payment is expected at the time of service. We accept cash, check, credit cards, or debit cards for your convenience."

Collecting Fees
Payment at the Time of Service

Collecting applicable copayments and other amounts due from the patient on each office visit is strongly recommended. To avoid difficulties in collecting at a future date, ask for fixed copayments before the patient is seen by the provider. This will alleviate billing for small amounts or possible problems with collection if statements are sent by mail after the visit. The importance of collecting outstanding bills, coinsurance amounts, and money from cash-paying patients up front should be communicated to office staff. One-on-one communication is the best way to motivate a **debtor.** Each patient's account **balance** (amount due) should be reviewed before his or her appointment. If the appointment schedule is on a computer system, print the account balance by each patient's name. If an appointment book is used, make a copy of the page showing the day's schedule. Write overdue balances by the patient's name after obtaining overdue amounts from each patient's financial accounting record card. This information also should be recorded on the transaction slip for that day's visit and may be "flagged" when the transaction slips are printed or written. Treat this information confidentially and keep it out of view of other patients. When a patient arrives whose name is "flagged," alert the patient accounts manager.

To do effective preappointment collection counseling, the patient should be taken to a quiet area away from the general activity of the office. Sit down with the patient and discuss the situation. Use an understanding attitude and helpful nature while verbalizing phrases such as "I understand" and "I can help." Ask direct questions to learn exactly what problems the patient is facing. Answers to questions such as "When do you expect your next paycheck?" and "How much are you able to pay today?" help determine the strategy. The goal should be to collect the full amount. If that is not possible, try to collect a portion of the balance. Get a promise to pay for the remaining balance by a specific date. If the patient is unable to comply, set up a payment plan. The chances of reaching a mutually satisfactory resolution are greatly improved when the two parties are face to face.

A personal interview is better than a telephone interview because a financial agreement can be signed when the debtor is present (Figure 10-7), resulting in a better follow-up response. Let the patient know that the practice is willing to help and that the debtor should inform the insurance specialist if he or she runs into further problems making the payment. This personal contact helps if a renegotiation of the agreement is necessary. A medical practice cannot refuse to let an established patient see the doctor because of a debt, but the office staff has every right to ask for payment while the patient is in the office.

Encounter Forms. Multipurpose billing forms (see Chapter 3) are known by many names, including the *encounter form.* These forms are helpful when collecting fees at the time of service. Encounter forms can be given to patients to bill their insurance companies, used to inform patients of current charges and outstanding balances, and used as receipts for payment (Figure 10-8).

Patient Excuses for Nonpayments. Nonpayers tend to dismiss financial arrangements with curt remarks. Look directly at the patient, confidently expecting payment. Demonstrate to the patient the right to request payment. Be ready if excuses are offered. Table 10-1 shows examples of patients' excuses and possible responses.

When a patient chatters nervously, it may be a way of setting up reasons to rationalize not paying. Do not let this be distracting. Pause after asking for payment and do not say another word until the patient responds. Many people feel uncomfortable with silence, but pauses may work to your advantage and help complete a transaction. The cash flow and collection ratio are increased by taking this approach, while decreasing billing chores and collection costs. The quick identification of nonpayers may be obtained, and the person responsible for collections notified.

Payment by Check

Check Verification. Check verification requires the insurance specialist to become familiar with the appearance of a good check. A personal check is the most common method of payment in most medical offices, but it is not a personal guarantee of payment. A driver's license and one other form of identification always should be required. Check these against existing records. Call the bank to verify all out-of-state and suspicious checks. A verification service (which is a private company with resources to quickly identify patient information over the telephone) or a check authorization system may be worthy of consideration for clinics and larger group practices.

Check Forgery. *Forgery* is false writing or alteration of a document to injure another person or with intent to deceive (e.g., signing another person's name on a check to obtain money or pay off a debt without permission). To guard against forgery, always check to be sure the endorsement on the back of the check matches the name on the front. Be suspicious if the beneficiary or provider states that he or she did not receive the check, but the

1. Total amount of the debt; wording "cash price" must be used according to Regulation Z.

2. Amount of down payment.

3. Interest rate expressed as an annual percentage; must be in capital letters and stand out.

4. Finance charge; must be in capital letters and stand out.

5. Amount of each payment.

6. Date each payment is due.

7. Signature of patient and physician with copies retained by both; narrative must be included.

College Clinic
4567 Broad Avenue
Woodland Hills, XY 12345-0001
Phone: 555/486-9002
Fax: 555/487-8976

FINANCIAL PAYMENT PLAN AGREEMENT

For medical professional services rendered to:

Patient Name _Keenan Kellog_　　　　　　　　Account No. _09-276_
Responsible Party _____

Address ____305 West Avenue____
____Woodland Hills, XY 12345____

Telephones:　Home ____555-461-2072____
　　　　　　　Mobile ____555-578-1000____
　　　　　　　Business ____555-486-0132____

1. Cash price of total medical treatment　　　　$ __5000.00__
2. Down payment (partial payment)　　　　　　$ __300.00__
3. Amount covered by insurance plan　　　　　$ __4000.00__
4. Unpaid balance due　　　　　　　　　　　$ __700.00__
5. **ANNUAL PERCENTAGE RATE** (interest rate)　　__-0-__ %
6. **FINANCE CHARGE** ($ amt of cost to patient)　$ __-0-__
7. Total amount of unpaid balance due　　　　　__700.00__
8. Monthly payment amount　　　　　　　　　$ __100.00__

TERMS:
1. ALL PAYMENTS ARE DUE ON OR BEFORE YOUR DUE DATE EACH MONTH.
2. The patient agrees to be fully responsible for the total payment of medical services performed in this office including any amounts not covered by any health insurance plan.
3. The patient has the right at any time to pay the unpaid balance due without penalty.
4. First payment due ___Feb / 15 / 20XX___ and subsequent payments on the same day of each consecutive month until paid in full.

Keenan Kellog　　　　　　　　　　_1/15/XX_
Signature of Patient/Responsible Party　　　　Date
Astro Parkinson, MD　　　　　　　　_1/15/XX_
Physician's signature or Authorized representative　　Date

FIGURE 10-7 Financial payment plan agreement that provides full disclosure of all information by the Truth in Lending Act, Regulation Z.

third-party payer shows it as being cashed, or if the payee of the check claims that the signature is not his or hers.

Payment Disputes. Problem checks appear in many forms. One is the check for partial payment when the debtor (the patient) writes "payment in full" on the check. If the **creditor** (the physician) cashes the check, it may be argued that the debt is paid in full. A legal theory called *accord and satisfaction* may apply to this situation if the debt is truly disputed by the debtor. If the check is retained (and cashed) by the physician, it can

be considered "accord and satisfaction," and the physician cannot procure the balance from the patient. The operative words are "truly disputed." If there is a legitimate, genuine dispute over the amount of the bill and an amount less than the full amount of the bill is accepted, the physician could be precluded from seeking the balance. However, acceptance of payment does not necessarily mean acceptance of the "paid in full" remark. Read the state's accord and satisfaction laws; the Uniform Commercial Code, Articles 3, 4, and 9; and the Retail Installment Sales Act and Escheats

TAX ID # 3664021CC
Medicaid #HSC12345F
Medicare DME #34007

COLLEGE CLINIC
4567 Broad Avenue, Woodland Hills, XY 12345-0001
Tel: (555) 486-8002 Fax: (555) 487-8976

CO-PAY: _$10.00_
CO. NAME: _Quality Care_
IPA: _____

1. Insurance identifying data

PATIENT INFO.

PATIENT'S LAST NAME	FIRST	INITIAL	FAMILY ACCT. NO.	BIRTHDATE	SEX	DATE OF SERVICE
McDonald	Lydia	P.	3794	01/06/80	☐ MALE ☒ FEMALE	05/06/XX

ADDRESS	CITY	STATE	ZIP
203 Base Street	Woodland Hills	XY	12345-0001

RESPONSIBLE PARTY INFORMATION	INS. ID	COVERAGE CODE	GROUP #
	215678	A2501	340

ASSIGNMENT: I hereby assign my insurance benefits be paid directly to the undersigned physician. I am financially responsible for non-covered services.
SIGNED: (Patient, or Parent, if Minor) _Lydia McDonald_   DATE: 05/06/XX

RELEASE: I authorize the undersigned physician to release to my insurance carriers any information required to process this claim.
SIGNED: (Patient, or Parent, if Minor) _Lydia McDonald_   DATE: 05/06/XX

2. Assignment of medical benefits

3. Procedure codes

✓	DESCRIPTION	CODE/MD	FEE	✓	DESCRIPTION	CODE/MD	FEE	✓	DESCRIPTION	CODE/MD	FEE
	OFFICE VISIT	NEW	ESTAB.		**PROCEDURES**				**HOSPITAL SERVICES (Cont'd.)**		
	Brief	99201	99211		Stress Test Phys Supv	93016			Replace Intracoronary Stent	92980	
	Focused	99202	99212		Stress Interp & Report	93018			Each Add'l. Vessel	92981	
	Expanded	99203	99213		Rhythm Strip	93040			PTCA	92982	
	Detailed	99204	99214		Holter (24) Interp & Report	93227			Each Add'l. Vessel	92984	
✓	Comprehensive	99205	99215 195.00		Echo M-Mode 2-D	93307-26			Right Heart Cath	93501	
	Post-Op Visit		99058	✓	Doppler	93320-26	250.00		Swanz-Ganz	93503	
					Color Flow Mapping	93352-26			Left Heart Cath	93510	
	HOSPITAL CONSULTATION								Comb Rt & Lf Heart Cath Sel	93526	
	For Dr.:				**HOSPITAL SERVICES**				Coronary & Lf Vent Angio		
					Endotracheal Intubation	31500			Comb RHC & Septal LHC	93527	
	Complex	99255			Thoracentesis	32421			(Intact Septum)		
	Comprehensive	99254			Insert/Replace Pacemaker	33206			Comb Rhc w/Lf Vent Puncture	93528	
	Limited	99253			Ventricular	33207			Comb RHC & LHC Thru	93529	
					AV Sequential	33208			Existing Septal Opening		
	HOSPITAL ADMISSION				Insert/Replace Pulse Gen	33212			Inj Proc (Internal Mammary)	93539	
	Comprehensive	99223			Repair Pacemaker (Single)	33218			Sel Opac Bypass Grafts	93540	
	Intermediate	99222			Rev/Reloc Skin Pocket	33222			1 Or More Arteries		
	Limited	99221			Remove Perm Pacemaker	33233			Pulmonary Angiography	93541	
					Unlisted Cardiac Procedure	33999			Sel Rf Vent/Atrial Angio	93542	
	HOSPITAL CARE				Arterial Cath Monitor	36620			Sel Lf Vent/Atrial Angio	93543	
	Extended	99233			Esophageal Lead	93615			For Aortography	93544	
	Intermediate	99232			IABP	33970			Sel Coronary Angiography	93545	
	Limited	99231			Aortogr Arch/Abdom	36200			S&I Cardiac Cath Vent	93555	
					Arterial Puncture	36600			And/Or Atrial Angio		
	CRITICAL CARE SERVICE				Cardiopulmonary Resuscitation	92950			Bil Sel Inj Incl Venous	93556	
	ICU/CCU 1st Hour	99291			Cardioversion	92960			Bypass Grafts		
	Each Add'l. 30 Minutes	99292			PTA (Complete) Perhipheral	75962			Indicator Studies Arterial	93561	
					PTA Complete	75964			w/Cardiac Output		
					PTA Renal	75966			Subsequent Measurement Of	93562	
					Thrombolysis	92975			Cardiac Output		

4. Diagnostic codes

ICD-9	DIAGNOSIS						
☐ 414.9	Ischemic Heart Disease	☐ 746.3	Congenital Aortic Stenosis	☐ 426.7	WPW Syndrome	☐ 278.00	Obesity
☐ 410.91	MI Acute (Unspec)	☒ 746.85	Coronary Artery Anomaly	☐ 428.0	Congestive Heart Failure	☐ 415.19	Pulm Embolism
☐ 411.0	Post MI Syndrome	☐ 746.86	Congenital Heart Block	☐ 429.1	Myocardial Degeneration	☐ 486	Pneumonia
☐ 411.1	Unstable Angina	☐ 785.51	Cardiogenic Shock	☐ 429.3	Cardiomegaly	☐ 491.22	Bronchitis
☐ 412	Old Myocardial Infarct	☐ 398.90	Rheumatic Heart Disease	☐ 780.2	Syncope / Collapse	☐ 492.8	Emphysema
☐ 413.9	Angina Pectoris	☐ 391.0	Rheum Pericarditis (Acute)	☐ 782.3	Edema	☐ 493.91	Asthma
☐ 413.1	Prinzmetal Angina	☐ 391.1	Rheum Endocarditis (Acute)	☐ 785.0	Tachycardia	☐ 531.90	Gastric Ulcer
☐ 414.10	Aneurysm (Heart)	☐ 427.9	Cardiac Dysrhythmias	☐ 785.1	Palpitations	☐ 532.91	Duodenal Ulcer
☐ 424.90	Valvular Heart Disease	☐ 427.81	Sick Sinus Syndrome	☐ 785.2	Heart Murmur	☐ 533.00	PUD
☐ 395.9	Aortic Stenosis	☐ 427.1	Ventricular Tachycardia	☐ 786.59	Chest Pain	☐ 593.9	Renal Disease
☐ 395.1	Aortic Regurgitation	☐ 427.31	Atrial Fibrillation	☐ 794.31	Abnormal ECG	☐ 581.9	Nephrotic Syndrome
☐ 394.0	Mitral Stenosis	☐ 427.32	Atrial Flutter	☐ 441.9	Aortic Aneurysm	☐ 584.9	Acute Renal Failure
☐ 397.0	Tricuspid Valve Disease	☐ 427.60	Premature Beats	☐ 443.81	Peripheral Vascular Disease	☐ 585.1	Chronic Renal Failure
☐ 424.0	Mitral Valve Disorders	☐ 427.61	Supraventricular	☐ 444.9	Arterial Embolism Throm	☐ 599.0	Urinary Tract Infection
☐ 401.9	Essential Hypertension	☐ 427.69	PVG	☐ 451.9	Phlebitis/ (Thrombo)	☐ 349.9	Neurological Disease
☐ 402.90	Hypertensive Ht Disease	☐ 312.9	Conduction Disorders	☐ 437.9	Cerebrovascular Disorder	☐ 259.9	Endocrine Disorders
☐ 746.9	Congenital Heart Disease	☐ 425.1	Hypertrop Subaortic Sten	☐ 433.11	OCC/Stenosis Bas/Car/Vert	☐ 714.0	Rheumatic Arthritis
☐ 745.4	Ventricle Septal Defect	☐ 425.4	Cardiomyopathy	☐ 435.9	Transient Ischemic Attack	☐ 715.00	Osteoarthritis
☐ 745.5	Atrial Septal Defect	☐ 426.0	Complete AV Block	☐ 436	CVA	☐ 716.99	Arthritis
☐ 746.02	Pulmonary Valve Stenosis	☐ 426.2	Lf Anterior Hemiblock	☐ 272.4	Hyperlipidemia	☐ 427.89	Bradycardia
☐ 746.2	Epstein's Anomaly	☐ 426.3	Lf Bundle Branch Block	☐ 250.00	Diabetes Mellitus		
		☐ 426.4	Rt Bundle Branch Block	☐ 274.9	Gout		

DIAGNOSIS: (IF NOT CHECKED ABOVE)

INSTRUCTIONS:

SERVICES PERFORMED AT: ☒ OFFICE ☐ IN PATIENT ☐ OUT PATIENT ☐ ER

☐ Hemet Valley Hospital   ☐ Menifee
116 Latham Avenue   28400 McCall Blvd.
Hemet, CA 92543   Sun City, CA 92381

DOCTOR'S SIGNATURE / DATE
P. Cardi, MD

ACCEPT ASSIGNMENT? ☒ YES ☐ NO

INSTRUCTIONS TO PATIENT FOR FILING INSURANCE CLAIMS:
1. COMPLETE THE "PATIENT INFORMATION" SECTION AT THE TOP OF THIS FORM.
2. SIGN AND DATE.
3. MAIL THIS FORM TO YOUR INSURANCE COMPANY FOR DIRECT REIMBURSEMENT.

REC'D. BY:		
☒ CASH	TOTAL TODAY'S FEE	445.00
☐ CR. CD.	OLD BALANCE	0
☐ CHECK	TOTAL DUE	445.00
	AMT. REC'D. TODAY	10.00
# _____	NEW BALANCE	335.00

5. Patient's previous balance

6. Total charges and payments received

INSUR-A-BILL ® BIBBERO SYSTEMS, INC. • PETALUMA, CA • © 03/06 EP005.SB CARDIO   (REV. 07/09)

FIGURE 10-8 Encounter form; diagnostic codes from *International Classification of Diseases, Ninth Revision, Clinical Modification* (ICD-9-CM), and procedural codes for professional services from Current Procedural Terminology (CPT). (Courtesy Bibbero Systems, Inc., Petaluma, CA; phone: 800-242-2376; fax: 800-242-9330; www.bibbero.com.)

Law. Even if a check marked "paid in full" is accidentally cashed, 90 days may be available to rectify the situation by returning the funds to the patient and informing him or her that the accord and satisfaction is not acceptable. A patient who is paying less may be dissatisfied with the practice in some way. This may help defuse any lurking issues and address the patient's underlying problem.

Postdated Checks. Checks dated to be payable 3 to 6 months in the future are not honored by the bank. Always read the date of every check. Federal collection law states that if a check dated more than 5 days in advance is accepted, the patient must be notified no more than 10 days and no less than 3 days before the check is deposited. State laws vary, but some states have regulations in addition to federal laws.

Table 10-1	Possible Responses to Patients' Excuses for Avoiding Payment
EXCUSE	**RESPONSE**
"Just bill me."	"As we explained when we made your appointment, Mr. Barkley, our practice bills for charges more than $50. Amounts under $50 are to be paid at the time of the visit. That will be $25 for today's visit, please."
"I have insurance to cover this."	"We will be billing your insurance for you, Miss Butler, but your policy shows a deductible in the amount of $300 that still must be met. We must collect the full fee for today's visit, which is $150 to meet that deductible responsibility."
"I get paid on Friday; you know how it is."	"I understand. Why don't you write the check today and postdate it for Saturday. We will hold the check and deposit it on the next business day" (depending on office policy).
"If I pay for this, I won't be able to pay for the prescription."	"Our payment policy is very much like the pharmacy's: we expect payment at the time of service. Let me check and see if the doctor can dispense some medication samples to last until you can get your prescription filled."
"I don't have that much with me."	"How much can you pay, Mrs. Fish? I can accept $10 now and give you an envelope to send us the balance within the week, or I can put it on your credit or debit card." (Get a commitment and write the balance due under the sealing flap of the envelope. Also write the date on a tickler calendar or the patient's financial accounting record while the patient is watching.)
"I'll take care of it."	"I know you will, Mr. Stone; I just need to know when that will be so that I can document your intentions for our bookkeeper." (Get a commitment and input the date in the patient's financial accounting record while in view of the patient. Hand him an envelope with the amount due written under the sealing flap.)
"I forgot my checkbook."	"We take Visa, MasterCard, and American Express, Mr. Storz." (If the patient still does not pay, provide him with a self-addressed envelope and write the patient's name, account number, date of service, amount due, and expected payment date under the sealing flap. Restate the expected payment date as you hand the patient the envelope. Input the date in the patient's financial accounting record while the patient is watching.)

Unsigned Checks. Another problem is unsigned checks. Ask the patient to come to the office and sign the check or send a new one. If you are unable to reach the patient or if there is a transportation or time limitation problem, write the word "over" or "see reverse" on the signature line on the front of the check. On the back of the check, where the endorsement should appear, write "lack of signature guaranteed," the practice's name, and one's own name and title. This endorsement in effect is a guarantee that the practice will absorb the loss if the patient's bank or the patient does not honor the check.

Returned Checks. When the physician's office receives notice that a check was not honored, the reason should be stated on the back of the check. The most common reason is nonsufficient funds (NSF). Call the bank to find out if there are adequate funds in the account to cover the check and take the NSF check to the bank immediately. You might telephone the patient to see if they suggest redepositing it. Check the state laws about NSF checks. There is a time limit for making the check good, and there are additional charges (up to 10% of the value of the check) that the patient must make to restore the check. If the patient does not respond, the matter may be turned over to a regional district attorney or satisfaction may be obtained through small claims court. An NSF demand letter (Figure 10-9) should be sent by certified mail with return receipt requested and include the following:

1. Check date
2. Check number
3. Name of the bank where the check is drawn
4. Name of person the check was payable to
5. Check amount
6. Any allowable service charge
7. Total amount due
8. Number of days the check writer has to take action

Future payments should be in the form of cash, money order, or a cashier's check. If the patient wants the check to be returned, be sure to photocopy it and keep it in the financial record because it serves as an acknowledgment of the debt. The bad check may be returned to the patient after it has been replaced with a valid payment. Place a notation on the patient's record to this effect.

If notified that the checking account is closed, send a demand letter immediately. In most states, legal action can be taken if the patient does not respond in 30 days. Consider filing a claim in small claims court. Most states have written codes or statutes pertaining to bad checks. Often, legislation allows the creditor to add punitive damages to the amount of the debt being collected, sometimes up to three times the amount of the check.

When a patient stops payment on a check, it is usually done to resolve a good faith dispute. In this case, the patient believes that he or she has legal entitlement to withhold payment. The physician may want to contact a

COLLEGE CLINIC
4567 Broad Avenue
Woodland Hills, XY 12345-0001
Tel. (555) 486-9002
FAX (555) 487-8976

August 15, 20XX

Mrs. Maxine Holt
444 Labina Lane
Woodland Hills, XY 12345-0001

Dear Mrs. Holt:

The following check has been dishonored by the bank and returned without payment:

Date:	08/04/20XX
Check No.:	755
Amount:	$106.11
Payable to:	Perry Cardi, MD
Bank:	Woodland Hills National Bank
Reason:	Nonsufficient funds

This is a formal notice demanding payment in the amount of $106.11 within 15 days from today's date or your account will be considered for legal action.

Please make payment immediately by cash, cashier's check, or money order at the above address. Your immediate attention will be appreciated.

Sincerely,

Delores Yee, CMA-A

Patient Accounts Manager
for Perry Cardi, MD

FIGURE 10-9 Demand letter for returned check. This letter serves as a formal notice to collect payment and notifies a patient of impending legal action.

lawyer to discuss his or her legal rights and responsibilities before sending a demand letter and trying to collect.

Itemized Patient Statements

Every patient receives an **itemized statement** (Figure 10-10) of his or her account showing the dates of service, a list of detailed charges, copayments and deductibles paid, the date insurance claim was filed (if appropriate), applicable adjustments, and the account balance. These items also are listed on the patient's account or financial accounting record card (see Figures 3-14 and 10-3). Timeliness, accuracy, and consistency have a significant effect on the cash flow and collection process when sending itemized statements. A credit card option should be printed on the statement to encourage easier and faster payment.

Professional bills are a reflection of the medical practice. The billing statement should be patient oriented and easy to read and understand. Avoid technical terms and abbreviations that might lead to misunderstandings and confusion. Enclose a return envelope. Addressed envelopes should contain the statement "Forwarding Service Requested" so that the postal service can forward the mail and provide the physician's office with a notice of the patient's new address. When this notice is received in the physician's office, it should be circulated to all necessary departments to record the new information.

Patients can be oriented to the billing process by having the insurance specialist electronically generate a printed statement as the patient leaves the office that explains pertinent information such as account number, dates of service, payments, procedures, interest fees, copayments, and deductibles. Patients may choose to receive their statements electronically, so ask software providers for this component. If using standard mail, patient information pamphlets about common health concerns, such as blood pressure, cholesterol, or back pain, can be sent with the bill to convey a caring attitude.

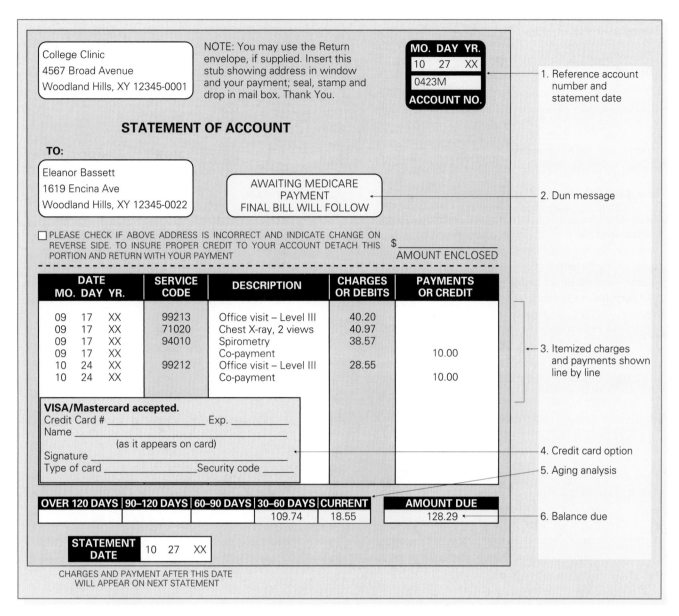

FIGURE 10-10 Computerized statement. A credit card option should be printed near the bottom of the statement to encourage payment. (Form adapted courtesy Bibbero Systems, Inc., Petaluma, CA; phone: 800-242-2376; fax: 800-242-9330; www.bibbero.com.)

The office is likely to experience an increase in telephone calls from inquiring patients when statements go out in the mail. One person or one department should handle all billing questions, ensuring a consistent response.

Accounts Receivable and Age Analysis by Aging Report. Age analysis is a term used for the procedure of systematically arranging the A/R by age from the date of service. Accounts are usually aged in time periods of 30, 60, 90, and 120 days and older, as shown at the bottom of Figure 10-10. An aging report can be generated by the practice management system or by use of

other software in a computer system. This helps collection follow-up by providing easy recognition of overdue accounts and allows the insurance specialist to determine which accounts need action in addition to a regular statement.

The formula for finding out the A/R ratio is to divide the month-end A/R balance by the monthly average charges for the prior 12-month period. An average total A/R (all monies not collected at the time of service) should be one and a half to two times the charges for 1 month of services (Examples 10-1 and 10-2).

Example 10-1	Formula	
Physician's Charges Monthly Total	$50,000 × 1.5 = $75,000 or $50,000 × 2.0 = $100,000	Total Outstanding Accounts Receivable

Total outstanding A/R should range from $75,000 to $100,000.

Example 10-2	Calculation of Accounts Receivable Ratio
Annual gross charges	$150,000
Average monthly gross charges (150,000 ÷ 12 months)	12,500
Current Accounts Receivable Balance	20,000
Accounts Receivable Ratio: 20,000 ÷ 12,500 = 1.60 months	

Accounts that are 90 days or older should not exceed 15% to 18% of the total A/R. To calculate this figure, divide the total amount of A/R by the amount of accounts that are 90 days old and older (Example 10-3). Practice management systems should calculate this automatically when an aging report is required.

Example 10-3	Formula for Determining Percentage of Accounts Over 90 Days		
Amount of A/R over 90 days		A/R Total	Percentage of A/R over 90 days
$12,000	÷	$75,000	= 16%

A decision tree showing time frames for sending statements and telephone calls is presented in Figure 10-11.

Collection Decision Tree

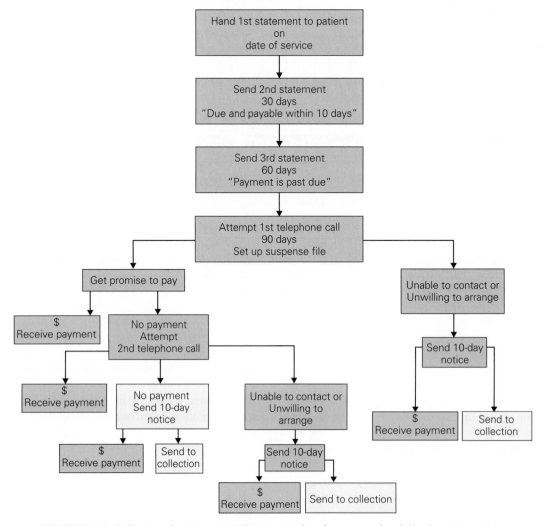

FIGURE 10-11 Collection decision tree. This is a quick reference used to help determine when to send statements, make telephone calls, and send accounts to a collection agency.

Dun Messages

Dun messages are phrases printed on statements to inform or remind a patient about a delinquent account and to promote payment (see Figures 10-3 and 10-10). The best and most effective collection statements include a handwritten note; however, this is seldom possible. Dun messages also can be printed by the computer system or applied with brightly colored labels. Examples of dun messages follow:

- "If there is a problem with your account, please call me at (555) 486-0000—Marlayn."
- "This bill is now 30 days past due. Please remit payment."
- "This bill is now 60 days past due. Please send payment immediately."
- "Your account is 90 days past due. Please remit payment now to avoid collection action."
- "FINAL NOTICE: If we do not hear from you within 10 days, this account will be turned over to our collection agency."

Do not send intimidating, impatient, or threatening statements. These only serve to antagonize patients. Dun messages should be printed in different languages and sent to patients who speak English as a second language. Examples are as follows;

- "No payment yet; your payment by return mail will be appreciated."
- "No hemos recibido pago. Agracieramos remita por correo."
- "Payment needed now. No further credit will be extended."
- "Se requiere pago hoy. No se le estendera mas credito."

Manual Billing. Manual billing is usually done by photocopying the patient's financial accounting record and placing it in a window envelope. The financial accounting record becomes the statement and should be clear and readable with nothing crossed out or misspelled. Typewritten statements may be used by small offices and generally are typed on continuous form paper. The completed statements are separated, folded, and placed into billing envelopes.

A coding system with metal clip-on tabs or peel-off labels that are placed on the financial accounting record card can be used with a manual system. Each time the account is billed, a different-colored tab or label is placed on the financial accounting record card, which shows at a glance how many times the account has been billed. It also provides aging of accounts, although if a report is desired it must be done manually in addition to this process.

 Computer Billing. Because most medical practices use the computer to generate billing statements, the manual system is not discussed in this edition. Computerized patient statements are generated by the practice management software. All charges, payments, and adjustments are reflected on hardcopy and made readily available to mail to the patient (see Figure 10-10). The computer program usually offers choices of billing types including patient billing, **insurance balance billing,** billing according to types of adjustments, and no bill. The insurance specialist can instruct the computer to print all bills of a specific type. The computer also can be instructed to print bills according to specific accounts, dates, and insurance types. Accounts are automatically aged, and standard messages can be printed on the statements for each of the aged dates (30, 60, 90, or 120 days). Some systems allow personalized messages to be inserted that override the standard messages.

Billing Services. Billing services are employed by many medical practices to reduce administrative paperwork by taking over the task of preparing and mailing patient statements. These services also may be employed to prepare and mail insurance claim forms or send them electronically. They may provide data entry of patients' demographic and billing information, charges, receipts, and adjustments; tracking of payments from patients and third-party payers; production of management reports; purging of inactive accounts; and collection of accounts.

Some advantages of billing services are advanced technology, professional and understandable bills, experts answering all billing-related telephone inquiries, and no downtime caused by vacations, or medical or personal leave. This service allows the medical office to have fewer disruptions and the freedom from worry about financial matters when trying to provide medical care.

The physician's office sends billing and receipt information into the system daily. This may be done in writing or through a computer system. The billing service then prepares the bills, mails them, and may also receive payments. Regular reports, whether weekly or monthly, are sent to the physician summarizing the transactions. Billing services may offer full account management services and in many cases customize a service that meets the needs of the provider. Using a billing service company is most commonly referred to as *outsourcing*. When choosing a billing service, make a list of important questions and visit the facility. Also ask for references so that you may obtain valuable feedback from other provider offices that have used the same billing service.

Have a written directive in place that gives the billing company permission to communicate directly with the insurance company and a Medicare Administrative Contractor (MAC) about denied or problem claims. When changing billing services, be sure to revoke such authorizations with each carrier and MAC.

Billing Guidelines

Billing procedures are determined by the size of the practice, number of accounts, and number of staff members assigned to the collection process. Adopt a specific method of handling accounts and decide which billing routine best fits the practice. Check insurance and managed care contracts carefully to determine which circumstances allow for patients to be billed. Be sure to conform to federal guidelines if there is a need to bill managed care patients. See Procedure 10-1 at the end of this chapter for the procedures for seven-step billing and collection guidelines.

CREDIT ARRANGEMENTS

Although payment at the time of service is ideal, many patients do not have funds available to pay at the time of the office visit. Alternative payment methods may be offered to help continuous cash flow and reduce collection costs.

Payment Options
Credit Card Billing

Credit card payment is an option that provides patients with an alternative to clear their account balances. Credit cards are issued by organizations that entitle the cardholder to credit at their establishments. This method of payment may be most useful as a down payment on uninsured or elective procedures. According to a survey by American Express, 33% of patients said they would use a credit card to pay for health care–related expenses if the option were given. Credit cards can help manage the A/R by improving cash flow, reducing billing costs, lowering overhead, and reducing the risk of bad debts. If a practice accepts credit cards, advise all patients in the following ways:

- Display a credit card acceptance sign.
- Include an insignia or message on the statement.
- Include the credit card policy in the new patient brochure.

- Have staff members verbalize to patients that this option is available.

Patients may prefer to clear a debt immediately and make monthly payments to the credit card company instead of owing money to their doctor.

Verifying Credit Cards. A one- or two-physician office may have a simple credit card imprinter in the office. The insurance specialist should check credit card warning bulletins to make sure that the card has not been canceled or stolen. Large practices may have an electronic credit card machine that allows the insurance specialist to swipe the card through the machine that is linked to the credit card company. Transactions are then approved, processed, and deposited into a bank account, usually in 2 working days. A receipt is generated for the patient. These machines may be rented or purchased.

VeriFone terminals are also used for credit card authorization. They are small computers with built-in software and modems for communicating with other computers over telephone lines. They have a small alphanumeric keypad and a small display screen that can show a line or two of data. This device reads the information off the magnetic card as it is swiped through the machine, dials a telephone number, connects with another computer, verifies the patient's credit, and displays a message.

Verifying Credit Card Holders. Always verify the cardholder by asking for photo identification such as a driver's license. Examine the card carefully and observe the following guidelines:

- Accept a credit card only from the person whose name is on the card.
- Match the name on the card with the patient's other identification and make sure the expiration date has not passed.
- Look on the back of the card for the word "void." This is an alert that the card has been heated, which is a method used to forge a signature.
- Check the "hot list" for problem cards.
- Verify all charges regardless of the amount and get approval from the credit card company.
- Complete the credit card voucher (Figure 10-12) before asking for a signature.
- Compare the signature on the credit card voucher against the signature on the card.

Credit Card Fees. Most banks directly deposit the credit card voucher and subtract the monthly fees from the practice's bank account. A statement from the bank indicates how much has been credited to the account. The fees can be negotiated on the basis of volume but usually range from 2% to 10% on each transaction. Some

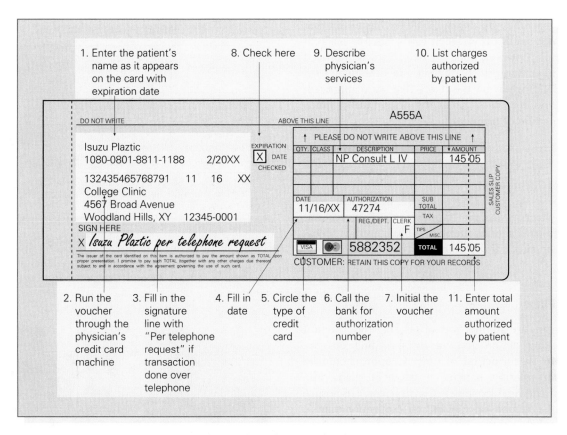

FIGURE 10-12 Credit card voucher completed in a physician's office.

medical practices charge patients a service fee for using credit cards. Do not issue cash or check refunds for any payments made by credit card. Credit vouchers (see Figure 10-12) used for crediting a credit card account are available at local banks. Patients who want to make payments may have their credit cards charged for each scheduled payment.

Credit Card Options. Online bill payment or e-payment, such as PayPal, is another way patients can pay their bills and use their credit cards to do so. It is done through the medical practice's secure website. Payment can be immediately verified and deposited directly into the physician's account.

Other cards are used for credit in a physician's office as well. Automated teller machine (ATM) cards are sometimes accepted for medical care if the practice has a credit card scanner. An ATM card is a magnetically encoded bank card used to make deposits and withdraw cash from checking or savings accounts. Private-label cards are credit vehicles that can be used only to pay for health care. Some large practices offer their own private-label health cards. Smart cards also are used in some locations. They are small credit or debit cards that contain a computer chip that can store money in the form of electronic data. Special-use smart cards for telephone

calls, gas stations, and fast food are now in use, as are common cards having multiple uses. These cards may also contain patient health care data.

Visa offers a credit card service unique to the health care market. It has a preauthorized health care form that allows patients to authorize the medical office to bill their account directly for copayments and the balance not covered by insurance. Patients who need a series of treatments, such as allergy injections or chemotherapy, can fill out one form designating these services, which authorizes the staff to charge the patient's account directly.

Debit Cards

A **debit card** is a card permitting bank customers to withdraw cash at any hour or for some ATMs until midnight from any affiliated ATM in the country. The holder may make cashless purchases from funds on deposit without incurring revolving finance charges for credit. A small fee may be charged to the customer's checking account when the card is used; however, this fee is usually applied only once a month (if the debit card is used), regardless of how many times the card is used during the month. Medical practices offering credit card payment may use the same electronic credit card machine to swipe the debit card for verification and approval. Separate debit card machines are also available for businesses that do not accept credit cards. Debit cards take the place of check writing; however, once the debit card is approved for a certain amount, the bank that issued the debit card is responsible for paying the funds that were approved. There are no returned checks for nonsufficient funds with this method of payment.

E-Checks

Another payment option that is becoming popular is payment by e-check. With an e-check, the patient gives his or her checking account information such as account number and bank routing number. No signature is necessary, and the check is deposited as if it was sent by the patient.

Payment Plans

Payment plans are another way of offering the patient a way of paying off an account by spreading out the amount due over a period of time. Caution should be taken when offering patients a payment plan. The Truth in Lending Consumer Credit Cost Disclosure Law (see the section on Credit and Collection Laws), also referred to as *Regulation Z*, requires full written disclosure about the finance charges for large payment plans involving four or more installments, excluding a down payment. However, this regulation does not apply if the patient agrees to pay in one sum or in fewer than four payments and then decides independently to make drawn-out partial payments. Patients often think that if they make any amount of payment, the physician is required to accept that payment and not take any additional action. This is incorrect. The physician can take action, including sending the account to a collection agency. Have a written payment plan schedule when working with accounts in which payment plans may be offered. Figure 10-13 illustrates sample guidelines that may be used or revised according to individual practice and management policies (Figure 10-14).

CREDIT AND COLLECTION LAWS

The following laws are important because they provide the legal framework within which the insurance specialist must execute the physician's collection policy. In addition, each state may have specific collection laws that are necessary to research and obey. Most states have *prompt payment laws* designed to govern actions of insurers and third-party payers to pay insurance claims in a timely manner. Box 10-1 includes names and descriptions of the federal credit and collection laws that affect medical practices.

PAYMENT PLAN SCHEDULE

Balance due amount	Minimum monthly payment	Time frame for full payment
$0 – $200	$35	6 months
$201 – $500	$50	1 year
$500 – $1000	$100	1 year
$1001 – $3000	$125	2 years
$3001 – $5000	$150	2 years
>$5001*	$200	5 years

*Accounts over $5000 must complete credit card application to certify minimum required payment and are subject to approval by office manager.

FIGURE 10-13 Payment plan schedule used in the physician's office to negotiate monthly payments shows balance due amounts, minimum monthly payment, and payment time frames.

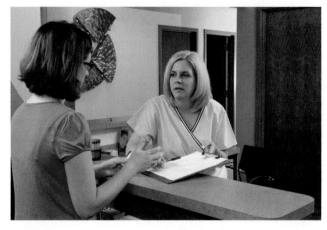

FIGURE 10-14 Insurance billing specialist setting up a payment plan with a patient.

The Red Flags Rule is a set of Federal Trade Commission requirements for businesses that have more than 20 employees and issue credit to their clients. These rules aim to prevent fraud and identity theft of a person's personal data for illegal use. A health care provider must create a plan to help recognize warning signs (or "red flags") associated with fraud and identity theft or face civil penalties for violation. A medical practice must notify patients if their data was stolen.

For additional information, see Internet Resources at the end of this chapter. The Evolve website has a link to individual state statutes of the articles of the Uniform Commercial Code.

Box 10-1   Federal Credit and Collection Laws

Equal Credit Opportunity Act (ECOA)

Prohibits discrimination in all areas of granting credit. Detailed credit information should be obtained before performing services to prevent accusations of impartiality. New patients should be informed that payment is due at the time of service and that they should arrive 20 minutes early to fill out a credit application if they wish to establish credit for treatment. Data, such as the patient's address, previous addresses, length of residence, employment history, and approximate wage, can be verified with a credit bureau. The report will also contain the patient's name changes, the patient's bill-paying history, and any history of bankruptcy. If the patient has a poor credit rating, credit may be denied and the patient then has 60 days to request the reason in writing. The law prohibits discrimination against any applicant for credit for the following reasons:
• Age, color, marital status, national origin, race, religion, or sex
• Receiving income from alimony or any public assistance program

Fair Credit Reporting Act (FCRA)

Regulates agencies that either issue or use reports on consumers (patients) in connection with the approval of credit. Credit reporting agencies can only provide reports when the following occurs:
• A court order is issued.
• The report is requested by the consumer (patient) or instructions are given by the patient to provide the report.
• There is a legitimate business need for the information.
   If credit is refused, the physician must provide the patient with a reason credit was denied and name and address of the agency from which the report came. Specific information about what the report contains is not necessary and should not be given. The patient must have an opportunity to correct any inaccuracies if they occur.

Fair and Accurate Credit Transactions (FACT) Act (Public Law 108-159)

Establishes (as of December 4, 2003) medical privacy provisions as part of consumer credit law. The bill amends the FCRA to include improved medical privacy protections and protections against identity theft. Credit bureaus and creditors must comply with a number of medical privacy restrictions that ban the sharing of medical information. Title IV of the FACT Act limits the use and sharing of medical information in the financial system and provides an expanded definition of medical information. For military personnel, it provides an active-duty alert that can be placed on the credit file for a year at the three major credit bureaus. This means that a creditor cannot issue new credit or a card without first contacting the active-duty individual whose name is on the card.

Fair Credit Billing Act (FCBA)

Applies to "open end" credit accounts such as credit cards and revolving charge accounts for department store accounts. It does not cover installment contracts such as loans or extensions of credit you repay on a fixed schedule. Consumers often buy cars, furniture, and major appliances on an installment basis, and they repay personal loans in installments as well. The FCBA settlement procedures apply only to disputes about "billing errors" such as unauthorized charges. Federal law limits the consumer's responsibility for unauthorized charges to $50; charges that list the wrong date or amount; charges for goods and services that the consumer did not accept or were not delivered as agreed; math errors; failure to post payments and other credits, such as returns; failure to send bills to the current address, provided the creditor receives the change of address, in writing, at least 20 days before the billing period ends; and charges for which an explanation or written proof of purchase along with a claimed error or request for clarification are requested. The consumer must write to the creditor at the address given for "billing inquiries," not the address for sending payments, and include one's name, address, account number, and a description of the billing error. Send the letter so that it reaches the creditor within 60 days after the first bill was mailed that contained the error. Send the letter by certified mail, return receipt requested, for proof of what the creditor received. Include copies (not originals) of sales slips or other documents that support the position. Keep a copy of the dispute letter. The creditor must acknowledge the complaint in writing within 30 days after receiving it, unless the problem has been resolved. The creditor must resolve the dispute within two billing cycles (but not more than 90 days) after receiving the letter. Payment may be withheld on the disputed amount (and related charges) during the investigation. Any part of the bill not in question must be paid including finance charges on the undisputed amount.
   The creditor may not take any legal or other action to collect the disputed amount and related charges (including finance charges) during the investigation. Although the account cannot be closed or restricted, the disputed amount may be applied against the credit limit. If the creditor's investigation determines the bill is correct, one must be told promptly and in writing how much is owed and why. Copies of relevant documents may be requested. At this point the disputed amount is owed plus any finance charges that accumulated while the amount was in dispute. The minimum amount that was missed because of the dispute may have to be paid. If the results of the investigation are disputed, the creditor may be written to within 10 days after receiving the explanation and the disputed amount may be refused. At this point the creditor may begin collection procedures. Any creditor who fails to follow the settlement procedure may not collect the amount in dispute, or any related finance charges, up to $50, even if the bill turns out to be correct. For example, if a creditor acknowledges the complaint in 45 days—15 days too late—or takes more than two billing cycles to resolve a dispute, the penalty applies. The penalty also applies if a creditor threatens to report, or improperly reports, one's failure to pay to anyone during the dispute period.

Electronic Fund Transfer Act (EFTA)

Limits consumers' liability if there has been an unauthorized use of an ATM card, debit card, or other electronic banking device.

Continued

Box 10-1   Federal Credit and Collection Laws—cont'd

Truth in Lending Act (TILA)

Applies to anyone who charges interest or agrees on payment of a bill in more than four installments, excluding a down payment. When a specific agreement is reached between patient and physician, Regulation Z of this consumer protection act requires that a written disclosure of all pertinent information be made, regardless of the existence of a finance charge (see Figure 10-7). This full disclosure must be discussed at the time the agreement is first reached between patient and physician and credit is extended. According to the Federal Trade Commission (FTC), the Truth in Lending provision is not applicable and no disclosures are necessary if a patient decides on his or her own to pay in installments or whenever convenient.

It is essential to include the following items:

1. Total amount of the debt
2. Amount of down payment
3. Finance charge
4. Interest rate expressed as an annual percentage
5. Amount of each payment
6. Date each payment is due
7. Date final payment is due
8. Signature of patient and physician with copies retained by both
9. Account balance with total interest and total amount paid by the patient at the end of the contract

Medical practices that implement late payment charges that meet the criteria defined in the TILA as a finance charge must comply with a host of requirements that revolve around proper disclosure to patients.

Charges must meet the following criteria to qualify as late payment charges:

1. The account balance must be paid in full at the time of initial billing.
2. The account is treated as delinquent when unpaid.
3. The charge is assessed to a patient's account only because of his or her failure to make timely payments.
4. Installments are limited to no more than three.
5. The creditor (physician or insurance specialist) makes a "commercially reasonable" effort to collect these accounts.

When a physician continues to treat a patient with an overdue account, the courts have viewed this as continuation of care and an extension of credit. Patients who fall into this delinquent status should be referred elsewhere. See Chapter 4 for instructions on sending a discharge letter. After the patient has paid the overdue amount, the patient can be taken back and treated on a cash-only basis.

Truth in Lending Consumer Credit Cost Disclosure

Requires businesses to disclose all direct and indirect costs and conditions related to the granting of credit. All interest charges, late charges, collection fees, finance charges, and so forth must be explained up front, before the time of service. Include the following on all statements to charge interest and bill the patient monthly:

• Amount of each payment
• Due date
• Unpaid balance at the beginning of the billing period
• Finance charges
• Date balance is due

Fair Debt Collection Practices Act (FDCPA)

Addresses the collection practices of third-party debt collectors and attorneys who regularly collect debts for others. Although this act does not apply directly to physician practices collecting for themselves, a professional health care collector must avoid the actions that are prohibited for collection agencies. The main intent of the act is to protect consumers from unfair, harassing, or deceptive collection practices. Refer to the guidelines in Box 10-2, which are taken from the FDCPA, to help avoid illegalities, enhance collections, and maintain positive patient relations. For more information about collection laws in your state, contact your state attorney general's office. The stricter law prevails if there is a conflict between state and federal laws.

Statute of Limitations

A formal regulation or law setting time limits on legal action is known as a **statute of limitations.** In regard to collections, the statute of limitations is the maximum time during which a legal collection suit may be rendered against a debtor. However, for a lawsuit to be successful, a concerted effort should be made to collect on an account from the time services are rendered. The patient should receive regular statements indicating that if the insurer does not pay, the patient will be held responsible.

Statutes vary according to the following three kinds of accounts:

1. *Open book accounts* (also called *open accounts*) are open to charges made from time to time. Payment is expected within a specific period, but credit has been extended without a formal written contract. Physicians' patient accounts are usually open book accounts.
2. *Written contract accounts* have a formal written agreement in which a patient signs to pay his or her bill in

more than four installments (see Truth in Lending Act).

3. *Single-entry accounts* have only one entry or charge, usually for a small amount.

THE COLLECTION PROCESS

For collections to be handled effectively, staff members should be trained in collection techniques. Most insurance specialists can be trained to be efficient collectors when given the correct tools. New collectors need time to gain confidence, which is an important aspect of being a good collector.

Telephone Collection Procedures

Telephone collections are made easier if the insurance billing specialist is convinced that he or she can collect before trying to convince the patient to pay. Two important factors to consider are the insurance specialist's ability to contact the patient and the patient's ability to pay the bill. The following are helpful suggestions for using the telephone to address a collection problem:

- Contact the patient in a timely manner at the first sign of payment delay. Prepare before making a telephone collection call by reviewing the account and noting anything unusual. Locate information as to where the patient is employed (or if unemployed) by reviewing the patient registration form.
- Decide what amount will be settled for if payment cannot be made in full. Make the first call count. Act in a calm, businesslike manner and combine empathy with diligence. Be positive and persuasive. Listen to what the patient has to say, even if he or she gets angry and raises his or her voice. Lower the volume of your own voice and respond in a composed manner. Try to pick up clues from what the patient is saying; he or she may be giving the real reason for nonpayment.
- Ask questions, show interest, and let the patient know that he or she is being listened to.
- Respond in a respectful manner and carefully word the reply; when patients are distressed they do not always make sense. The goal is to encourage the patient to pay, not agitate the patient.
- Use all resources and learn to negotiate.

Office Policy

Use an organized approach to determine which collection calls to make first. Print out the A/R by age and target the accounts that are in the 60- to 90-day category. The most effective results come from this group. If financial accounting record cards are used, pull all the cards with tabs or labels that indicate the patient has received two or three statements, depending on office protocol. Start with the largest amount owed and work the accounts in decreasing amounts owed. After this category has been completed, move on to the 90- to 120-day accounts. Finally, go after accounts that are more than 120 days old.

Most state collection laws allow telephone calls to the debtor between 8 AM and 9 PM. Never call between 9 PM and 8 AM because to do so may be considered harassment. However, according to collection experts, the best time to telephone is between 5:30 PM and 8:30 PM on Tuesdays and Thursdays and between 9 AM and 1 PM on Saturdays. However, regardless of when the call is made, track the times when the most patients are contacted and adjust the calling schedule accordingly. Perhaps the physician's office hours should be increased to include one evening a week or Saturday mornings to make collection calls. Another option is the use of flex time in which the employee can choose his or her own working hours from within a broad range of hours approved by management. Use a private telephone away from the busy operations of the office to eliminate interruptions. Patients may be embarrassed about not being able to pay their bills, and patient confidentiality must be maintained. Follow the guidelines stated in the Fair Debt Collection Practices Act (Box 10-2).

Be alert for new ideas or approaches to collection by watching how banks and other retailers implement sophisticated collection skills. Decide whether any of these could be used to the medical practice's advantage and present the techniques to the office manager. Keep abreast of improvements made to collection software that improve collection results and allow more collectors to work from their homes. Other advances (e.g., call block, which is an expanded telephone service) have made it more difficult to make collection calls. This service was originally intended to screen out unwanted telemarketing calls by intercepting blocked, unlisted, or unknown numbers. Standard numbers are usually allowed to go through. The key to averting a block is to make sure the number the call is being placed from is listed and within the patient's area. Telephone company services vary, so research to discover all expanded services used in your area.

For step-by-step procedures on making telephone collection calls, see Procedure 10-2 at the end of this chapter.

Telephone "Don'ts." Communication is important, especially when trying to work with a patient through difficulties in making payments. Remain professional at all times and treat the patient with respect. The following is a list of *do nots* for telephone collections:

- Do not raise your voice and antagonize the patient.
- Do not accuse the patient of dishonesty or lying.

Box 10-2   Fair Debt Collection Practices Act Guidelines

1. Contact debtors only once a day; in some states, repeated calls in 1 day or the same week could be considered harassment.
2. Place calls after 8 AM and before 9 PM.
3. Do not contact debtors on Sunday or any other day that the debtor recognizes as a Sabbath.
4. Identify yourself and the medical practice represented; do not mislead the patient.
5. Contact the debtor at work only if unable to contact the debtor elsewhere; no contact should be made if the employer or debtor disapproves.
6. Contact the attorney if an attorney represents the debtor; contact the debtor only if the attorney does not respond.
7. Do not threaten or use obscene language.
8. Do not send postcards for collection purposes; keep all correspondence strictly private.
9. Do not call collect or cause additional expense to the patient.
10. Do not leave a message on an answering machine indicating that you are calling about a bill.
11. Do not contact a third party more than once unless requested to do so by the party or the response was erroneous or incomplete.
12. Do not convey to a third party that the call is about a debt.
13. Do not contact the debtor when notified in writing that a debtor refuses to pay and would like contact to stop, except to notify the debtor in writing that there will be no further contact or that there will be legal action.
14. Stick to the facts; do not use false statements.
15. Do not prepare a list of "bad debtors" or "credit risks" to share with other health care providers.
16. Take action immediately when stating that a certain action will be taken (e.g., filing a claim in small claims court or sending the patient's case to a collection agency).
17. Send the patient written verification of the name of the creditor and the amount of debt within 5 days of the initial contact.

- Do not act like a "tough guy" or threaten a patient.
- Do not consent to partial payments until payment in full has been asked for and do not agree to a long string of small partial payments.
- Do not engage in a debate.
- Do not report a disputed account to a collection agency or bureau until the patient's dispute is disclosed as part of the record.

Telephone collection calls are effective the day before patients are due for their appointments. State the date and time of the appointment and then remind the patient of the balance owed and ask whether he or she would please bring payment to the appointment.

Telephone Collection Scenarios

The most difficult part of one-on-one collections is preparing for the many situations that may be encountered

and the various responses the patient may make. Table 10-2 shows some statements that patients make for not paying an account and examples of responses the insurance specialist can make.

Collection Letters

Collection letters are another method of reaching patients and reminding them of their debt. Knowledge of the patient base and of individual patients may help determine the effectiveness of collection letters. Every medical practice is unique, and the number of accounts, the geographic spread of patients, the staff size, and the amount of time collectors have to spend on individual accounts helps determine which collection method best suits the practice.

The positive aspect of collection letters is that they can reach a large number of patients rapidly and the cost is relatively low, especially if form letters are used (Figure 10-15).

Collection letters have some negative aspects such as the following:

- Letters usually take 2 or 3 days to reach the patient and may lie unopened for a week or more.
- Letters are one-way communication, thus lacking the ability to provide the reason for nonpayment.
- The response and recovery through letters are relatively poor.
- Manual preparation takes time (especially if a decision must be made before sending each letter).

The insurance specialist is often the one to compose collection letters and devise a plan for collection follow-up. A series of collection letters may be written using varying degrees of forcefulness, starting with a gentle reminder. When a collection letter is written, use a friendly tone and ask why payment has not been made. Imply that the patient has good intentions to pay. This may be done by suggesting that the patient has overlooked a previous statement. Communicate the doctor's sincere interest in the patient. Always invite the patient to explain the reason for nonpayment in a letter, telephone call, or office visit. It should sound as though the patient is eager to clear the debt.

When collection letters are sent toward the end of the year, include a statement letting the patient know that if the account is paid in full by the end of the year, the medical expense may be used as an income tax deduction. Another tactic is to send a notice advising the patient that he or she may skip December's payment because of increased expenses during the holidays. This tactic may be used as an opportunity to build patient relationships,

Table 10-2 | **Telephone Collection Scenarios**

STATEMENT	RESPONSE
"I can't pay anything now."	"Are you employed? Are you receiving unemployment compensation, welfare, or Social Security benefits?" You are determining the patient's ability to pay.
"I can't pay the whole bill now."	"How long will it take you to pay this bill?" Ask this question instead of "How much can you pay?"
"I can pay, but not until next month."	"When do you get paid?" Ask for payment the day after payday. "Do you have a checking account?" Ask for a postdated check.
"I have other bills."	"This is also one of your bills that should be paid now. Let's talk about exactly how you plan payment."
"How about $10 a month (on a $300 bill)?"	"I'd like to accept that, but our accountant does not allow us to stretch out payments beyond 90 days, which would be $100 a month." This adheres to (Truth in Lending Law) regulations for collecting payment in installments without a written agreement. If the patient tries to cooperate, then compromise. If not, turn the account over to a collection agency.
"I sent in the payment."	"When was the payment sent? To what address was it sent? Was it a check? On what bank was it drawn and for what amount? What is the canceled check number?" Investigate to determine whether the check was posted to a wrong account. If not, call the patient back and ask if he or she would call his or her bank to see if it cleared; if it has not, the patient should stop payment. Ask the patient to call back and verify the status of the check. If the patient is lying, he or she will not follow through. Ask for a new check and tell the patient that a refund will be made if the other one shows up.
"I cannot make a payment this month."	"The collection agency picks up all our delinquent accounts next Monday. I don't want to include yours, but I need a check today."
"The check's in the mail."	"May I have the check number and date it was mailed?" Call back in 3 days if not received.
"I'm not going to pay the bill because the doctor didn't spend any time with me."	"May I confirm the doctor you saw, the date, and time? For what reason did you see the doctor? Do you still have the problem for which you saw the doctor?" Get as much information as possible and research the office schedule the day the patient was seen. Let the doctor know about the patient's complaint and inquire how he or she would like to handle the complaint.
"I thought the insurance company was paying this."	"Your insurance paid most of the bill; now the balance is your responsibility. Please send your check before Friday to keep your account current." Explain why (deductible, copayment benefit) the service is not covered under the insurance plan.

but the collector must be firm and clear when offering such leeway. Collection letters sent after the first of the year can suggest that the patient clear the debt by using an income tax refund check.

Types of Collection Letters

A form letter saves time and can go out automatically at specific times during the billing cycle (see Figure 10-15). Letters with checklists are a type of form letter (Figure 10-16) that makes it easier for the patient to choose a payment option. Personally typed letters can be individualized to suit any situation. Collection letters should contain the following information:

- Full amount owed
- Services performed
- What action the patient should take
- Time frame in which the patient should respond
- How the patient should take care of the bill
- Why the patient should take care of the bill

- Address to which patients send payment
- Telephone number to contact the office
- Contact person's name
- Signature, which can be listed as "Financial Secretary," "Insurance Specialist," "Assistant to Doctor _____," or one's name and title with the physician's name below

When pursuing collection, the insurance specialist should stay within the authorization of the physician. All letters should be noted on the back of the financial accounting record, in the collection log, or in the computer comment area. Abbreviations can be used to indicate which letter was sent (Table 10-3), as well as the date the letter was mailed. Letters can be sent in brightly colored envelopes to attract attention. The envelope should include "Address Service Requested" or "Forwarding Service Requested" on the outside to ensure the letter is forwarded if the patient has moved so that the office will be notified of the patient's new address. Always include a self-addressed stamped envelope.

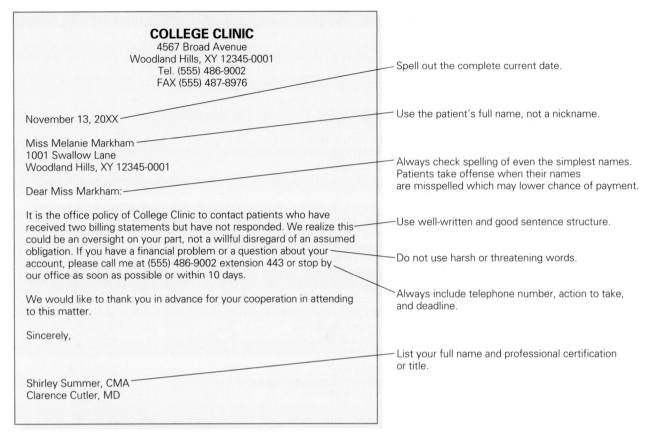

COLLEGE CLINIC
4567 Broad Avenue
Woodland Hills, XY 12345-0001
Tel. (555) 486-9002
FAX (555) 487-8976

— Spell out the complete current date.

November 13, 20XX

— Use the patient's full name, not a nickname.

Miss Melanie Markham
1001 Swallow Lane
Woodland Hills, XY 12345-0001

— Always check spelling of even the simplest names. Patients take offense when their names are misspelled which may lower chance of payment.

Dear Miss Markham:

It is the office policy of College Clinic to contact patients who have received two billing statements but have not responded. We realize this could be an oversight on your part, not a willful disregard of an assumed obligation. If you have a financial problem or a question about your account, please call me at (555) 486-9002 extension 443 or stop by our office as soon as possible or within 10 days.

— Use well-written and good sentence structure.

— Do not use harsh or threatening words.

— Always include telephone number, action to take, and deadline.

We would like to thank you in advance for your cooperation in attending to this matter.

Sincerely,

— List your full name and professional certification or title.

Shirley Summer, CMA
Clarence Cutler, MD

FIGURE 10-15 Collection form letter sent to all patients who have not responded after two billing cycles.

Collection Abbreviations

Collection abbreviations can be used to save time and space while documenting efforts to collect and patients' responses. A few of the most common abbreviations are listed in Table 10-3. Always use standard abbreviations so that anyone working on the account will know exactly what attempts have been made to collect and what action has been taken.

Insurance Collection

Most patients carry some form of insurance; however, filing an insurance claim is only the first step in collecting fees owed. Good follow-up techniques (see Chapter 9) are necessary to ensure payment from the third-party payer and copayment or coinsurance payment from the patient.

First, affirm that a clean insurance claim was sent with all necessary precertification, preauthorization, and documentation for services. Next, follow up in a timely manner with telephone calls and written tracers. Track all denials to learn what services are being denied and which insurance companies are denying payment. It is worth investing money and staff resources to identify the cause of claim denials. Send all high-dollar claims by certified mail to alleviate the problem of the third-party payer saying that "it was never received." This saves time and is cost effective.

History of Accounts

If the third-party payer seems to be ignoring all efforts to trace the claim, an exact history of the account may be the best weapon with which to proceed. A history of the account is a chronologic record of all events that have occurred. Keep all communications received from the third-party payer, note all telephone calls, and keep copies of all documents sent. Send a copy of the history of the account directly to the third-party payer and demand a reply. This may also be done in the case of an insurance company dispute or a refusal to pay.

Coinsurance Payments

Use a letter or statement to collect from patients who have insurance coverage. Clearly indicate to the patient that the insurance biller has submitted an insurance claim and advise the patient what action is expected. The status of the insurance claim should be noted on all statements. Notify patients promptly when insurance payment has been received. Ask patients to get involved in the

COLLEGE CLINIC
4567 Broad Avenue
Woodland Hills, XY 12345-0001
Tel. (555) 486-9002
FAX (555) 487-8976

March 16, 20XX

Mr. Frank Lincoln
3397 Westminster Avenue
Woodland Hills, XY 12345-0001

Account No.   593287
Amount Due: $ _____

Dear Mr. Lincoln:

The care of our patients is more important than writing letters about overdue accounts. Yet, as you must realize, the expense of furnishing care can only be met by payments from appreciative patients.

Your account is seriously past due and has been removed from our current files because of its delinquent status. Our office policy indicates that your account should be placed with a collection agency. However, we would prefer to hear from you regarding your preference in this matter.

Enclosed is a current statement of your account. Please indicate your payment choice.

☐ I would prefer to settle this account immediately. Please find payment in full enclosed.

☐ I would prefer to make monthly payments (up to six months). To exercise this option please call and make arrangements to come into our office to sign a financial agreement.

☐ Please charge the full amount to my credit card. (We accept American Express, MasterCard, and Visa). To exercise this option, please telephone our office or fill in the enclosed form and return it with the envelope provided.

_____   _____
Signature   Date

Please select one of the three options above, sign the form, and return this notice within 10 days from the date indicated in the letter. A postmarked return envelope is provided. Failure to respond will result in an automatic referral to our collection agency. Please do not hesitate to call if you have any questions regarding this matter.

Sincerely,

Gil Steinberg
Office Manager

Enc. Envelope, Credit Card Agreement Form

FIGURE 10-16 Multipurpose collection letter with checklist. This advises the patient of a seriously past due account, offers the patient three payment options, and warns the patient that failure to respond will result in a referral to a collection agency.

insurance process or to pay the bill within 10 days if a problem exists. Following are examples of notations on statements for patients with insurance coverage:

- "We have received payment from your insurance company. The balance of $_____ is now your responsibility."
- "Your insurance company has paid its share of your bill. This statement is for the amount payable directly by you."
- "Your insurance company has paid $_____ for the above services. The remaining portion of $_____ is now your responsibility."
- "The balance of this account is your share of the cost. Please remit today. For questions, call 486-9002."
- "Your insurance company has not responded. The account is due and payable. Please contact your insurance company about payment. Thank you for your assistance."

Table 10-3	**Collection Abbreviations**		
Atty	Attorney	NSN	No such number
B	Bankrupt	OFC	Office
Bal	Balance	OOT	Out of town
Bk*	Bank	OOW	Out of work
BLG	Belligerent	PA	Payment arrangement
BTTR	Best time to reach	PH or PH'D	Phoned
CB	Call back	Ph/Dsc*	Phone disconnected
CLM	Claim	PIF	Payment in full
DA*	Directory assistance	PIM	Payment in mail
DFB	Demand for balance	PMT	Payment
DNK	Did not know	POE	Place of employment
DSC	Disconnected	POLK†	Polk directory
EMP	Employment	POW	Payment on way
EOM	End of month	PP	Promise to pay or partial payment
EOW	End of week	PT	Patient
FA	Further action	RCD	Received
FN	Final notice	R/D*	Reverse directory
H	He (or husband)	RE	About
HHCO	Have husband call office	RES	Residence
HSB	Husband	S	She (or wife)
HTO	He telephoned office	SEP	Separated
HU	Hung up	SK*	Skip or skipped
INS	Insurance	SOS	Same old story
L1, L2	Letter one, letter two (sent)	SP/DEL*	Special delivery
LB	Line busy	STO	She telephoned office
LD	Long distance	T	Telephoned
LM	Left message	TB	Telephoned business
LMCO	Left message, call office	TR	Telephoned residence
LMVM	Left message, voice mail	TT	Talked to
LTR	Letter	TTA	Turned to agency
MR	Mail return	UE	Unemployed
N1, N2	Note one, note two (sent)	U/Emp	Unemployed
NA	No answer	UTC	Unable to contact
N/B*	Nearby or neighbors (no phone listing)	VFD	Verified
NFA*	No forwarding address	Vfd/E	Verified employment
NHD*	Never heard of debtor	Vfd/I	Verified insurance
NI	Not in	W/	Will
NLE	No longer employed	WCO	Will call office
NPL	No phone listed	WCIO	Will come in office
NPN	Nonpublished number	W/I	Walk-in
NR	No record	WVO	Will visit office
NSF	Nonsufficient funds	X	By

*Used in skip tracing.
†Directories used to locate patients by street address or telephone number.

Insurance Checks Sent to Patients

Send a letter immediately to notify patients who receive insurance checks (see Chapter 9). Advise such patients that they have received payment from their insurance company and that their account is due and payable within 10 days. Do not send continuous monthly bills; instead speed up the collection process. If the patient refuses to pay and the physician does not want the patient to return, send a 10-day notification advising the patient that the account will go to a collection agency. If there is no response, ask the physician whether he or she wishes to discharge the patient from the practice.

Managed Care Organizations

When a medical practice deals with several managed care organizations, trying to remember all the contract information can be confusing. A managed care desk reference (see Chapter 11) can help staff members find information quickly. "Promised payment date" along with all the other information on the desk reference grid or matrix can be easily referred to by the insurance specialist when trying to collect from managed care organizations.

Make sure all referral authorizations are in place before the patient is to be seen. If a patient shows up without a referral, offer to reschedule or inform the patient that the visit must be paid for in cash before leaving the office. If the patient has no money, a promissory note may be executed, but this action is not preferred and would be carried out as a last option.

When dealing with managed care contracts, do not sign any contract that holds a third party "harmless." The "hold harmless" clause is a way for one party to shift financial responsibilities to another party. Such "hold harmless" clauses often include phrases that state that the third party is "held harmless" to pay claims, liabilities, costs, expenses, judgments, or damages awarded by any court to all patients who bring any legal action against the medical practice. If the third party goes out of business or goes bankrupt before the contract is honored, the physician cannot collect any money from the patient that the third party was to have paid. To avoid such possibilities, make sure payments from all managed care organizations are current.

Check to see that all third-party payers are insured by a federal agency. Such insurance would pay the physician in the event the managed care organization could not. Managed care bankruptcy is discussed in Chapter 11.

Medicare

A provider must make genuine collection efforts to collect the unpaid deductible and coinsurance amounts from all Medicare patients. Reasonable efforts must include subsequent billings, telephone calls, and in-person collection efforts done in the same manner as with all patients. Accounts may not be written off until sequential statements (spaced 15 to 30 days apart) have been sent with an increasing intensity in the collection message. A telephone call should be placed to the debtor asking for payment; a request for payment should be made when the patient is seen in person as well.

Medigap Insurance

When a patient has Medigap insurance, make sure the patient's signature appears in Block 13 of the CMS-1500 (08-05) insurance claim form. Do not routinely enter "signature on file" unless the insured has signed an insurance-specific statement authorizing assignment of benefits to the physician named on the claim form. A signed statement allowing the physician to bill for and receive payment for Medigap-covered services until the beneficiary revokes authorization is preferred. A Medicare "signature on file" is not sufficient.

Workers' Compensation

Verify the validity of work-related injury and illness through the patient's employer and obtain accurate billing information. Send timely bills and reports using the correct coding system and fee schedule. Always keep the adjuster assigned to the case informed of ongoing treatment. The patient and employer should both be notified if a problem exists. Document all correspondence including telephone authorizations for treatment and any tracing efforts. Any disputed or unresolved workers' compensation cases may be revised to self-pay or be referred to a financial service representative or the proper state-level authority. The physician may file for mediation on behalf of the patient if proper authorization was obtained and a claim form sent at the time of the patient's treatment. A claim may also be filed with the state labor board naming the patient's employer and workers' compensation carrier whenever there is difficulty getting full payment. The industrial board has the employer pressure the carrier to resolve the matter. If an insurance company has not paid or has sent a written notice of nonpayment, the provider may file a request for default judgment from the state authority. If the judgment is in the provider's favor, the payer is ordered to pay in full. See Chapter 15 for more information on delinquent workers' compensation claims.

Suing a Third-Party Payer

As stated in the section on Statute of Limitations, there are time periods during which an insured person may sue the insurance company to collect the amount the claimant believes is owed. An insured person may not initiate a legal action against the insurer until 60 days after the initial claim has been submitted. A lawsuit against the insurer must be filed within 3 years of the date the initial claim was submitted for payment.

When the insurance company does not respond to reason or negotiation after the physician's office has tried to collect from an insurance plan, the only alternatives are surrender or litigation. A lawsuit may be worthwhile if a high-dollar claim is in question. Third-party payers may be sued for payment under two circumstances: claim for plan benefits or breach of contract and claim for damages.

Claim for plan benefits is used when the claim is governed by the Employee Retirement Income Security Act (ERISA), a Federal Employee Health Benefit Act (FEHBA). ERISA governs health insurance that is provided as a benefit of employment. FEHBA governs all health insurance provided as a benefit to federal employees. An insured person is entitled to appeal a denied claim under these two federal laws. A timely request must be filed to sue for payment. The time limit for ERISA is within 60 days of denial; the time limit for FEHBA is within 6 months. Federal laws apply across the country and overrule all state laws. Suits based on claims for plan benefits may be made when denial is based on the following:

- Medical necessity
- Preexisting condition
- Usual and customary rate issues
- Providers or facilities that are not covered
- Services that fall within an exclusion to coverage
- Failure to offer Consolidated Omnibus Budget Reconciliation Act (COBRA) coverage by a plan administrator

When the claim falls outside of the scope of these federal laws, it is possible to sue if the conduct of the payer constitutes a violation of state laws relating to unfair insurance practices.

Suing based on claim for damages falls entirely under state law. This is most likely to occur if the patient has no plan benefit but the patient or physician's office is led to believe so by the insurer or plan administrator. Examples may include the following:

- Insurer misquoting benefits during a verification of those benefits
- Denial of payment because of lack of medical necessity when preauthorization of treatment was obtained

Collection Agencies

Delinquent accounts should be turned over to a collection agency only after all reasonable attempts have been made to collect by the physician's office. Knowing when to turn accounts over helps determine the success of the collection agency. The longer the unpaid balance remains in the physician's office, the less chance the agency has to collect the account, so the determination that an account is uncollectable should be made quickly. Some guidelines follow:

- When a patient states that he or she will not pay or there is a denial of responsibility
- When a patient breaks a promise to pay
- When a patient makes partial payments and 60 days have lapsed without payment
- When a patient fails to respond to the physician's letters or telephone calls
- When payment terms fail for no valid reason
- When a check is returned by the bank because of NSF and the patient does not make an effort to rectify the situation within 1 week of notification
- When delinquency coexists with marital problems, divorce proceedings, or child support agreements

- When a patient is paid by the insurance company and does not forward the payment to the physician (this constitutes fraud and may be pursued with legal action)
- When a patient gives false information
- When a patient moves and the office has used all resources to locate the patient

Not all accounts should go to a collection agency. Such accounts include those of personal friends, elderly widows or widowers living on pensions, and accounts with balances under $25. Many physicians prefer to adjust small bad debts off of the books rather than increase administrative costs. All disputed accounts should be reviewed and approved by the physician before they are sent to collection. There should be a systematized approach for turning accounts over to a collection agency that still allows room for exceptions.

Choosing an Agency

A collection agency should be chosen with great care because it is a reflection of the medical practice. Choose a reputable agency that is considerate and efficient with a high standard of ethics. The agency should specialize in physician accounts and have an attitude toward debtors with which the physician agrees. Find out how long the agency has been in business and request a list of at least 10 references and statistics on their collection effectiveness. The average collection rate varies greatly but falls between 20% and 60% on assigned accounts. Be sure the report rate includes all accounts more than 1 year old and does not exclude accounts with small balances.

An agency's performance can be evaluated by the amount collected, less the agency's fees, which is called the **netback.** For instance, if a collector recovered 25% of $5000 ($1250) and takes a 50% commission, the physician's netback is $625. If a different collector recovered 25% of the $5000 ($1250) and charged a 30% commission, the netback is $375. Although the second agency collected less, its lower commission afforded the physician more money.

When choosing a collection agency, make sure (1) to set up a separate post office box or lock box for the collection project; (2) to set up a separate bank account for the collection project; (3) that the contract stipulates that all correspondence be sent to the post office box (no correspondence is to be sent to the collection agency's physical or payment address); (4) that all e-checks and credit card receipts are deposited into the physician's bank account; and (5) that under no circumstance is the collection agency to receive any payments.

If money goes to the collection agency (whether insured, bonded, registered, or licensed), there is nothing to stop the collection agency from stealing the physician's money. The collection agency also could have a hidden lawsuit against it or an income tax lien, and the physician may lose all of his or her money if the money goes to the agency's bank account. Do not put "hold harmless" clauses in contracts. Hold the collection agency responsible for its actions. Many states do not regulate collection agencies and simply require that collection agencies be registered. In addition to checking references, check with the state's Department of Corporations to determine whose name is on the collection agency's registration, if the tax identification number is correct and current, and if the address listed is different than the one the agency gave. Contact the circuit court to determine whether there are any lawsuits or judgments against the collection agency. Find out how many of the collection agency's employees will be assigned to the account, then monitor them once the contract is signed. They may have the best credentials and references and belong to all the correct organizations, but if they acquire an increasing number of accounts and the amount of recoupment remains constant each month or is less than the national average, they may be picking and choosing the accounts. This is especially true when they are overanxious to receive a new file. If this happens, consider looking for another collection agency. Make sure an account can be recalled without a penalty. The patient may have coverage with a carrier already contracted with, so find out if the collection agency has the ability to resend a claim or if the billing company or office staff handles this. If so, does the contract have provisions for this, and does the collection agency receive recoupment for obtaining insurance information?

The biggest key to the agency's effectiveness is the doctor's own credit and collection policy. A comprehensive patient registration form, along with verifying employment, turning accounts over quickly when they qualify, and giving the agency all the available information, helps the agency pick up the paper trail and secure payment. A good collection agency has membership in a national collection society and the approval of the local medical society. Review the agency's financial statement and make sure the agency is licensed, bonded, and carries "hold harmless clause" insurance. If a patient should sue because of harassment, this insurance will protect the physician from being sued as well. The local bar association and state licensing bureaus can be contacted to determine whether any complaints have been lodged against the agency or law firm. Find out if the agency reports uncollectable debtors ("deadbeats") to a credit bureau and investigate which one is used.

Types of Agencies

There are local, regional, and national agencies. National agencies and ones that use the Internet may have better results tracing skips (patients who owe balances on their accounts and move without leaving a forwarding address). Local agencies are more aware of the socioeconomic status of patients. Some agencies pay their staff commissions and bonuses for high productivity, and others are low key and more customer oriented. Find out the experience level of the staff and make sure the agency values the physician's business.

Another option is to use a collection service, such as CollectNet, which gives small and midsized facilities with limited budgets the collection capabilities of large collection systems by connecting to databases. The medical practice is able to make calling lists, print collection letters, search for telephone numbers and addresses, access patient credit reports, write and format reports, monitor collection progress, and set automatic callback reminders. Optional features include BankruptcyNet, SkipNet, LetterNet, and BureauNet. Collection agencies use this service, but it is also available to large groups and clinics.

Agency Operating Techniques

Collection agencies must follow all the laws stated in the Fair Debt Collection Practices Act. They may not "harass" the debtor or make false threats, and they may not use letters that appear to be legal documents. A provision should be included for the agency to seek permission from the physician's office before suing a debtor in municipal court and charging a percent of the judgment. A progress report should be provided to the physician's office on a regular basis at least monthly. The agency also should return any uncollectable accounts to the physician's office within a reasonable time and not charge for these accounts. If a debtor moves, ask if the account is forwarded to another collection office. All procedures used to make collections should be shown to the physician's office, including collection letters and telephone script. The physician's office should be aware if the agency uses a personalized or standard approach. A personal visit to the premises of the collection agency can provide a first-hand view of its operating techniques.

Agency Charges

Agencies may be paid a flat rate on all accounts according to volume. Some agencies may leave the accounts in the control of the physician's office where the staff speaks with the patient and posts all delinquent incoming monies. Other agencies charge a commission on the basis of a percentage of an account, and the physician's office refers all calls to the agency once the account is turned over to it. A standard rate for most agencies to break even is one-third of all monies collected, and an average rate charged is 50%. Make sure the commission is based on how much is collected on the overdue accounts and not the total amount of overdue accounts turned over to the agency.

Agency Assigned Accounts

Patients' accounts turned over to a collection agency should have a letter of withdrawal sent by certified mail (see Figure 4-21). Place a note on all financial accounting records indicating the date the account was assigned. Once an account has been given to a collection agency, it is illegal to send the patient a monthly statement. Financial management consultants usually recommend that the patient's balances be written off the A/R at the time the account is assigned. A portion of the account balance can be written back on if and when the agency collects on the debt. Accounts also should be listed in a separate journal to help track the effectiveness of the agency. Allow enough columns to show the future date, amount, and percentage of an account collected by the agency, as well as the total account balance.

Flag or insert a full sheet of brightly colored paper in the patient's chart noting the date the account was assigned to collection. This will alert all medical staff of the situation if the patient calls on short notice or walks in to be seen. If the patient sends payment to the physician's office after the account has been turned over to an agency, notify the collection agency immediately. Any calls about accounts that have gone to collection should be referred to the agency.

Credit Bureaus

Collection agencies also can offer the services of a credit bureau. Credit bureaus gather credit information from many sources and make it available for a fee to members of a credit bureau service. Credit reports can be issued on new patients, enabling the physician's office to verify credit. The information may consist of the patient's residence and moving habits (a measure of permanency), number of dependents, verification of employment and approximate salary, the patient's payment history on other merchant accounts, and any history of bankruptcy or use of an alias. This report can be obtained over the telephone or provided in written form.

The Fair Credit Reporting Act (FCRA) of 1970 allows a person to see and correct his or her credit report. The credit report can be checked for negative credit information, disputed information, mistakes, and out-of-date information. If credit is denied in whole or in part on the basis of an adverse credit report, a letter should be sent advising the patient of the name and address of the agency and stating that credit has been denied because credit requirements have not been met. The insurance specialist need not reveal data or specify the exact nature of the information obtained from the credit bureau but must name the bureau. A copy of the letter should be kept in the patient's file.

Credit Counseling

A consumer credit counseling service is a nonprofit agency that assists people in paying off their debts. The insurance specialist may have to refer patients for this service if continued medical care is being provided and the patient becomes overwhelmed by the cost. The patient may also contact his or her own bank or credit union, which may provide counseling at no charge. Care must be given with such referrals; use only legitimate agencies and warn patients that many private commercial debt consolidators may charge high fees. Dissatisfied patients may blame the physician or the insurance specialist if satisfactory financial arrangements are not made.

A patient seeking medical care who is unable to pay for services and is ineligible for state aid should be directed to the local hospital that services recipients under the Hill-Burton Act of 1946. These hospitals obtained federal construction grants to enlarge their facilities in exchange for their provision of health care for needy patients. The Department of Health and Human Services will furnish the names of local hospitals that participate in this service. Patients must complete financial applications to determine eligibility before care is rendered.

Small Claims Court

Small claims court is a part of our legal system that allows lay people access to a court system without the use of an attorney. Some advantages are a modest filing fee, minimal paperwork, exclusion of costly lawyers, and a short time frame from filing the action to trial date. Incorporated physicians are usually represented by an attorney, and the agency must file in a municipal or justice court if an account has already been sent to a collection agency.

Most states have small claims courts (also called *conciliation courts*, *common pleas*, *general sessions*, *justice courts*, or *people's courts*). Each state has monetary limits on the amount that can be handled in small claims court, and accounts should be reviewed for eligibility. The dollar amount varies from state to state and sometimes from one county to another. The national median small claims jurisdiction is $5300. Several legislative bills being considered by United States (US) Senate and House committees address raising the dollar limit. Several states have already had such bills signed into law. The new limits in these states vary from $3000 to $25,000. There may also be limits on the number of claims filed per year that are more than a specific dollar amount.

When filing a claim, the person filing the petition (the physician's office) is referred to as the *plaintiff* and the party being brought to suit (the patient) is called the *defendant.* It is generally recommended that the plaintiff send a written demand to the defendant before filing a lawsuit to give the defendant a last opportunity to resolve the claim.

For step-by-step procedures on filing a claim, see Procedure 10-4 at the end of this chapter.

After filing a claim, a trial date will be set, and both plaintiff and defendant will be ordered to appear before the judge. Often a postcard is sent notifying the plaintiff when the defendant has been served. If the amount of delinquent debt is more than the monetary limit for the small claims court, consider "cutting the claim to fit" the limit. For example, if the amount of debt is $2757 and the state limit is $2500, consider waiving (giving up) the $257 (difference) to bring the amount down to the limit. The claim cannot be divided into two different suits of $1378.50, and one cannot sue twice on the same claim.

Claim Resolutions

The defendant has the following four options after he or she is served:

1. Pay the claim. The court clerk will receive the money and forward it to the physician's office, but the filing fee or service charges will not be refunded.
2. Ignore the claim. The judge may ask the physician's representative to state the physician's side, but the physician will win by default and the judgment will be awarded in the physician's favor, usually including court costs.
3. Answer the petition. A contested court hearing will be held. The plaintiff (physician) has the burden of proving his or her claim to the court. A counterclaim may be filed by the patient at this time.
4. Demand a jury trial. The case will be taken out of small claims court and the physician will be notified by the county clerk to file a formal complaint in a higher court. An attorney must represent the physician if this occurs.

Trial Preparation

The plaintiff and defendant must both appear on the trial date or the claim will be dismissed and cannot be refiled.

Instead of attending the trial in person, the doctor may send a representative such as his or her assistant or bookkeeper. If the claim is settled before trial, a dismissal form should be dated, signed, and filed with the clerk.

Preparation for the trial is essential and can mean the difference between success and failure. Decide what the judge should hear to conclude in the physician's favor. Although one cannot be represented in court by a lawyer, a lawyer can be asked for advice before going to court. Recommendations to help prepare for trial are as follows:

1. Be on time; otherwise, the court may give a judgment in the defendant's favor.
2. Be ready to submit the basic data required by the court: the physician's name, address, and telephone number; the patient's name and address; the delinquent amount being claimed; and a brief summary of the claim.
3. Show all dates of service and amounts owed, the date the physician's bill was due (if a series of treatments is involved), the date of the last visit, the date of the last payment (if any payment was made), and the amount still unpaid.
4. Include all attempts to collect the debt and organize all exhibits in chronologic order. Include documentation such as copies of statements, letters, notes, receipts, contracts, dishonored checks, telephone calls, other discussions with the patient, and other evidence to present to the court. A timeline showing the sequence of events may be useful.
5. Speak slowly and clearly, present the case in a concise manner, and use a business-like approach. Answer all questions accurately but briefly.
6. Present a witness if live testimony is relevant. A notarized statement from a witness is admissible but not as effective.
7. Try to anticipate the opposing party's evidence and arguments so that a rebuttal may be prepared. Keep in mind that a third party will be making the decision.

The judge will question the physician or representative and the patient, review the evidence, and then make a ruling. Winning the case gives the physician the right to attach a debtor's bank assets, salary, car, personal assets, or real property. The small claims office can show the assistant how to execute a judgment. Judgments are usually effective for many years. There is a small charge if the physician decides to execute against the patient's assets, but the charge is recoverable from the defendant.

A losing defendant may appeal and request a new trial in superior court. The defendant may ask the judge to make small installment payments, but not all judges order this alternative. If the defendant fails to pay, a writ of execution may be obtained from the clerk's office to enforce judgment. This writ of execution permits the marshal to obtain funds from a losing party's bank account or take items of the losing party's property to satisfy the judgment.

Federal Wage Garnishment Laws

Federal wage garnishment laws provide a limit on the amount of employee earnings withheld in a work week or pay period when a debtor's future wage is seized to pay off a debt. It also protects the employee from being dismissed if his or her pay is garnished for only one debt regardless of the number of levies that must be made to collect. This law is enforced by the compliance officers of the Wage and Hour Office of the US Department of Labor. The law does not apply to federal government employees, court-ordered support of any person, court orders in personal bankruptcy cases, or state or federal tax levies. The patient's employer becomes involved as the "trustee" because the employer owes money to the debtor for wages earned.

Once a **garnishment** has been ordered by the court, an employer has to honor it by satisfying the terms of garnishment before wages can be paid to the debtor. Only a percentage of the wage (usually 25%) is garnished and paid to the creditor. This amount is determined from the employee's disposable earnings. Disposable earnings are the amount left after Social Security and federal, state, and local taxes are deducted. The statute resulting in the smaller garnishment applies when state garnishment laws conflict with federal laws. This method of collection should be considered a last resort for the medical office and used only with large bills.

Tracing a Skip

A patient who owes a balance on his or her account and moves but leaves no forwarding address is called a **skip.** In these cases, an unopened envelope is returned to the office marked "Returned to Sender, Addressee Unknown." Place the words "Forwarding Service Requested" below the doctor's return address on the envelope, and the post office will make a search and forward the mail to the new address. The physician's office will be informed of this new address for a nominal fee. Complete a Freedom of Information Act form at the post office if the address is a rural delivery box number, and the US Postal Service will provide the physical location of a person's residence. When patients send payments by mail, precautions must be taken to avoid discarding envelopes with a change of address. Always match the address on the envelope, along with the check, against the patient's account. One staff person should have the responsibility of updating all patients' addresses in all locations to prevent this problem.

Skip Tracing Techniques

Once it is determined that a patient is a skip, tracing should begin immediately. Office policies should be established stating how the skip should be traced, whether he or she is to be traced in the office, or at what point the account should be sent to a collection agency. Some offices choose to make only one attempt, whereas others prefer to do most of the detective work themselves. Box 10-3 lists techniques that can be used to initiate the search for the debtor.

Box 10-3 Search Techniques Used to Trace a Debtor

1. Cross-check the address on the returned envelope with the patient registration form and account to ensure it was mailed correctly.
2. Check the ZIP code directory to determine whether the ZIP code corresponds with the patient's street address or post office box.
3. File a request with the local post office to obtain a new or corrected address.
4. Look in the local telephone directory. Call people with names that are spelled the same. Check directory assistance for a new or current listing.
5. Call the primary care physician for updated information when investigating for a physician specialist or any referring practice.
6. Determine whether the patient has been seen at the hospital; if so, speak to someone in the accounts department.
7. Inquire at the patient's place of employment. If the patient is no longer employed, ask to speak to the personnel department in an effort to locate the patient. Do not divulge the reason for the call.
8. Contact persons listed on the patient registration form including personal referrals.
9. Request information from the Department of Motor Vehicles if a driver's license number is available.
10. Obtain information from street directories, city directories, and cross-index directories (available at many public libraries) for a new address or the names and telephone numbers of neighbors, relatives, or landlords.
11. Telephone the local moving company or moving rental service and ask for the patient's new address.
12. Request information from utility companies.
13. Inquire at the patient's bank to determine whether he or she is still a customer.
14. Obtain the services of a local credit bureau to check reports and receive notification if the patient's Social Security number shows up under a different name or at a new address.
15. Contact the Board of Education when the patient has children or is a student to find out the patient's school district and the school closest to his or her former residence. Request a forwarding address.
16. Call the police department if it is suspected that the patient may have a criminal record.
17. Check public records such as tax records, voter registration, court records, death and probate records, hunting and fishing licenses, and marriage licenses.

Never state one's business with the patient when trying to make any of these contacts. Keep all information confidential. A good skip tracer must be patient and have the ability to pursue all necessary steps with tenacity and tact. A good imagination, a detective's instincts, and the ability to get along with people help in this tedious job.

Skip Tracing Services

There are several outside services from which to choose. Some agencies offer customized service with several levels of skip tracing available. Each level is more extensive and costly. The physician's office decides at which level it would like the search conducted. The first level usually involves verifying the patient's information and checking for typographical errors. The highest level uses every resource available to find the patient. The age of the account, the account balance, and the cost of the level of skip tracing service are all considerations when deciding which level to choose. A collection agency or credit bureau (as mentioned) may offer the services of skip tracing as well.

Search via Computer

Another method of skip tracing is to use electronic databases or online services. "Information wholesalers" also exist. They cater to bill collectors and similar interested parties. Currently there are a number of bills pending in Congress aimed at restricting the flow of personal data in cyberspace. Perhaps in the future this information will not be so easy to obtain; however, conducting a successful electronic search is relatively easy at present. Following are several methods used to search electronic databases to locate a debtor's address and home telephone number.

- *Surname scan* can be done locally, regionally, or nationally using data banks that have been compiled from public source documents.
- *Address search* provides property search and any change of address from all suppliers of data to the database, including the US Postal Service. Names of other adults in the household who may have the debtor's telephone number listed under their name may be included.
- *Electronic directory* allows access to the regional telephone operating company's screen of information.
- *Credit holder search* is used to establish occupation.
- *Phone number search* permits access to the names of other adults within the same household who have a telephone number.
- *Neighbor search* displays the names, addresses, and telephone numbers of the debtor's former neighbors.
- *ZIP code search* provides the names, addresses, and telephone numbers of everyone within that ZIP code who has the same last name as the debtor.

- *City search* locates everyone with the same last and first name within a given city, as well as all people who live in that city.
- *State search* finds all people with the same last name or same last and first name within the state and lists their addresses and telephone numbers.
- *National search* operates the same way as the state search. It is recommended for people with unusual last names.
- *Business search* lists all the names of the businesses in the neighborhood of the patient's last known residence. This search may help find where the patient has relocated or verify the patient's place of employment.

Refer to the Internet Resources at the end of the chapter for active links using the Evolve website. Explore several directories to cross-check results because data change frequently. Information is not secure when using the Internet. The patient's right to privacy must never be violated.

Special Collection Issues
Bankruptcy

Bankruptcy laws are federal laws applicable in all states that ensure equal distribution of the assets of an individual among the individual's creditors. There are two kinds of bankruptcy petitions: voluntary and involuntary. A voluntary petition is one filed by a person asking for relief under the Bankruptcy Reform Act (the Code). An involuntary petition is one filed against a person by his or her creditors requesting that a person obtain relief under the Code.

When a patient files for bankruptcy, he or she becomes a ward of the court and has its protection. The patient is granted an **automatic stay** against creditors, which means that the physician may contact patients only for the name, address, and telephone number of their attorney. The insurance specialist should no longer send statements, make telephone calls, or attempt to collect the account. A creditor can be fined for contempt of court if he or she continues to proceed against the debtor. If a collection agency has the account and has been notified of the bankruptcy, the situation is the same as if the physician has been notified. If the physician is notified first, the collection agency should be called and informed of the fact. Notification of bankruptcy does not have to be in writing; verbal communication is valid (e.g., if a patient telephones the doctor's office to inform him or her of the bankruptcy). Bankruptcy remains part of the debtor's permanent credit record for 10 years.

After a patient informs the physician's office of the bankruptcy, determine what type of bankruptcy the debtor has filed. Refer to Box 10-4 for a listing of the five types of bankruptcy cases.

Bankruptcy Rules. Under the bankruptcy rules effective October 17, 2005, debtors have to meet an income test and must have insufficient assets to be

---

Box 10-4   Types of Bankruptcy Cases

Chapter 7 Case

This is sometimes called a *straight petition in bankruptcy* or *absolute bankruptcy*. In this case, all of the **nonexempt assets** of the bankrupt person are liquidated and are distributed according to the law to the creditors. Secured creditors are first in line for payment of all **secured debt.** Unsecured creditors are last. A person declares those to whom he or she owes money and is not required to make payment, thus eliminating all of the debtor's outstanding legal obligations for **unsecured debt.** Most medical bills are considered unsecured debt because they are not backed by any form of **collateral**. The only debt that is discharged in Chapter 7 bankruptcy is the debt that had been incurred up to the point of filing for protection under Chapter 7. So, if a patient files before services are rendered, the bankruptcy laws do not apply for the treatment provided. A Chapter 7 bankruptcy does not necessarily result in the discharge of all debts. If the patient lies about his or her financial status, the debt may not be dischargeable. If the debt incurred was for a luxury service (e.g., facelift), immediately preceding the filing, it is possible that it may not be discharged. Consult the practice's attorney before adjusting the debt off the books in such a situation. All creditors are notified by the Administrator in Bankruptcy as to the proceedings and may choose either to attend the proceedings or make a claim against whatever assets remain.

Chapter 9 Case

This case is used for reorganization proceedings when a city or town is insolvent or unable to meet its debts. A plan is put into effect to adjust such debts.

Chapter 11 Case

This case is used for reorganization of a business enterprise when the company is unable to meet its debts but would like to continue business and would be unable to do so if creditors took away its assets. A plan of arrangement is confirmed by the court, and each class of creditor must accept the plan or receive at least that which it would receive on liquidation of the company.

Chapter 12 Case

This case is used for reorganization when a farmer is unable to meet his or her debts.

Chapter 13 Case

This is sometimes called a *wage earner's bankruptcy.* It is designed to protect the wage earner from creditors while allowing the wage earner to make arrangements to repay a portion of his or her bills (about 70%) over a 3- or 5-year period. The debtor pays a fixed amount agreed on by the court to the trustee in bankruptcy. A claim needs to be filed as directed by the debtor's attorney.

---

eligible for filing a Chapter 7 bankruptcy. Otherwise, they are forced into Chapter 13, in which a debt repayment plan is ordered.

When filing a claim, the proper form may be obtained from a stationery store or by writing to the presiding judge of the bankruptcy court. If a creditor fails to file a claim, the creditor will lose his or her right to any proceeds from the bankruptcy. A plan for payment will be approved by the court. The trustee may be contacted from time to time to check the status of the claim and the payments that should be expected. Once a patient has obtained credit counseling and petitioned for bankruptcy, there must be a time lapse of 6 years before he or she can file again. The only exception to this is Chapter 13 bankruptcy.

Terminally Ill Patients

Although it may be difficult to collect from patients who are terminally ill, it is usually harder to collect from the estate after they have died. When a patient is too sick or scared to communicate necessary information, consult the physician about whether to obtain the patient's permission to speak to family members and stress the need for help. Usually, terminally ill patients want to do the right thing. Call the patient before he or she comes in to receive service. Make sure the patient is aware of the existing balance and try to work with the patient to eliminate at least a portion of the balance before the next appointment. Estimate costs and prepare a plan that is agreeable to both the physician and the patient.

Estate Claims

Great care and sensitivity should be taken when trying to collect on a deceased patient's account. When you discover that a patient has died, first pursue insurance or managed care plan coverage. The entire probate system was set up to help protect families from painful involvement in estate settlements. Do not offend the deceased's family by making contact during the time of bereavement. However, file a claim after the first or second week so that the physician's name can be added to the list of creditors.

Refer to Procedure 10-5 at the end of this chapter for filing an estate claim.

After filing, the claim is then denied or accepted. If accepted, an acknowledgment of the debt is sent to the physician's office. Many delays arise because of the legal complications of settling an estate, but the debts are paid according to a priority system when the estate is settled. Usually funeral expenses are paid first; following in order are estate administration expenses, claims due for the deceased person's last illness, and taxes and other debts. Any amounts left are divided among family members. A lien or lawsuit may be filed against the estate in the rare case of a rejection of the claim.

Various state time limits and statutes govern the filing of a claim against an estate. Check with the county court in your state to obtain filing deadlines. Deadlines may range from 2 months to 3 years but must be adhered to for successful collection from an estate.

Litigation

A difficult question arises when the physician is advised that a patient is involved in a pending litigation related to the services provided to the patient. It may not be necessary to wait until the litigation is resolved to pursue payment. Assess whether the patient has the ability to pay before possibly receiving a settlement in a lawsuit. Before withholding collection activity, the medical practice should get a guarantee that the physician will be paid in full before the patient (debtor) receives money out of a settlement. The agreement must be guaranteed by the lawyer representing the patient. If the patient is working, regular payments should be required pending the settlement of the patient's litigation. It is always advisable to contact a malpractice attorney in such cases.

Liens. A **lien** is a claim on the property of another as security for a debt. This may include a claim on a future settlement of a lawsuit. The physician may be asked to accept a lien by a patient or the patient's attorney when the patient has been involved in an automobile accident and is awaiting a settlement (Figure 10-17). In litigation cases, a lien is a legal promise to satisfy a debt owed by the patient to the physician out of any proceeds received on the case. See Chapter 15 for further details about industrial cases.

Patient Complaints

It is generally in the physician's best interest to resolve patient complaints and billing disputes quickly, accurately, and amicably. Always address collection complaints seriously. Listen to the patient with an open mind. Note specifically what the patient is saying and what the patient wants to do. Look beyond the complaint to determine what caused the problem. The source of the problem should be resolved, not just the result of the problem. A patient complaint form may be adapted to prompt staff to pay close attention to positive customer relations. This form may help screen poor collection techniques by staff members, pinpoint billing department problems, and identify policies and procedures that need improvement.

The patient may refuse to pay the physician if the patient's complaint is not addressed. Some guidelines to follow when a patient calls or writes a letter complaining about the physician or the medical practice are as follows:

1. Listen carefully (or read the letter carefully) and establish exactly what the patient complaint is and what the patient wants done about it.
2. Thank the person for calling (or writing); demonstrate appreciation of his or her input into the situation.
3. Apologize, regardless of whether the patient is right or wrong.
4. Answer the complaint. Explain what happened, if applicable, and state what is being done about it.
5. Use a professional and sincere approach. If the patient is wrong, state that the complaint is unjustified, but first explain your estimation of the situation and its resolution. Otherwise, he or she is likely to become quite upset. Do not be sarcastic, condescending, or insulting.
6. Take all complaints seriously. Do not respond in a lighthearted manner or use humor; it will only serve to upset the patient.
7. Respond in letter form. Whether the complaint has been received by telephone or by letter, take the time to write to answer the complaint. This indicates that the matter is not being taken lightly.
8. Be cordial and sincere. Express to the patient the hope of continuing a friendly relationship, but that payment is necessary. Treat the patient with respect, good will, and sincere appreciation. Often, kindness can turn a negative into a positive. The complaint can be turned into a payment.
9. Follow-up after the complaint has been resolved by looking at the root of the problem and taking the necessary time to communicate this to the office manager. This follow-up allows creation of a plan of action that can help prevent the same type of problem from recurring.

Collection Controls

All collections should be carefully controlled to prevent lost checks and embezzlement.

Embezzlement

Embezzlement is stealing money that has been entrusted in one's care. In many cases of insurance claims embezzlement, the physician is held as the guilty party and has to pay huge sums of money to the third-party payer when false claims are submitted by an employee. If an undiscovered embezzler leaves the employer and you are hired to replace that person, you could be accused some months down the line of doing something that you did not do. Take precautions as an employee and to protect the medical practice.

**REQUEST FOR ALLOWANCE OF LIEN
ASSIGNMENT AND AUTHORIZATION**

WHEREAS, I have a right or cause of action out of personal injury,
to wit:

I, _____ hereby authorize_____ ,
      patient's name   physician's name

to furnish upon request, to my attorney,_____ , any
and all medical records, or reports of examination, diagnosis, treatment, or
prognosis but not necessarily limited to those items as set forth herein, in addition
to an itemized statement of accounts for services rendered therefore or in
connection therewith, which my attorney may from time to time request in
connection with the injuries described above and sustained by me on
the_____ day of_____, 20XX.

I hereby irrevocably authorize and direct my said attorney set forth herein to pay
to _____ all charges for attendance in court,
           patient's name

if required as an expert witness whether he testifies or not; reports or other data
supplied by him; depositions given by said doctor; medical services rendered or
drugs supplied; and any other responsible and customary charges incurred by my
attorney as submitted by_____ and in
                        physician's name

connection with said injury. Said payment or payments are to be made from any
money or monies received by my attorney whether by judgment, decree, or
settlement of this case, prior to disbursement to me and payment of the amount as
herein directed shall be the same as if paid by me. This authorization to pay the
aforementioned doctor shall constitute and be deemed as assignment of so much
of my recovery I receive. It is agreed that nothing herein relieves me of the primary
responsibility and obligation of paying my doctor for services rendered, and I shall at
all times remain personally liable for such indebtedness unless released by the
aforementioned doctor or by payment disbursed by my attorney. I accept the above
assignment:

Dated:_____ Patient:_____

As the attorney of record for the above-named, I hereby agree to observe the terms
of this agreement, and to withhold from any award in this case such sums as are
required for the adequate protection of Dr._____

Date:_____ Attorney:_____

FIGURE 10-17 A patient's authorization to release information to an attorney and grant lien to the physician against proceeds of settlement in connection with accident, industrial, or third-party litigation cases.

Precautions for Financial Protection

To prevent the temptation to steal from a medical practice, these office policies should be routinely practiced. The physician or supervisor must approve of all entries posted about adjustments, discounts, and write-offs. If a patient owes money to the physician that is uncollectable and adjusted off, be sure the physician has approved and the balance due has been brought to zero. Ask the physician, an auditor, or an outside consultant to occasionally check an entire day's records (the patient sign-in log and appointment schedule) with the daysheet, patients' financial accounting records, encounter forms, and cash receipt slips. A daily trail of the balance of A/R, including daily deposit of checks and cash, can assist in reviewing monthly income and aid in discovering embezzlement. Review the

monthly bank statement to verify that all deposits tally with the receipts for each business day (Figure 10-18). If poor bookkeeping and record keeping are noticed, bring this to your employer's attention.

All insurance payment checks should be immediately stamped within the endorsement area on the back "For Deposit Only," called a *restrictive endorsement*. The bank should be given instructions never to cash a check made payable to the physician.

Encounter forms, transaction slips, and cash receipts should be prenumbered. If a mistake is made when completing one, void it and keep the slip as part of the financial records. It is especially imperative to have prenumbered insurance forms if the physician's practice allows the use of a signature stamp when submitting claims. Thus filing of fictitious insurance claims can be totally eliminated.

As a precautionary measure, always type your initials at the bottom left or top right corner of the insurance claim forms that you submit. This will indicate to office personnel who did the work. Always retain the Explanation of Benefits or Remittance Advice documents that accompany checks from insurance companies.

Only a few of the many precautions for protection are mentioned here; embezzlement can occur in A/R, accounts payable, with petty cash, use of computers, and in various other aspects of a medical practice.

Bonding

Insurance billers, claims assistance professionals, or anyone who handles checks or cash should be bonded or insured. A practice that carries a fidelity or honesty bond means that an insurance company will prosecute any

guilty employees. **Bonding** is an insurance contract by which a bonding agency guarantees payment of a certain sum to a physician in case of a financial loss caused by an employee or some contingency over which the payee has no control. Bonding methods for a practice with three or more office employees are as follows:

- *Position-schedule bond* covers a designated job, such as a bookkeeper or nurse, rather than a named individual. If one employee in a category leaves, the replacement is automatically covered.
- *Blanket-position bond* provides coverage for all employees regardless of job title.
- *Personal bond* provides coverage for those who handle large sums of money. A thorough background investigation is required.

Such bonding contracts may be obtained from a casualty insurance agent or broker. Bond coverage should be reviewed periodically with the insurance agent to ensure that coverage is keeping pace with the expansion of the business.

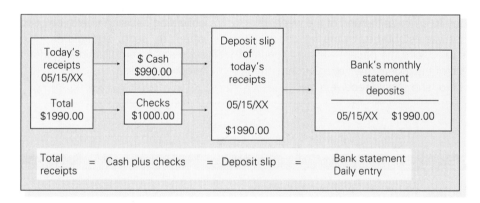

FIGURE 10-18 Explanation of an audit trail to review monies received by a medical practice and monies deposited into a bank account.

PROCEDURE 10-1

Seven-Step Billing and Collection Guidelines

OBJECTIVE: To properly bill and collect payments for professional services rendered to patients

EQUIPMENT/SUPPLIES: Patients' financial accounting statements, envelopes, calendar, and telephone

DIRECTIONS: Follow these step-by-step procedures and guidelines, which include rationales, to learn this job skill.

1. Present the first statement at the time of service. This can be a formal statement or an encounter form (multipurpose billing form).

2. Mail the second itemized statement within 30 days of treatment. The phrase "due and payable within 10 days" should be printed on each statement. Local paycheck issuing patterns should be considered before selecting a date for statements to be mailed. Choose which billing routine the office will use:

   a. Monthly billing. Using the monthly billing system, all statements are mailed at the same time during the month. Choose a mail-out day at the beginning of the month so that the patient will receive

Continued

PROCEDURE 10-1—cont'd

Seven-Step Billing and Collection Guidelines

the bill near the 15th, or send statements near the end of the month so that the patient receives the bill on the 1st.

b. Cycle billing. **Cycle billing** is a system of billing accounts at spaced intervals during the month based on a breakdown of accounts by alphabet, account number, insurance type, or date of first service. This relieves the pressure of having to get all the statements out at one time and allows collection at a faster, more organized rate than accounts collected at random. It also allows continuous cash flow throughout the month and distributes the influx of incoming calls from patients about problem accounts. The number of cycles may be determined by how the collector wishes to divide the workload. Using two cycles per month, statements would be sent on the 25th to arrive by the 1st, and on the 10th to arrive by the 15th of the month. Using four cycles per month, statements should be sent every Tuesday or Wednesday to arrive at the end of the week. If a cycle that was established by the first date of service is used, and the patient was first seen on the 11th of the month, then every month on the 11th he or she should receive a bill.

3. Send the third statement 30 days after the second statement was sent. Indicate that the payment is past due.

4. If there is no response to the third statement, place the first telephone call to the patient depending on office policy (7 to 14 days). Ask if there is a problem. Ask for a payment commitment and set up a suspense file. Accounts are put in a suspense file for active follow-up. Action must be taken within the time frame mentioned, after the patient has been so advised.

5. Check for payment as promised. Allow 1 day for mail delay. Place the second telephone call to the patient and ask for payment. Set up a new payment date. Allow 5 days.

6. Check for payment as promised. Send a 10-day notice advising the patient that unless payment is received in 10 days, the account will be turned over for legal action.

7. Check for payment. Promptly surrender the account for collection or legal action. Figure 10-11 shows a collection decision tree to be used when determining when to send statements, 10-day notices, and accounts to a collection agency and when to make telephone calls.

PROCEDURE 10-2

Telephone Collection Plan

OBJECTIVE: To obtain payment of a delinquent account balance due by making the first collection telephone call

EQUIPMENT/SUPPLIES: Telephone, pen or pencil, patient's financial accounting record, computerized account, or collection telephone log

DIRECTIONS: Follow these step-by-step procedures and guidelines, which include rationales, to learn this job skill.

1. Set the mood of the call by the manner of speech and tone of voice. The first 30 seconds of the call set the scene for the relationship with the patient. Follow the Fair Debt Collection Practices Act when making a telephone call.

2. State the name of the caller, the practice represented, and identify the patient. Be certain the debtor is being spoken to before revealing the nature of the call.

3. Identify oneself and the facility.

4. Verify the debtor's address and any telephone numbers.

5. State the reason for the call by asking for full payment and stating the total amount owed. Ask for payment courteously but firmly.

6. Take control of the conversation and establish urgency by asking for full payment now. Speak slowly in a low voice; staying calm and polite prevents quarreling.

7. Ask when payment will be made, how it will be made, and if it will be sent by mail or in person.

8. Pause for effect. This turns the conversation back to the patient to respond to the demand or explain why payment has not been made. Never assume that if a patient does not respond, it means "no."

9. Find out if the patient needs clarification of the bill.

PROCEDURE 10-2—cont'd

Telephone Collection Plan

10. Inquire if the patient has a problem. Ask if the practice can be of assistance, especially when the patient is unable to give a reason for nonpayment.

11. If the patient is reluctant to agree to an amount, question him or her by asking one of the following: "How much are you willing to pay?" "Do you have a regular paycheck?" "Will payment be made through a checking account?"

12. Obtain a promise to pay with an agreeable amount and a due date; be clear how and when payment is expected, but give the patient a choice of action. Set immediate deadlines for payment.

13. Ask for half of the amount if full payment is not possible.

14. Discuss a payment plan if the patient is not able to pay half of the balance owed. Be realistic and reasonable. It is self-defeating to set up payment arrangements the patient cannot afford. Advise the patient that the entire balance will become due and payable if the payment is even 1 day late. Ask the patient to please call before the due date with an explanation if any problems arise to prevent payment.

15. Restate the importance of the agreement.

16. Tell the patient to write down the amount and due date.

17. Document the agreement on the patient's financial accounting record by inserting the date of the call and abbreviated notations, in the computer system, or in a collection telephone log. Note the time the patient was spoken to.

18. Send confirmation of the agreement (Figure 10-19) as a follow-up to the telephone call.

19. Check the account the day after the payment was due; allow 1 day for mail delay. If the patient fails to make payment as promised, make another telephone call and ask the patient if there is still a problem. Get a new commitment to pay and confirm again. If the patient continues to avoid payment, advise the patient that the account will be turned over to a collection agency and follow through as stated.

COLLEGE CLINIC
4567 Broad Avenue
Woodland Hills, XY 12345-0001
Tel. (555) 486-9002
FAX (555) 487-8976

October 2, 20XX

Mr. Leonard Blabalot
981 McCort Circle
Woodland Hills, XY 12345-0001

Dear Mr. Blabalot:

I am glad we had an opportunity to discuss your outstanding balance with our practice during our phone conversation on October 1, 20XX. This will confirm and remind you that you agreed to pay $100 on your account on or before October 15, 20XX.

A return envelope is enclosed for your convenience.

Sincerely,

Charlotte Rose Routingham
Business Office

Enc. envelope

FIGURE 10-19 Telephone confirmation letter sent to remind patient of the payment terms agreed to in a telephone conversation.

PROCEDURE 10-3

Create a Financial Agreement with a Patient

OBJECTIVE: To assist the patient in making credit arrangements by completing and signing a Truth in Lending form

EQUIPMENT/SUPPLIES: Patient's financial accounting record (ledger), calendar, Truth in Lending form, typewriter or computer, calculator, and quiet private room

DIRECTIONS: Follow the step-by-step procedures that include rationale to learn this job skill. An assignment is presented in the *Workbook* to practice this skill.

1. Explain the patient's balance due and answer questions about credit.
2. Inform the patient of the medical practice's office policy about extending credit payments.
3. Discuss an installment plan concerning the amount of the total debt, the down payment, amount and date of each installment, and the date of final payment.
4. Subtract the down payment from the total debt. Decide the remaining amount by the number of months the debt is being carried to determine the monthly installment amounts and date of final payment.
5. Complete a Truth in Lending form after mutually agreeing on the terms if the payments require more than four installments. This procedure complies with Regulation Z.
6. Review the completed Truth in Lending form with the patient.
7. Ask the patient to sign the Truth in Lending form.
8. Make a photocopy of the form for the patient to retain.
9. File the original Truth in Lending form in the patient's financial files in the office.

PROCEDURE 10-4

File a Claim in Small Claims Court

OBJECTIVE: To file a claim to obtain payment for a delinquent or uncollectable financial account in small claims court

EQUIPMENT/SUPPLIES: Small claims court filing form, photocopy of the patient's financial accounting record, computer or typewriter, pen or pencil, envelope, and check for filing fee

DIRECTIONS: Follow these step-by-step procedures and guidelines, which include rationales, to learn this job skill.

1. Obtain a Claim of Plaintiff or Plaintiff's Original Petition form to notify the patient that action is being filed. This can be obtained from the clerk's office located at the municipal or justice court. Obtain booklets and material to help guide the claimant through the process.
2. Complete and file the papers with the small claims court; make sure to have the patient's correct name and street address.
3. Make a photocopy of the small claims court form for the office files.
4. Pay the clerk the small filing fee. Filing fees vary by state, by county within some states, and by the amount of the claim.
5. Make arrangements to serve the defendant. The summons or citation can be served on the patient by a sheriff or court-appointed officer by paying a small fee plus mileage for the constable who serves it. The person serving the defendant must fill out a proof of service form.
6. After being served, a patient has one of four options:
   a. Pay the claim to the court clerk. This will be forwarded to the physician, but the filing fee or service charge will not be refunded.
   b. Ignore the claim. The physician will win by default. In some states a judgment may be requested in writing, but in other states the physician or the physician's representative (medical employee) must appear on a specified date. If the patient does not appear, the judgment is granted in the physician's favor and usually court costs are included in the judgment.
   c. Request a small claims hearing. The court clerk will let both parties know when to appear. The patient may file a counterclaim against the physician at this time.
   d. Demand a jury trial. The case will be taken out of small claims court. The physician will be notified by the court clerk to file a formal complaint in a higher court, and an attorney must represent the physician.
7. Appear in court (physician or the physician's medical employee or representative) on the specified date; claim will be dismissed and cannot be refiled.

PROCEDURE 10-4—cont'd

File a Claim in Small Claims Court

8. Basic information required by the court follows:
   a. Physician's name, address, and telephone number
   b. Patient's name and address
   c. Delinquent amount
   d. Summary of the claim including the date the physician's bill was due, date of the last visit, date of the last payment, unpaid amount, and all records of telephone contacts and letters sent.
9. Determine what the judge needs to hear to decide a favorable case. Good preparation for the trial can make the difference between success or failure.
10. Organize all the exhibits in a notebook, in chronologic order. A timeline showing the sequence of events can be useful.
11. Take a businesslike professional approach at the hearing by giving concise and accurate answers to the judge's questions, speaking slowly and clearly. The physician or assistant must bring any witnesses, statements, receipts, contracts, notes, dishonored checks, or other evidence to court. The judge will question the physician's medical employee or representative or physician and the patient, review the evidence, and then make a ruling.
12. Put a lien on the debtor's wages, automobile, bank or personal assets, or real property if the judgment, which is usually effective for many years, is in the physician's favor. This is the physician's legal right. The small claims office will show the physician's medical employee or physician how to execute a judgment.
13. Pay a small fee if the physician decides to execute against the patient's assets. It is recoverable from the patient.

PROCEDURE 10-5

File an Estate Claim

OBJECTIVE: To file a claim on an estate for a deceased patient who has an outstanding balance on his or her financial accounting record
EQUIPMENT/SUPPLIES: Statement of Claim form, computer or typewriter, pen or pencil, photocopy machine, patient's financial accounting record, US Postal Service certified mail forms, and envelope
DIRECTIONS: Follow these step-by-step procedures and guidelines, which include rationales, to learn this job skill.

1. Confirm the date and place of death with the hospital, nursing home, or funeral home.
2. Pursue payment from all third-party payers first.
3. Contact the Register of Wills' office in the county where the patient lived or the probate department of the superior court, County Recorder's Office. Request a Statement of Claim form or the county's proper document to formally register a claim against an estate.
4. File the claim according to the instructions received with the claim form. When probate is filed, a notification will be sent advising the court of probate, the attorney representing the estate, and the **estate executor** or **estate administrator.** Perhaps a small fee should be included for court costs.
5. Send a photocopy of the patient's financial accounting record (itemized statement) by certified mail, return receipt, to the attorney and copies to the executor and the court. If the physician treated the deceased patient's last illness, that fact should be clearly indicated on the statement.
6. Allow the legal system to take its course. A call to the executor can be made periodically to check on the status of the estate.

KEY POINTS

This is a brief chapter review or summary of the key issues presented. To further enhance your knowledge of the technical subject matter, review the key terms and key abbreviations for this chapter by locating the meanings in the glossary at the end of this book that appear in a section before the index.

1. The physician, the practice administrator responsible for financial affairs, and the patient must understand insurance contracts, which list payment provisions, medical services not covered, the portion of the bill the patient is responsible for, and the process for reimbursing the office.

2. The insurance billing specialist must monitor the A/R weekly to find out the effectiveness of collection. An average A/R should be one and a half to two times the charges for 1 month of services.

3. Collect copayments and deductibles from patients at the time service is rendered.

4. Under HIPAA, physicians are free to use whatever policies they want on charity care, discounts, write-offs, and collections, but this must be done consistently and the reasons must be documented. Professional courtesy should be kept to a minimum.

5. When payments are made by check, require two forms of verification. Always take immediate action when the bank returns a check for NSF.

6. Recognize overdue accounts to determine when to send dun messages on statements, make telephone calls, or send to a collection agency.

7. Use alternative payment methods to help cash flow and reduce collection costs such as credit card payments, debit cards, e-checks, and payment plans.

8. Follow all federal and state laws that affect collection of delinquent accounts.

9. Contact the patient in a timely manner by telephone at the first sign of payment delay and then send a collection letter as a reminder.

10. Delinquent accounts should be turned over to a collection agency only after all reasonable attempts have been made to collect.

11. Learn and use all techniques in skip tracing a debtor.

12. It is in the physician's best interest to resolve patient complaints and billing disputes quickly, accurately, and amicably.

evolve INTERNET RESOURCES

For active links to the following resources, visit the Evolve website at
http://evolve.elsevier.com/fordney/handbook

Websites to learn more about bankruptcy laws:

- American Bar Association
- Nolo

Websites to help you search for a debtor:

- Anywho
- Bigfoot
- InfoSpace
- Info USA

- SearchBug
- Switchboard
- WhoWhere?
- Yahoo People Search
- 411Locate

Websites for small claims court:

- Small claims court.com
- Website for the Fair and Accurate Credit Transactions (FACT) Act
- State statutes that correspond to the Articles of the Uniform Commercial Code Locator

STUDENT ASSIGNMENT

✓ Study Chapter 10.

✓ Answer the fill-in-the blank, multiple choice, and true/false review questions in the *Workbook* to reinforce the theory learned in this chapter and to help prepare you for a future test.

✓ Complete the assignment in the *Workbook* to give you hands-on experience in selecting a dun message, posting a courtesy adjustment and insurance or patient payment, composing a collection letter, and completing a credit card voucher and financial agreement.

✓ Turn to the glossary at the end of this textbook for a further understanding of the key terms and key abbreviations used in the chapter.

UNIT 3
Health Care Payers

KEY TERMS*

ancillary services
buffing
capitation
carve outs
churning
claims-review type of
    foundation
closed panel program
comprehensive type of
    foundation
copayment
deductible
direct referral
disenrollment

exclusive provider organization
fee-for-service
formal referral
foundation for medical care
gatekeeper
health maintenance
    organization
in-area
independent (or individual)
    practice association
managed care organizations
participating physician
per capita
physician provider group

point-of-service plan
preferred provider organization
prepaid group practice model
primary care physician
self-referral
service area
staff model
stop-loss
tertiary care
turfing
utilization review
verbal referral
withhold

KEY ABBREVIATIONS*

copay
EBP
EPO
ERISA
FMC

HEDIS
HMO
IPA
MCO
NCQA

PCP
POS
PPG
PPO
QIO

QISMC
UR

*Definitions for the key terms and key abbreviations are located near the back of this textbook in the glossary.

The Blue Plans, Private Insurance, and Managed Care Plans

OBJECTIVES

After reading this chapter, you should be able to:

- State the difference between a traditional indemnity insurance plan and a managed care plan.
- Explain health maintenance organization (HMO) benefits and eligibility requirements.
- State the provisions of the Health Maintenance Organization Act of 1973.
- Explain major provisions of the Patient Protection and Affordable Care Act of 2010.
- List features of an exclusive provider organization (EPO).
- List two types and two different functions of foundations.
- Define independent practice associations.

- Name the features of preferred provider organizations (PPOs).
- Explain the features of a point-of-service (POS) plan.
- Explain how the Employee Retirement Income Security Act (ERISA) affects managed care insurance.
- State reasons for a Quality Improvement Organization (QIO) program.
- Identify four types of referrals for medical services, tests, and procedures.
- State the purpose of creating a managed care plan reference guide.
- Describe types of payment mechanisms used for managed care plans.

Service to Patients

Carefully follow guidelines for each managed care contract in regard to preauthorization for certain tests and services, hospital admissions, inpatient or outpatient surgeries, elective procedures, or when the patient must be seen by someone other than the primary care physician. If authorization is obtained in a timely manner, the patient's health care will not be delayed and payment will be forthcoming. These policies and procedures provide good service to the patient.

PRIVATE INSURANCE

Numerous private insurance companies across the United States (US) offer health insurance to individuals and groups. Most offer a variety of managed care plans. This chapter describes the difference between private insurance and managed care. Fee-for-service reimbursement was discussed in previous chapters. This chapter explains managed care capitation as a form of reimbursement.

Performance objectives, testing and review material, and hands-on practical exercises for this chapter are available in these resources

 The Insurance Handbook Student Workbook   The Insurance Handbook Evolve Site

403

Blue Cross and Blue Shield Plans

Blue Cross/Blue Shield plans are pioneers in private insurance and had a nonprofit status that made them unique among all private insurance carriers for many years. Blue Cross/Blue Shield is the largest insurance company in the US. Each plan is independently owned and operated in each state. The plans work together in a network similar to a spider web. Originally, Blue Cross plans were developed to cover hospital expenses and Blue Shield plans were primarily established to cover physician services. Different plans have been developed to allow members to seek treatment from Blue Cross/Blue Shield providers anywhere in the US. With so many different plans, it is difficult for the medical biller to know which type the member is enrolled in. However, the patient's identification card is important and helpful in obtaining the correct information needed for billing purposes. The identification number consists of 9 to 12 numbers with one to three alpha characters. The patient may have a traditional plan or a managed care plan (e.g., preferred provider organization [PPO], point-of-service [POS] plan, independent [or individual] practice association [IPA], health maintenance organization [HMO], or Medicare HMO). Plans are different and may have diverse names in each state (e.g., Premera in Alaska and Washington state; Care First in Maryland, northern Virginia, Washington, DC, and Delaware; and Horizon in New Jersey). This chapter describes these managed care systems.

Nationally, the Blue Cross/Blue Shield Association is a single corporation administering the rules and regulations for the regional plans to follow. The regional plans process claims for members who have plan coverage for hospital expenses, outpatient care, other institutional services, home care, dental benefits, and vision care. Most of the affiliated organizations have converted to for-profit status and operate in much the same way as other private insurance carriers. In some areas, Blue Cross and Blue Shield are separate organizations, and in some situations they may compete against each other. They have plans that are similar to other private insurance companies and they do not have standardized claim form guidelines. In addition, Blue Cross/Blue Shield may act as a Medicare administrative contractor (fiscal intermediary) in certain regions. An experienced medical biller should be aware of the many problems these circumstances cause. For example, the policy number may require the claim to be sent to the home plan, or the policy number may require the claim to be sent through the provider's state carrier. Blue Cross/Blue Shield realizes this is a problem, so the organization is developing a product called Blue Plan that incorporates all products. The intent is to help the patient avoid making payments. Always verify the mailing address for claims, as well as the address for sending appeals,

because these may not always be the same. Some plans may have a form to be used as a cover sheet when submitting an appeal.

There are other unique situations with Blue Cross/Blue Shield in regard to contracts. Blue Cross/Blue Shield would like to have contracts with both medical groups and the providers that work for the group. This poses unique problems when the group and provider are contracted, when the group is contracted and the provider is not, and when there is no contract with either the provider or group. Each situation has a different effect on claims processing and payment. A provider must be individually contracted with Blue Cross/Blue Shield to receive reimbursement as a member physician. Deductibles and copayments vary according to the patient's plan.

Because Blue Cross/Blue Shield contracts are like other types of private and managed care plans, in this textbook the organization is not listed separately in the description of types of fee structures, network physicians, managed care plans, and guidelines for completing the CMS-1500 (08-05) insurance claim form or electronic claims processing. A medical practice should have available for reference the current provider manual for its state's Blue Cross/Blue Shield plans.

MANAGED CARE

Until the early 1970s, most health insurance was delivered through traditional fee-for-service plans. This scenario has changed from indemnity plans to managed health care plans such as health maintenance organizations (HMOs). In an indemnity plan also referred to as *traditional insurance*, the insured pays a fixed monthly premium and 100% of all medical bills until he or she reaches the annual deductible and then the insurance company pays a percentage of covered benefits up to a maximum amount. The insured may obtain care from any health care provider, and the provider is paid each time a service is rendered on a fee-for-service basis. In a managed care plan, a specified set of health benefits is provided in exchange for a yearly fee or fixed periodic payments to the provider by the plan. The patient pays a smaller monthly premium and may be restricted as to which health care provider to seek care from. In this chapter, the health care reforms of the past and present are defined and explained. In addition to HMOs, other types of prepaid group practice models that use a managed care approach and are operated by **managed care organizations (MCOs)** are discussed.

In prepaid group plans, patients join the plan and pay monthly medical insurance premiums individually or through their employer. The physician renders service to the patient, and the patient usually pays a small copayment and occasionally a deductible as required by the plan. Providers that join the plan are paid using the capitation method. **Capitation** is a system of payment used by managed care plans in which physicians and hospitals are paid a fixed per capita amount for each patient enrolled over a stated period of time, regardless of the type and number of services provided.

Prepaid Group Practice Health Plans

The *Ross-Loos Medical Group* in Los Angeles was America's oldest privately owned prepaid medical group. It was founded in 1929 by Drs. Donald E. Ross and H. Clifford Loos and existed only in southern California, where it expanded to 17 medical group locations. In 1975 the Ross-Loos Medical Group formed a corporation and received a federal grant to develop a health care system under the federal Health Maintenance Organization Act of 1973. In 1980, INA Healthplan, Inc., of Philadelphia merged with Ross-Loos. Ross-Loos is now known as *CIGNA Healthplans of California.*

Most CIGNA patients are served under a prepayment group plan by which they pay a monthly premium and receive hospital, surgical, and professional benefits from a CIGNA staff physician or CIGNA Health Care Center. Several thousand other CIGNA patients are private and are treated on a fee-for-service basis. In the case of an emergency when the patient is outside the area of a CIGNA Health Care Center, he or she may seek professional or hospital care in other facilities, but CIGNA must be notified as soon as possible. A dental plan and Medicare supplemental plan are available through CIGNA as well.

Another pioneer of the prepaid group practice concept is the *Kaiser Permanente Medical Care Program*. It began in 1933 when Dr. Sidney R. Garfield and a few physicians working for him gave combined industrial accident and personal medical care to approximately 5000 workers building a fresh-water aqueduct across the California desert to Los Angeles. Dr. Garfield charged the insurance carriers $1.50 per man per month and the workers 5 cents a day. In return, he provided comprehensive health care. Then in 1938, Henry J. Kaiser and his son Edgar started a joint venture to complete the Grand Coulee Dam in Washington and invited Dr. Garfield to form a medical group to furnish care to the workers for 7 cents a day prepaid by the employer. The group expanded to include the workers' wives and children.

Kaiser Permanente now has centers in 12 regions covering 16 states. Patients are served under a prepayment group plan and receive hospital, surgical, and professional benefits from physicians located at the Kaiser Permanente Medical Care Centers. In most regions the Kaiser Permanente Medical Plan is a **closed panel program** composed of multispecialty physicians, and the plan limits the patient's choice of personal physicians to those practicing in one of the 12 geographic regions.

In January 1994 Kaiser Permanente announced a venture with Pacific Mutual Life Insurance Company to give Kaiser's 4.6 million California patients an option of using physicians and medical facilities outside the vast Kaiser network. This was the first time that Kaiser allowed certain member groups of its two California HMOs to seek medical help from non-Kaiser physicians, and it was termed a *POS option* (see discussion later in this chapter). In this option, Kaiser pays up to a specified amount and the patient pays the rest, depending on the contract. Kaiser does not provide care on a fee-for-service or cost reimbursement basis.

In emergency situations when patients cannot reach a Kaiser Center, they may seek the services of outside facilities or physicians. They are transferred to a Kaiser facility when their condition stabilizes.

Health Maintenance Organization Act of 1973

An HMO is a prepaid group practice that can be sponsored and operated by the government, medical schools, clinics, foundations, hospitals, employers, labor unions, community or consumer groups, insurance companies, hospital medical plans, or the US Department of Veterans Affairs (VA).

In 1973 Congress passed the Health Maintenance Organization Act of 1973 (Public Law 93-222), creating authority for the federal government to assist HMO development in a number of ways, including (1) providing grants, loans, and loan guarantees to offset the initial operating deficits of new HMOs that meet federal standards (e.g., are federally qualified) and (2) requiring most employers to offer an HMO to their employees as an alternative to traditional health insurance.

Accreditation

The National Committee for Quality Assurance (NCQA) is a not-for-profit organization that accredits HMOs including traditional staff and group model HMOs, network and IPA model HMOs, mixed models, and open-ended HMOs. NCQA developed HEDIS (Health Plan Employer Data Information Set), which is a set of data reporting standards that compares performance between plans. For further information, go to the Evolve website listed in Internet Resources at the end of this chapter. The website has an active link to NCQA.

Eligibility

Those who have voluntarily enrolled in an HMO plan from a specific geographic area (**in-area** or **service area**) or who are covered by an employer who has paid an established sum per person to be covered by the plan are eligible. The law states that an employer employing 25 or more persons may offer the services of an HMO as an alternative health treatment plan for employees. Medicare and Medicaid beneficiaries also may become members of managed care plans whether retired or employed. The federal government reimburses the HMOs on a per capita basis, depending on the size of the enrollment. This means that the HMO is paid a fixed **per capita** amount (also known as capitation) for each patient served without considering the actual number or nature of services provided to each person.

To qualify as an HMO, an organization must present proof of its ability to provide comprehensive health care. To retain eligibility, an HMO must render periodic performance reports to the offices of the Department of Health and Human Services. Thus accurate and complete medical records are imperative to the survival and cost control of an HMO.

Primary Care Physician. Most managed care plans use a **primary care physician (PCP)** as a gatekeeper. A **gatekeeper** is a physician who controls patient access to specialists and diagnostic testing services. Usually, PCPs are physicians who practice in the fields of internal medicine, family practice, general practice, or pediatrics. Although obstetrics/gynecology is considered specialty care, the obstetrician/gynecologist may be contracted as a PCP, and when not, it is common for MCOs to allow self-referral by members to obstetricians/gynecologists for certain services (e.g., Pap smears).

Identification Card. Each enrollee of a managed care plan is given an identification card as shown in Figure 3-9. The card usually lists the patient's name, member number, group number, and primary care physician's name. The name of the MCO and type of plan with the amount of copayment for various outpatient services (e.g., office visit, emergency department, urgent care center, and pharmacy) may be included by some plans.

Both sides of the patient's card should be photocopied because the insurance address, telephone numbers used for inquiries and authorizations, or other important information may be listed on the front or back of the card.

Benefits

Benefits under the HMO Act fall under two categories: basic and supplemental health service, which are listed in Box 11-1.

Health Care Reform

Over the past 75 years, leaders of the US, from President Roosevelt to President Obama, have announced reforms of the health care system. Medical practices have made transitions from rural to urban, generalist to specialist, solo to group practice, and fee-for-service to capitation and have expanded to a number of health care delivery systems that try to manage the cost of health care. Before capitation, **fee-for-service** was the usual method of billing by physicians in private practice. A professional service was rendered by the physician to the patient, and the physician made a separate charge for each service and expected to receive a fee for each service provided. Early insurance contracts were indemnity plans. They paid a flat fee for covered services and the patient paid the full balance. There were no participating agreements with physicians or hospitals.

Box 11-1   Health Maintenance Organization Act Benefits of 1973

Basic Health Services

Alcohol, drug abuse, and addiction medical treatment
Dental services (preventive) for children younger than age 12 years
Diagnostic laboratory, x-ray, and therapeutic radiology services
Emergency health services in or out of the HMO service area
Family planning and infertility services
Health education and medical social services
Home health services
Hospital services (inpatient and outpatient)
Mental health services on an outpatient basis, short-term (not to exceed 20 visits) ambulatory, evaluative, and crisis intervention
Physicians' services and consultant or referral services without time or cost limits

Preventive health services (e.g., physical examinations for adults, vision and hearing tests for children through age 17 years, well-baby care, immunizations, health education)

Supplemental Health Services

Dental care not included in basic benefits
Extended mental health services not included in basic benefits
Eye examinations for adults
Intermediate and long-term care (nursing facilities and nursing homes)
Prescription drugs
Rehabilitative services and long-term physical medicine (e.g., physical therapy)

A major restructuring of the US health care system was necessary during the 1990s for the following reasons:

- A growing percentage of Americans were not covered by private or government insurance.
- Employers had to pay escalating health care premiums and did not want to cut wages to cover these costs.
- Government needed to reduce the deficit by keeping down increases in the Medicare and Medicaid programs.
- Physicians and hospital costs soared with no end in sight because of inflation, high-tech equipment, expensive medications, and so on.
- Patients spent more and more money for less and less care and coped with a system riddled with inefficiency and fraud.
- Services were overused by patients.

Integrated health care delivery systems have been formed in many states in the past decade to reduce costs. These have included MCOs, physician-hospital organizations, and group practices accepting a variety of MCOs and fee-for-service patients. These systems allow for better negotiations for contracts with large employers and managed care plans, as well as with medical and office suppliers for discounts. Each type of organization differs in ownership, purpose, governance, management, and type of services provided. Even before the government released its health care reform proposal, some states began establishing laws implementing managed care for the general populations, as well as for Medicaid patients and those injured on the job (workers' compensation cases). Hawaii has had a statewide universal health insurance plan since 1974. Many regions have large groups of Medicare-eligible people who have opted to belong to an HMO or other prepaid plans.

In 1994 California put together the first working alliance in the nation, followed by Florida's voluntary purchasing group, the Community Health Purchasing Alliances. In California the alliance is formally known as the Health Insurance Plan of California. This allows firms with 5 to 50 workers to offer their employees a wide choice of different insurance programs. All plans must offer the same benefits, but some physicians and hospitals are more desirable than others. The company must pay an amount equal to at least half of the cost of the lowest-priced plan; the worker pays the remainder.

On March 21, 2010, the House of Representatives passed national health care reform legislation, H.R. 3590, the Patient Protection and Affordable Care Act (the Affordable Care Act), and H.R. 4872, the Health Care and Education Reconciliation Act of 2010 (the Reconciliation Act). Provisions effective within a year include: forbids insurers from canceling insurance coverage (*rescission*), eliminates preexisting condition exclusions, ends lifetime limits on benefits, gives tax credits to small businesses that offer coverage, provides temporary insurance until 2014 for people who have been denied because of their health status, allows young people to remain on their parents' insurance until age 26, requires insurers to use a high percentage of premiums for benefits instead of profits or overhead, and makes preventive measures free to Medicare beneficiaries, such as screenings for colon, prostate, and breast cancer. Beginning in 2014, almost everyone is required to be insured or they will pay a fine. Small businesses, the self-employed, and the uninsured may pick plans offered through state-based purchasing pools. This legislation also has an impact on Medicare and Medicaid programs, and this information is explained in Chapters 12 and 13.

At the time of the printing of this edition, the health care reform legislation has not been completely finalized. To keep you up to date as legislation is passed, additional provisions are on the Evolve website.

MANAGED CARE SYSTEMS

Health Maintenance Organizations

The oldest of all the prepaid health plans is the **health maintenance organization (HMO)**. An HMO is a plan or program by which specified health services are rendered by participating physicians to an enrolled group of persons. Fixed periodic payments are made in advance to providers of services **(participating physicians)** by or on behalf of each person or family. If a health insurance carrier administers and manages the HMO, it contracts to pay in advance for the full range of health services to which the insured is entitled under the terms of the health insurance contract.

HMO Models

There are important differences in the structure of various HMOs that influence the way physicians practice and perhaps the quality of medical care delivered. Following are several types of HMO models.

Prepaid Group Practice Model. The **prepaid group practice model** delivers services at one or more locations through a group of physicians who contract with the HMO to provide care or through its own physicians who are employees of the HMO. For example, Kaiser Permanente is a prepaid group practice model wherein physicians form an independent group (Permanente) and contract with a health plan (Kaiser) to provide medical treatment to members enrolled by the plan. Although the physicians work for a salary, it is paid by their own independent group, not by the administrators of the health plan. This design permits the physicians to concentrate on medicine.

Staff Model. The **staff model** is a type of HMO in which the health plan hires physicians directly and pays them a salary instead of contracting with a medical group.

Network HMO. A *network HMO* contracts with two or more group practices to provide health services. It is common for those physicians to see both HMO and non-HMO patients in their own offices. Network physicians are typically paid a capitation amount for the care of each HMO patient in their panel of patients, regardless of whether the patient is actually seen by the physician in any given month.

Direct Contract Model. A common type of model in open-panel HMOs is the *direct contract model*. This type of managed care health plan contracts directly with private practice physicians in the community rather than through an intermediary such as an IPA or a medical group. Contracted health care services are delivered to subscribers by individual physicians in the community.

The Office of Health Maintenance Organizations can provide further information on HMOs.*

Exclusive Provider Organizations

An **exclusive provider organization (EPO)** is a type of managed care plan that combines features of HMOs (e.g., enrolled population, limited provider panel, gatekeepers, utilization management, capitated provider reimbursement, and authorization system) and PPOs (e.g., flexible benefit design, negotiated fees, and fee-for-service payments). It is referred to as exclusive because employers agree not to contract with any other plan. The member must choose medical care from network providers with certain exceptions for emergency or out-of-area services. If a patient decides to seek care outside the network, generally he or she is not reimbursed for the cost of the treatment. Technically, many HMOs can be considered EPOs. However, EPOs are regulated under insurance statutes rather than federal and state HMO regulations.

Foundations for Medical Care

A **foundation for medical care (FMC)** is an organization of physicians sponsored by a state or local medical association concerned with the development and delivery of medical services and the cost of health care. The first foundation for medical care was established in 1954 in Stockton, CA. Foundations have sprung up across the US, and some comprehensive foundations have assumed a portion of the underwriting risk for a defined population. Foundations deal primarily with various

groups—employer groups, government groups, and county and city employees. Some plans are open to individual subscribers, but these instances usually represent a small percentage of the foundation activity.

Two basic types of foundations for medical care operations exist, and each functions differently: (1) a **comprehensive type of foundation,** which designs and sponsors prepaid health programs or sets minimum benefits of coverage, and (2) a **claims-review type of foundation,** which provides evaluation of the quality and efficiency of services by a panel of physicians to the numerous fiscal agents or carriers involved in its area, including the ones processing Medicare and Medicaid. Reviews are done for services or fees that exceed local community guidelines.

A key feature of the foundation is its dedication to an incentive reimbursement system. For a participating physician, income is received in direct proportion to the number of medical services delivered (e.g., fee-for-service) rather than payment through capitation. The FMC offers a managed care plan fee schedule to be used by member physicians. In some areas, foundation physicians agree to accept the foundation allowance as payment in full for covered services. The patient is not billed for the balance. However, the patient is billed for nonbenefit items, a deductible, and coinsurance.

The patient may select any member or nonmember physician he or she wishes. Member physicians agree to bill the foundation directly, and a nonmember physician may wish to collect directly from the patient. Many foundations submit claims on the CMS-1500 (08-05) form, and others transmit data electronically. The foundation movement has a national society, the American Managed Care and Review Association (AMCRA), which can provide further information on AMCRA or foundations in an individual state.*

Independent Practice Associations

Another type of MCO is the **independent (or individual) practice association (IPA),** in which the physicians are not employees and are not paid salaries. Instead, they are paid for their services on a capitation or fee-for-service basis out of a fund drawn from the premiums collected from the subscriber, union, or corporation by an organization that markets the health plan. A withheld amount of up to 30% is used to cover costs of operating the IPA. IPA physicians make contractual arrangements to treat HMO members out of their own offices. A participating physician may also treat non-HMO patients.

---

*Centers for Medicaid and Medicare Services, Room 4350, Cohen Building, 330 Independence Ave., SW, Washington, DC 20201.

*1227 25th St., NW, #610, Washington, DC 20037 (formerly known as the American Association of Foundations for Medical Care).

Preferred Provider Organizations

A **preferred provider organization (PPO)** is another type of managed care plan. A PPO contracts with a group of providers (designated as "preferred") to deliver care to members. PPO members have the freedom to choose any physician or hospital for services, but they receive a high level of benefits if the preferred providers are used. There are usually coinsurance requirements and deductibles, and claims have to be filed. Occasionally, the PPOs pay 100% of the cost of care, but most do not. As with major medical policies, coinsurance requires the patient to pay 20% to 25% of the allowed amount up to a certain point and then the PPO pays 80% to 100% of the balance. Predetermination of benefits may be required, as well as fee limits, quality control, and utilization review. Some hospital indemnity plans pay fixed fees for various services. The patient pays the difference if the charges are higher.

Silent Preferred Provider Organizations

Sometimes, preferred provider payers and plan administrators purchase existing preferred provider networks without talking to those providers who have signed contracts. These may be referred to as *silent, blind, or phantom PPOs, discounted indemnity plans, nondirected PPOs,* or *wraparound PPOs*. They gain the ability to limit reimbursement (lower or discount payments) without the provider's knowledge or consent. Providers that are taken in by silent PPOs are unable to get paid out of network, which reduces their income. Silent PPOs complicate the appeal process because it may be difficult to contact another payer directly and claims may be lost because of timely filing laws. Silent PPOs are considered legitimate in most states. Whenever you see "network discount applied" on an explanation of benefits document, investigate further into the claim to determine whether a silent PPO is operating. To discover silent PPOs, always precertify procedures and look at patients' insurance cards even if the patients are established.

Physician Provider Groups

A **physician provider group (PPG)** is a physician-owned business entity that has the flexibility to deal with all forms of contract medicine and still offer its own packages to business groups, unions, and the general public. One division may function as an IPA under contract to an HMO. Another section may act as the broker or provider in a PPO that contracts with hospitals, as well as other physicians, to market services or medical supplies to employers and other third parties. Still another portion might participate in joint ventures with hospitals, freestanding imaging centers and laboratories, purchase of diagnostic equipment, retail medical equipment as a

corporate subsidiary, and so on. The sideline businesses do not pay dividends but provide income to make future assessments to participating physicians unnecessary. The difference between an IPA and a PPG is that an IPA may not be owned by its member physicians, whereas a PPG is physician owned.

The ability of the PPGs to combine services (joint purchasing, marketing, billing, collections, attorneys, and accountant fees) is an advantage because it cuts down on the cost of running a business and allows each physician to retain his or her own practice in addition to these joint ventures. The physicians turn over a small percentage of their income to the PPG for expenses. Patients call one telephone number to make appointments, and the billing is done in one location.

Point-of-Service Plans

The typical **point-of-service (POS) plan** combines elements of an HMO and a PPO while offering some unique features. It is basically an HMO consisting of a network of physicians and hospitals that provides an insurance company or an employer with discounts on its services. In a POS program, members choose a primary care physician who manages specialty care and referrals. A POS plan allows the covered individual to choose service from a participating or nonparticipating provider, with different benefit levels. The POS program pays members a higher level of benefits when they use program (network) providers. The member may use providers outside the network, but higher deductibles and coinsurance percentages for out-of-network services give members incentives to stay within the network.

The POS plan may also provide nonparticipating benefits through a supplemental major medical policy. The key advantage of POS programs is the combination of HMO-style cost management and PPO-style freedom of choice.

Triple-Option Health Plans

Triple option health plans allow members to select from three choices: HMOs, PPOs, or "traditional" indemnity insurance. Some of these plans allow the employee to change plans more often than traditional arrangements. They incorporate cost containment measures such as precertification for hospital admission, hospital stays, and second surgical opinions.

Provider-Sponsored Organization

A *provider-sponsored organization* (PSO) is a managed care plan that is owned and operated by a hospital and provider group instead of an insurance company.

Table 11-1	Types of Managed Care Organizations and Their Characteristics	
PLAN TYPE	**MEMBER ADVANTAGES**	**MEMBER DISADVANTAGES**
HMO (Health Maintenance Organization)	• Low cost for benefits • Preventive health care • No claim forms • Fixed, low copayments • Low monthly premium • Less out-of-pocket regardless of usage	• Restricted access to providers, tests, hospitals, and treatments except in emergencies or pay a penalty
Group model (open or closed panel)	• Providers care only for plan members	• Must use gatekeeper, approved providers
Staff model	• Providers on staff of HMO	• Must use gatekeeper, approved providers
Network model	• Providers see plan and non-plan patients • Small copayment/office visit • Providers receive capitation fee	• Must use gatekeeper, approved providers
Direct contract model	• Contracted health care services to members by private practice physicians in the community	
EPO (Exclusive Provider Organization)	• Flexible benefit design • Providers give negotiated discounts	• Must use gatekeeper, approved providers except in emergencies • Employer contracts only with one plan • Patient who seeks care outside the network is not reimbursed
IPA (Independent Practice Association)	• Can use services from several affiliated providers, hospitals, or facilities • Out-of-pocket expenses minor	• Must use gatekeeper, approved providers
POS (Point-of-Service Plan)	• Patients choose network or non-network providers • Providers give negotiated discounts • More flexible than basic HMO • Can bypass gatekeeper to see specialist	• Pay more if member sees non-network provider
PPO (Preferred Provider Organization)	• More flexible than HMO • Does not require gatekeeper • Patients may choose network or non-network providers • Providers give negotiated discounts for each service and patients pay a small percentage • Pay less for network provider • Reduced costs for drugs	• Pay more if member sees non-network provider • Preventive services may not be covered • Patients pay a deductible • Claims must be filed • Possible predetermination of benefits • Pay fixed fees and patient pays the difference if bill is higher

Religious Fraternal Benefit Society

A *religious fraternal benefit society* (RFBS) is a managed care option that is associated with a church, group of churches, or convention. Membership is restricted to church members and is allowed regardless of the person's health status.

Tables 11-1 and 11-2 give an overview or summary of five of the most common types of managed care plans.

Employee Retirement Income Security Act

The medical biller should be aware that no matter what the type of plan, coverage is either purchased by an individual or paid by an employer. This is extremely important to know because if the plan is paid by the employer it is regulated by the Employee Retirement Income Security Act (ERISA). However, the passing of the federal legislation known as the Patient Protection and Affordable Care Act (the Affordable Care Act), and H.R. 4872, the Health Care and Education Reconciliation Act of 2010 (the Reconciliation Act) beginning in 2014, almost everyone is required to be insured or they will pay a fine. Small businesses, the self-employed, and the uninsured may pick plans offered through state-based purchasing pools. Large employers with more than 50 employees must pay a $2,000-per-employee fee excluding the first 30 employees from the assessment if the government subsidizes their workers' coverage. ERISA regulates all managed care insurance paid by the employer or supplemented by the employee for the employee's spouse or children, which today is about 85% of the claims that are non-Medicare/Medicaid/workers' compensation. ERISA is regulated by the Department of Labor, and if the plan is an ERISA plan, the State Insurance Commissioners have no power to help with insurance carrier issues. Consequently, if the managed care organization is "related to" an employee benefit plan (EBP), the requirements of ERISA and its regulations are of overriding importance and severely restrict patient rights.

No employer is obligated to establish an EBP. To encourage them to do so, Congress has given them, their

Table 11-2	Financial Systems of Managed Care Plans				
	Network				
PLAN	IN	OUT	COPAY DEDUCTIBLE	PAYMENT METHOD	AUTHORIZATION REQUIRED
HMO	X		Fixed copay	Capitated Fee-for-service (carve outs)	X
PPO	75/25% 80/20% 90/10%	 60/40% 70/30%	Fixed copay Deductible	Fee-for-service	X
IPA	Limit Large group		Fixed copay	Capitated Fee-for-service (carve outs)	X
EPO	X		Fixed copay	Fee-for-service Capitated	X
POS	X	X	Fixed copay Deductible	Fee-for-service Capitated	X

plans, their HMOs and insurers, and their administrators substantial immunities from liability. State regulation of HMOs administered by self-insured EBPs is preempted by ERISA; therefore employees cannot be protected by those state laws that limit the excesses of other HMOs not subject to ERISA.

Any case "relating to" an EBP falls under federal jurisdiction and is always moved from state court to federal court when a lawsuit is initiated. There the patient and provider will find that the usual state law tort claims are also preempted by ERISA; therefore any claims against the HMO or EBP for medical malpractice, wrongful death, fraud, nonpayment or incorrect payment of claims, and so on will be summarily dismissed if filed in state courts. Effective January 1, 2003, changes to ERISA took effect regarding time limitations on claims processing and the appeals process. Therefore you should know whether the policy is paid for by the patient or employer. Refer to the resources at the end of this chapter for more information on ERISA.

At the time of the printing of this edition, the health care reform legislation has not been completely finalized and its impact on ERISA has not been stated. To keep you up to date as legislation is passed, additional provisions will be placed on the Evolve website.

MEDICAL REVIEW

Quality Improvement Organization

A *Quality Improvement Organization* (QIO) program (formerly known as *professional* or *peer review organization*) contracts with CMS to review medical necessity, reasonableness, appropriateness, and completeness and adequacy of inpatient hospital care for which additional payment is sought under the outlier provisions of the Prospective Payment System. Generally, it operates at the state level. A review addresses whether the services met professionally recognized standards of health care and may include whether the appropriate services were provided in appropriate settings. The QIO's professional medical staff performs these reviews. The results of the reviews are submitted to CMS. A review is an evaluation of the quality and efficiency of services rendered by a practicing physician or physicians within the specialty group. Practitioners in a managed care program may come under peer review by a QIO. A review may be used to examine evidence for admission and discharge of a hospital patient and to settle disputes over fees (see Chapter 17). QIOs are not restricted to MCO programs but also play a role in Medicare inpatient cases.

Quality Improvement System for Managed Care

Quality Improvement System for Managed Care (QISMC) is a CMS initiative to strengthen managed care organization efforts to protect and improve the health and satisfaction of Medicare and Medicaid beneficiaries. QISMC adopts a broad definition of "quality" to include the "measurement of health outcomes, consumer satisfaction, accountability of managed care organizations for achieving ongoing quality improvement, the need for intervention to achieve this improvement, and the importance of data collection, analysis, and reporting."

Utilization Review of Management

A management system called **utilization review (UR)** is necessary to control costs in a managed care setting. UR is a formal assessment of the cost and use of components of the health care system. The utilization review committee reviews individual cases to determine medical necessity for medical tests and procedures. It also watches over how providers use medical care resources. If medical care, tests, or procedures are denied, the patient must be informed of the need for the denied service and the risks of not having it. The written reasons for denial let the patient know his or her rights to receive the service and obligation to pay before obtaining such services.

Emphasis is placed on seeing a high volume of patients in a performance-based reimbursement system. **Churning** occurs when a physician sees a patient more than medically necessary, thus increasing revenue through an increased number of services. Churning may be seen in fee-for-service practices, as well as some managed care environments. **Turfing** is the term used when the sickest, high-cost patients are transferred to other physicians so that the provider appears to be a low utilizer. **Buffing** is the term for making this practice look justifiable to the plan. All of these situations may affect UR.

MANAGEMENT OF PLANS

Contracts

Nationwide data from Medirisk, Inc.* can be used to make a knowledgeable financial decision on how a managed care plan will affect an existing medical practice. Data supplied by this company can evaluate existing fees, negotiate with managed care firms, and weigh practice expansions (e.g., add partners or a satellite office). A physician should have the contract reviewed by an attorney before signing a contract with a managed care plan.

Carve Outs

When an MCO contracts with a physician group, the following important considerations should be known:

1. How many patients will the MCO provide?
2. What is the per capita rate (capitation amount per patient)?
3. What services are included in the capitated amount?

Medical services not included in the contract benefits are called **carve outs** (not included within the capitation rate) and may be contracted for separately. For example, if an internist contracts with an MCO, all evaluation and management services, as well as electrocardiograms, spirometries, hematocrits, fasting blood sugar tests, and urinalyses, might be included in the capitation amount that is received per person, per month, regardless of whether any of these services were rendered. However, sigmoidoscopies and hospital visits might be "carved out" of the contract and paid on a fee-for-service basis. Generally, physicians prefer carve outs for expensive procedures when contracting with MCOs.

---

*5901 Peachtree Dunwoody Road, NE, Suite 455, Building B, Atlanta, GA 30328.

PLAN ADMINISTRATION

Patient Information Letter

Inform managed care subscribers in writing what is expected from them and what they can expect in turn. The patient information letter should outline possible restrictions, noncovered items, expectations for copayment, and names of the managed care plans in which the physician is currently participating. Note that if the patient neglects to notify the office of any change about eligibility status in the plan, such as **disenrollment**, the patient is then held personally responsible for the bill. Also mention that the managed care patient must inform the office if hospitalization, surgery, or referral to a specialist is necessary. State that because of restrictions, failure to do so will make the patient liable for denied services. This letter may be referred to as a *waiver of liability* and in the Medicare program is called an *Advance Beneficiary Notice* (ABN). Post a sign in the waiting room advising managed care patients to check with the receptionist about participating plans.

Figure 11-1 is a sample letter of appropriate wording and content. File a copy of the letter given to the patient in the patient's medical record. If the patient refuses to agree with managed care policy, document this in the medical record. Reimbursement may depend on the documentation.

RIGHT TO AUDIT RECORDS

When patients are members of a managed care organization (MCO) and the physician has signed a contract with the MCO that has a clause stating "for quality care purposes, the MCO has a right to access the medical records of their patients and for utilization management purposes," the MCO has a right to audit those patients' financial records that only relate to the medical services provided to the member by the physician.

Medical Records

Manual medical record management may differ when handling multiple managed care contracts. Place colored adhesive dots on patient file folder labels or color-code managed care files by using a different-colored chart for each EPO, HMO, IPA, and PPO patient. This decreases confusion and saves time in identifying individual plans so that coverage, copayment, billing, and authorization requirements are met.

When using an electronic medical record system, the patient's account may be identified with a patient type

---

XYZ MEDICAL GROUP, INC.
1400 Avon Road, Suite 200
Woodland Hills, XY 12345

January 1, 20XX

TO: OUR PATIENTS

RE: PREFERRED PROVIDER ORGANIZATIONS

The following is a list of the PPOs and health insurance plans that we are members of and, therefore, will bill for you:

1. Georgia County Foundation
2. VIP Health Plan
3. Blue Cross Prudent Buyer Plan
4. Georgia County PPO
5. Northwest PPO
6. Blue Shield PPO

We are participating providers in several different PPOs. In order that we may maintain proper records for referrals and/or hospitalization, we request that each patient who is enrolled in a specific PPO keep our office currently informed regarding his or her eligibility status in that plan. Each time you are in the office for a visit, please verify with the receptionist that we have the correct coverage information.

If you have not informed us of changes in the status of your eligibility within the plan, you will be held responsible for any outstanding balance on your account due to that change.

Additionally, when your physician feels it is necessary to either hospitalize you or refer you to another physician outside this group, it is your responsibility to inform your physician that you belong to a specific PPO, as there may be restrictions imposed by that PPO regarding admission and referrals. If you fail to inform your physician at the time of referral or admission, our group may not be held responsible for noncoverage charges due to these restrictions.

If you have any questions regarding the above, please ask to speak to our insurance specialist.

I have read and understand the above text.

Signed: _____ Date: _____
Patient (subscriber)

FIGURE 11-1 Letter to preferred provider organization (PPO) subscribers outlining restrictions and noncovered services.

that corresponds with the insurance plan the patient has joined.

Scheduling Appointments

Screen patients when they call for appointments to determine whether they belong to the same prepaid health plan as the physician. Ask the patient to read from the insurance card to determine whether the physician's name is listed as the patient's primary care physician. Keep on hand an alphabetic list and profile of all plans with which the practice has a signed contract. It might also be useful to have a list of plans to which the practice does not belong. If the patient is not in a participating plan and still wishes to schedule a visit, inform him or her that payment at the time of the appointment is

necessary and the amount is determined by the private fee schedule. This is an excellent idea if the patient is not a member of an HMO. In some states, Florida for example, an HMO patient cannot be billed for services that are covered. The provider must obtain authorization to treat the patient if the person is an HMO patient and the provider is not a participating provider because collecting from the HMO patient could "backfire" on the provider. The patient will pay for the visit, then send a copy of the receipt to his or her HMO. The HMO could file a complaint with the appropriate HMO regulatory agency because the provider treated its client without authorization and billed the client for the balance. The HMO could request a claim form from the provider and the provider would enter his or her private fee, which is more than the provider billed the HMO for another patient. This would open the door to possible fraud and abuse charges. The HMO could contact the patient, stating it should not have had to pay for the visit because the patient was in an HMO. Finally, the patient could demand a refund, and the provider would have no choice but to refund the money because the patient could turn the provider over to the HMO regulatory agency. The assignment of benefits must be checked on the claim form either to the provider or the patient.

Encounter Form

Many managed care plans use an internal document on which the services rendered to the patient are checked off (charge ticket, encounter form, routing slip). It also may be used as a billing statement. The original is forwarded to the health plan's administrative office, and a copy is retained in the physician's files. Some plans require data from such documentation on a CMS-1500 (08-05) Health Insurance Claim form. Examples of encounter forms are shown in Figures 3-11, 8-3, and 10-8.

Preauthorization or Prior Approval

Some managed care plans require preauthorization for certain services or referral of a patient to see a specialist. The following are several types of referrals that a plan may use.

1. **Formal referral.** An authorization request is required by the MCO contract to determine medical necessity. This may be obtained via telephone or a completed authorization form mailed or transmitted via fax (Figure 11-2) or e-mail.
2. **Direct referral.** An authorization request form is completed and signed by the physician and handed to the patient. Certain services may not require completion of a form and may be directly referred (e.g., obstetric care, dermatology).
3. **Verbal referral.** Primary care physician informs the patient and telephones the referring physician that the patient is being referred for an appointment.
4. **Self-referral.** The patient refers himself or herself to a specialist. The patient may be required to inform the primary care physician.

Patients may be unaware of preapproval requirements. A good precaution is to ask the patient about insurance coverage at the time the appointment is made. If the patient is a member of a managed care plan, carefully review the patient's preauthorization requirements. If approval is necessary for certain situations, inform the patient of this before he or she sees the physician. If a patient has obtained the written authorization approval, ask the patient to fax or mail you a copy because it may have an expiration date noted on it. Even if preapproved,

the treatment must be medically necessary or payment may be denied after submission of a claim. If an authorization is delayed and the patient comes in for the appointment, the plan should be called to obtain a verbal authorization. The date, time, and name of the authorizing person should be documented; otherwise, the patient's appointment should be rescheduled. A referral recommendation must be documented in the patient's record and, if applicable, sent to the referring physician.

A tracking system, such as a referral tracking log, should be in place for pending referrals so that care may be rendered in a timely manner and patients do not get "lost" in the system (Figure 11-3). This log should include the date the authorization is requested, the patient's name, procedure or consultant requested, insurance plan, effective and expiration dates, dates of follow-up, name of person who approved or denied the request, and appointment date for consult or procedure. Sometimes, authorization approvals are sent to the primary care physician and not to the referring or ordering physician. In these cases, follow-up must be made with the primary care physician. A maximum 2-week turnaround time should be allowed, and all authorization requests should be tracked.

If a managed care plan refuses to authorize payment for a recommended treatment, tests, or procedures, have the primary care physician send a letter to the plan that is worded similarly to that shown in Figure 11-4. Include medical documentation such as office visit notes, laboratory reports, and x-ray reports to support the insurance claim. Then, after all efforts have been exhausted, send a letter such as that shown in Figure 11-5 to the patient informing him or her of this fact and asking the patient to appeal the denial of benefits.

In some managed care plans, when a primary care physician sends a patient to a specialist for consultation who is not in the managed care plan, the specialist bills the primary care physician. This is done because the primary care physician receives a monthly capitation check from the plan and any care for the patient must come from the capitation pool. This type of plan encourages primary care physicians not to refer patients so that he or she can retain profits.

If a specialist recommends referral to another specialist **(tertiary care)**, be sure the recommendation is in writing. Call the specialist at a later date to determine whether the recommendation was acted on. If the patient refuses to be referred, be sure this is documented. If a referral form is necessary, do not telephone or write a letter. The managed care plan may refuse payment if the proper form is not completed.

College Clinic
4567 Broad Avenue
Woodland Hills, XY 12345-0001
Telephone: (555) 486-9002
Fax: (555) 487-8976

MANAGED CARE PLAN AUTHORIZATION REQUEST

**TO BE COMPLETED BY PRIMARY CARE PHYSICIAN
OR OUTSIDE PROVIDER**

☐ Health Net   ☐ Met Life
☒ Pacificare   ☐ Travelers
☐ Secure Horizons   ☐ Pru Care
☐ Other

Member/Group No.: __54098XX__

Patient Name: __Louann Campbell__   Date: __7-14-20XX__

☐ Male   ☐ Female   Birthdate: __4-7-1952__   Home Telephone Number: __(555) 450-1666__

Address: __2516 Encina Avenue, Woodland Hills, XY 12345-0439__

Primary Care Physician: __Gerald Practon, MD__   Provider ID #: __TC 14021__

Referring Physician: __Gerald Practon, MD__   Provider ID #: __TC 14021__

Referred to: __Raymond Skeleton, MD__   Office Telephone number: __(555) 486-9002__

Address: __4567 Broad Avenue, Woodland Hills, XY 12345__

Diagnosis Code: __724.2__   Diagnosis __Low back pain__

Diagnosis Code: __722.10__   Diagnosis __Sciatica__

Treatment Plan: __Orthopedic consultation and evaluation of lumbar spine; R/O herniated disc L4-5__

Authorization requested for: ☐ Consult only   ☐ Treatment only   ☐ Consult/Treatment
☐ Consult/Procedure/Surgery   ☐ Diagnostic Tests

Procedure Code: __99244__   Description: __New patient consultation__

Procedure Code: _____   Description: _____

Place of service: ☒ Office ☐ Outpatient ☐ Inpatient ☐ Other   Number of Visits: __1__

Facility: _____   Length of Stay: _____

List of potential future consultants (i.e., anesthetists, surgical assistants, or medical/surgical):

Physician's Signature: __Gerald Practon, MD__

TO BE COMPLETED BY PRIMARY CARE PHYSICIAN

PCP Recommendations: __See above__   PCP Initials: __GP__

Date eligibility checked: __7-14-20XX__   Effective Date: __1-15-20XX__

TO BE COMPLETED BY UTILIZATION MANAGEMENT

Authorized: _____ Auth. No. _____ Not Authorized _____

Deferred: _____ Modified: _____

Effective date: _____ Expiration date: _____ Number of visits: _____

FIGURE 11-2 A managed care plan treatment authorization request form completed by a primary care physician for preauthorization of a professional service.

When a referral authorization form is received, make a copy of the form for each approved office visit, laboratory test, or series of treatments. Then use the form as a reference to bill for the service. All copies being used indicates that all services the patient's plan has approved are completed. Ask the primary care physician or the managed care plan for a new authorization to continue treatment on the patient. The request should be generated in a timely manner so that treatment is not delayed.

AUTHORIZATION REQUEST LOG

Date requested	Patient name	Procedure/ consult	Insurance plan	1st F/U	2nd F/U	3rd F/U	Approved	Scheduled date
2/8/XX	Juan Percy	Bone scan- full body	Health Net	2/20			J. Smith	2/23/XX
2/8/XX	Nathan Takai	MRI-L-knee	Pru-Care	2/20	3/3			
2/9/XX	Lori Smythe	Consult Neuro G. Frankel MD	FHP	2/22			T. Hope	2/26/XX
2/10/XX	Bob Mason	Cervical collar	Secure Horizons	2/22	3/5	3/19		

FIGURE 11-3 An authorization request log to be used as a system for tracing referral of patients for diagnostic testing, procedures, and consultations.

Ms. Jane Smith
Chairperson
Utilization Review Committee
ABC Managed Care Plan
111 Main Street
Anytown, XY 12345-0122

Dear Ms. Smith:

On _____ I prescribed_____ for_____ .
     Date   List treatment, test, procedure Patient's name

On _____ you refused to authorize for that treatment. I find that I
     Date
must take issue with your determination for the following reasons:

In my medical judgment, the treatment is a very important part of my overall care of _____
_____ . This patient suffers from _____ . The treatment is
Patient's name   Describe condition
necessary to _____ . Failure to perform the treatment could
          Describe why necessary
result in the following problem(s):

Enclosed are copies of the laboratory and radiological reports. For these reasons, I urge you to reconsider your refusal to authorize payment for the procedure I have prescribed.

By copy of this letter to_____ I am reiterating my suggestion that
          Patient's name
he/she obtain the treatment despite your refusal to authorize payment, for the reasons I have set forth in this letter and in prior discussions with _____ .
                                   Patient's name

Yours truly,

John Doe, MD
Enclosures
cc: (Name of patient)

FIGURE 11-4 A letter to a managed care plan when there is a refusal to authorize payment for a recommended treatment, test, or procedure.

Mr. Avery Johnson
130 Sylvia Street
Anytown, XY 12345-0022

Dear Mr. Johnson:

On _____ I prescribed _____ for you. On _____ ,
    Date   Treatment, test, procedure   Date

_____ refused to authorize for same. On that basis,
   Name of Managed Care Plan
you have informed me of your decision to forego the treatment I have prescribed. I
expressed my concerns regarding your decision during our discussion on _____ about
                                                        Date
the potential ramifications of your refusal to undergo the treatment.

The purpose of this letter is to recommend that you appeal_____
                                              Name of Managed Care Plan's
denial of benefits and reconsider your decision to forego the treatment in light of the
potential consequences of your refusal.

Should you wish to discuss this further, please do not hesitate to contact me.

Sincerely yours,

John Doe, MD

FIGURE 11-5 A letter sent by the provider to inform the patient about refusal of payment for treatment, test, or procedure by the managed care plan.

Diagnostic Tests

Many managed care plans require that patients have laboratory and radiology tests performed at plan-specified facilities. These are referred to as *network facilities*. Obtain the necessary authorizations for such services and allow sufficient time to receive the test or x-ray results before the patient's return appointment. When verifying benefits, ask if the deductible applies; that is, if a provider orders a radiology service that is on site, the deductible may not apply, but if the patient is sent to an outside facility, the deductible applies.

Inform the patient ahead of time when there is doubt about coverage for a test or the managed care plan indicates a test is not covered. Disclose the cost and have the patient sign a waiver agreement to pay for the service, thus enabling the billing of the patient for the service. If an authorization is denied because a test is deemed "medically unnecessary" and the physician wishes to appeal, the physician can present clinical reasons to the MCO's medical director to receive approval and bring attention to possible expansion of benefits for future patients.

Managed Care Guide

Creating a grid or matrix of all MCOs with which the practice has contracts can help you keep up with the growth of local managed care plans and remember which physician belongs to which plan in the practice. Use a sheet of paper and list each plan with billing address vertically in a column to the left, and then list significant data horizontally across the top. Suggested titles for column categories are as follows: eligibility telephone numbers, copayment amounts, preauthorization requirements, restrictions on tests frequently ordered, participating laboratories, participating hospitals, and the contract's time limit for promised payment. Referring to this grid can provide specifics at a glance about each plan's coverage and copayment amounts (Figure 11-6). Some practices keep this information in a three-ring binder with dividers for each insurance plan. A good procedure is to include this information on each patient's data sheet when benefits are verified.

FINANCIAL MANAGEMENT

Payment
Deductibles

Usually there is no **deductible** for a managed care plan. However, if there is one, be sure to verify with the insurance company, ask patients if they have met their deductibles, and collect them in the early months of the year (January through April). Deductibles are applied to claims as they are received and processed by the plan.

MANAGED CARE PLAN REFERENCE GUIDE

Plan name/address	Telephone eligibility	Copay	Preauthorization requirements	Test restrictions	Contracted lab(s) radiology	Contracted hospital(s)	Promised payment
Aetna PPO POB 43 WH XY 12345	555-239-0067	$5	hosp/surg/all dx tests	PE 1/yr	ABC Labs	College Hosp	30 days
Blue PPO POB 24335 WH XY 12345	555-245-0899	$8	referral specialist	PE 1/yr	Main St. Lab	St. John MC	30 days
Health Net POB 54000 WH XY 12345	555-408-5466	$5	hosp/surg see check list referrals	Mammo-gram 1/yr	Valley Lab	St. Joseph MC	45 days
Travelers MCO POB 1200 WH XY 12345	555-435-9877	$10	surg/hosp admit referrals	Pap >50 q3yr <50 q1yr	College Hosp Metro Lab	College Hosp	30 days

FIGURE 11-6 Managed care plan quick reference guide to help keep track of specifics for each managed care plan in which the physician participates.

Copayments

In a managed care plan, a **copayment** is a predetermined fee paid by the patient to the provider at the time service is rendered. It is commonly referred to as a *copay* and is a form of cost sharing because the managed care plan or insurance company pays the remaining cost. Remember to verify the copayment amount when inquiring about insurance plan benefits. Always collect the copay at the time of the patient's office visit. Billing for small amounts is not cost effective. Copays are commonly made for office visits, prescription drugs, inpatient mental health services, urgent care visits, and emergency department visits. However, the amount may vary according to the type of service. In some plans, there may be a separate copayment for x-ray studies and durable medical equipment.

Payment Mechanisms

Payment mechanisms in managed care plans vary and can range from fee-for-service and capitation to salaried physicians. Following are some details about other payment mechanisms.

Contact Capitation. Contact capitation is based on the concept of paying physicians for actual patient visits or "contacts." A scenario under this payment method is when a patient is referred to a specialist for care. A "contact" occurs when the patient visits the specialist for treatment. The patient is assigned to the specialist for a defined period of time called the contact period. The

length of the contact period is set in advance for each type of specialty by the participating specialty physician panel and MCO and may be tailored to the demographic and practice needs of the group. Each new patient visit during a contact period initiates a "contact point." Contact points determine how much to pay each physician. The average contact point value is determined by dividing the net specialty capitation pool or total amount of money set aside to be used for a particular specialty by the number of contacts in a certain time period. The average contact value is used to determine the amount paid to each specialist during each month in the contact period.

Case Rate Pricing. For specialists, another payment method is case rate pricing. This means the specialist contracts with the managed care plan for an entire episode of care. This may be done for certain high-volume, expensive surgical procedures (e.g., knee surgery, cataracts, bypass surgery).

Stop-Loss Limit. Some contracts have a **stop-loss** section, which means that if the patient's services are more than a certain amount, the physician can begin asking the patient to pay (fee for service). Monitor each patient's financial accounting record in those instances.

Contract Payment Time Limits

Usually state laws dictate the time limit within which a managed care plan must pay. The contract may or may not state the terms of payment, time limits, and late payment penalties, all of which can vary from one plan to another. Prompt payment laws require payment within 30, 45, 55, or 60 days. To diminish late payment of claims, a contract can specify that late claims accrue interest (e.g., 5% interest for claims paid after the payment time limit has elapsed). Some states have enacted laws enforcing interest penalties for late payment for either or both private payers, as well as managed care plans. Therefore know the laws for the pertinent state. A time limit payment provision is an important factor to consider when reviewing a contract before a medical practice participates.

Monitoring Payment

Monitor payments made from all managed care plans and note whether the payment received is less than the agreed amount as stated in the contract. If payment has been reduced, send a letter to the plan citing, "As per contract, see page xx about the fee for the consultation."

Sometimes a procedure (e.g., angioplasty with an assistant) may be done and the plan will not pay for an assistant, stating that it is not usual practice. However, perhaps the standard practice in a specific region is to always use an assistant for an angioplasty. When this is emphasized, the plan may remit additional payment.

Some states may have screening fees for emergency services and may or may not require prior approval for such services as defined by the Consolidated Omnibus Budget Reconciliation Act of 1985 (COBRA). Some states have adjudication laws with penalties if the managed care plan does not pay promptly. The following steps should be taken if claims are not paid in a timely manner (30 days):

1. Write to the plan representative and list the unpaid claims, claims paid after the payment time limit, and claims paid in error.
2. Send a statement to the director of the managed care plan notifying him or her that if the bill is not paid, the employer's benefits manager or patient will be contacted and alerted to outstanding, slow-paying accounts. Explain that this will prevent the physician from renewing the plan's contract, and ask the recipient to contact the plan's representative. The consumer has a choice of managed care plans; if the present plan does not fulfill his or her expectations, then the managed care plan loses members because of dissatisfaction.
3. Take examples and statistics to the next renegotiating session when the physician's contract is expiring.

Chapters 9 and 10 present information on how to handle slow or delinquent managed care plan payers.

Statement of Remittance

Managed care plans pay by either a capitation system (monthly check for the number of patients in the plan) or on the basis of the services given to the patient (monthly check with a statement of remittance or explanation of benefits [EOB]).

In the capitation system, a monthly check arrives written out for the total amount of monthly capitation. The accompanying paperwork lists all eligible patients being paid for on a per capita basis divided into two groups, commercial and senior. Patients categorized as commercial are usually younger than age 65 and are paid at a lesser rate because their risk is lower (e.g., they do not need to see the doctor frequently). The senior patient category includes those older than 65 years of age; these are paid at a higher rate because of the increased risk. Always verify the individual capitated amounts listed by each name on the accompanying paperwork against the monthly eligibility list to balance the amount of the check. Contact the MCO if an error appears. If a specialist is capitated, there may be thousands of patients on the capitation plan and a list of patients will not be provided. The capitation amount for a specialist may be only a few cents per month calculated according to the risk of the patient needing specialty services.

In the system when payment is based on services rendered and a statement of remittance or EOB is generated, such statements itemize services that have been rendered to patients and usually indicate the amount billed, amount allowed, amount paid, and any copayment to be made by the patient (Figure 11-7). Generally patients under managed care plans do not receive an EOB. Payments are checked against the managed care contract for verification and then posted to the patients' accounts. An error should be brought to the attention of the plan's administrator and, depending on the circumstances, appealed.

Accounting

Managed care plans vary in their financial reimbursement structure, and careful accounting procedures are required. Accounting can become a confusing issue because of mixture of private and managed care patients with copayment requirements, coinsurance amounts, deductibles, and withholds. Good practice management software is designed to separately handle each plan in the computer to eliminate mistakes.

Fee-for-Service

Some medical practices handle managed care patient accounts the same as fee-for-service patient accounts. If

STATEMENT OF REMITTANCE

PATIENT NAME (ID NUMBER)	SERVICE DATE MO. DAY YR	P O S	NO SVC	PROCEDURE NUMBER AND DESCRIPTION	AMOUNT BILLED	AMOUNT ALLOWED	RISK WITHHELD	CO PAY	AMOUNT PAID	ADJ. CODE
380224171-01 ALAN E.				CLAIM NO. 62730406 ACCOUNT NO.						
	092620XX	03	1 81000 URINALYSIS-ROUTINE		1000	1000	100	0	900	
	092620XX	03	1 82270 OCCULT BLOOD ANY S		1200	1200	120	0	1080	
	092620XX	03	1 99243 COMPRE RE-EXAM OR		6500	6500	650	0	5850	
	092620XX	03	1 36415 VENIPUNCTURE W/CEN		1700	1700	170	0	1530	
			CLAIM TOTALS =		10400	10400	1040	0	9360	
558700321-01 RONALD B.				CLAIM NO. 62730407 ACCOUNT NO.						
	092520XX	03	1 90050 LIM EXAM EVAL A/O		3000	3000	300	300	2400	
			CLAIM TOTALS =		3000	3000	300	300	2400	
473760096-01 DORMA L.				CLAIM NO. 62730408 ACCOUNT NO.						
	092520XX	03	1 90050 LIM EXAM EVAL A/O		3000	3000	300	300	2400	
			CLAIM TOTALS =		3800	3000	300	380	3120	

VENDOR SUMMARY: TOTAL AMOUNT PAID $1,638.96 TOTAL WITHHELD $194.39

AMOUNT PAID YEAR-TO-DATE: $42,411.95 AMOUNT WITHHELD YEAR-TO-DATE $5,109.94

Adjustment Code Legend
A = Adjusted: Billed amount exceeds VIP allowed.
O = Claim for service denied. Charges for this service included in other benefit payment. No patient liability.

FIGURE 11-7 Statement of remittance or explanation of benefits for noncapitated patients or contracted fee for service indicating the amount billed, amount allowed, amount paid, and any copayment that is to be made by the patient.

coinsurance payment is necessary at the time of service, post first the charge and then the coinsurance prepayment, either calculated based on the percentage of the charge the plan allows or the flat copayment amount (e.g., $15 for each office visit). After receiving the EOB document from the insurance plan, post an adjustment entry of the disallowed amount, which is calculated on a percentage of the MCO's allowable charge to balance the account (Figure 11-8). An overpayment should be shown as a refund or credit to the account.

Year-End Evaluation
Withhold

Depending on the contract, a managed care plan may retain a percentage of the monthly capitation payment or a percentage of the allowable charges to physicians until the end of the year to cover operating expenses. This is known as **withhold**. A statement of remittance from the MCO shows the risk amounts withheld for each patient's visit in the eighth column of Figure 11-7. The withhold plus interest is returned to the physician at the end of the plan-year if the budgeted services for the plan are not overused. However, the withhold or a portion of it is retained by the plan if services are overused. Thus the

physicians share in any surplus or pay part of any deficit at year's end. This risk sharing creates an incentive for limiting care by the gatekeeper and limiting referrals to specialists, thereby keeping medical costs down. The withhold can cover all services or be specific to hospital care, **ancillary services** (laboratory/x-ray use), or specialty referrals.

A managed care plan that withholds a percentage of the allowable charge must be tracked in the physician's accounts receivable so that it is not prematurely written off as a bad debt. To do this, develop a capitation accounting worksheet listing the dates of service, patients' names, CPT code for the service rendered, fee-for-service charges, withheld amounts, and disallowed amounts (Figure 11-9). Then total all columns. The total of the withheld column is a debit entry that indicates what the managed care plan owes to the medical practice pending its year-end reconciliation. If and when the withheld amount arrives, the accounting worksheet can be compared with the amount withheld during the year. The amount of withholds that are not returned to the physician is adjusted once withholds are settled. The total of the column for disallowed amounts shows the amount written off by the medical practice. Combine the withheld returned amount with the

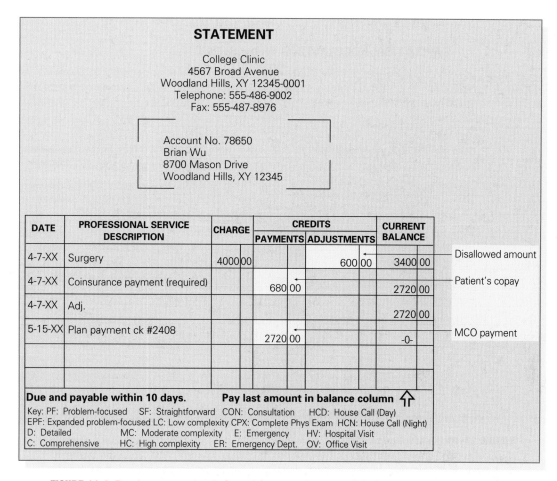

STATEMENT

College Clinic
4567 Broad Avenue
Woodland Hills, XY 12345-0001
Telephone: 555-486-9002
Fax: 555-487-8976

Account No. 78650
Brian Wu
8700 Mason Drive
Woodland Hills, XY 12345

DATE	PROFESSIONAL SERVICE DESCRIPTION	CHARGE	CREDITS PAYMENTS	CREDITS ADJUSTMENTS	CURRENT BALANCE	
4-7-XX	Surgery	4000 00		600 00	3400 00	Disallowed amount
4-7-XX	Coinsurance payment (required)		680 00		2720 00	Patient's copay
4-7-XX	Adj.				2720 00	
5-15-XX	Plan payment ck #2408		2720 00		-0-	MCO payment

Due and payable within 10 days.   **Pay last amount in balance column** ⇑

Key: PF: Problem-focused   SF: Straightforward CON: Consultation   HCD: House Call (Day)
EPF: Expanded problem-focused LC: Low complexity CPX: Complete Phys Exam HCN: House Call (Night)
D: Detailed   MC: Moderate complexity   E: Emergency   HV: Hospital Visit
C: Comprehensive   HC: High complexity   ER: Emergency Dept.   OV: Office Visit

FIGURE 11-8 Posting to a patient's financial accounting record (ledger card) showing charge of $4000. The plan allows $3400; therefore the patient's prepaid coinsurance amount is $680 (20% of $3400). The managed care plan sent a check for $2720 (80% of $3400), and the disallowed amount ($600) is adjusted off the account, which brings the account balance to zero.

DEBIT

Date	Patient	Service	Charge	Withhold	Disallow	
5/15/20XX	Mason	99204	106.11	5.94	21.22	Disallowed amounts
5/15/20XX	Mason	93000	34.26	1.92	3.43	
5/15/20XX	Mason	81000	8.00	.38	2.40	
5/15/20XX	Self	93501	1500.00	240.00	300.00	
Total			1648.38	248.24	327.05	Total withheld amount owed by MCO

FIGURE 11-9 A managed care plan when payment is on a fee-for-service basis. Note the disallowed portion of the charge, which is based on the plan's allowable charge. A portion of the allowable charge is withheld.

managed care payment for the year to determine whether it is worthwhile for the practice to participate in the plan. Some practices can use the information to renegotiate increased fees when the managed care contract is to be renewed.

Capitation Versus Fee-for-Service

Financial management reports are generated via computer and are the responsibility of the manager or accountant in most medical practices. However, it can be an asset for an insurance biller to have some knowledge of

CAPITATION ACCOUNTING WORKSHEET

NAME OF PLAN ABC Managed Care Plan

DATE OF SERVICE	PROFESSIONAL SERVICE DESCRIPTION	CHARGES Services Fees	PAYMENTS Capitation	Copay	
20XX 1/15	Capitation (105 members) @ $8 ea		840.00*		Capitation payment
2/15	Capitation (115 members)		920.00		
2/20	Sanchez OV/Copay	35.00		5.00*	Copayment amount
2/22	Jones OV/Copay	35.00		5.00	
2/23	Davis OV/Copay	35.00*		5.00	Actual fee-for-service charge
3/6	Evans OV/Copay	35.00		5.00	
3/15	Capitation (130 members)		1040.00		
4/10	Wu OV/Copay	35.00		5.00	
4/15	Capitation (135 members)		1080.00		
	May through December are not shown				
END OF YEAR TOTALS		3500.00	6880.00	500.00	

FIGURE 11-10 An accounting sheet for a capitation plan from January through April showing dates of service, professional service descriptions, members' charges, and capitation payments and copayments received by the medical practice. Charges and payments columns may be totaled at the end of the year to compare capitation with fee-for-service earnings.

the content of these reports. Most medical practices monitor plan payments for profit or loss by comparing actual income from managed care patients with what would have been received from fee-for-service plans. To do this, one designs a capitation accounting sheet for each capitated plan. This sheet shows a listing of dates of service and professional service descriptions (procedures, injections, and laboratory work), as well as charges and payments (Figure 11-10). As managed care plan patients receive services, actual service fees are posted in a charge column from the office fee schedule as if the patient were a private payer. In a payment column, office visit, copayments, and the monthly capitation payment are posted. Then all columns are totaled. It is necessary to apply a discount to the total charged amount for a realistic comparison because the physician is usually paid on an allowed amount rather than an actual charge. Calculate the difference between the actual charge and the average allowed amount to do this.

Compare the capitated payment amounts plus copayment amounts with the total discounted charges at the end of the year. This gives an accurate idea of whether the capitated payment received is adequate for the services the physician performed. Compiling monthly records and reviewing them at the end of the year helps a medical practice assess the gain or loss of each capitation plan.

Bankruptcy

If an MCO declares bankruptcy, such as a Chapter 11 filing, it is obligated to pay all bills incurred before the filing. However, in some situations, another entity may take over the plan and all services incurred after filing are paid by the new payer. If the patient had treatment before the filing, a delay in getting reimbursed may occur because the MCO cannot repay debts incurred before its filing until it has worked out a reorganization plan. Physicians under contract with the MCO are obligated to honor their contractual commitments. If their contracts expire or if they have escape clauses, they may be required to continue accepting patients, depending on the contract provisions.

Some clauses allow a physician to withdraw from seeing managed care patients or leave if the MCO is in bankruptcy proceedings for more than 4 months. However, bankruptcy courts have broad powers to prevent physicians from leaving MCOs in bankruptcy proceedings if the court deems such actions to be detrimental to the rehabilitation of the debtor.

For additional information on the topic of bankruptcy, see Chapter 10.

KEY POINTS

This is a brief chapter review or summary of the key issues presented. To further enhance your knowledge of the technical subject matter, review the key terms and key abbreviations for this chapter by locating the meanings in the glossary at the end of this book that appear in a section before the index.

1. Providers must be contracted with Blue Cross/Blue Shield to receive payment as a member physician. Patients may have a traditional fee-for-service or one of many types of managed care plans. Plan benefits and coverage, as well as deductibles and copayments, vary.

2. Managed care plans are prepayment health care programs in which a specified set of health benefits are provided in exchange for a yearly fee or fixed periodic payments to the provider of service. Patients join the plan and pay monthly medical insurance premiums individually or through their employer. Patients pay a small copayment and sometimes a deductible for medical services.

3. Primary care physicians act as gatekeepers who control patient access to specialists and diagnostic testing services.

4. Health maintenance organizations have models such as prepaid group practice model, staff model, network HMO, and direct contract model.

5. The Patient Protection and Affordable Care Act (the Affordable Care Act), and H.R. 4872, the Health Care and Education Reconciliation Act of 2010 (the Reconciliation Act) have provisions effective within a year that include the following: forbids insurers from canceling insurance coverage *(rescission)*, eliminates preexisting condition exclusions, ends lifetime limits on benefits, gives tax credits to small businesses that offer coverage, provides temporary insurance until 2014 for people who have been denied because of their health status, allows young people to remain on their parents' insurance until age 26, requires insurers to use a high percentage of premiums for benefits instead of profits or overhead, makes some preventive measures free, and almost everyone is required to be insured or they will pay a fine.

6. Types of managed care plans are the EPO, FMC, IPA, PPO, silent preferred provider organization, PPG, POS plan, triple-option health plan, PSO, and RFBS.

7. Managed care plans, such as employee benefit plans (EBPs) purchased by employers, must comply with the federal regulations of ERISA and do not fall under state laws.

8. The QIO program, formerly the peer review organization, evaluates cases to determine appropriateness, medical necessity, and quality of care.

9. UR is a process based on established criteria for evaluating and controlling the medical necessity of services and providers' use of medical care resources to curb expenditures.

10. Some managed care plans may require prior approval for certain medical services or referral of a patient to a specialist. Four types of referrals are formal referral, direct referral, verbal referral, and self-referral.

11. If a contract has a stop-loss limit, it means that the provider can begin asking the patient to pay the fee for the service when the patient's services are more than a specific amount.

12. A managed care plan that has a withhold provision may retain a percentage of the monthly capitation payment or a percentage of the allowable charges to physicians until the end of the year to cover operating expenses.

⊖volve INTERNET RESOURCES

For active links to the following resources, visit the Evolve website at
http://evolve.elsevier.com/fordney/handbook

- America's Health Insurance Plans (AHIP), formerly known as American Association of Health Plans (AAHP), American Managed Care and Review Association, and American Association of Foundations for Medical Care.

- Employee Retirement Income Security Act (ERISA). Do a search and select "E." ERISA is listed as a selection.
- *Federal Register*
- *Glossary of Managed Care Terminology*
- *Managed Care Museum*
- National Committee for Quality Assurance

STUDENT ASSIGNMENT

✓ Study Chapter 11.

✓ Answer the fill-in-the-blank, multiple choice, and true/false review questions in the *Workbook* to reinforce the theory learned in this chapter and to help prepare you for a future test.

✓ Complete the assignments in the *Workbook* to give you hands-on experience in abstracting information from a medical record to complete treatment authorization forms for prepaid health insurance cases.

✓ Turn to the glossary at the end of this textbook for a further understanding of the key terms and key abbreviations used in this chapter.

KEY TERMS*

Advance Beneficiary Notice of
  Noncoverage
approved charges
assignment
benefit period
Centers for Medicare and
  Medicaid Services
Correct Coding Initiative
crossover claim
diagnostic cost groups
disabled
end-stage renal disease
formulary
hospice
hospital insurance
intermediate care facilities
limiting charge
medical necessity

Medicare
Medicare administrative
  contractors
Medicare Part A
Medicare Part B
Medicare Part C
Medicare Part D
Medicare/Medicaid
Medicare Secondary Payer
Medicare Summary Notice
Medigap
national alphanumeric codes
nonparticipating physician
nursing facility
participating physician
Physician Quality Reporting
  Initiative
premium

prospective payment system
Quality Improvement
  Organization
qui tam action
reasonable fee
Recovery Audit Contractor
  Initiative
relative value unit
remittance advice
resource-based relative value
  scale
respite care
Supplemental Security Income
supplementary medical
  insurance
volume performance standard
whistleblowers

KEY ABBREVIATIONS*

ABN	ICFs	NEMB	PSO
CAP	ICU	NF	QIO
CCI	LCD	nonpar provider	RA
CLIA	LGHP	OASDI	RAC initiative
CMS	LMRP	OBRA	RBRVS
COBRA	MAAC	OCNA	RFBS
DC	MACs	OIG	RVU
DCGs	Medi-Medi	OR	SMI
DEFRA	MG	par provider	SOF
DME	MMA	PAYRID	SSI
EGHP	MSA	PFFS plan	TEFRA
ERA	MSN	PIN	VPS
ESRD	MSP	PPS	
GPCI	NCDs	PQRI	

---

*Definitions for the key terms and key abbreviations are located near the back of this textbook in the glossary.

CHAPTER

12

Medicare

OBJECTIVES

After reading this chapter, you should be able to:

- Explain eligibility criteria for Medicare.
- Name important information to abstract from a patient's Medicare card.
- Identify the benefits and nonbenefits of Medicare.
- Calculate a payment for a procedure using the current conversion factor.
- List five federal laws adopted to increase health benefits for employed elderly individuals.
- Name the conditions when an HMO-Medicare patient can be seen by a nonmember HMO physician.
- Differentiate between an HMO risk plan and an HMO cost plan.
- Name the federal program that relates to utilization and quality control of health services.
- State the name of the federal act applicable to reducing fraud and abuse.

- State the benefits for a participating versus nonparticipating physician.
- Explain when to obtain a patient's signature on an Advance Beneficiary Notice of Noncoverage or waiver of liability agreement.
- Define a Medicare-mandated prepayment screen.
- List situations for obtaining an annual patient's signature authorization.
- Determine the time limit requirements for transmitting a Medicare claim.
- Explain claims submission for individuals who have Medicare with other insurance.
- List CMS-1500 (08-05) block numbers that require Medigap information when transmitting a Medicare/Medigap claim.
- Post information on the patient's financial accounting record after a Medicare payment has been received.

Service to Patients

Remind the patient to bring in his or her insurance identification card or cards. Give assistance to patients who may be visually impaired or have hearing impairment and need to complete registration forms for filing insurance claims. Work closely with caregivers and be aware of each patient's limitations, caring for each one with dignity.

Answer the patient's questions about Medicare Summary Notice documents because these can be confusing to elderly patients and can lead to misunderstandings about payments for services rendered.

BACKGROUND

Although Social Security is one of the United States' most important domestic programs, this system is by no means the first. A number of social insurance programs existed throughout Europe and Latin America before the Social Security Act was signed into law in 1935. Before the United States had Social Security, 20 other nations already had similar systems in operation. Another 30 countries had different social insurance programs in place, such as workers' compensation.

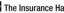

POLICIES AND REGULATIONS

Medicare is administered by the **Centers for Medicare and Medicaid Services (CMS).** It is subdivided into three divisions with the following responsibilities:

1. The Center for Medicare Management oversees traditional fee-for-service Medicare, including development of payment policy and management of fee-for-service contractors.
2. The Center for Beneficiary Choices provides beneficiaries with information on Medicare, Medicare Select, and Medicare Plus (+) Choice programs and Medigap (MG) options. It also manages the Medicare+Choice plans, consumer research, and grievance and appeals functions.
3. The Center for Medicaid and State Operations focuses on federal-state programs such as Medicaid, the State Children's Health Insurance Program, insurance regulations, and the Clinical Laboratory Improvement Amendments (CLIA).
4. CMS also enforces the insurance portability and transaction and code set requirements of the Health Insurance Portability and Accountability Act (HIPAA).

Eligibility Requirements

The Social Security Administration (SSA) offices take applications for Social Security, control the eligibility process, and provide information about the Medicare program. If an individual already receives Social Security or Railroad Retirement benefits, he or she is automatically enrolled in Medicare Parts A and B starting the first day of the month that the individual turns 65 years of age. In the year 2000, the retirement age gradually increased for people born in the year 1938 or later. By 2027, full-time retirement age will be 67 for people born after 1959. Benefits may increase if retirement is delayed beyond full-retirement age. As of this edition, Medicare still may begin at age 65. Those who apply for Social Security early (at age 62 years) do not receive Medicare but receive monthly reduced Social Security benefits. If an individual is younger than 65 years of age and disabled, he or she will automatically get Medicare Parts A and B after getting Social Security disability or Railroad Retirement benefits for 24 months. An individual does not have to be retired to receive Medicare benefits.

Medicare is a federal health insurance program for the following categories of people:

1. People 65 years of age or older who are on Social Security
2. People 65 years of age or older who are retired from the railroad or Civil Service

3. **Disabled** individuals who are eligible for Social Security disability benefits* and who are in the following categories:
   a. Disabled workers of any age
   b. Disabled widows of workers who are fully or currently insured through the federal government, Civil Service, SSA, **Supplemental Security Income (SSI),** or the Railroad Retirement Act and whose husbands qualified for benefits under one of these programs
   c. Adults disabled before age 18 years whose parents are eligible for or retired on Social Security benefits
4. Children and adults who have chronic kidney disease requiring dialysis or **end-stage renal disease (ESRD)** requiring a kidney transplant
5. Kidney donors (all expenses related to the kidney transplantation are covered)

All persons who meet one of the previously stated eligibility requirements determined by SSA are eligible for **Medicare Part A** (hospital coverage) at no charge. Those who qualify for full Medicare benefits may also elect to take **Medicare Part B** (outpatient coverage). Medicare Part B recipients pay annually increasing basic premiums to the SSA, and some pay a Medicare surtax on federal income tax payments. This premium may be deducted automatically from the patient's monthly Social Security check if he or she wishes. Those individuals not eligible for Medicare Part A (hospital insurance) at 65 years of age may purchase Part B from the SSA.

Aliens

An alien (may be referred to as an immigrant when a person from another country comes to settle) is an individual who is not a citizen or national of the United States but belongs to another country or people. In the Medicare program, an alien may be eligible for Part A or B coverage. To be eligible, the applicant must have lived in the United States as a permanent resident for 5 consecutive years. It is usually not necessary to state on the CMS-1500 (08-05) form that the patient is an alien when billing Medicare.

Health Insurance Card

The patient should present his or her Medicare health insurance card. It indicates the patient's name and insurance claim number (Figures 12-1 and 12-2) that must be abstracted from the card and used when transmitting a

---

*In the disabled categories, a person must be disabled for not less than 12 months to apply for disability benefits. A disabled beneficiary must receive disability benefits for 24 months before Medicare benefits begin. See Chapter 16 for further information on this topic.

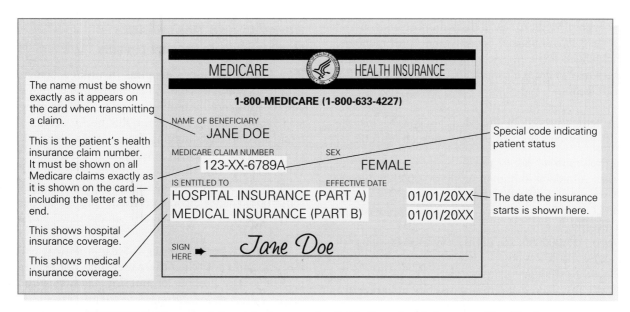

The name must be shown exactly as it appears on the card when transmitting a claim.

This is the patient's health insurance claim number. It must be shown on all Medicare claims exactly as it is shown on the card — including the letter at the end.

This shows hospital insurance coverage.

This shows medical insurance coverage.

MEDICARE ✦ HEALTH INSURANCE

1-800-MEDICARE (1-800-633-4227)

NAME OF BENEFICIARY
JANE DOE

MEDICARE CLAIM NUMBER   SEX
123-XX-6789A   FEMALE

IS ENTITLED TO   EFFECTIVE DATE
HOSPITAL INSURANCE (PART A) 01/01/20XX
MEDICAL INSURANCE (PART B)   01/01/20XX

SIGN HERE ➡ *Jane Doe*

Special code indicating patient status

The date the insurance starts is shown here.

FIGURE 12-1 Important information on a patient's Medicare health insurance identification card.

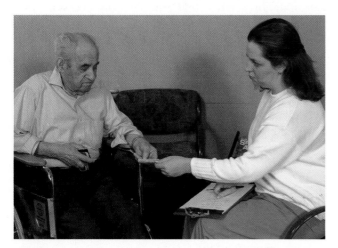

FIGURE 12-2 Insurance billing specialist obtaining the identification card from a disabled Medicare patient.

claim. The claim number is the Social Security number of the wage earner with an alpha suffix. The card indicates hospital and medical coverage, effective date, and patient status. Verify effective date because Part A and Part B may have different effective dates. If a beneficiary applies after his or her eligibility date, Part B could have a future date shown on the card. When a husband and wife both have Medicare, they receive separate cards and claim numbers. However, a spouse's card might have the husband's claim number if she has never worked and has no SSA work credits. Medicare cards are red, white, and blue, and cards issued after 1990 are plastic. In addition, ask to see the patient's Part D card for prescription coverage. If it shows a health maintenance organization (e.g., Kaiser or Secure Horizons), then you know that the

patient signed up and is covered by a managed care plan and not the Medicare standard program. The physician may or may not have a contract with that plan, so coverage for services would be in question. Then ask to see the insurance card for the managed care plan.

The Centers for Medicare and Medicaid Services (CMS) discourages the transmission of Social Security numbers in whole on documents that pertain to a Medicare beneficiary. Some medical practices use only the last four digits of the Social Security number or a medical record number to protect the patient's identity.

The letters after the Medicare number on the patient's identification card indicate the patient's status as follows (this is only a partial listing):

A = wage earner (shown in Figure 12-1)
B = husband's number (wife 62 years or older)
D = widow
HAD = disabled adult
C = disabled child
J, Kl, or Jl = special monthly benefits, never worked under Social Security
M = Part B benefits only
T = entitled to hospital and/or medical insurance benefits but is not entitled to monthly Social Security benefits

A patient whose Medicare card claim number ends in "A" has the same Social Security and claim numbers. A patient whose Medicare card claim number ends in "B" or "D" has *different* Social Security and claim numbers. A quick check between Social Security and card claim numbers may identify a submission error and forestall a claims rejection.

The letters preceding the Medicare number on the patient's identification card indicate railroad retirees:

A = retired railroad employee
Examples: A 000000 (6 digits); A 000-00-0000 (9 digits)
MA = spouse of a retired railroad employee
WA/WD = widow or widower of deceased employee (age or disability)
Examples: WA000000 (6 digits); WA000-00-0000 (9 digits)
CA = child or student
WCA/WCD = widow of retiree with child in her care or disabled child of deceased employee
PA/PD = parent of deceased employee (male or female)
H = Railroad Retirement Board pensioner before 1937
MH = wife of Railroad Retirement Board pensioner before 1937
WH = widowed wife of Railroad Retirement Board pensioner before 1937
WCH = widow of Railroad Retirement Board pensioner with child in her care
PH = parent of Railroad Retirement Board pensioner before 1937
JA = widow receiving a joint and survivor annuity
X = divorced spouse's annuity, for use on forms AA-3 and AA-7 only
Example: CA 123-45-6789C

Enrollment Status

Under Medicare Part B, if an individual receiving Social Security or Railroad Retirement benefits did not sign up for Medicare at the time of eligibility, then an individual is eligible to enroll in Medicare 3 months before his or her 65th birthday. The enrollment period ends 3 months after the month in which the person turns 65. If the enrollment period is missed, the individual must wait until the next general enrollment period, January 1 through March 31, of the following year.

A telephone hotline, or in some states, a modem connection, is available to verify the enrollment status. This is useful because patients can switch coverage to a senior managed care plan on a month-to-month basis. Most carriers also allow information on deductible status. The patient's numeric information (Medicare number and date of birth) is entered into the telephone system, and the digital response indicates how much of the deductible has been satisfied. Contact the local Medicare administrative contractor (MAC) for information about this service.

Benefits and Nonbenefits
Medicare Part A: Hospital Benefits

Part A of Medicare is **hospital insurance** benefits for people 65 years of age or older, for people younger than age 65 with certain disabilities, or for people with end-stage renal disease. Funds for this health service come from special contributions from employees and self-employed persons, with employers matching contributions. These contributions are collected along with regular Social Security contributions from wages and self-employment income earned during a person's working years.

A **benefit period** begins the day a patient enters a hospital and ends when the patient has not been a bed patient in any hospital or **nursing facility (NF)** (formerly called *skilled nursing facility*) for 60 consecutive days. It also ends if a patient has been in a nursing facility but has not received skilled nursing care for 60 consecutive days. A nursing facility offers nursing or rehabilitation services that are medically necessary to a patient's recovery. Services provided are not custodial. Custodial services are those that assist the patient with personal needs (e.g., dressing, eating, bathing, and getting in and out of bed). Hospital insurance protection is renewed every time the patient begins a new benefit period. There is no limit to the number of benefit periods a patient can have for hospital or nursing facility care. However, special limited benefit periods apply to hospice care.

Medicare Part A provides benefits to applicants in any of the following situations:

1. A bed patient in a hospital (up to 90 hospital days for each benefit period)
2. A bed patient in a nursing facility receiving skilled nursing care (up to 100 extended-care days for each benefit period)
3. A patient receiving home health care services
4. A patient who needs care in a psychiatric hospital (up to 190 days in a lifetime)
5. A terminally ill patient diagnosed as having 6 months or less to live who needs hospice care. A **hospice** is a public agency or private organization that is primarily engaged in providing pain relief, symptom management, and supportive services to terminally ill people and their families.
6. A terminally ill patient who needs respite care. **Respite care** is a short-term inpatient stay that may be necessary for the terminally ill patient to give temporary relief to the person who regularly assists with home care. Inpatient respite care is limited to stays of no more than 5 consecutive days for each respite period.

MEDICARE (PART A): HOSPITAL INSURANCE–COVERED SERVICES FOR 2011

Services	Benefit	Medicare Pays	Patient Pays
HOSPITALIZATION Semiprivate room and board, general nursing and miscellaneous hospital services and supplies. (Medicare payments based on benefit periods.)	First 60 days	All but $1132	$1132 deductible
	61st to 90th day 91st to 150th day[1]	All but $283 a day	$283 a day
	60-reserve-days benefit	All but $566 a day	$566 a day
	Beyond 150 days	Nothing	All costs
NURSING FACILITY CARE Patient must have been in a hospital for at least 3 days and enter a Medicare-approved facility generally within 30 days after hospital discharge.[2] (Medicare payments based on benefit periods.)	First 20 days	100% of approved amount	Nothing
	21st to 100th day	All but $141.50 a day	Up to $141.50 a day
	Beyond 100 days	Nothing	All costs
HOME HEALTH CARE Part-time or intermittent skilled care, home health aide services, durable medical equipment and supplies, and other services.	Unlimited as long as Medicare conditions are met and services are declared "medically necessary."	100% of approved amount; 80% of approved amount for durable medical equipment.	Nothing for services; 20% of approved amount for durable medical equipment.
HOSPICE CARE Pain relief, symptom management, and support services for the terminally ill.	If patient elects the hospice option and as long as doctor certifies need.	All but limited costs for outpatient drugs and inpatient respite care.	Limited cost sharing for outpatient drugs and inpatient respite care.
BLOOD	Unlimited if medically necessary.	All but first 3 pints per calendar year.	For first 3 pints.[3]

[1] This 60-reserve-days benefit may be used only once in a lifetime.
[2] Neither Medicare nor private Medigap insurance will pay for most long-term nursing home care.
[3] To the extent the blood deductible is met under Part B of Medicare during the calendar year, it does not have to be met under Part A.

FIGURE 12-3 Five major classifications of Medicare Part A benefits. (Updated from Medicare and You 2011, US Government Printing Office.)

Figure 12-3 contains information on five major classifications of inpatient hospital cost-sharing benefits for Medicare Part A. Miscellaneous hospital services and supplies might consist of intensive care unit (ICU) costs, blood transfusions, drugs, x-ray and laboratory tests, medical supplies (casts, surgical dressings, and splints), use of wheelchair, operating room (OR) and recovery room costs, and therapy (physical, occupational, and speech language). There are no benefits for personal convenience items (television, radio, and telephone), private duty nurses, or a private room unless the private room is determined medically necessary. Similar benefits also relate to nursing facilities.

Benefits for hospice and respite care consist of nursing and physicians' services, drugs, therapy (physical, occupational, and speech-language pathology), home health aide, homemaker services, medical social services, medical supplies and appliances, short-term inpatient care, and counseling.

Medicare Part B: Medical and Preventive Care Benefits

Part B of Medicare is **supplementary medical insurance (SMI)** benefits for the aged and disabled. Funds for this program come equally from those who sign up for it and the federal government. A medical insurance **premium** is automatically deducted from monthly checks for those who receive Social Security benefits, Railroad Retirement benefits, or a Civil Service annuity. Others pay the premium directly to the SSA. In some states, when a person is eligible for Medicare Part B and Medicaid, Medicaid pays for the monthly Part B premiums.

Table 12-1 contains information on medical and preventive care benefits for Medicare Part B. In addition to medical and surgical services by a doctor of medicine (MD), doctor of osteopathy (DO or MD), or a doctor of dental medicine or dental surgery (DDS), certain services by a doctor of podiatric medicine (DPM) and limited

Table 12-1	Medicare (Part B): Medical Insurance–Covered Services and Preventive Care Benefits for 2011		
SERVICES	**COVERAGE REQUIREMENTS AND LIMITATIONS**	**MEDICARE PAYS**	**PATIENT PAYS**
Ambulance services	For transportation to a hospital or skilled nursing facility	80% of approved amount after deductible	$162 deductible* plus 20% of approved amount or limited charges†
Ambulatory surgery center	Facility fees are covered for approved services	80% of approved amount after deductible	$162 deductible plus 20% of approved amount
Blood	Pints of blood as an outpatient or as part of a Part B–covered service	80% of approved amount	First 3 pints plus 20% of approved amounts for additional pints (after $162 deductible)‡
Bone mass measurement	Once every 24 months for qualified individuals and more frequently if medically necessary	100% of approved amount	Nothing for test
Cardiovascular screening	Every 5 years to test cholesterol, lipid, and triglyceride levels for heart attack or stroke prevention	100% of approved amount	Nothing for tests
Chiropractic services	Limited services to correct subluxation using manipulation	80% of approved amount after deductible	$162 deductible plus 20% of approved amount
Clinical laboratory services	Includes blood tests, urinalysis, and some screening tests	100% of approved amount	Nothing for tests
Clinical trials	Tests new types of medical care to prevent, diagnose, or treat diseases	80% of approved amount after deductible	$162 deductible plus 20% of approved amount
Colorectal cancer screening (one or more of the following tests may be covered)§			
Fecal occult blood test	Once every 12 months	100% of approved amount	Nothing for test
Flexible sigmoidoscopy	Once every 48 months if age 50 or older, or every 120 months when used instead of a colonoscopy for those not at high risk	100% of approved amount	Nothing for test
Screening colonoscopy	Once every 120 months (high risk every 24 months)	100% of approved amount	Nothing for test
Barium enema	Once every 48 months if age 50 or older (high risk every 24 months) when used instead of sigmoidoscopy or colonoscopy	80% of approved amount after deductible	Part B deductible does not apply; 20% of approved amount
Diabetes screening	Twice a year for glucose monitors, test strips, and lancets	100% of approved amount	Nothing for screening
Diabetes self-management training	Provider must issue a written order	80% of approved amount after deductible	$162 deductible plus 20% of approved amount
Diabetic supplies	Includes glucose testing monitors, test strips, lancet devices, lancets, glucose control solutions, and therapeutic shoes. Syringes and insulin covered if used with an insulin pump or if patient has Part D coverage	80% of approved amount after deductible	$162 deductible plus 20% of approved amount
Doctor services	No coverage for routine physical examinations except for one-time "Welcome to Medicare" physical examination	80% of approved amount after deductible	$162 deductible plus 20% of approved amount
Durable medical equipment	Oxygen, wheelchairs, walkers, and hospital beds for home use	80% of approved amount	20% of approved amount
Emergency department services	Bad injury or sudden illness when patient is in serious danger	80% of approved amount after deductible	$162 deductible plus 20% of approved amount
Eyeglasses	One pair of glasses with standard frames after cataract surgery that implants an intraocular lens	80% of approved amount after deductible	$162 deductible plus 20% of approved amount
Flu shots	Annually to prevent influenza or flu virus	100% of approved amount	Nothing for flu shots
Foot examinations and treatment	For diabetes-related nerve damage	80% of approved amount after deductible	$162 deductible plus 20% of approved amount
Glaucoma screening	Once every 12 months	80% of approved amount after deductible	$162 deductible plus 20% of approved amount

Table 12-1	Medicare (Part B): Medical Insurance–Covered Services and Preventive Care Benefits for 2011—cont'd		
SERVICES	**COVERAGE REQUIREMENTS AND LIMITATIONS**	**MEDICARE PAYS**	**PATIENT PAYS**
Hearing and balance examination	Ordered by a doctor to determine whether medical treatment is necessary. Hearing aids and examinations for fitting hearing aids are not covered	80% of approved amount after deductible	$162 deductible plus 20% of approved amount
Hepatitis B shots	Three shots for people with high or intermediate risk	100% of approved amount	Nothing for shots
HIV screening	Once every 12 months	80% of approved amount for office visit	Nothing for test; 20% of approved amount for office visit
Home health services	Limited to reasonable and necessary part-time or intermittent skilled nursing care, home health aide services, physical therapy, and speech-language pathology. Also includes durable medical equipment	100% of approved amount; 80% of approved amount for durable medical equipment	Nothing for services; 20% of approved amount for durable medical equipment
Kidney dialysis services and supplies	In a facility or at home	80% of approved amount after deductible	$162 deductible plus 20% of approved amount
Mammogram screening§	Once every 12 months also covers digital technologies	100% of approved amount	Nothing for screening
Medical nutrition therapy services	For people who have diabetes or renal disease not on dialysis or with a doctor's referral 3 years after a kidney transplantation	80% of approved amount after deductible	$162 deductible plus 20% of approved amount
Mental health care (outpatient)	Certain limits and conditions apply	50% of approved amount after deductible	$162 deductible plus 20% of approved amount
Occupational therapy	To help patients return to usual activities after an illness (e.g., bathing)	100% of approved amount after deductible	$162 deductible plus 20% of approved amount
Outpatient hospital services	When received as part of a doctor's care	Medicare payment to hospital based on hospital cost	$162 deductible plus 20% of whatever the hospital charges
Outpatient medical and surgical services and supplies	For approved procedures	80% of approved amount after deductible	$162 deductible plus 20% of approved amount
Papanicolaou (Pap) test/pelvic§	Once every 24 months (low risk) and once every 12 months (high risk)	100% of approved amount	Nothing for test
Physical examination	One-time "Welcome to Medicare" physical examination within first 12 months patient is on Part B	80% of approved amount after deductible	$162 deductible plus 20% of approved amount
Physical therapy	Heat, light, exercise, and massage treatment of injuries and disease	100% of approved amount after deductible	$162 deductible plus 20% of approved amount
Pneumococcal pneumonia vaccine (PPV)	Once in a lifetime	100% of approved amount	Nothing for flu and PPV if doctor accepts assignment
Practitioner services	Clinical social worker, physician assistant, and nurse practitioner	80% of approved amount after deductible	$162 deductible plus 20% of approved amount
Prescription drugs	Certain injectable cancer drugs. Drug coverage for patients who have Part D	80% of approved amount	$162 deductible plus 20% after deductible of approved amount
Prostate cancer screening§	Prostate-specific antigen (PSA) test and digital rectal examination once every 12 months	100% of approved amount	Nothing for test
Prosthetic/orthotic items	Arm, leg, back, and neck braces; artificial eyes; artificial limbs and replacement parts; breast prostheses after mastectomy; prosthetic devices to replace an internal body part or function (includes ostomy supplies and parenteral and enteral nutrition therapy)	80% of approved amount after deductible	$162 deductible plus 20% of approved amount
Second surgical opinions	Covered in some cases. Some third surgical opinions are covered for surgery that is not an emergency	80% of approved amount after deductible	$162 deductible plus 20% of approved amount

Table 12-1	Medicare (Part B): Medical Insurance–Covered Services and Preventive Care Benefits for 2011—cont'd		
SERVICES	COVERAGE REQUIREMENTS AND LIMITATIONS	MEDICARE PAYS	PATIENT PAYS
Smoking cessation counseling	Eight face-to-face visits during a 12-month period if diagnosed with a smoking-related illness or if taking medicine that is affected by tobacco	100% of approved amount	Nothing for counseling sessions
Speech-language pathology services	To regain and strengthen speech skills	100% of approved amount after deductible	$162 deductible plus 20% of approved amount
Surgical dressings	For surgical or surgically treated wound	80% of approved amount after deductible	$162 deductible plus 20% of approved amount
Telemedicine	For some rural areas in a practitioner's office, hospital, or federally qualified health center	80% of approved amount after deductible	$162 deductible plus 20% of approved amount
Tests	X-rays, magnetic resonance imaging, computed tomography scans, electrocardiograms, and some other diagnostic tests	80% of approved amount after deductible	$162 deductible plus 20% of approved amount
Transplant services	Heart, lung, kidney, pancreas, intestine, and liver transplants; bone marrow and cornea transplants; immunosuppressive drugs	80% of approved amount after deductible	$162 deductible plus 20% of approved amount
Travel	Services in United States, District of Columbia, Puerto Rico, Virgin Islands, Guam, Northern Mariana Islands, American Samoa, and Canada or on board a ship within U.S. territorial waters	80% of approved amount after deductible	$162 deductible plus 20% of approved amount

*Once the patient has had $162 of expenses for covered services in the year, the Part B deductible does not apply to any further covered services received for the rest of the year.
†See Figure 12-7 for an explanation of approved amount for participating physicians and limited charges for nonparticipating physicians.
‡To the extent the blood deductible is met under Part A of Medicare during the calendar year, it does not have to be met under Part B.
§Patient Protection and Affordable Care Act of 2010 made this preventive test free.

services by a doctor of chiropractic (DC) are paid for. Dental care is covered only for fractures or surgery of the jaw. Optometric examinations are provided if a person has aphakia (absence of the natural lens of the eye). In 2010, the Patient Protection and Affordable Care Act (the Affordable Care Act) makes preventive measures free to Medicare beneficiaries such as screenings for colon, prostate, and breast cancer.

Nonbenefits. Nonbenefits, also referred to as *noncovered services*, consist of routine physical examination, routine foot care, eye or hearing examinations, and cosmetic surgery unless caused by injury or performed to improve functioning of a malformed part. A physician may bill a patient separately for noncovered services.

Other benefits and nonbenefits are too numerous to list here. Refer to Medicare newsletters or contact the Medicare carrier to find out whether a particular procedure qualifies for payment.

Medicare Part C: Medicare Advantage Plan

The Balanced Budget Act of 1997 created **Medicare Part C**, commonly referred to as *Medicare Advantage Plan* (MA plan), formerly called *Medicare+Choice*. The program

was introduced in 2004 and by 2006 replaced Medicare+Choice. This program was formed to increase the number of health care options in addition to those that are available under Part A and Part B. A Medicare beneficiary can join an MA plan if he or she has both Parts A and B and lives in the service area of the plan. Individuals who have ESRD must meet special situational requirements to join an MA plan. Individuals who sign up for MA plans are issued an insurance card and do not use the Medicare Part A and B card. Medicare Advantage Plans receive a fixed amount of money from Medicare to spend on their Medicare members. Some plans may require members to pay a premium similar to the Medicare Part B premium. In 2010, national health care reform legislation froze payments to these plans with cuts in the following years. It is predicted that enrollees may lose some benefits such as free eyeglasses and hearing aides.

Plans available under this program may include the following: health maintenance organization (HMO), point-of-service (POS) plan, preferred provider organization (PPO), private fee-for-service (PFFS) plan, provider-sponsored organization (PSO), religious fraternal benefit society (RFBS), and a pilot program, Medicare medical savings account (MSA). In an MSA plan, the patient chooses an insurance policy approved by Medicare that has a high annual deductible. Medicare pays the premiums for this policy and deposits the dollar amount difference between what it pays for the average beneficiary in the patient's area and the cost of the premium into the patient's MSA. The patient uses the MSA money to pay medical expenses until the high deductible is reached. If the MSA money becomes depleted, the patient pays out of pocket until the deductible is reached. Unused funds roll over for use the next year.

Medicare Part D

The Medicare Prescription Drug Improvement and Modernization Act (MMA) became effective in 2003, but drug benefits began January 1, 2006. This legislation known as **Medicare Part D** provides seniors and people living with disabilities with a prescription drug benefit. It covers prescription drugs used for conditions not already covered by Parts A and B. It is a stand-alone prescription drug plan offered by insurance companies and other private companies providing drug coverage that meet standards established by Medicare. Other names for these plans are *Part D private prescription drug plans* (PDPs) and *Medicare Advantage prescription drug plans* (MA-PDs).

The two ways to get Medicare prescription drug coverage are as follows:

1. Join a Medicare prescription drug plan that adds drug coverage to the original Medicare plan, some Medicare cost plans, some Medicare private fee-for-service plans, and Medicare medical savings account plans.
2. Join a Medicare Advantage plan, such as an HMO or PPO, that includes prescription drug coverage as part of the plan.

Individuals who enroll pay a monthly premium. Those who decide not to enroll in a Medicare drug plan when they are first eligible may pay a penalty if they decide to join later. Beginning in 2007, enrollees pay an annual deductible of $310 with an estimated premium of $38.94 a month (varies, depending on plan) and a copayment of drug costs up to $2830 in a year. After that, enrollees pay all drug costs until they have spent $4550 out-of-pocket, which is sometimes referred to as the *doughnut hole*. This does not include the drug plan's premium. At that point, the coverage gap ends and the enrollees pay a small coinsurance (5%) or a small copayment ($5 to $10) for each prescription until the end of the year. In 2010, national health care reform legislation provided a $250 rebate for all Medicare Part D enrollees who cross into the doughnut hole to help pay for the drugs. In addition, patients in the coverage gap receive a 50% discount on brand-name drugs. The federal government will close the doughnut hole by providing subsidies for brand-name drugs beginning at 2.5% and will increase to 25% by 2020. In 2011, it will begin subsidies for generic name drugs at 7% of the cost.

People eligible for Medicaid and Medicare pay no premium or deductible and have no gap in coverage. They pay $1 per prescription for generics and $3 for brand names. Copayments are waived for those in nursing homes. In addition, several programs help people who have limited income and resources, and the programs, qualifications, and copayments vary by areas.

Prescription drug plans refer to the drugs in their formularies by tier numbers. A **formulary** is a list of the drugs that a plan covers. Tier one represents generic drugs and has a low copayment associated with it. Tier two covers preferred brand drugs and has a copayment, but higher than tier one. Tier three drugs are the non-preferred drugs and could have either a copayment or a percentage of full drug cost associated with it. The fourth classification, identified as "S," represents specialty drugs and requires a percentage of total cost of the drug. Following are several classes of drugs excluded from coverage:

- Barbiturates
- Benzodiazepines
- Drugs for cosmetic purposes
- Drugs for symptomatic relief of cough and colds
- Drugs for weight loss or gain
- Erectile dysfunction drugs
- Fertility drugs
- Prescription vitamins or minerals except prenatal

A provider who prescribes a drug that can be covered by either Part B or Part D must clarify the condition and part coverage on the prescription form (Example 12-1). A bonus is given to providers who electronically prescribe drugs and as of 2010, Healthcare Common Procedure Coding System (HCPCS) code G8553 should be used for reporting.

Example 12-1 **Prescription Note Clarifying Medical Use of Drug and Coverage Determination**

Patient with psoriasis (autoimmune disorder) is prescribed methotrexate. Generally, this immunosuppressive drug is prescribed for transplant patients and is covered under Part B.

Added prescription note should read: "Psoriasis for Part D."

When a patient has coverage under a Part D plan, obtain a photocopy of either the patient's Medicare supplement or the patient's Medicare Advantage plan card. Then check whether the drug that the patient needs is covered by the plan, which generic drugs are available, and whether a drug needs prior authorization. Either telephone the number listed on the card or use a free software program—Epocrates—that is available to providers to help with these needs. Refer to the Internet Resources at the end of this chapter. To learn more about Epocrates, go to the Evolve website and click on the link for Epocrates.

Railroad Retirement Benefits

Railroad Retirement Board offices maintain eligibility records for Medicare and provide information about the program for railroad workers and their beneficiaries. Medical insurance premiums are automatically deducted from the monthly checks of people who receive Railroad Retirement benefits. Those who do not receive a monthly check pay their premiums directly or in some cases, have premiums paid on their behalf under a state assistance program. If the allowed fees differ from those allowed by the regular Medicare carrier, write or fax the Medicare railroad retiree carrier, asking that fees be based on fee data from the local carrier.

Railroad Retirement beneficiaries generally are entitled to benefits for covered services received from a qualified American facility. However, under certain circumstances, a Medicare beneficiary may receive care in Canada or Mexico. Benefits and deductibles under Parts A and B are the same as for other Medicare recipients.

Some railroad retirees are members of a railroad hospital association or a prepayment plan. These members pay regular premiums to the plan and then receive health services that the plan provides without additional charges. In some plans, small charges are made for certain services such as drugs or home visits. Many prepayment plans make arrangements with Medicare to receive direct payments for services they furnish that are covered under Medicare Part B. Some prepayment plans have contracts with Medicare as HMOs or competitive medical plans and can receive direct payment for services covered by either hospital or medical insurance. After a claim is transmitted to the Medicare railroad retiree carrier, which is usually to a different regional MAC, a remittance advice (RA) document is generated explaining the decision made on the claim and what services Medicare paid for.

Employed Elderly Benefits

To understand various types of scenarios that may be encountered when transmitting claims for elderly individuals, one must know about several federal laws that regulate health care coverage of those age 65 and older who are employed. Such individuals may have group insurance or a Medigap (MG) policy and may fall under billing categories of Medicare first payer or Medicare secondary payer (all are presented in detail later in this chapter). The federal laws that affect employed elderly individuals are shown in Box 12-1.

ADDITIONAL INSURANCE PROGRAMS

Many Medicare recipients have Medicare in combination with other insurance plans. This section explains various coverage combinations. Guidelines for processing claims for these plans are presented later in this chapter.

Medicare/Medicaid

Patients designated as **Medicare/Medicaid (Medi-Medi)** are on both Medicare and Medicaid simultaneously. These patients qualify for Old Age, Survivors, and Disability Insurance (OASDI) assistance benefits (older than age 65), are severely disabled, or are blind.

Medicare/Medigap

A specialized insurance policy devised for the Medicare beneficiary is called **Medigap (MG)** or *Medifill*. This type of policy is designed to supplement coverage under a fee-for-service Medicare plan. It may cover prescription costs and the deductible and copayment (e.g., 20% of the Medicare allowed amount) that are typically the patient's responsibility under Medicare. These plans are offered by private third-party payers to Medicare beneficiaries who pay the monthly premiums for this supplemental insurance.

The federal government in conjunction with the insurance industry established predefined minimum benefits for 10 MG policies categorized by alpha letters A through J (Figure 12-4). Basic benefits are found in policy A. Each subsequent letter represents basic benefits plus other coverage, with the most comprehensive benefits in policy J. Sale of all policies are not available in all states, so individuals in some states have fewer options than others.

A slightly different variation of the MG policy is *Medicare Select*. This policy has the same coverage as regular MG policies, but there is a restriction in that the beneficiary must obtain medical care from a list of specified network doctors and providers.

Medicare Secondary Payer

In some instances, Medicare is considered secondary and classifies the situation as **Medicare Secondary Payer (MSP)**. MSP may involve aged or disabled patients with the following qualities:

Box 12-1 Federal Laws Affecting Employed Elderly Individuals

Omnibus Budget Reconciliation Act

The Omnibus Budget Reconciliation Act (OBRA) of 1981 required that in the case of a current or former employee or dependent younger than age 65 years and eligible for Medicare solely because of ESRD, the employer's group coverage is primary for up to 30 months. The Balanced Budget Act of 1997 mandated this change in the length of the coordination period. OBRA applies to all employers regardless of the number of employees. OBRA of 1986, effective in 1987, required that, if an employee or dependent younger than age 65 years has Medicare coverage because of a disability other than ESRD, the group coverage is primary and Medicare is secondary. This act applies only to large group health plans having at least 100 full- or part-time employees.

Tax Equity and Fiscal Responsibility Act

The Tax Equity and Fiscal Responsibility Act (TEFRA) of 1982 established that an employee or spouse age 65 to 69 years is entitled to the same health insurance benefits offered under the same conditions to younger employees and their spouses. The group insurance is primary and Medicare is secondary. TEFRA applies to employers with at least 20 full- or part-time employees.

Deficit Reduction Act

The Deficit Reduction Act (DEFRA) of 1984, effective 1985, was an amendment to TEFRA and stated that a spouse age 65 to 69 years or an employee of any age is entitled to the same group health plan offered to younger employees and their spouses. The group's coverage is primary and Medicare is secondary. DEFRA applies to employers with at least 20 full- or part-time employees.

Consolidated Omnibus Budget Reconciliation Act

The Consolidated Omnibus Budget Reconciliation Act (COBRA) of 1985, effective 1986, is another amendment to TEFRA eliminating the age ceiling of 69 years. An employee or spouse age 65 or older is entitled to the same group health plan offered to younger employees and their spouses. COBRA requires that third-party payers reimburse for certain care rendered in government-run veteran and military hospitals. The group's coverage is primary and Medicare is secondary. COBRA applies to employers with at least 20 full- or part-time employees.

Tax Reform Act

The Tax Reform Act was passed in 1986 and clarified certain aspects of COBRA. A spouse and dependents may elect to receive continued coverage even if the employee does not wish insurance coverage and terminates the plan. However, the spouse and dependents must have been covered under the plan before the covered employee terminates it. Spouses who are widowed or divorced while receiving continued coverage must report such changes to the benefit plan administrator within 60 days of the employee's death to determine how many additional months of coverage are available.

ESRD, End-stage renal disease.

Medigap Plans Effective on or after June 1, 2010

If a checkmark appears in a column of this chart, the Medigap policy covers 100% of the described benefit. If a column lists a percentage, the policy covers that percentage of the described benefit. If a column is blank, the policy doesn't cover that benefit. NOTE: The Medigap policy covers coinsurance only after the insured has paid the deductible (unless the Medigap policy also covers the deductible).

Medigap Benefits	A	B	C	D	F*	G	K	L	M	N
Medicare Part A Coinsurance hospital costs up to an additional 365 days after Medicare benefits are used up	√	√	√	√	√	√	√	√	√	√
Medicare Part B Coinsurance or Copayment	√	√	√	√	√	√	50%	75%	√	√***
Blood (First 3 Pints)	√	√	√	√	√	√	50%	75%	√	√
Part A Hospice Care Coinsurance or Copayment	√	√	√	√	√	√	50%	75%	√	√
Skilled Nursing Facility Care Coinsurance			√	√	√	√	50%	75%	√	√
Medicare Part A Deductible		√	√	√	√	√	50%	75%	50%	√
Medicare Part B Deductible			√		√					
Medicare Part B Excess Charges					√	√				
Foreign Travel Emergency (Up to Plan Limits)			√	√	√	√			√	√
Medicare Preventive Care Part B Coinsurance	√	√	√	√	√	√	√	√	√	√

Out-of pocket limit**: $4,620 $2,310

*Plan F also offers a high-deductible plan. This means the insured must pay for Medicare-covered costs up to the deductible amount $2,000 in 2010 before your Medigap plan pays anything.

**After meeting the out-of-pocket yearly limit and the yearly Part B deductible ($162 in 2011), the Medigap plan pays 100% of covered services for the rest of the calendar year. Out-of-pocket limit is the maximum amount the insured would pay for coinsurance and copayments.

***Plan N pays 100% of the Part B coinsurance except up to $20 copayment for office visits and up to $50 for emergency department visits.

FIGURE 12-4 Medigap Plans effective June 1, 2010 from a Medicare government publication.

- Aged workers under group health plans with more than 20 covered employees
- Disabled individuals age 64 and younger who are covered under a group health plan with more than 100 covered employees or covered under a family member's current employment
- Medicare beneficiaries under an employer-sponsored group health plan that have end-stage renal disease during the first 18 months of the patient's eligibility for Medicare
- Cases of workers' compensation when the injury or illness occurs at work
- Individuals either currently or formerly employed with black lung disease who fall under the Federal Black Lung Program
- Individuals receiving benefits under the Department of Veterans Affairs (VA) and Medicare
- Individuals covered under a Federal Research Grant Program
- Automobile accident cases such as medical no-fault cases and third-party liability insurance cases

Follow the suggested steps in the procedure at the end of the chapter to identify whether Medicare is primary or secondary and to determine what additional benefits the patient might have.

Managed Care and Medicare

When a patient's primary insurance is a managed care plan that requires fixed copayments, it is possible to obtain reimbursement from Medicare for those amounts. An assigned MSP claim must be filed with Medicare after the managed care organization (MCO) has paid. When Medicare's copayment reimbursement has been received, the provider must refund to the patient the copayment amount previously collected.

The practice is paid a capitated amount and there is no explanation of benefits (EOB) document. Have the patient sign a statement that explains the situation. Attach the statement and the copayment receipts to the claim. The statement may read as shown in the following box:

Patient Name _____

Medicare Number _____

There is no Explanation of Benefits documentation available for the attached billed services. I am currently enrolled with _____ managed care plan for my health care. My physician, _____ MD, is paid on a capitated basis, and the copayment that I pay is $ _____ for each service or visit.

Patient's signature_____

Date _____

A nonparticipating physician (nonpar) must file an unassigned MSP claim. The patient is directly reimbursed by Medicare and no refund is necessary.

Automobile or Liability Insurance Coverage

Liability insurance is not secondary to Medicare because there is no contractual relationship between the injured party and third-party payer. A physician who treats a Medicare patient who has filed a liability claim must bill the liability insurer first unless the insurer will not pay promptly (e.g., within 120 days after the liability insurance claim is filed). After 120 days have gone by without a payment from the liability insurer and if the services performed are covered Medicare benefits, a participating (par) or nonpar physician may seek conditional payment from Medicare. However, if a claim is filed with Medicare, the provider must drop the claim against the liability insurer.

If the payment made by the liability insurer is less than the physician's full charge, the physician may file an assigned claim and must accept as full payment the greater of either the Medicare-approved charge or sum of the liability insurance primary payment and the Medicare secondary payment.

A nonpar physician may file an unassigned claim for Medicare secondary payment only if the payment by the liability insurer is less than the Medicare limiting charge. If the payment equals or exceeds the limiting charge, the physician must accept the disbursement as full payment.

If Medicare payments have been made but should not have been because the services are excluded under this provision, or if the payments were made on a conditional basis, they are subject to recovery. A copy of the notice of payment or denial form from the other insurer should be included when sending in the CMS-1500 (08-05) claim form. Medicare is secondary even if a state law or a private contract of insurance states that Medicare is primary. The physician must bill the other insurer first. A claim for secondary benefits may be transmitted to Medicare only after payment or denial has been made by the primary coverage. Liability insurance is not considered an MSP.

MEDICARE MANAGED CARE PLANS

Health Maintenance Organizations

During the spring of 1984, the Department of Health and Human Services published regulations giving Medicare enrollees the right to join and assign their Medicare benefits to HMOs. HMOs had been in operation for

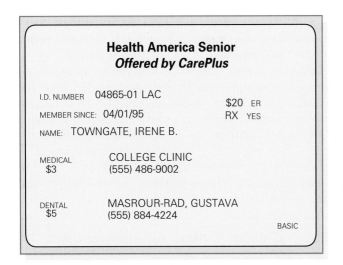

FIGURE 12-5 A senior managed care plan card.

nearly 50 years when they became available as an option for Medicare enrollees. With a Medicare HMO (also known as a senior HMO or senior plan), the patient does not need a Medicare supplemental insurance plan. On enrollment, the Medicare beneficiary is sent an insurance card from the managed care plan (Figure 12-5). However, Medicare cards are not forfeited, and an elderly patient may show two cards, leading to confusion about what the coverage is and whom to bill.

Medicare makes payments directly to the HMO on a monthly basis for Medicare enrollees who use the HMO option. Enrollees pay the HMO a monthly premium, which is an estimate of the coinsurance amounts for which the enrollee would be responsible plus the Medicare deductible. It appears that HMOs contracting to provide services for Medicare patients will be converted to a Medicare Advantage Plan (MA plan) as their contract renewal dates occur.

Some HMOs provide services not usually covered by Medicare such as eyeglasses, prescription drugs, and routine physical examinations. Once a person has converted from Medicare to an HMO, he or she cannot go back to a former physician of personal choice and expect Medicare to pay the bill. The patient should receive services from a physician and hospital facility that are contracted with the HMO plan.

If a Medicare patient has switched over to a managed care plan and wishes to disenroll, the patient must do the following:

1. Notify the plan in writing of disenrollment.
2. Complete Medicare form Medicare Managed Care Disenrollment CMS-566, attach a copy of the disenrollment letter, and take it to the Social Security office.

Many plans allow the patient to enroll and disenroll at any time during the year. It may take the plan 30 days for disenrollment, and Medicare may take as long as 60 days to reenroll a patient. Patients who disenroll may have to requalify for supplemental coverage at a higher cost.

Two types of HMO plans may have Medicare Part B contracts: HMO risk plans and HMO cost plans.

Risk Plan

As a condition of enrollment in an HMO risk plan, beneficiaries receive Medicare-covered services (except emergency, urgent need, and prior authorized services) only from providers who are contracted members of the HMO network. Enrollees of HMO risk plans are referred to as *restricted beneficiaries*. Usually services rendered by "out-of-plan" physicians are not covered when the same services are available through the organization unless a referral or prior authorization is obtained. The only exception is for emergency care. Claims for HMO risk plan beneficiaries must be sent directly to the organization.

A system of Medicare reimbursement for HMOs with risk contracts is called **diagnostic cost groups** (DCGs). The HMO enrollees are classified into various DCGs on the basis of each beneficiary's prior 12-month history of hospitalization, and payments are adjusted accordingly. This payment system does not apply to disabled and hospice patients, those on renal dialysis, or those enrolled only in Medicare Part B. Patients are reclassified each year according to their previous year's use of hospital service. This is further discussed in Chapter 17.

Cost Plan

Under an HMO cost plan, beneficiaries receive Medicare-covered services from sources in or outside of the HMO network. Enrollees are referred to as *unrestricted beneficiaries*. Claims for cost plan beneficiaries may be sent to the HMO plan or the regular Medicare carrier.

Noncontract Physician

If a noncontract physician treats a Medicare HMO patient, the services are considered "out-of-plan" services. The claim must be submitted to the managed care plan, which determines whether it is responsible to pay for the services. Conditions that must be met are as follows:

1. The service was an emergency, and the patient was not able to get to an HMO facility or member physician (patient was out of the HMO area).
2. The service was covered by Medicare.

3. The service was medically necessary.
4. The service was authorized previously or was an approved referral.

The patient is responsible for the fee if the HMO determines there was no emergency and denies payment. The HMO reimburses according to the Medicare Fee Schedule Allowable Amount, so the physician cannot bill the patient for the balance. If the physician does not receive 100% of the allowable, steps must be taken through the HMO's appeals process. If this fails, contact the Medicare Managed Care Department at the Medicare Regional CMS Operations Office. Denied services can be billed to the patient (no more than the Medicare fee schedule or limiting charge) after the HMO EOB is received.

Carrier Dealing Prepayment Organization

A Carrier Dealing Prepayment Organization may be set up by a medical practice under contract to the government. Such plans are considered a service contract rather than insurance. In the past, such plans were run by HMOs, but now practices of 12 to 15 physicians are opting to run their own plans. These organizations must be incorporated and have their own Medicare provider number. The organization must furnish physicians' services through employees and partners or under formal arrangement with medical groups, independent practice associations, or individual physicians. Part B services must be provided through qualified hospitals or physicians. When operating this type of organization, the physician accepts Medicare assignment and agrees to deal with the Medicare carrier instead of CMS. Patients sign a contract agreeing to pay a monthly fee (usually $20 to $25). This is supposed to cover all Medicare copayments, deductibles, and nonreimbursable expenses (annual physical examinations and preventive care). The patient is not responsible for paying for noncovered services.

UTILIZATION AND QUALITY CONTROL

Quality Improvement Organizations

As explained in detail in Chapter 11, a **Quality Improvement Organization (QIO)** program (formerly known as *professional* or *peer review organization*) contracts with CMS to review medical necessity, reasonableness, appropriateness, and completeness and adequacy of care given in inpatient, outpatient, and emergency department hospitals, nursing facilities, home health agencies, private fee-for-service plans, and ambulatory surgical centers for which additional payment is sought under the outlier provisions of the prospective payment system (PPS).

CMS has assigned a point system for medical documentation as discussed in Chapter 4. If sufficient points are lacking, penalties can lead to fines or forfeiture of the physician's license. Therefore it is extremely important that each patient's care be well documented from the treatment standpoint, as well as for justifying maximum reimbursement. A physician who receives a letter from a QIO about quality of care should consult his or her attorney before responding by letter or personal appeal. A photocopy of the patient's health record can be used to substantiate the claim if there is detailed clinical documentation.

Federal False Claims Amendment Act

Another federal law to prevent overuse of services and to spot Medicare fraud is the Federal Claims Amendment Act of 1986. This act offers financial incentives of 15% to 25% of any judgment to informants **(whistleblowers)** who report physicians suspected of defrauding the federal government. This is called a **qui tam action.** The laws are intended to help catch Medicare and Medicaid cheaters. The health insurance companies that process Medicare claims have a Medicare fraud unit whose job is to catch people who steal from Medicare. The Office of the Inspector General (OIG), Department of Health and Human Services, is the law enforcement agency that investigates and prosecutes people who steal from Medicare. The OIG works closely with Medicare insurance companies, the Federal Bureau of Investigation (FBI), the Postal Inspection Service, and other federal law enforcement agencies. If the physician is on an optical disk retrieval (ODR) A-1000 system, it is possible for the OIG to obtain procedure codes that show comparison billing with peers in the area. The CMS alerts the OIG of offices to investigate. To reduce the chances of a Medicare beneficiary complaining to the government, take the following actions:

- Listen to the patient's complaint and follow-up.
- Publicize the provider's hotline.
- Route a beneficiary's complaint to a compliance officer or office manager.

For information on fraud and abuse, see Boxes 2-11 and 2-12. See Chapter 15 for information about fraud in the workers' compensation program.

Clinical Laboratory Improvement Amendments

The CLIA of 1988 established federal standards, quality control, and safety measures for all freestanding laboratories including physician office laboratories (POLs). Various laboratory procedures fall within CLIA categories depending on the complexity of each test. If a physician performs only tests that pose no risk to the patient, the laboratory may be eligible for a certificate of waiver that exempts it from CLIA regulations' quality control and personnel standards; however, a registration fee must still be paid for the waived category. The other two categories are moderate or high-complexity laboratory services. Each category level requires a yearly licensing fee

MEDICARE BILLING COMPLIANCE ISSUES

Because Medicare is a federal program, legislation sets down the policies that must be followed. Therefore whoever participates in the program must comply with all the regulations. Billing issues about which medical practices should be aware may include, but are not limited to, the following:

- Release of medical information
- Reassignment of payment
- Limiting charges for nonparticipating providers
- Correct procedural code assignment and service utilization
- Accurate diagnostic code assignment
- Medical necessity of services performed
- Billing for ancillary employees (physician assistants and nurse practitioners) called "incident-to" billing
- Documentation related to selection of procedural codes for services performed
- Ancillary orders and supervision requirements
- Teaching physician and resident billing
- Routine waiver of copayments, deductibles, or professional courtesy discounts
- Stark I and II antireferral and compensation regulations
- Credit balance refunds
- Correct coding initiative edits

to be paid by the physician. A certificate is then issued and must be posted in the laboratory. Various levels of quality control measures are necessary for each CLIA level and must be performed in a timely manner (e.g., daily or weekly). Fines may be levied if federal standards are not maintained. This has had an impact on office laboratories, and because of the strict requirements, many physicians send patients to independent laboratories for tests (e.g., blood cell counts, cytology specimens, or cultures). However, some physicians prefer to draw blood from a patient, particularly if the patient has a history of difficult venous access.

When claims to Medicare administrative contractors are submitted for laboratory services performed in the physician's office, the 10-digit CLIA certificate number should be entered in Block 23 of the CMS-1500 (08-05) claim form (Figure 12-6). Physicians billing patients for outside laboratory work are not held to these standards but may charge the patient only what the laboratory charges (based on a fee schedule), plus any additional services the physician provides (e.g., drawing, handling, shipping, interpretation of the blood, or office visit).

PAYMENT FUNDAMENTALS

Provider
Participating Physician

In a **participating physician (par)** agreement, a physician agrees to accept payment from Medicare (80% of the **approved charges**) plus payment from the patient (20% of approved charge) after the $162 deductible (2011) has been met (Figure 12-7). The Medicare annual deductible is based on the calendar year, January 1 through December 31. This agreement is referred to as accepting **assignment.** The physician must complete and transmit the CMS-1500 (08-05) claim form to the fiscal

FIGURE 12-6 Section of the CMS-1500 (08-05) claim form with Block 23 emphasized indicating where to insert a certificate number for laboratory services (CLIA No.) or a prior authorization number for a procedure when permission has been granted.

PAYMENT EXAMPLES

	Actual charge	Medicare approved amount*	Deductible	Medicare pays	Beneficiary responsible for	Medicare courtesy adjustment†
Doctor A accepts assignment	$480	$400	$162 already satisfied	$320 (80% of approved amount)	$80 (20% of approved amount)	$80 (difference between actual charge and approved amount)
Doctor B does not accept assignment and charges the limiting amount	$437	$380	$162 already satisfied	$304 (80% of approved amount)	$133 (20% of approved amount [$76] plus difference between limiting charge [actual charge] and approved amount [$57] = $133)	None
Doctor C accepts assignment; however, the patient has not met the deductible amount	$480	$238 ($400 minus the deductible)	$162 has not been met	$190.40 (80% of approved amount determined after subtracting the deductible)	$209.60 (deductible plus 20% of approved amount)	$80 (difference between actual charge and approved amount)

*The Medicare approved amount is less for nonparticipating physicians than for participating physicians.
†The courtesy adjustment is the amount credited to the patient's account in the adjustment column. The word "courtesy" implies that Medicare patients are treated well and is preferred to phrases like "not allowed."

FIGURE 12-7 Payment examples for three physicians showing a physician accepting assignment versus not accepting assignment, and the amounts the patient is responsible for paying with deductible satisfied and not met.

intermediary. The assignment of benefits, Block 12, is signed by the patient, the physician indicates that assignment is being accepted by checking "Yes" in Block 27, and the payment goes directly to the physician (Figure 12-8). Physicians, practitioners, and suppliers who fail to electronically transmit or manually submit claims are subject to civil monetary penalties up to $2500 for each claim.

Nonparticipating Physician

A **nonparticipating physician (nonpar)** does not have a signed agreement with Medicare and has an option about assignment. The physician may decline assignment for all services or accept assignment for some services and collect from the patient for other services performed at the same time and place. An exception to this policy is mandatory assignment for clinical laboratory tests and services by physician assistants. Unassigned electronic claims that are denied have no appeal rights.

Nonpar physicians receive only 95% of the Medicare-approved amount. Nonpar physicians may decide on a case-by-case basis whether to accept assignment. If the nonpar physician accepts assignment for a claim, Medicare pays 80% of the nonpar Medicare-approved amount directly to the physician and the physician collects the remaining 20% from the patient. If the nonpar physician does not take assignment on a particular claim, he or she

may "balance bill" the patient 115% of the nonpar rate because Medicare will send the payment to the patient. For example, if the nonpar rate is $100, the provider can "balance bill" the patient for $115. However, in this case, even though the physician is required to transmit the claim to Medicare, the carrier pays the patient directly and the physician therefore must collect his or her entire fee from the patient; thus physicians must "chase the money." Consequently, physicians should evaluate whether the ability to "balance bill" and collect a higher fee from the patient is worth the potential extra billing and collection costs. Furthermore, some hospitals and states, including Minnesota, Pennsylvania, Vermont, and New York, prohibit or limit balance billing, so physicians must ascertain whether these restrictions apply before making a Medicare participation or nonparticipation decision.

Limiting charge is a percentage limit on fees, specified by legislation, that nonpar physicians may bill Medicare beneficiaries above the allowed amount. Nonpar physicians may submit usual and customary fees for assigned claims. Because of these two situations, nonpar physicians usually have a fee schedule that lists both usual fees and limiting charges. Some states have set limiting charges that are more restrictive than Medicare policies. These states are Connecticut, Massachusetts, New York, Ohio, Pennsylvania, Rhode Island, and Vermont. Inquire from the fiscal intermediary of those states for guidelines.

FIGURE 12-8 Block 12 of the CMS-1500 (08-05) claim form where the patient signs authorizing payment to be sent to the physician, and Block 27 marked with an X showing that the physician accepts Medicare assignment of benefits.

Prior Authorization

For Medicare patients who have additional insurance, many insurance carrier group plans and MCO senior plans require prior authorization for surgical procedures, diagnostic testing, and referrals to specialists. Some of these procedures requiring authorization are on a mandatory list, whereas others are chosen by the regional carrier. The mandatory list is composed of procedures such as the following:

● Bunionectomy
● Carotid endarterectomy
● Cataract extractions
● Cholecystectomy
● Complex peripheral revascularization
● Coronary artery bypass graft surgery
● Hysterectomy
● Inguinal hernia repair
● Joint replacements (hip, shoulder, or knee)
● Transurethral prostatectomy

Carriers may have a toll-free line to call for authorization, require the completion of a preauthorization form, or require a letter only if there is a dispute over claims payment. Check with the local carrier on its policy for preauthorization.

The prior authorization number is used when billing the Medicare carrier and is entered on the CMS-1500 (08-05) claim form in Block 23 (see Figure 12-6). If the procedure is not approved, the carrier sends a denial to the physician, patient, and hospital, if applicable. If the procedure is done as an emergency, notify the carrier within the time frame designated by the insurance plan so that an authorization can be arranged.

 ADVANCE BENEFICIARY NOTICE OF NONCOVERAGE

Medicare considers the appropriate use of an Advance Beneficiary Notice of Noncoverage (ABN) document as a compliance issue. Ask the patient to sign an ABN document if you know the service is not covered or if there is a possibility that a service may be denied for medical necessity or limitation of Medicare benefits. A step-by-step procedure of how to complete an ABN form is presented at the end of this chapter.

Waiver of Liability Provision
Limited Liability

When a patient is to receive a service from a participating physician that might be denied for **medical necessity** or because of *limitation of liability* by Medicare, inform the patient and have him or her agree to pay for the denied service in advance. If the Medicare guidelines or parameters are not known for a certain procedure or service, refer to *Medicare transmittals* (formerly called *program memorandums*) or call the Medicare carrier and ask. Some medical practices use a computerized method to screen for the medical necessity of a service but must have access to national coverage determinations (NCDs) and local coverage decisions (LCDs; formerly called *local medical review policies* [LMRPs]) to find out if there is limited coverage.

If you expect Medicare to deny payment (entirely or in part), instruct the patient to sign an **Advance Beneficiary Notice of Noncoverage (ABN),** also known as a *waiver of liability agreement* or *responsibility statement,* as shown in Figures 12-9 and 12-10. This form should not be given to someone who is in a medical emergency, confused, legally incompetent, or otherwise under great duress. It cannot be signed after a patient has received the service and must specifically state what service or procedure is being waived. Write the specific time frequency limitation for a particular service such as screening colonoscopy once every 10 years. Each space on the ABN must be completed before providing the ABN to the patient. Blank or partially completed ABNs, even with the patient's signature, are not acceptable. An ABN may be mailed to a patient when presenting it face to face is not possible, but the patient must have an opportunity to ask questions. When the ABN is mailed, it should be sent with a cover letter explaining that the procedure will be denied by Medicare and include contact information so that the patient can ask questions before the procedure.

To determine which services require an ABN, refer to the NCDs and the LCDs from the insurance carrier. An office policy should be in place for handling patients who refuse to sign an ABN. When sending in a claim, the HCPCS level II modifier -GA (waiver of liability on file) must be added to pertinent codes to indicate a patient has signed the waiver. The Medicare carrier then informs the patient that he or she is responsible for the fee. Keep this signed waiver with other patient financial documents and not with the patient's health record.

If the service was not reasonable because of Medicare guidelines, but the patient thought it was covered and there is no advance notice given with signed waiver of liability agreement, then the following apply:

● The provider cannot bill the patient.
● The patient does not have to pay the deductible or coinsurance.
● The patient is refunded any amount paid to the provider on the item or service.

A. Notifier: John Doe, MD, College Clinic, 4567 Broad Avenue, Woodland Hills, XY 12345 555-486-9002

B. Patient Name: Mary Judd   **C. Identification Number:** 0920XX7291

Advance Beneficiary Notice of Noncoverage (ABN)

NOTE: If Medicare doesn't pay for **D.** _B12 injections_ below, you may have to pay.
Medicare does not pay for everything, even some care that you or your health care provider have good reason to think you need. We expect Medicare may not pay for the **D.** _B12 injections_ below.

D.	E. Reason Medicare May Not Pay:	F. Estimated Cost
B12 injections	Medicare does not usually pay for this injection or this many injections	$35.00

WHAT YOU NEED TO DO NOW:
- Read this notice, so you can make an informed decision about your care.
- Ask us any questions that you may have after you finish reading.
- Choose an option below about whether to receive the **D.** _B12 injections_ listed above.
  Note: If you choose Option 1 or 2, we may help you to use any other insurance that you might have, but Medicare cannot require us to do this.

G. OPTIONS: Check only one box. We cannot choose a box for you.

☑ **OPTION 1.** I want the **D.** _B12 injections_ listed above. You may ask to be paid now, but I also want Medicare billed for an official decision on payment, which is sent to me on a Medicare Summary Notice (MSN). I understand that if Medicare doesn't pay, I am responsible for payment, but **I can appeal to Medicare** by following the directions on the MSN. If Medicare does pay, you will refund any payments I made to you, less co-pays or deductibles.

☐ **OPTION 2.** I want the **D.** _____ listed above, but do not bill Medicare. You may ask to be paid now as I am responsible for payment. **I cannot appeal if Medicare is not billed.**

☐ **OPTION 3.** I don't want the **D.** _____ listed above. I understand with this choice I am **not** responsible for payment, and **I cannot appeal to see if Medicare would pay.**

H. Additional Information:

This notice gives our opinion, not an official Medicare decision. If you have other questions on this notice or Medicare billing, call **1-800-MEDICARE** (1-800-633-4227/**TTY:** 1-877-486-2048). Signing below means that you have received and understand this notice. You also receive a copy.

I. Signature: *Mary Judd*	J. Date: *March 20, 20XX*

According to the Paperwork Reduction Act of 1995, no persons are required to respond to a collection of information unless it displays a valid OMB control number. The valid OMB control number for this information collection is 0938-0566. The time required to complete this information collection is estimated to average 7 minutes per response, including the time to review instructions, search existing data resources, gather the data needed, and complete and review the information collection. If you have comments concerning the accuracy of the time estimate or suggestions for improving this form, please write to: CMS, 7500 Security Boulevard, Attn: PRA Reports Clearance Officer, Baltimore, Maryland 21244-1850.

Form CMS-R-131 (03/11)   Form Approved OMB No. 0938-0566

FIGURE 12-9 Advance Beneficiary Notice of Noncoverage (ABN), Form CMS-R-131, which is also referred to as a *responsibility statement* or *waiver of liability agreement*.

FIGURE 12-10 Insurance billing specialist instructing an elderly patient to sign an Advance Beneficiary Notice of Noncoverage (ABN) form for services not covered.

If assignment is accepted and the physician and patient thought the service was covered under reasonable assumptions, then the following apply:

● Medicare is billed to pay for the service.
● The patient must pay the deductible and coinsurance.
● Medicare will not seek a refund of money already paid to the physician.

Nonpar providers must refund any amount collected from the beneficiary when services are later found to be not reasonable and necessary.

Noncovered Services

Do not get confused with the issue of noncovered Medicare services because these may always be billed to the patient. Do not give a patient an ABN when a service is never covered by Medicare. Instead give those patients a different form, the Notice of Exclusions from Medicare Benefits (NEMB) (Figure 12-11). This form clearly states that the service is never covered by Medicare and the patient is responsible for payment. It is not a requirement to give the patient an NEMB for a never-covered service to bill the patient, but use of the form makes it clear before the procedure is done that he or she must pay for it. Services denied as inclusive of another service (a payment already made for the other service) are not considered a noncovered item and may not be billed to the patient. If a formal denial is necessary to bill the patient or another insurer, a claim should be sent with a letter attached stating the need for the denial to bill another payer.

Elective Surgery Estimate

Effective October 1, 1987, under the Tax Reform Act, a nonparticipating physician who does not accept

assignment for an elective surgery for which the actual charge will be $500 or more must provide the beneficiary with the following in writing: (1) the estimated fee for the procedure, (2) the estimated Medicare-approved allowance for the procedure, and (3) the difference in the physician's actual charge (limiting charge and the allowed amount) (Figure 12-12). The term *elective surgery* means a surgical procedure that can be scheduled in advance, is not an emergency, and is discretionary on the part of the physician and the patient. Failure to undergo elective surgery does not pose a mortality threat. Give a copy of the estimation letter to the Medicare patient and keep the original for the files. Document the patient's acknowledgment by obtaining his or her signature at the bottom of the letter.

Prepayment Screens

On some procedures, Medicare limits the number of times a given procedure can be billed during a specific time frame (e.g., one treatment every 60 days for routine foot care). This is known as a *Medicare prepayment screen*. The screens or flags are computer triggers that suspend processing. These screens are used to identify and review claims for medical necessity and determine compliance with other appropriate criteria. The suspended claim is checked by a reviewer who decides whether the services are medically necessary. If the claim was previously submitted for the procedure performed in the allotted time frame by another physician, the claim will be downcoded or denied. Refer to the local Medicare administrator contractor's transmittals (formerly known as *program memorandums*) or contact the contractor for a complete list of the Medicare prepayment screens that are applicable locally.

To avoid problems, use good procedure code guidelines discussed in Chapter 6 and adhere to the following criteria:

● The level of service is appropriate to documentation.
● The procedure is accurate to the gender of the patient.
● The frequency is appropriate.
● The diagnosis and procedure match.
● The provider has certification for performing services (e.g., laboratories).
● The fee is within the Medicare-approved charge.

Correct Coding Initiative

Medicare's **Correct Coding Initiative (CCI)** is implemented by CMS in an attempt to eliminate unbundling or other inappropriate reporting of *Current Procedural Terminology* (CPT) codes. As you may recall, unbundling is coding and billing numerous CPT codes to identify procedures that usually are described by a single code. Coding conflicts are picked up and claims are reviewed,

NOTICE OF EXCLUSIONS FROM MEDICARE BENEFITS (NEMB)

There are items and services for which Medicare <u>will not pay</u>.

- Medicare does **not** pay for all of your health care costs. Medicare only pays for covered benefits. **Some items and services are not Medicare benefits and Medicare will not pay for them.**

- When you receive an item or service that is **not** a Medicare benefit, **you are responsible to pay for it,** personally or through any other insurance that you may have.

  The purpose of this notice is to help you make an informed choice about whether or not you want to receive these items or services, knowing that you will have to pay for them yourself. **Before you make a decision, you should read this entire notice carefully.**
  Ask us to explain, if you don't understand why Medicare won't pay.
  Ask us how much these items or services will cost you (**Estimated Cost: $_____**).

Medicare will not pay for: _____
_____ ;

☐ **1.** **Because it does not meet the definition of any Medicare benefit.**

☐ **2.** **Because of the following exclusion * from Medicare benefits:**

- ☐ Personal comfort items.
- ☐ Most shots (vaccinations).
- ☐ Hearing aids and hearing examinations.
- ☐ Most outpatient prescription drugs.
- ☐ Orthopedic shoes and foot supports (orthotics).
- ☐ Health care received outside of the USA.
- ☐ Services required as a result of war.
- ☐ Routine physicals and most tests for screening.
- ☐ Routine eye care, eyeglasses and examinations.
- ☐ Cosmetic surgery.
- ☐ Dental care and dentures (in most cases).
- ☐ Routine foot care and flat foot care.
- ☐ Services by immediate relatives.
- ☐ Services under a physician's private contract.
- ☐ Services paid for by a governmental entity that is not Medicare.
- ☐ Services for which the patient has no legal obligation to pay.
- ☐ Home health services furnished under a plan of care, if the agency does not submit the claim.
- ☐ Items and services excluded under the Assisted Suicide Funding Restriction Act of 1997.
- ☐ Items or services furnished in a competitive acquisition area by any entity that does not have a contract with the Department of Health and Human Services (except in a case of urgent need).
- ☐ Physicians' services performed by a physician assistant, midwife, psychologist, or nurse anesthetist, when furnished to an inpatient, unless they are furnished under arrangements by the hospital.
- ☐ Items and services furnished to an individual who is a resident of a skilled nursing facility (a SNF) or of a part of a facility that includes a SNF, unless they are furnished under arrangements by the SNF.
- ☐ Services of an assistant at surgery without prior approval from the peer review organization.
- ☐ Outpatient occupational and physical therapy services furnished incident to a physician's services.

* This is only a general summary of exclusions from Medicare benefits. It is not a legal document. The official Medicare program provisions are contained in relevant laws, regulations, and rulings.

FIGURE 12-11 Notice of Exclusions from Medicare Benefits (NEMB) form.

suspended, or denied when conflicts occur. Software is available to give physicians, private insurance companies, and billing services access to the same government database used in auditing physicians for improper use of CPT codes. It is currently available on the CMS website at no charge. Refer to the Internet Resources at the end of this chapter.

MEDICARE REIMBURSEMENT

Chronology of Prospective Payment System

For many years, Medicare payments were based on reasonable fees (e.g., the amounts approved by the Medicare administrative contractor). Medicare paid 80% of the

WORKSHEET FOR ESTIMATED MEDICARE PAYMENT FOR ELECTIVE SURGERY

Worksheet

1. Physician's actual fee (limiting charge) $ 1248.03
2. Medicare approved or allowed amount $ 1085.24
3. Difference between physician's actual fee and Medicare approved or allowed amount (1 − 2 = 0)   − 162.79
4. Twenty percent coinsurance (0.20 × 2 = 0)   + 217.05
5. Beneficiary's out-of-pocket expense (3 + 4 + 0) $ 379.84
   Assume the $131 deductible has been met

Items 1, 2, and 5 must be included in the letter to the beneficiary

A

Beneficiary Letter

Dear Patient:

Because I do not accept assignment for elective surgery, Medicare requires that I give you certain information before surgery when my charges are $500 or more.

The following information concerns the surgery we have discussed. These estimates assume that you have already met the $131 deductible.

Type of surgery ... Osteotomy, proximal left tibia
Limiting charge $ 1248.03
Medicare estimated payment $ 868.19
Patient's estimated payment $ 379.84

This estimate is based upon our present expectations of what surgical procedure(s) will be required. Please remember that this is only an estimate of charges; we cannot be sure that additional procedures will or will not be necessary.

Sincerely,

John Doe, M.D.
Medicare Provider Number ... 126XX5479

I understand the foregoing physician charges and my financial responsibility with respect to those estimated charges.

Patient's Signature ... *Jane Doe*   Date 5-18-20XX
Jane Doe

B

FIGURE 12-12 **A,** Worksheet. **B,** Sample beneficiary letter for estimated Medicare payment for elective surgery.

approved charge. On October 1, 1983, an important development in the Medicare Part A program, the **prospective payment system (PPS),** became effective. Under the regulations enacted by the Social Security Amendments of 1983, hospitals treating Medicare patients are reimbursed according to preestablished rates for each type of illness treated on the basis of diagnosis. Payments to hospitals for Medicare services are classified according to more than 700 diagnosis-related group (DRG) numbers. Beneficiaries (patients) cannot be billed beyond the preestablished DRG rate except for normal deductible and copayment amounts. (See Chapter 17 for an in-depth discussion of DRGs.)

In 1984 the Deficit Reduction Act established a participating physician program that offered incentives to participating physicians and froze the fees of nonparticipating physicians. The 1987 Omnibus Budget Reconciliation Act (OBRA) introduced the maximum allowable actual charge (MAAC) formula, which developed the maximum fee (limiting charge) that a nonpar physician could charge Medicare patients for each service.

Reasonable Fee

Reasonable fee is the amount that Medicare participating providers agree to accept. It is listed on the RA, formerly known as the EOB, as an allowed (approved) charge for a procedure. This charge may be higher or lower than the fee the physician lists on the claim. When a physician accepts assignment, he or she may bill the patient only 20% of the Medicare-allowed charge. Charging for completion and submission of a claim form on an assignment claim violates the terms of the assignment. Interest fees cannot be assessed to Medicare patients. It is permissible to collect the deductible at the time of service if you know how much of the deductible has already been paid, but the Medicare copayment should not be collected until Medicare pays.

Mandatory assignment laws have been adopted in several states, and legislation is under consideration and pending in many more states. These state laws would require physicians to accept the approved charge for their Medicare patients as a condition for being licensed to practice medicine in the state. Arkansas, Florida, Illinois, Maryland, Montana, and New Hampshire have rejected mandatory assignment proposals.

Resource-Based Relative Value Scale

As mentioned in Chapter 6, a **resource-based relative value scale (RBRVS)** is the system Medicare uses for establishing fees. This system takes into account work, overhead expense, and malpractice values for all CPT codes that are published in the *Federal Register* each November. These are adjusted for each Medicare local carrier by geographic practice cost indices (GPCI) by using a formula that gives the total value for a code. To access the Medicare fee schedule, refer to the Internet Resources at the end of this chapter and visit the Evolve website, which has an active link to the CMS.

The formula for obtaining the allowed amount of a given service or procedure is to choose an HCPCS/CPT code and use the **relative value unit (RVU)** amounts listed in the *Federal Register* for work value, practice expense, and malpractice value and multiply each of those by the GPCI. Then to obtain the total adjusted RVU, add the three amounts together. Finally, to discover the allowed amount for this code, multiply the annual Medicare conversion factor (CF) by the HCPCS/CPT code's total adjusted RVU amount. For a graphic illustration of this formula, see Figure 6-2. To give you experience in using this formula, do the assignments relating to RBRVS for this chapter in the *Workbook*.

To eliminate having to spend time in establishing fees and using the formula, many medical practices use a fee analyzer for their geographic area.

Healthcare Common Procedure Coding System (HCPCS)

As mentioned in Chapter 6, the federal government developed the HCPCS for the Medicare program. To obtain correct payment for a procedure or service, a code number must be selected from level I or II of the HCPCS coding system. To review, the Medicare HCPCS levels of coding are as follows:

- Level I: American Medical Association (AMA) CPT codes and modifiers (national codes)
- Level II: CMS-designated codes and alpha modifiers (national codes)

When transmitting a claim, be sure to use the level II HCPCS **national alphanumeric codes** and modifiers rather than CPT procedure codes for certain appliances and procedures when indicated. When billing CPT modifiers, a good reference is presented in Table 6-5, as helpful hints entitled "Medicare Payment Rule."

Physician Quality Reporting Initiative

The Tax Relief and Health Care Act of 2006 authorized the **Physician Quality Reporting Initiative (PQRI)**, which is a pay-for-reporting program for providers who bill under Medicare Part B. This financial incentive program is for eligible professionals who choose to participate and successfully report on a designated set of quality measures for services paid under the Medicare Physician Fee Schedule and furnished between specific dates. The services must be reported using temporary G-codes and/or CPT category 2 codes. These codes should be added to claims to reflect elements of quality of care delivered during the encounter with the patient. Participants may receive a bonus payment of 1.5% of their charges, subject to a cap. No enrollment or registration is required. To find additional information about the PQRI, such as eligible professionals, G-codes, and forms used for documenting patient encounters, refer to the Internet Resources at the end of this chapter and visit the Evolve website, which has an active link to the CMS.

Recovery Audit Contractor (RAC) Program

The **Recovery Audit Contractor (RAC) Initiative** originally created a demonstration program that became permanently implemented when Congress enacted the Tax Relief and Health Care Act of 2006 (TRHCA). This extended the RAC program to all fifty states by 2010. Its goals are to identify Medicare underpayments and overpayments and recover overpayments using automated review and complex review. An automated review is done electronically without human review and complex review is done using human review of the medical record. A single RAC will serve one of four geographic regions (Regions A, B, C, and D) and perform recovery audit services for all Medicare claim types in that region. RACs may identify improper payments from claims they review that may show incorrect payment amounts, non-covered services, incorrectly coded services, DRG miscoding, and duplicate services. RAC contractors are paid a percentage of the incorrect payments they recover. When an underpayment is found, a RAC will communicate this to the MAC. If both underpayments and overpayments are found, the RAC will offset the underpayment from the overpayment. On overpayments, interest accrues from the date of the final determination. Claims identified as overpayments are subject to the Medicare appeals process.

CLAIM SUBMISSION

Local Coverage Determination

LCD, formerly known as LMRP, is a decision by the MAC whether to cover a particular service on a contractor-wide basis in accordance with the SSA (i.e., a determination as to whether the service is reasonable and necessary). LCD is an educational and administrative tool to assist physicians, providers, and suppliers in transmitting correct claims for payment. Contractor medical directors and staff develop LCDs with input from the public. LCDs list covered and noncovered codes for a given Medicare policy but do not include any of the coding guidance that were found in LMRPs. LCDs outline how contractors review claims to determine whether Medicare coverage requirements have been met. CMS requires that local policies be consistent with national guidance. Use of LCDs helps avoid situations in which claims are paid or denied without a full understanding of the basis for payment and denial. LCDs may be obtained from the Medicare carrier website at www.cms.hhs.gov/mcd.

Medicare Administrative Contractors and Fiscal Intermediaries

An organization handling claims from hospitals, NFs, **intermediate care facilities (ICFs),** long-term care facilities (LTCFs), and home health agencies is called a *fiscal intermediary* (FI). The National Blue Cross Association holds the fiscal intermediary contract for Medicare Part A; in turn, it subcontracts it out to member agencies.

Organizations handling claims from physicians and other suppliers of services covered under Medicare Part B are called **Medicare administrative contractors (MACs),** formerly called *fiscal agents*. Medicare Part B payments are handled by private insurance organizations under contract with the government. Since January 1, 1992, the rule for where to send a Medicare claim is to bill the carrier who covers the area where the service occurred or was furnished, not the carrier who services the physician's office.

See Internet Resources at the end of this chapter to go to the Evolve website to access the active link for the names and addresses for claims submission in each state and to obtain further information about this program.

Provider Identification Numbers

Another requirement of the Tax Reform Act was the establishment of several types of identification numbers for each physician and non-physician practitioner providing services paid by Medicare. Because there are so many numbers, they are easily confused and end up being the source of many errors when completing blocks on the CMS-1500 (08-05) claim form. The numbers defined and shown in template examples with correct placement in Chapter 7 follow:

- Provider identification numbers (PINs), group and individual. With the implementation of the National Provider Identifier (NPI) on May 23, 2007, PINs are no longer used.
- Unique physician identification numbers (UPINs). With the implementation of the NPI on May 23, 2007, UPINs are no longer used.
- NPI assigned by the CMS was implemented on May 23, 2007.
- Durable medical equipment (DME) supplier number.

Patient's Signature Authorization

Signatures for transmitting electronic claims and acceptance of financial responsibility must be obtained and retained in the office records because there are no handwritten signatures on electronic claims. A form created by the medical practice may be used or a Medicare patient's signature may be obtained in Block 12 of the CMS-1500 (08-05) claim form. This block should be signed regardless of whether the physician is a participating or nonparticipating physician. The signed authorization should be kept on file in the patient's health record for an episode of care or for a designated time frame (e.g., 1 year). Claims may indicate "Signature on file" or "SOF" in Block 12 of the claim form. Further information on this topic may be found in Chapters 3, 7, and 8.

SOF situations that may occur in a medical practice are as follows:

- Illiterate or physically handicapped. When an illiterate or physically handicapped enrollee signs by mark (X), a witness should sign his or her name and address next to the mark. If the claim is filed for the patient by another person, that person should enter the patient's name and write "By," sign his or her own name and address, indicate relationship to the patient, and state why the patient cannot sign.
- Confinement in a facility. Sometimes it is not possible to obtain the signature of a Medicare patient because of confinement in a nursing facility, hospital, or home. In such cases, physicians should obtain an annual signature authorization from the patient.
- Medigap claim. When transmitting a crossover claim to a Medigap carrier, annually obtain a signature authorization for the Medigap carrier.
- Deceased patient. Refer to the section on Claims for Deceased Patient later in this chapter for signature requirements.
- Medi-Medi claim. These crossover claims do not require the patient's signature.

Time Limit

The Health Care Reform of 2010 changed the filing deadline for claims. Beginning October 1, 2009, providers no longer have 15 to 24 months to file and must submit claims within 12 months of the date of service. Claims for services rendered before October 1, 2009 must be sent in by the end of the calendar year after the fiscal year in which services were furnished. The fiscal year for claims begins October 1 and ends September 30 (see the box).

For services furnished on:	The time limit for filing is :
October 1, 2010, to September 30, 2011	December 31, 2012
October 1, 2011, to September 30, 2012	December 31, 2013

On assigned claims, the provider may file without penalty up to 27 months after providing service if reasonable cause for the delay is shown to the insurance carrier. Otherwise, there is a 10% reduction in the reimbursement. On unassigned claims, the provider may be fined up to $2000 for delinquent claim submission or be dropped from Medicare. When transmitting a late claim, ask the fiscal intermediary for the guidelines that CMS considers reasonable cause for delay.

Paper Claims

The form that physicians use to submit paper claims to Medicare is the CMS-1500 (08-05). Refer to Chapter 7 for instructions on how to complete the CMS-1500 (08-05) claim form for the Medicare program. The reference templates (samples of completed claim forms) for Medicare and supplemental coverage shown at the end of that chapter are as follows:

- Medicare, no secondary coverage: Figure 7-6
- Medi/Medi, crossover: Figure 7-7
- Medicare/MG, crossover: Figure 7-8
- Other insurance/Medicare MSP: Figure 7-9

Patients are not allowed to submit claims to Medicare (with four exceptions). Situations when a patient may file a claim are the following:

- Services covered by Medicare for which the patient has other insurance that should pay first, called *MSP*
- Services provided by a physician who refuses to transmit the claim
- Services provided outside the United States
- Situations in which durable medical equipment is purchased from a private source

Medicare claim status is also explained in detail in Chapter 7 (e.g., clean, incomplete, rejected, dirty, or other claims). To obtain the mailing address for sending Medicare claim forms for your state or county, go to the Internet website http://www.cms.hhs.gov/apps/contacts/. For further information and booklets, pamphlets, and the annual *Medicare & You* handbook, contact the nearest Social Security office.

Electronic Claims

Medicare requests that all providers transmit claims electronically. All electronic transmission formats are standardized by the use of ANSI ASC X12N (837) Version 4010. On January 1, 2012, providers, payers, and clearinghouses will begin using upgraded standards ASC X12N Version 5010. Refer to Chapter 8 for information on how to transmit claims electronically to the Medicare carrier.

Medicare/Medicaid Claims

Medi-Medi patients qualify for the benefits of Medicare and Medicaid. Use the CMS-1500 (08-05) claim form and check "Yes" for the assignment in Block 27. If the physician does not accept assignment, then payment goes to the patient and Medicaid (in California Medi-Cal) will not pick up the residual. The CMS-1500 (08-05) claim form will be crossed over and processed automatically by Medicaid after processing is completed by Medicare. The fiscal intermediary may refer to this as a **crossover claim,** or *claims transfer.* It is not necessary to submit another form. Claims should be sent according to the time limit designated by the Medicaid program in the state. Generally, the Medicare payment exceeds the Medicaid fee schedule, and little or no payment is received except when the patient has not met his or her annual Medicare deductible.

In some states, the fiscal intermediary for a crossover claim may have a different address from that used for the processing of a patient who is on Medicare only. Write or call the nearest Medicare fiscal intermediary for the guidelines pertinent to the state.

Medicare/Medigap Claims

Medicare has streamlined the processing of Medicare/Medigap claims in most states. Medicare carriers transmit Medigap claims electronically for participating physicians, thus eliminating the need to file an additional claim. This is also called a *crossover claim.* Medigap payments go directly to the participating physicians, and a Medicare Summary Notice is sent to the patient that states, "This claim has been referred to your supplemental carrier for any additional benefits."

To ensure the crossover of the Medicare/Medigap claim, complete Blocks 9 through 9d of the CMS-1500 (08-05) claim form and list the PAYRID number of the Medigap plan in Block 9d. The PAYRID for Medigap plans is referred to as the *Other Carrier Name and Address* (OCNA) number, and a list of all OCNAs is published in the Medicare newsletter.

If automatic crossover capabilities are not offered in one's state, attach the Medicare RA to the claim form and electronically transmit or submit a claim to the Medigap plan separately.

Refer to Figure 7-8 for submitting claims when Medicare is primary and the patient has a Medigap (supplemental) policy.

Medicare/Employer Supplemental Insurance Claims

Some individuals have supplemental coverage with complementary benefits by employment plans even after retirement. In some cases, this coverage may be paid by a former employer after retirement. Usually, crossover relationships exist with many insurance carriers who insure Medicare beneficiaries.

Medicare/Supplemental and Medicare Supplementary Payer Claims

Completing the CMS-1500 (08-05) claim form for a Medicare patient who has supplemental insurance can be confusing. First, decide whether the case is Medicare primary or secondary payer. The procedure on determining whether Medicare is primary or secondary is presented at the end of this chapter. If Medicare is primary and the secondary payer is a Medigap policy, follow Medi/Medi processing guidelines. After determining which insurance is primary, follow the directions on what should be entered in each block of the CMS-1500 claim form, depending on the primary payer, or follow MSP guidelines.

Templates (samples of completed claim forms) shown at the end of Chapter 7 make it easier to learn which blocks to complete and which to ignore, depending on the primary and secondary payer. Figure 7-9 is for billing other insurance primary and Medicare secondary (MSP). A copy of the front and back sides of the primary insurance's EOB document must be attached to the claim when billing Medicare.

See Chapter 7 for general instructions for completing claims in Medicare and Medicare secondary payer cases.

Claims for Deceased Patients

The following are two ways in which to submit billing for a patient who has died:

1. Participating physician accepts assignment on the claim form. This results in the quickest payment. No signature by a family member is necessary on the CMS-1500 (08-05) claim form. Type "Patient died on (indicate date)" in Block 12 where the patient's signature is necessary.
2. The nonparticipating physician does not accept assignment, bills Medicare, and submits the following:
   a. A CMS-1500 (08-05) claim form signed by the estate representative who is responsible for the bill
   b. A statement or claim for all services provided
   c. Name and address of the responsible party
   d. Provider's statement, signed and dated, refusing to accept assignment

Nothing can be done about the open balance on the account until the estate is settled, and then Medicare will pay.

Physician Substitute Coverage

Many times, special substitute coverage arrangements are made between physicians (e.g., on-call, vacation, or unavailable because of another commitment). These arrangements are referred to as either *reciprocal* for on-call situations or *locum tenens* for a vacation situation. Specific modifiers are used to distinguish these situations, and special billing guidelines are stated as follows:

- *Reciprocal arrangement.* When transmitting Medicare claims, the regular physician must identify the service provided by the substitute doctor by listing the -Q5 modifier after the procedure code.

- *Locum tenens arrangement.* When transmitting Medicare claims, the regular physician must identify the service provided by the substitute doctor by listing the -Q6 modifier after the procedure code.

AFTER CLAIM SUBMISSION

Remittance Advice

Medicare sends a payment check and a nationally standardized document to participating physicians called a Medicare **remittance advice (RA),** formerly known as an *explanation of Medicare benefits (EOMB).* The front side of the RA lists status codes that are the same nationwide, representing the reason a claim may not have been paid in full, was denied, and so forth. These codes are defined on the reverse side of the RA. If the patient has Medigap, supplementary, or complementary crossover coverage, the "other payer" statement states whether the claim has been transferred to the supplemental insurer.

Nonpar physicians also receive an RA with payment information about unassigned claims. The RA separates payment information about assigned claims from unassigned claims to avoid posting errors by the practice. Check the payment against the fee schedule to determine whether the benefits are for the correct amount. On each claim form, note the date the payment is posted for reference. Optional items to document are amount of payment, RA processing data, and batch number.

Offices transmitting claims electronically receive an electronic remittance advice (ERA) showing payment data, and this may be automatically uploaded into the office computer system. The ERA electronically posts payments, and the provider does not have to manually post them. Paper and electronic remittance notices have the same format.

Medicare Summary Notice

A patient is mailed a similar document called a **Medicare Summary Notice (MSN).** This document is designed to be easier for the patient to understand, but because many patients do not know what is meant by amount charged, Medicare approved, deductible, and coinsurance, it often becomes necessary for the insurance billing specialist to educate the patient. First, photocopy an RA to be used as an example, deleting the patient's name to ensure confidentiality. Then use the RA to illustrate to future patients what various terms mean. This will increase patient understanding and save time.

When a claim is denied, the MSN will identify the number of the LCD or NCD used in denial of the claim.

BENEFICIARY REPRESENTATIVE/ REPRESENTATIVE PAYEE

Medicare beneficiaries may have memory impairment or may be confined to a wheelchair or bed, so they have a legal right to appoint an individual to serve as their representative.

Claims assistance professionals (CAPs) act as client representatives. They have some legal standing and are recognized by Medicare to act on the beneficiary's behalf if the beneficiary completes a Beneficiary Representative Form SSA-1696. This form is available from the SSA district office. Copies of the completed form should be sent to the Medicare intermediary or carrier when appropriate.

In contrast, a representative payee is an individual or organization chosen by the SSA to receive and administer SSA benefit funds on behalf of the beneficiary. Other duties consist of assisting the beneficiary with check writing for financial obligations, such as personal care and maintenance, housing, and medical service expenses, and investing any surplus monies for the beneficiary's benefit. A representative payee is responsible for using payments received only for the benefit of the beneficiary, accounting for the benefits received on request, and contacting SSA when anything affects eligibility for SSA benefits or prevents the representative payee's ability to perform these responsibilities. Additional information on CAPs is found in Chapters 1 and 18.

Posting Payments

Usually a physician's charge is higher than the charge approved by the MAC. This does not mean that his or her charges are unreasonable. As mentioned, payments are established using a fee schedule based on an RBRVS, a **volume performance standard (VPS)** for expenditure increases, and a limiting charge for nonparticipating physicians. VPS is the desired growth rate for spending on Medicare Part B physician services that is set each year by Congress.

Because some services may be disallowed or the payments on them may be lower than those charged by the physician, know how to post payments to the patient's financial accounting record card or computerized account. Figure 12-13 illustrates how payments and contractual or courtesy adjustments are posted. The word courtesy implies that Medicare patients are treated well and is preferred to phrases such as "not allowed" or "write-off."

Medicare does not allow for the standardized waiving of copayments. Medicare regulations require that a patient be billed for the copayment at least three times

FIGURE 12-13 Electronically generated financial accounting record (ledger card) illustrating how payments and contractual or courtesy adjustments should be posted.

before the balance is adjusted off as uncollectable. Document this as further justification if the patient is suffering financial hardship.

When an RA is received, it may list many patients (Figure 12-14). Do not post the entire payment made in a lump sum to the daysheet. Individually post each line item paid to the patient's financial accounting record card or computerized account and to the daysheet (Figure 12-15). To prevent funds from going astray, some offices prefer to post Medicare payments to a separate daysheet and deposit each multiple reimbursement check separately. The daysheet totals will then agree with the deposit slip totals and not get confused with other monies collected.

Figure 12-16, *A*, illustrates an example of a Medicare/Medicaid case after payment by Medicare. Medicare applied the patient's full $162 deductible amount to the

Medicare-allowed amount, reducing payment to $4. The Medicaid RA (Figure 12-16, *B*) shows reimbursement of the coinsurance and deductible amounts dual-billed to Medicaid.

Calculations are shown in the following box:

Medicare		Medicaid	
$180	Allowed amount	$180	Medicare allowed
−162	Deductible		amount
$ 18	Balance on which	−32	Medicaid cutback
	payment is	$148	Medicaid allowed
×.80	calculated		
$14.40		−4	Medicare paid
		$144	Medicaid payment

When referring to the Medicaid program, a cutback means a reduction, which is reducing Medicare's allowable

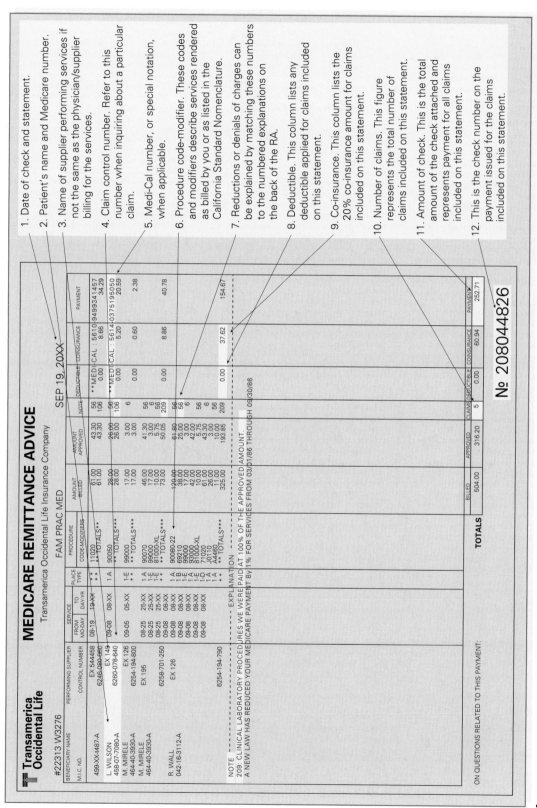

FIGURE 12-14 Medicare remittance advice (RA) document. **A,** Front. Insurance carriers are required to use Centers for Medicare and Medicaid Services (CMS) messages for Medicare RA, but each carrier has its own code numbers to denote the messages.

Continued

EXPLANATION OF NOTES   Additional notes may be listed on the front of this form.

1 – See enclosed letter.

2 – Claim was filed after the time limit.

4 – These bills are handled by a special intermediary.

5 – This payment is for an adjustment of a previous claim.

6 – Charges over the maximum Medicare allowance are not covered.

7 – Services before Medicare entitlement are not covered.

8 – Services after Medicare entitlement ended are not covered.

10 – Other charges submitted with this claim may be on a separate statement which you have received or will receive soon.

12 – Routine examinations and related services are not covered.

13 – Immunizations or other routine and preventative services are not covered.

16 – We need an itemization of this charge. Please resubmit your claim with this information.

17 – Prescription drugs are not covered.

18 – Charges for this physician/supplier are not covered.

19 – We need a full description of the service or supply to consider this charge. Please resubmit your claim with this information.

23 – We need a written report for this service. Please resubmit your claim with this information.

26 – More than $312.50 annual psychiatric expense is not covered.

27 – We need from the prescribing physician the specific length of time this medical equipment is needed. Please resubmit your claim with this information.

30 – This charge was previously considered.

37 – Claims for these services will be made by a home health agency or hospital.

39 – Equipment that is not medically necessary is not covered. (See Note 89)

42 – These supplies or services are not covered.

45 – Over $62\frac{1}{2}\%$ of psychiatric expenses is not covered.

46 – Routine foot care is not covered.

47 – Routine eye examinations or eye refractions are not covered.

48 – Partial payment of this claim was made to the beneficiary.

49 – This service cannot be considered until the hospital makes the necessary arrangement with the carrier for its processing.

50 – The beneficiary is not responsible for this reduction/denial under the assignment agreement.

54 – Care before and/or after surgery is included in the surgery benefit. (See Note 50)

56 – This is the full charge allowed based upon the prevailing or usual and customary rate.

62 – Payment has been reduced because this test is commonly part of an automated test group. (See Note 50)

66 – This service is not covered when done by this laboratory.

70 – There were no charges or bills with your claim form. Please resubmit your claim with this information.

72 – We need a signed and dated prescription showing medical necessity and specific length of time needed. Please resubmit your claim with this information.

73 – Before another month's payment can be made, we need a new signed and dated prescription showing further necessity of the medical equipment and specific length of time needed.

80 – We need to know the place of service to consider this charge. Please resubmit your claim with this information.

83 – SSA advises us that they are unable to verify the patient's eligibility for Part B Medical Insurance Plan. For this reason, no payment can be made on this claim.

84 – The patient's HIC number shown on this claim was incorrect. Please use the correct HIC number on all future claims.

85 – The patient's name shown on this claim was incorrect. Please use the correct name on all future claims.

86 – Over $62\frac{1}{2}\%$ of the allowable charges for psychiatric services is not covered.

89 – If you did not know that Medicare does not pay for this medical service, you may request a review of this decision. See below paragraph entitled "Your right to review of a case."

90 – This service by a chiropractor is not covered.

93 – Over $500.00 annual expense billed by a physical therapist is not covered.

95 – These specific services by this supplier are not covered.

96 – Please verify the date of this service. Resubmit your claim with this information.

99 – We need a complete diagnosis before the claim can be considered. Please resubmit your claim with this information.

106 – The Medicare covered services on this claim have been forwarded for additional processing under Medi-Cal.

107 – This claim was not forwarded for Medi-Cal processing. Please bill Medi-Cal directly and attach a copy of this statement.

108 – The bills for these services have been transferred to Blue Shield of California Medicare Claims, Chico, CA 95976. You will hear from them.

129 – Payment for services prior to July 1 is based on the previous year's payment rate.

131 – Payment for this physician service in a hospital department is reduced since this service is commonly performed in the physician's office. (See Note 50)

138 – This amount is more than Medicare pays for maintenance treatment of renal disease.

147 – This charge is not covered because an allowance for purchase of the same equipment was previously made.

151 – Your claim was transferred to a Health Maintenance Organization for processing.

153 – These are more visits (treatments) for this diagnosis than Medicare covers unless there were unusual circumstances. (See Note 89)

154 – This service is not covered for your patient's reported condition. (See Note 89)

155 – Only one visit per month to a nursing home is covered unless special need is indicated. (See Note 89)

156 – This laboratory test for the reported condition and/or illness is not covered. (See Note 89)

158 – Procedures whose effectiveness has not been proven are not covered. (See Note 89)

161 – The frequency of services for this condition are not covered. (See Note 89)

162 – More than one visit per day for this condition are not covered. (See Note 89)

172 – This type of services billed by a psychologist are not covered.

179 – The amount for this service is included in the approved amount for the consultation/office/hospital visit.

181 – Payment for this service is included in the major surgical fee.

187 – We need the name and address of the individual doctor who performed this service. Please resubmit your claim with this information.

192 – Medicare benefits have been reduced because the patient's employer group health plan has paid some of these expenses.

198 – A claim must be sent to the patient's employer group health plan first. After the claim has been processed by that plan, resubmit this claim with the bills and the notice the other insurance company sent you.

203 – Clinical laboratory services. Blood Gas Studies and Rhythm Strips (1–3 leads) furnished in a hospital setting are reimbursed through the hospital.

205 – The date of this service is after the patient's expiration date provided to us by SSA. If service was rendered to this patient on this date, have the patient's estate contact the local Social Security Office for assistance.

206 – For payment, these services must be billed by the performing laboratory with the assignment accepted.

213 – We did not send this claim to Medicaid. Please send this statement and a copy of the claim to the agency that handles Medicaid in your area.

216 – This service or item cannot be processed until your application for a Medicare provider identification number is received and approved.

218 – Since you are Medicare participating, we have processed this claim as assigned. Future claims must be billed on assignment. If the bill was paid in full, you must immediately refund the amount due to the beneficiary.

219 – We need this charge submitted on your letterhead bill. Please resubmit your claim with this information.

221 – The name and Medicare number submitted on this claim do not match. Please verify for whom these services were rendered and provide the correct name and number on the claim and resubmit.

223 – We did not consider this for payment because you did not send the extra information we asked for. Payment can be requested again by sending us another claim form and all the information.

226 – Medicare will pay rent for the prescribed number of months or until the equipment is no longer needed, whichever occurs first. This is the first monthly rental payment.

227 – You will receive a notice each month when additional rental payments are paid.

231 – Medicare will no longer pay for rental on this item since the purchase price has been paid.

237 – The amount of this payment is the difference between the approved purchase allowance and the rental payments you have received.

YOUR RIGHT TO REVIEW OF A CASE

If you have a problem or question about the way a claim was handled or about the amount paid, please write Transamerica Occidental Life, Box 54905, Terminal Annex, Los Angeles, California 90054, within 6 months of the date of this notice. We will give your request full consideration.

Your Social Security office will help you file a request for review of a claim if it is more convenient for you.

WHERE TO SEND REFUNDS

When refunding a payment you should send a check with a letter of explanation. The letter should include your Transamcrica Occidental/Medicare check number, beneficiary name and Medicare identification number (HICNo.), control number to which the payment relates, and any other information which may be pertinent to the refund. Send this information to:

Transamerica Occidental Life
C/O Check and Payment Control
Box 54905, Terminal Annex
Los Angeles, CA 90054-0905

KEY TO CODES FOR PLACE AND TYPE OF SERVICE

Place of service	Type of service
1. Office	A. Medical care
2. Home	B. Surgery (includes treatment of fractures)
3. Inpatient hospital	C. Consultation
4. Skilled nursing facility	D. Diagnostic X-ray
5. Outpatient hospital	E. Diagnostic laboratory
6. Independent laboratory	F. Radiation therapy
7. Other	G. Anesthesia
8. Independent kidney disease treatment center	H. Assistance at surgery
	I. Other medical service
	J. Whole blood or packed red cells

B

FIGURE 12-14, cont'd B, Back of Medicare RA document.

charges to Medicaid's allowable charges. This would require an adjustment entry on the patient's financial accounting record. Cutbacks are common on Medicaid claims.

Medicare overpayments can occur in the following situations:

● The carrier processes the charge more than once.
● The physician receives duplicate payments from Medicare and a secondary payer.

FIGURE 12-15 Insurance billing specialist explaining a Medicare remittance advice document that the physician's office has received.

● The physician is paid directly on an unassigned claim.
● The item is not covered but is paid.
● The payment is made on erroneous information.
● If an overpayment check is received, providers have 60 days to report and return any overpayments discovered. Deposit the check and then write to Medicare notifying them of the overpayment. Include a copy of the check and the RA. Depending on the policy of the carrier, the provider can either write a check or this overpayment will be deducted from the next Medicare payment and will be shown on the RA. If the physician wishes to repay a Medicare overpayment on the installment plan, Financial Statement of Debtor CMS-379 form may be used. This form is sent to the physician when the carrier notifies the physician that money is due back.

Refer to Chapter 9 for additional information about EOB documents from private insurance carriers.

Review and Redetermination Process

Chapter 9 outlines in detail the steps to take for having a claim reviewed and the process of appealing a claim in the Medicare program.

MEDICARE REMITTANCE ADVICE
XYZ Insurance Company

Physician or supplier name	Dates of service From MMDD To MMDDYY	See back serv typl	Sub code (alwcode)	Billed amount	Amount allowed	See ** act cde	Beneficiary obligation Deductible Co-ins		Medicare payment to Beneficiary provider

BENEFICIARY: BILL HUTCH   HIC NUMBER: 5432-112-34
CONTROL NO.: 92106-30810-00   DE/MI: 2121D52

John Doe MD 0310	0310XX	D 03	120101	145.00	105.00	101	110.00	1.00	0.00 4.00
CLAIM TOTALS:				145.00	105.00	101	110.00	1.00	0.00 4.00

A

MEDICAID REMITTANCE ADVICE

RECIPIENT NAME	RECIPIENT MEDICAID ID NO.	CLAIM CONTROL NUMBER	SERVICE DATE MO DAY YR	PROCEDURE CODE	PATIENT ACCT. NO.	QTY.	MEDICARE ALLOWED	MEDICAID ALLOWED	PATIENT LIABILITY	COMPUTED MCR AMT.	MEDICAID PAID	EOB MESSAGE
BILL HUTCH	521345678	4006984891200	03 10 XX	49555–80		001	105.00	73.00		4.00	.00	
		4006984891200	00 00 XX			000	105.00	73.00		4.00	69.00	
BLOOD DEDUCT 00 DEDUCTIBLE 110.00 COINSUR 1.00 CUTBACK 32.00												CUTBACK 443

B

FIGURE 12-16 A, A Medicare/Medicaid case after payment by Medicare. **B,** The Medicaid remittance advice shows reimbursement of the coinsurance and deductible amounts dual billed to Medicaid.

PROCEDURE 12-1

Determine Whether Medicare Is Primary or Secondary and Determine Additional Benefits

1. Inquire whether the patient is covered under one or more of the following plans or situations:

    • *Automobile liability insurance, no-fault insurance,* and *self-insured liability insurance.* An individual injured or ill because of an automobile accident may be covered by liability insurance or no-fault insurance.

    • *Disability insurance.* Disability insurance coverage offered through an employer-sponsored large group health plan (LGHP).

    • *Employee group health plan* (EGHP). Insurance policies for individuals 65 years of age or older who are still employed. Employers with 20 or more employees are required to offer workers and their spouses ages 65 through 69 years the same health benefits offered to younger workers. Workers may accept or reject the employer's health insurance plan. If they accept it, Medicare becomes the secondary insurance carrier.

    • *Employer supplemental insurance.* A Medicare beneficiary has this plan through a former employer. Some people are covered by employment plans even after retirement, as long as the plan allows it and the insured informs the insurance company that he or she wishes to maintain coverage. These are known as *conversion policies.* Complementary benefits can vary in these supplemental plans, and these policies are not considered "Medigap" as defined by federal law. Note: When an employee retires and Medicare becomes the primary coverage, the company's group health plan coordinates benefits with Medicare.

    • *Federal Black Lung Act.* This act was formed to cover employees or former coal miner employees who have illness related to black lung disorder and have acceptable diagnoses that occur on the Department of Labor's list.

    • *Veterans Affairs* (VA). A Medicare beneficiary is also receiving benefits from the Department of Veterans Affairs. In this situation, there must be a decision made as to where to send the claim. Medicare is not secondary to the VA, and the VA is not secondary to Medicare. The claim is sent where specified by the patient. The claim can be sent to Medicare, where, if the claim is processed, the patient must satisfy his or her contractual requirement to pay any deductible and copayment amounts. If the patient asks that the claim be sent to the VA instead of Medicare, the claim is processed and any payments issued are considered as payment in full. Many veterans want the claim sent to the VA.

    • *Workers' compensation.* An individual suffers a disease or injury connected with employment.

    These plans are billed as primary (first) payer and Medicare second. Payments for these types of policies may not necessarily go to the physician but may go to the insured.

2. Ask to see the Medicare card, as well as any other insurance cards, and make photocopies of both sides of each card.

3. Inquire of the patient whether the supplemental coverage was carried over (conversion policy) from his or her employer.

4. Call both carriers if the type of plan is not clearly identified.

5. Bill the correct insurance plan.

    For Medigap (MG) cases, nonparticipating physicians may collect copayments and deductibles up to their limiting charge (unless the state forbids collection of more than the allowed amount) from patients at the time of service. Participating physicians may not collect copayments/deductibles from patients covered by MG if the patient requests the physician to submit the claim to the MG insurer. Collect copayments after receiving the Medicare/MG remittance advice (RA) document.

    For other secondary insurance, write the patient's group and policy (or certificate) numbers on the Medicare RA, attach it to either a new CMS-1500 (08-05) or a copy of the original Health Insurance Claim Form CMS-1500 (08-05), and electronically transmit or submit it to the secondary carrier. Then copy the physician's billing statement that shows date of treatment, description of service(s) rendered, fees, and diagnosis.

PROCEDURE 12-2

Complete an Advance Beneficiary Notice of Noncoverage (ABN) Form CMS-R-131

THERE ARE 10 BLANKS FOR COMPLETION LABELED A THROUGH J:

A. Notifier(s): Enter the name, address, and telephone number of the provider.

B. Patient Name: Enter the first and last name and middle initial of the Medicare beneficiary.

C. Identification Number: Enter a number for the Medicare beneficiary that helps to link the notice with a related claim. However, this field is optional and choosing not to enter a number does not invalidate the ABN. The beneficiary's Medicare health insurance claim number will no longer be used.

D. Enter name of item(s), service(s), tests, or procedures. If not enough space, use an attached sheet noting it in the box.

E. Reason Medicare May Not Pay: Explain the reason why you think the service may not be covered by Medicare (e.g., Medicare does not pay for this test for the condition or Medicare does not pay for these tests as often as this [denied as too frequent]).

F. Estimated Cost: Enter a cost estimate for any item or service described in field D.

G. Options: Patient should choose and check one of the three boxes. If the beneficiary cannot make a choice, the notice should be annotated.

H. Additional Information: Insert more comments for clarification (e.g., provide context on Medicare payment policy applicable to a specific benefit or other payer information).

I. Signature: Medicare beneficiary should sign the notice.

J. Date: Insert the date the beneficiary signed the ABN.

KEY POINTS

This is a brief chapter review or summary of the key issues presented. To further enhance your knowledge of the technical subject matter, review the key terms and key abbreviations for this chapter by locating the meanings in the glossary at the end of this book that appear in a section before the index.

1. Medicare is administered by the CMS.

2. Medicare is a health insurance program for people age 65 or older, people younger than age 65 with certain disabilities, and people of all ages with end-stage renal disease.

3. The patient's complete name exactly as shown on his or her insurance card and Medicare claim number including the letter at the end must appear on all Medicare claims.

4. Medicare Part A is for hospital insurance benefits, and Part B is for SMI benefits.

5. Medicare Part C is referred to as Medicare Advantage Plan. These plans offer a number of health care options in addition to those available under Medicare Part A and Part B.

6. Medicare Part D Prescription Drug Plan is a stand-alone drug plan, presented by insurance and other private companies, that offers drug coverage that meets the standards established by Medicare.

7. Several federal acts regulate health care coverage of persons age 65 and older who are employed.

8. MG is a specialized Medicare supplemental insurance policy whose predefined minimum benefits are regulated by the federal government and devised for the Medicare beneficiary.

9. MSP is a primary insurance plan of a Medicare beneficiary who must pay for any medical care or services first before a Medicare fiscal intermediary is sent a claim.

10. To prevent overuse of services and spot fraud, the Federal Claims Amendment Act was enacted in 1986. It offers financial incentives to informants (whistleblowers).

11. CLIA is a federal act established in 1988 that regulates laboratory certification and accreditation standards, quality control, proficiency testing, personnel standards, program administration, and safety measures for all freestanding laboratories, including POLs.

12. Because Medicare is a federal program, providers that transmit claims to Medicare must comply with billing and coding regulations issued by CMS.

13. Participating physicians agree to accept assignment on all Medicare claims and may bill the patient only for the Medicare deductible ($155 in 2010) and coinsurance amounts.

14. An ABN is an agreement given to the patient to read and sign before rendering a service if the

participating physician thinks that it may be denied for payment because of medical necessity or limitation of liability by Medicare. ABNs apply if the patient is in an original Medicare program and do not apply for patients in private fee-for-service or managed care plans.

15. CCI is federal legislation that attempts to eliminate unbundling or other inappropriate reporting of procedural codes for services to Medicare patients.

16. To obtain correct payment for a procedure or service, a code number must be selected from level I or II of the HCPCS coding system and transmitted to the Medicare administrative contractor.

17. The time limit for sending in Medicare claims is the end of the calendar year after the fiscal year in which services were furnished.

18. Medicare sends a payment check and a nationally standardized document to participating physicians called a *Medicare RA* and a similar document to the patient called an MSN.

℮volve INTERNET RESOURCES

For active links to the following resources, visit the Evolve website at
http://evolve.elsevier.com/fordney/handbook

- Centers for Medicare and Medicaid Services (CMS) Forms, Publications, Regulations, Transmittals (formerly called Program Memorandums)
- CLIA-waived tests
- CMS Manual System
- Education and training
- Epocrates freeware
- *Federal Register*
- Intermediary Carrier Directory
- Social Security Online

STUDENT ASSIGNMENT

✓ Study Chapter 12.

✓ Answer the multiple choice, fill-in-the-blank, and true/false review questions in the *Workbook* to reinforce the theory learned in this chapter and to help prepare you for a future test.

✓ Complete the assignments in the *Workbook* to give you experience in computing Medicare in mathematic calculations, selecting HCPCS code numbers, abstracting from patients' health records, preparing financial accounting record cards, and completing forms pertinent to the Medicare program.

✓ Turn to the glossary at the end of this textbook for a further understanding of the key terms and key abbreviations used in this chapter.

KEY TERMS*

categorically needy
coinsurance
copayment
covered services
Early and Periodic Screening,
  Diagnosis, and Treatment

fiscal agent
Maternal and Child Health
  Program
Medicaid
Medi-Cal
medically needy

prior approval
recipient
share of cost
State Children's Health
  Insurance Program
Supplemental Security Income

KEY ABBREVIATIONS*

DEFRA
EPSDT
FPL
MCHP
MN

MQMB
OBRA
OOY claims
POS machine
QI program

QMB
RA
SCHIP
SLMB
SSI

TANF
TEFRA

---

*Definitions for the key terms and key abbreviations are located near the back of this textbook in the glossary.

CHAPTER 13

Medicaid and Other State Programs

OBJECTIVES

After reading this chapter, you should be able to:

- Define terminology relating to Medicaid.
- Interpret Medicaid abbreviations.
- Discuss the history of Medicaid.
- Describe added benefits for Medicaid recipients afforded by the Patient Protection and Affordable Care Act and the Health Care and Education Reconciliation Act of 2010.
- Identify those eligible for the Medicaid Qualified Medicare Beneficiaries program.
- Name the two Medicaid eligibility classifications.

- State eligibility requirements and claims procedures for the Maternal and Child Health Program.
- List important information to abstract from the patient's Medicaid card.
- Describe the Medicaid basic benefits.
- Explain basic operations of a Medicaid-managed care system.
- Explain basic Medicaid claim procedure guidelines.
- File claims for patients who have Medicaid and other coverage.

Service to Patients

Avoid stereotyping patients. Provide the same quality of service regardless of the patient's age, sex, race, nationality, economic level, education, occupation, religion, or diagnosis. Signs of discrimination and prejudice have no place in the health care field.

HISTORY

Federal participation in providing medical care to needy persons began between 1933 and 1935 when the Federal Emergency Relief Administration made funds available to pay the medical expenses of the needy unemployed. The Social Security Act of 1935 set up the public assistance programs. Although no special provision was made for medical assistance, the federal government paid a share of the monthly assistance payments, which could

be used to meet the costs of medical care. However, the payment was made to the assistance recipient rather than the provider of medical care.

In 1950 Congress passed a law mandating that all states set up a health care program of assistance, which meant that the states had to meet minimum requirements. As a result of this mandate, the states set up **Medicaid** programs. Congress authorized vendor payments for medical care—payments from the welfare agency directly to physicians, health care institutions, and other providers of medical services. By 1960, four-fifths of the states had made provisions for medical vendor payments.

A new category of assistance recipient was established for the medically needy aged population. The incomes of these individuals were too high to qualify them for cash

Performance objectives, testing and review material, and hands-on practical exercises for this chapter are available in these resources

The Insurance Handbook Student Workbook   The Insurance Handbook Evolve Site

assistance payments, but they needed help in meeting the costs of medical care. The federal government financially supports the minimum assistance level, and the states must wholly support any part of the program that goes beyond the federal minimum. This is referred to as *state share*.

In 1965 Title XIX of the Social Security Act became federal law, and Medicaid legally came into being. To a large extent it was the result of various attempts during the previous 30 years to provide medical care to the needy. The program has always had somewhat of a split personality. On one hand, it is viewed as an attempt on the part of the government to provide comprehensive quality health care to those unable to afford it. On the other hand, Medicaid has been seen as merely a bill-paying mechanism that uses the most efficient and economic system possible to administer the provision of health care.

In 1982 the Tax Equity and Fiscal Responsibility Act (TEFRA) set down laws affecting those under the Medicare program, as well as Medicaid medically needy recipients and those in certain other categories. See Chapter 12 for information about how TEFRA affects Medicare recipients.

Since 1983, the trend in many states has been to expand Medicaid eligibility requirements and services. Changes in Medicaid eligibility allowing more people into the program were made by many states after the passage by the federal government of the Deficit Reduction Act of 1984 (DEFRA) and the Child Health Assurance Program (CHAP). On July 1, 2006, as part of DEFRA, a federal law became effective requiring new applicants and current beneficiaries renewing their benefits (except seniors and people with disabilities) to submit birth certificates, passports, or other documents to establish their legal right as United States (US) citizens to benefits. If no documentation of citizenship can be found, sworn affidavits from the beneficiary and at least one or two other individuals can be used.

In 2002 and 2003, states across the nation faced steep budget shortfalls. A vast majority of them made cuts of some kind in their Medicaid programs by either instituting or boosting copayments for certain types of services or eliminating some services. **Copayment** (copay) is a required specific dollar amount that must be collected at each office visit for medical services received by an individual. Under Medicaid, different copayment amounts may be set for each patient type and for certain medical procedures.

Health care reform legislation, known as the Patient Protection and Affordable Care Act and the Health Care and Education Reconciliation Act, was passed in 2010. These Acts impact the Medicaid program by expanding access for childless adults, nonelderly, and non-pregnant individuals and include preventive services and long-term care benefits. Additional funds were allocated for maternal and child health services. Community First Choice was made available for states to offer medical assistance for home- and community-based attendant services and supports for individuals eligible for medical assistance under a state Medicaid plan.

MEDICAID PROGRAMS

Title XIX of the Social Security Act provides for a program of medical assistance for certain low-income individuals and families. The program is known as Medicaid in 49 states and **Medi-Cal** in California. In 2010 health plans were established as the result of a state mandate to transform Medi-Cal from a state-run insurance system to a locally run managed care program. Arizona is the only state without a Medicaid program similar to those existing in other states. Since 1982, Arizona has received federal funds under a demonstration waiver for an alternative medical assistance program (prepaid care) for low-income persons called the *Arizona Health Care Cost Containment System* (AHCCCS). In 2006 a "Waiver Renewal Proposal" gave an extension until September 30, 2011.

Medicaid is administered by state governments with partial federal funding. Coverage and benefits vary widely from state to state because the federal government sets minimum requirements and the states are free to enact more benefits. Thus each state designs its own Medicaid program within federal guidelines. The Centers for Medicaid and Medicare Services (CMS) of the Bureau of Program Operations of the US Department of Health and Human Services is responsible for the federal aspects of Medicaid. Medicaid is not so much an insurance program as it is an assistance program.

Maternal and Child Health Program

 Each state and certain other jurisdictions including territories and the District of Columbia (56 programs total) operate a **State Children's Health Insurance Program (SCHIP)** with federal grant support under Title V of the Social Security Act. In some states, this program may be known as **Maternal and Child Health Program (MCHP)** or Children's Special Health Care Services (CSHCS). Although Title V has been amended on a number of occasions, notably between 1981 and 1987, no changes have been as sweeping as those in the Omnibus Budget Reconciliation Act (OBRA) of 1989. SCHIP insures children from families whose income is below 200% of the federal poverty level or whose family has an income 50% higher than the state's Medicaid eligibility threshold. However, some states have expanded SCHIP eligibility beyond the 200% federal poverty limit and others are covering entire families and not just children. States have three options in designing their program. The state can do one of the following:

- Use SCHIP funds to expand Medicaid eligibility to children who previously did not qualify for the program.
- Design a separate children's health insurance program entirely separate from Medicaid.
- Combine both the Medicaid and separate program options.

Federal funds are granted to states, enabling them to:

- Provide low-income mothers and children access to quality maternal and child health services.
- Reduce infant mortality and the incidence of preventable diseases and handicapping conditions among children.
- Increase the number of children immunized against disease and the number of low-income children receiving health assessments and follow-up diagnostic and treatment services.
- Promote the health of mothers and infants by providing prenatal, delivery, and postpartum care for low-income, at-risk pregnant women.
- Provide preventive and primary care services for low-income children.
- Provide rehabilitation services for the blind and disabled younger than age 16 years.
- Provide, promote, and develop family-centered, community-based, coordinated care for children with special health care needs.

The state agency tries to locate mothers, infants, and children younger than 21 years of age who may have conditions eligible for treatment under the MCHP. The conditions are diagnosed, and the necessary medical and other health-related care, any hospitalization, and any continuing follow-up care are given.

After a child is examined at an MCHP clinic and a diagnosis is made, the parents are advised about the treatment that will benefit the child. The state agency then helps them locate this care. If the parents cannot afford this care, the agency assists them with financial planning and may assume part or all of the cost of treatment, depending on the child's condition and the family's resources.

Individuals who work in a physician's office need to be aware of these services in the event a patient needs to be referred to a state agency for assistance.

Low-Income Medicare Recipients

There are three aid programs for Medicare patients who have low incomes and have difficulty paying Medicare premiums, copayments, and deductibles. Each program addresses a different financial category, and the monthly income figures are adjusted each year. The titles of the three programs follow:

- Medicaid Qualified Medicare Beneficiary Program
- Specified Low-Income Medicare Beneficiary Program
- Qualifying Individuals Program

The programs are usually administered through county social services departments, the same ones that administer Medicaid. One application is completed that pertains to all three programs, and an individual is placed in one of the programs depending on how he or she qualifies financially.

Medicaid Qualified Medicare Beneficiary Program

The Medicaid Qualified Medicare Beneficiary (MQMB) program was introduced in the Medicare Catastrophic Act of 1988 as an amendment to the Social Security Act. In 1990 the Omnibus Budget Reconciliation Act allowed for assistance to qualified Medicare beneficiaries (QMBs, pronounced "kwim-bees") who are aged and disabled and are receiving Medicare and have annual incomes below the federal poverty level. Eligibility also depends on what other financial resources an individual might have.

Under this act, states must provide limited Medicaid coverage for QMBs. They must pay Medicare Part B premiums (and Part A premiums if applicable), along with necessary Medicare deductibles and coinsurance amounts. **Coinsurance** is the dollar amount of payment that is above the rate that Medicare pays for medical services. When discussing Medicaid, the terms *copayment* and *coinsurance* do not have the same meaning as they do when talking about private insurance coverage issues. MQMB coverage is restricted to Medicare cost sharing unless the beneficiary qualifies for Medicaid in some other way. Medicaid will not pay for the service if Medicare does not cover the service to the patient.

States are also required to pay Part A premiums but no other expenses for qualified disabled and working individuals. It is optional for states to provide full Medicaid benefits to QMBs who meet a state-established income standard.

Specified Low-Income Medicare Beneficiary Program

The Specified Low-Income Medicare Beneficiary (SLMB, pronounced "slim-bee") program was established in 1993 for elderly individuals whose income is 20% above the federal poverty level. It pays the entire Medicare Part B premium. The patient must pay the deductible and copay and must pay for noncovered items.

Qualifying Individuals Program

The Qualifying Individuals (QI) program was created in 1997 for qualifying individuals whose income is at least 135% but less than 175% of the federal poverty level (FPL). It also pays for the Medicare Part B premium.

MEDICAID ELIGIBILITY

Medicaid is available to certain needy and low-income people such as the elderly (65 years or older), blind, disabled, and members of families with dependent children deprived of the support of at least one parent and financially eligible on the basis of income and resources. In general, Medicaid is available only to US citizens and certain "qualified immigrants." Passports and birth certificates must be submitted for proof of citizenship. If a person may be eligible for Medicaid, he or she goes to the local public service welfare office, human service, or family independence agency and applies for benefits.

Verifying Eligibility

After acceptance into the program, the patient brings a form or card to the physician's office that verifies acceptance into the program (Figure 13-1), but this does not indicate proof of eligibility. It is the provider's responsibility to verify at each visit that the person to receive care is eligible on the date the service is rendered and is the individual to whom the card was issued.

FIGURE 13-1 Medicaid patient checking in with the receptionist.

Each state decides which services are covered and what the payments are for each service. There are two classifications that contain several basic groups of needy and low-income individuals.

Categorically Needy

The first classification, the **categorically needy** group, includes all cash recipients of the Temporary Assistance to Needy Families (TANF), certain other TANF-related groups, most cash recipients of the **Supplemental Security Income (SSI)** program, other SSI-related groups, QMBs, and institutional and long-term care and intermediate-care facility patients (Box 13-1).

A **recipient** is an individual certified by the local welfare department to receive benefits of Medicaid under one of the specific aid categories. TANF was instituted by the *Personal Responsibility and Work Opportunity Act*, also known as the *Welfare Reform Act of 1996*. This federal law ended welfare as an entitlement program and requires recipients to work after receiving benefits for 2 years, with a lifetime limit of 5 years of benefits paid by federal funds. This Act aims to encourage two-parent families, discourages out-of-wedlock births, and helps enforce child support. It replaced the federal program of Aid to Dependent Children (ADC), later known as Aid to Families with Dependent Children (AFDC).

Medically Needy

The second classification involves state general assistance programs for low-income people, the medically indigent, and individuals losing employer health insurance. This classification is sometimes referred to as the **medically needy (MN)** class. A Medicaid recipient in this category may or may not pay a copayment or a deductible, which must be met within the eligibility month or other specified time frame before he or she can receive state benefits (also known as *share of cost* or *spend down*). Emergency care and pregnancy services are exempt by law from copayment requirements. This may be a component of a state's general assistance program for low-income people. Another method to meet Medicaid eligibility requirements is to spend down to or below the state's medically needy income level by incurring medical expenses that reduce excess income. This then makes it low enough to make him or her eligible for the program.

For those individuals who may become medically indigent as a result of high medical care expenses and inadequate health insurance coverage, a number of states have adopted a State Program of Assistance for the Medically Indigent. Box 13-1 lists the classes and basic groups for Medicaid eligibility.

Box 13-1   Groups Eligible for Medicaid Benefits

Mandatory Eligibility Groups

- Families, pregnant women, and children
- Temporary Assistance to Needy Families (TANF)-related groups
- Non-TANF pregnant women and children
- Infants born to Medicaid-eligible pregnant women
- Children younger than age 6 and pregnant women whose family income is at or below 135% of the federal poverty level (FPL)
- Recipients of adoption assistance or foster care assistance under Title IV-E of the Social Security Act
- Aged and disabled
- Supplemental Security Income (SSI)-related groups
- Qualified Medicare Beneficiaries (QMBs)
- Persons who receive institutional or other long-term care in nursing facilities (NFs) and intermediate care facilities (ICFs)
- Certain Medicaid beneficiaries
- Medicare-Medicaid beneficiaries

Optional Eligibility Groups

Low-income persons losing employer health insurance coverage (Medicaid purchase if person has Consolidated Omnibus Budget Reconciliation Act [COBRA] coverage)

Infants up to age 1 and pregnant women not covered under the mandatory rules whose family income is not more than 185% of the FPL (note that percent may be modified by each state)

Children younger than age 21 who meet TANF income and resource requirements but who are otherwise not eligible for TANF

Persons who would be eligible if institutionalized, but receive care under home- and community-based service waivers

Persons infected with tuberculosis who would be financially eligible for Medicaid at the SSI income level if they were within a Medicaid-covered category (limited coverage)

Low-income children with the State Children's Health Insurance Program (SCHIP)

Low-income, uninsured women who are diagnosed through the Centers for Disease Control and Prevention's National Breast and Cervical Cancer Early Detection program and who are in need of treatment for breast or cervical cancer

Medically Needy Eligibility Group

Medically indigent low-income individuals and families who have too much income to qualify under mandatory or optional eligibility Medicaid groups

Maternal and Child Health Program Eligibility

 Specific conditions qualify a child for benefits under the MCHP. The state law under which each agency operates either defines the conditions to be included or directs the children's agency to define them. All state laws include children who have some kind of handicap that requires orthopedic treatment or plastic surgery; a few states add other conditions. A list of both types of conditions that qualify children for MCHP follows:

- Cerebral palsy
- Chronic conditions affecting bones and joints
- Cleft lip
- Cleft palate
- Clubfoot
- Cystic fibrosis*
- Epilepsy*
- Hearing problems*
- Mental retardation*
- Multiple handicaps*
- Paralyzed muscles
- Rheumatic and congenital heart disease*
- Vision problems requiring surgery*

---

*Only some states include this item in their MCHP.

Spousal Impoverishment Protection Law

Spousal Impoverishment Protection refers to federal legislation that affects special financial provisions in Medicaid for the Elderly, Blind, or Disabled (EBD) law. It has rules affecting income and assets for certain elderly married or disabled couples that receive or apply for nursing home or community waiver services. Formerly, if one partner (institutionalized spouse) needed to be in a nursing facility, a couples' income and assets would become so depleted to qualify that the other spouse (community spouse) did not have a sufficient amount to live on. This protection counts assets such as cash, checking and savings accounts, life insurance policies, and certificates of deposits. It does not count the couples' home, car, household furnishings, burial assets (insurance, trust funds, or plots), clothing, or other personal items. This prevents the community spouse from being impoverished by his or her spouse's institutionalization.

New Freedom Initiative

The New Freedom Initiative (NFI), federal legislation passed in 2001, aims to remove barriers to community living for people of all ages with disabilities and long-term illnesses. NFI ensures opportunities so disabled individuals can learn and develop skills, engage in productive work, make choices about their daily lives, and participate fully in community life. Several departments in the federal government partner with states and communities in the areas of employment, education, housing, transportation, assistive technology, community integration, and health. Their goal is to give necessary support to allow elderly and disabled people to fully participate in community life at all those levels.

Accepting Medicaid Patients
Program Participation

A provider must enroll for participation in the Medicaid program by signing a written provider agreement, depending on state guidelines, with the fiscal agent, local public service welfare office, human service agency, or family independence agency.

Individual physicians have their own office procedures for handling Medicaid patients. A patient can be on Medicaid one month and then off the following month, or the patient could be on the program for several months or years; each case is different. The physician may accept or refuse to treat Medicaid patients but must make the decision on the basis of the entire Medicaid program, not an individual patient's personality, medical situation, or other discriminating factor. The patient must receive quality care and be treated the same as the paying patient. If the physician decides to take Medicaid patients, he or she must accept the Medicaid allowance as payment in full. The Medicaid allowance is the maximum dollar amount to be considered for payment for a service or procedure by the program.

When obtaining personal information from the patient at the time of the first visit or a follow-up visit, always check and/or update the patient's name and address by asking for photo identification such as a driver's license. If you wish to verify the patient's telephone number, use a reverse address directory to substantiate that it is correct. Another type of directory, such as City Directory, is one that lists everyone on a given block or even in an apartment building who has a telephone. These easy reference guides cut verification time in half. They may be too expensive for a small office, but the information may be accessible via the Internet or through a local library or hospital library if there is an online service. Some Medicaid individuals are homeless and may list fake addresses, which makes locating them difficult. Always follow the same policies for processing Medicaid patients as those used for private patients so that the office cannot be accused of using prejudicial procedures.

Identification Card

A plastic or paper Medicaid identification card (or coupons in some states) is usually issued monthly (Figure 13-2). Under certain classifications of eligibility, identification cards are issued in some states on the 1st and 15th of each month, every 2 months, every 3 months, or every 6 months. Sometimes an unborn child can be issued an identification card that is used for services promoting the life and health of the fetus. Obtain a photocopy of the front and back of the card. Carefully check the expiration date of the card each time the patient visits the physician's office to see whether eligibility is indicated for the month of service. Note whether the patient has other insurance, copayment requirements, or restrictions such as being eligible for only certain types of medical services. The items that must be abstracted from the card for claim submission are (1) the patient's name exactly as shown, (2) Medicaid identification number, (3) gender, and (4) the date of birth.

Point-of-Service Machine

When professional services are rendered, eligibility for that month must be verified, which may be done in a number of ways. The Potomac Group, Inc., in Nashville, TN, has developed MediFAX for some states. This is a machine that allows the user to verify coverage in seconds and is available for several states. Some states provide their own electronic system for Medicaid verification via touch-tone telephone, modem, or specialized Medicaid terminal equipment such as a point-of-service (POS) machine (Figure 13-3). Some states issue cards that contain adhesive labels listing the month of eligibility that must be used on the billing claim form.

Retroactive Eligibility

Retroactive eligibility may be granted to a patient in some cases. In a situation when the patient has been referred to apply for Medicaid, the patient must ask for retroactive status; otherwise, the approval effective date is the date of the application. When patients are seeking medical care who are in hope of qualifying for Medicaid but have not done so at the time of service, the account must be set up as a cash account until retroactive eligibility has been established. Retroactive eligibility status must be decided within 90 days of filing of the application. If the patient has documentation or a retroactive card confirming this and has paid for any services during the retroactive period, a refund must be made and Medicaid billed. As described and shown in the previous chapter, a waiver of liability agreement rewritten to the Medicaid program and signed by the patient might be used in such cases.

MEDICAID BENEFITS

Covered Services

Under federal guidelines, the state Medicaid basic benefits offered to eligible recipients include the types of

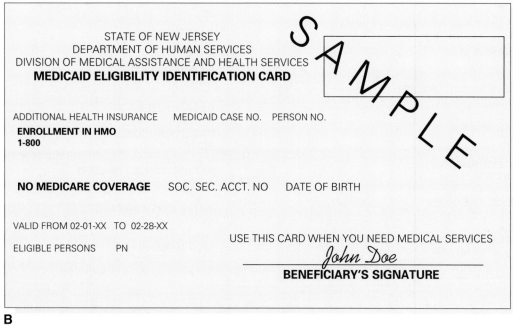

FIGURE 13-2 A, Plastic Medi-Cal benefits identification card. **B,** Medicaid eligibility identification card issued in the State of New Jersey.

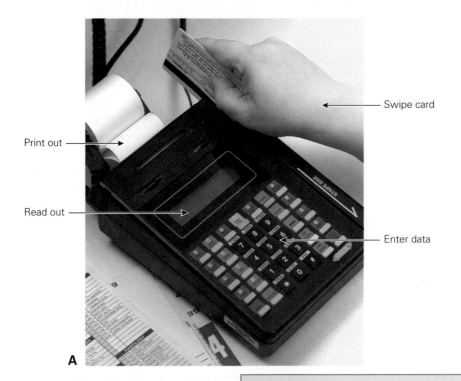

A

POS Device: Medi-Service Printout

EDS BROAD AVENUE TERMINAL T309006
XX-02-15
17:16:36

PROVIDER NUMBER:
12345F

TRANSACTION TYPE: MEDI-SERVICES

RECIPIENT ID:
5077534XX

YEAR & MONTH OF BIRTH:
1975-12

DATE OF ISSUE:
XX-02-15

DATE OF SERVICE:
XX-02-15

PROCEDURE CODE:
45339

LAST NAME: MORRISON MEDI SVC
RESERVATION APPLIED

B

POS Device: Share of Cost Printout

EDS BROAD AVENUE TERMINAL T309006
XX-02-15
17:16:36

PROVIDER NUMBER:
12345F

TRANSACTION TYPE: SHARE OF COST

RECIPIENT ID:
5077534XX

YEAR & MONTH OF BIRTH:
1984-10

DATE OF ISSUE:
XX-02-15

DATE OF SERVICE:
XX-02-15

CASE NUMBER:

PROCEDURE CODE:
90945

PATIENT APPLIED AMOUNT:
$50.00

TOTAL BILLED AMOUNT:
$100.00

LAST NAME: ADAMS
AMOUNT DEDUCTED: $50.00
SHARE OF COST HAS BEEN MET

C

FIGURE 13-3 A, Insurance biller using a point-of-service (POS) device machine to check a patient's Medicaid eligibility. **B,** Printout from a POS device for Medi-Service. **C,** Printout from a POS device for share of cost.

Box 13-2 Medicaid Basic Benefits

Family planning
Home health care
Immunizations
Inpatient hospital care
Laboratory and x-ray
Outpatient hospital care
Physicians' care
Screening, diagnosis, and treatment of children younger than 21 years of age
Skilled nursing care
Transportation to and from health care providers
In some states, additional services included might be the following:
  Allergy care
  Ambulance services
  Certain medical cosmetic procedures
  Chiropractic care
  Clinic care
  Dental care
  Dermatologic care
  Diagnostic, screening, preventive, and rehabilitative services (e.g., physical therapy)
  Emergency department care
  Eyeglasses and eye refractions
  Hospice care
  Intermediate care
  Occupational therapy
  Optometric services
  Podiatric care
  Prescription drugs
  Private duty nursing
  Prosthetic devices
  Psychiatric care
  Respiratory care
  Speech therapy

covered services listed in Box 13-2. Consult state regulations for additional benefits. **Covered services** are specific mandatory and optional services and supplies that Medicaid provides.

Early and Periodic Screening, Diagnosis, and Treatment

Another benefit of the Medicaid program is the **Early and Periodic Screening, Diagnosis, and Treatment (EPSDT)** service. This is a program of prevention, early detection, and treatment of welfare children (younger than age 21). In California (Medi-Cal), it is known as the Child Health and Disability Prevention (CHDP) program and in Ohio as Healthchek. Because many states are changing the name of EPSDT and the services offered under the program, check with the state Medicaid vendor.

The EPSDT guidelines include a medical history and physical examination; immunization status assessment; dental, hearing, and vision screening; developmental assessment; and screening for anemia and lead

absorption, tuberculosis, bacteriuria, and sickle cell disease and trait. States are required to provide necessary health care, diagnostic services, treatment, and other services to correct physical or mental defects found.

Disallowed Services

If a service is totally disallowed by Medicaid (denied claim), a physician is within legal rights in many states to bill the patient; consult state regulations before deciding to bill. However, it is wise to have the patient sign a waiver of liability agreement if the service to be provided may be a denied service from known past claim submission experience. An example of a waiver of liability agreement is shown in Figure 12-9. Write or telephone the state agency to obtain up-to-date information and details on the Medicaid program in a particular state (see Internet Resources at the end of this chapter for an active link from the Evolve website).

MEDICAID MANAGED CARE

As early as 1967, some states began bringing managed care to their Medicaid programs. In the past decade, many states adopted pilot projects to determine whether a managed care system would work and what benefits might be received. Mainly this was done to control escalating health care costs by curbing unnecessary emergency department visits and emphasizing preventive care.

When the last state, Arizona, joined Medicaid, it began with prepaid care rather than adhering to the way most states have structured their programs. By then, most states had been struggling with Medicaid for nearly 20 years. In these systems, the Medicaid recipient enrolls either in an existing or specifically formed plan similar to a health maintenance organization (HMO). Some plans are run by independent commissions appointed by county boards of supervisors. The patient may be either assigned or may choose a gatekeeper (clinic or primary care physician) who must approve all specialty care and inpatient or outpatient hospital treatment. Patients must use physicians, clinics, and hospitals participating in their assigned plan. Some doctors prefer to operate on a contract-to-contract, per-patient basis, rather than to be a participating provider.

Patients can be cared for side by side with private-paying patients. Some states have adopted capitation (a flat fee per patient) rather than fee-for-service reimbursement. There may be a small copayment for services. In programs run for a number of years, it has been found that there is better access to primary health care and savings of monies in delivering the care if the programs are well managed.

CLAIM PROCEDURES

Medicaid policies and claim procedures about identification cards, prior approval regulations, claim forms, and time limits vary from state to state. General guidelines for submitting claims are stated here.

For specific state guidelines, consult the current *Medicaid Handbook* online at the state fiscal agent's website (see Internet Resources at the end of this chapter for an active link from the Evolve website).

Copayment

There are two types of copayment requirements that may apply to a state. Some states require a small fixed copayment paid to the provider at the time services are rendered. This policy was instituted to help pay some of the administrative costs of physicians participating in the Medicaid program.

Another requirement is the **share of cost** or *spend down* copayment. Some Medicaid recipients must meet this copayment requirement each month before Medicaid benefits can be claimed. The amount may change from month to month, so be sure to verify the copayment each time it is collected. Obtain this copayment amount when the patient comes in for medical care and report on the claim form that it has been collected.

Prior Approval

Many times, **prior approval** is necessary for various services, except in a bona fide emergency. Some of these goods and services are the following:

● Durable medical equipment
● Hearing aids
● Hemodialysis
● Home health care
● Inpatient hospital care
● Long-term care facility services
● Medical supplies
● Medications
● Prosthetic or orthotic appliances
● Surgical procedures
● Transportation
● Some vision care

Usually prior authorization forms are completed to obtain permission for a specific service or hospitalization (Figure 13-4) and mailed or faxed to the Department of Health or a certain office in a region for approval. In some cases, time does not allow for a written request to be sent for prior approval, so an immediate authorization can be obtained via a telephone call to the proper department in any locale. Note the date and time that the authorization was given, the name of the person who gave authorization, and any verbal number given by the field office. Usually, a treatment authorization form indicating that the service was already authorized must be sent in as follow-up to the telephone call.

Time Limit

Each state has its own time limit for the submission of a claim. The time limit can vary from 2 months to 12 or 18 months from the date that the service was rendered. A bill can be rejected if it is submitted after the time limit unless the state recognizes some valid justification. Some states have separate procedures for billing over-one-year (OOY) claims. A percent of the claim may be reduced according to the date of a delinquent submission. Prescription drugs and dental services are often billed to a different intermediary than are services performed by a physician, depending on the state guidelines.

Reciprocity

Most states have reciprocity for Medicaid payments if a patient requires medical care while out of state. Contact the Medicaid fiscal intermediary in the patient's home state and ask for the appropriate forms. If the case was an emergency, state this on the form. File the papers with Medicaid in the patient's home state. Reimbursement will be at that state's rate.

Claim Form

As of October 1, 1986, federal law has mandated that the CMS-1500 Insurance Claim Form be adopted for the processing of Medicaid claims in all states.

Physicians either submit a claim form to a **fiscal agent,** which might be an insurance company, or the bill is sent directly to the local public service welfare office, human service, or family independence agency. These agencies have different names in each state. Refer to Internet Resources at the end of this chapter to locate the website for your local Medicaid fiscal agent.

Chapter 7 includes general instructions for block-by-block entries on how to complete the CMS-1500 (08-05) claim form for the Medicaid program. Because guidelines for completing the form vary among all Medicaid intermediaries, refer to the local Medicaid intermediary for their directions. Figure 7-5 is a template emphasizing placement of basic elements on the claim form and shaded blocks that do not require completion. Note that when questions about "insured" are asked on the claim form, the patient is always the insured even if a minor.

FIGURE 13-4 Completed treatment authorization request form used in California for the Medi-Cal program.

To keep up to date, always read the current bulletins or program memos on the Medicaid or Medi-Cal program at the state fiscal agent's website. Read and implement the rule changes and updates to avoid rejected claims.

Medicaid Managed Care

When filing a claim for a Medicaid managed care patient, send the bill or claim form to the managed care organization (MCO) and not the Medicaid fiscal agent. The MCO receives payment for services rendered to eligible members via either the capitation or other managed care method.

Maternal and Child Health Program

Each state's jurisdiction operates its own MCHP with its own unique administrative characteristics. Thus each has its own system and forms for billing and related procedures. The official plans and documents are retained in the individual state offices and are not available on either a regional or national office basis. For specific information about a state's policies, contact your local Department of Health to locate the office near you or go to Internet Resources at the end of this chapter for the website address.

Medicaid and Other Plans

It is possible that a person can be eligible for Medicaid and also have group health insurance coverage through an employer. When Medicaid and a third-party payer cover the patient, Medicaid is always considered the payer of last resort. The third-party payer (other insurance) is billed first.

Third-party liability occurs if any entity is liable to pay all or part of the medical cost of injury, disease, or disability. In these cases the primary carrier is the other program or insurance carrier, and it is sent the claim first. After a remittance advice/explanation of benefits (RA/EOB) or check voucher is received from the primary carrier, Medicaid (the secondary carrier) is billed. A copy of the RA/EOB or check voucher is enclosed.

Government Programs and Medicaid. When a Medicaid patient has Medicare (sometimes referred to as a *crossover case*), TRICARE, or CHAMPVA, always send the insurance claim first to the federal program fiscal agent servicing the region. Usually the Medicare fiscal agent automatically forwards the claim to the secondary payer, Medicaid. If this does not occur, then bill Medicaid second and attach to the claim form the RA/EOB or check voucher that has been received from the federal program. Only send in a claim if the other coverage denies payment or pays less than the Medicaid fee

schedule, or if Medicaid covers services not covered by the other policy.

Electronic claims may be automatically crossed over from primary government programs. Chapter 12 gives additional information on crossover claim submission. Figures 7-7 and 7-8 are templates emphasizing placement of basic elements on the claim form and shaded blocks that do not require completion for crossover claims. Chapter 14 gives further information on patients who receive benefits from TRICARE and CHAMPVA.

Medicaid and Immigrants

Some immigrants may have Medicare Part A or Part B or both (see Chapter 12). If an immigrant is older than 65 years, is on Medicaid (Medi-Cal in California), and is not eligible for Medicare benefits, then bill the Medicaid processing agent and use the proper Medicaid claim form for the region. On the CMS-1500 (08-05) claim form in Block 19, indicate "Immigrant is older than 65 years and not eligible for Medicare benefits." Your *Medicaid Handbook* should provide specifics for your region or state.

AFTER CLAIM SUBMISSION

Remittance Advice

If a provider wants to receive an electronic remittance advice, a form must be completed and submitted to the fiscal agent (Figure 13-5). However, a provider that relies on the paper system is sent an RA or check voucher that accompanies all Medicaid payment checks. Sometimes, five categories of adjudicated claims appear on an RA—adjustments, approvals, denials, suspends, and audit/refund (A/R) transactions—although this terminology may vary from one fiscal agent to another (Figure 13-6). *Adjudication* or *claim settlement* is the processing of an insurance claim through a series of edits for final determination of coverage (benefits) for possible payment.

Adjustments occur from overpayments or underpayments by the fiscal agent. Approval is when an original claim or a previously denied claim is approved for payment. Denied claims are listed with a reason code on the RA. Claims in suspense for a certain period of time may be listed on the RA. Accounts receivable A/R transactions are miscellaneous transactions as a result of cost settlements, state audits, or refund checks received. RAs for a Medicare case and a Medicaid case are illustrated in Figure 12-16.

Appeals

The time limit to appeal a claim varies from state to state, but it is usually 30 to 60 days from the date listed on the

FIGURE 13-5 Electronic Explanation of Payment (EOP) Agreement used by the Medicaid program in Alabama. It must be completed by a provider and authorizes the fiscal agent to transmit EOPs to the physician's electronic mail box.

RA. Most Medicaid offices consider an appeal filed when they receive it, not when it is sent. Usually appeals are sent on a special form or with a cover letter along with photocopies of documents applicable to the appeal (e.g., claim form, RA, and preauthorization forms). Appeals go first to either the regional fiscal agent or Medicaid bureau, next to the Department of Social Welfare or Human Services, and then to an appellate court that evaluates decisions by local and government agencies. At each level, an examiner looks at the case and makes a decision. If not satisfied, the physician may ask for further review at the next level.

MEDICAID REMITTANCE ADVICE

TO: ANYBODY, FERNANDO G.
1000 ELM STREET
ANYTOWN, XY 12345-0001

REFER TO PROVIDER MANUAL FOR DEFINITION OF RAD CODES

PROVIDER NUMBER 00AX65800	CLAIM TYPE MEDICAL	WARRANT NO 39248026	EDS SEQ NO 20000617	DATE 06/01/20XX	PAGE 1 of 1 pages

RECIPIENT NAME	RECIPIENT MEDICAID I.D. NO.	CLAIM CONTROL NUMBER	SERVICE DATES FROM MMDDYY	SERVICE DATES TO MMDDYY	PROCED CODE MODIFIER	PATIENT ACCOUNT NUMBER	QTY	BILLED AMT	PAYABLE AMT			PAID AMT	RAD CODE
APPROVES (RECONCILE TO FINANCIAL SUMMARY)													
TORRES R	559978557	5079350917901	030720XX	030720XX	Z4802		0001	20.00	16.22			16.22	0401
		5079350917901	030720XX	030720XX	Z4802		0001	20.00	16.22			16.22	0401
						TOTAL		40.00	32.44			32.44	
CHAN B	561198435	5044351314501	020320XX	020320XX	Z4800		0001	30.00	27.03			27.03	0401
		5044351314501	020320XX	020320XX	Z4800		0001	20.00	16.22			16.22	0401
						TOTAL		50.00	43.25			43.25	
	TOTALS FOR APPROVES							90.00	75.69			75.69	
												75.69	AMT PAID
DENIES (DO NOT RECONCILE TO FINANCIAL SUMMARY)													
GOMEZ M	624163192	501134031900	122720XX	122720XX	Z4800		0001	30.00					0036
	TOTAL NUMBER OF DENIES						0001						
SUSPENDS (DO NOT RECONCILE TO FINANCIAL SUMMARY)													
HERN D	562416373	5034270703001	010520XX	010520XX	Z4800		0001	20.00					0602
MART E	623105478	5034270712305	010520XX	010520XX	Z4800		0001	20.00					0602
		5034270712305	010520XX	010520XX	Z4800		0001	20.00					0602
						TOTAL		40.00					0602
LOPEZ C	560291467	5034270712502	012420XX	012420XX	Z4800		0001	20.00					0602
		PAT LIAB 932.00 OTH COVG			0.00	SALES TX		0.00					
	TOTAL NUMBER OF SUSPENDS						0004	80.00					

EXPLANATION OF DENIAL/ADJUSTMENT CODES

0401 PAYMENT ADJUSTED TO MAXIMUM ALLOWABLE
0036 RESUBMISSION TURNAROUND DOCUMENT WAS EITHER NOT RETURNED OR WAS RETURNED UNCORRECTED, THEREFOR YOUR CLAIM IS FORMALLY DENIED
0602 PENDING ADJUDICATION

OHC CARRIER NAME AND ADDRESS
N049 NORTHWESTERN NATIONAL LIFE   111 WASHINGTON AVE. FL 3   MINNEAPOLIS MN 55401

FIGURE 13-6 Medicaid remittance advice form showing adjustments, cutbacks, denied claims, and claims in suspense.

MEDICAID FRAUD CONTROL

Each state has a Medicaid Fraud Control Unit (MFCU), which is a federally funded state law enforcement entity usually located in the state attorney general's office. The MFCU investigates and prosecutes cases of fraud and other violations including complaints of mistreatment in long-term care facilities. The state Medicaid agency must cooperate and ensure access to records by the MFCU and agree to refer suspected cases of provider fraud to this division of the attorney general's office for investigation.

KEY POINTS

This is a brief chapter review or summary of the key issues presented. To further enhance your knowledge of the technical subject matter, review the key terms and key abbreviations for this chapter by locating the meanings in the glossary at the end of this book that appear in a section before the index.

1. Medicaid was established by Title XIX of the Social Security Act, a federally aided, state-operated, and state-administered program that provides medical benefits for certain low-income persons in need of health and medical care.

2. Medicaid is administered by each state's government with partial federal funding.

3. The Patient Protection and Affordable Care Act and the Health Care and Education Reconciliation Act passed in 2010 impact the Medicaid program by expanding access for childless adults, nonelderly, and non-pregnant individuals and include preventive services and long-term care benefits.

4. Coverage and benefits vary widely from state to state.

5. Each state operates a children's health insurance program with federal support under Title V of the Social Security Act.

6. Some federal acts allow assistance to QMBs and SLMBs who are aged and/or disabled and receiving Medicare but have annual incomes below the federal poverty level.

7. A medically needy Medicaid classification may or may not pay a deductible, copayment, or share of cost (spend down) within a specific time frame before receiving state benefits.

8. Providers must enroll for participation in the Medicaid program with the fiscal agent or local public service welfare office.

9. Medicaid benefits identification cards are issued monthly to recipients.

10. Medicaid eligibility must be verified before providing medical services to patients. Some patients may have retroactive eligibility.

11. Sometimes prior approval is required for medical services and procedures.

12. Each state may have a different time limit for submitting a claim for reimbursement.

13. The CMS-1500 (08-05) insurance claim form has been adopted for processing Medicaid claims in all states to a regional fiscal agent.

14. An RA or check voucher accompanies all Medicaid payment checks sent by the fiscal agent to the provider of services.

15. Each state has an MFCU that investigates and prosecutes cases of fraud and other violations including complaints of mistreatment in long-term care facilities.

evolve INTERNET RESOURCES

For active links to the following resources, visit the Evolve website at
http://evolve.elsevier.com/fordney/handbook

• To obtain general Medicaid program data, contact the Centers for Medicaid and Medicare Service.
• Information about each state's Medicaid plan.

• To find out who the current fiscal agent is for your state, go to the website and drop down to the link section. Click on "fiscal agents" to download the file.
• To obtain information about State Children's Health Insurance Program (SCHIP), which in some states is known as Maternal and Child Health Program or Children's Special Health Care Services.

STUDENT ASSIGNMENT

✓ Study Chapter 13.
✓ Answer the fill-in-the-blank, multiple choice, and true/false review questions in the *Workbook* to reinforce the theory learned in this chapter and to help prepare you for a future test.
✓ Complete the assignments in the *Workbook* to give you hands-on experience in abstracting from case histories, posting to financial accounting record

cards, and completing forms pertinent to the Medicaid program in your state. As an option, obtain Medicaid forms for your locale to use for your assignments.
✓ Turn to the glossary at the end of this textbook for a further understanding of the key terms and key abbreviations used in this chapter.

KEY TERMS*

active duty service member
allowable charge
authorized provider
beneficiary
catastrophic cap
catchment area
Civilian Health and Medical
  Program of the Department
  of Veterans Affairs
cooperative care
coordination of benefits
cost share
Defense Enrollment Eligibility
  Reporting System

emergency
health benefits advisor
health care finder
medically (or psychologically)
  necessary
military treatment facility
nonparticipating provider
other health insurance
participating provider
partnership program
point-of-service option
preauthorization
primary care manager
quality assurance program

regional contractor
service benefit program
service-connected injury
service retiree (military retiree)
sponsor
summary payment voucher
total, permanent service-
  connected disability
TRICARE Extra
TRICARE for Life
TRICARE Prime
TRICARE service center
urgent care
veteran

KEY ABBREVIATIONS*

ADSM
CHAMPVA
DEERS
FTM
HAC
HBA

HCF
MHS
MTF
NAS
nonpar
OHI

par
PCM
POS option
SHCP
TFL
TMA

TPR
TPRADFM
TSC
USFHP
VA

---

*Definitions for the key terms and key abbreviations are located near the back of this textbook in the glossary.

TRICARE *and* CHAMPVA

OBJECTIVES

After reading this chapter, you should be able to:

- Define pertinent TRICARE and CHAMPVA terminology and abbreviations.
- State who is eligible for TRICARE.
- Explain the benefits of the TRICARE Standard government program.
- List the circumstances when a nonavailability statement is necessary.
- State the TRICARE fiscal year.
- Name authorized providers who may treat a TRICARE Standard patient.

- List the managed care features of TRICARE Extra.
- State the managed care features of TRICARE Prime.
- Explain TRICARE for Life benefits and those who are eligible individuals.
- Name individuals eligible for TRICARE Plus.
- Define individuals who may enroll in the TRICARE Prime Remote program.
- Identify individuals who are eligible for CHAMPVA.
- Describe how to process a claim for an individual who is covered by the TRICARE Standard program.

Service to Patients

Know what types of health care services require prior approval from the TRICARE health contractor so that you can promptly assist patients by obtaining necessary permissions for scheduling procedures or hospital admission.

HISTORY OF TRICARE

The United States (US) Congress created CHAMPUS (Civilian Health and Medical Program of the Uniformed Services) in 1966 under Public Law 89-614 because individuals in the military were finding it increasingly difficult to pay for the medical care required by their families. CHAMPUS is a federally funded comprehensive health benefits program. Beginning in 1988, CHAMPUS beneficiaries had a choice of retaining their benefits under CHAMPUS or enrolling in a regional managed care plan called CHAMPUS Prime, a plan to control escalating medical costs and standardize benefits. Enrollees may be dependents of personnel who are actively serving in the armed services and military retirees and their dependents. In January 1994, TRICARE became the new title for CHAMPUS. TRICARE Management Activity (TMA) is the current name of the administrative office that was formerly known as the Office of Civilian Health and Medical Programs of the Uniformed Services (OCHAMPUS). Individuals have the following three choices to obtain health care under TRICARE:

- TRICARE Standard (fee-for-service cost-sharing type of option)
- TRICARE Extra (preferred provider organization type of option)
- TRICARE Prime (health maintenance organization type of option)

Performance objectives, testing and review material, and hands-on practical exercises for this chapter are available in these resources

 The Insurance Handbook Student Workbook　　　⊜ The Insurance Handbook Evolve Site

479

In 2005, the former 11 TRICARE regions in the US consolidated and merged to form the following: Region West, Region North, and Region South. In addition, there is TRICARE Europe, Canada/Latin America, and Puerto Rico/Virgin Islands. Figure 14-1 shows the locations of the states merged into these regions.

The TRICARE programs meet standards set by the 2010 health care reform federal legislation.

TRICARE PROGRAMS

Eligibility

The following individuals are entitled to medical benefits under TRICARE:

- Active duty uniformed service members in a program called TRICARE Prime Remote for members of Army, Navy, Air Force, Marines, Coast Guard, Public Health Service, and National Oceanic and Atmospheric Administration
- Eligible family members of active duty service members
- Military retirees and their eligible family members
- Surviving eligible family members of deceased active or retired service members
- Wards and preadoptive children
- Former spouses of active or retired service members who meet certain length-of-marriage rules and other requirements
- Family members of active duty service members who were court-martialed and separated from their families for spouse or child abuse
- Abused spouses, former spouses, or dependent children of service members who were eligible for retirement but lost that eligibility as a result of abuse of the spouse or child
- Spouses and children of North Atlantic Treaty Organization (NATO) nation representatives, under certain circumstances
- Families of activated Reserve and National Guard members if the military sponsor's active duty orders are for 30 consecutive days or an indefinite period
- Disabled beneficiaries younger than 65 years of age who have Medicare Parts A and B and who qualify under one of the aforementioned categories
- Medicare-eligible beneficiaries in a program called *TRICARE for Life*

An individual who qualifies for TRICARE is known as a **beneficiary;** the active duty service member is called the **sponsor.** A person who is retired from a career in the armed forces is known as a **service retiree (military retiree)** and remains in a TRICARE program until age 65, at which time the individual becomes eligible for the Medicare program. No further family benefits are provided in the event that an active duty military person served from 4 to 6 years and then chose to leave the armed services, thereby giving up a military career. CHAMPVA beneficiaries are not eligible for TRICARE.

Defense Enrollment Eligibility Reporting System

All TRICARE-eligible persons must be enrolled in the **Defense Enrollment Eligibility Reporting System (DEERS)** computerized database. TRICARE claims processors check DEERS before processing claims to verify beneficiary eligibility. A TRICARE beneficiary may check his or her status by contacting the nearest

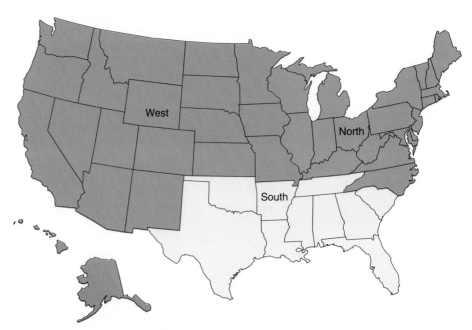

FIGURE 14-1 Map of TRICARE West Region, North Region, and South Region, which shows states that have been merged into each of the regions.

personnel office of any branch of the service or by calling the toll-free number of the DEERS center.

Nonavailability Statement

A Nonavailability Statement (NAS) is a certification from a military hospital stating that it cannot provide the care needed. As of December 2003, this type of certification is no longer necessary for TRICARE and CHAMPVA beneficiaries for outpatient procedures or for those who wish to receive treatment as inpatients at a civilian hospital and who live within a catchment area surrounding a **military treatment facility (MTF).** An MTF is a uniformed services hospital sometimes referred to as a *military hospital,* formerly called a US Public Health Service (USPHS) hospital. The only exception is that an NAS is still required for nonemergency inpatient mental health care services.

Catchment Area

The **catchment area** is a specific geographic region defined by ZIP codes and is based on an area of approximately 40 miles in radius surrounding each MTF in the US. Individuals whose home address ZIP code falls outside the local military hospital's service area do not need an NAS before seeking civilian health care under TRICARE.

TRICARE STANDARD

TRICARE Standard is a health care program offered to spouses and dependents of service personnel with uniform benefits and fees implemented nationwide by the federal government.

Enrollment

Those entitled to medical benefits under TRICARE are automatically enrolled in the TRICARE Standard program.

Identification Card

All dependents 10 years of age or older are required to have a Uniformed Services (military) identification and privilege card for TRICARE Standard. Dependents and survivors of active duty personnel and retirees carry a military identification card DD Form 1173 (Figure 14-2). Dependents younger than 10 years of age are not normally issued Uniformed Services identification cards; information for their claims should be provided from either parent's card. Refer to the back of the card under "medical" to ensure that the card authorizes civilian medical benefits. Essential information must be abstracted from the front and back of the card; therefore photocopy both sides to retain in the patient's medical record.

Benefits

In the TRICARE Standard program, beneficiaries may receive a wide range of civilian health care services, with a significant portion of the cost paid by the federal government. Patients are not limited to using network providers, and benefits include medical or psychological services or supplies that are considered appropriate care. Such services are generally accepted by qualified professionals to be reasonable and adequate for the diagnosis and treatment of illness, injury, pregnancy, and mental disorders, or are reasonable and adequate for well-baby care. These services are referred to as **medically (or psychologically) necessary**.

Beneficiaries also may receive urgent care and emergency care services. **Urgent care** is medically necessary treatment needed for an immediate illness or injury that would not result in further disability or death if not treated immediately. Treatment should not be delayed but should occur within 24 hours to avoid development of further complications. An **emergency** is a sudden and unexpected medical condition, or the worsening of a condition, which poses a threat to life, losing a limb, or sight and requires immediate treatment to alleviate suffering (e.g., shortness of breath, chest pain, or drug overdose). Emergency care is usually obtained at a hospital emergency department.

TRICARE Standard patients usually seek care from a military hospital near their home. The military physician may refer the patient to a civilian source if the service hospital that is managing the TRICARE Standard patient cannot provide a particular service or medical supplies. **Cooperative care** consists of services or supplies that may be cost shared by TRICARE Standard under certain conditions.

A **partnership program** is another option that lets TRICARE Standard–eligible persons receive inpatient or outpatient treatment from civilian providers of care in a military hospital, or from uniformed services providers of care in civilian facilities. Whether a partnership program is instituted at a particular military hospital is up to the facility's commander, who makes the decision on the basis of economics.

In addition, there are times when there is no service hospital in the catchment area and a TRICARE Standard beneficiary may seek care through a private physician's office or hospital. Delivery of care through the private physician is emphasized in this chapter.

Read carefully through Figures 14-3 and 14-4 to see the overall picture of TRICARE benefits, which includes cost sharing (deductibles and copayments).

FIGURE 14-2 A, TRICARE Standard active duty dependent's identification card (DD Form 1173) from which essential information must be abstracted. **B,** Sample identification card (DD Form 1173) for a retiree's widowed spouse. Cards indicate *1,* sponsor's status and rank; *2,* authorization status for treatment by a civilian provider; and *3,* expiration date.

Fiscal Year

The TRICARE fiscal year begins October 1 and ends September 30. It is different from most programs; therefore office staff should be alert when collecting deductibles.

Authorized Providers of Health Care

An **authorized provider** is a physician or other individual authorized provider of care or a hospital or supplier approved by TRICARE to provide medical care and supplies. These providers may treat a TRICARE Standard patient. This means the provider can be reimbursed by TRICARE for its share of costs for medical benefits and the provider is qualified to provide certain health services to TRICARE beneficiaries. Only "certified"

providers, those who have passed a credentialing process, can be authorized by TRICARE. Verify with the physician that he or she is certified to treat TRICARE beneficiaries before rendering medical services. Authorized providers include the following:

- Doctor of medicine (MD)
- Doctor of osteopathy (DO or MD)
- Doctor of dental surgery (DDS)
- Doctor of dental medicine (DDM)
- Doctor of podiatric medicine or surgical chiropody (DPM or DSC)
- Doctor of optometry (OD)
- Psychologist (PhD)

Other authorized nonphysician providers include audiologists, certified nurse midwives, clinical social workers, licensed practical nurses, licensed vocational

TRICARE Costs for Active Duty Family Members

Deductibles	TRICARE Prime	TRICARE Standard/Extra	
	No deductibles (Unless Point of Service is used)	E4 and Below: $50/person, $100/family E5 and Above: $150/person, $300/family	

Outpatient Services	TRICARE Prime	TRICARE Extra	TRICARE Standard
■ Ambulance Services ■ Durable Medical Equipment (DME) ■ Emergency Room Services ■ Enhanced Clinical Preventive Services ■ Laboratory and X-ray Services ■ Medical Supplies ■ Medication Management ■ Mental Health (Behavioral Health) ■ Occupational Therapy ■ Office Visits ■ Physical Therapy ■ Prosthetic Devices ■ Radiology/Pathology/Cardio Studies ■ Urgent Care	No copay	15%	20%
■ Ambulatory Surgery (Same Day)	No copay	$25*	$25*
■ Clinical Preventive Services: (Effective 10/01/2008 no cost for Standard beneficiaries) ■ Breast MRIs† ■ Clinical Preventive Exams† (Except School Physicals) ■ Colonoscopies/Other Colon Cancer Screening† ■ Immunizations† ■ Mammograms† ■ Pap Smears† ■ Well Child Care Visits† ■ Home Health Care ■ Hospice Care ■ Outpatient Maternity Office Visits	No copay	No cost share	No cost share

Inpatient Services	TRICARE Prime	TRICARE Extra	TRICARE Standard
■ Hospitalization for Medical/Surgical Care ■ Inpatient Maternity ■ Skilled Nursing Facility (SNF) Care	No copay	$16.88/day ($25 min. charge)	$16.88/day ($25 min. charge)
■ Hospitalization for Mental Illness ■ Substance Use Treatment ■ Partial Hospitalization Program (PHP) - Mental Health ■ Residential Treatment Center (RTC)	No copay	$20/day ($25 min. charge)	$20/day ($25 min. charge)

Pharmacy	Generic (Tier 1)	Brand Name‡ (Tier 2)	Non-Formulary (Tier 3)
Military Pharmacy (up to 90-day supply)	$0	$0	Not Applicable
Mail Order (up to 90-day supply)	$3	$9	$22
Network Retail (up to 30-day supply)	$3	$9	$22
Non-Network Retail (up to 30-day supply)	Prime: POS fees apply Standard: Greater of $9 or 20%		Prime: POS fees apply Standard: Greater of $22 or 20%

* The copay is for facility fees; there is no separate copay for professional fees, and deductibles are not applied to the facility or professional claims.

† Clinical Preventive Services are screenings or treatment with no symptoms. Diagnostic services due to a symptom will have outpatient office visit or ancillary service copay/cost shares.

‡ Prescription for a brand name needs to document one or more of the following: Patient must experience, or would likely experience, significant adverse effects from the generic medicine; generic medicine has resulted in, or is likely to result in, therapeutic failure; patient previously responded to the brand name medicine and a change to a generic medicine would incur unacceptable clinical risk.

FIGURE 14-3 TRICARE Prime, Extra, and Standard benefits and costs for active duty family members.

TRICARE Costs for Retirees, Their Family, and Others

- Cost-shares for TRICARE Standard and Extra are applied after the deductible has been satisfied.
- TRICARE Extra is when a TRICARE Standard beneficiary uses a network provider.
- TRICARE Standard beneficiaries may be required to pay up to 15% above the TRICARE allowed amount when using a provider that does not participate in TRICARE.
- Cost-shares are subject to change at the beginning of each fiscal year (October 1).
- Copayments below are per occurrence or per visit.
- Percentage cost shares are based on the TRICARE allowed amount or negotiated rate.

Deductibles	TRICARE Prime	TRICARE Standard/Extra
	No deductibles (Unless Point of Service is used)	$150/person, $300/family

Deductibles are applied each fiscal year, which begins October 1.

Outpatient Services	TRICARE Prime	TRICARE Extra	TRICARE Standard
■ Laboratory and X-ray Services ■ Medication Management Visits ■ Occupational Therapy ■ Office Visits/Consultations ■ Physical Therapy ■ Urgent Care	$12	20%	25%
■ Ambulatory Surgery (Same Day)	$25*	20%	25%
■ Ambulance Services	$20	20%	25%
■ Home Health Care ■ Hospice Care	No copay	No cost	No cost
■ Radiology/Pathology/Cardio Studies ■ Maternity Care Office Visits	No copay	20%	25%
■ Durable Medical Equipment (DME) ■ Medical Supplies ■ Prosthetic Devices	20%	20%	25%
■ Emergency Room Services	$30*	20%	25%
■ Mental Health (Behavioral Health)	Individual/Family therapy $25 Group Therapy $17	20%	25%

*The copay is for the facility fees, there is no separate copay for professional fees.

Inpatient Services	TRICARE Prime	TRICARE Extra	TRICARE Standard
■ Hospitalization for Medical/Surgical Care ■ Inpatient Maternity	$11/day ($25 min. charge)**	Lesser of $250/day or 25%; plus 20% of professional fees**	Lesser of $535/day or 25%; plus 25% of professional fees**
■ Skilled Nursing Facility (SNF) Care	$11/day ($25 min. charge)**	Lesser of $250/day or 20%; plus 20% of professional fees**	25%**
■ Hospitalization for Mental Illness ■ Substance Use Treatment	$40/day	20%	High Volume Hospital: 25% Low Volume Hospital: lesser of $197/day or 25%; plus 25% of professional fees
■ Partial Hospitalization Program (PHP)-Mental Health ■ Residential Treatment Center (RTC)	$40/day	20%	25%

**Inpatient care at a Military Treatment Facility (MTF) has a copay of $14.80 per day.

Pharmacy	Generic (Tier 1)	Brand Name (Tier 2)	Non-Formulary (Tier 3)
Military Pharmacy (up to 90-day supply)	$0	$0	Not Applicable
Mail Order (up to 90-day supply)	$3	$9	$22
Network Retail (up to 30-day supply)	$3	$9	$22
Non-Network Retail (up to 30-day supply)	Prime: POS fees apply Standard: Greater of $9 or 20%		Prime: POS fees apply Standard: Greater of $22 or 20%

FIGURE 14-4 TRICARE Prime, Extra, and Standard benefits and costs for retirees, their families, and others.

nurses, nurse practitioners, physician assistants, psychiatric social workers, registered nurses, registered physical therapists, and speech therapists.

Beneficiaries who use nonauthorized providers may be responsible for their entire bill, and there are no legal limits on the amounts these providers can bill beneficiaries. Examples of nonauthorized providers are most chiropractors and acupuncturists and those physicians who do not meet state licensing or training requirements or who were rejected for authorization by TRICARE.

Preauthorization

There are certain referral and **preauthorization** requirements for TRICARE Standard patients. When specialty care or hospitalization is necessary, the MTF must be used if services are available. If services are not available, the **health care finder (HCF)** can assist with the referral or preauthorization process. A TRICARE referral/authorization form is shown in Figure 14-5. An HCF is a health care professional, usually a registered nurse, who helps the patient work with his or her primary care physician

FIGURE 14-5 TRICARE Patient Referral/Authorization Form.

to locate a specialist or obtain a preauthorization for care. HCFs are found at a **TRICARE service center (TSC)**, which is an office staffed by HCFs and beneficiary service representatives. All admissions, ambulatory surgical procedures, and other selected procedures require preauthorization. Certain types of health care services requiring prior approval from the TRICARE health contractor follow:

- Arthroscopy
- Breast mass or tumor removal
- Cardiac catheterization
- Cataract removal
- Cystoscopy
- Dental care
- Dilatation and curettage
- Durable medical equipment (DME) purchases
- Gastrointestinal endoscopy
- Gynecologic laparoscopy
- Hernia repairs
- Laparoscopic cholecystectomy
- Ligation or transection of fallopian tubes
- Magnetic resonance imaging (MRI)
- Mental health care
- Myringotomy or tympanostomy
- Neuroplasty
- Nose repair (rhinoplasty and septoplasty)
- Strabismus repair
- Tonsillectomy or adenoidectomy

Payment
Deductible and Copayment

Deductibles and copayments are determined according to two groups: (1) active duty family members and (2) retirees, their family members, and survivors.

Spouses and Children of Active Duty Members. For inpatient (hospitalized) care, the beneficiary pays the first $25 of the hospital charge or a small fee for each day, whichever is greater, and TRICARE pays the remainder of the allowable charges for authorized care.

For outpatient (nonhospitalized) care, the beneficiary pays the first $150 (deductible) plus a 20% coinsurance (charges more than the $150 deductible). A family with two or more eligible beneficiaries pays a maximum of $300 (deductible) plus a 20% coinsurance (charges in excess of $300). TRICARE pays the remainder of the allowable charges, which is 80%.

All Other Eligible Beneficiaries. The all other eligible beneficiaries category consists of retired members, dependents of retired members, dependents of deceased members who died in active duty, and so forth.

For inpatient (hospitalized) care, the beneficiary pays 25% of the hospital charges and fees of professional personnel. TRICARE pays the remaining allowable charges for authorized care, or 75%.

For outpatient (nonhospitalized) care, the beneficiary pays $150 (deductible) plus a 25% coinsurance (charges more than the $150 deductible). A family with two or more eligible beneficiaries pays a maximum of $300 plus a 25% coinsurance (charges in excess of $300). TRICARE pays the remainder of the allowable charges for authorized care, which is 75%.

Refer to Figures 14-3 and 14-4 for further clarification and to see the differences in benefits between the three TRICARE program options.

Participating Provider

A **participating provider (par)** is a physician who has signed a participating provider contractural agreement with TRICARE to give medical care to TRICARE beneficiaries. Some provisions of the participating provider agreement are that the provider agrees to accept assignment, agrees to accept the TRICARE-determined **allowable charge** as payment in full, and transmits claims to the regional contractor directly. Assignment status (yes or no) is indicated when the CMS-1500 (08-05) claim form is transmitted to the regional contractor. The provider may bill the patient for his or her **cost share** or coinsurance (20% to 25% of the allowable charge after the deductible has been met) and for any uncovered services or supplies. The provider may not bill for the difference between the provider's usual charge and the allowable charge.

Beneficiaries pay only a certain amount each year for the cost share and annual deductible. This amount is known as the **catastrophic cap**. After this cap is reached, TRICARE pays 100% of the allowable charges for the rest of the year. A note should be attached to the claim when the patient has met the catastrophic cap; this may help expedite claims processing and payment. After the claim is completed and sent to the regional contractor, the payment goes directly to the physician.

Nonparticipating Provider

A health care provider who chooses not to participate in TRICARE is called a **nonparticipating provider (nonpar)** and as of November 1, 1993, may not bill the patient more than 115% of the TRICARE allowable charge, which is referred to as the *limiting charge*.

For example, if the TRICARE allowable charge for a procedure is $100, providers who decide not to participate in TRICARE may charge TRICARE patients no more than $115 for that procedure. The patient pays the deductible (20% or 25% of the charges determined to be allowable) and any amount more than the allowable charge up to 115% when the physician does not accept assignment. Nonpar providers may choose to accept TRICARE assignment on a case-by-case basis. Assignment should always be accepted when the service member is transferring within 6 months because this avoids collection problems.

TRICARE EXTRA

Enrollment

TRICARE Extra is a preferred provider organization type of option in which the individual does not have to enroll or pay an annual fee. On a visit-by-visit basis, the individual may seek care from an authorized network provider and receive a discount on services and reduced cost share (copayment). An unenrolled beneficiary automatically becomes a TRICARE Extra beneficiary when care is rendered by a network provider. If an unenrolled beneficiary receives care from a non-network provider, the services received are covered under TRICARE Standard. Providers receive a contract rate for giving care.

Identification Card

A TRICARE Extra beneficiary must present the military identification card when receiving care as proof of eligibility. The military identification card indicates a "Yes" in Box 15B (back of card) if the beneficiary is eligible. Children younger than 10 years of age may use the sponsor's identification card (attach a copy of the child's card to the claim). Individuals older than 10 years must have their own identification card. Contact the local HCF to verify eligibility. Active duty and retiree dependents and survivors carry an orange or brown military identification card (see Figure 14-2). Retirees carry a blue-gray military identification card.

Benefits

See Figures 14-3 and 14-4 for outpatient and inpatient benefits and deductible and copayment amounts.

Network Provider

The network provider is the physician who provides medical care to TRICARE beneficiaries under the TRICARE Extra program at contracted rates. They have discount agreements with the TRICARE program.

Preauthorization

Referrals from other network providers are coordinated through the HCF. The network provider refers the beneficiary for additional services, when necessary, after precertification requirements and completing a referral form.

Payments
Deductible and Copayment

Deductibles and copayments are determined by group: (1) active duty family members and (2) retirees, their family members, and survivors.

Spouses and Children of Active Duty Members. No copayment is required for inpatient (hospitalized) care.

For outpatient (nonhospitalized) care, the beneficiary pays the first $150 (deductible) plus a 15% coinsurance (charges more than the $150 deductible). A family with two or more eligible beneficiaries pays a maximum of $300 (deductible) plus a 15% coinsurance (charges in excess of $300). TRICARE pays the remainder of the allowable charges (85%).

All Other Eligible Beneficiaries. For inpatient (hospitalized) care, the copayment is $250 per day or 25% of the plan's allowable charges, whichever is less, plus 20% of separately billed professional charges at the plan's allowable rate.

For outpatient (nonhospitalized) care, the beneficiary pays $150 (deductible) plus a 20% coinsurance (charges more than the $150 deductible). A family with two or more eligible beneficiaries pays a maximum of $300 plus a 20% coinsurance (charges in excess of $300). TRICARE pays the remainder of the allowable charges for authorized care (80%).

See Figures 14-3 and 14-4 for further clarification of deductibles and copayments.

TRICARE PRIME

TRICARE Prime is a voluntary health maintenance organization (HMO)–type option. Participation in TRICARE Prime is optional. Beneficiaries who are not enrolled as members in TRICARE Prime may continue to receive services through TRICARE Extra from network providers or through TRICARE Standard using non-network providers. The beneficiary may no longer use the TRICARE Standard program once enrolled in TRICARE Prime.

Enrollment

An individual must complete an application and enroll for a minimum of 12 months to become a TRICARE Prime member. An annual enrollment fee is charged per person or family except for active duty families, who may enroll free. Active duty service members are enrolled automatically in TRICARE Prime and are not eligible for benefits under TRICARE Standard or TRICARE Extra. These members are able to use the local military and civilian provider network with necessary authorization.

Enrollees normally receive care from within the Prime network of civilian and military providers. The beneficiary has the option of choosing or being assigned a **primary care manager (PCM)** for each family member. The PCM manages all aspects of the patient's health care (except emergencies) including referrals to specialists. Enrolled beneficiaries may not use a non-network provider, except in emergencies or for pharmaceuticals, without a specific referral from an HCF.

Identification Card

Individuals who enroll are issued a TRICARE Prime identification card, as shown in Figure 14-6. This card does not guarantee TRICARE eligibility; therefore providers must check the TRICARE Uniformed Services military identification card for the effective and expiration dates or call the local HCF. Copies of the military identification card and the TRICARE Prime card should always be made and retained in the patient's file. For TRICARE Prime patients, both cards should be checked at every visit.

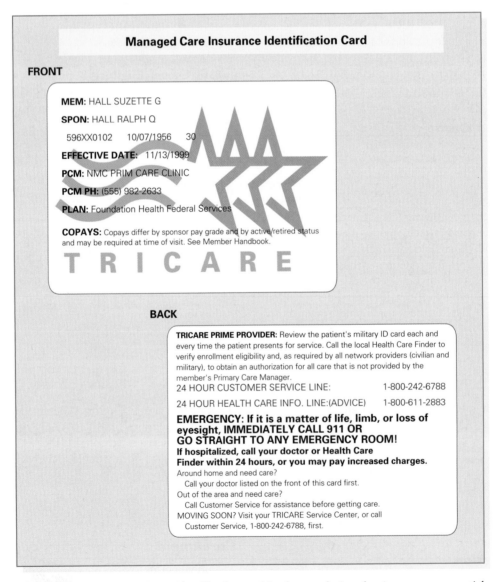

FIGURE 14-6 TRICARE Prime identification card has been redesigned to incorporate essential contact information to help enrollees access health care.

Benefits

Covered services are the same as those for TRICARE Standard patients plus additional preventive and primary care services. For example, periodic physical examinations are covered at no charge under TRICARE Prime but are not covered under TRICARE Extra or TRICARE Standard. Prime also covers certain immunizations and annual eye examinations for dependent children of retirees that are not a benefit under Extra or Standard. A dental plan is available for an additional monthly premium. An NAS is necessary for certain inpatient services if the beneficiary resides within the designated MTF catchment area. See Figures 14-3 and 14-4 for outpatient and inpatient benefits and deductible and copayment amounts.

Primary Care Manager

The PCM is a physician who is responsible for coordinating and managing the entire beneficiary's health care unless there is an emergency. A provider who decides to participate in a managed care program goes through a credentialing process. This is done approximately every 2 years for all physicians who participate as providers. The PCM may refer the beneficiary for additional services, when necessary, but specific referral and preauthorization requirements must be carried out. Referral patterns are evaluated to determine excessive or inappropriate referrals to specialists. A pattern of such referrals could result in termination of participation in TRICARE Prime.

Preauthorization

All admissions, ambulatory surgical procedures, and other selected procedures require preauthorization. Outpatient or ambulatory surgery must be on the approved procedure list before it is performed. The list is in the *TRICARE Handbook* available on the website: http://www.tricare.osd.mil.

The **health benefits advisor (HBA)** at the nearest military medical facility should be called to determine whether an NAS statement is necessary for the procedure before the surgery is scheduled in the approved facility. An HBA is a person at a military hospital or clinic who is there to help beneficiaries obtain medical care needed through the military and TRICARE. A **point-of-service (POS) option** is available if no authorization is obtained. This means that the individual can choose to get TRICARE-covered nonemergency services outside the Prime network of providers without a referral from the PCM and without authorization from the HCF. There is an annual deductible and 50% cost share if the POS option is used.

Payments
Copayment

TRICARE Prime copayments for inpatient hospital services vary for active duty family members and for retirees and their family members and survivors. For outpatient services, copayments are the same for active duty family members and for retirees and their family members and survivors but vary in amounts depending on the type of service received. Copayments should be collected at the time services are rendered. Refer to Figures 14-3 and 14-4 for further clarification of copayments.

TRICARE RESERVE SELECT

TRICARE Reserve Select (TRS) is a premium-based health plan available for purchase by qualified members of the Selected Reserve and their families who are not eligible for or enrolled in the Federal Employee Health Benefits (FEHB) program or currently covered under FEHB, either under their own eligibility or through a family member. These can include the Army National Guard, Army Reserve, Navy Reserve, Marine Corps Reserve, Air National Guard, Air Force Reserve, and Coast Guard Reserve. TRS healthcare benefits are similar to TRICARE Standard and Extra.

TRICARE FOR LIFE

In October 2001, **TRICARE for Life (TFL)** was enacted and offered additional TRICARE benefits as a supplementary payer to Medicare for uniformed service retirees, their spouses, and survivors age 65 or older. This plan was originally introduced as TRICARE Senior Prime. When beneficiaries become entitled to receive Medicare Part A and Medicare Part B on attaining the age of 65, they experience no break in TRICARE coverage. The only change is that TRICARE will pay secondary to Medicare beginning on the first day of the month they turn 65.

TRICARE for Life is provided to the following beneficiaries:

- Medicare-eligible uniformed service retirees including retired National Guard and Reservists
- Medicare-eligible family members including widows and widowers
- Certain former spouses if they were eligible for TRICARE before age 65

Dependent parents and parents-in-law are not eligible for TRICARE benefits. They may continue to receive services within an MTF on a space-available basis.

Enrollment

Most beneficiaries must be eligible for Medicare Part A and enrolled in Medicare Part B to qualify for TFL. An exception is Uniformed Services Family Health Plan (USFHP) members. Prospective TFL beneficiaries do not have to sign up or enroll for the program; however, they should be enrolled in DEERS. TFL has no enrollment fees. The member is required to enroll in Medicare Part B but without surcharge.

The DEERS notifies a beneficiary within 90 days before his or her 65th birthday that the medical benefits are about to change. They ask the beneficiary to contact the nearest Social Security Administration office about enrollment in Medicare. The beneficiary must elect to enroll in Medicare Part B to be eligible for TFL benefits. If the beneficiary is age 65 or older and only has Medicare Part A, he or she can enroll in Medicare Part B during the annual general enrollment period, which runs from January 1 to March 31 every year. Medicare Part B coverage then begins on July 1 of the year in which the beneficiary enrolls.

Refer to Internet Resources at the end of this chapter, access the Evolve website, and click on the active link to Medicare for more information about enrolling in Medicare Part B and monthly fees that apply.

Identification Card

Beneficiaries who qualify for TFL do not need a TRICARE enrollment card.

Benefits

Each beneficiary receives a matrix comparing Medicare benefits to TRICARE benefits. Refer to Internet Resources at the end of this chapter and access the Evolve website. Click on the active link for the TRICARE Management Activity website address to download this information. Certain benefits (e.g., prescription medications) are covered under the TRICARE Senior Pharmacy Program. Pharmacy benefits provide Medicare-eligible retirees of the uniformed service, their family members, and survivors the same pharmacy benefit as retirees who are younger than age 65. This includes access to prescription drugs at MTFs, retail pharmacies, and through the National Mail Order Pharmacy. Medicare Part B enrollment is not mandatory to receive TRICARE Senior Pharmacy Program benefits.

Referral and Preauthorization

There are no preauthorization requirements for the TFL program. All services and supplies must be benefits of the Medicare or TRICARE programs to be covered.

Payment

The following four scenarios represent most cases and explain the payment mechanism:

1. Services covered under both Medicare and TRICARE. Medicare pays first at the Medicare rate and the remaining is paid by TRICARE, which covers the beneficiary's cost share and deductible. No copayment, cost share, or deductible is paid by the TFL beneficiary.
2. Services covered under Medicare but not TRICARE. Medicare pays the Medicare rate and the beneficiary pays the Medicare cost share and deductible amounts. TRICARE pays nothing.
3. Services covered under TRICARE but not Medicare. TRICARE pays the allowed amount and Medicare pays nothing. The beneficiary is responsible for the TRICARE cost share and the deductible amounts.
4. Services not payable by TRICARE or Medicare. The beneficiary is entirely responsible for the medical bill.

TRICARE PLUS

Enrollment

TRICARE Plus is open to persons eligible for care in military facilities and not enrolled in TRICARE Prime or a commercial HMO. TRICARE Plus allows some Military Health System (MHS) beneficiaries to enroll with a military primary care provider. TRICARE Plus has no enrollment fee.

Identification Card

Persons enrolled in TRICARE Plus are issued an identification card and identified in the DEERS.

Benefits

The TRICARE Plus program is designed to function in the following ways:

● Enrollees use the MTF as their source of primary care; it is not a comprehensive health plan.
● Enrollees may seek care from a civilian provider but are discouraged from obtaining nonemergency primary care from sources outside the MTF.
● Enrollees are not guaranteed access to specialty providers at the MTF.
● Enrollees may not use their enrollment at another facility.
● The MTF's commander determines the enrollment capacity at each MTF.

Payment

TRICARE Plus offers the same benefits as TRICARE Prime when using an MTF. It has no effect on the enrollees' use or payment of civilian health care benefits; therefore TRICARE Standard, TRICARE Extra, or Medicare may pay for civilian health care services obtained by a TRICARE Plus enrollee.

TRICARE PRIME REMOTE PROGRAM

Enrollment

TRICARE Prime Remote (TPR) is a program designed for **active duty service members (ADSMs)** who work and live more than 50 miles or 1 hour from military treatment facilities (military hospitals and clinics). An ADSM is an active member of the US government military services (e.g., Army, Navy, Air Force, Marines, or Coast Guard). ADSMs must enroll for this program, which enables them to receive care from any civilian provider. TRICARE Prime Remote for Active Duty Family Members (TPRADFM) is the TPR benefit for family members with similar benefits and program requirements. TPR and TPRADFM are offered in the 50 United States only, and both require enrollment.

Identification Card

Active duty service members must present their military identification card to receive care from providers (Figure 14-7). Photocopy front and reverse sides of the card so that information is available for reference when completing the insurance claim form.

Benefits

TPR program benefits are similar to TRICARE Prime. Services may be received from an MTF when available or from any civilian provider. Primary routine care does

not require prior authorization (e.g., office visits, preventive health care). The HCF must be contacted to receive authorization for referrals, inpatient admissions, maternity, physical therapy, orthotics, hearing appliances, family planning (tubal ligation or vasectomy), outpatient and inpatient behavioral health services, and transplants. Table 14-1 is a summary of the unique aspects of TPR.

Referral and Preauthorization

Routine primary care does not require prior authorization (e.g., office visits, preventive health care). The PCM must initiate all specialty referrals and coordinate requests through the HBA for certain outpatient services, all inpatient surgical or medical services, maternity services, physical therapy, orthotics, hearing appliances, family planning, transplants, and inpatient or outpatient behavioral health services. The HBA is a government employee who is responsible for helping all MHS beneficiaries to obtain medical care.

Payments

Those persons covered and receiving benefits under TPR are not responsible for any out-of-pocket costs. ADSM claims for services provided by a TRICARE network provider are paid at the same contracted rate as other TRICARE beneficiary claims.

SUPPLEMENTAL HEALTH CARE PROGRAM

Enrollment

The Supplemental Health Care Program (SHCP) covers both MTF-referred care, as well as civilian health care

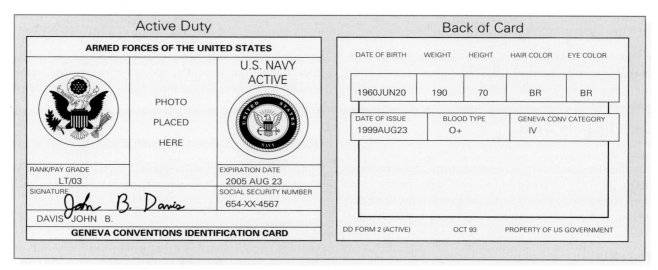

FIGURE 14-7 Military identification card for an active duty individual in the Armed Forces. It is used as the identification card for the TRICARE Prime Remote Program and is considered a sponsor identification card.

Table 14-1	Summary of Unique Aspects of TRICARE Prime Remote Program and Supplemental Health Care Program	
	TRICARE PRIME REMOTE (TPR)	**SUPPLEMENTAL HEALTH CARE PROGRAM (SHCP)**
Plan description	TPR is a program for Active Duty Service Members (ADSMs) who live and work more than 50 miles or 1 hour from a military treatment facility (MTF). ADSMs must enroll.	SHCP is a program for • Active Duty Service Members (ADSMs). • Inpatients at military treatment facilities who are not TRICARE eligible (e.g., eligible parents, parents-in-law) referred by an MTF to a civilian provider for care (usually for a specific test, procedure, or consultation). • Non-MTF referred ADSMs (e.g., ROTC students, cadets/midshipmen, eligible foreign military).
Provider type	Any civilian provider.	Any civilian provider.
Beneficiary access to care	TPR ADSMs receive from any civilian provider, or from a military treatment facility when available. Under TPR, ADSMs will have the same priority to care as other ADSMs at the MTF.	The beneficiary may receive services from any civilian provider, in accordance with referral and preauthorization requirements, below.
Beneficiary responsibility	TPR ADSMs have no annual deductible, cost shares, or copayments. The TPR ADSM must present his or her Military ID card at the time care is received.	ADSMs and others eligible for SHCP referred to civilian providers have no copayment, deductible, or cost share. Beneficiary must present his or her Military ID card at the time care is received.
Point-of-Service (POS)	Point-of-Service does not apply. If the ADSM receives care without a referral or preauthorization, the claim will be processed if it meets all other TRICARE requirements on a case-by-case basis.	The Point-of-Service option does not apply.
Program benefits	Offers benefits similar to TRICARE Prime. Some benefits (including all behavioral health care) require preauthorization.	Offers benefits similar to TRICARE Prime. Some benefits (including all behavioral health care) require preauthorization.
Referrals and preauthorizations	Primary care: ADSMs can receive primary care from a provider without a referral or preauthorization. ADSMs with an assigned PCM will receive primary care from their PCM. ADSMs with no PCM can use any TRICARE-certified provider. Or, he or she can contact an HCF for assistance in locating a provider. Specialty and inpatient care: The SPOC will review requests for specialty and inpatient care.	Specialty and inpatient care: The MTF will review all requests for specialty and inpatient care for ADSMs. **The MTF Commander or designee signature on a DD Form 2161 is required for** designated patients **referred** for civilian care. Preauthorization for **nonreferred** ADSMs for specialty, inpatient, and behavioral health care must **be obtained from the SPOC or the health care finder.**

ADSMs, Active Duty Service Members; *MTF,* military treatment facility; *POS,* point-of-service; *SPOC,* service point of contact.

provided to ADSMs. The MTF always administers routine care (e.g., routine office visits, preventive health care).

Identification Card

Active duty service members must present their military identification card to receive care from providers (see Figure 14-7). The front and reverse sides of the card should be photocopied so that information is available for reference when the insurance claim form is completed.

Benefits

See Table 14-1 for a summary of the unique aspects of SHCP. SHCP enables beneficiaries to be referred to a civilian provider for care. The MTF must initiate all referrals to civilian providers and use a DD Form 2161 signed by the facility commander. There is no deductible, copayment, or cost share for services provided by a civilian provider.

Referral and Preauthorization

The MTF initiates all referrals for ADSMs and other designated patients to civilian specialists when needed.

Payments

Those covered and receiving benefits under SHCP are not responsible for any out-of-pocket costs. ADSMs claims for services provided by a TRICARE network provider are paid at the same contracted rate as other TRICARE beneficiary claims.

TRICARE HOSPICE PROGRAM

The TRICARE hospice program is based on Medicare's hospice program. It is designed to provide care and comfort to patients who are expected to live less than 6 months if the terminal illness runs its normal course. Those persons who receive care under the hospice program cannot receive other services under the TRICARE basic programs (treatments aimed at a cure) unless the hospice care has been formally revoked. Many additional rules and limits apply to the hospice program; therefore the HBA at the nearest military medical facility should be called and a copy of the guidelines requested.

TRICARE AND HMO COVERAGE

TRICARE considers HMO coverage to be the same as any other primary health insurance coverage. TRICARE shares the cost of covered care received from an HMO (including the HMO's user fees), after the HMO has paid all it is going to pay, under the following conditions:

- The provider must meet TRICARE provider certification standards.
- The type of care must be a TRICARE benefit and medically necessary.
- TRICARE does not pay for emergency services received outside the HMO's normal service area.

TRICARE does not cost share services an individual obtains outside the HMO if the services are available through the HMO. For example, if an HMO provides psychiatric services but the patient does not like the HMO's psychiatrist and obtains services outside the HMO, TRICARE will not pay anything on the claim.

CHAMPVA PROGRAM

The Veterans Health Care Expansion Act of 1973 (PL93-82) authorized a CHAMPUS-like program called **CHAMPVA (Civilian Health and Medical Program of the Veterans Administration**; now known as the Department of Veterans Affairs [VA]), which became effective on September 1, 1973. CHAMPVA is not an insurance program in that it does not involve a contract guaranteeing the indemnification of an insured party against a specified loss in return for a premium paid. It is considered a **service benefit program;** therefore there are no premiums.

This program is for the spouse and children of a veteran with a **total, permanent service-connected disability** or for the surviving spouse and children of a veteran who died as a result of a service-connected disability. A **veteran** is any person who has served in the armed forces of the United States, is no longer in the service, and has received an honorable discharge. Just as in the TRICARE program, individuals who qualify for CHAMPVA are known as *beneficiaries* and the veteran is called the *sponsor.*

Examples of service-connected total, permanent disabilities include an injury with paraplegic results, a bullet wound with neurologic damage, and loss of a limb. This contrasts with a chronic or temporary service-connected disability, which might exist if an individual improperly lifts a heavy object while in the Navy, suffers a back injury with ongoing sporadic symptoms, and requires continuing medical care after leaving the service. Both scenarios present service-connected disabilities; however, the first example illustrates a person permanently disabled, whereas the second illustrates what may be a chronic or temporary disability.

Eligibility

The following persons are eligible for CHAMPVA benefits as long as they are not eligible for TRICARE Standard and not eligible for Medicare Part A as a result of reaching age 65:

- The husband, wife, or unmarried child of a veteran with a total disability, permanent in nature, resulting from a **service-connected injury**
- The husband, wife, or unmarried child of a veteran who died as the result of a service-connected disability or who, at the time of death, had a total disability, permanent in nature, resulting from a service-connected injury
- The husband, wife, or unmarried child of an individual who died in the line of duty while in active service

Qualifying children are those unmarried and younger than age 18, regardless of whether dependent or not, or those up to age 23 who are enrolled in a course of instruction at an approved educational institution.

Determination of eligibility is the responsibility of the VA. The prospective beneficiary visits the nearest VA medical center and receives a VA identification card if eligible.

Enrollment

Dependents of veterans must have a Social Security number and must have contacted the local VA regional office to establish dependency on the veteran sponsor. The individual obtains and completes an application by telephone, fax, or downloading from the VA's website (see Internet Resources at the end of this chapter and access the Evolve website, which has an active link to the Department of Veterans Affairs).

Identification Card

The issuing station's number appears on the identification card to identify the home station where the beneficiary's case file is kept. The identification card number is the veteran's VA file number with an alpha suffix. The suffix is different for each beneficiary of a sponsor. All dependents 10 years of age or older are required to have a uniformed services (military) identification and privilege card for CHAMPVA, as shown in Figure 14-8.

Benefits

The VA elected to provide these beneficiaries with benefits and cost-sharing plans similar to those received by dependents of retired and deceased uniformed services personnel under TRICARE Standard. An overall picture of CHAMPVA benefits, which includes cost sharing (deductibles and copayments), can be seen in Table 14-2.

FIGURE 14-8 CHAMPVA card.

Table 14-2	CHAMPVA Service Benefits and Cost Share Summary Chart		
	Beneficiary Pays*		
BENEFIT (COVERED SERVICES)	**DEDUCTIBLE ($50/INDIVIDUAL OR $100/FAMILY PER CALENDAR YEAR)**	**COST SHARE†**	**CHAMPVA PAYS**
Outpatient Services			
Ambulatory			
Family services	No	25% of allowable	75% of allowable
Professional services	Yes	25% of allowable	75% of allowable
Pharmacy services	Yes	25% of allowable	75% of allowable
DME			
Non–VA source	Yes	25% of allowable	75% of allowable
VA source	No	NONE	100% of VA cost
Inpatient Services			
Facility services			
DRG based	No	Lesser of (1) per day amount × number of inpatient days; (2) 25% of billed amount; or (3) DRG rate	DRG rate less beneficiary cost share
Non–DRG based	No	25% of allowable	75% of allowable
Mental Health Services			
High-volume/RTC	No	Lesser of (1) per day amount × number of inpatient days or (2) 25% of billed amount	Balance of allowable AFTER beneficiary cost share
Low-volume	No		
Professional services	No	25% of allowable	75% of allowable

DME, Durable medical equipment; *DRG*, diagnosis-related group; *RTC*, residential treatment center.
*Services received at VA health care facilities under the CHAMPVA Inhouse Treatment Initiative (CITI) program are exempt from beneficiary cost sharing.
†Under catastrophic protection plan (Cat Cap), annual beneficiary cost sharing is limited to $7500.

Provider

The beneficiaries of the CHAMPVA program have complete freedom of choice in selecting their civilian health care providers.

Preauthorization

Preauthorization is necessary for organ and bone marrow transplantation, hospice services, most mental health or substance abuse services, all dental care, and all DME with a purchase price or total rental cost of $300 or more. Preauthorization requests are made directly to CHAMPVA at 800-733-8387 or by mail to VA Health Administration Center, CHAMPVA, Attn: Preauthorization, PO Box 65023, Denver, CO 80206-9023.

CLAIMS PROCEDURE

Regional Contractor

TRICARE Standard is governed by the Department of Defense (DoD). As such, it is not subject to those state regulatory bodies or agencies that control the insurance business. The DoD and the VA have agreed to use the Office of the Assistant Secretary of Defense and the TRICARE Standard system of fiscal intermediaries and hospital contractors to receive, process, and pay CHAMPVA claims, following the same procedures currently used for TRICARE Standard.

A **regional contractor** (also known as a *fiscal intermediary [FI]* or *claims processor*) is an organization under contract to the government that handles insurance claims for care received under the TRICARE Standard or CHAMPVA program.

TRICARE Standard and CHAMPVA

The most efficient way to file claims for TRICARE Standard and CHAMPVA is electronic transmission of 837P (Professional) Health Insurance Portability and Accountability Act (HIPAA) claim transaction and format to the Health Administration Center (HAC). Paper claims on the CMS-1500 (08-05) claim form are also accepted, but the turnaround time to payment is, on average, an additional 20 days. Remember to abstract the correct information from the front and back of the patient's identification card. Service members move often, and it is common for providers to have an old or temporary address on file. Always ask beneficiaries to update their information during each office visit. Refer to Chapter 6 and follow the TRICARE or CHAMPVA instructions for completing the CMS-1500 (08-05) claim form. Refer to Figure 7-10 for an example of a completed TRICARE case with no other insurance and Figure 7-11 for an example of a completed CHAMPVA case. If electing to complete the VA Form 10-1759A for a CHAMPVA case, refer to the instructions presented later in this chapter.

If the physician is nonparticipating and does not accept assignment, the patient completes the top portion of the CMS-1500 (08-05) claim form, attaches the physician's itemized statement, and submits the claim. Alternatively, the patient may submit the claim on the white TRICARE claim DD Form 2642 Patient's Request for Medical Payment. Patients and providers of care for health services in foreign countries must use DD Form 2520. The Uniform Bill (UB-04) form is used for inpatient hospital billing.

Time Limit

Effective January 1, 1993, claims must be filed within 1 year from the date a service is provided or (for inpatient care) within 1 year from the patient's date of discharge from the inpatient facility.

Claims Office

The TRICARE program is administered by the DoD, TRICARE Management Activity, 16401 East Centretech Parkway, Aurora, CO 80011-9043, but claims are not processed in Colorado. The medical biller must understand that when transmitting or sending the claim to TRICARE, the claim goes to the TRICARE claims office nearest to the residence of the military sponsor. For example, if the patient is a child who was treated in California, but the sponsor is an active duty service member stationed in Florida, the claim should be transmitted to the TRICARE claims office in the south region and not a claims office in the west region. Refer to the Internet Resources at the end of this chapter and access the Evolve website to link to the TRICARE website to locate the address of the regional claims processor for submitting a TRICARE Standard claim in each state. Write to the TRICARE Support Office or contact the HBA at the nearest MTF to obtain a current *TRICARE Standard Handbook* or for answers to any questions about the name of the regional claims processor, benefits, nonbenefits, the need for an NAS, and so on.

Because of the September 11, 2001, attack in New York City and the activation of the US National Guard and Reserve components to the Middle East, the provider's office may come into contact with members of the National Guard or Reserve component. The members of these two organizations normally join a unit located near their place of residence. The National Guard and Reserve are only called to active duty in certain circumstances. Otherwise, they are required to

MEDICAL RECORD ACCESS

Privacy Act of 1974

The Privacy Act of 1974 became effective on September 27, 1975, and establishes an individual's right to review his or her medical records maintained by a federal medical care facility such as a VA medical center or US Public Health Service facility, and to contest inaccuracies in such records. The act directs each agency to make its own rules establishing access procedures. Agencies are allowed to adopt special procedures when it is believed that direct access could be harmful to a person. The act requires that an individual from whom personal information is requested be informed of (1) the authority for the request, (2) the principal purpose of the information requested, (3) routine use of the information, and (4) the effect on an individual who does not provide the information.

Some federal agencies or federally funded institutions may be regulated by both the Privacy Act and HIPAA standards. Such entities are required to comply with both sets of regulations. Although the HIPAA standards generally provide more restrictive regulations, entities are advised to revise their policies and procedures to comply with both the HIPAA standards and the Privacy Act. Under certain situations, HIPAA standards are likely to prevail and require regulated entities to obtain individual authorization for some disclosures that they now make without authorization under the "routine uses" exception. HIPAA compliance managers should make a determination of the effects of the interplay between the federal laws and the HIPAA standards, consult with legal counsel, and plan an entity's compliance initiatives accordingly.

Computer Matching and Privacy Protection Act of 1988

The Computer Matching and Privacy Protection Act of 1988 was established and is specific to TRICARE. It permits the government to verify information by way of computer matches. By law, the provider must tell a TRICARE member that he or she is calling TRICARE, which is governed by the DoD, and only information to determine eligibility and to learn what services are covered is to be obtained.

Both of these acts are mentioned on the back of the CMS-1500 (08-05) claim form. TRICARE patients must be made aware of this information by physicians who treat them so that they are knowledgeable about routine use and disclosure of medical data. Providers must follow both HIPAA and the Computer Matching and Privacy Protection Act of 1988. Patients may make a Privacy Protection Act request in writing, in person, or by telephone. Individuals should call the facility to determine the required procedures to obtain access to the records and what to include in making a written request.

---

perform their duties once in "drill status" and to participate in "annual training." Drill status occurs on a Saturday and a Sunday. Annual training occurs for 2 weeks, normally during the summer. While these service members are on drill status or in annual training, they are entitled to medical care at government expense. The government pays for an illness or injury incurred while on the way to drill status, during drill status, and on the way home from drill status. If the service member stops anywhere on the way to or from drill (e.g., to put gas in the car), any injury received is not paid for by the government. Sometimes, when a service member is injured or becomes ill, he or she may have medical personnel available within the unit to provide medical care. If not, the service member is sent to a clinic or hospital near the drill center. This injury or illness is not covered by workers' compensation. The military unit must be contacted to be compensated for the medical care. Each unit has a staff member called a *full-time manager* (FTM). This person is assigned to the unit and works full-time during the week and attends drills with the unit on weekends. He or she processes all medical claims for unit members. Medical records must accompany the claim for it to be paid. The unit also may require the physician to prepare additional forms that must accompany the claim. The payment is not paid by the unit. The claim is sent to a higher command where the illness or injury is investigated. This is a time-consuming procedure, and it could take months for the claim to be paid. It is better to bill the service member for payment if payment is not received with 60 to 90 days.

The CHAMPVA program is administered by the VA, Health Administration Center, PO Box 65023, Denver, CO 80206-9023.

TRICARE Extra and TRICARE Prime

The beneficiary does not file any claim forms under TRICARE Extra or TRICARE Prime programs when using network providers. Providers must electronically transmit 837P claims to TRICARE subcontractors for services given to beneficiaries. Referral and preauthorization numbers are required when applicable.

Time Limit

For outpatient care, a claim must be transmitted to the state or region's TRICARE contractor within 1 year of the date that the provider rendered the service to the patient. For inpatient care, a claim must be received by the contractor within 1 year from the date that the patient was discharged from the facility. If a claim covers several different medical services or supplies that were provided at different times, the 1-year deadline applies to each item on the claim.

When a claim is electronically transmitted on time but the contractor returns it for more information, the claim should be retransmitted with the requested information so that it is received by the contractor no later than 1 year after the medical services or supplies were provided or 90 days from the date the claim was returned to the provider, whichever is later.

A contractor may grant exemptions from the filing deadlines for several reasons. A request that includes a complete explanation of the circumstances of the late filing, all available documentation supporting the request, and the claim denied for late filing should be electronically transmitted to the contractor.

Claims Office

See the Internet Resources and access the Evolve website to link to the TRICARE website to find where claims should be electronically transmitted and to obtain more information about this program.

TRICARE Prime Remote and Supplemental Health Care Program

Outpatient professional services are electronically transmitted using an 837P HIPAA transaction and format, or paper claims may be submitted using a CMS-1500 (08-05) claim form. Primary care service claims are processed and paid without a referral or preauthorization from a network or non-network provider. A referral number provided by the HCF must be included for specialty medical or surgical care and for behavioral health counseling and therapy sessions. The POS option and NAS requirements do not apply to TPR and SHCP claims.

Time Limit

A claim must be electronically transmitted within 1 year from the date a service is provided or (for inpatient care) within 1 year from the patient's date of discharge from the inpatient facility.

Claims Office

Claims of ADSM patients should not be transmitted electronically to TRICARE. Claims for patients on active duty must be received by the specific branch of service (i.e., Army, Navy, Air Force, or Marines). Claims are submitted to Palmetto Government Benefits Administrators (PGBAs) for processing and payment (see Internet Resources at the end of this chapter and access the Evolve website to link to the TRICARE Prime website to locate the address).

TRICARE for Life

If the beneficiary receives care from a civilian provider, the provider electronically transmits claims to Medicare. Medicare pays its portion and then electronically forwards the claim to TRICARE for the remaining amount. TRICARE sends its payment directly to the provider. The beneficiary receives a TRICARE summary payment voucher that indicates the amount paid to the provider.

TRICARE/CHAMPVA and Other Insurance

By law, TRICARE/CHAMPVA is usually the second payer when a beneficiary is enrolled in **other health insurance (OHI)** or a civilian health plan, or belongs to an HMO or preferred provider organization. OHI may be coverage through an employer, an association, or a private insurer. However, two exceptions are as follows:

- When a plan is administered under Title XIX of the Social Security Act (Medicaid), electronically transmit TRICARE or CHAMPVA claims first if the beneficiary is a recipient of the Medicaid program.
- When coverage is specifically designed to supplement TRICARE benefits (e.g., Medigap health plan)

When the patient has other health insurance that is primary (meaning that it pays before TRICARE Standard or CHAMPVA), electronically transmit or send a paper claim using the CMS-1500 (08-05) insurance claim form. Attach the explanation of benefits from the primary carrier. If the patient is submitting his or her claim to the other insurance, take these steps:

1. Bill the other insurance carrier with the form it has supplied.
2. Bill TRICARE or CHAMPVA by completing the top section of the CMS-1500 (08-05) after receiving payment and an explanation of benefits from the other third-party payer. Submit the physician's itemized statement, which must contain the following:
   a. Provider's name
   b. Date the services or supplies were provided
   c. Description of each service or supply

d. Place of treatment
e. Number or frequency of each service
f. Fee for each item of service or supply
g. Procedure code numbers
h. Diagnostic code number or description of condition for which treatment is being received
i. Billing statements showing only total charges, canceled checks, or cash register receipts (or similar-type receipts) are not acceptable as itemized statements
3. Attach a photocopy of the explanation of benefits from the other third-party payer.
4. Electronically transmit the TRICARE or CHAMPVA claim to the local contractor (claims processor/regional contractor).

Medicare and TRICARE

TRICARE is considered secondary to Medicare for persons younger than age 65 who have Medicare Part A as a result of a disability and who have enrolled in Medicare Part B. Those eligible for Medicare Part A are not covered by TRICARE unless disabled. Claims should be electronically transmitted to Medicare, then to TRICARE with a copy of the Medicare remittance advice. Services covered by TRICARE but not covered by Medicare (e.g., prescriptions) are paid by TRICARE. Participating providers may obtain a TRICARE fee schedule by contacting their regional contractor.

Medicare and CHAMPVA

Effective December 5, 1991, CHAMPVA became secondary payer to Medicare for persons younger than age 65 who are enrolled in Medicare Parts A and B and who are otherwise eligible for CHAMPVA. Claims first must be electronically transmitted to Medicare because CHAMPVA is a secondary payer.

Dual or Double Coverage

A claim must be filed if a patient has an additional private insurance policy that provides double coverage. Refusal by the beneficiary to claim benefits from other health insurance coverage results in a denial of TRICARE benefits. In double coverage situations, TRICARE pays the lower of the following:

- The amount of TRICARE-allowable charges remaining after the double coverage plan has paid its benefits
- The amount TRICARE would have paid as primary payer

There must be **coordination of benefits** so that there is no duplication of benefits paid between the double coverage plan and TRICARE.

Third-Party Liability

If the patient is in an automobile accident or receives an injury that may have third-party involvement, the following two options are available for reimbursement:

Option 1: TRICARE Form DD 2527 (Statement of Personal Injury, Possible Third-Party Liability) must be sent in with the regular claim form for cost sharing of the civilian medical care. All five sections of the form should be completed by the patient. This form allows TRICARE to evaluate the circumstances of the accident and the possibility that the government may recover money for medical care from the person who injured the patient. If a CMS-1500 (08-05) claim form is submitted without TRICARE Form DD 2527, a request is made to complete it. This form must be returned within 35 days of the request, or the claims processor will deny the original and all related claims. Then the regional contractor submits a claim to the third party for reimbursement or files a lien for reimbursement with the liability insurance carrier, the liable party, or the attorneys or court involved.

Option 2: The provider can submit claims exclusively to the third-party liability carrier for reimbursement. Claims submitted with ICD-9-CM diagnostic codes between 800 and 999 (Injury and Poisoning) trigger the fact that there might be third-party litigation, and the claims processor may request the completion of DD Form 2527.

Workers' Compensation

If a TRICARE or CHAMPVA beneficiary is injured on the job or becomes ill because of his or her work, a workers' compensation claim must be filed with the compensation insurance carrier. TRICARE or CHAMPVA can be billed when all workers' compensation benefits have been exhausted.

In some situations it must be decided whether a case that involves an accident or illness is work related, and the claim might be electronically transmitted to the TRICARE or CHAMPVA claims regional contractor. In those instances, the claims processor files a lien with the workers' compensation carrier for recovery when the case is settled.

AFTER CLAIM SUBMISSION

TRICARE Summary Payment Voucher

For each TRICARE claim, the claims processor issues a **summary payment voucher** (Figure 14-9) that details the payment of the claim. When the provider participates (accepts assignment), the voucher is sent to him or her

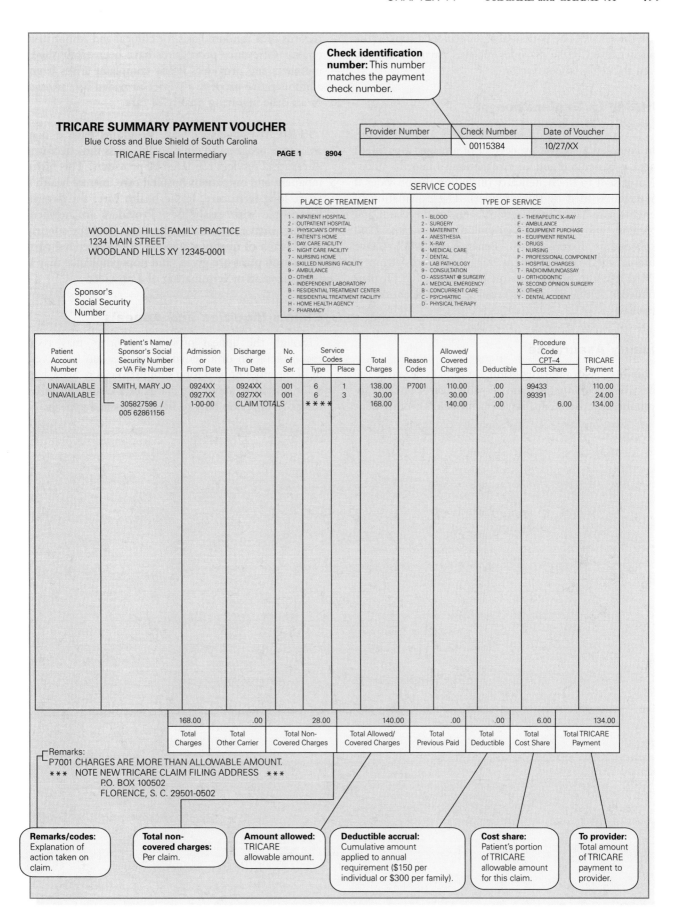

FIGURE 14-9 TRICARE summary payment voucher.

with the check. The patient always receives a copy of the voucher, even if the provider receives payment directly from the regional contractor.

CHAMPVA Explanation of Benefits Document

On completion of the processing of a claim, a payment check is generated and an explanation of benefits document is sent to the beneficiary (including the provider if the claim is filed by the provider). The explanation of benefits summarizes the action taken on the claim and contains information as graphically illustrated and explained in Figure 14-10. Beneficiaries who receive durable medical equipment or VA services from a CHAMPVA In-house Treatment Initiative (CITI, pronounced "city") do not receive an explanation of benefits.

Quality Assurance

A **quality assurance program** continually assesses the effectiveness of inpatient and outpatient care. The quality assurance department reviews providers' outpatient records on a random basis for clinical and administrative quality. Grievance procedures have been established for members and providers if any complaint arises from an administrative process, a service provided by a physician, or an issue involving quality of care.

TRICARE–managed care programs have a quality assurance program to continually assess the effectiveness of care and services rendered by providers. This includes inpatient and outpatient hospital care, mental health services, long-term care, home health care, and programs for people with disabilities. Providers are notified in writing when a potential quality issue has been confirmed as a breach of quality standards. Recommended corrective action plans are given, and noncompliance may lead to suspension or termination of a provider.

Claims Inquiries and Appeals

Through the appeal process, providers may request reconsideration of a denial of certification for coverage or of the amount paid for a submitted claim. See Chapter 9 for inquiring about the status of a claim and to learn the procedures on how to file reviews and appeals.

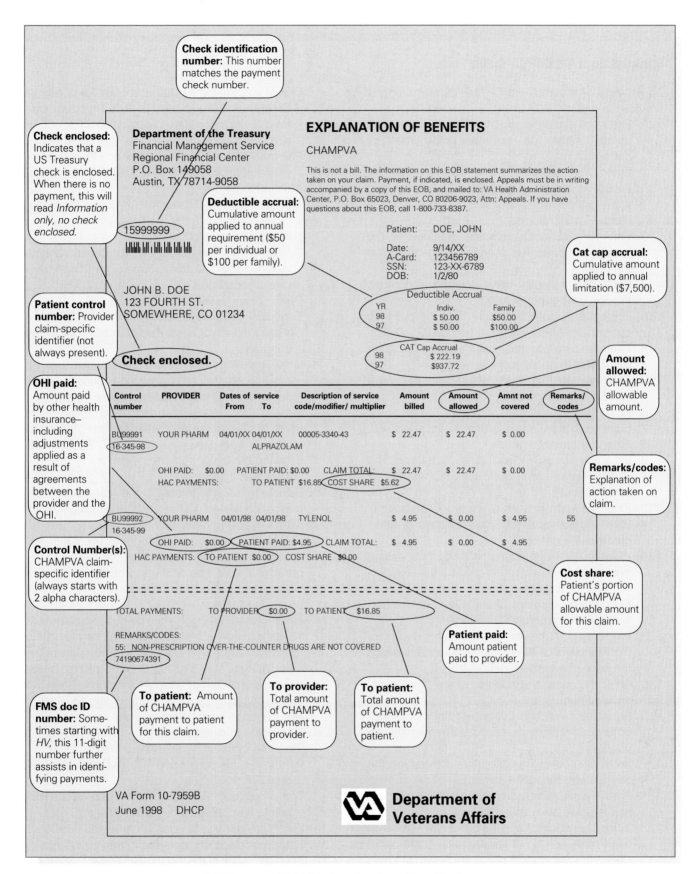

FIGURE 14-10 CHAMPVA explanation of benefits document.

PROCEDURE 14-1

Completing a CHAMPVA Claim Form

An example of a completed CHAMPVA claim form is provided in Figure 14-11.

1. Enter the patient's last name, first name, and middle initial (do not use nicknames or abbreviations).
2. Enter the patient's Social Security number exactly as it appears on the Social Security card. If the patient does not have a Social Security number, print "None."
3. Enter the patient's complete address. If the patient's address has changed, place an "X" in the box.
4. Enter the patient's home telephone number. Include the area code.
5A. Enter the number from Item 6 of the patient's current CHAMPVA Authorization Card.
5B. Enter the date from Item 4 of the patient's current CHAMPVA Authorization Card.
5C. Enter the date from Item 5 of the patient's current CHAMPVA Authorization Card.
6. Enter the patient's date of birth.
7. Enter the patient's relationship to the sponsor.
8. Enter the patient's gender.
9. Enter the sponsor's last name, first name, and middle initial (do not use nicknames or abbreviations).
10. Enter the sponsor's VA Claim or File Number.
11. Enter the sponsor's complete address (if different from the patient's).
12A. Place an "X" in the appropriate box if the patient is covered under any other medical benefits plan or health insurance coverage. CHAMPVA does not duplicate benefits of any other health insurance plan or program.
12B. Place an "X" beside all applicable types of medical plans or other health insurance to which the patient is entitled.
12C. Enter the name and address of the other insurance carrier.
12D. Enter the name and address of the employer if other health insurance is provided by the patient's employer.
12E. Enter the policy identification number of the other health insurance carrier.
12F. Enter the insurance agent's name. If this information is not known, enter "Unknown."
12G. Enter the insurance agent's telephone number. If this information is not known, enter "Unknown."
13. Check the appropriate box according to the type of medical care the patient received.
    Inpatient: Check the Inpatient box for admission to a civilian hospital.

Outpatient: Check the Outpatient box for all eligible CHAMPVA beneficiaries provided medical care from civilian facilities unless otherwise authorized by the VA.
Pharmacy: Check the Pharmacy box for claims for payment of drugs and medicines requiring a prescription by law.
Travel: Check the Travel box for claims for ambulance travel to, from, or between hospitals for inpatient care.
Dental: Check the Dental box for dental care for which the patient has an approved preauthorization.
DME: Check the DME box for payment of durable medical equipment costing more than $100.
College Infirmary: Check the Other box for College Infirmary.
Other Inpatient Care: Check the Inpatient box for admissions to an approved nursing facility (including a Christian Science sanatorium).

14. If the patient needs treatment for any kind of an injury (e.g., broken toe, sprained knee, lacerated forehead, back injury), check "YES" and briefly describe the injury and circumstances of how the patient was injured.
15. Be sure to read the release of medical record information contained in this item and complete the blanks, if appropriate.
16. CHAMPVA is a benefit program. As such, the patient (or sponsor) must assign the benefit to the provider of care if he or she wishes the payment to be made to the provider. Otherwise payment will be made to the patient.
17A. Every CHAMPVA claim must be signed by a patient 18 years of age or older. If the beneficiary is unable to sign on his or her own behalf, the sponsor (or other parent) may sign. In the absence of either parent, a guardian or fiduciary may sign. (note: For privacy reasons a patient younger than 18 years of age may sign his or her own claim form.)
17B. Insert date of signature.
17C. Enter the claimant's relationship to sponsor.
    Part V: To be completed by physician or other provider.
    Top of page II: Enter patient and sponsor's last name, first name, and middle initial.
18. Enter provider's (physician's) name and title.
19. Enter provider's tax identification number.
20. Enter the name of the referring physician or agency.
21. Enter the admission and discharge dates if the patient is hospitalized.

Completing a CHAMPVA Claim Form

OMB NC: 2900-
Estimated burden: 30 min

VA Department of Veterans Affairs	**CHAMPVA CLAIM FORM**

CHAMPVA CENTER, 4500 Cherry Creek Drive South, Box 300, Denver CO 80222

WARNING: IF YOU KNOWINGLY MAKE A FALSE STATEMENT OF ANY MATERIAL FACT IN OR IN CONNECTION WITH THIS CLAIM, YOU ARE SUBJECT TO PROSECUTION IN A U.S. COURT

PART 1 - PATIENT INFORMATION (To be completed by the beneficiary, patient or sponsor)

1. PATIENT'S NAME
CHIEU, MARION W.

2. PATIENT'S SOCIAL SECURITY NUMBER
742-XX-0491

3. PATIENT'S ADDRESS (Street, City, State, ZIP) (Check if new address)
321 OAK STREET, WOODLAND HILLS, XY 12345

4. TELEPHONE NUMBER (Include area code)
(555)492-7800

	5B. EFFECTIVE DATE			5C. EXPIRATION DATE		
	MONTH	DAY	YEAR	MONTH	DAY	YEAR
5A. CHAMPVA IDENTIFICATION CARD/AUTHORIZATION NUMBER 49-467-081C	09	01	XX	12	19	XX

6. PATIENT'S DATE OF BIRTH (Month, day, year)
12-01-77

7. PATIENT'S RELATIONSHIP TO SPONSOR (Check one)
☒ SPOUSE ☐ CHILD

8. PATIENT'S SEX (Check one)
☐ MALE ☒ FEMALE

PART II - SPONSOR INFORMATION (To be completed by the beneficiary, patient or sponsor)

9. SPONSOR'S NAME (Last, first, middle initial)
CHIEU, FRANK T.

10. VA CLAIM/FILE NUMBER
421-05-0129

11. SPONSOR'S ADDRESS IF DIFFERENT FROM PATIENT'S (Street, City, State, Zip)

PART III - PATIENT INSURANCE INFORMATION (To be completed by the beneficiary, patient or sponsor)

12A. IS PATIENT'S TREATMENT COVERED BY OTHER HEALTH INSURANCE
☐ YES ☒ NO IF YES, PLEASE COMPLETE ITEMS 12B THROUGH 12G BELOW

12B. TYPE OF COVERAGE
☐ GROUP HEALTH ☐ PRIVATE (NON–GROUP)
☐ MEDICARE ☐ CHAMPVA SUPPLEMENTAL
☐ MEDICAID ☐ WORKERS COMPENSATION
☐ OTHER ☐ NONE

12C. NAME AND ADDRESS OF INSURANCE CARRIER

12D. IF COVERAGE IS THROUGH WORK, NAME AND ADDRESS OF EMPLOYER

12E. POLICY IDENTIFICATION NUMBER

12F. INSURANCE AGENT'S NAME

12G. AGENT'S TELEPHONE NUMBER

PART IV - TREATMENT INFORMATION (To be completed by the beneficiary, patient or sponsor)

13. TYPE OF CLAIM (Check one)
☐ INPATIENT ☐ DENTAL
☒ OUTPATIENT ☐ DME
☐ PHARMACY ☐ OTHER
☐ TRAVEL

14. WAS NEED OF TREATMENT DUE TO A PHYSICAL INJURY? YES☐ NO☒
(If "Yes", briefly describe injuries and give a statement of circumstances)

15. I authorize the identified provider of service to disclose to CHAMPVA medical record information that pertains to the medical services described on this form. Unless limitations are shown below, this consent pertains to all of my medical records, including records related to treatment for medical or dental conditions, psychological or psychiatric impairments, drug or alcohol abuse, acquired immune deficiency syndrome (AIDS) or infection with the human immunodeficiency virus (HIV), and sickle cell disease.
The information will be used to process my CHAMPVA claim and determine my (or the patient identified above) eligibility for medical benefits. I also authorize the release of or obtaining of medical and/or other coverage information to and from another organization with which I have other medical benefits plan or health insurance coverage. I understand that I may revoke this authorization at any time, except to the extent that action has already been taken to comply with it. Without my express revocation, this consent will automatically expire: (1) upon satisfaction of the need for disclosure; (2) on February 2, 20XX (date supplied by the beneficiary); or (3) under the following conditions:

LIMITATIONS:

16. I assign payment to the provider(s) of these claim services ☐ YES ☒ NO

17. I CERTIFY THAT THE ABOVE STATEMENTS AND ATTACHMENTS ARE CORRECT AND REPRESENT ACTUAL SERVICES, DATES AND FEES CHARGED TO ME OR MY ELIGIBLE DEPENDENTS.

17A. CLAIMANT'S SIGNATURE	17B. DATE 2–2–XX	17C. RELATIONSHIP TO SPONSOR WIFE

FIGURE 14-11 Completed CHAMPVA claim form VA Form 10-7959A, used when billing for professional services.

Completing a CHAMPVA Claim Form

PATIENT'S NAME (Last, first, middle initial)	SPONSOR'S NAME (Last, first, middle initial)
CHIEU, MARION W.	CHIEU, FRANK T.

PART V - PHYSICIAN/OTHER PROVIDER (To be completed by physician or other provider)

18. PROVIDER'S NAME	19. PROVIDER'S TAX I.D. NUMBER	20. NAME OF REFERRING PHYSICIAN OR OTHER SOURCE (e.g. public health agency)
DOE, JOHN M.D.	93-4267890	

21. WHEN SERVICES ARE RELATED TO A PERIOD OF HOSPITALIZATION, GIVE DATES	22. NAME AND ADDRESS OF FACILITY WHERE SERVICES RENDERED (if other than home office)
ADMITTED / DISCHARGED	

23. DIAGNOSIS OR NATURE OF ILLNESS OR INJURY. RELATE DIAGNOSIS TO PROCEDURE BY USING PROCEDURE NUMBER IN COLUMN 24E BELOW.

A. Dysfunctional uterine bleeding.

B.

C.

24A DATE OF SERVICE	24B * PLACE OF SERVICE	24C PROCEDURE CODE	24D DESCRIBE UNUSUAL SERVICE OR CIRCUMSTANCES	24E DIAGNOSIS CODE	24F CHARGES	24G DAYS OR UNITS	24H TYPE OF SERVICE
02-02-XX	0	99213	Ofc visit Eval & Mgmt Level 3	626.8	45 00	1	1

25. I certify that the statements on the reverse of this bill apply and are made a part hereto.	26. PROVIDER'S SOCIAL SECURITY NO	27. TOTAL CHARGES	
John Doe, MD 02-02-XX	272-XX-5731	45.00	
SIGNATURE OF PROVIDER DATE	28. PROVIDER'S ADDRESS, ZIP CODE AND TELEPHONE NUMBER 123 MAIN STREET, WOODLAND HILLS, XY 12345 013/486-9002		

* PLACE OF SERVICE CODE FOR ITEM 24B

IN -INPATIENT HOSPITAL	NCF -NIGHT CARE FACILITY (PSY)	IL -INDEPENDENT LABORATORY
OH -OUTPATIENT HOSPITAL	NH -NURSING HOME	OF -OTHER MEDICAL/SURGICAL FACILITY
O -DOCTOR'S OFFICE	SNF -SKILLED NURSING FACILITY	RTC -RESIDENTIAL TREATMENT CENTER
H -PATIENT'S HOME	AMB -AMBULANCE	STF - SPECIALIZED TREATMENT FACILITY
DCF -DAY CARE FACILITY (PSY)	OL -OTHER LOCATIONS	

PART VI- PHARMACY INFORMATION (To be completed by pharmacist)	PATIENT'S NAME

29A. NATIONAL DRUG CODE	29B. RX NUMBER	29C. PHARMACY NAME	29D. FILL DATE (Month, day, year)	29E. PHYSICIAN NAME	29F. CHARGES

30. TOTAL CHARGES – $

VA FORM 10-7959A
DEC 1990

Pg II

reference initials

FIGURE 14-11, cont'd

PROCEDURE 14-1—cont'd

Completing a CHAMPVA Claim Form

22. Enter the name and address of the facility where services were rendered if other than home or office.
23. Enter diagnostic description or nature of illness or injury.
24A. Enter the date of service.
24B. Enter the place of service using one of the codes shown midway down on this page of the form.
24C. Enter the CPT procedure code number with modifier.
24D. Insert a description of the service or procedure.
24E. Enter the ICD-9-CM diagnostic code number for each diagnosis as described in Item 23.
24F. Enter the fee for each service, procedure, or test described in 24D.
24G. Enter the number of days or units. This block is commonly used for multiple visits, number of miles, and units of supplies including drugs, anesthesia minutes, or oxygen volume.
24H. Enter the type of service code from the following list:
   1 Medical care
   2 Surgery
   3 Consultation

4 Diagnostic x-ray
5 Diagnostic laboratory dialysis
6 Radiation therapy
7 Anesthesia
8 Assistance at surgery
9 Other medical service
0 Blood or packed red cells
A Used DME
F Ambulatory surgical center
H Hospice
L Renal supply in home
M Alternate payment for maintenance
N Kidney donor
V Pneumococcal vaccine
Y Second opinion on elective surgery
Z Third opinion on elective surgery

25. Show the signature of the physician, or his or her representative, and the date the form was signed.
26. Enter the provider's Social Security number.
27. Enter the total of all charges.
28. Enter the provider's street address, city, state, ZIP code, and telephone number including area code.
29. Items 29A through 30 may be completed if the patient is receiving prescription drugs.

KEY POINTS

This is a brief chapter review or summary of the key issues presented. To further enhance your knowledge of the technical subject matter, review the key terms and key abbreviations for this chapter by locating the meanings in the glossary at the end of this book that appear in a section before the index.

1. TRICARE is a three-option managed health care program offered to spouses and dependents of service personnel with uniform benefits and fees implemented nationwide by the federal government. It also covers retirees, reservists on active duty after 30 days, widows, and widowers.
2. An electronic database used to verify beneficiary eligibility for those individuals in the TRICARE programs is called *DEERS*.
3. The TRICARE fiscal year begins October 1 and ends September 30.
4. Under the TRICARE Standard program, the annual fiscal year deductible is $150 per person and $300 per family.
5. There are certain referral and preauthorization requirements for TRICARE Standard patients.
6. If the physician agrees to accept assignment in a TRICARE Standard case, the participating provider agrees to accept the TRICARE-determined allowable charge as payment in full. The provider may bill the patient for his or her cost share or coinsurance (20% to 25% of the allowable charge after the deductible has been met) and for any noncovered services or supplies.
7. TRICARE Extra is a preferred provider organization type of option in which the individual does not have to enroll or pay an annual fee.
8. TRICARE Prime is a voluntary HMO-type option.

9. TFL is a health care program that offers additional TRICARE benefits as a supplementary payer to Medicare for uniformed service retirees, their spouses and survivors age 65 or older, and certain former spouses.
10. TPR is a program designed for active duty service members who work and live more than 50 miles or 1 hour from military treatment facilities (military hospitals and clinics).
11. CHAMPVA is a service benefit program similar to TRICARE and is for veterans with total, permanent, service-connected disabilities or surviving spouses and dependents of veterans who died of service-connected disabilities.

12. TRICARE Standard and CHAMPVA claims must be billed on the CMS-1500 (08-05) claim form and submitted to the regional contractor for processing within 1 year from the date a service is provided or (for inpatient care) within 1 year from the patient's date of discharge from a facility.
13. The Computer Matching and Privacy Protection Act of 1988 permits the government to verify TRICARE patients' information by way of computer matches.
14. For each TRICARE claim, the claims processor issues a summary payment voucher that details the payment of the claim to the provider and a copy to the patient.

evolve INTERNET RESOURCES

For active links to the following resources, visit the Evolve website at
http://evolve.elsevier.com/fordney/handbook

- CHAMPVA website
- Medicare website
- Social Security Administration (for information about enrolling in Medicare Part B)

- TRICARE (for download of a TRICARE manual)
- TRICARE regional contractor directory (Click on Your TRICARE Benefit, click on Claims from the pop-up menu, then click on your state on the map for the name and address of the regional contractor.)
- TRICARE military health care beneficiary
- VA government forms

STUDENT ASSIGNMENT

✓ Study Chapter 14.

✓ Answer the fill-in-the-blank, multiple choice, and true/false review questions in the *Workbook* to reinforce the theory learned in this chapter and help prepare you for a future test.

✓ Complete the assignments in the *Workbook* for computing mathematic calculations and giving you hands-on experience in completing TRICARE and CHAMPVA insurance claim forms and proficiency in procedural and diagnostic coding.

✓ Turn to the glossary at the end of this textbook for a further understanding of the key terms and key abbreviations used in this chapter.

KEY TERMS*

accident
adjudication
by report
claims examiner
compromise and release
deposition
ergonomic
extraterritorial
Federal Employees'
    Compensation Act
fee schedule
injury

insurance adjuster
lien
medical service order
nondisability claim
occupational illness or disease
Occupational Safety and Health
    Administration
permanent and stationary
permanent disability
petition
second-injury fund
sequelae

sub rosa films
subsequent-injury fund
temporary disability
third-party liability
third-party subrogation
waiting period
work hardening
Workers' Compensation
    Appeals Board
workers' compensation
    insurance

KEY ABBREVIATIONS*

AME
BR
C and R
ERISA
FECA

IAIABC
IME
LHWCA
MSDS
ND claim

OSHA
P and S
PD
QME
ROM

SIF
TD
WC
WCAB
WP

---

*Definitions for the key terms and key abbreviations are located near the back of this textbook in the glossary.

CHAPTER 15

Workers' Compensation

OBJECTIVES

After reading this chapter, you should be able to:

- State the purposes of workers' compensation laws.
- Specify who is eligible for insurance coverage under federal workers' compensation laws.
- Name persons entitled to be insured under state workers' compensation laws.
- Differentiate between workers' compensation insurance and employers' liability insurance.
- Define second-injury fund.
- Determine the waiting period in each state before benefits begin.
- Describe the types of compensation benefits.
- Define nondisability, temporary disability, and permanent disability claims.
- List signs of fraud and abuse involving employees, employers, insurers, medical providers, and lawyers.

- State when to report fraud or abuse involving a workers' compensation claim.
- Explain OSHA's role in protecting employees.
- Explain two ways in which depositions are used.
- Explain the advantages of filing a lien.
- Define third-party subrogation.
- Describe workers' compensation health and financial record-keeping in a medical practice.
- Name the contents of a progress or supplemental medical report.
- Complete workers' compensation forms properly.
- Explain how to handle out-of-state claims.
- Describe actions to take in following up on delinquent workers' compensation claims.
- Explain the procedure of completing the doctor's first report of occupational injury or illness.

Service to Patients

If a patient who has a work-related injury or illness arrives for an appointment without the employer's signed permission for treatment, telephone the employer and ask to have an official person fax the authorization. This will expedite the medical care and necessary documents and/or forms that must be completed for the patient in a workers' compensation case.

Always educate the patient with regard to the medical practice's billing policies for workers' compensation cases by having him or her complete a patient agreement form to pay the physician's fees if the case is declared non–work related or an illness is discovered that is not work related.

Performance objectives, testing and review material, and hands-on practical exercises for this chapter are available in these resources

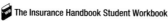 The Insurance Handbook Student Workbook

 The Insurance Handbook Evolve Site

HISTORY

Before the establishment of a workers' compensation program in the United States (US), either the employer was responsible for any injury or death to his or her employees resulting from administrative negligence or employees paid for medical expenses. Employees are individuals employed by another, generally for wages, in exchange for labor or services. A physician whose practice is incorporated is also considered an employee under workers' compensation laws.

Originally the worker had to prove legally that injury was caused by negligence on the part of the employer. By the close of the nineteenth century, the number of accidents had increased and legal processes were uncertain; therefore federal and state legal provisions were required. In the early 1900s, employers' liability laws were adopted by many states, but there was still a great need for improvement. In 1911 the first workers' compensation laws that allowed injured employees to receive medical care without first taking employers to court were enacted. All states currently have workers' compensation laws.

Workers' compensation insurance is the most important coverage written to insure industrial accidents. Previously, this form of insurance was known as "workmen's compensation." The term *workmen* was changed to *workers* for a more generic title and to avoid sexual bias in language. Employers use employers' liability coverage occasionally to protect themselves when their employees do not come within the scope of a compensation law.

Workers' Compensation Statutes

There are two kinds of statutes under workers' compensation: federal compensation laws and state compensation laws. Federal laws apply to miners, maritime workers, and those who work for the government; they do not apply to state and private business employees. State compensation laws apply to employers and employees within each state, but the laws vary for each state.

The workers' compensation statutes relieve the employer of liability for injury received or illness contracted by an employee in a work situation, except in gross negligence cases. They also enable the employee to be more easily and quickly compensated for loss of wages, medical expenses, and permanent disability. Before these statutes were passed, the employer could be found legally responsible for the employees' injuries or illnesses, and frequently there were delays in the employee's attempt to recover damages.

WORKERS' COMPENSATION AND HIPAA COMPLIANCE

It is important to note that workers' compensation programs are not included under the definition of a "health plan" as identified in the HIPAA statutes. Therefore workers' compensation programs are not required to comply with HIPAA standards; however, it is beneficial to workers' compensation insurance payers and health care providers to use the adopted HIPAA transaction and code set (TCS) to work harmoniously within the claims processing activities used throughout the industry.

Workers' Compensation Reform

By 1994, dysfunctional workers' compensation systems were costing companies more than $65 billion annually in many US cities, driving insurers to deny insurance to businesses and causing companies to close their doors. Some employers began moving their businesses to states requiring lower premiums. Widespread legal and medical corruption and abuse had evolved throughout the system in the form of record-high medical treatment and legal expenses. Reforms of the compensation of health care workers became necessary because of these problems. Reform laws have been introduced in a number of states that deal with the following issues:

- Antifraud legislation and increased penalties for workers' compensation fraud
- Antireferral provisions (e.g., restrictions of physicians referring patients for diagnostic studies to sites where the physician has a financial interest)
- Proof of the medical necessity for treatment (or tests), as well as appropriate documentation. If guidelines are not adhered to, the carrier may refuse to pay the entire fee (e.g., utilization review of inpatient and outpatient claims and treatment plans)
- Preauthorization for major operations and expensive tests (e.g., computed tomography and magnetic resonance imaging)
- Caps on vocational rehabilitation
- Utilization of a disabled worker in another division of the company where he or she was employed so that the worker may be gainfully employed while not using the injured part of the body
- Increase in occupational safety measures
- Employers offering a variety of managed care plans from which employees can choose, with some of these restricting their choice of provider (e.g., health maintenance organizations [HMOs] and preferred provider organizations [PPOs])
- Development of fee schedules

- Medical bill review (mandatory review by law or payers' voluntary review identifying duplicate claims and billing errors)
- Use of mediators instead of lawyers to reach agreement between employers and the injured employee
- Prosecuting of physicians, lawyers, and employees who abuse the system

Although the system is far from perfect or complete, much progress has been made toward reducing high costs by trimming reimbursement for medical services and minimizing abuses of the system.

WORKERS' COMPENSATION LAWS AND INSURANCE

Purposes of Workers' Compensation Laws

Workers' compensation laws have been developed for a variety of reasons and accomplish much, including the following:

1. Provide the best available medical care necessary to ensure a prompt return to work of any injured or ill employee, as well as achieving maximum recovery.
2. Provide income to the injured or ill worker or to his or her dependents, regardless of fault.
3. Provide a single remedy and reduce court delays, costs, and workloads arising out of personal injury litigation.
4. Relieve public and private charities of financial drains resulting from uncompensated industrial accidents.
5. Eliminate payment of fees to attorneys and witnesses, as well as time-consuming trials and appeals.
6. Encourage maximum employer interest in safety and rehabilitation through an appropriate experience-rating mechanism.
7. Promote the study of causes of accidents and reduce preventable accidents and human suffering rather than concealing fault.

Self-Insurance

Self-insurance is another way that employers can fight high medical costs after an accident. A large employer can save money by self-insuring employees for a predetermined amount of money and then purchasing policies with large deductibles to cover catastrophic problems. A self-insuring company pays for medical expenses instead of insurance premiums. Benefits are variable from plan to plan, and precertification for certain services may be required. Because of health reform in 2010, companies that offer health plans must allow their employees to keep their children on their plans until the children are 26 years old. Employers are prohibited from putting lifetime caps and some annual caps on benefits for their

employees. Employers that have existing plans for their employees at the time of the passing of this legislation may be able to change medical benefits, such as copayments and deductibles, or reduce what their plans cover.

Self-insured employers are covered by the Employee Retirement Income Security Act (ERISA). This federal law mandates reporting and disclosure requirements for group life and health plans, with guidelines for administration, servicing of plans, some claims processing, and appeals; therefore the state insurance commissioner does not have jurisdiction over such plans. Because they are not state regulated, they often overlook timely payment. ERISA regulations state that a claim must be paid or denied within 90 days of receipt or submission; however, this regulation is not helpful because there is no penalty for violation of the 90-day deadline. Thus physicians who care for individuals under such plans may wish to negotiate payment terms to be 60 days or less.

Sometimes, a self-insured plan may have stop-loss or reinsurance that becomes active on large claims, or a set dollar limit per policy year or employee, depending on how it is structured. Such provisions give them an excuse to delay claims until the reinsurer decides to fund the claim. In such cases, it may be necessary to become aggressive and ask for the name, address, and telephone number of the reinsurer to learn the claim status. Prompt processing and payment should be demanded because delaying claims is a violation of federal laws and ERISA regulations.

With the passing of the federal legislation, known as the Patient Protection and Affordable Care Act (the Affordable Care Act) and H.R. 4872, the Health Care and Education Reconciliation Act of 2010 (the Reconciliation Act), beginning in 2014, almost everyone is required to be insured or they will pay a fine. Large employers with more than 50 employees must pay a $2,000-per-employee fee excluding the first 30 employees from the assessment if the government subsidizes their workers' coverage.

At the time of the printing of this edition, the health care reform legislation and its impact on ERISA is not completely known. To keep you up to date, information will be placed on the Evolve web site as it is released (see the ERISA section in Chapter 11 for additional information).

A form of self-insurance designed to serve a small manufacturing company is known as *captive insurance*. This is best for companies that have good safety records and those willing to implement worker safety programs to keep claims to a minimum. Members of captive self-insurance programs may hire an outside firm to process claims and purchase extra insurance for major claims. They share overhead expenses and investment income if any remains after paying expenses and claims. Most captive programs are based in Bermuda or the Cayman Islands to take advantage of favorable tax benefits.

Managed Care

Increasing numbers of employers are seeking managed care contracts with PPOs and HMOs to insure their workers against industrial accidents and illnesses. Some states have adopted laws authorizing managed care programs, and other states are conducting pilot programs to test the effectiveness of managed care networks. Managed care contracts are not uniform and may limit the choice of providers, use fee schedule-based payments, require precertification for certain procedures, implement hospital and medical bill review, and incorporate utilization review of medical services.

ELIGIBILITY

Individuals entitled to workers' compensation insurance coverage are private business employees, state employees, and federal employees (e.g., postal workers, Internal Revenue Service [IRS] employees, coal miners, and maritime workers). **Workers' compensation (WC) insurance** coverage provides benefits to employees and their dependents if employees suffer work-related injury, illness, or death.

Industrial Accident

An **accident** is an unplanned and unexpected happening traceable to a definite time and place and causing **injury** (damage or loss).

Workers' compensation (industrial) accidents do not necessarily occur at the customary work site. For example, an individual may be asked to obtain cash for the petty cash reserve during the lunch hour. He or she may misstep off the curb while walking to the bank and suffer a fractured ankle. This person is considered to be working, although not at the customary work site, and the injury is covered under workers' compensation insurance.

Occupational Illness

Occupational illness or disease is any abnormal condition or disorder caused by exposure to environmental factors associated with employment including acute and chronic illnesses or diseases that may be caused by inhalation, absorption, ingestion, or direct contact. Occupational diseases usually become apparent soon after exposure. However, some diseases may be latent for a considerable amount of time. Therefore some states have

extended periods during which claims may be filed for certain slowly developing occupational diseases. These diseases include silicosis, asbestosis, pneumoconiosis, berylliosis, anthracosilicosis, radiation disability, loss of hearing, cumulative trauma, and repetitive motion illnesses (e.g., carpal tunnel syndrome).

COVERAGE

Federal Laws

Employees who work for federal agencies are covered by a number of federal workers' compensation laws:

- Workmen's Compensation Law of the District of Columbia. This law became effective on May 17, 1928, and provides benefits for those working in Washington, DC.
- Federal Coal Mine Health and Safety Act. This act, also referred to as the *Black Lung Benefits Act*, became effective on May 7, 1941. The act provides benefits to coal miners and is administered through the national headquarters in Washington, D.C.
- Federal Employees' Compensation Act. The **Federal Employees' Compensation Act (FECA)** was instituted on May 30, 1908, to provide benefits for on-the-job injuries to all federal employees. The insurance is provided through an exclusive fund system. Many different claim forms are used depending on the type of injury. Payment is based on a schedule of maximum allowable charges. The time limit for submitting a bill is by December 31 of the year after the year in which services were rendered (or by December 31 of the year after the year the condition was accepted as work compensable, whichever is later). For further information, locate your regional office of the FECA by going to the Evolve website listed in Internet Resources at the end of this chapter.
- Longshoremen's and Harbor Workers' Compensation Act (LHWCA). This act became effective on March 4, 1927, and provides benefits for private or public employees engaged in maritime work nationwide. It is administered through regional offices in Boston, Chicago, Cleveland, Denver, Honolulu, Jacksonville, Kansas City, New Orleans, New York City, Philadelphia, San Francisco, Seattle, and Washington, DC. This type of insurance corresponds to that available through the private insurance system. Locate the nearest district office by going to the Evolve website listed in Internet Resources at the end of this chapter.

State Laws

State compensation laws cover those workers not protected by the previously mentioned federal statutes. Federal law mandates that states set up laws to meet minimum requirements. If an employer does not purchase workers' compensation insurance from a private insurance company, the employer must self-insure and have enough cash in reserve to cover the cost of medical care for all workers who suffer work-related injuries. An employer may be reluctant to file a workers' compensation report with the state in some instances, preferring to pay medical expenses out of pocket rather than have premium rates increase. It is illegal for an employer to fail to report a work-related accident when reporting is required by state law, and some states consider it a misdemeanor. Different penalties can be imposed, depending on state law, such as imprisonment or assessment of fines of from $50 to $2500 or more.

Statutes require that employers have employers' liability insurance in addition to workers' compensation protection. The difference between workers' compensation insurance and employers' liability insurance is that the latter is coverage that protects against claims arising out of bodily injury to others (nonemployees) or damage to their property when someone is on business premises. It is not considered insurance coverage for someone who is working at a business site.

State compensation laws are compulsory or elective, which may be defined as follows:

1. Compulsory law. Each employer is required to accept its provisions and provide for specified benefits.
2. Elective law. The employer may accept or reject the law. If the statute of the law is rejected, the employer loses the three common-law defenses, which are the following:
   a. Assumption of risk
   b. Negligence of fellow employees
   c. Contributory negligence

Coverage is elective in only one state, New Jersey. This means that, in effect, all laws are "compulsory."

Minors

Minors are covered by workers' compensation; in some states, double compensation or added penalties are provided. Minors also receive special legal benefit provisions in many states.

Interstate Laws

Questions may arise as to which state's law determines payment of compensation benefits if a worker's occupation takes him or her into another state (e.g., truck drivers). Most compensation laws are **extraterritorial** (effective outside of the state) by either specific provisions or court decisions. When billing, follow the rules and fee schedule of the state in which the workers' compensation claim was originally filed. This may or may not be the same as the patient's current state of residence. The only exception is workers' compensation for federal employees, which has nationwide rules. For railroad workers, most states abide by nationwide rules, but some states have their own. Claims submission for out-of-state claims is discussed later in this chapter.

Volunteer Workers

Several states have laws to compensate civil defense and other volunteer workers such as firefighters who are injured in the line of duty.

Funding

Six states (Nevada, North Dakota, Ohio, Washington, West Virginia, and Wyoming), two US territories, and most provinces require employers to insure through a monopolistic state or provincial fund. Puerto Rico and the Virgin Islands require employers to insure through a territorial fund. Employers may qualify as self-insurers in 48 states and territories. A number of states permit employers to purchase insurance from either a competitive state fund or a private insurance company.

The employer pays the premiums for workers' compensation insurance, the amount depending on the employee's job and the risk involved in job performance. The physician usually must supply comprehensive information, and the reporting requirements vary from state to state (Table 15-1). The state bureau or individual insurance carrier should be contacted to obtain instructions and proper forms. State bureaus may be found by going to the Evolve website listed in Internet Resources at the end of this chapter.

Second-Injury Fund (Subsequent-Injury Fund)

The **second-injury fund,** also known as the **subsequent-injury fund (SIF),** was established to meet problems arising when an employee has a preexisting injury or condition and is subsequently injured at work. The preexisting injury combines with the second injury to produce disability that is greater than that caused by the latter alone.

Two functions of the fund are (1) to encourage hiring of the physically handicapped and (2) to allocate more equitably the costs of providing benefits to such employees. Second-injury employers pay compensation related primarily to the disability caused by the second injury, even though the employee receives benefits relating to the combined disability. The difference is made up from the subsequent-injury fund.

Table 15-1 Employers' or Physicians' Report of Accident[1]

JURISDICTION	TIME LIMIT	INJURIES COVERED
Alabama	Within 15 days	Death or disability exceeding 3 days
Alaska	Within 10 days	Death, injury, disease, or infection
American Samoa	Within 10 days of employer	Death, injury, or disease
Arizona	Within 10 days	All injuries
Arkansas	10 days from notice of injury	Indemnity, injuries, or death[2]
California	Immediately[3] (employer)	Death or serious injuries
	As prescribed	Disability of 1 day or more, other than first aid
	Within 5 days	Occupational diseases or pesticide poisoning
Colorado	Immediately[4]	Death
	Within 10 days[4]	Injuries causing lost time of 3 days or more or 3 shifts
	Immediately[4]	Any accident in which three or more employees are injured
	10 days[4]	Occupational disease cases
	10 days[4]	Cases of permanent physical impairment
Connecticut	7 days or as directed	Disability of 1 day or more
Delaware	Within 48 hours[5]	Death or injuries requiring hospitalization
	Within 10 days	Other injuries
District of Columbia	Within 10 days	All injuries
Florida	Within 24 hours[6]	Death
	Within 7 days to carrier	All injuries requiring medical treatment
Georgia	Within 21 days[7]	All injuries requiring medical or surgical treatment or causing more than 7 days of absence
Guam	Within 10 days[8]	Injury, illness, or death
Hawaii	Within 48 hours	Death
	Within 7 working days	All injuries
Idaho	As soon as practicable but not later than 10 days after the accident[9]	All injuries requiring medical treatment or causing 1 day's absence
Illinois	Within 2 working days	Death or serious injuries
	Between 15th and 25th of month	Disability of more than 3 days
	As soon as determinable	Permanent disability
Indiana	Within 7 working days[9]	Disability of more than 1 day
Iowa	Within 4 days	Disability of more than 3 days, permanent partial disability or death
Kansas	Within 28 days[10]	Death
	Within 28 days	Disability of more than remainder of day or shift
Kentucky	Within 7 days[11]	Disability of more than 1 day
Louisiana	Within 10 days of employer's actual knowledge of injury[12]	Lost time over 1 week or death
Maine	Within 7 days[13]	Only injuries causing 1 day or more of lost time[13]
Maryland	Within 10 days	Disability of more than 3 days
Massachusetts	Within 7 days, except Sundays and holidays	Disability of 5 or more calendar days
Michigan	Immediately	Death, disability of 7 days or more, and specific losses
Minnesota	Within 48 hours	Death or serious injury
	Within 14 days	Disability of 3 days or more
Mississippi	Within 10 days[14]	Death or disability of more than 5 days[14]
Missouri	Within 30 days[15]	Death or injury
Montana	Within 6 days	All injuries

[1]Federal Occupational Safety and Health Act of 1970 established uniform requirements and forms to meet its criteria for all businesses affecting interstate commerce to be used for statistical purposes and compliance with the Act. 12 U.S.C. §651.

[2]Arkansas. Medical only claims reported monthly.

[3]California. To Division of Occupational Safety and Health. Within 5 days of employer's notice or knowledge of employee death, employer must report death to the Department of Industrial Relations.

[4]Colorado. Failure to report tolls time limit for claims.

[5]Delaware. Supplemental report on termination of disability.

[6]Florida. Death cases—by telephone to workers' compensation division within 24 hours. All injuries—carrier to send first report form to division, if injury involved lost time.

[7]Georgia. Supplemental report on first payment and suspension of payment and within 30 days after final payment.

[8]Guam. Failure to report tolls time limits for claims.

[9]Idaho and Indiana. Supplemental report within 10 days after termination of compensation period.

[10]Kansas. Failure to report tolls time limit for claims. *Childress v. Childress Painting Co., 1979.*

[11]Kentucky. Supplemental report required after 60 days or on termination of disability.

[12]Louisiana. Employers with more than 10 employees must also report, within 90 days, death, any nonfatal occupational illness or injury causing loss of consciousness, restriction of work or motion, job transfer, or medical treatment other than first aid. Violation of confidentiality of any record, subject to $500 fine.

[13]Maine. Up to $1000 for individual and $25,000 for corporation for willful violation, fraud, or intentional misrepresentation.

[14]Mississippi. Permanent disability, serious head or facial disfigurement also covered; $2000 may be added to any award and $2000 may be ordered payable to the workers' compensation commission.

[15]Missouri. A report of medical costs and temporary benefits paid pursuant to sections 287.170 and 287.180 RS Mo shall be filed within 30 days of the date of original notification of the injury. If medical treatment or temporary benefits will continue past 30 days, a status report including estimated dates of completion of medical treatment and temporary benefits shall be provided to the division at that time. A final report shall be filed on conclusion or termination of medical treatment and medical benefits. A final medical report shall be filed with the final report.

Table 15-1 Employers' or Physicians' Report of Accident—cont'd

JURISDICTION	TIME LIMIT	INJURIES COVERED
Nebraska	Within 10 days[16]	All injuries or diagnosed occupational diseases that result in death, time away from work, restricted work, or termination of employment; loss of consciousness; or medical treatment other than first aid
Nevada	Within 6 working days after report from physician[17]	All injuries requiring medical treatment
New Hampshire	Within 5 calendar days	All injuries involving lost time or medical expenses
New Jersey	Within 3 weeks of learning of occupational disease	All injuries, other than those requiring first aid
New Mexico	Within 10 days of employer notification[18]	Any injury or illness resulting in 7 or more days of lost time
New York	Within 10 days[19]	Disability of 1 day beyond working day or shift on which accident occurred or requiring medical care beyond 2 first aid treatments
North Carolina	Within 10 days[20]	Disability of more than 1 day or charges for medical compensation exceeding the amount set by the commission
North Dakota	Within 7 days	All injuries
Ohio	Within 1 week	Injuries causing total disability of 7 days or more
Oklahoma	Within 10 days or a reasonable time	Fatalities; all injuries causing lost time or requiring treatment away from worksite
Oregon	Within 5 days[21]	All claims or injuries that may result in compensable inquiry claims injuries
Pennsylvania	Within 48 hours[22]	Death
	After 7 days but not later than 10 days	Disability of 1 day or more
Puerto Rico	Within 5 days	All injuries
Rhode Island	Within 48 hours	Death
	Within 10 days	Disability of 3 days of more and all injuries requiring medical treatment Any claim resulting in medical expense
South Carolina	Within 10 days[23]	All injuries requiring medical attention costing more than $500, more than 1 day disability or permanency
South Dakota	Within 7 days[24]	Disability of 7 days or more, other than first aid or injuries requiring medical treatment
Tennessee	Within 14 days	Report of Injury must be filed when employee receives medical care outside of employer's premises
Texas	Within 8 days[25]	Disability of more than 1 day, or occupational disease
Utah	Within 7 days	All injuries requiring medical attention
Vermont	Within 72 hours	Disability of 1 day or more requiring medical care
Virgin Islands	Within 8 days	Injury or disease
Virginia	Within 10 days[26]	All injuries
Washington	Immediately	Deaths and accidents resulting in workers' hospitalizations or inability to work
West Virginia	Within 5 days	All injuries
Wisconsin	Within 14 days[27]	Disability beyond 3-day waiting period
Wyoming	Within 10 days	All injuries
Federal Employees' Compensation Act (FECA)	Within 10 days	All injuries involving medical expenses, disability, or death
Longshoremen's and Harbor Workers' Compensation Act (LHWCA)	10 days	Injuries that cause loss of 1 or more shifts of work or death

[16]Nebraska. Report may be made by insurance carrier or employer. Failure to report tolls time limits.
[17]Nevada. For minor injuries not requiring medical treatment, the employee may file a "Notice of Injury," which must be retained by the employer for 3 years.
[18]New Mexico. For EDI filings all injuries having more than $300 of expenses must be reported to the administration. A subsequent report from the claims administrator is required on payment of any claim.
[19]New York. Carrier or employer, if self-insured, is required to provide a written statement of rights under the law to injured employee or dependent if worker deceased.
[20]North Carolina. Supplemental report required after 60 days or on termination of disability.
[21]Oregon. Insurers to send initial disabling claims acceptance, aggravation claim acceptance, and claim denial to WC Division within 14 days.
[22]Pennsylvania. Late filing of accident report may be penalized by sum up to 10% of compensation awarded plus interest accrued and payable. In cases of excessive delay, penalty can be increased to 50%.
[23]South Carolina. Supplemental report every 6 months or on termination of disability.
[24]South Dakota. Any injury that requires treatment other than first aid or that incapacitates employee for at least 7 calendar days.
[25]Texas. Supplemental report required upon termination of disability or change in postinjury earnings.
[26]Virginia Accident reports to commission must be submitted electronically through EDI or WebFile.
[27]Wisconsin. 10% of first payment goes to injured employee.

Scenario: Second-Injury Fund

Bob Evans lost his left thumb while working a lathe. Then, 2 years later, Bob lost his left index finger in a second work-related accident. A question could arise of whether the second injury added to a preexisting condition or was related to the prior injury. This case illustrates that the existence of the former injury or disability substantially increased (added to) the disability caused by the latter injury. The employer would pay compensation related to the second injury, and funds would come from a second-injury fund to pay for the difference between the first and second injuries.

Minimum Number of Employees

Each state requires a minimum number of employees at one business before the state workers' compensation law comes into effect. The majority of the states require at least one employee, but the exceptions are American Samoa (2); Arkansas, Georgia, Michigan, New Mexico, North Carolina, and Virginia (3); Florida and South Carolina (4); and Alabama, Mississippi, Missouri, and Tennessee (5). Many states have exemptions for certain occupations such as domestic or casual employees,

laborers, babysitters, newspaper vendors or distributors, charity workers, and gardeners. Some states do not require compensation insurance for farm laborers or may specify a larger number of farm employees than the number shown in the table.

Waiting Periods

The laws state that a **waiting period (WP)** must elapse before income benefits are payable. This waiting period affects only wage compensation because medical and hospital care are provided immediately. See Table 15-2 to find the waiting period of each state.

State Disability and Workers' Compensation

Five states and one US territory have state disability insurance (also known as *unemployment compensation disability insurance*): California, Hawaii, New Jersey, New York, Rhode Island, and Puerto Rico. If a recipient is collecting benefits from a workers' compensation insurance carrier and the amount that the compensation carrier pays is less than that allowed by the state disability

Table 15-2	Waiting Period for Income and Medical Benefits*		
JURISDICTION	**WAITING PERIOD (DAYS)**	**JURISDICTION**	**WAITING PERIOD (DAYS)**
Alabama	3	Nebraska	7
Alaska	3	Nevada	5
Arizona	7	New Hampshire	3
Arkansas	7	New Jersey	7
California	3	New Mexico	7
Colorado	3	New York	7
Connecticut	3	North Carolina	7
Delaware	3	North Dakota	5
District of Columbia	3	Ohio	7
Florida	7	Oklahoma	3
Georgia	7	Oregon	3
Guam	3	Pennsylvania	7
Hawaii	3	Puerto Rico	3
Idaho	5	Rhode Island	3
Illinois	3	South Carolina	7
Indiana	7	South Dakota	7
Iowa	3	Tennessee	7
Kansas	7	Texas	7
Kentucky	7	Utah	3
Louisiana	7	Vermont	3
Maine	7	Virgin Islands	0
Maryland	3	Virginia	7
Massachusetts	5	Washington	3
Michigan	7	West Virginia	3
Minnesota	3	Wisconsin	3
Mississippi	5	Wyoming	3
Missouri	3	FECA	3
Montana	4 days or 32 hours, whichever is less	LHWCA	3

FECA, Federal Employees' Compensation Act; *LHWCA*, Longshoremen's and Harbor Workers' Compensation Act.
*These are statutory provisions for waiting periods. Statutes provide that a waiting period must elapse, during which income benefits are not payable. This waiting period affects only compensation because medical and hospital care are provided immediately.

insurance program, then the latter pays the balance. See Chapter 16 for further information on state disability insurance.

BENEFITS

Five principal types of state compensation benefits that may apply in ordinary cases are the following:

1. *Medical treatment.* This includes hospital, medical and surgical services, medications, and prosthetic devices. Treatment may be rendered by a medical doctor, osteopath, dentist, or chiropractor.
2. *Temporary disability indemnity.* This is in the form of weekly cash payments made directly to the injured or ill person.
3. *Permanent disability indemnity.* This may consist of either weekly or monthly cash payments based on a rating system that determines the percentage of permanent disability or a lump sum award. California has a unique system of permanent disability evaluation that requires a separate determination by the disability rating bureau in San Francisco. No other state has this system.
4. *Death benefits for survivors.* This consists of cash payments to dependents of employees who are fatally injured. A burial allowance is also given in some states.
5. *Rehabilitation benefits.* This can be medical or vocational rehabilitation in cases of severe disabilities.

TYPES OF STATE CLAIMS

There are three types of state workers' compensation claims: nondisability (ND) claims, temporary disability claims, and permanent disability claims. Each type is discussed in detail for a clear definition and understanding of the determination process.

Nondisability Claim

The simplest type of claim is a **nondisability (ND) claim,** which generally involves a minor injury in which the patient is seen by the physician but is able to continue working (Figure 15-1). This type of case does not require weekly temporary disability payments.

Temporary Disability Claim

Temporary disability (TD) occurs when a worker has a work-related injury or illness and is unable to perform the duties of his or her occupation for a specific time or range of time. The time period of temporary disability can extend from the date of injury until the worker either returns to full duty without residual ratable disability (discussed later), returns to modified work, or has ratable residual disability that the physician states is permanent and stationary.

FIGURE 15-1 Physician interacting with an injured worker in the examination room.

An **insurance adjuster** is the person at the workers' compensation insurance carrier who oversees the industrial case. He or she is responsible for keeping in contact with the physician's office about the patient's ongoing progress. The insurance adjuster's most important function is adjusting an industrial claim. This means that the insurance adjuster must evaluate the injury or illness, predict in advance the amount of money reserves needed to cover medical expenses, and calculate as accurate a reserve as possible for weekly TD payments to the injured. This is frequently a difficult task because a seemingly minor back strain ultimately may require fusion, or a small cut may become gangrenous and lead to an amputation. The insurance carrier wants to provide the best possible medical care for the patient. The patient is immediately referred to the specialist if a specialist is necessary.

Usually workers' compensation weekly TD payments are based on a percentage of the employee's earnings at the time of the injury. Compensation benefits are not subject to income tax.

Sometimes a patient is released to modified work to effect a transition between the period of inactivity caused by disability and a return to full duty, especially when heavy work is involved. Other times an employee is returned to the company and placed in a different department or division so that he or she is gainfully employed while not using the injured body part. This topic is further detailed in the next section.

Vocational Rehabilitation

Many states provide vocational rehabilitation in the form of retraining, education, job guidance, and placement to assist an injured individual in finding work before temporary disability compensation benefits expire. In any successful rehabilitation program, the insurance carrier, physician, physical therapist, employer supervisor, and personnel department must act as a team with the common goal of getting an injured employee back to light duty or regular work as soon as possible. It is believed that the longer a person remains out of work, the less chance there is that he or she will return to the workplace. The employer and insurance adjuster must remain in communication with rehabilitation center therapists to determine when the injured person will be able to resume some form of work. The physician may suggest a rehabilitation center that provides good care, or the employer may have an in-house program.

Work Hardening

Sports medicine therapy and physical medicine rehabilitation are often used to strengthen the injured worker. Physical medicine/therapy CPT codes 97001 to 97542 are used to report these services. Another type of therapy, called **work hardening,** is an individualized program using simulated or real work tasks to build up strength and improve the worker's endurance toward a full day's work. *Current Procedure Terminology* (CPT) codes 97545 and 97546 are used to report work hardening conditioning.

Ergonomics

In some cases an **ergonomic** evaluation of the work site is performed and modifications may be instituted to the job or work site to lessen the possibility of future injury and to get the employee back to gainful employment. CPT code 97537 may be used to report a work site modification analysis. Injured individuals may also be retrained into another career field if their disability prevents them from returning to their former occupation.

Permanent Disability Claim

In this type of claim, the patient or injured party is usually on TD benefits for a time and then concludes that he or she is unable to return to his or her former occupation. The physician states in the report that the patient has residual disability that will hamper his or her opportunity to compete in the open job market. Examples of residual disability include loss of a hand, an eye, or a leg and neurologic problems. Each patient who has **permanent disability (PD)** is rated according to the severity of the injury, the age of the injured person, and the patient's occupation at the time of the injury. The older the person, the greater the PD benefit. One might think that a younger person deserves higher compensation because he or she will be disabled for a longer portion of his or her working career. However, the workers' compensation laws assume that a young person has a better chance of being rehabilitated into another occupation.

In a PD claim, the physician's final report must include the words **"permanent and stationary" (P and S).** This phrase means that damage from the injury or illness is permanent, the patient has recovered to the fullest extent possible, the physician is unable to do anything more for the patient, and the patient will be hampered by the disability to some extent for the rest of his or her life. The P and S examination is usually comprehensive, and a level 5 CPT code may be appropriate. Depending on the fee schedule, a modifier indicating that the evaluation and management service is a P and S examination may also be used. The case is rated for PD, and a settlement, called a **compromise and release (C and R),** is made. This is an agreement between the injured party and insurance company on a total sum. The case can then be closed.

Reasons that may delay closing a workers' compensation case include the following:

1. Unanswered questions or incomplete answers to data required on workers' compensation forms by the employee, employer, or physician
2. Vague terminology used by the physician in medical reports
3. Omitted signatures on forms or written reports by the employee, employer, or physician
4. Incorrect billing by the physician's office
5. Inadequate progress reports (e.g., the physician fails to send in a medical report routinely to update the insurance carrier when the injured employee is seen in subsequent visits)

Rating

Final determination of the issues involving settlement of an industrial accident is known as **adjudication,** or the rating of a case. A physician does not rate disability but renders a professional opinion on whether the injured individual has temporary or permanent disability that prevents him or her from gainful employment. Rating itself is carried out by the state's industrial accident commission or workers' compensation board. Wage loss, earning capacity, and physical impairment are three categories that may be taken into consideration to rate temporary partial, permanent partial, or total disabilities.

In addition, permanent partial disabilities may be rated by using a scheduled or nonscheduled injury award system. This system is based on a set number of weeks of compensation for a specific loss such as 288 weeks for the loss of a leg. Scheduled injuries may be loss of a body part, disfigurement, permanent hearing loss, and so on. Nonscheduled injuries are more general, such as disability caused by injury to the back or neck.

If an injured person is dissatisfied with the rating after the case has been declared P and S, he or she may appeal the case (by **petition**—formal written request) to the **Workers' Compensation Appeals Board (WCAB)** or the Industrial Accident Commission.

Surveillance

Sub rosa films are provided occasionally when rating a case to document the extent of a patient's permanent disability. Sub rosa means "under the rose." In ancient times the rose was a symbol of silence or secrecy. Videotapes are made over a period of 2 to 3 days without the patient's knowledge. This surveillance is expensive and is used as a last resort, especially in a case in which a person receiving workers' compensation benefits is suspected of making exaggerated complaints. It is also used in cases when a worker has been off work for a long time and supposedly is unable to perform any work activity, even light duty.

Investigators have been known to carry a camera in a gym bag and videotape a supposedly disabled claimant bench pressing at the gym. Patients also have been videotaped going into the physician's office for an appointment wearing a neck brace and removing the brace after returning to their car.

FRAUD AND ABUSE

Increases in the number of fraudulent workers' compensation claims were noted throughout many large metropolitan cities in the 1990s. These problems involved employers, employees, insurers, medical providers, and lawyers. An increasing number of states have enacted some kind of antifraud legislation and stiffened penalties for workers' compensation fraud, making it a felony. Some states require reporting suspected insurance fraud and have forms to incorporate wording in regard to fraudulent statements. An example is shown in Figure 15-2.

Physicians are responsible for determining the legitimacy of work injuries and reporting findings accurately. If a report is prepared with the intent to use it in support of a fraudulent claim, or if a fraudulent claim is knowingly submitted for payment under an insurance contract, the physician may be subject to fines or imprisonment and the revocation or suspension of his or her medical license. Some physicians sign and send a disclosure statement with the medical report certifying that they personally performed an evaluation. The physician may list the total time spent in reviewing records, face-to-face time with the patient, preparation of a report, and other relevant activities.

It is the responsibility of all individuals who deal with workers' compensation cases to notify the insurance carrier of any suspicious situation. By doing so, action can be taken to have the case investigated further by personnel from the fraud divisions or referred to the district attorney's office. Perpetrators and signs of workers' compensation fraud and abuse are listed in Box 15-1.

See Chapters 2, 12, and 13 for further information on fraud and abuse in the medical setting.

OCCUPATIONAL SAFETY AND HEALTH ADMINISTRATION ACT OF 1970

Background

Congress has established an office known as the **Occupational Safety and Health Administration (OSHA)** to protect employees against on-the-job health and safety hazards. This program includes strict health and safety standards and a sensible complaint procedure enabling individual workers to trigger enforcement measures.

Work standards are designed to minimize exposure to on-the-job hazards such as faulty machinery, noise, dust, and toxic chemical fumes. Employers are required by law to meet these health and safety standards. Failure to do so can result in fines against the employer that could run into thousands of dollars.

Coverage

The act provides that if a state submits an OSHA plan and it is approved by the government, the state may assume responsibility for carrying out OSHA policies and procedures and is excluded from federal jurisdiction.

The act applies to almost all businesses, large or small. It applies to heavy, light, and service industries, nonprofit and charitable institutions, churches' secular activities in hospitals, farmers, and retailers. Employees of state and local governments are also covered. Federal employees, a farmer's immediate family, church employees engaged in religious activities, independent contractors, and household domestic workers are not covered.

EMPLOYEE'S CLAIM FOR WORKERS' COMPENSATION BENEFITS

If you are injured or become ill because of your job, you may be entitled to workers' compensation benefits.

Complete the **"Employee"** section and give the form to your employer. Keep the copy marked **"Employee's Temporary Receipt"** until you receive the dated copy from your employer. You may call the Division of Workers' Compensation at **1-800-736-7401** if you need help in filling out this form or in obtaining your benefits. An explanation of workers' compensation benefits is included on the back of this form.

You should also have received a pamphlet from your employer describing workers' compensation benefits and the procedures to obtain them.

Any person who makes or causes to be made any knowingly false or fraudulent material statement or material representation for the purpose of obtaining or denying workers' compensation benefits or payments is guilty of a felony.

PETICION DEL EMPLEADO PARA BENEFICIOS DE COMPENSACIÓN DEL TRABAJADOR

Si Ud. se ha lesionado o se ha enfermado a causa de su trabajo, Ud. tiene derecho a recibir beneficios de compensación al trabajador.
Complete la sección **"Empleado"** y entregue la forma a su empleador. Quédese con la copia designada **"Recibo Temporal del Empleado"** hasta que Ud. reciba la copia fechada de su empleador. Si Ud. necesita ayuda para completar esta forma o para obtener sus beneficios, Ud. puede hablar con la Division de Compensación al Trabajador llamando al **1-800-736-7401**. En la parte de atrás de esta forma se encuentra una explicación de los beneficios de la compensación al trabajador.

Ud. también debería haber recibido de su empleador un folleto describiendo los beneficios de compensación al trabajador lesionado y los procedimientos para obtenerlos.

Toda aquella persona que a propósito haga o cause que se produzca cualquier declaración o representación material falsa o fraudulenta con el fin de obtener o negar beneficios o pagos de compensación a trabajadores lesionados es culpable de un crimen mayor "felonía".

Employee: Empleado

1. Name. Nombre. Ima B. Hurt   Today's date. Fecha de hoy. 4-3-20XX
2. Home address. Dirección residencial. 300 East Central Avenue
3. City. Ciudad. Woodland Hills   State. Estado. XY   Zip. Código postal 12345-0001
4. Date of injury. Fecha de la lesión (accidente). 4-3-XX   Time of injury. Hora en que ocurrió. _____ a.m. 2:00 p.m.
5. Address and description of where injury happened. Dirección/lugar dónde occurió el accidente. The Conk Out Company
   45 South Gorman Street, Woodland Hills, XY 12345   injured in stock room
6. Describe injury and part of body affected. Describa la lesión y parte dél cuerpo afectada. Fell off ladder in stock room.
   Injured left ankle.
7. Social Security Number. Número de Seguro Social del Empleado. 120 XX 6542
8. Signature of employees. Firma del empleado. Ima B. Hurt

Employer—complete this section and give the employee a copy immediately as a receipt.
Empleador—complete esta sección y déle inmediatamente una copia al empleado como recibo.

9. Name of employer. Nombre del empleador. The Conk Out Company
10. Address. Dirección. 45 South Gorman Street, Woodland Hills, XY 12345
11. Date employer first knew of injury. Fecha en que el empleador supo por primera vez de la lesión o accidente. 4-3-20XX
12. Date claim form was provided to employee. Fecha en que se le entregó al empleado la petición. 4-3-20XX
13. Date employer received claim form. Fecha en que el empleado devolvió la petición al empleador. 4-3-20XX
14. Name and address of insurance carrier or adjusting agency. Nombre y dirección de la compañía de seguros o agencia administradora de seguros. XYZ Insurance Company, P.O. Box 5, Woodland Hills, XY 12345
15. Insurance policy number. El número de la poliza del Seguro. B 12345
16. Signature of employer representative. Firma del representante del empleador. J. D. Hawkins
17. Title. Título. Owner   18. Telephone. Teléfono. 555-430-3488

Employer: You are required to date this form and provide copies to your insurer or claims administrator and to the employee, dependent or representative who filed the claim within **one working day** of receipt of the form from the employee.

SIGNING THIS FORM IS NOT AN ADMISSION OF LIABILITY

Empleador: Se requiere que Ud. feche esta forma y que provéa copias a su compañía de seguros, administrador de reclamos, o dependiente/répresentante de reclamos y al empleado que hayan presentado esta petición dentro del plazo de **un día hábil** desde el momento de haber sido recibida la forma del empleado.

EL FIRMAR ESTA FORMA NO SIGNIFICA ADMISION DE RESPONSABILIDAD

FIGURE 15-2 Employee's Claim for Workers' Compensation Benefits. Notice the insert about fraudulent material.

Box 15-1 Perpetrators and Signs of Workers' Compensation Fraud and Abuse

Employee

- Symptoms are all subjective.
- Misses the first physician's visit or cancels or repeatedly reschedules appointments.
- Cannot describe the pain or is overly dramatic such as an employee who comes into the physician's office limping on the left leg, suddenly starts limping on the right leg, and then goes back to limping on the left leg.
- Delays in reporting the injury.
- Does not report Friday's injury until Monday morning.
- First reports an injury to a legal or regulatory agency.
- Reports an injury after missing several days of work.
- Changes physicians frequently.
- Is a short-term worker.
- Has a curious claim history.
- Fabricates an injury.
- Exaggerates a work-related injury to obtain larger benefits such as an injured employee who has a back pain and claims inability to bend over or lift. Surveillance cameras capture the individual at work on weekends repairing cars in the driveway at home—a task he is supposedly unable to perform.
- Blames an injury that occurred off the job on the employer.
- Adds symptoms in response to efforts to return the person to work.

Employer

- Misrepresents the annual payroll to get lower premium rates.
- Misrepresents the number of workers employed.
- Gives a false address with the least expensive premium rates.
- Falsely classifies the job duties of workers (as not hazardous) such as stating the job title as a clerical worker when, in fact, the employee is using a lathe every day.
- Conspires with the employee to defraud.

Insurer

- Refuses to pay valid medical claims.
- Forces the injured worker to settle by using unethical tactics. For example, an insurance agent tells an employee that he has a back sprain. Relying on that information, the

worker settles the case. Later, a myelogram reveals a herniated intervertebral disk. The patient is left with a permanent partial disability.

Medical Provider

- Makes immediate referral for psychiatric care despite the worker's report of a trauma injury.
- Orders or performs unnecessary tests.
- Treatment dates fall on weekends and holidays.
- Renders unnecessary treatment.
- Lists a diagnosis that is not consistent with the course of treatment.
- Charges the insurance carrier for services never rendered.
- Prolongs treatment for what appears to be a minor injury.
- Participates in a provider mill scheme (see explanation under "Lawyer").
- Makes multiple referrals from a clinic practice regardless of type of injury.
- Sends medical reports that look photocopied with the same information typed in (e.g., employer's address, description of injury) or that read almost identical to other reports.
- Sends in many claims in which injuries are of a subjective nature such as stress, emotional distress, headaches, inability to sleep.
- Sends in claims from one employer showing several employees with similar injuries, using the same physicians and/or attorneys.
- Bills both the workers' compensation carrier and the health insurer for the same service.

Lawyer

- Overbills clients.
- Participates in a medical provider mill scheme. For example, an individual is solicited while in the unemployment line by a recruiter known as a "capper." The capper tells the worker it is possible to obtain more money on disability than through unemployment. The worker is referred to an attorney and a "provider mill" clinic, which help the individual fabricate a claim by claiming stress or an on-the-job injury. In some states, such acts may be considered a public offense and are punishable as a misdemeanor or felony.

Regulations

Specific regulations that affect the medical setting are those aimed at minimizing exposure to hepatitis B virus (HBV), human immunodeficiency virus (HIV), and other bloodborne pathogens. Any worker who comes in contact with human blood and infectious materials must receive proper information and training and use universal precautions (protective safety measures) to avoid infection. Vaccinations must be provided for those who are at risk for exposure to hepatitis B, and comprehensive records must be maintained. For fact sheets, booklets, and guidelines on bloodborne pathogens, contact the nearest OSHA office or write to OSHA Publications Office, 200 Constitution Avenue, NW, Room N3101, Washington, DC 20210.

Chemicals and hazardous substances that impose dangers in many work settings are used. Businesses are required to obtain material safety data sheets (MSDSs) for each hazardous chemical used on site. Employers that produce a hazardous chemical must develop MSDSs. A compliance kit is available from the Superintendent of Documents, US Government Printing Office, Washington, DC 20402.

Filing a Complaint

To file a complaint, the proper form is obtained from the federal Division of Industrial Safety or a state OSHA office and completed by the employee. It is against the law for an employer to take any adverse action against an employee who files such a complaint.

Inspection

A compliance officer (inspector) may call for an appointment or may be sent unannounced to the place of employment. If an officer arrives unannounced, the office manager must be notified so that an appointment may be arranged for the inspection to take place. A court warrant may be required to search a company's premises if the employer does not consent to OSHA entry. A business may be cited and, depending on the violation, fines or criminal penalties may be imposed.

Record Keeping and Reporting

Employers must keep records of their employees' work-related injuries and illnesses on OSHA Form No. 200. Forms may be obtained from the OSHA office or from any office of the U.S. Department of Labor. This document must be on file at the workplace and available to employees and OSHA compliance officers on request. Form 200 must be retained in the file for 5 years. After 6 days, a case recorded on Form 200 must have a supplementary record (OSHA Form 101) completed and kept in the files. Some states have modified their workers' compensation forms so that they may be used as substitutes for Form 101. Certain low-hazard industries are exempt from having to complete and retain Forms 200 and 101.

Companies with fewer than 11 employees must complete safety survey OSHA Form 200-S. Companies are also required to display OSHA posters to inform employees of their job safety rights. Federal law states that an accident that results in the death or hospitalization of five or more employees must be reported to OSHA.

LEGAL SITUATIONS

Medical Evaluator

Physicians who conduct medical-legal (ML) evaluations of injured workers must pass a complex medical examination. They are then certified by the Industrial Medical Council (IMC) and may be referred to as one of the following titles:

- Agreed medical evaluator (AME)
- Independent medical evaluator (IME)
- Qualified medical evaluator (QME)

The medical evaluator is hired by the insurance company or appointed by the referee or appeals board to examine an individual, independent from the attending physician, and render an unbiased opinion about the degree of disability of an injured worker. When the physician performs an evaluation on an injured worker, the workers' compensation fee schedule may have specific procedure codes to bill for the examination. Evaluation

and management consultation codes or the CPT code for work-related evaluation by "other" physician (99456) may be used. Some state fee schedules may have specific ML procedure codes to bill for various levels of examination. When a case involves a medical evaluation, a deposition may be taken of his or her testimony.

Depositions

A **deposition** is a proceeding in which an attorney asks a witness questions about a case, and the witness answers under oath but not in open court. It may take place in the attorney's office or often in the physician's office. In permanent disability workers' compensation cases, depositions are usually taken from the physician and the injured party by the attorney representing the workers' compensation insurance company. The injured party's attorney is also present if the witness is the defendant. Direct questioning and cross-examination may be done by both attorneys.

The session may be recorded on a stenotype machine, in shorthand, or by audiotape or videotape. Video depositions are used in several instances. For example, if a plaintiff in a case is terminally ill and the plaintiff's attorney wishes to preserve the plaintiff's testimony, a video deposition may be used as substantive (essential) evidence. A video deposition may also be taken if a witness cannot be present at the trial. In a case in which a witness may be in Arizona and cannot appear in Pennsylvania, the attorney takes the deposition in Arizona and proves to the court that the witness is beyond its jurisdiction. The same is true for a physician defendant who is not available for some reason.

Exhibits may be entered into evidence. The witness is allowed to read the transcript and make corrections or changes. The witness may be asked to sign the transcript but can waive a signature if his or her attorney recommends against signing it. The deposition is used when the case comes to trial.

Depositions may be taken to find out additional information, the physician's version of the facts, the patient's version of the facts, what kind of witnesses the physician and patient will be, and so on. Another use for a deposition is to impeach (challenge the credibility or validity of) a witness on cross-examination. If the witness takes the stand and the testimony is inconsistent with the deposition, the attorney will make this known to the jury.

Medical Testimony

In the instance of an accident case with third-party liability, the physician may have to testify as an expert witness, take time to give a deposition, or attend a pretrial conference. There should be a clear understanding of the terms

---

MEDICAL TESTIMONY AGREEMENT

AGREEMENT made this _____ day of _____ 20XX, between _____
herein referred to as attorney, and _____,
of _____ , _____ , _____ , _____ , a licensed _____ .
          (street address)   (city)   (state)   (ZIP code)

In consideration of their mutual covenants set forth herein, the parties agree as follows:

1. The doctor will give medical testimony in the case of:

_____

as a treating physician or as an expert witness (delete the unwanted phrase).

2. The doctor agrees to appear promptly when called and to present his or her medical testimony in a well-prepared professional manner.

3. The doctor will be compensated for time away from the practice of his or her medical duties in accordance with the following:
    (a) $_____ per hour for reports and preparation of medical testimony.
    (b) $_____ per hour for pretrial conferences.
    (c) $_____ per hour for court appearance, including travel time to and from the office.
    (d) $_____ per hour for deposition.
    (e) $_____ per hour for being on call with cancellation of appointments but not appearing in court.

4. The doctor will appear in court on _____ hour's notice from the attorney, unless prior arrangements have been made for the exact time of appearance.

5. The doctor will be compensated on completion of his or her medical testimony, and payment will not be contingent upon the outcome of the case. However, if the case is settled before reaching the court, the doctor will be compensated for being on call as noted above.

This contract shall be binding upon the parties.

IN WITNESS WHEREOF, the said parties hereto have subscribed their respective signatures.

_____
    (physician)

_____
    (attorney)

Date: _____

FIGURE 15-3 Example of a medical testimony agreement between physician and attorney. This is signed by the physician and sent to the attorney for signature. A copy is retained by the attorney and the original is kept by the physician.

of testimony and payment to eliminate future misunderstandings. A written agreement from the patient's lawyer should be obtained stating exactly what compensation the physician will receive for research (preparation), time spent waiting to testify (if appointments must be canceled), and actual testimony time (Figure 15-3). In some cases the physician may want to ask for partial payment in advance. If the physician is subpoenaed, he or she must appear in court regardless of whether an agreement exists. The correct CPT code for medical testimony is 99075. This agreement should be signed by the physician and sent to the attorney. The attorney should return the original to the physician, retaining a copy for his or her files.

Liens

The word **lien** derives from the same origin as the word *liable*, and the right of lien expresses legal claim on the property of another for the payment of a debt (Figure 15-4). Liens sometimes are called *encumbrances* and may be filed for a number of reasons.

The advantages of filing a lien are as follows:

- It is a written agreement and is recognized in court.
- It is a source of protection in the event of litigation.
- It ensures that payment for previously rendered medical services are received when the attorney and patient have reached a settlement with the insurance company in an accident case.
- It is an inexpensive method of collecting the fee. The physician can file suit and try to get a judgment against the patient, but this is relatively expensive when compared to filing a lien.
- The physician will collect the full fee. If the physician assigns such a delinquent account to a collection agency, he or she may lose as much as 50% of the fee when it is collected.

**REQUEST FOR ALLOWANCE OF LIEN
ASSIGNMENT AND AUTHORIZATION**

WHEREAS, I have a right or cause of action arising out of personal injury, to wit:

I,_____ hereby authorize _____ ,
   patient's name   physician's name

to furnish, upon request, to my attorney,_____ ,
any and all medical records, or reports of examination, diagnosis, treatment, or prognosis but not necessarily limited to those items as set forth herein, in addition to an itemized statement of account for services rendered therefore or in connection therewith, which my attorney may from time to time request in connection with the injuries described above and sustained by me on the _____ day of _____ , 20XX.

I, hereby irrevocably authorize and direct my said attorney set forth herein to pay to_____ all charges for attendance in court,
                       physician's name

if required as an expert witness whether he testifies or not; reports or other data supplied by him; depositions given by said doctor; medical services rendered or drugs supplied; and any other reasonable and customary charges incurred by my attorney as submitted by_____ and in
                              physician's name

connection with said injury. Said payment or payments are to be made from any money or monies received by my attorney whether by judgment, decree, or settlement of this case, prior to disbursement to me and payment of the amount as herein directed shall be the same as if paid by me. This authorization to pay the aforementioned doctor shall constitute and be deemed as assignment of so much of my recovery I receive. It is agreed that nothing herein relieves me of the primary responsibility and obligation of paying my doctor for services rendered, and I shall at all times remain personally liable for such indebtedness unless released by the aforementioned doctor or by payment disbursed by my attorney.
I accept the above assignment:
Dated: _____ Patient:_____

As the attorney of record for the above-named patient, I hereby agree to observe the terms of this agreement, and to withhold from any award in this case such sums as are required for the adequate protection of Dr._____ .

Date: _____ Attorney:_____

FIGURE 15-4 Patient's authorization to release information to an attorney and grant lien to the physician against proceeds of settlement in connection with accident, industrial, or third-party litigation cases.

- If the physician wishes to bill more than what is allowed for a given service or services, a lien can be filed and the judge will determine whether it is reasonable.
- It avoids harassment in trying to collect the bill.

The chief disadvantage of not filing a lien is that there is no legal documentation if the case goes to court as far as collecting monies owed to the physician. A case could be settled, the attorney would get his or her fee, and the physician's fee may be placed last on the list for payment or remain unpaid.

A time limit should be specified when a lien form is completed; reaching a settlement may involve several years of litigation. Some patients may be persuaded to pay before a legal settlement is made or at least make payments until a settlement is reached. The lien becomes null and void at the end of the time limit. If the patient's

financial status has changed, one might be able to collect because the patient can then be billed. If not, an amended or subsequent lien should be filed that states the actual balance of the patient's account. The word "amended" should be typed on the new lien below the Workers' Compensation Appeals Board case number.

The physician's fee should be protected by having the attorney sign the lien, thereby indicating that he or she will pay the physician directly from any money received in a settlement. This makes the attorney responsible for the fee. The patient's file must be placed in a Hold for Settlement category until the case comes up in court. In some states the physician's fee owed by the patient constitutes a first lien against any such money settlement, and the attorney must first satisfy the lien of the physician before the patient or attorney receives any money from the settlement. State laws should be checked. The office of the patient's attorney should be called at least quarterly for an update.

Problem 1. Suppose Attorney Blake advises client Roger Reed not to pay the physician until after the trial. Or what happens if payment is not made for Dr. Practon's courtroom testimony and the case is lost? Suppose medical reports are ordered and Attorney Blake neglects to pay for them. What happens if Roger Reed forgets about the physician's bill?

Solution. If a lien had been signed, then once the case has been settled, the money would be paid to the physician; otherwise, the settlement would belong to the patient, Roger Reed, and he could take any action with the money that he wanted.

Problem 2. Suppose Dr. Practon had an oral agreement covering his fee. The patient, Katie Crest, was unable to pay for medical treatment except on legal monetary recovery. When Katie Crest settled her case, the proceeds went almost entirely to welfare agencies because she received retroactive Medicaid. Dr. Practon sued the patient's attorney and lost.

Solution. If Dr. Practon had gotten a written assignment of the proceeds, the lawyer could have been held liable for the fee.

If there is a third-party litigation involved in an industrial case or a decision has not been reached as to whether an accident is caused by industrial or nonindustrial causes, both a regular lien and a workers' compensation lien should be filed. In most states a special lien form for workers' compensation filing is available and should be used. A copy of the lien should be completed and sent to all concerned parties:

- Appeals board
- Employer of the patient
- Employee (the patient)
- Insurance carrier
- Physician's files (lien claimant or one who is filing for the lien)

The patient/employee consents to the lien by his or her signature. Do not accept a lien form unless it is also signed by the patient's attorney. Check with the local Division of Industrial Accidents for forms pertinent to filing a lien and instructions on the formalities, number of copies required, and where they are to be sent.

Third-Party Subrogation

The legal term *subrogation* is the process of initiating a legal claim against either another individual, an individual's insurer, or, in the case of a car accident, one's own automobile insurance company to pay health insurance bills. **Third-party subrogation** means "to substitute" one party for another. When applied to workers' compensation cases, it means a transfer of the claims and rights from the original creditor (workers' compensation insurance carrier) to the **third-party liability** carrier. In

a compensation case the insurance carrier that is "subrogated" to the legal claims has a right to be paid all of the monies they paid out for the injuries. That reimbursement is obtained from any money the injured collects either from a legal claim, directly from the individual who caused the injury, or from another insurer.

Scenario. As Monica Valdez, a secretary, went to the bank to deposit some money for her employer, her car was rear-ended by another automobile and she was injured.

Subrogation solution. In such a case, there is no question of fault and no question of cause. Monica was hurt during the performance of her work, and the workers' compensation insurance carrier is liable. The carrier must adjust the claim, provide all medical treatment, and pay all TD and PD benefits.

However, the insurance carrier does have legal recourse. It may send a representative to visit with Monica, explain to her that she has a good subrogation case, encourage her to seek the advice of an attorney, and sue the third party (other automobile driver) in civil court. This is sometimes referred to as litigation, which is the process of carrying on a lawsuit. If Monica agrees to sue, the insurance carrier files a demand with the court for repayment of all the money that it has paid out. This is called a lien, which is discussed earlier in the chapter. When the case is settled, if an award is made to Monica, the insurance carrier is reimbursed for all that it has paid and Monica receives the balance. In some states such as California, the patient is legally prevented from collecting twice.

MEDICAL REPORTS

Health Information Record Keeping

If a private patient comes to the office with an industrial injury, a separate health record (chart) and financial record (ledger) should be set up for the work-related injury. A private health record should never be combined with an industrial case record because separate disclosure laws apply to each, and the workers' compensation case may go to court. Some medical practices use a colored file folder or tabs for the industrial health record, which makes filing of all private and workers' compensation documents easier for the insurance billing specialist. If two charts are maintained, it is easy to pull the industrial health record and financial accounting record quickly without having to go through the patient's previously unrelated private health records.

It is preferable that a patient not be scheduled to see a physician for a workers' compensation follow-up examination and an unrelated complaint during the same appointment time. Separate appointments (back to back, if necessary) should be arranged. This allows for separate dictation without intermixing the required documentation for each chart.

PRIVACY AND CONFIDENTIALITY

The HIPAA Privacy Rule allows for the disclosure of personal health information (PHI) to workers' compensation insurers, state administrators, and employers to the extent necessary to comply with laws relating to workers' compensation. The HIPAA Privacy Rule recognizes the legitimate need of insurers and other entities involved in the workers' compensation systems to have access to individuals' health information as authorized by state or other law. Because of the significant variability among such laws, the HIPAA Privacy Rule permits disclosures of health information for workers' compensation purposes in a number of different ways:

1. *Disclosures without Individual Authorization.* The HIPAA Privacy Rule permits covered entities to disclose protected health information to workers' compensation insurers, state administrators, employers, and other persons or entities involved in workers' compensation systems, without the individual's authorization. This relates to workers' compensation injuries or illnesses and federal programs such as Black Lung Benefits Act, Federal Employees' Compensation Act, the Longshoremen's and Harbor Workers' Compensation Act, and Energy Employees' Occupational Illness Compensation Program Act. The disclosure must comply with and be limited to what the state law requires. Disclosure is allowed for purposes of obtaining payment for any health care provided to the injured or ill worker.

2. *Disclosures with Individual Authorization.* Covered entities may disclose PHI to workers' compensation insurers and others involved in workers' compensation systems to which the individual has provided his or her authorization for the release of the information to the entity. For example, if a patient's attorney calls the physician's office for information, it is only ethical and legal to get a signed authorization from the patient and to ask permission from the insurance carrier before giving out any medical information. The contract exists between the physician and insurance carrier, not the physician and patient.

3. *Minimum Necessary.* Covered entities are required to limit the amount of PHI disclosed to the minimum necessary to accomplish the workers' compensation purpose. Under this requirement, PHI may be shared for such purposes to the full extent authorized by state or other law.

If you get the patient's authorization to disclose the information, then you do not need to include it or track it for accounting because the disclosures that are made following somebody's authorization do not need to be accounted for.

Documentation

Documentation must show the necessity for the procedures performed. If there is no accurate diagnostic code to explain the patient's condition, a report that describes the details of the diagnosis should be sent.

As learned in Chapter 5, the ICD-9-CM code book has a section that lists E codes, which are categorized by external causes of injuries, poisonings, and adverse effects. E codes describe how injuries occur. In workers' compensation cases, it is important to use E codes because they indicate the external cause of injury such as E849.3 (place of occurrence; industrial place and premises). Some cases may need two E codes, one for the circumstance of the event and one for its location. E codes are never used as a primary diagnosis, but they give supplemental information to the insurance carrier. This may help the insurance carrier to differentiate between the claims and get a claim paid quicker.

CPT code 99080 may be used to bill for workers' compensation reports. The monetary value assigned to the code is usually determined by the number of pages in the report. If health records are reviewed before consulting or treating a workers' compensation patient, a bill should be submitted for this service. Refer to Chapter 4 for comprehensive information on the topic of documentation.

Terminology

Most workers' compensation cases involve accidents causing bodily injuries. Therefore one should become familiar with anatomic terms, directional and range-of-motion words, types of fractures, body activity terms, and words that describe pain and symptoms (Box 15-2). This terminology appears in progress chart notes and industrial injury reports. The more knowledgeable one becomes about the meaning of the documentation, the more proficient he or she will be in knowing whether the procedure and diagnostic codes assigned are substantiated or if code selection is deficient and should be enhanced for better payment. One should learn how to spell the words and find the definitions of the words in the dictionary.

Box 15-2	Terms That Describe Intensity of Pain and Frequency of Occurrence of Symptoms

Definitions that describe intensity of pain and frequency of symptoms were developed to assist the physician when documenting subjective complaints.

A *severe* pain would preclude the activity causing the pain.

A *moderate* pain could be tolerated but would cause marked handicap in the performance of the activity precipitating the pain.

A *slight pain* could be tolerated but would cause some handicap in the performance of the activity precipitating the pain.

A *minimal* (mild) pain would constitute an annoyance but would cause no handicap in the performance of the particular activity. It would be considered a nonratable permanent disability.

Occasional means approximately 25% of the time.

Intermittent means approximately 50% of the time.

Frequent means approximately 75% of the time.

Constant means 90% to 100% of the time.

Directional terms are commonly used when a case is being rated for permanent disability. A range-of-motion (ROM) test determines whether the body part is able to move to the full extent possible. Often, after an injury to an extremity or joint, there is restriction of motion and loss of strength (e.g., grip). ROM can be improved with activity and therapy. It is measured with special measurement devices and documented each time a patient is examined. Fractures can occur from falling, blows, impact hits, a disease process, or direct violence such as in an automobile accident. Healing may take months and depends on the location and severity of the injured part, associated injury, and complications or infections. To view graphics and terminology that shows directional words, ROM, body activity words, bones and joints of the skeletal anatomy, and different types of fractures, visit the Evolve website (see Box 15-2).

REPORTING REQUIREMENTS

Employer's Report

The laws clearly state that the injured person must promptly report the industrial injury or illness to his or her employer or immediate supervisor, which may be a safety officer in some businesses. By law in most states, the employer must send an Employer's Report of Occupational Injury or Illness Form (Figure 15-5) to the insurance company. The time limit on submission of this form varies from immediately to as long as 30 days in different states (see Table 15-1). Many states have adopted the form shown in Figure 15-5 to meet the requirements of the federal OSHA of 1970 and for state statistical purposes.

Medical Service Order

In addition to the employer's report, the employer may complete and sign a **medical service order,** giving this to the injured employee to take to the physician's office (Figure 15-6). This authorizes the physician to treat the injured employee. The form should be photocopied and the copy retained for the physician's files. The original should be attached to the Doctor's First Report of Occupational Injury or Illness (preliminary report). An employer may prefer to write the service order on his or her business letterhead, on billhead, or simply on a piece of scratch paper.

Authorizations may also be obtained over the telephone. However, if a patient arrives for an appointment without written authorization, some offices prefer that the employer be telephoned and asked to have the authorized person fax the permission for treatment. Subsequently, if payment is not received or the claim is disputed, it may be easier to collect if a copy of the written authorization is included when sending collection follow-up correspondence.

However, copayment should be collected when the patient has a managed care plan and neglects to bring in an authorization. It is the patient's responsibility to get the authorization if injured on the job (Figure 15-7).

A charge can be made if an appointment was arranged by the employer or insurance company for a workers' compensation patient and was not canceled 72 hours before the appointment time. Check with the insurance company because this policy may vary depending on state laws.

If outside testing or treatment is necessary, authorization should be obtained from the employer or the adjuster for the insurance company. When this is done by telephone, the name of the procedure or test and the medical necessity for it should be stated. The name and title of the person giving authorization should be obtained and written in the patient's chart and on the order form along with the date. No authorization numbers are issued in workers' compensation cases.

The insurance adjuster handling the case should be contacted if a translator is necessary for a workers' compensation patient. He or she should make arrangements for an official translator to be present for all appointments. A member of the patient's family or the patient's friend should not be allowed to serve as a translator because there may be no legal recourse for the physician if miscommunicated information leads to a bad outcome.

FIGURE 15-5 Employer's Report of Occupational Injury or Illness. This form complies with OSHA requirements and California State Workers' Compensation laws.

**WORKERS' COMPENSATION
MEDICAL SERVICE ORDER**

To: Dr./Clinic _____ Martin Feelgood, MD _____

Address _____ 4567 Broad Avenue, Woodland Hills, XY 12345 _____

We are sending _____ Mrs. Ima Hurt _____

Address _____ 300 East Central Ave. Woodland Hills, XY 12345 _____

Social Security No. _____ 120-XX-6542 _____ Date of birth 3-4-1966 _____
        to you for treatment in accordance with the terms of the Workers'
        Compensation Laws. Please submit your report to the
        _____ XYZ Insurance Company _____
        at once. Compensation cannot be paid without complete medical
        information.
Insurance carrier _____ XYZ Insurance Company _____

Address _P.O. Box 5, Woodland Hills, XY 12345_ Telephone _555-271-0562_

Employer _____ The Conk Out Company _____

Address _45 S. Gorman St. Woodland Hills, XY 12345_ Telephone _555-430-3488_

Signature _____ *J.D. HAWKINS, MD* _____ Date _____ 4-3-20XX _____
        If patient is able to return to work today or tomorrow, please
        show date and time below — sign and give to patient to return to
        employer. If there are any work restrictions indicate on the back
        of this form. Please submit your usual first report in any case.

Date/Time _____ By_____

FIGURE 15-6 Medical service order.

FIGURE 15-7 Receptionist receiving a medical service order via telephone for the worker to receive medical services.

Physician's First Report

After the physician sees the injured person, he or she sends in either a medical report detailing the injury together with a CMS-1500 (08-05) claim form (Figure 15-8) or a Doctor's First Report of Occupational Injury or Illness form (used in California; see Figure 15-15) as soon as possible. Some states either have modified the CMS-1500 (08-05) claim form, which allows for additional data so that an accompanying medical report may not be required, or have created a first treatment medical report form. Bill using CPT code 99455 (work-related or medical disability examination by the treating physician).

If the physician prefers to submit a narrative letter, the medical report should include the components, if relevant, shown in Table 15-3. The time limit for filing this report varies; state requirements are provided in Table 15-1. Failure to file the report can be a misdemeanor. Copies of the report form go to the insurance carrier and the state. Some physicians also send a copy to the employer.

Because the report is a legal document, each copy *must be signed in ink* by the physician. The insurance company waits for the physician's report and bill, then issues

(1500) HEALTH INSURANCE CLAIM FORM

APPROVED BY NATIONAL UNIFORM CLAIM COMMITTEE 08/05

☐☐ PICA   PICA ☐☐

1. MEDICARE / MEDICAID / TRICARE CHAMPUS / CHAMPVA / GROUP HEALTH PLAN / FECA BLK LUNG / OTHER [X] (ID)	1a. INSURED'S I.D. NUMBER (For Program in Item 1)
	B785700

2. PATIENT'S NAME (Last Name, First Name, Middle Initial)
TASK LESTER M

3. PATIENT'S BIRTH DATE 05 06 1990 SEX M [X] F

4. INSURED'S NAME (Last Name, First Name, Middle Initial)
JONAS CONSTRUCTION COMPANY

5. PATIENT'S ADDRESS (No., Street)
5400 HOLLY STREET

6. PATIENT RELATIONSHIP TO INSURED
Self ☐ Spouse ☐ Child ☐ Other [X]

7. INSURED'S ADDRESS (No., Street)
300 MAIN STREET

CITY WOODLAND HILLS **STATE** XY

8. PATIENT STATUS
Single ☐ Married ☐ Other ☐
Employed [X] Full-Time Student ☐ Part-Time Student ☐

CITY WOODLAND HILLS **STATE** XY

ZIP CODE 12345 **TELEPHONE (Include Area Code)** (555) 783 3200

ZIP CODE 12345 **TELEPHONE (INCLUDE AREA CODE)** (555) 309 9800

9. OTHER INSURED'S NAME (Last Name, First Name, Middle Initial)

10. IS PATIENT'S CONDITION RELATED TO:

11. INSURED'S POLICY GROUP OR FECA NUMBER

a. OTHER INSURED'S POLICY OR GROUP NUMBER

a. EMPLOYMENT? (CURRENT OR PREVIOUS) [X] YES ☐ NO

a. INSURED'S DATE OF BIRTH MM DD YY SEX M ☐ F ☐

b. OTHER INSURED'S DATE OF BIRTH MM DD YY SEX M ☐ F ☐

b. AUTO ACCIDENT? ☐ YES [X] NO PLACE (State)

b. EMPLOYER'S NAME OR SCHOOL NAME

c. EMPLOYER'S NAME OR SCHOOL NAME

c. OTHER ACCIDENT? ☐ YES [X] NO

c. INSURANCE PLAN NAME OR PROGRAM NAME

d. INSURANCE PLAN NAME OR PROGRAM NAME

10d. RESERVED FOR LOCAL USE

d. IS THERE ANOTHER HEALTH BENEFIT PLAN? ☐ YES ☐ NO *If yes,* return to and complete item 9 a-d.

READ BACK OF FORM BEFORE COMPLETING & SIGNING THIS FORM.

12. PATIENT'S OR AUTHORIZED PERSON'S SIGNATURE I authorize the release of any medical or other information necessary to process this claim. I also request payment of government benefits either to myself or to the party who accepts assignment below.

SIGNED _____ DATE _____

13. INSURED'S OR AUTHORIZED PERSON'S SIGNATURE I authorize payment of medical benefits to the undersigned physician or supplier for services described below.

SIGNED _____

14. DATE OF CURRENT: 08 11 20XX ILLNESS (First symptom) OR INJURY (Accident) OR PREGNANCY(LMP)

15. IF PATIENT HAS HAD SAME OR SIMILAR ILLNESS. GIVE FIRST DATE MM DD YY

16. DATES PATIENT UNABLE TO WORK IN CURRENT OCCUPATION FROM 11 08 20XX TO 12 08 20XX

17. NAME OF REFERRING PHYSICIAN OR OTHER SOURCE
17a.
17b. NPI

18. HOSPITALIZATION DATES RELATED TO CURRENT SERVICES FROM 11 08 20XX TO 11 10 20XX

19. RESERVED FOR LOCAL USE

20. OUTSIDE LAB? ☐ YES [X] NO $ CHARGES

21. DIAGNOSIS OR NATURE OF ILLNESS OR INJURY. (RELATE ITEMS 1,2,3 OR 4 TO ITEM 24E BY LINE)
1. 822.1
2. ____
3. ____
4. ____

22. MEDICAID RESUBMISSION CODE ____ ORIGINAL REF. NO.

23. PRIOR AUTHORIZATION NUMBER

24. A. DATE(S) OF SERVICE From MM DD YY To MM DD YY	B. PLACE OF SERVICE	C. EMG	D. PROCEDURES, SERVICES, OR SUPPLIES (Explain Unusual Circumstances) CPT/HCPCS MODIFIER	E. DIAGNOSIS POINTER	F. $ CHARGES	G. DAYS OR UNITS	H. EPSDT Family Plan	I. ID. QUAL.	J. RENDERING PROVIDER ID. #
1 11 08 20XX	21		99222	21	125 00	1		NPI	46789377XX
2 11 08 20XX	21		27524	21	600 00	1		NPI	46789377XX
3								NPI	
4								NPI	
5								NPI	
6								NPI	

25. FEDERAL TAX I.D. NUMBER 7544530XX SSN EIN [X]

26. PATIENT'S ACCOUNT NO. 1577

27. ACCEPT ASSIGNMENT? (For govt. claims, see back) ☐ YES ☐ NO

28. TOTAL CHARGE $ 725 00

29. AMOUNT PAID $

30. BALANCE DUE $ 725 00

31. SIGNATURE OF PHYSICIAN OR SUPPLIER INCLUDING DEGREES OR CREDENTIALS (I certify that the statements on the reverse apply to this bill and are made a part thereof.)
GREGORY GETWELL MD
SIGNED 110820XX DATE

32. SERVICE FACILITY LOCATION INFORMATION
COLLEGE HOSPITAL
4500 BROAD AVE
WOODLAND HILLS XY 12345
a. X950731067 b.

33. BILLING PROVIDER INFO & PH # (555)459 0087
GREGORY T GETWELL MD
60 NORTH STATE STREET
WOODLAND HILLS XY 12345
a. 36644021CC b.

NUCC Instruction Manual available at: www.nucc.org   **PLEASE PRINT OR TYPE**   APPROVED OMB-0938-0999 FORM CMS-1500 (08-05)

FIGURE 15-8 Example of a completed CMS-1500 (08-05) Health Insurance Claim Form for a workers' compensation case.

Table 15-3	Narrative Medical Report Issues, If Relevant
History	Outline all specific details of accident, injury, or illness. Physician should state whether there is a causal connection between the accident and conditions that may appear subsequently but are not obvious **sequelae** (diseased conditions following, and usually resulting from, a previous disease). If facts were obtained by reviewing prior records or x-ray films, the source should be mentioned. When a history is obtained through an interpreter, include that person's name.
Present complaints	Usually given as subjective complaints. Subjective refers to statements made by the patient about symptoms and how he or she feels. Subjective disability is evaluated by: • A description of the activity that produces the disability • The duration of the disability • The activities that are precluded by, and those that can be performed with, the disability • The means necessary for relief
Past history	Description of any previous, current, or subsequent medical information relevant to this injury or illness and whether there is a preexisting defect that might entitle the injured person to benefits from the subsequent injury fund or represent the actual cause of the present condition.
Examination findings	Usually given as objective findings. State all significant physical or psychiatric examination, testing, laboratory, or imaging findings.
Diagnostic impression	State all diagnostic findings and opinion as to relationship, if any, between the injury or disease and the condition diagnosed. Use diagnostic terminology that corresponds to the diagnostic code book.
Disability/ prognosis	• Period during which the patient has been unable to work because of the injury or illness. • Opinion as to probable further temporary disability and a statement as to when the patient will be able to return to work or has returned to work. • Statement indicating whether the condition is currently permanent and stationary, as well as the probability of future permanent disability. • Statement indicating "All objective tests for organic pathology are negative. There is obviously a strong functional or emotional overlay," when a patient has multiple complaints but no clinical objective findings.
Work limitations	Description of any limitations to all activities.
Causation	Description of how the permanent disability is related to the patient's occupation and the specific injury or cumulative events causing the illness.

payment to the physician. The case can be closed if there is no further treatment or disability.

Progress or Supplemental Report

In a TD case, a supplemental report is sent to the insurance carrier after 2 to 4 weeks of treatment to give information on the current status of the patient. If there is a significant change in the prognosis, a detailed progress report (sometimes called a *reexamination report*) is sent to the insurance carrier. Subsequent progress or supplemental reports should be sent to the insurance carrier after each hospitalization and office visit to update the progress of a case. They may be narrative and are not necessarily completed on the special forms available in most states (Figure 15-9). If the disability is ongoing over a period of time, monthly progress reports should be submitted. A follow-up report must contain the following information:

1. Date of most recent examination
2. Present condition and progress since last report
3. Measurements of function
4. X-ray or laboratory report since last examination
5. Treatment (give type and duration)
6. Work status (patient working or estimated date of return to work if patient is still temporarily disabled)
7. Permanent disability to be anticipated

The insurance carrier authorizing the examination should be furnished with the report in triplicate or quadruplicate, depending on its needs. A copy should be retained for the physician's files.

Final Report

TD ends when the physician tells the insurance carrier that the patient is able to return to work. Sometimes a physician submits a final report at the time of discharge. When the patient resumes work, the insurance carrier closes the case and the TD benefits cease.

A physician's final report indicating any impairment or permanent disability should be sent, accompanied by a statement listing total expenses incurred (Figure 15-10).

CLAIM SUBMISSION

Financial Responsibility

As discussed in Chapter 3, the contract for treatment in a personal illness or injury case is between the physician and patient, who is responsible for the entire bill. However, when a business is self-insured, a person is under a state program for care, or an individual is being treated as a workers' compensation case, the financial

ATTENDING PHYSICIAN'S REPORT

Employee: __Mrs. Ima B. Hurt__   Claim number: __120 XX 6542__

Employer: __The Conk Out Company__   Date of injury(ies): __4-3-20XX__   Date of next exam: __4-24-20XX__

Date of this exam: __4-10-XX__   Patient Social Security No: __120 XX 6542__

Current diagnosis: __824.6 closed fracture; L. trimalleolar ankle__
(include ICD•9 code)

PATIENT STATUS

Since the last exam, this patient's condition has:

☒ improved as expected.   ☐ improved, but slower than expected.   ☐ not improved significantly.

☐ worsened.   ☐ plateaued, no further improvement is expected.   ☐ has been determined to be non-work related.

Briefly, describe any change in objective or subjective complaint: _____

TREATMENT

Treatment plan: (only list changes from prior status)   ☐ No change   ☐ Patient is/was discharged from care on _____

Est. discharge date: __5-18-20XX__   Medications: __Tylenol for pain__

Therapy: Type _____   Times per week _____ Estimated date of completion _____

Diagnostic studies: __X-ray, L. ankle 3 views__

Hospitalization/surgery: _____

Consult/other service: _____

WORK STATUS

The patient has been instructed to:

☐ return to full duty with no limitations or restrictions.

☐ remain off the rest of the day and return to work tomorrow:

_____ with no limits or restrictions. _____ with limits listed below.

☐ return to work on _____

    work limitations: _____

☒ remain off work until __5-17-20XX — discharge exam scheduled__

Estimated date patient can return full duty: __5-18-20XX__

DISABILITY STATUS

☐ Patient discharged as cured.

Please supply a brief narrative report if any of the below apply:

☐ Patient will be permanently precluded from engaging in his/her usual and customary occupation.

☐ Patient's condition is permanent and stationary.

☐ Patient will have permanent residuals   ☐ Patient will require future medical care.

Physician name: __Martin Feelgood, MD__   Address: __4567 Broad Avenue, Woodland Hills, XY 12345__

Date: __April 10, 20XX__   Telephone: __(555)__ __482-9002__

Signature: __Martin Feelgood, MD__

reference initials

FIGURE 15-9 Physician's supplemental report form.

XYZ INSURANCE COMPANY

DOCTOR'S FINAL (OR MONTHLY) REPORT AND BILL

Monthly itemized bills required on all cases under continuing treatment.
Services beginning late in month and extending into succeeding month may be itemized on one statement.

120 XX 6542

EMPLOYEE _____ Mrs. Ima B. Hurt
DATE OF INJURY _____ April 3, 20XX
EMPLOYER _____ The Conk Out Company

May _____ XX

Patient refused treatment _____ 20 _____		Patient able to return to work _____ May 18, _____ 20 XX	
Patient stopped treatment		Patient discharged as cured _____ 20 _____	
without orders _____ 20 _____		Condition at time of last visit _____ fracture healed	
Patient entered hospital _____ 20 _____			
Further treatment anticipated? _____ X _____			
(Yes) (No)			

P.T L. Ankle 2 x wk 3 wks

Any other charges authorized such as drugs? _____ (Check) Hospital? _____ (Check)

Code: O—Office: V—Home Visit: H—Hospital Visit: N—Night Visit: S—Operation: X—X-ray.

Month	1	2	3	4	5	6	7	8	9	10	11	12	13	14	15	16	17	18	19	20	21	22	23	24	25	26	27	28	29	30	31
May							O										O														

	RVS CODE	TOTALS
First aid treatment *(describe)* _____	# _____	$ _____
Office Visits _____ 5/7/XX and 5/17/XX	# 99213	$ 40.20
Home Visits _____	# 99213	$ 40.20
Hospital Visits _____	# _____	$ _____
Operations _____	# _____	$ _____
MATERIAL *(Itemize at cost)* _____ Left ankle films; complete 5/7/xx	# 73610	$ 34.26
5/17/xx	# 73610	$ 34.26
	# _____	$ _____

Any charges shown above which are in excess of the scheduled fee must
be explained regarding nature of such services, indicating the date rendered.   TOTAL $ _____ 148.92

Make check payable to:

Doctor _____ Martin Feelgood, MD

Signature _____ *Martin Feelgood, MD*

Address _____ 4567 Broad Avenue
          (Street)

Date _____ May 18, 20XX

_____ Woodland Hills, XY 12345
      (City)   (Zip)

Internal Revenue Code Section 6109
requires you to furnish your Internal
Revenue Service Employer Identification
Number or Social Security Number.
Please enter the Identification Number
here _____ 95-36640XX

LEAVE BLANK	
	APPROVED
	BY _____
(Dollars) (Cents)	DATE _____

IMPORTANT—
Bills Must Be Submitted in Duplicate
MAIL ADDRESS: P.O. BOX S, WOODLAND HILLS, XY 12345

SCIF FORM 60 REV 5 78

FIGURE 15-10 Doctor's Final (or Monthly) Report and Bill form.

responsibility exists between the physician and insurance company or state program. As long as treatment is authorized by the insurance carrier, the insurance company is responsible for payment. A physician who agrees to treat a workers' compensation case must agree to accept payment in full according to the workers' compensation fee schedule. A copayment amount cannot be collected or the balance billed to the patient for any amount not covered. However, an exception to this may occur when a patient is under a managed care plan and does not give the physician an authorization for medical treatment.

If an injured worker refuses to accept the physician retained by the insurance company for the employer, the patient may be responsible for the cost of medical treatment. The employee should first contact the employer and then the insurance company to find out if there are any provisions for a change of physicians.

Some states have a medical program wherein employers can reduce their workers' compensation rates by paying the first $1000 in medical bills. This is similar to a deductible for the employer's policy. The statement should be sent to the employer for payment in this situation.

When billing a workers' compensation case for the initial visit, always check your state regulations about how to bill for the physician's service. If a physician sees an established patient who comes in with an injury sustained while working, some states do not issue payment based on new or established patient criteria but ask for the correct level of evaluation and management service verified by the documentation. Other states require physicians to bill a patient as new for each new injury, even when the patient is an established patient.

Health insurance information should always be obtained in case services provided are not work related or should be billed for, or the injury or illness is declared nonindustrial. To assist in informing patients of financial responsibility for nonrelated illness, the worker should sign an agreement for nonrelated medical expenses, as shown in Figure 15-11. If the workers' compensation carrier declares the case is nonindustrial, bill the patient's health insurance, attaching a copy of the refusal by the workers' compensation carrier.

Sometimes a physician discovers a problem unrelated to the industrial injury or illness (e.g., high blood pressure) while examining an injured worker. The physician may bill the workers' compensation carrier for the examination but should code the claim carefully with regard to treatment of the injury. If treatment is initiated for the patient's high blood pressure, that portion of the examination becomes the financial obligation of the patient (or his or her private insurance plan) and not the workers' compensation carrier.

Fee Schedules

Some states have developed and adopted a workers' compensation **fee schedule,** whereas other states pay medical claims on the basis of the Medicare fee schedule plus a certain percentage. The insurance carrier is sent the bill and no billing statements are sent to the patient. Fee schedules assist with the following:

1. They limit the fees providers can charge for standard medical procedures paid by workers' compensation companies.
2. They limit the amount that providers will be paid.
3. They make the allowable charges and procedures more consistent.
4. They provide follow-up procedures in case of a fee dispute.

Some workers' compensation fee schedules list maximum reimbursement levels for physicians and other nonhospital providers. However, the physician is generally expected to accept payment by the insurance company as payment in full when reimbursement is based on a fee schedule. If the fee charged is more than the amount listed, the following factors may be considered:

- Provider's medical training, qualifications, and time in practice
- Nature of services provided
- Fees usually charged by the provider
- Fees usually charged by others in the region where services were given
- Other relevant economic factors of the provider's practice
- Any unusual circumstances in the case

The insurance carrier may pay the additional amount if documentation is sent validating the fee and noting the aforementioned facts.

Types of Fee Schedules

Types of fee schedules include the following:

- *Percentile of charge schedule*, which is designed to set fees at a percentile of the providers' usual and customary fee.
- *Relative value scale schedule*, which takes into account the time, skills, and extent of the service provided by the physician. Each procedure is rated on how difficult it is, how long it takes, the training a physician must have to perform it, and expenses the physician incurs

PATIENT AGREEMENT

Patient's Name ___James Doland___ Soc. Sec. # _431-XX-1942_

Address _67 Blyth Dr., Woodland Hills, XY 12345_ Tel. No. _555-372-0101_

WC Insurance Carrier ___Industrial Indemnity Company___

Address ___30 North Dr., Woodland Hills___ Telephone No. _555-731-7707_

Date of illness _2-13-20XX_ Date of first visit _2-13-20XX_

Emergency Yes _X_ No _____

Is this condition related to employment Yes _X_ No _____

If accident: Auto _____ Other _____

Where did injury occur? ___Construction site___

How did injury happen? _fell 8 ft from scaffold suffering fractured right tibia_

Employee/employer who verified this information ___Scott McPherson___

Employer's name and address ___Willow Construction Company___

Employer's telephone No. _555-526-0611_

In the event the claim for workers' compensation is declared fraudulent for this illness or condition or it is determined by the Workers' Compensation Board that the illness or injury is not a compensable workers' compensation case, I _James Doland_ , hereby agree to pay the physician's fee for services rendered.

I have been informed that I am responsible to pay any services rendered by Dr. _Raymond Skeleton_ with regard to the discovery and treatment of any condition not related to the workers' compensation injury or illness. I agree to pay for all services not covered by workers' compensation and all charges for treatment and personal items unrelated to my workers' compensation illness or injury.

Signed _James Doland_ Date _2-13-20XX_

FIGURE 15-11 Patient agreement to pay the physician's fees if the case is declared not work related or an illness is discovered and treated that is not work related.

including the cost of malpractice insurance. Many of the fee schedules are similar to the CPT format in regard to sections (e.g., evaluation and management; anesthesia; surgery; radiology, nuclear medicine, and diagnostic ultrasound; pathology and laboratory; and medicine).

A *conversion factor* that uses a specific dollar amount is used for each of the sections of the fee schedule.

2011 Conversion Factors of the Physicians' and Pharmaceutical Fee Schedule Adopted by the Industrial Commission of Arizona Effective October 1, 2010, through September 30, 2011

$53.83/unit	Anesthesia
$142.24/unit	Surgery
$17.46/unit	Radiology (total services)
$3.43/unit	Radiology (professional components)
$1.21/unit	Pathology
$6.10/unit	Medicine
$5.46/unit	Physical Medicine
$6.10/unit	Evaluation and Management

Conversion factors may be adjusted to reflect regional differences and in some states are recalculated annually.

Actual covered procedures, descriptions, modifiers, global periods, and other elements of a fee guideline may significantly differ from those used for other plans or programs. Sometimes a schedule includes modifiers and code numbers not listed in the CPT code book. The workers' compensation codes should be used regardless of what is done for other insurance plans. Some states have their fee schedules posted at their state website. If it is not available online, telephone your state's program to obtain a copy.

Reviews or audits may be performed by the following entities to enforce fee schedules:

- The state agency or state fund responsible for overseeing workers' compensation (bill review)
- The payer, employer, or insurance carrier (bill review)
- The payer (bill review) and state agency (compliance audit)

Helpful Billing Tips

The following are helpful hints for billing workers' compensation claims.

1. Ask whether the injury occurred within the scope of employment and verify insurance information with the benefits coordinator for the employer. This will promote filing initial claims with the correct insurance carrier.
2. Either ask the employer the name of the claims adjuster or request that the patient obtain the claim number of his or her case when he or she comes in for the initial visit.
3. Ask the workers' compensation carrier who is going to review the claim. Sometimes independent third-party billing vendors work for the insurance carriers. Get the name and contact information.
4. Educate the patient with regard to the medical practice's billing policies for workers' compensation cases by having him or her complete the patient agreement form shown in Figure 15-11.
5. Verify whether prior authorization is necessary before a surgical procedure is performed.
6. Document in a telephone log or patient's record all data for authorization of examination, diagnostic studies, or surgery (e.g., date, name of individual who authorizes, response).
7. Obtain the workers' compensation fee schedule for the relevant state.
8. Use appropriate five-digit code numbers and modifiers to ensure prompt and accurate payment for services rendered.
9. Include a diagnostic E code as secondary to the primary diagnosis to report the cause of the injury.
10. Complete the Doctor's First Report of Occupational Injury or Illness form for the relevant state. Refer to the instructions presented near the end of this chapter. Submit it within the time limit shown in Table 15-1. Some states (e.g., California) allow a late fee if payment is not received within 30 to 45 days.
11. Ask whether there is a state-specific insurance form or if the CMS-1500 (08-05) form is acceptable.
12. Ask what year CPT and ICD-9-CM code books the insurance carrier uses. Some carriers use 2009 or earlier books, which means they do not reflect the deletion or addition of some procedure and diagnostic codes.
13. Submit a monthly itemized statement or bill on the termination of treatment for nondisability claims.
14. Clearly define any charges in excess of the fee schedule. Attach any x-ray reports, operative reports, discharge summaries, pathology reports, and so on to clarify such excess charges or when **by report (BR)** is shown for a code selected from the workers' compensation procedure code book.
15. Itemize in detail and send invoices for drugs and dressings furnished by the physician. Bill medical supplies on a separate claim or statement and do not bill with services because this may be routed to a different claims processing department.
16. Call the insurance carrier and talk with the **claims examiner** (also known as the *claims adjuster* or *claims representative*) who is familiar with the patient's case if there is a question about the fee.
17. Search the Internet for a website or write to the workers' compensation state plan office in each state for booklets, bulletins, forms, and legislation information. Refer to the Internet Resources at the end of this chapter and access the Evolve website for an active link to locate the workers' compensation address in each state.
18. Find out if the insurance carrier uses "usual and customary" payments tied to the physician's ZIP code. Most carriers use fee schedules.
19. Follow up and track the date the claim was filed. If no payment has been received or payment has been received beyond the 30- to 45-day deadline, determine whether it meets eligibility requirements for interest.

Billing Claims

For efficiency in processing industrial claims, many insurance carriers have developed their own forms for workers' compensation cases, whereas others allow use of the CMS-1500 (08-05) claim form. Some carriers have made slight modifications to the CMS-1500 (08-05) claim form as depicted in Figure 15-8.

Figure 7-12 is an illustration of a completed workers' compensation case on a nonmodified CMS-1500 (08-05) claim form.

Electronic Claims Submission and Reports

Uniform data processing codes and universal electronic injury report forms have been developed by the American National Standards Institute (ANSI) and the International Association of Industrial Accident Boards and Commissions (IAIABC). ANSI is a national organization founded in 1918 to coordinate the development of voluntary business standards in the US. Texas is one of the first states to establish an insurance regulation requiring workers' compensation carriers to use universal electronic transmission for first report of injury forms and subsequent reports developed by IAIABC.

Electronic Data Systems, Inc. (EDS) in Dallas, and Insurance Value-Added Network Services (IVANS) in Greenwich, CT, introduced the nation's first coast-to-coast electronic claims processing and report-filing network, called Workers' Compensation Reporting

Service. EDS processes all claims and follow-up reports. IVANS provides the network service and marketing of software to employers. This system is operational in many states.

Some workers' compensation insurance companies are using telephone reporting of claims. Employers report injuries occurring on the job by calling a toll-free number. Calls go to a regional center where service representatives document the first report of injury and electronically transmit it to the local claims office handling workers' compensation insurance. Employers avoid tardiness of reporting when using this system. Employers neglecting prompt reporting of injuries could delay payments to physicians.

Because workers' compensation is operated under state laws, each state is required to report financial data, statistics on injuries and illnesses, and other information to state insurance regulators. In the states that use telephone reporting service, workers' compensation payers use the system to reduce the paper processing costs that have escalated out of proportion and to improve administrative efficiency.

Out-of-State Claims

When billing for an out-of-state claim, insurance billing specialists must follow all workers' compensation regulations from the jurisdiction (state) in which the injured person's claim was originally filed.

However, companies that have employees who travel to other states are required to obtain workers' compensation insurance in those states unless they have a policy that covers out-of-state employees. Sometimes a patient may seek care from a physician in an adjacent state because he or she feels the physician provides a higher quality of care or the patient needs a specialized type of surgery, expensive diagnostic tests, or treatment. Referral requirements should be met before the patient is seen (e.g., letter of referral or preauthorization from the managing doctor with a copy to the workers' compensation carrier). Nine states hold the injured employee responsible for unauthorized care (Alabama, Alaska, Arkansas, New Jersey, North Dakota, Ohio, Washington, West Virginia, and Wisconsin). When a patient crosses a state line for treatment, he or she may be liable for some balance billing and the patient should be informed of this fact. The date the employer subcontracts with another company to have the work performed must be researched. Many times the injured employee states that he or she works for ABC Company.

The claim is denied because the employee is actually working for XYZ Company, which has subcontracted

with ABC Company. This also happens with hospitals. One may think a hospital employee is being treated when an employee working for a company hired by the hospital is actually being treated. In these cases, extra time is spent identifying the subcontractor, and it may be discovered that the subcontractor does not have workers' compensation insurance and expected the hiring company to provide the coverage. In another scenario, a cruise ship employee injured at sea does not fall under state workers' compensation laws and is not required to have insurance in the state. Many cruise ships have maritime companies that settle these types of claims. Normally the claim should be paid in full, but many of these companies try to negotiate a much lower rate. This rate can be accepted in lieu of futile attempts to collect from the patient.

When the claim is billed, the out-of-state fee schedule should be obtained to determine the proper procedure codes, modifiers, and amounts. It should be determined whether the claimant's jurisdiction accepts electronic submission of the CMS-1500 (08-05) claim form or another form and whether other documents (e.g., the operative report) are required to be submitted with the bill.

Delinquent or Slow Pay Claims

If payment of a workers' compensation claim is slow or the claim becomes delinquent, the insurance billing specialist should use an organized standard follow-up procedure:

1. Telephone the patient's employer. Note the name of the person with whom you spoke; the name, address, and telephone number of the workers' compensation carrier; and the claim number. Verify the employer's address.
2. Send a copy of the claim form and an itemized copy of the financial account statement to the carrier. Send a letter and include details of the accident if necessary (Figure 15-12). For problem claims it may be wise to obtain and complete a Certificate of Mailing form from the U.S. Postal Service. The form is initialed and postmarked at the post office and returned to the insurance biller for the office file. Because the post office does not keep a record of the mailing, this certificate costs less than certified mail. It shows proof that a special communication was mailed or sent on a certain date if a deadline is in question.
3. Telephone the insurance carrier after 45 working days and request the expected date of payment.
4. Be reminded of that payment date by using a computer-automated reminder or a note on the desk calendar. If payment is not received on or before that day, call the carrier again and ask for payment on a day determined by the facility's expectations.

```
                    Martin Feelgood, MD
                    4567 Broad Avenue
                    Woodland Hills, XY 12345
                    555-486-9002


June 20, 20XX


XYZ Insurance Company
P. O. Box S
Woodland Hills, XY 12345

Dear Madam or Sir:

Re:    Case No.:          120 XX 6542
       Injured:           Mrs. Ima B. Hurt
       Date of Injury:    April 3, 20XX
       Employer:          The Conk Out Company
       Amount:            $148.92

Our records indicate that our final statement for the above case
dated ___5/18/20XX___ remains unpaid.

Your cooperation in furnishing us the present status of this
statement will be appreciated.  A notation on the bottom of
this letter will be sufficient.

Very truly yours,

___Martin Feelgood___,MD

ref initials

- - - - - - - - - - - - - - - - - - - - - - - - - - - - - - -

_____No Employer's Report on file
_____No Doctor's First Report on file
_____Did not receive itemized billing statement
_____Payment was made.  Check No.____Date_____
_____Other reason(s) _____
```

FIGURE 15-12 Letter sent to the insurance carrier when a workers' compensation claim becomes 45 days delinquent.

```
                    Martin Feelgood, MD
                    4567 Broad Avenue
                    Woodland Hills, XY 12345
                    555-486-9002


June 20, 20XX


The Conk Out Company
45 South Gorman Street
Woodland Hills, XY 12345

Dear Madam or Sir:

Re:    Case No.:          120 XX 6542
       Injured:           Mrs. Ima B. Hurt
       Date of Injury:    April 3, 20XX

I have been informed by your workers' compensation insurance
carrier that they have not as yet received the employer's report
in regard to the above injured person.

Unless you have already done so, may I ask your cooperation in
completing and sending this report so that the case may be
closed.

Should you have any questions or if I can be of assistance to
you in any way, please do not hesitate to call on me.

Very truly yours,

___Martin Feelgood___ , MD

ref initials
```

FIGURE 15-13 Letter sent to the employer when the insurance company notifies the physician's office that the employer's preliminary report of injury has not been received.

5. Telephone the patient's employer and explain that there is difficulty with the carrier. Ask the employer to contact the carrier and have the carrier send payment immediately. You might talk to the patient and suggest that he or she discuss the problem with his or her employer to see if doing so will bring positive action.

6. Send the employer a copy of the financial account statement showing the outstanding balance. If the carrier is not paying, ask the employer for payment. An employer's legal obligation to pay may vary from case to case.

7. Contact the patient only if given information by the carrier or employer that the injury is not work related.

8. Develop office policies that address when an outstanding account should be reviewed (perhaps after 90 or 120 days), whether to continue collection efforts internally, and at which point the account should be turned over to a collection agency.

It may be necessary to send subsequent letters to the employer after receiving a response from the insurance carrier. For example, a letter should be sent to the employer (Figure 15-13) if the insurance company notifies the physician's office that the employer's preliminary report of injury has not been received.

If 30 days have elapsed from the date the letter was sent requesting the Employer's Report of Work Injury and the employer has not responded, a letter should be sent to the state Workers' Compensation Board or Industrial Accidents Commission (Figure 15-14).

Refer to Chapter 9 for additional information and helpful suggestions on following up on delinquent claims.

Martin Feelgood, MD
4567 Broad Avenue
Woodland Hills, XY 12345
555-486-9002

July 15, 20XX

Division of Industrial Accidents
State Office Building
107 South Broadway, Room 4107
Woodland Hills, XY 12345

Dear Madam or Sir:

Re: Failure of employer to follow Section No. 3760

Your office is being solicited to help secure an Employer's
Report of Work Injury from the employer listed below.

Case No.:	120 XX 6542
Name of Employer:	The Conk Out Company
Address:	45 South Gorman Street
	Woodland Hills, XY 12345
Name of Injured:	Mrs. Ima B. Hurt
Address:	300 East Central Avenue
	Woodland Hills, XY 12345
Date of Injury:	April 3, 20XX
Name of Insurance Carrier:	XYZ Insurance Company
Amount of Unpaid Bill:	$148.92

Your cooperation in this matter will be greatly appreciated. If you
need further information, please feel free to contact my office.

Sincerely yours,

Martin Feelgood , MD

ref initials

FIGURE 15-14 Letter sent to the Workers' Compensation Board or Industrial Accident Commission in your state if the employer does not respond to your letter requesting the Employer's Report of Work Injury after 30 days have elapsed from the date of the letter.

PROCEDURE 15-1

Completing the Doctor's First Report of Occupational Injury or Illness

The submission of this form (Figure 15-15) has a deadline, from immediately to within 5 days after the patient has been seen by the physician, depending on each state's law. An original and three or four copies should be distributed as follows:

- Original to the insurance carrier (unless more copies are required)
- One copy to the state agency
- One copy to the patient's employer
- One copy retained for the physician's files in the patient's workers' compensation file folder

In some states, attending physicians may file a single report directly to the insurer or self-insured employer within a specified number of days from initial treatment. The insurer or self-insured employer, in turn, is required to send a report to the state agency. This reduces paperwork and postage. Table 15-1 provides the time limit in each state during which the physician must submit the initial report.

1. Enter the insurance carrier's complete name, street address, city, state, and ZIP code.

Continued

PROCEDURE 15-1—cont'd

Completing the Doctor's First Report of Occupational Injury or Illness

STATE OF CALIFORNIA	**DOCTOR'S FIRST REPORT OF OCCUPATIONAL INJURY OR ILLNESS**

Within 5 days of your initial examination, for every occupational injury or illness, send two copies of this report to the **employer's workers' compensation insurance carrier** or the **self-insured employer.** Failure to file a timely doctor's report may result in assessment of a civil penalty. **In the case of diagnosed or suspected pesticide poisoning,** send a copy of this report to Division of Labor Statistics and Research, P.O. Box 420603, San Francisco, CA 94142-0603, and notify your local health officer by telephone within 24 hours.

	PLEASE DO NOT USE THIS COLUMN
1. **INSURER NAME AND ADDRESS** XYZ Insurance Company, P.O. Box 5, Woodland Hills, XY 12345	
2. **EMPLOYER NAME** The Conk Out Company Policy# B12345	Case No.
3. Address No. and Street City Zip 45 So. Gorman St. Woodland Hills, XY 12345	Industry
4. Nature of business (e.g., food manufacturing, building construction, retailer of women's clothes) plumbing repair	County
5. **PATIENT NAME** (first name, middle initial, last name) Ima B. Hurt 6. Sex ☐ Male ☒ Female 7. Date of birth Mo. Day Yr. 3-4-1966	Age
8. Address: No. and Street City Zip 300 East Central Ave., Woodland Hills, XY 12345 9. Telephone number (555) 476-9899	Hazard
10. Occupation (Specific job title) clerk typist 11. Social Security Number 120-XX-6542	Disease
12. Injured at: No. and street City County 45 So. Gorman St., Woodland Hills, XY 12345 Humboldt	Hospitalization
13. Date and hour of injury or onset of illness Mo. Day Yr. 4-3-20XX Hour ____a.m. 2:00 p.m. 14. Date last worked Mo. Day Yr. 4-3-20XX	Occupation
15. Date and hour of first examination or treatment Mo. Day Yr. 4-3-20XX Hour ____a.m. 4:00 p.m. 16. Have you (or your office) previously treated patient? ☐ Yes ☒ NO	Return date/Code

Patient please complete this portion, if able to do so. Otherwise, doctor please complete immediately. Inability or failure of a patient to complete this portion shall not affect his/her rights to workers' compensation under the California Labor Code.

17. **DESCRIBE HOW THE ACCIDENT OR EXPOSURE HAPPENED** (Give specific object, machinery or chemical. Use reverse side if more space is required.)

I climbed a ladder in the stock room and while I was coming down I missed a step, lost my balance, and fell hurting my left ankle.

18. **SUBJECTIVE COMPLAINTS** (Describe fully. Use reverse side if more space is required.)

Pain in left ankle.

19. **OBJECTIVE FINDINGS** (Use reverse side if more space is required.)
A. Physical examination

Pain, swelling and discoloration of l. ankle.

B. X-ray and laboratory results (state if none or pending). Ankle x-ray (left) 3 views

20. **DIAGNOSIS** (if occupational illness specify etiologic agent and duration of exposure.) Chemical or toxic compounds involved? ☐ Yes ☒ No

Trimalleolar ankle fracture (left)   ICD-9 Code ___824.6___

21. Are your findings and diagnosis consistent with patient's account of injury or onset of illness?   ☒ Yes   ☐ No if "no", please explain.

22. Is there any other current condition that will impede or delay the patient's recovery?   ☐ Yes   ☒ No if "yes", please explain.

23. **TREATMENT RENDERED** (Use reverse side if more space is required.)

Examination, x-rays, closed treatment of trimalleolar ankle fracture (left) without manipulation. Return in one week for recheck.

24. If further treatment required, specify treatment plan/estimated duration.

25. If hospitalized as inpatient, give hospital name and location   Date admitted   Mo. Day Yr.   Estimated stay

26. WORK STATUS–Is patient able to perform usual work?   ☐ Yes ☒ No
If "no", date when patient can return to: Regular work _5_ / _17_ / _20XX_
Modified work__ /__ /__   Specify restrictions_____

Doctor's signature___ *Martin Feelgood, MD*___ 4-8-20XX___ CA license number __A 12345__
Doctor name and degree (please type) Martin Feelgood, MD___ IRS number __95-36640XX__
Address___ 4567 Broad Avenue, Woodland Hills, XY 12345 __ Telephone number __(555) 486-9002__

FORM 5021 (REV. 4) 1992

Any person who makes or causes to be made any knowingly false or fraudulent material statement or material representation for the purpose of obtaining or denying workers' compensation benefits or payments is guilty of a felony.

reference initials

FIGURE 15-15 Doctor's First Report of Occupational Injury or Illness form, used in California.

PROCEDURE 15-1—cont'd

Completing the Doctor's First Report of Occupational Injury or Illness

2. Enter the employer's full name and policy number if known. Some insurance carriers file by employer and then by policy number. Sometimes the employer's telephone number is necessary on this line.
3. Enter the employer's street address, city, state, and ZIP code.
4. Enter the type of business (e.g., repairing shoes, building construction, retailing men's clothes).
5. Enter the patient's complete first name, middle initial, and last name.
6. Enter a check mark in the appropriate box to indicate the patient's gender.
7. Enter the patient's birth date and list the year as four digits.
8. Enter the patient's street address, city, state, and ZIP code.
9. Enter the patient's home telephone number.
10. Enter the patient's specific job title. Be accurate in listing the occupation with the job title so that the insurance carrier may be certain the patient was doing the job for which he or she was insured.
11. Enter the patient's Social Security number. Some insurance carriers use the Social Security number as the industrial case number.
12. Enter the exact location where the patient was injured. Many times the injury may occur off the premises of the company or factory, depending on the type of job on which the employee was working. List the county where the patient was injured.
13. Enter the date the patient was injured and time of the injury. List the year as four digits.
14. Enter the date the patient last worked. This date should coincide with the date the patient reported to work and worked any portion of his or her shift (work day). This may be the same date of injury. This item is important because it informs the insurance carrier of the working status of the patient or whether the patient has been disabled and cannot return to work. List the year as four digits.
15. Enter the date and hour of the physician's first examination. The insurance carrier should know how soon after the accident the patient sought medical attention. List the year as four digits.
16. Enter a check mark in the appropriate box indicating whether the physician or an associate treated the patient previously.

17. Have the patient complete this section if possible in his or her own words, stating how the illness or injury occurred. The physician also may dictate this information after obtaining it from the patient.
18. Enter the answers to these questions about the patient's complaints and medical findings, which may be found in the patient's health record. List all of the patient's subjective complaints.
19A. Enter all objective findings from physical examination.
19B. Enter all x-ray and laboratory results. If none, state "none" or "pending."
20. Enter a check mark in "yes" or "no" to indicate if chemical or toxic compounds are involved. Enter the diagnosis and diagnostic code number. Specify etiologic agent and duration of exposure if occupational illness.
21. Enter a check mark in "yes" or "no" to indicate if the findings and diagnosis are consistent with the history of injury or onset of illness. Insert an explanation if "yes."
22. Enter a check mark in "yes" or "no" to indicate if there is any other current condition that will impede or delay the patient's recovery. Insert an explanation if "yes."
23. Enter a full description of what treatment was rendered.
24. Enter an explanation if further treatment is necessary and, if so, specify the treatment plan. Indicate if physical therapy is necessary and its frequency and duration.
25. Enter the name and location of the hospital, admission date, and estimated stay if the patient is to be hospitalized.
26. Enter a check mark in "yes" or "no" to indicate whether the patient is able to work as usual. If the answer is "no," give the date when it is estimated that the patient will be able to return to regular or modified work. List the year as four digits. Specify any work restrictions. It is very important for the insurance company to anticipate how long the patient will be off work so that money may be set aside for temporary disability benefits, medical benefits, and, if necessary, permanent disability benefits. If the estimated date of return to work should change after the form is submitted, a supplemental report or progress note should be sent to the insurance carrier to change the date of the disability.

Continued

PROCEDURE 15-1—cont'd

Completing the Doctor's First Report of Occupational Injury or Illness

Bottom of Form: If not preprinted, enter the physician's name and degree (e.g., MD, DC), complete address, state license number, federal tax identification number, and telephone number. Indicate the date the report is submitted. The insurance billing specialist should type reference initials in the lower left-hand corner of the form. This form must be signed in ink by the physician. Any carbon copies or photocopies must be signed in ink, too. A stamped signature will not be accepted because sometimes these cases go into litigation or are presented for a permanent disability rating. Only those documents considered original health records are acceptable; this means a handwritten signature by the attending physician is necessary.

KEY POINTS

This is a brief chapter review or summary of the key issues presented. To further enhance your knowledge of the technical subject matter, review the key terms and key abbreviations for this chapter by locating the meanings in the glossary at the end of this book that appear in a section before the index.

1. Federal and state regulations require that employers have workers' compensation insurance coverage against on-the-job injury or illness and pay the premium for each of their employees.

2. Workers' compensation programs are not included under the definition of a health plan as identified in the HIPAA statutes.

3. Employees who work for federal agencies are covered by a number of federal workers' compensation laws.

4. The second-injury fund, also known as the *subsequent injury fund*, was established to meet problems arising when an employee has a preexisting injury or condition and is subsequently injured at work.

5. Each state's legislation lists a waiting period that must elapse before income benefits are paid. However, medical and hospital care for industrial injuries is provided immediately.

6. Workers' compensation benefits consist of medical treatment, temporary disability indemnity, permanent disability indemnity, death benefits for survivors, and rehabilitation benefits.

7. A nondisability claim involves a minor injury in which the patient is seen by the physician but is able to continue to work.

8. A temporary disability claim occurs when a worker has a work-related injury or illness and is unable to perform the duties of his or her occupation for a specific time.

9. A PD consists of an illness or injury (impairment of the normal use of a body part) that is expected to continue for the lifetime of the injured worker and prevents the person from performing the functions of his or her occupation, therefore impairing his or her earning capacity.

10. In a permanent disability case, the physician's final report must contain the words "permanent and stationary" so that the case can be adjudicated or rated, settlement can be reached (called a compromise and release), and the case can be closed.

11. It is the responsibility of all individuals who handle workers' compensation cases to notify the insurance carrier of any fraudulent or suspicious situation.

12. OSHA is the federal agency that regulates and investigates safety and health standards at work sites for the protection of employees.

13. Depositions from the physician and the injured individual by the attorney representing the workers' compensation insurance company are usually taken in permanent disability cases.

14. The physician should file a lien in a workers' compensation case that has gone into third-party litigation or if there is a question whether the case is compensable or not.

15. A private health record should never be combined with an industrial case record because separate disclosure laws apply to each, and the workers' compensation case may go to court.

16. The first report of an industrial injury must be completed by the employer and the physician and is required by law in most states.

17. A medical service order given to the employee by the employer authorizes the physician to treat the injured worker.

18. In industrial cases, all medical reports and forms are legal documents and must be signed in ink by the physician.

evolve INTERNET RESOURCES

For active links to the following resources, visit the Evolve website at
http://evolve.elsevier.com/fordney/handbook

● Website for Division of Coal Mine Workers' Compensation; Division of Federal Employees'

Compensation; Division of Longshoremen's and Harbor Workers' Compensation
● Website providing information about state benefits (forms, statutes, news bulletins, links to all states)

STUDENT ASSIGNMENT

✓ Study Chapter 15.
✓ Answer the fill-in-the-blank, multiple choice, and true/false review questions in the *Workbook* to reinforce the theory learned in this chapter and to help prepare you for a future test.
✓ Complete the assignments in the *Workbook* for hands-on experience in completing workers'

compensation insurance claim forms and reports, as well as enhanced proficiency in procedural and diagnostic coding.
✓ Turn to the glossary at the end of this textbook for a further understanding of the key terms and key abbreviations used in this chapter.

KEY TERMS*†

accidental death and dismemberment

Armed Services Disability

benefit period

Civil Service Retirement System

consultative examiner

cost-of-living adjustment

Disability Determination Services

disability income insurance

double indemnity

exclusions

Federal Employees Retirement System

future purchase option

guaranteed renewable

hearing

long-term disability insurance

noncancelable clause

partial disability

reconsideration

regional office

residual benefits

residual disability

short-term disability insurance

Social Security Administration

Social Security Disability Insurance program

State Disability Insurance

supplemental benefits

Supplemental Security Income

temporary disability

temporary disability insurance

total disability

unemployment compensation disability

Veterans Affairs disability program

Veterans Affairs outpatient clinic card

voluntary disability insurance

waiting period

waiver of premium

KEY ABBREVIATIONS*

AIDS	FERS	SDI	TDI
CE	HIV	SSA	UCD
CSRS	OASDHI	SSDI program	VA
DDS	RO	SSI	

---

*Definitions for the key terms and key abbreviations are located near the back of this textbook in the glossary.

†Some of the insurance terms presented in this list are italicized and may seem familiar from previous chapters. However, their meanings may have a slightly different connotation when referring to disability income insurance.

Disability Income Insurance and Disability Benefit Programs

OBJECTIVES

After reading this chapter, you should be able to:

- Define terminology and abbreviations pertinent to disability insurance and disability benefit programs.
- Describe benefits and exclusions contained in individual and group disability income insurance.
- Name federal disability benefit programs.
- Differentiate between SSDI and SSI.
- State eligibility requirements, benefits, and limitations of SSDI and SSI.
- Explain disability benefit programs for disabled active military personnel, veterans, and their dependents.

- Name states that have state disability insurance plans.
- State eligibility requirements, benefits, and limitations of state disability plans.
- Explain voluntary disability insurance plans.
- Recognize forms used for processing state disability plans.
- Describe topics and contents of a medical report.
- List guidelines for federal disability claims.
- Explain procedures for state disability claims.

Service to Patients

Efficiently and quickly completing the attending physician's portion of the disability insurance form assists the patient in obtaining disability income when he or she is unable to work because of a non–work-related illness or injury.

Describe How Your Disability Occurred

"A hernia from pulling cork out of bottle."
"Put tire patch on Playtex girdle and it caused infection on right thigh."
"While waving goodnight to friends, fell out a two-story window."
"Back injury received from jumping off a ladder to escape being hit by a train."
One victim graphically described an experience most of us have had: "Getting on a bus, the driver started before I was all on." Can you hear them asking at the hospital, "Was this your assigned seat?"
Another victim stated, "I dislocated my shoulder swatting a fly." When asked, "Have you ever dislocated a shoulder at this sport?" He stated, "I have—I knocked over two table lamps, several high-balls, and skinned an elbow."

DISABILITY CLAIMS

Not everyone has disability insurance, but when working with patients who do have it, one may encounter some interesting and unique accidents, injuries, or illnesses. After reading these extracts or direct quotations from disability insurance claim applications, one may ask, "How in the world could something like this happen?" The following gems show just how funny some situations can appear.

Performance objectives, testing and review material, and hands-on practical exercises for this chapter are available in these resources

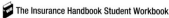 The Insurance Handbook Student Workbook   The Insurance Handbook Evolve Site

---

Describe How Your Disability Occurred—cont'd

Because this is near the end of the course on insurance billing and a great deal of information has been covered, one may feel a bit overwhelmed by the many rules and regulations and their ever-changing nature. This introduction was intended to add a bit of levity before one delves into the world of disability insurance.

This chapter introduces various types of disability income insurance plans, as well as a number of disability benefit programs. The first topic, **disability income insurance,** is a form of insurance providing periodic payments under certain conditions when the insured is unable to work because of illness, disease, or injury—not as a result of a work-related accident or condition.

The second section describes major programs administered by the United States (US) government related to industrial accidents and other disability benefit programs unrelated to work injuries.

The third part of the chapter deals with nonindustrial state disability programs administered in five states and Puerto Rico, as well as voluntary disability insurance plans.

Guidelines for federal, state, individual, and group disability claim procedures are presented at the end of the chapter.

HISTORY

Before the late 1800s, disability income insurance provided only accident protection. Some life insurance contracts had disability income riders attached to them that offered limited benefits. In the early 1880s, insurance companies began selling disability income policies that offered coverage for accident and illness. The Paul Revere Life Insurance Company introduced the first "noncancelable" disability income policy in the early 1900s. The noncancelable clause guaranteed that the contract would be in force for a certain period of time and the premium would not be increased. By 1956, Congress had enacted legislation under the Social Security program that provided disability income protection to disabled individuals older than 50 years of age. This program was expanded in 1965 to cover workers without regard to age as long as certain eligibility standards were met.

Today, disability income insurance is available from private insurance companies (individual policies) and employer-sponsored plans (group policies). Government-funded and state benefit programs are also available for disabled persons. All of these plans and programs are discussed in this chapter, along with the role of the insurance billing specialist in dealing with this type of insurance.

DISABILITY INCOME INSURANCE

Individual

Individual disability income insurance is coverage that provides a specific monthly or weekly income when a person becomes unable to work, temporarily or totally, because of an illness or injury. Disability income policies do not provide medical expense benefits. The disability cannot be work related. As explained in the previous chapter, an illness or accident that is work related is covered by workers' compensation insurance.

For individuals who are self-employed, this insurance is particularly important because a business could not meet its financial obligations if the owner became injured or too ill to work. For example, if an individual is self-employed with a home-based business, repetitive stress injuries (RSIs) would not allow that individual to use the computer for several months. The main purpose of these policies is to provide some benefits while the person is unable to work. To collect benefits, the individual must meet the policy's criteria of what constitutes partial, temporary, or total disability. These policies terminate when the individual retires or reaches a certain age, usually 65 years.

Waiting Period

The time period from the beginning of disability to receiving the first payment of benefits is called an *elimination period* or **waiting period.** During this initial period, a disabled individual is not eligible to receive benefits even though he or she is unable to work.

Benefit Period

A **benefit period** is the maximum amount of time that benefits will be paid to the injured or ill person for the disability (e.g., 2 years, 5 years, to age 65, or lifetime).

Benefits

Compensation paid to the insured disabled person is called *indemnity benefits* and can be received daily, weekly, monthly, or semiannually, depending on the policy. Premiums and benefits depend on several risk factors such as age, gender, health history and physical state, income, and occupational duties. Some policies include residual or partial disability income benefits. Benefits are not taxable if premiums are paid by the individual.

Residual benefits pay a partial benefit when the insured is not totally disabled. If one becomes partially disabled or can work only part time or in a limited capacity, the residual benefits make up the difference between what an individual can earn at present and what he or she would have earned working full time.

Supplemental benefits may consist of insurance provisions that will increase monthly indemnity such as a **future purchase option** or a **cost-of-living adjustment.** Provisions also distribute a percentage of the policy premiums if an individual keeps a policy in force for 5 or 10 years or does not file any claims.

An **accidental death and dismemberment** benefit is written into some contracts. This offers the insured person protection when loss of sight or loss of limb occurs. In some policies (e.g., life insurance), a special provision known as **double indemnity** applies if an unintended, unexpected, and unforeseeable accident results in death. This feature provides for twice the face amount of the policy to be paid if death results from accidental causes.

Types of Disability

A disability may be partial, temporary, or total. There is no standard definition for **total disability,** and the definition stated in each disability income policy varies. For example, a liberal definition might read as follows: "The insured must be unable to perform the major duties of his or her specific occupation." Social Security has a restrictive definition presented later in this chapter.

The terms **residual disability** and **partial disability** are defined as occurring "when an illness or injury prevents an insured person from performing one or more of the functions of his or her regular job"—in other words, when a person cannot perform all of his or her job duties.

Temporary disability exists when a person cannot perform all the functions of his or her regular job for a limited period of time.

Clauses

With a **guaranteed renewable** policy, the insurer is required to renew the policy as long as premium payments are made for a specified number of years or to a specified age, such as 60, 65, or 70 years, or for life. However, the premium may be increased when it is renewed. When the policy has a **noncancelable clause,** the premium cannot be increased.

If a **waiver of premium** is included in the insurance contract, the policy pays all premiums while the employee is disabled; the employee does not have to pay. Usually, this provision is used as a total and permanent disability benefit and may be available in certain other cases.

Exclusions

Exclusions are provisions written into the insurance contract denying coverage or limiting the scope of coverage. Examples are preexisting conditions; disability because of war, riot, self-inflicted injury, or attempted suicide; mental or nervous conditions; disability while legally intoxicated or under the influence of narcotics (unless prescribed by a licensed physician); conditions arising from normal pregnancy; conditions arising during the act of committing a felony; or if benefits are being received under workers' compensation or a government program. The phrase "legally intoxicated" means intoxication in an individual whose blood alcohol level, when tested, exceeds limits set by state law.

Acquired Immunodeficiency Syndrome and Human Immunodeficiency Virus Infection

States have statutes governing questions that can and cannot be asked on insurance application forms about acquired immunodeficiency syndrome (AIDS) and human immunodeficiency virus (HIV) testing; therefore each state has developed its own forms. If a private insurance company wishes to test an applicant, a consent or notice form, including acceptance of pretest and posttest counseling, must be signed.

Group

Some employers elect to offer group disability income insurance as a fringe benefit. These contracts are drawn up between the insurer and employer. Premiums may be paid by the employer with or without contributions from the employee. Employees hold certificates of insurance and are covered under the employer's policy; therefore they are not called policyholders. When the employee leaves the company, the insurance terminates unless the employee is disabled. A few group policies allow conversion to a limited benefit individual policy.

Benefits

Benefits vary from one plan to another but are usually for **short-term disability insurance** (13 weeks to 24 months) or **long-term disability insurance** (to age 65). To qualify for benefits, an individual must be unable to perform the major duties of his or her occupation during the initial period of disability (e.g., the first 2 years). Benefits cease when the employee returns to work, even part time. However, some of these policies offer the worker partial disability income benefits to motivate a disabled individual to return to work on a part-time basis. Monthly benefits are usually paid directly to the employee and are taxable if the employee is not making any contribution toward the premiums.

Exclusions

Disabilities commonly excluded from coverage include those seen in individual disability income insurance policies, as previously described.

FEDERAL DISABILITY PROGRAMS

Workers' Compensation

The federal government has a number of programs that cover workers from loss of income because of work-related disability. These programs are mentioned in Chapter 15 because work-related disabilities fall under workers' compensation laws. When an individual is eligible under more than one program, coordination of benefits is used so that a worker cannot receive benefits that result in an amount greater than what the person receives when working. Coordination of benefits is a provision preventing double payment for expenses by making one of the programs the primary payer and ensuring that no more than 100% of the costs are covered.

Disability Benefit Programs

The government's major disability programs are as follows:

- Social Security Disability Insurance (SSDI) program
- Supplemental Security Income (SSI)
- Civil Service Retirement System (CSRS)
- Federal Employees Retirement System (FERS)
- **Armed Services Disability**
- **Veterans Affairs (VA) disability program**

The **Social Security Administration (SSA)** manages two programs that pay monthly disability benefits to people younger than age 65 who cannot work for at least a year because of a severe disability: SSDI and SSI. Medical requirements are the same for both programs.

Social Security Disability Insurance Program

Background. In 1935 the Social Security Act, the Old-Age, Survivors, Disability, and Health Insurance (OASDHI) Program, was enacted. It provided benefits for death, retirement, disability, and medical care. In 1956, Congress established a program for long-term disability known as **Social Security Disability Insurance (SSDI)** under Title II of the Social Security Act. This is an entitlement (not welfare) program that provides monthly benefits to workers and those self-employed who meet certain conditions.

Disability Definition. *Disability* under Social Security has a strict definition: "inability to engage in any substantial gainful activity by reason of any medically determinable physical or mental impairment which can be expected to result in death or which has lasted or can be expected to last for a continuous period of not less than 12 months."

Eligibility. The following is a list of individuals who meet eligibility requirements for SSDI:

- Disabled workers younger than age 65 years and their families
- Individuals who become disabled before age 22 years, if a parent (or in certain cases, a grandparent) who is covered under Social Security retires, becomes disabled, or dies
- Disabled widows or widowers, age 50 years or older, if the deceased spouse worked at least 10 years under Social Security
- Disabled surviving divorced spouses older than age 50 years, if the ex-spouse was married to the disabled person for at least 10 years
- Blind workers whose vision in the better eye cannot be corrected to better than 20/200 or whose visual field in the better eye, even with corrective lenses, is 20 degrees or less

Workers must be fully insured in accordance with standards set by the SSA in terms of age, number of quarters worked, and amount of wages earned per quarter. The processing of eligibility application forms may take up to 2 months.

Benefits. Monthly benefits are paid to qualified individuals. After 24 months of disability payments, the disabled individual also becomes eligible for Medicare. The benefits convert to retirement benefits when an individual reaches age 65.

Supplemental Security Income

Eligibility. The **Supplemental Security Income (SSI)** program is under Title XVI of the Social Security Act and provides disability payments to people (adults and children) with limited income and few resources. No prior employment is necessary. Many SSI recipients also qualify for Medicaid, a state assistance program. The following individuals may qualify for SSI disability payments:

- Disabled persons younger than 65 years who have limited income and resources
- Disabled children younger than age 18 years, if the disability compares in severity with one that would keep an adult from working and has lasted or is expected to last at least 12 months or result in death

- Blind adults or children who have a visual acuity no better than 20/100 or have a visual field of 20 degrees or less in the better eye, with the use of corrective lenses

Disability Determination Process. To establish disability under SSDI or SSI, an individual calls or visits any Social Security office and completes application forms with the help of a social worker. This triggers a determination process. A physician may be involved in the determination process in one of three ways: (1) as a treating source who provides medical evidence on behalf of his or her patient, (2) as a **consultative examiner (CE)** who is paid a fee and examines or tests the applicant, or (3) as a full- or part-time medical or psychologic consultant reviewing claims for a state or **regional office (RO).**

In addition to a medical report from one of these sources, other criteria taken into consideration are the individual's age and vocational and educational factors that may contribute to the person's ability to work. It is possible that a person may be eligible for disability payments under one government program and not be eligible under Social Security because the rules differ. The SSA may use reports that an applicant has from another agency to determine whether the person is eligible for Social Security disability payments. Many SSA state agencies have a division known as **Disability Determination Services (DDS).** Determination of disability is made by a DDS team composed of a physician or psychologist and disability examiner (DE), not by the applicant's physician.

Appeals Evaluation Process. If a claimant does not agree with the determination of disability, the following four-level appeals process is available.

1. A **reconsideration,** which is a complete review of the claim by a medical or psychologic consultant or disability examiner team that did not take part in the original disability determination.
2. A **hearing** before an administrative law judge who had no part in the initial or reconsideration determinations of the claim. The hearing is held within 75 miles of the claimant's home. The claimant and his or her representative are permitted to present their case in person and present a written statement. They are also permitted to review information the judge will use to make a decision and question any witnesses.
3. A review by the Appeals Council, which considers all requests for review but may deny a request if it believes the decision by the administrative law judge was correct. If the Appeals Council decides the case should be reviewed, it will make a decision on the case or return it to an administrative law judge for further review.

4. A review by the federal court for which the claimant may file an action where he or she resides.

Disability cases are reviewed from time to time to be sure the individuals are still disabled. The frequency depends on the nature and severity of the impairment, the likelihood of improvement, rehabilitation, ability to work, and so on.

Benefits. Social Security disability programs are designed to give long-term protection and benefits to individuals totally disabled who are unable to do any type of work in the national economy. In contrast, short-term disability may be provided through workers' compensation, insurance, savings, and investments.

Work Incentives. Special rules allow disabled or blind people presently receiving Social Security or SSI to work and still receive monthly benefits, as well as Medicare or Medicaid (e.g., an SSDI recipient who is given a 90-day trial of work and at the end of that time either continues to work and lose SSDI coverage or leaves the temporary employment and remains on SSDI). A limit exists as to how much the person can earn in a calendar year. These are referred to as "work incentives"; the rules are different for Social Security beneficiaries and SSI recipients. Occasionally, a patient may be working and receiving SSDI benefits, as illustrated by the earlier example.

Civil Service and Federal Employees Retirement System Disability

Background. There are two types of federal retirement, **Civil Service Retirement System (CSRS)** and the **Federal Employees Retirement System (FERS).** CSRS began in 1920 until a second system, FERS, was introduced in 1984. People who began working for the Federal government in 1984 or later are covered by FERS instead of CSRS. Some workers who had been covered by the CSRS program changed to the FERS program when it became available.

Eligibility. Federal employees who work in civil service fall under the CSRS. This system has provisions for those who become totally disabled. This program is a combination of federal disability and Social Security disability. Both portions of the program must be applied for by the worker. The disability cannot be work related, and 5 years of service are necessary before benefits are payable. Eighteen months of service are necessary under the FERS.

Benefits. Those who qualify are entitled to benefits that are payable for life. For example, an individual who works for the Internal Revenue Service performing clerical and filing job duties is involved in an automobile accident on the weekend. The head injuries are so severe that the person is unable to return to gainful employment at any job. He or she could apply for benefits under either the CSRS or FERS, depending on his or her eligibility status.

Armed Services Disability

Eligibility. Individuals covered under this program must be members of the armed services on active duty who suffer a disability or illness.

Benefits. Monthly benefits are payable for life if a disability occurs or is aggravated while the individual is serving in the military service. Benefit amounts are based on years of service, base pay, and severity of disability. This is also subject to review.

Veterans Affairs Disability

Eligibility. The VA is authorized by law to provide a wide range of benefits to both those who have served their country in the armed forces and their dependents. If a veteran who is honorably discharged files a claim for a service-connected disability within 1 year of sustaining that injury, he or she is eligible for outpatient treatment. Veterans with non–service-connected disabilities who are in receipt of housebound or aid-in-attendance benefits are eligible for treatment from a private physician if they are unable to travel to a VA facility because of geographic inaccessibility. Their identification card, benefits, and claims procedures are identical to those of veterans with service-connected disabilities who receive outpatient medical care.

Benefits. The following is a general list of veterans' medical benefits. Each benefit requires that certain criteria be met. These criteria are ever-changing and are not mentioned here. A complete up-to-date booklet listing all the benefits is available.*

● Hospital care in a VA hospital
● Nursing home care in a VA facility
● Domiciliary care
● Outpatient medical treatment at a VA facility or by a private physician
● Emergency treatment in a hospital for a service-connected condition
● Prescription drugs and medication issued by a VA pharmacy or other participating pharmacy. Only bona

---

*Federal Benefits for Veterans and Dependents. Department of Veterans Affairs, Washington, DC 20420. The booklet is published annually and is available for a small fee from the Superintendent of Documents, US Government Printing Office, Mail Stop: SSOP, Washington, DC 20402-9328.

fide emergency prescriptions can be filled by a private pharmacy.
● Certain medical equipment, such as oxygen and prosthetics
● Travel expenses when receiving VA medical care
● Outpatient dental treatment (if the veteran files a claim within 90 days from the date that he or she was discharged from the service)
● Treatment for Agent Orange or nuclear radiation exposure
● Alcohol and drug dependence outpatient care
● Readjustment counseling services

The physician must accept what the VA pays as payment in full for treatment of a service-connected disability and cannot bill the patient for any additional charges, even if there is a balance after the VA pays the claim. If the treatment is likely to cost more than $40 per month, the physician must obtain prior authorization from the nearest VA facility. A separate financial accounting record card must be prepared for VA benefits if the physician is also treating the patient for ailments other than a service-connected disability. Any professional service that is not related to a service-connected disability must be paid for by the veteran out of his or her own pocket. For example, a Vietnam veteran who has a long history of stump pain at the site of an amputation or suffers from old shrapnel wounds as the result of stepping on a land mine during active duty is seen and treated for acute gastroenteritis. The VA disability benefits do not apply to the episode of acute gastroenteritis, and the veteran must personally pay for professional services related to that diagnosis.

Veterans with non–service-connected disabilities may have copayments when they seek treatment. For example, individuals on Medicare may be responsible for the deductible for the first 90 days of care during any 365-day period. For each additional 90 days of hospital care, the patient is charged half of the Medicare deductible, $10 a day of hospital care, and $5 a day for VA nursing home care. For outpatient care, the copayment is 20% of the cost of an average outpatient visit.

Outpatient Treatment. Veterans eligible for outpatient treatment may obtain outpatient medical care only for the disability as listed on the **VA outpatient clinic card** (Figure 16-1). Usually a veteran seeks care at the nearest VA outpatient clinic. However, when a VA facility is not within reasonable distance, when the veteran is too ill to travel to the nearest location, or when the condition needs prompt attention, the veteran can apply for and be granted medical care by a private physician through the Home Town Care Program. The VA outpatient clinic must be notified within 15 days of the treatment rendered. In such cases the treating physician

BILLING AND REPORTS. Bill the Station of Jurisdiction monthly. Please itemize your usual statement to include (1) patient's name; (2) identification number; (3) condition treated; (4) treatment and dates rendered; and (5) your usual and customary fee. Bills for auxiliary medical services must reflect the name of the prescribing doctor of medicine or osteopathy. Submit a brief treatment report only when the cost of urgent treatment causes the $30.00 limitation to be exceeded, or when a significant clinical change in a disability occurs.

PAYMENT. Payment by the VA for services rendered is payment in full.

IMPORTANT: Direct inquiries and any change of address to the Station of Jurisdiction.

Station of Jurisdiction:

FOLD

VETERANS ADMINISTRATION
OUTPATIENT C 9044/136A6
428 SOUTH HILL ST.
LOS ANGELES CA 90013

VA OUTPATIENT MEDICAL TREATMENT INFORMATION CARD

E. Z. Slipdisk
Beneficiary's name

012-XX-5678
Identification No.

DISABILITY FOR WHICH TREATMENT IS AUTHORIZED–VALID UNTIL CANCELLED BY VA

X P. O. HERNIATED NUC. PULPOSUS

VA FORM 10-1174, FEB 1971

Front

PLEASE READ CAREFULLY

TO VETERAN — You are authorized to obtain treatment within a reasonable distance from your permanent or temporary residence for the disability shown. When treatment is required, select a doctor of medicine or osteopathy who is licensed in the State in which treatment will be rendered. This card constitutes an agreement to provide care to you as a VA beneficiary within the limitations stated. Please alert the doctor to the instructions printed on the card and be sure he has your NAME, IDENTIFICATION NO. and the ADDRESS OF THE STATION OF JURISDICTION. If a specific therapy is authorized in lieu of listing disabilities, this card authorizes ONLY that therapy. IT MAY NOT BE USED TO OBTAIN OTHER MEDICAL SERVICES, SURGICAL PROCEDURES, NON-VA HOSPITALIZATION, OR PROSTHETIC APPLIANCES. Prescriptions of a recurring nature and others not needed at once should be brought or mailed to the VA station of jurisdiction. They will be filled promptly. When it is necessary to obtain medication immediately, PLEASE REQUEST THE PRIVATE PHARMACIST TO BILL THE STATION OF JURISDICTION SHOWN ON THIS CARD.

The VA may reimburse local, round trip, travel expenses between your permanent or temporary residence and the place treatment is obtained. A mileage allowance will be paid in lieu of actual and necessary expenses of travel (including lodging and subsistence).

Your one-time, written request for travel expenses, when received within 30 days from the date you first obtain medical services, will be approved to be effective with the first visit. A claim received after that 30-day-period will be effective from the date received. Generally, travel expenses are paid for a 3-month period.
TO PHYSICIAN — The beneficiary named on this card is authorized OUT-PATIENT TREATMENT for the disabilities shown by a doctor of medicine or osteopathy licensed in the state in which medical services are rendered. When treatment of these conditions requires eyeglasses, hearing aids, other prostheses, home nursing services, and/or dental services, notify the station of Jurisdiction. Items or services of this nature will be provided by the Veterans Administration. Please request additional medical or other information from the station of jurisdiction, if required.
MEDICAL SERVICES includes prescription and referral for auxiliary medical services when required. All routine treatment may not exceed a total cost of $30.00 per month without prior VA approval.
PHARMACY SERVICES: Please have Rxs filled by VA unless needed at once. Veteran may obtain stat Rx from private pharmacy if you certify Rx, "The VA has authorized me to treat the disability for which this prescription is written."

Back

FIGURE 16-1 Veterans Affairs outpatient clinic card.

must submit evidence of medical necessity (e.g., detailed justification on the invoice) to the VA outpatient clinic. Form 10-583, Claim for Payment of Cost of Unauthorized Medical Services (Figure 16-2), generally used for hospital emergency care, can also be used for professional care if the doctor is billing after the 15-day period has elapsed. Some patients have both Medicare and medical coverage from the VA. In such cases Medicare is not secondary to the VA and the VA is not secondary to Medicare. The claim is to be sent where specified by the patient. The claim can be sent to Medicare, where, if the claim is processed, the patient must satisfy his or her contractual requirement to pay any deductible and copayment amounts. If the patient asks that the claim be sent to the VA instead of Medicare, the claim is processed and any payments issued are considered as payment in full. Many veterans prefer to have the claim sent to the VA.

Veterans Affairs Installations. For information on veterans' benefits or assistance in locating VA installations, go to the Evolve website listed in Internet Resources at the end of this chapter for a link to the VA home website.

STATE DISABILITY INSURANCE

Background

In 1944, Rhode Island began a **State Disability Insurance (SDI)** program that proved successful. This form of insurance is part of an employment security program that provides temporary cash benefits for workers suffering a wage loss because of off-the-job illness or injury. It can be referred to as **unemployment compensation**

Form Approved
Budget Bureau No. 76-H0325

VETERANS ADMINISTRATION
CLAIM FOR PAYMENT OF COST OF
UNAUTHORIZED MEDICAL SERVICES

Each person, firm or institution claiming payments or reimbursements must complete this form. No carbon paper is necessary.
Please use typewriter or ball point pen, and submit both copies.

1A. VETERAN'S LAST NAME – FIRST – MIDDLE INITIAL	1B. CLAIM NO.	1C. SOCIAL SECURITY NO.
Thornberg, Joey T.	c–	421-XX-4182

1D. PRESENT ADDRESS (*include zip code*)

4628 Image Street, Woodland Hills, XY 12345-1290

2. NAME AND ADDRESS OF PERSON, FIRM OR INSTITUTION MAKING CLAIM (*Leave blank if same as above*)

Gerald Practon, MD 4567 Broad Ave., Woodland Hills, XY 12345-0001

3. STATEMENT OF CIRCUMSTANCES UNDER WHICH THE SERVICES WERE RENDERED (Include diagnosis, symptoms, whether emergency existed, and reason VA facilities were not used)

Patient fell on sidewalk in front of home and suffered traumatic injury of right arm.
Symptoms: Localized pain, swelling, and bruising of right arm near elbow.
AP and lateral x-rays of right elbow show anterior dislocation right radius. Negative for fracture.
Medical care rendered in Emergency Dept. at College Hospital (99282).
Patient unable to go to VA facility as this is 60 miles away.
Treatment of closed elbow dislocation without anesthesia (23400).
Diagnosis: Anterior closed dislocation right radius (Dx code No. 832.01).

4. AMOUNT CLAIMED	*Attach bills or receipts showing services furnished, dates, and charges*
$ 237.02	attached

5. COMPLETE A OR B, AS APPROPRIATE

A. Amount claimed does not exceed that charged the general public for similar services, and payment has not been received.	B. I certify that the amount claimed has been paid and reimbursement has not been made.
Gerald Practon, MD 5/11/XX	
SIGNATURE AND TITLE OF PROVIDER OF SERVICE, AND DATE	SIGNATURE OF VETERAN OR REPRESENTATIVE, AND DATE

FOR VETERANS ADMINISTRATION USE ONLY

6. ACTION ☐ APPROVED $ _____ ☐ DISAPPROVED	Treatment was provided in an emergency for a service-connected or adjunct disability, any disability of a veteran who has a total disability permanent in nature from a service-connected disability, or for any illness, injury, dental condition in the case of a veteran eligible under Chapter 31 (Vocational Rehabilitation) Title 38, U. S. Code. VA facilities were not feasibly available and delay would have been hazardous.

7. SIGNATURE, CHIEF, MEDICAL ADMINISTRATION SERVICE	8. DATE	9. ADMINISTRATION VOUCHER NO.

VA FORM   10-583
MAY 1974

SUPERSEDES VA FORM 10-583 FEB 1966 AND
WHICH WILL NOT BE USED.

FIGURE 16-2 Veterans Affairs Form 10-583, Claim for Payment of Cost of Unauthorized Medical Services.

disability (UCD) or **temporary disability insurance (TDI).** California became the second state to add nonindustrial disability coverage to the Social Security protection afforded to its citizens by appending Article 10 to the Unemployment Insurance Act. This became law on May 21, 1946; when the legislation took effect on December 1, 1946, this article diverted the 1% tax formerly paid by workers for unemployment insurance to a disability insurance fund. New York and New Jersey soon followed with similar programs. Two decades later, in 1969, Puerto Rico and Hawaii passed nonindustrial disability insurance laws.

Some accidents that occur are quite serious at the time but can appear rather humorous on review.

Unique Accident

The patient was under the kitchen sink repairing a leak when the family cat came along, watched for awhile, then playfully—but painfully—reached up and clawed him. Startled, the man threw his head back, cracked it on the bottom of the sink, and was knocked out cold. He came to as he was being carried out on a stretcher and explained to the attendants what had happened. One stretcher bearer laughed so hard that he relaxed his hold and the patient fell to the ground and broke his arm.

State Programs

Nonindustrial disability insurance programs existed in only five states and Puerto Rico as of 2010. The law is known by a different name in each area.

Active links to websites for most of these programs can be found by going to the Evolve website listed in Internet Resources at the end of this chapter.

Funding

To fund state disability insurance, a small percentage of the wage is deducted from employees' paychecks each month, or the employer may elect to pay all or part of the cost of the plan as a fringe benefit for employees. The money is then sent in quarterly installments to the state and put into a special fund.

Eligibility

To receive state disability insurance benefits, an employee must be as follows:

- Employed full or part time or actively looking for work when disability begins
- Suffering a loss of wages because of disability
- Eligible for benefits, depending on the amount withheld during a previous period before disability began
- Under the care and treatment of a physician who certifies that the employee is disabled
- Disabled at least 7 calendar days
- Filing a claim within the time limit

If the worker was employed at the time of disability, benefits are not subject to federal income tax. An employee who retires is no longer eligible for the insurance. A worker may file a claim with the state seeking exemption from program participation on religious grounds.

Types of workers not covered are employees of school districts, community college districts, and churches; state workers; federal employees; interstate railroad workers; nonprofit organization employees; and domestic workers.

Benefits

Weekly benefits are determined by the wages earned in a base period or based on a percentage of average weekly wages (Table 16-1). Benefits begin after the seventh consecutive day of disability. There is no provision under the law for hospital or other medical benefits.

Limited Benefits

In some states, a patient may qualify for benefits if he or she is a resident of an approved alcoholic recovery facility or an approved drug-free residential facility.

Table 16-1 State Disability Information Summary

STATE	NAME OF STATE LAW	MAXIMUM BENEFIT PERIOD (WK)	TIME LIMIT FOR FILING CLAIMS	2010 DEDUCTIONS FROM SALARY (%)	BENEFITS
California	California Unemployment Insurance Code	52	49 days from disability	1.1 of first $93,316 ($1026.48)	Based on earnings in a 12-mo base period, which begins approximately 18 mo before disability
Hawaii	Temporary Disability Insurance Law	26	90 days from disability	0.5	Based on 58% of average weekly wage
New Jersey	Temporary Disability Benefits Law	26	30 days from disability	0.5	Based on average weekly wage (max $561/wk)
New York	Disability Benefits Law	26	30 days from disability	0.5 (max. 60 cents/wk)	Based on 50% of average weekly wage (max $170/wk)
Puerto Rico	Disability Benefits Act	26	3 mo from disability	0.3 employee; 0.3 employer	Based on wages earned during base yr
Rhode Island	Temporary Disability Insurance Act	30	1 yr from disability	1.2	Based on taxable wage base of $57,900

Reduced Benefits

An individual may be entitled to partial benefits if he or she is receiving certain types of income such as the following:

- Sick leave
- Vacation
- Wages paid by employer
- Insurance settlement for the disability
- Workers' compensation benefits
- Unemployment benefits

Time Limits

A claim for state disability insurance should be filed within the time limit of the state laws (see Table 16-1). There is usually a grace period of 7 or 8 days after the deadline. After the claim is approved, basic benefits become payable after the seventh day of disability. A person may continue to draw disability insurance for a maximum of 26 weeks in Hawaii, New Jersey, New York, and Puerto Rico, and for 52 weeks in California on the same illness or injury or overlapping disabilities. An employee is also entitled to disability benefits 15 days after recovery from a previous disability or illness. For example, if a patient is discharged by the physician to return to work and is on the job 15 calendar days and then becomes ill with the same ailment, he or she may file a new claim.

Medical Examinations

The claimant may be required to submit to an examination or examinations by an independent medical examiner to determine any mental or physical disability. Fees for such examinations are paid by the state department that handles disability insurance. Code 99450 for billing these medical examinations may be found in the Special Evaluation and Management Services section of *Current Procedural Terminology* (CPT).

Restrictions

Disability insurance has many restrictions. A few of the major situations in which a claim could be denied are listed here.

1. Conditions covered by workers' compensation unless the rate is less than the disability insurance rate. In that case the state pays the difference between the two rates.
2. Applicants receiving unemployment insurance benefits more than a certain specified amount. **Exception:** If the applicant is on unemployment insurance and then becomes ill or injured, he or she is put on temporary disability insurance until able to go on a job interview.

3. Disabilities beginning during a trade dispute. If an employee is on strike and is injured while walking a picket line, he or she is considered to still be employed. If injured while picketing, it may be considered workers' compensation. However, if the union is on strike and an individual member remains at home and then becomes ill or injured, he or she can claim disability and will receive benefits.
4. Confinement by court order or certification in a public or private institution as an alcoholic, drug addict, or sexual psychopath.
5. When legal custody is the cause of unemployment.
6. When the employing company has a voluntary disability plan and is not paying into a state fund.
7. Religious exemption certificate on file by employee or company with no payment being made into a state fund.
8. Pregnancy-related disability, unless the pregnancy is complicated (e.g., cases in which the patient has diabetes, varicose veins, ectopic pregnancy, or cesarean section). **Exceptions:** California, Hawaii, New Jersey, and Rhode Island have maternity benefits that may be applied for at the time the physician tells the patient to stop working.

VOLUNTARY DISABILITY INSURANCE

Persons residing and working in states that do not have state disability insurance programs may elect to contact a local private insurance carrier to arrange for coverage under a **voluntary disability insurance** plan. If these persons become ill or disabled, they receive a fixed weekly or monthly income, usually for approximately 6 months. If the disability or illness is permanent and the individual is unable to return to work, there is sometimes a small monthly income for the duration of the person's life. Some of the state laws provide that a "voluntary plan" may be adopted instead of the "state plan" if a majority of company employees consent to private coverage.

CLAIMS SUBMISSION GUIDELINES

Disability Income Claims

When the insurance billing specialist is handling disability income claim forms, he or she should note that the insured (claimant) is responsible to notify the insurance company of the disability. A proof of loss form is completed to establish disability.

The necessary facts are as follows:

- Date the disability occurred
- Date the disabled is expected to be well enough to return to work

- Description of how the disability occurred
- Name of treating physician
- Explanation of how the disability prevents the insured from work

The report must show that the patient's disability meets the policy's definition of disability, or benefits will be denied. Because the definition of disability varies among policies, the critical issues are the content and wording on the claim form.

A portion of this form is usually completed by the attending physician. The following data are necessary:

- Medical history
- Dates patient became disabled
- Subjective symptoms (patient's own words about his or her chief complaints)
- Objective findings on physical examination (e.g., rashes, lacerations, abrasions, or contusions)
- Severity of the illness or injury (range-of-motion tests)
- Photocopies of laboratory tests, x-ray studies, or hospital discharge report
- Medication
- Treatment dates
- Diagnosis
- Prognosis (outcome of the disease or injury)
- Names of any other treating physician
- Date patient expected to return to work
- Description of job duties and patient's ability to perform work

Providing this information helps verify the disability. In some cases the physician may wish to dictate a medical report and attach it to the claim form instead of completing a portion of the form. The insurance billing specialist must be prepared to extract data from source documents such as medical and financial records to complete the claim form. In such situations the physician should be asked to read the information carefully before signing the document. The patient should always be asked to sign an authorization form to release medical information. Reasons for denial of benefits often include improper choice of words or inadequate medical information.

The insurance company may request information from other places to justify payment of benefits such as employer's records, employee's wage statements or tax forms, or the patient's health records from the attending physician. A company representative may interview the insured if conflicting information exists.

If disability continues, additional claim forms should be completed monthly, or more frequently, by the insured and attending physician. Other sources of information may be requested; for example, records from medical specialists or Social Security records.

If the validity of the case is in question, an independent medical examiner may be asked by the insurance company to examine the disabled individual. If the claimant neglects to return claim forms, refuses telephone calls, misses appointments, or engages in questionable activities, the insurance company will discreetly engage in surveillance of the insured through the services of a professional investigation firm.

Federal Disability Claims

The SSA division called *DDS* has a teledictation service so that the physician or psychologist can dictate the medical report over the telephone instead of completing a medical report form. The service is available at any time, including nights and weekends. A typed transcript is sent to the physician to review, sign, and return to the SSA state agency, or a report may be typed on the physician's stationery. The physician may photocopy relevant portions of the patient's chart and submit that information, but it should be legible. An authorization signed by the patient to release information should be on file. Copies of consultation reports and hospital summaries are also helpful. By law, only data no more than 1 year old are allowed.

A medical report must include the following:

- Relevant medical history, past history, social history, and family history
- Subjective complaints (patient's symptoms)
- Objective findings on physical examination (e.g., results of physical or mental status examination, blood pressure)
- Laboratory and x-ray findings
- Diagnostic studies (e.g., treadmill tests, pulmonary function tests, and electrocardiographic [ECG] tracings)
- Diagnosis (statement of disease or injury based on signs and symptoms)
- Treatment prescribed, with patient's response and prognosis
- Medical prognosis about disability based on medical findings. A description of the individual's ability to perform work-related activities, such as standing, sitting, lifting, carrying, walking, handling objects, hearing, speaking, and traveling, is necessary. For cases of mental impairment, the statement should present the individual's capacity for understanding and remembering, sustained concentration and persistence, social interaction, and adaptation.

Veterans Affairs Disability Outpatient Clinic Claims

The processing of invoices from private physicians is a somewhat lengthy procedure as required by VA regulations and involves several steps. To keep the delay in payment to a minimum, private physicians are urged to bill the VA monthly. To ensure prompt processing, invoices should contain the following information:

- Patient's name as shown on the ID card, VA Form 10-1174 (see Figure 16-1).
- Patient's Social Security number.
- Condition treated, shown on every invoice, because this is the basis for approval of payment.
- Diagnosis being treated must be listed on the ID card or authorized by the statement "for any condition." Abstract the diagnosis exactly as it is stated on the ID card.
- Treatment given and dates rendered.
- Physician's usual and customary fee for services rendered.
- Name and address of private physician and his or her Social Security or Federal Taxpayer ID number. If the ID number is assigned to a group and the physician desires to be paid individually, the VA outpatient clinic must be so advised.

Private physicians, as well as veterans, are urged to read the instructions on the ID card carefully. This is sometimes neglected and can lead to misunderstanding.

If the physician does not wish to bill the VA outpatient clinic, the patient can pay the physician and then be reimbursed, but the veteran must carefully follow the instructions on the back of the VA outpatient clinic card.

State Disability Claims

Residents of a state that provides state disability benefits may call or write to the nearest office that handles state disability insurance to obtain a claim form and insurance pamphlet. See Internet Resources at the end of this chapter and go to the Evolve website to link to the state disability websites.

In some states, the claim form is in three parts and must be completed by the claimant, employer, and physician. In other states the form is in two parts and is completed by the claimant and physician (Figures 16-3 and 16-4). In either instance, the case must be substantiated by a physician before the applicant may begin receiving benefits. All information from the state disability insurance office should be read carefully and the directions followed precisely. The data requested should be provided, and the physician and patient should sign the forms. The form should be submitted within the stated time limits.

After the claim has been completed by all parties concerned, it is submitted to the nearest local office for processing. The most important items on the claim form are the following:

- The claimant's Social Security number; without it the claim cannot be researched properly to establish wages earned in the base period.
- The first day the patient was too sick to perform all of his or her regular work duties (item 3). This cannot be the same day the patient worked, even if the patient went home sick.
- The last day the patient worked (item 4). List the last day the patient worked even if for only part of the day.

NOTE: The two dates listed in items 3 and 4 cannot be the same; for example, if the patient went home sick on October 4, that would be considered the last day worked; October 5 would be the first day the patient was unable to work.

California has been selected as the model state for examples of the different forms used in the processing of disability insurance. To establish a claim, the First Claim for Disability Insurance Form DE 2501 must be completed by both the patient (see Figure 16-3) and the attending physician (see Figure 16-4). If an extension of disability is necessary, the Physician's Supplementary Certificate Form DE 2525XX must be completed by the physician (Figure 16-5). This accompanies the last check issued to the patient. For additional medical information that might be necessary, Forms DE 2547 and DE 2547A are sometimes sent to the attending physician for completion (Figures 16-6 and 16-7).

All follow-up correspondence should include the patient's name and Social Security number. The insurance billing specialist should promptly report any change of address, telephone number, or return-to-work date to the state disability insurance office. Patients must report any income received to the state disability insurance office because income received may affect benefits.

CONCLUSION

This chapter ends as it began—with a bit of levity. The following were taken from actual disability insurance application forms, completed by employees, that came across the desk of a claims adjuster.

Spelled as:	Should have been:
yellow "jonders"	yellow jaundice
"goalstones"	gallstones
"limp glands"	lymph glands
"falls teeth"	false teeth
"high pretension"	hypertension
"Pabst smear"	Pap smear
"wrecktum"	rectum

Claim for Disability Insurance Benefits –
Claim Statement of Employee

TYPE or PRINT with BLACK INK.

1A. YOUR SOCIAL SECURITY NUMBER	1B. IF YOU HAVE EVER USED OTHER SOCIAL SECURITY NUMBERS, SHOW THOSE NUMBERS BELOW	2. STATE GOVERNMENT EMPLOYEE (IF YES, INDICATE BARGAINING UNIT #.)
540 - XX - 9881	- - - -	☐ YES (UNIT #) ☒ NO

3. DATE YOUR DISABILITY BEGAN	4. LAST DATE YOU WORKED	5. HAVE YOU WORKED ANY FULL OR PARTIAL DAYS SINCE YOUR DISABILITY BEGAN?	6. DATE YOU RECOVERED OR RETURNED TO WORK (IF ANY)
10 / 10 / 20XX MM DD YY	10 / 09 / 20XX MM DD YY	☐ YES ☒ NO	/ / MM DD YY

7. GENDER	8. YOUR LEGAL NAME	9. YOUR DATE OF BIRTH
☐ MALE ☒ FEMALE	MARCIA (FIRST NAME) M (MIDDLE NAME OR INITIAL) MONROE (LAST NAME)	03 / 04 / 1972 MM DD YY

10. OTHER NAMES, IF ANY, UNDER WHICH YOU HAVE WORKED

11. LANGUAGE YOU PREFER TO USE ☒ ENGLISH ☐ ESPAÑOL ☐ OTHER _____

12. YOUR MAILING ADDRESS (IF YOU WISH TO RECEIVE MAIL AT A PRIVATE MAIL BOX—NOT A US POSTAL SERVICE BOX—YOU MUST SHOW THE NUMBER IN THE "PMB#" SPACE.)

NUMBER / STREET / P.O. BOX / APARTMENT OR SPACE #	PMB # (PRIVATE MAIL BOX #)
3501 MAPLE STREET	

CITY	STATE	COUNTRY (IF NOT UNITED STATES OF AMERICA)	ZIP CODE
WOODLAND HILLS	XY		12345

13. YOUR AREA CODE AND TELEPHONE NUMBER	14. YOUR RESIDENCE ADDRESS, IF DIFFERENT FROM YOUR MAILING ADDRESS
(555) 412-0731	NUMBER / STREET / APARTMENT OR SPACE #

CITY	STATE	COUNTRY (IF NOT UNITED STATES OF AMERICA)	ZIP CODE

15. WHY DID YOU STOP WORKING?

DEVELOPED LUNG PROBLEM ON RIGHT AND LEFT

16. YOUR LAST OR CURRENT EMPLOYER – IF YOUR LAST OR CURRENT EMPLOYMENT WAS SELF-EMPLOYMENT, ENTER "SELF"

EMPLOYER'S AREA CODE AND TELEPHONE NUMBER	NAME OF EMPLOYER [STATE GOVERNMENT EMPLOYEES: PROVIDE THE AGENCY OR DEPARTMENT NAME (FOR EXAMPLE: CALTRANS)]
(555) 487-9980	A AND B COMPANY

NUMBER / STREET / SUITE # (STATE GOVERNMENT EMPLOYEES: PLEASE PROVIDE THE ADDRESS OF YOUR PERSONNEL OFFICE)
401 STATE STREET

CITY	STATE	COUNTRY (IF NOT UNITED STATES OF AMERICA)	ZIP CODE
WOODLAND HILLS	XY		12345

17. YOUR REGULAR OCCUPATION	18. IF YOUR EMPLOYER CONTINUED TO PAY YOU, INDICATE TYPE OF PAY	19. MAY WE DISCLOSE BENEFIT PAYMENT INFORMATION TO YOUR EMPLOYER?
SECRETARY	☐ SICK ☐ VACATION ☐ OTHER _____	☒ YES ☐ NO

20. SECOND EMPLOYER (IF YOU HAVE MORE THAN ONE EMPLOYER)

EMPLOYER'S AREA CODE AND TELEPHONE NUMBER	NAME OF EMPLOYER
( )	

NUMBER / STREET / SUITE #

CITY	STATE	COUNTRY (IF NOT UNITED STATES OF AMERICA)	ZIP CODE

21. AT ANY TIME DURING YOUR DISABILITY WERE YOU IN THE CUSTODY OF LAW ENFORCEMENT AUTHORITIES BECAUSE YOU WERE CONVICTED OF VIOLATING A LAW OR ORDINANCE?

☐ YES ☒ NO   IF "YES," INDICATE NAME OF FACILITY: _____

FIGURE 16-3 Form DE 2501, Claim Statement of Employee. This side of the three-part form is completed by the claimant. *Continued*

Claim Statement of Employee - continued

22. PLEASE RE-ENTER YOUR SOCIAL SECURITY NUMBER.. 540 - XX - 9881

23. IF YOU ARE A RESIDENT OF AN ALCOHOLIC RECOVERY HOME OR A DRUG-FREE RESIDENTIAL FACILITY, SHOW THE NAME, TELEPHONE NUMBER, AND ADDRESS

NAME OF FACILITY	FACILITY AREA CODE AND TELEPHONE NUMBER ( )

ADDRESS OF FACILITY (NUMBER AND STREET / CITY / STATE / ZIP CODE)

24. HAVE YOU FILED OR DO YOU INTEND TO FILE FOR WORKERS' COMPENSATION BENEFITS? ☐ YES–COMPLETE ITEMS 25 THROUGH 32 ☒ NO– COMPLETE ITEMS 25, 31 AND 32	25. WAS THIS DISABILITY CAUSED BY YOUR JOB? ☐ YES ☒ NO	26. DATE(S) OF INJURY SHOWN ON YOUR WORKERS' COMPENSATION CLAIM

27. WORKERS' COMPENSATION INSURANCE COMPANY

COMPANY NAME	COMPANY AREA CODE AND TELEPHONE NUMBER ( )

NUMBER / STREET / SUITE #

CITY	STATE	ZIP CODE	YOUR WORKERS' COMPENSATION CLAIM NUMBER

28. WORKERS' COMPENSATION ADJUSTER

ADJUSTER NAME	ADJUSTER AREA CODE AND TELEPHONE NUMBER ( )

29. EMPLOYER SHOWN ON YOUR WORKERS' COMPENSATION CLAIM

EMPLOYER NAME	EMPLOYER AREA CODE AND TELEPHONE NUMBER ( )

30. YOUR ATTORNEY (IF ANY) FOR YOUR WORKERS' COMPENSATION CASE

ATTORNEY NAME	ATTORNEY AREA CODE AND TELEPHONE NUMBER ( )

NUMBER / STREET / SUITE #

CITY	STATE	ZIP CODE	WORKERS' COMPENSATION APPEALS BOARD CASE NUMBER

PLEASE REVIEW, SIGN, AND DATE BOTH NO. 31 AND NO. 32.

31. Health Insurance Portability and Accountability Act Authorization. I authorize any physician, practitioner, hospital, vocational rehabilitation counselor, or workers' compensation insurance carrier to furnish and disclose to employees of California Employment Development Department (EDD) all facts concerning my disability that are within their knowledge and to allow inspection of and provide copies of any medical, vocational rehabilitation, and billing records concerning my disability that are under their control. I understand that EDD may disclose information as authorized by the California Unemployment Insurance Code and that such redisclosed information may no longer be protected by this rule. I agree that photocopies of this authorization shall be as valid as the original. I understand that, unless revoked by me in writing, this authorization is valid for fifteen years from the date received by EDD or the effective date of the claim, whichever is later. I understand that I may not revoke this authorization to avoid prosecution or to prevent EDD's recovery of monies to which it is legally entitled.

Claimant's Signature (DO NOT PRINT) *Marcia M. Monroe*	Date Signed *October 12, 20XX*

32. Declaration and Signature. By my signature on this claim statement, I claim benefits and certify that for the period covered by this claim I was unemployed and disabled. I understand that willfully making a false statement or concealing a material fact in order to obtain payment of benefits is a violation of California law and that such violation is punishable by imprisonment or fine or both. I declare under penalty of perjury that the foregoing statement, including any accompanying statements, is to the best of my knowledge and belief true, correct, and complete. By my signature on this claim statement, I authorize the California Department of Industrial Relations and my employer to furnish and disclose to State Disability Insurance all facts concerning my disability, wages or earnings, and benefit payments that are within their knowledge. By my signature on this claim statement, I authorize release and use of information as stated in the "Information Collection and Access" portion of this form. I agree that photocopies of this authorization shall be as valid as the original, and I understand that authorizations contained in this claim statement are granted for a period of fifteen years from the date of my signature or the effective date of the claim, whichever is later.

Claimant's Signature (DO NOT PRINT) *Marcia M. Monroe*	Date Signed *October 12, 20XX*

If your signature is made by mark (X), it must be attested by two witnesses with their addresses

1st Witness Signature and Address	2nd Witness Signature and Address

33. Personal Representative signing on behalf of claimant must complete the following: I,_____, represent the claimant in this matter as authorized by ☐ power of attorney (attach copy)   ☐ Declaration of Individual Claiming Disability Insurance Benefits Due an Incapacitated or Deceased Claimant, DE 2522 (see pg. A,#4)

Personal Representative's Signature (DO NOT PRINT)	Date Signed

FIGURE 16-3, cont'd

Claim for Disability Insurance Benefits – Doctor's Certificate

TYPE or PRINT with BLACK INK.

34. PATIENT'S FILE NUMBER	35. PATIENT'S SOCIAL SECURITY NO.	36. PATIENT'S LAST NAME
	540 - XX -9881	MONROE

37. DOCTOR'S NAME AS SHOWN ON LICENSE	38. DOCTOR'S TELEPHONE NUMBER	39. DOCTOR'S STATE LICENSE NO.
DAVID W. SMITH, MD	(555) 486-9002	C 14020

40. DOCTOR'S ADDRESS – NUMBER AND STREET, CITY, STATE, COUNTRY (IF NOT USA), ZIP CODE. POST OFFICE BOX NUMBER IS NOT ACCEPTED AS THE SOLE ADDRESS

4567 BROAD AVENUE, WOODLAND HILLS, XY 12345

41. THIS PATIENT HAS BEEN UNDER MY CARE AND TREATMENT FOR THIS MEDICAL PROBLEM
FROM 10 / 12 / 20XX TO PRESENT   AT INTERVALS OF ☐ DAILY ☒ WEEKLY ☐ MONTHLY ☐ AS NEEDED   TWO VISITS TO DATE

42. AT ANY TIME DURING YOUR ATTENDANCE FOR THIS MEDICAL PROBLEM, HAS THE PATIENT BEEN INCAPABLE OF PERFORMING HIS/HER REGULAR OR CUSTOMARY WORK?
☐ NO – SKIP TO THE DOCTOR'S CERTIFICATION SECTION   ☒ YES – ENTER DATE DISABILITY BEGAN: 10 / 10 / 20XX

43. DATE YOU RELEASED OR ANTICIPATE RELEASING PATIENT TO RETURN TO HIS/HER REGULAR / CUSTOMARY WORK ("UNKNOWN," "INDEFINITE," ETC., NOT ACCEPTED.) 10 / 30 / 20XX

44. ICD9 DISEASE CODE, PRIMARY (REQUIRED UNLESS DIAGNOSIS NOT YET OBTAINED)
486 . ___

45. ICD9 DISEASE CODE(S), SECONDARY
_____ . ___ , _____ . ___ , _____ . ___

46. DIAGNOSIS (REQUIRED) – IF NO DIAGNOSIS HAS BEEN DETERMINED, ENTER OBJECTIVE FINDINGS OR A DETAILED STATEMENT OF SYMPTOMS

BILATERAL PNEUMONITIS

47. FINDINGS – STATE NATURE, SEVERITY, AND EXTENT OF THE INCAPACITATING DISEASE OR INJURY. INCLUDE ANY OTHER DISABLING CONDITIONS

BILATERAL PNEUMONITIS CONFIRMED BY AP AND LATERAL CHEST X-RAYS

48. TYPE OF TREATMENT / MEDICATION RENDERED TO PATIENT
BED REST   R℞ ANTIBIOTICS

49. IF PATIENT WAS HOSPITALIZED, PROVIDE DATES OF ENTRY AND DISCHARGE
____/____/____ TO ____/____/____

50. DATE AND TYPE OF SURGERY / PROCEDURE PERFORMED OR TO BE PERFORMED
____/____/____

ICD9 PROCEDURE CODE(S)

51. IF PATIENT IS NOW PREGNANT OR HAS BEEN PREGNANT, WHAT DATE DID PREGNANCY TERMINATE OR WHAT DATE DO YOU EXPECT DELIVERY?
____/____/____

52. IF PREGNANCY IS / WAS ABNORMAL, STATE THE ABNORMAL AND INVOLUNTARY COMPLICATION CAUSING MATERNAL DISABILITY

53. BASED ON YOUR EXAMINATION OF PATIENT, IS THIS DISABILITY THE RESULT OF "OCCUPATION," EITHER AS AN "INDUSTRIAL ACCIDENT" OR AS AN "OCCUPATIONAL DISEASE"? (INCLUDE SITUATIONS WHERE PATIENT'S OCCUPATION HAS AGGRAVATED PRE-EXISTING CONDITIONS.)	54. ARE YOU COMPLETING THIS FORM FOR THE SOLE PURPOSE OF REFERRAL / RECOMMENDATION TO AN ALCOHOLIC RECOVERY HOME OR DRUG-FREE RESIDENTIAL FACILITY AS INDICATED BY THE PATIENT IN QUESTION 23?	55. WOULD DISCLOSURE OF THIS INFORMATION TO YOUR PATIENT BE MEDICALLY OR PSYCHOLOGICALLY DETRIMENTAL?
☐ YES ☒ NO	☐ YES ☒ NO	☐ YES ☒ NO

Doctor's Certification and Signature (REQUIRED): Having considered the patient's regular or customary work, I certify under penalty of perjury that, based on my examination, this Doctor's Certificate truly describes the patient's disability (if any) and the estimated duration thereof.

I further certify that I am a   M.D.   GENERAL PRACTICE   licensed to practice in the State of   CALIFORNIA   .
(TYPE OF DOCTOR)   (SPECIALTY, IF ANY)

► *David W. Smith, MD*
ORIGINAL SIGNATURE OF ATTENDING DOCTOR – RUBBER STAMP IS NOT ACCEPTABLE

► *10 - 19 - 20XX*
DATE SIGNED

FIGURE 16-4 Form DE 2501, Doctor's Certificate. This side of the form is completed by the attending physician. It is submitted within a set time period, determined by the beginning date of disability, to initiate benefits. If the patient is seen by a second physician, this form is mailed to the claimant to secure the certification of a new physician or to clarify a specific claimed period of disability.

NOTICE OF FINAL PAYMENT

The information contained in your claim for Disability Insurance indicates that you are now able to work; therefore, this is the final check that you will receive on this claim.

IF YOU ARE **STILL** DISABLED: You should complete the Claimant's Certification portion of this form and contact your doctor immediately to have him/her complete the Physician's Supplementary Certificate below.

IF YOU BECOME DISABLED **AGAIN:** File a new Disability Insurance claim form.

IF YOU ARE UNEMPLOYED AND AVAILABLE FOR WORK: Report to the nearest Unemployment Insurance office of the Department for assistance in finding work and to determine your entitlement to Unemployment Insurance Benefits.

This determination is final unless you file an appeal within twenty (20) days from the date of mailing of this notification. You may appeal by giving a detailed statement as to why you believe the determination is in error. All communications regarding this Disability Insurance claim should include your Social Security Account Number and be addressed to the office shown.

CLAIMANT'S CERTIFICATION

I certify that I continue to be disabled and incapable of doing my regular work, and that I have reported all wages, Workers' Compensation benefits and other monies received during the claim period to the Employment Development Department.

ENTER YOUR SOCIAL SECURITY NUMBER *540* *XX* *9881*

Sign Your Name *Marcia M. Monroe* Date signed *October* *29* 20 *xx*

PHYSICIAN'S SUPPLEMENTARY CERTIFICATE

Department Use Only

1. Are you still treating patient? *Yes* Date of last treatment *October* *29* 20 *xx*

2. What present condition continues to make the patient disabled?
bilateral pneumonitis; infiltrate still present

3. Date patient recovered, or will recover sufficiently (even if under treatment) to be able to perform his/her regular and customary work *November* *7* 20 *xx* Please enter a specific or estimated recovery date.

4. Would the disclosure of this information to your patient be medically or psychologically detrimental to the patient?
Yes ☐ No ☒

I hereby certify that the above statements in my opinion truly describe the claimant's condition and the estimated duration thereof.

Date *October* *29* 20 *xx*

Doctor's Signature *David W. Smith M.D.*

Phone Number *555-486-9002*

DE 2525XX Rev. 13 (3-86) —Version en español el dorso—

FIGURE 16-5 Notice of Final Payment/Physician's Supplementary Certificate Form DE 2525XX. This form indicates that the period of disability is "closed" or terminated with the accompanying check on the basis of the information in the claim records. Benefits will cease unless the reverse side of the form is completed by the claimant's physician, extending the duration of disability. This form is pink. One side of the form is in English and the other is in Spanish.

STATE OF CALIFORNIA
EMPLOYMENT DEVELOPMENT DEPARTMENT

FOR DEPT. USE ONLY

REFER TO

4920 — Our File No.
Marcia M. Monroe — Your Patient
Secretary — Regular or Customary Work

REQUEST FOR ADDITIONAL
MEDICAL INFORMATION

David W. Smith, MD
4567 Broad Avenue
Woodland Hills, XY 12345

The original basic information and estimate of duration of your patient's disability have been carefully evaluated. At the present time, the following additional information based upon the progress and present condition of this patient is requested. This will assist the Department in determining eligibility for further disability insurance benefits. Return of the completed form as soon as possible will be appreciated.

WM. C. SCHMIDT, M.D., MEDICAL DIRECTOR

CLAIMS EXAMINER **DOCTOR: Please complete either Part A or B, date and sign.**

PART A IF YOUR PATIENT HAS RECOVERED SUFFICIENTLY TO BE ABLE TO RETURN TO HIS/HER REGULAR OR CUSTOMARY WORK LISTED ABOVE, PLEASE GIVE THE DATE, _____20_____.

PART B THIS PART REFERS TO PATIENT WHO IS STILL DISABLED.

Are you still treating the patient? YES ☒ NO ☐ November 15 , 20 xx
DATE OF LAST TREATMENT

What are the medical circumstances which continue to make your patient disabled?
Bilateral pneumonitis. Patient has had continual fever 100°F to 102°F, productive cough, chest pains, and lethargy

What is your present estimate of the date your patient will be able to perform his/her regular or customary work listed above? Date November 30 20 xx .

Further Comments: _____

Would the disclosure of this information to your patient be medically or psychologically detrimental to the patient? YES ☐ NO ☒

Date November 17 20 xx

David W. Smith M.D.
DOCTOR'S SIGNATURE

SE David W. Smith, MD
ENCLOSED IS A STAMPED PREADDRESSED ENVELOPE FOR YOUR CONVENIENCE.

DE 2547 R v. 18 (8-84)

FIGURE 16-6 Request for Additional Medical Information Form DE 2547. This form is mailed to the physician when the normal expectancy date of the disability is reached, provided that the physician has requested a longer than normal duration without complications as indicated.

STATE OF CALIFORNIA

EMPLOYMENT DEVELOPMENT DEPARTMENT
P.O. Box 1529, Santa Barbara, CA 93102
(555) 963-9611

For Dept. Use Only

REFER TO

4920
Marcia M. Monroe
Secretary

- Our File No.
- Your Patient
- Regular Work

MEDICAL INQUIRY

David W. Smith, MD
4567 Broad Avenue
Woodland Hills, XY 12345

A review of the medical certificate received in conjunction with a claim
for disability insurance benefits filed by your patient, named above,
reveals that some additional information is needed in order to evaluate
the claim properly. Your cooperation in answering the question or
questions below and returning the form in the enclosed stamped and
addressed envelope will be appreciated.

WM. C. SCHMIDT, MD, MEDICAL DIRECTOR

CLAIMS EXAMINER

What is the name and address of the facility that took the x-rays on
this patient?

Speedy Radiology Service
4598 Main Street
Woodland Hills, XY 12345

Would the disclosure of this information to your patient be medically or
psychologically detrimental to the patient: Yes ☐   No ☒

October 24	20XX	*David W. Smith MD*
Date		Doctor's Signature
SE		David W. Smith, MD

DE 2547A Rev. 10 (9-84)

FIGURE 16-7 Medical Inquiry Form DE 2547A. This form is mailed to the physician at any
time during the life of the claim if any questions need to be answered or if the physician has
failed to enter a prognosis date.

KEY POINTS

This is a brief chapter review or summary of the key issues presented. To further enhance your knowledge of the technical subject matter, review the key terms and key abbreviations for this chapter by locating the meanings in the glossary at the end of this book that appear in a section before the index.

1. Disability income insurance is a type of insurance that provides periodic payments under certain conditions when the insured is unable to work because of illness, disease, or injury, not as a result of a work-related accident or condition.

2. While disabled, benefits begin after an elimination or waiting period.

3. The types of disability are temporary, residual or partial, and total.

4. Disability policies may be guaranteed renewable for a specific number of years to a certain age.

5. The SSA manages two programs that pay monthly disability benefits to people younger than age 65 who cannot work for at least a year because of a severe disability: SSDI program and SSI program.

6. Federal employees who have put in a certain number of years of service and who become disabled not by work-related means may be eligible for Civil Service and FERS programs.

7. Individuals on active duty fall under the Armed Services Disability program if they become disabled while serving in the military.

8. The VA disability program provides benefits for veterans who have suffered a service-connected disability.

9. Six states have a state disability insurance program for those who suffer a wage loss because of off-the-job illness or injury.

10. Claims for state disability insurance must be filed within the time limits of each state's laws.

11. For disability income claims, the insured must file a proof of loss form and the attending physician must also complete a section to verify the disability.

12. For federal disability cases, the physician must submit details about the individual's disabled condition.

13. State disability claim forms must be completed by the attending physician to substantiate the claimant's condition to receive benefits.

evolve INTERNET RESOURCES

For active links to the following resources, visit the Evolve website at
http://evolve.elsevier.com/fordney/handbook

- California Unemployment Insurance Code
- Hawaii Temporary Disability Laws

- New Jersey Temporary Disability Benefits Law
- New York Disability Benefits Law
- Rhode Island Temporary Disability Insurance Act
- Department of Veterans Affairs Facility Directory

STUDENT ASSIGNMENT

✓ Study Chapter 16.
✓ Answer the fill-in-the-blank, multiple choice, and true/false review questions in the *Workbook* to reinforce the theory learned in this chapter and to help prepare you for a future test. Complete the assignments in the *Workbook*. These assignments will provide you with hands-on experience in working with patient histories and completing disability insurance claim forms described in this chapter.

✓ Turn to the glossary at the end of this textbook for a further understanding of the key terms and key abbreviations used in this chapter.

UNIT 4
Inpatient and Outpatient Billing

KEY TERMS*

admission review

ambulatory payment classifications

appropriateness evaluation protocols

capitation

case rate

charge description master

charges

clinical outliers

code sequence

comorbidity

cost outlier

cost outlier review

day outlier review

diagnosis-related groups

DRG creep

DRG validation

elective surgery

grouper

inpatient

International Classification of Diseases, Ninth Revision, Clinical Modification

International Classification of Diseases, Tenth Revision, Procedure Classification System

looping

major diagnostic categories

outpatient

percentage of revenue

per diem

preadmission testing

principal diagnosis

procedure review

Quality Improvement Organization program

readmission review

scrubbing

stop loss

transfer review

Uniform Bill CMS-1450 paper or electronic claim form

utilization review

KEY ABBREVIATIONS*

AEPs

APCs

APGs

ASCs

AVGs

CC

CDM

CMHCs

CMS-1450

DRGs

FL

GAO

HSI

ICD-9-CM

ICD-10-PCS

LOS

MCC

MDCs

MCE

MS-DRGs

OCE

OPPS

PAT

QIO program

RHIA

RHIT

RN

TJC

UB-04 paper or electronic claim form

UR

---

*Definitions for the key terms and key abbreviations are located near the back of this textbook in the glossary.

CHAPTER
17

Hospital Billing

OBJECTIVES

After reading this chapter, you should be able to:

- Define common terms related to hospital billing.
- Name qualifications necessary to work in the financial section of a hospital.
- List instances of breach of confidentiality in a hospital setting.
- Explain the purpose of the appropriateness evaluation protocols.
- Describe criteria used for admission screening.
- Define the 72-hour rule.
- Describe the quality improvement organization and its role in the hospital reimbursement system.
- State the role of *International Classification of Diseases, Ninth Revision, Clinical Modification* (ICD-9-CM) volume 3 in hospital billing.
- Identify categories in ICD-9-CM volume 3.
- Describe the *International Classification of Diseases, Tenth Revision, Procedure Classification System* (ICD-10-PCS)
- Explain the basic flow of the inpatient hospital stay from billing through receipt of payment.

- Describe the charge description master.
- State reimbursement methods used when paying for hospital services under managed care contracts.
- State when the CMS-1450 (UB-04) paper or electronic claim form may and may not be used.
- Describe the history and purpose of diagnosis-related groups.
- Identify how payment is made on the basis of diagnosis-related groups.
- State how payment is made on the basis of the ambulatory payment classification system.
- Name the four types of ambulatory payment classifications.
- Edit and complete insurance claims in both hospital inpatient and outpatient settings to minimize their rejection by insurance carriers.
- State the general guidelines for completion of the paper CMS-1450 (Uniform Bill [UB-04]) and transmission of the electronic claim form.

Service to Patients

Learn to be courteous in all interactions with co-workers and patients so that patients sense an atmosphere of high morale in the working environment. Be watchful about observing how patients and co-workers react to you and to hospital policies and procedures so that communication ends up as a positive patient encounter. Make sure you are educated about your job duties and hospital policy; otherwise, responses to the patient may vary from employee to employee when training is not thorough. Always look and act as a professional and respond immediately to patients' questions and problems.

Performance objectives, testing and review material, and hands-on practical exercises for this chapter are available in these resources

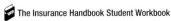 The Insurance Handbook Student Workbook   The Insurance Handbook Evolve Site

567

PATIENT SERVICE REPRESENTATIVE

Qualifications

A variety of jobs are available in the financial department and health information management (HIM) department, formerly known as the *medical record department*, of hospitals; therefore this chapter focuses on hospital inpatient and outpatient insurance billing and coding. Individuals who desire a position in a hospital facility business department should have knowledge and competence in the following subjects:

- ICD-9-CM, ICD-10-CM, and ICD-10-PCS diagnostic codes
- CPT and HCPCS procedure codes
- Paper or electronic CMS-1500 (08-05)/837P insurance claim form
- Paper or electronic CMS-1450/UB-04 insurance claim form
- Explanation of benefits and remittance advice document
- Medical terminology (i.e., anatomy and physiology, diseases, and treatments)
- Major health insurance programs
- Managed care plans
- Insurance claim submission
- Denied and delinquent claims

A hospital facility is larger than a clinic or private physician's office, so there is greater opportunity for advancement. An individual may be hired as a file clerk or insurance verifier and advance from junior to senior clerk, insurance clerk, or patient service representative. He or she may continue to advance to an administrative position. Most hospital facilities have policies that encourage career growth by promoting jobs from within. Usually a coder must have some working diagnostic and/or procedural code experience before being hired as an entry-level coder. Additional personal and physical qualifications are shown in Figure 17-1. See Chapter 1 for details on educational and training requirements and ethics and Chapter 18 for information on certification.

Primary Functions and Competencies

A generic job description for a patient service representative in a hospital business office whose primary function is to file hospital inpatient and outpatient claims with third-party payers is shown in Figure 17-1. Competencies for inpatient coding that were approved by the American Hospital Association (AHA), American Health Information Management Association (AHIMA), Centers for Medicare and Medicaid Services (CMS; formerly Health Care Financing Administration), and the National Center for Health Statistics are shown in Box 17-1.

Principal Responsibilities

Because of the diversity in reimbursement methods, ideally the insurance billing specialist must have basic knowledge of insurance programs and know how to use summary sheets, which give main provisions of the contracts to correctly process each insurance claim. Accurate claim processing is essential for obtaining maximum reimbursement from the insurance company and when collecting payment from the patient. However, in reality many hospitals function by submitting insurance claims, receiving payment, and writing off the difference, which is subject to huge numbers of errors and loss of many dollars. To remain an asset to employers, an insurance billing specialist must continually update his or her knowledge of coding and insurance program policies by attending seminars, workshops, classes, and in-house training.

MEDICOLEGAL CONFIDENTIALITY ISSUES

Documents

The patient's financial and medical records and any photographs are legal documents and must be kept confidential. This means they must not be disclosed to other individuals and may not be released unless a patient has signed an authorization form to make the information public. An exception is when a medical record is subpoenaed by the court. Chapter 4 contains information on confidentiality when facsimile communication is used. When work is done in a sensitive area of a facility, document shredders should be used to destroy unwanted documents and prevent violations of confidentiality.

Examples 17-1 and 17-2 show breaches of confidentiality with medical and financial records.

Computer Security

As you learned in Chapter 8 in regard to computer security, when using a computer, adhere to hospital policies with respect to the following:

- Use of passwords and other encryption methods
- Policies for composition and transmission of electronic mail
- Policies for use of the fax machine
- Downloading of computer data from one department to another
- Length of time that documents may be retained on computer hard drives by employees
- Procedures for deletion of confidential information
- Procedures for archiving of data
- Closing out when leaving a workstation or desk

MEDICOLEGAL CONFIDENTIALITY ISSUES—cont'd

Example 17-1   Medical Record Scenario

An insurance billing specialist working at home has a sister who was hospitalized to undergo major surgery and wants to help his or her parents better understand the medical condition. The specialist calls a friend in the hospital billing department and asks that person to make photocopies of a document in the medical record.

Comment

Remember that all medical reports are confidential, so the employee must deny the request unless the sister signs a release of information that would authorize her family to have copies of the document.

Example 17-2   Financial Record Scenario

An experienced insurance billing specialist applies for a job. At an interview, he or she presents some samples of typed insurance claims that include hospital and patient names.

Comment

This indicates that the prospective employee has taken data from a former employer's facility and violated the patient's confidentiality by not removing the names in the samples.

Verbal Communication

Verbal breaches of confidentiality in a hospital setting, much like in a provider's office, could result in an insurance billing specialist being held liable and the facility being sued by a patient. A breach of confidential communication is the unauthorized release of confidential information about a patient to a third party. Also, Health Insurance Portability and Accountability Act (HIPAA) violations carry monetary penalties and may include a jail sentence. New employees must be trained in confidentiality and asked to sign an understanding of confidentiality statement. This statement should emphasize that the employee may be subject to immediate termination in the event of a violation. Any one of the following scenarios in which the patient's right to privacy has been breached in the hospital setting may be encountered by an insurance billing specialist such as an employee overhearing employees discussing a patient's case, an employee who talks to family about a patient's case, an employee who discusses a diagnosis with a co-worker, or a physician who talks on a cell phone about a patient's diagnosis (Examples 17-3 through 17-6).

Example 17-3   Verbal Breach of Confidentiality Scenario

A coding clerk overhears two hospital employees discussing a patient by name. Because the clerk had been working on the medical record of that patient and is now familiar with the patient's history, he or she realizes that the information being discussed is not accurate. The coding clerk then interrupts, making a comment about the patient's diagnosis.

Comment

Information should not be discussed with co-workers or other hospital employees and must never be related to anyone other than a person who has a valid need to provide care for the patient.

Example 17-4   Verbal Breach of Confidentiality Scenario

A Marilyn Monroe impersonator is discharged from the hospital after receiving plastic surgery. Over dinner at home, an insurance billing specialist relates the diagnosis and name of the surgery to his or her spouse.

Comment

Never discuss confidential information about patients to family or friends.

Example 17-5   Verbal Breach of Confidentiality Scenario

In reviewing an insurance claim before it is mailed, the insurance billing specialist realizes that he or she knows the individual who has a diagnosis that indicates a mental condition. The specialist discusses this with a co-worker.

Comment

This is a violation because a hospital employee must never give anyone information on a patient's diagnosis.

Example 17-6   Verbal Breach of Confidentiality Scenario

A physician in private practice calls via cellular telephone to the billing clerk to answer a question about the diagnosis to be listed on a patient's insurance claim.

Comment

Cellular transmission may be intercepted by anyone with inexpensive eavesdropping equipment. In this scenario, a traditional telephone line must be used when relating confidential information about a patient's diagnosis. The physician should verify whether he or she is speaking to the billing clerk.

POSITION DESCRIPTION

Title: Patient Service Representative
Department: Business Office
Reports to: Patient Accounts Supervisor

Job Number: 215
Effective Date: 3/1/07
Revision Date: 11/1/07

Primary Function:

To promptly file hospital inpatient and outpatient claims with third-party payers, following up in a timely and efficient manner, to ensure maximum reimbursement is received for services provided. To assist the public in obtaining full benefits from their coverage and in understanding billing procedures, always maintaining good public relations.

Principal Responsibilities:

1. Processes claims within assigned responsibility in a timely and efficient manner, performing all associated duties in order to ensure completeness and correctness of all claims information, facilitating maximum reimbursement.
   a. Analyzes, updates and corrects claim data according to established procedure.
   b. Inputs data accurately, efficiently and consistently.
   c. Performs work as scheduled, prioritizing as required for maximizing cash flow.
   d. Demonstrates thorough knowledge of third-party payers, claims requirements, UB-92 requirements by payer, computer capabilities as related to claims production, and admitting/medical records input as it affects claims.
2. Handles phone, mail and personal inquiries from and regarding patient accounts.
   a. Assists each person promptly, efficiently and courteously.
   b. Follows through on all issues identified as requiring action as a result of inquiry.
   c. Performs duties with a minimum of supervision, exhibits innovation and good judgment as well as thorough knowledge of ethical and legal billing procedures.
3. Performs related business office responsibilities as assigned by patient accounts manager.
   a. Follows hospital and department policies and procedures.
   b. Observes confidentiality in all matters.
   c. Maintains all documentation and records in accordance with federal and state regulations.
   d. Maintains good interdepartmental relations.
4. Provides coverage for A/R specialist 2 position for vacation and illness.
   a. Demonstrates knowledge of and ability to perform all duties and functions.
5. Participates in educational opportunities offered by hospital for job and personal development.
   a. Attends classes, workshops and seminars relating to billing/collection functions.
   b. Participates actively in such seminars, classes and workshops.
   c. Takes advantage of opportunities for personal growth and development as offered.
6. Takes an active role in facilitating team approach to functions within the department.
   a. Attends departmental meetings.
   b. Actively participates as team member in resolution of problems as they are identified.
   c. Analyzes current procedures, bringing suggestions for improvement to the attention of team members and supervisor for consideration.

Direction of Others:

Provides some direction to student learner. Number of persons supervised —1.

Qualifications:

High school graduation with 1–3 years experience in claims processing, business or accounting. Experience in health care field desirable.

Physical Qualifications:

These requirements may be met with the aid of mechanical devices and are those minimally necessary for safe completion of duties. They are not intended to discriminate against handicapped persons, only to ensure safe working conditions for all persons.
1. Must be able to enter data into a computer and effectively operate a 10-key adding machine.
2. Must be able to communicate in a pleasant and tactful manner to other employees and patients.
3. Must pass a pre-employment physical examination.

Working Conditions:

Normal office working conditions.

Department approval: _____ Date: _____

Administrative approval: _____ Date: _____

Human resources approval: _____ Date: _____

FIGURE 17-1 Job description for patient service representative (hospital biller). (From Goselin L: *Questions and answers: job descriptions provide guidelines for employees/managers: get it in writing, health care biller,* volume 4, no 6, New York, 1995, Aspen Publishers.)

Box 17-1   American Health Information Management Association Certified Coding Specialist Coding Competencies—ICD-9-CM and CPT/HCPCS Procedural Coding

Data Identification

1. Read and interpret health record documentation to identify all diagnoses and procedures that affect the current inpatient stay or outpatient encounter visit.
2. Assess the adequacy of health record documentation to ensure that it supports all diagnoses and procedures to which codes are assigned.
3. Apply knowledge of anatomy and physiology, clinical disease processes, pharmacology, and diagnostic and procedural terminology to assign accurate codes to diagnoses and procedures.
4. Apply knowledge of disease processes and surgical procedures to assign nonindexed medical terms to the appropriate class in the classification/nomenclature system.

Coding Guidelines

1. Apply knowledge of current approved ICD-9-CM coding guidelines to assign and sequence the correct diagnosis and procedure codes for hospital inpatient services.
2. Apply knowledge of current diagnostic coding and reporting guidelines for outpatient services.
3. Apply knowledge of CPT format, guidelines, and notes to locate the correct codes for all services and procedures performed during the encounter/visit and sequence them correctly.
4. Apply knowledge of procedural terminology to recognize when an unlisted procedure code must be used in CPT.

Regulatory Guidelines

1. Apply Uniform Hospital Discharge Data Set definitions to select the principal diagnosis, principal procedure, complications and comorbid conditions, other diagnoses, and significant procedures that require coding.
2. Select the appropriate principal diagnosis for episodes of care in which determination of the principal diagnosis is not clear because the patient has multiple problems.
3. Apply knowledge of the PPS to confirm DRG assignment that ensures optimal reimbursement.
4. Refuse to fraudulently maximize reimbursement by assigning codes that do not conform to approved coding principles/guidelines.

5. Refuse to unfairly maximize reimbursement by unbundling services and codes that do not conform to CPT basic coding principles.
6. Apply knowledge of the Ambulatory Surgery Center Payment Groups to confirm ASC assignment that ensures optimal reimbursement.
7. Apply policies and procedures on health record documentation, coding and claims processing, and appeal.
8. Use the HCPCS to appropriately assign HCPCS codes for outpatient Medicare reimbursement.

Coding

1. Exclude from coding diagnoses, conditions, problems, and procedures related to an earlier episode of care that has no bearing on the current episode of care.
2. Exclude from coding ICD-9-CM nonsurgical, noninvasive procedures that carry no operative or anesthetic risk.
3. Exclude from coding information such as symptoms or signs characteristic of the diagnosis, findings from diagnostic studies, or localized conditions that have no bearing on the current management of the patient.
4. Apply knowledge of ICD-9-CM instructional notations and conventions to locate and assign the correct diagnostic and procedural codes and sequence them correctly.
5. Assist data retrieval by recognizing when more than one code is required to adequately classify a given condition.
6. Exclude from coding procedures that are component parts of an already assigned CPT procedure code.

Data Quality

1. Clarify conflicting, ambiguous, or nonspecific information appearing in a health record by consulting the appropriate physician.
2. Participate in quality assessment to ensure continuous improvement in ICD-9-CM and CPT coding and collection of quality health data.
3. Demonstrate ability to recognize potential coding quality issues from an array of data.
4. Apply policies and procedures on health record documentation and coding that are consistent with official coding guidelines.
5. Contribute to development of facility-specific coding policies and procedures.

ASC, Ambulatory Surgery Category; *CPT, Current Procedural Terminology; HCPCS,* Healthcare Common Procedure Coding System; *PPS,* prospective payment system.

ADMISSIONS PROCEDURES

Appropriateness Evaluation Protocols

The definition of admission from a hospital perspective is the act of accepting an individual for inpatient services. A patient is considered an **inpatient** on admission to the hospital for an overnight stay for observation care or for an extended stay for medical services. Hospitals must follow specific procedures so that quality patient care for preadmission tests, such as laboratory tests, x-rays, and electrocardiogram (ECG), is given. Hospitals must meet **appropriateness evaluation protocols (AEPs)** by the

hospital's **utilization review (UR)** department to certify that the patient's complaints warrant admittance to the hospital. UR is done to evaluate compliance with AEPs and other standards. In addition, the hospital may have specific rules for observation status dictated by the American Hospital Association (AHA), the hospital administration, and the hospital medical staff's specific rules. Specific criteria are used by the insurance company for admission screening. It is the hospital's responsibility to obtain the approved utilization review of the case with the insurance carrier. The Medicare Prospective Payment System (PPS) requires that all patients meet at least one

FIGURE 17-2 Illustration that depicts referral of the patient to the hospital and the basic flow after inpatient admission. It shows various services a patient might encounter during a hospital stay and ends with the patient's discharge, the billing process, and accounts receivable management.

severity of illness (SI) or intensity of service (IS) criterion, unless otherwise indicated, to be certified for reimbursement. Within the first 24 hours, the hospital's UR department analyzes the documentation on the medical record, which must reflect how the patient meets these criteria. UR is discussed in detail later in this chapter. Figure 17-2 shows the basic flow of the inpatient admission process after discharge of the patient. A list of AEPs is provided in Figure 17-3.

Admitting Procedures for Major Insurance Programs

The admitting process varies according to rules set down by the patient's insurance plan and hospital rules on the basis of guidelines from the AHA. Following are basic admitting procedures and preadmission authorization requirements for the major insurance programs.

Private Insurance (Group or Individual)

It is the responsibility of the outpatient and inpatient admitting personnel to obtain complete and accurate information during initial registration of the patient. The patient must provide a current insurance card or cards. Obtain photocopies of the front and back of all cards. Some hospital facilities employ an insurance verification clerk. He or she has the responsibility of contacting the insurance company (within 24 hours or the next working day) or the insured individual's employer in workers' compensation cases to verify the type of health insurance. The clerk also must

call the insurance company to verify eligibility and benefits and determine whether prior authorization is necessary. Some facilities use the Internet to obtain insurance verification from an insurance company or use a point-of-service (POS) machine. These methods are quicker and less expensive than telephone verification.

Managed Care

There may be restrictions and various policies and procedures to follow when admitting a patient who has a managed care health maintenance organization (HMO) or preferred provider organization (PPO) type of insurance. Obtain photocopies of the front and back sides of the identification card. Several types of patient admissions to the hospital are recognized by managed care plans. See Chapter 11 for further information on this subject.

Emergency Inpatient Admission. *Hospital with Contract.* A patient is seen in the emergency department (formerly called *emergency room [ER]*), and the physician determines that it is necessary to admit the patient to the hospital. The managed care program should be notified the next working day or within 48 hours to obtain an authorization number. The plan authorizes the first days of the admission and approves subsequent days based on UR. The review organization determines the emergency status and may send written notification to the hospital and physician. The patient may have a deductible and copayment requirement. Emergency department charges are billed with charges for the inpatient stay on the

APPROPRIATENESS EVALUATION PROTOCOL CRITERIA FOR ADMISSION CERTIFICATION

An admission may be certified if one of the following criteria is met:

SEVERITY OF ILLNESS (SI)

1. Sudden onset of unconsciousness or disorientation (coma or unresponsiveness).
2. Pulse rate <50 or >140.
3. Systolic blood pressure <80 or >200 mm Hg. Diastolic blood pressure <60 or >120 mm Hg.
4. Sudden onset of loss of sight or hearing.
5. History of persistent fever ≥ 100° F (orally) or 101° F (rectally) for more than 5 days or with white blood cell count >15,000/mm³.
6. Sudden onset of motor function loss of any body part.
7. Active, uncontrolled bleeding.
8. Electrolyte or blood gas abnormality of serum K+: <2.5, >6.0; serum Na+ <123, >156; CO_2 <20 mEq/L, >36 mEq/L (new findings).
9. Acute or progressive sensory, motor, circulatory, or respiratory embarrassment sufficient to incapacitate the patient (one of the IS criteria must also be met).
10. Electrocardiographic evidence of acute ischemia with suspicion of new myocardial infarction.
11. Wound dehiscence or evisceration.

INTENSITY OF SERVICE (IS)

12. Administration and monitoring of intravenous medications and/or fluid replacement (does not include tube feeding).
13. Surgery or procedure scheduled within 24 hours requiring general or regional anesthesia with use of equipment and facilities available only in a hospital.
14. Vital sign monitoring at least every 2 hours, including telemetry and bedside cardiac monitoring.
15. Use of chemotherapeutic agents that require continuous observation for a life-threatening toxic reaction.
16. Treatment in intensive/coronary care unit.
17. Administration of intramuscular antibiotics at least every 8 hours.
18. Intermittent or continuous respirator use at least every 8 hours.
19. Documentation on the medical record by the attending physician that the patient has been unsuccessfully treated as an outpatient *with* further documentation of how the patient is now to be treated as an inpatient.

FIGURE 17-3 Appropriateness evaluation protocol criteria for admission certification listing severity of illness and intensity of service.

electronic or paper (Uniform Bill [UB-04]) claim form. This form is also known as the *837i (institutional)* and has been redesigned. An employed physician's professional services for a patient seen in the emergency department are submitted as outpatient billing on the CMS-1500 (08-05) insurance claim form. This form is also known, though less commonly, as the *837p (professional)*.

Hospital without Contract. The managed care program of emergency admission should be notified on the next working day to obtain an authorization number. The patient should be prepared for transfer to a contracting hospital if necessary. The patient may have the option of staying and paying the deductible, copayment, or entire bill and not file a claim with the managed care plan.

Nonemergency Inpatient Admission. *Hospital with Contract.* The patient must be referred by his or her primary care physician and obtain preliminary authorization for the length of the hospital stay. The patient may have a copayment requirement.

Hospital without Contract. The patient may request authorization with a noncontracted hospital; however, the patient may be responsible for a higher deductible and copayment or the entire bill.

Elective Admission to a Participating Hospital. An attending participating physician contacts the insurance plan at least 3 days before admission to give notification of a member's proposed elective admission. If a preadmission review is necessary, the physician is responsible for obtaining prior authorization from the review organization or the managed care plan. The physician calls the hospital to relay information about the patient for admitting purposes.

Elective Admission to a Nonparticipating Hospital. An attending physician contacts the designated review organization for admission approval in a nonemergency situation. Within 1 working day of approved requests for prior authorization, the review organization calls the physician and hospital and assigns a control number that certifies approval of the admission. The review organization furnishes the physician and hospital with an approved preadmission or referral request form.

Medicaid

 In most states a treatment authorization request form should be approved before elective admissions. For an emergency, preapproval is not necessary; however, a retroactive form is necessary before the claim is billed. Photocopies of the front and back of the patient's identification card should be obtained or eligibility verified via touchtone telephone, modem, or specialized Medicaid terminal equipment. See Chapter 13 for additional information.

Medicare

Medicare patients do not need prior approval for admission to a hospital. However, their admittance should be certified by AEPs, as previously discussed in this chapter. Photocopies of the front and back of the patient's identification cards should be obtained for Medicare and any supplemental or secondary insurance policies. A common working file is used to verify coverage, look up information, and bill Medicare. For patients who receive both Medicare and Medicaid or other secondary insurance benefits, the claims are considered crossover claims. The claim form is processed automatically by Medicaid (in California Medi-Cal) after processing is completed by Medicare. See Chapter 12 for detailed data on the Medicare program.

TRICARE and CHAMPVA

As stated in Chapter 14, all admissions to a civilian hospital and ambulatory surgical facility except emergency cases require precertification. The health care finder assists with this process when a military treatment hospital is not available. Precertification should be verified; photocopies of the front and back of the patient's identification card should be obtained or eligibility verified via touchtone telephone or modem. See Chapter 14 for additional information.

Workers' Compensation

The patient does not have an insurance card in a workers' compensation case. When the patient is seen on an emergency basis, an employer's report of injury must be completed and sent to the insurance company and the state industrial accident board before a hospital or physician's insurance claim may be submitted. A case number is assigned. Appropriate information relating to the injured patient, industrial accident, insurance carrier, and employer must be obtained. The insurance adjuster must authorize admission, length of stay, and all surgical procedures for an elective admission. See Chapter 15 for further details on this subject.

Preadmission Testing

To obtain necessary diagnostic information, reduce inpatient expenses, and eliminate extra hospital days, a patient is usually sent to the hospital for **preadmission testing (PAT)** before being admitted for major surgery. Preadmission tests include diagnostic studies such as laboratory tests, chest x-ray films, and ECG. When a laboratory panel of tests is performed, each separate test must be itemized and must show the clinical benefit for each test performed on the basis of the patient's diagnosis. In elective surgical cases, preadmission services (e.g., history and physical examination) are done in the physician's office and are bundled with hospital services instead of appearing as separate charges on inpatient or outpatient bills.

Medicare 3-Day Payment Window Rule or 72-Hour Rule

One of the most important regulations in hospital billing is compliance with the CMS's 72-hour rule, also called the *3-day payment window rule*, because it is 3 calendar days rather than 72 hours. The Medicare rule states that if a patient receives diagnostic tests and hospital outpatient services within 72 hours of admission to a hospital (3-day payment window), then all such tests and services are combined (bundled) with inpatient services only if services are related to the admission. However, unrelated therapeutic service is paid. The preadmission services become part of the diagnosis-related group (DRG) payment to the hospital and may not be billed or paid separately. DRG payment is one of several methods of reimbursement for hospital services that are discussed later in this chapter. This is valid if the services (including emergency department services) are considered related to the reason for admission. If a hospital owns or operates a physician's office that provides diagnostic or other services related to the admission within 3 days of subsequent inpatient admission, the services must be included in the DRG payment. If this rule is not followed, fraud and abuse may be considered and a penalty in the form of a fine or imprisonment may be carried out.

Exceptions to the 72-Hour Rule. The following are exceptions to the 72-hour rule:

- Services provided by home health agencies, hospice, nursing facilities (NFs), and ambulance services
- Physician's professional portion of a diagnostic service (the technical portion of a diagnostic service must be included in the inpatient bill)
- Preadmission testing at an independent laboratory when the laboratory has no formal agreement with the health care facility

For patients with private insurance (non-Medicare) receiving tests within 24 hours of hospital admission, include such tests with inpatient billing.

Present on Admission

Hospitals were required to begin reporting the present-on-admission (POA) indicator code on claims with discharges beginning on or after October 1, 2007. POA was implemented because CMS was trying to reduce costly medical errors. Medicare no longer pays hospitals for preventable medical errors in patient care, such as object left in during surgery, catheter-associated urinary tract infection, hospital acquired injury, and so on. POA refers to a diagnosis that is present at the time of the inpatient admission. It can include conditions known at the time of admission, present at admission but not diagnosed until later, and conditions that develop during outpatient encounters such as emergency department, observation, or outpatient surgery. This requirement is discussed later in this chapter for Field 67 when completing the UB-04 (CMS-1450) paper or 837i electronic claim form.

COMPLIANCE SAFEGUARDS

Many times a patient is seen in the physician's office (outpatient service), which leads the provider to admit the patient to the hospital as an inpatient; therefore services related to both outpatient and inpatient cases are performed. Problems may develop when billing for the physician's office is done on a separate billing system, making it difficult to match the outpatient services with subsequent inpatient hospital admission billed by the hospital's system. Ideally a facility should have a computer editing program that searches for any outpatient services given within the time frame before admission, or both sides (provider and hospital) should have integrated information systems. If not an integrated system, the hospital should have a relationship with the provider's office to obtain the minimum necessary information to treat the patient and bill for services. The hospital admitting clerk can also ask patients if they have received any medical service in the past 3 days; however, a patient may not be feeling well and not be able to recall or communicate the correct dates. Another solution is to use a post-claim submission review program that searches outpatient claims and generates a weekly report identifying the outpatient and inpatient accounts that overlap. This should be manually reviewed by a billing department supervisor or manager. Identified overpayments must be promptly documented and refunded to the insurance program.

UTILIZATION REVIEW

Each hospital should have a UR department that conducts an admission and concurrent review and prepares a discharge plan on all cases. An admission review is a review for appropriateness and necessity of admissions. A concurrent review is an evaluation of health care services to determine medical necessity and appropriateness of medical care during the time services are being provided. It is done by a health care provider other than the one giving the care. This process anticipates length of stay

(LOS) and concludes the expected discharge date. If the admission is found to be necessary, it is certified.

UR companies provide utilization review and case management services for self-insured employers, third-party administrators, and insurance companies. They furnish data to the person who buys their services to achieve cost savings, and they generate reports on how much money has been saved.

Quality Improvement Organization Program

CMS administers the **Quality Improvement Organization (QIO) program,** which is designed to monitor and improve the usage and quality of care for Medicare beneficiaries. The program consists of a national network of 53 QIOs (formerly known as *professional* or *peer review organizations [PROs]*) responsible for each state, territory, and the District of Columbia. QIO is governed by Titles XI and XVIII of the Social Security Act and is an organization contracting with CMS to review medical necessity, reasonableness, appropriateness, and completeness and adequacy of inpatient hospital care for which additional payment is sought under the outlier provisions of the PPS. QIOs are required to review all written quality of service complaints submitted by Medicare beneficiaries. The review addresses whether the services met professionally recognized standards of health care and may include whether the appropriate services were or were not provided in appropriate settings. The QIO's professional medical staff performs these reviews. The results of the reviews are submitted to CMS. The QIOs are responsible for the following types of review:

- **Admission review** for appropriateness and necessity of admissions.
- **Readmission review** on patients readmitted within 7 days with problems related to the first admission to determine whether the first discharge was premature or the second admission is medically necessary.
- **Procedure review** of diagnostic and therapeutic procedures in cases in which past abuses have been found, to determine appropriateness.
- **Day outlier review** of short or unusually long length of hospital stays to determine the number of days before the day outlier threshold is reached, as well as the number of days beyond the threshold. This process is done to certify necessity of admission and medical necessity of services for additional Medicare reimbursement.
- **Cost outlier review** of cases not eligible for day outlier review to determine the necessity of admission and the necessity and appropriateness of services rendered.
- **DRG validation** to find out whether the diagnostic and procedural information affecting DRG assignment

is substantiated by the clinical information in the patient's chart. DRGs are discussed later in this chapter.

- **Transfer review** of cases involving a transfer to a distinct part or unit of the same hospital or other hospitals.

CODING HOSPITAL DIAGNOSES AND PROCEDURES

Current Procedural Terminology (CPT), Medicare's Healthcare Common Procedure Coding System (HCPCS), and the three volumes of *International Classification of Diseases, Ninth Revision, Clinical Modification* (**ICD-9-CM**) are used to list codes on hospital insurance claims. Beginning in 2013, the code system will be *International Classification of Diseases, Tenth Revision, Clinical Modification* (ICD-10-CM) and *International Classification of Diseases, Tenth Revision, Procedure Classification System* (**ICD-10-PCS**). In lieu of the books, computer software programs contain the same data to locate the codes accurately, quickly, and easily. Different code books are used to code an insurance claim when a patient receives services as an outpatient or inpatient. They are the following:

- *Outpatient* hospital insurance claims use CPT and HCPCS codes for procedures and ICD-9-CM volumes 1 and 2 for diagnoses (in 2013 ICD-10-CM volumes 1 and 2).
- *Inpatient* hospital insurance claims use ICD-9-CM volumes 1 and 2 to code diagnostic conditions and volume 3 for coding procedures (in 2013 ICD-10-PCS). (Some private insurance companies request CPT codes.)

Chapter 5 provides basic information and instructions on how to use ICD-9-CM and ICD-10-CM volumes 1 and 2. This chapter explains the use of volume 3 and ICD-10-PCS. Chapter 6 gives information on CPT and HCPCS procedure codes.

Outpatient—Reason for Visit

The patient's reason for the visit is listed for outpatient claims rather than the patient's principal diagnosis (e.g., the reason for the outpatient visit may be chest pain, but anxiety could be listed as the final outpatient diagnosis).

Inpatient—Principal Diagnosis

The **principal diagnosis** is the condition that is assigned a code representing the diagnosis established after study that is chiefly responsible for the admission of the patient to the hospital. This is the most important code, so be sure the code for the principal diagnosis is listed first. For example, heart disease is the principal diagnosis if a patient initially comes in for heart transplantation. However, pneumonia is the principal diagnosis if the heart transplant patient goes home and then comes back to the hospital with pneumonia. Subsequent diagnostic codes should be used for any current condition that coexists with the principal condition, complicating the treatment and management of the principal disorder and that is documented in the record. These codes are sequenced after the principal diagnosis. Codes for conditions that were previously treated and no longer exist should not be included. A secondary diagnosis is one that may contribute to the condition, treatment, or recovery from the condition shown as the principal diagnosis. It also may define the need for a higher level of care but is not the underlying cause. The diagnostic **code sequence** (correct order) is important in billing of hospital inpatient cases because maximum reimbursement is based on the DRG system. This is explained in detail at the end of this chapter.

Rules for Coding Inpatient Diagnoses

Coding diagnoses for inpatient and outpatient cases can differ. One important difference is how uncertain diagnoses are coded. For inpatient cases, code all "rule out," "suspected," "likely," "questionable," "possible," or "still to be ruled out" as if it existed. For example, the physician documents *upper abdominal pain, rule out cholecystitis.* Assign code 575.0 (cholecystitis) for this diagnosis. This rule applies to inpatient records only.

In addition, the following rules and examples should be noted about the principal diagnosis.

- Codes for signs and symptoms of ICD-9-CM are not reported as principal diagnoses (Example 17-7).
- When two or more conditions meet the definition of principal diagnosis, either condition may be sequenced first unless otherwise indicated by the circumstances of admission or the therapy provided (Example 17-8).
- When a symptom is followed by a contrasting comparative diagnosis, sequence the symptom code first (Example 17-9).

Example 17-7 Principal Diagnosis/Signs and Symptoms

Mr. Brown was admitted to the hospital with fever, severe abdominal pain, nausea, and vomiting.

Diagnosis:	Acute appendicitis
ICD-9-CM Dx Code:	540.9 (acute appendicitis without peritonitis)
ICD-10-CM Dx Code:	K35.9 (acute appendicitis without generalized peritonitis)

NOTE: Symptoms are considered integral to the condition, so the condition should be coded.

Example 17-8 Two Medical Conditions

Mrs. Sanchez was admitted with acute congestive heart failure (CHF) and unstable angina. Both conditions are treated.

Diagnosis: CHF and unstable angina

ICD-9-CM Dx Code: 428.0 (CHF) or 411.1 (unstable angina). Either code may be used.

ICD-10-CM Dx Code: I50.9 (Congestive heart failure NOS) and I20.0 (unstable angina)

NOTE: This is the focus of many compliance reviews.

Example 17-9 Symptom as Principal Diagnosis

Miss Chan was admitted with acute epigastric abdominal pain.

Diagnosis: Epigastric abdominal pain, acute pyelonephritis versus acute gastritis.

ICD-9-CM Dx Code: 789.06 (epigastric abdominal pain)
                    590.10 (acute pyelonephritis)
                    535.00 (acute gastritis without hemorrhage)

ICD-10-CM Dx Code: R10.13 (epigastric pain)
                    N10 (acute pyelonephritis)
                    K29.00 (acute gastritis without bleeding)

NOTE: Code symptoms first followed by conditional diagnoses.

Conditions that are an integral part of a documented disease process should not be coded, and abnormal findings should not be coded unless the physician indicates their clinical significance.

The physician should be made aware that certain principal diagnoses are subject to 100% review by the review agency. The physician should pay special attention when using the following as principal diagnoses:

• Arteriosclerotic heart disease (ASHD)—acceptable as a diagnosis only when cardiac catheterization or open heart surgery is performed
• Diabetes mellitus without complications
• Right or left bundle branch block
• Coronary atherosclerosis

Local hospital health information management personnel should be contacted periodically to find out whether new items have been added to this list.

CODING INPATIENT PROCEDURES

ICD-9-CM Volume 3 Procedures

ICD-9-CM volume 3, which is not used in physician's offices, is used for the inpatient hospital setting and some payers require the codes on ambulatory surgical claims. This volume combines both the alphabetic and tabular lists for the classification of surgical and nonsurgical procedures and miscellaneous therapeutic and diagnostic procedures. Some editions of ICD-9-CM may contain volumes 1, 2, and 3 in one book.

ICD-9-CM Volume 3 Tabular List

The Tabular List is divided into chapters that relate to operations or procedures for various body systems, with the last chapter referring to miscellaneous diagnostic, therapeutic, and prophylactic procedures. Procedure codes are two digits at the category code level with one or two digits beyond the decimal point. The third and fourth digits differentiate unilateral or bilateral, surgical approach or technique, and condition type (e.g., indirect and direct hernia). No alphabetic characters are used. All four digits must be listed when a three-digit code is followed by a fourth digit. Remember to always code to the highest level of specificity. Chapter categories are as follows:

Chapter	Codes
Chapter 1 Operations on the Nervous System	Codes 01-05
Chapter 2 Operations on the Endocrine System	Codes 06-07
Chapter 3 Operations on the Eye	Codes 08-16
Chapter 4 Operations on the Ear	Codes 18-20
Chapter 5 Operations on the Nose, Mouth, and Pharynx	Codes 21-29
Chapter 6 Operations on the Respiratory System	Codes 30-34
Chapter 7 Operations on the Cardiovascular System	Codes 35-39
Chapter 8 Operations on the Hemic and Lymphatic System	Codes 40-41
Chapter 9 Operations on the Digestive System	Codes 42-54
Chapter 10 Operations on the Urinary System	Codes 55-59
Chapter 11 Operations on the Male Genital System	Codes 60-64
Chapter 12 Operations on the Female Genital System	Codes 65-71
Chapter 13 Obstetrical Procedures	Codes 72-75
Chapter 14 Operations on the Musculoskeletal System	Codes 76-84
Chapter 15 Operations on the Integumentary System	Codes 85-86
Chapter 16 Miscellaneous Diagnostic and Therapeutic Procedures	Codes 87-99

Alphabetic Index. The Alphabetic Index is arranged by procedure (e.g., incision, excision, graft, or implant) and not anatomic site. It is used to locate the procedure that is referred to as the main term. Read any notations that appear under the main term in bold type. A main term may be followed by modifiers (e.g., a series of subterms in parentheses) that give differences in site or surgical technique (Example 17-10).

Example 17-10 Main Diagnostic Term

Amputation (cineplastic) (closed flap) (guillotine) (kineplastic) (open) 84.91

An operation named for a person is termed an *eponym*. Such names are listed both as main terms and under the main term "operation." The description of the procedure or anatomic site follows the eponym (Example 17-11).

Example 17-11 Eponyms

Billroth II operation (partial gastrectomy with gastrojejunostomy) 43.7
Operation
Billroth II (partial gastrectomy with gastroduodenostomy) 43.6

Refer to the end of this chapter to learn the step-by-step procedure for coding from ICD-9-CM volume 3.

ICD-10-PCS

In 2013, when submitting diagnostic codes for inpatient hospital claims, ICD-10-PCS will replace ICD-9-CM volume 3 Procedures and Tabular List. Download free rough-draft versions of 2011 ICD-10-PCS Reference Manual, 2011 Code Tables and Index, and 2011 Development of ICD-10-PCS from the Internet to a flash drive or computer hard drive. Once downloaded, they are easily navigated. You must have Acrobat Reader (available at no charge from www.adobe.com) to open and read these files.

Code Structure

Because ICD-10-PCS codes have individual values and not lists of fixed codes with descriptions, each code in the system has a unique definition. ICD-10-PCS has a seven-character alphanumeric code structure. Each character contains up to 34 possible values. The 10 digits 0-9 and the 24 letters A-H, J-N, and P-Z may be used in each character. To avoid confusion with digits 0 and 1, the letters O and I are not used. There are 16 sections of the manual. The structure may be defined as follows:

Alphabetic Index

Locate codes in the index by the general type of procedure (e.g., drainage, dilation, or resection). It is not possible to construct a procedure code from the alphabetic index. The index gives the first three or four values of the code or directs you to see another term. Then, go to the appropriate table.

Tables

Each table has rows that specify the valid combination of code values, and a valid procedure code is chosen directly from the table.

Character Meaning

In each section, each of the 7 characters has a certain meaning.

Guidelines

Coding guidelines appear near the beginning of the codebook and must be read before locating a code. The three main sections of guidelines are: General, Medical and Surgical Section, and Other Medical and Surgical-Related Sections. In addition, each section, body system, root operation, body part, approach, device, and qualifier has specific guidelines that must be read before coding.

Procedure Coding

It is recommended that an individual have a high level of anatomy and physiology, medical terminology, and clinical knowledge to competently locate ICD-10-PCS codes. Therefore, step-by-step procedures for locating codes from the ICD-10-PCS codebook are not detailed in this Handbook. It is recommended that a separate course on ICD-10-PCS be undertaken to become skillful and proficient.

CODING OUTPATIENT PROCEDURES

HCPCS Level I CPT Coding System

The Medicare HCPCS (pronounced "hick-picks") consists of the following two levels of coding:

- Level I: the AMA CPT codes and modifiers (national codes)
- Level II: CMS-designated codes and alpha modifiers (national codes)

	Section	Body System	Root Operation	Body Part	Approach	Device	Qualifier
Characters:	1	2	3	4	5	6	7

An up-to-date edition of CPT, the code book published by the American Medical Association, is used to list procedural codes on outpatient hospital insurance claims for hospital services. Chapter 6 gives basic information and instruction on how to use the code book. These five-digit codes and two-digit modifiers are updated during each year. Billing software must be updated with new codes to receive maximum reimbursement.

HCPCS Level II Medicare National Coding System

The HCPCS Level II codebook is used to obtain procedural codes for Medicare and some non-Medicare patients on outpatient hospital insurance claims that are not in the CPT code book (e.g., supplies, equipment rental, and drugs administered other than oral method [injectables, inhalants, and chemotherapeutics]). Chapters 6 and 12 give basic information on this code system.

Modifiers

HCPCS Level I and II code systems contain modifiers. HCPCS Level I modifiers cannot be used with HCPCS Level II codes. HCPCS Level II modifiers may be used with HCPCS Level I or Level II codes. They can be used with a CPT or Medicare national code. When doing hospital billing, diagnosis codes, procedure codes, and modifiers are recorded on a worksheet and entered into a grouper program with other clinical information for either outpatient APC or inpatient DRG assignment. However, only specific CPT modifiers have been approved for hospital outpatient use as listed in Table 17-1. See Appendix A of the CPT manual or Chapter 6 of this textbook for a detailed explanation of CPT modifier use. Selected HCPCS/National Level II and CPT Level I modifiers that are generally approved and used for outpatient hospital billing are listed in Tables 17-1 and 17-2.

INPATIENT BILLING PROCESS

The insurance billing division is often part of the hospital's business office and may be placed near the admission department, hospital cashier, or main lobby (entry and exit) of the hospital because patients need easy access. In some facilities, the financial department may be so large that it is relocated to a building at another site. The inpatient billing process involves many people and departments in the hospital. As an introduction, Figure 17-4 shows which main departments of the hospital interact as the billing process flows from beginning to end. Explanations of each hospital employee's role in this process are included in the following.

Admitting Clerk

An admitting clerk registers the patient by interviewing and obtaining personal (demographic) and insurance information and admitting diagnosis or symptoms. There is no law requiring that a person give his or her real name

Table 17-1	HCPCS Level I CPT Modifiers for Hospital Outpatient Use					
MODIFIER	DESCRIPTION	E/M	SURGERY	RADIOLOGY	PATHOLOGY AND LABORATORY	MEDICINE
-25	Significant, separately identifiable E/M service by the same physician on the same day of the procedure or other service	•				
-27	Multiple outpatient hospital E/M encounters on the same date	•				
-50	Bilateral procedure		•			
-52	Reduced services		•	•	•	•
-58	Staged or related procedure or service by the same physician during the postoperative period		•			
-59	Distinct procedural service		•	•		•
-73	Discontinued outpatient procedure before anesthesia administration		•			
-74	Discontinued outpatient procedure after anesthesia administration		•			
-76	Repeat procedure by same physician		•	•		•
-77	Repeat procedure by another physician		•	•		•
-78	Return to the operating room for a related procedure during the postoperative period		•			•
-79	Unrelated procedure or service by the same physician during the postoperative period		•			
-91	Repeat clinical diagnostic laboratory test				•	

CPT, Current Procedural Terminology; E/M, evaluation and management; HCPCS, Healthcare Common Procedure Coding System.

Table 17-2	HCPCS Level II Medicare National Code Modifiers for Hospital Outpatient Use
MODIFIER	**DESCRIPTION**
-LT	Left side (used to identify procedures performed on the left side of the body)
-RT	Right side (used to identify procedures performed on the right side of the body)
-CA	Procedure payable only in the inpatient setting when performed emergently on an outpatient who expires before admission
-E1	Upper left, eyelid
-E2	Lower left, eyelid
-E3	Upper right, eyelid
-E4	Lower right, eyelid
-FA	Left hand, thumb
-F1	Left hand, second digit
-F2	Left hand, third digit
-F3	Left hand, fourth digit
-F4	Left hand, fifth digit
-F5	Right hand, thumb
-F6	Right hand, second digit
-F7	Right hand, third digit
-F8	Right hand, fourth digit
-F9	Right hand, fifth digit
-GA	Waiver of liability statement on file
-GG	Performance and payment of a screening mammogram and diagnostic mammogram on the same patient, same day
-GH	Diagnostic mammogram converted from screening mammogram on same day
-LC	Left circumflex, coronary artery (hospitals use with codes 92980-92984, 92995, 92996)
-LD	Left anterior descending coronary artery (hospitals use with codes 92980-92984, 92995, 92996)
-RC	Right coronary artery (hospitals used with codes 92980-92984, 92995, 92996)
-QM	Ambulance service provided under arrangement by a provider of services
-QN	Ambulance service furnished directly by a provider of services
-TA	Left foot, great toe
-T1	Left foot, second digit
-T2	Left foot, third digit
-T3	Left foot, fourth digit
-T4	Left foot, fifth digit
-T5	Right foot, great toe
-T6	Right foot, second digit
-T7	Right foot, third digit
-T8	Right foot, fourth digit
-T9	Right foot, fifth digit

on admission. High-profile individuals often give fictitious names. In some facilities, there may be a preadmission surgery form from which data are obtained for elective surgery. The admitting clerk position may be outsourced, and he or she may gather information via telephone from home for patients being admitted for elective procedures.

HIPAA Compliance Alert

The admitting clerk has the patient sign various legal documents (e.g., consent form for an invasive procedure, insurance assignment form, blanket form for routine hospital procedures, release of information forms, arbitration agreement, verification of acknowledgment of privacy information hospital policies, or responsibility for payment form). Patients must be reminded that they may be excluded from the hospital's daily patient census, which prohibits hospital workers from releasing their condition to the media. Also, a password can be selected by or assigned to each patient being admitted, thereby allowing disclosure to family members and friends who know the password given to them by the patient.

The patient is assigned a patient control number at this time. This is a unique number given for each hospital admission, and a new number is assigned for subsequent admissions. The patient's account contains this number and all charges and payments are posted to this number for the account. Copies of the admitting face sheet, which is similar to the patient registration information form, are sent to the primary care physician or surgeon's office. Registration information, copies of all authorization and signature documents, a copy of the insurance card or cards, and a copy of the emergency department report if the patient is admitted through the emergency department are scanned in paperless facilities or assembled in a financial folder in facilities using a traditional system.

Insurance Verifier

An insurance verifier, who may work either at the hospital or from home, reads the photocopied insurance identification card and may telephone the patient or physician for additional data. During or after admission, the insurance verifier's primary responsibility is to either swipe the card through scan equipment or contact the insurance plan by either a computer or telephone to verify eligibility, predetermine coverage, and obtain authorization if necessary. In a workers' compensation case, the verifier may telephone the employer or insurance adjuster for needed data.

Attending Physician, Nursing Staff, and Medical Transcriptionist

The patient is taken to the hospital department that is providing the outpatient service or, if an inpatient, to his or her hospital room. Generally, it is the attending physician's responsibility to dictate a history and physical (H

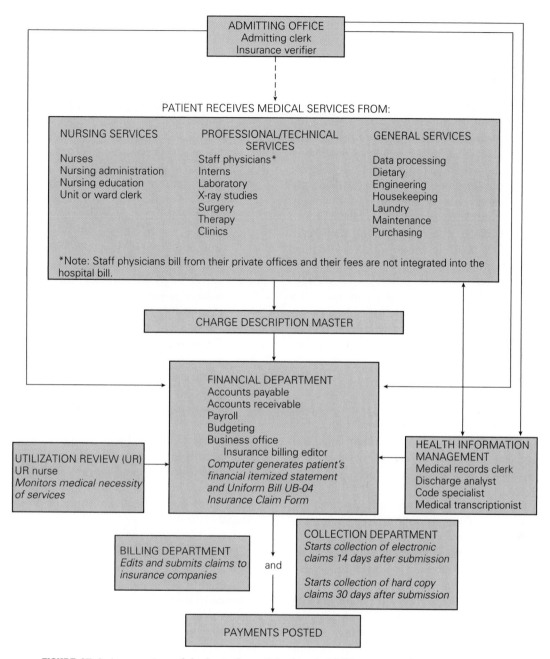

FIGURE 17-4 An overview of the basic flow of the hospital billing process for an inpatient.

& P) on admission that lists the admitting diagnosis. A medical transcriptionist transcribes the dictation into a report form. The attending physician and nurses enter daily notations on the patient's medical record as the patient receives medical services. A unit secretary or ward clerk inputs the physician's orders by use of a computer that electronically transmits them to other departments (e.g., pharmacy, laboratory, or radiology). A handheld computer may be used in some hospitals. If supplies are used, stickers are removed from the supply item and scanned to record data. The attending physician supplies documentation for all medical and surgical reports,

ending the patient's stay with a discharge summary that is sometimes known as a *clinical resume*. A final progress note may be substituted for a discharge summary under specific instances, that is, when the inpatient stay does not exceed 48 hours for an uncomplicated condition. This document is transcribed by the medical transcriptionist and includes the course of treatment during the hospital stay, all diagnostic studies, consultations, admission and discharge diagnoses, operations performed, condition of patient at the time of discharge, instructions for continuing care and follow-up treatment, and time frame for postoperative office visit.

Discharge Analyst

A discharge analyst, usually in the Health Information Management (medical records) department, checks the completeness of each patient's medical record for dictated reports and signatures. He or she completes a deficiency sheet that is put on the medical record indicating any documentation deficiencies. The office receptionist (administrative medical assistant) can help by scheduling the physician's time so that medical records can be completed. Hospitals bill for services only after the discharge summary is completed and signed by the physician. Many hospitals strive to complete charts within 3 to 4 days, and no more than 14 days, after a patient is discharged; otherwise a cash flow problem will result. Per The Joint Commission (TJC) (formerly the Joint Commission on Accreditation of Healthcare Organizations [JCAHO]), hospital charts may be completed up to 30 days after discharge. TJC is an accrediting body for clinics, hospitals, and other federal and military facilities. It reviews the policies, patient records, credentialing procedures, and quality assurance programs of the facility.

Charge Description Master

All services and items provided to the patient are keyed into a computer system to assist with a high volume of billing for services received by hospital patients. This may occur in one of the following two ways:

1. A designated person in each hospital department keys in (posts) all services and procedures using an internal code. This is referred to as *order entry*. The order entry automatically goes to the data processing department.
2. A charge sheet that has services and procedures checked off may be sent to the data processing department, where a data processor keys in the information using the internal code. These services, coded with an internal code, link up in a computer system called a **charge description master (CDM)**. This is commonly referred to as a *charge master* and includes the following data:
   a. *Procedure code.* CPT and HCPCS codes appear on detail bill, outpatient bill, outpatient paper or electronic 837i claim form, but not usually on the inpatient CMS-1450 (UB-04) claim form.
   b. *Charge.* Dollar amount for each CPT procedure or service. This is a standard fee for the item and not the actual amount paid by a third-party payer.
   c. *Revenue code.* A four-digit code number represents a specific accommodation, ancillary service, or billing calculation related to service that is inserted in Form Locator 42 of the CMS-1450 (UB-04) claim form. Examples are where the service was performed (0320 = Radiology), where the service may have been provided (0450 = ER), or the total

dollar amount of the services provided for a particular time frame/bill/claim (0001 = last entry on the bill). The revenue code must be coded to the highest level of specificity. You may see a code 030X with the "X" indicating that further breakdown is necessary to best identify the service or supply being provided. Before using a fourth digit, confirm that the code is accepted by the payer. Some payers require the general code (three digit) instead of the four-digit code. Some revenue codes may indicate that a service should be put on a CMS-1500 (08-05) claim form instead of a CMS-1450 (UB-04) claim form. For example, durable medical equipment (DME) code 0292 must be submitted on a CMS-1500 (08-05) claim form, not on a CMS-1450 (UB-04), with the correct HCPCS and facility DME provider number. For Medicare, some revenue codes can only be used on an outpatient claim. The facility software should be able to hard-code a revenue code for inpatient but a different revenue code for outpatient for the same service/supply by financial class. An HIPAA compliance issue is that it would be fraudulent for a biller to change a revenue code so that a claim would pass edits.

The master charge list or charge description list is a computer file unique to each hospital that accommodates the charges for items and services that may be provided to patients. The content and format of the charge master varies among facilities, but the function remains the same.

Thus charges may be easily compiled via computer from all hospital departments that furnished services to the patient. For institutional facilities (e.g., inpatient and outpatient departments, rural health clinics, chronic dialysis services, or adult day health care), each patient's data consisting of revenue codes, procedure codes, descriptions, charges, and medical record data are organized by the charge description master and printed onto a hospital paper CMS-1450 (UB-04) or stored electronically for future claim transmission.

The charge master database must be kept current and accurate to obtain proper reimbursement. It must be regularly audited; otherwise, negative impacts such as overpayment, underpayment, undercharging for services, claims rejections, fines, or penalties may result. A committee may oversee maintenance of the charge master composed of experts in coding, billing regulations, clinical procedures, and health record documentation. Because this system is often accomplished without human intervention, there is a high risk that a single coding or data mapping error could replicate and many errors could occur before being identified and corrected. Data mapping is a method of matching one set of data elements or individual code values to the nearest equivalents in another set, also known as *crosswalk*. Duplicate reports of CPT or HCPCS level II codes for the same service, both by the department performing the service and by the HIM coding specialists, are common billing problems. These problems may be prevented by regularly reviewing the charge master (sorted by CPT code number) with the coding staff so that they are aware of the codes reported via the charge master. Category III CPT codes should be reported by only one source, either the department that charges for the service or the code specialist. *Category III codes* are temporary codes for emergency technology, services, and procedures and are used instead of a category I unlisted code number.

In a direct data entry (DDE) system, there is usually a lag time (e.g., from 1 to 4 days after patient discharge) before the bill is "dropped" by the charge master to be sure that all charges have been entered. The word *dropped* refers to the dropped time, which is the time between the discharge of the patient from the hospital and the input of the late charges to the time when the final bill is printed.

Code Specialist

The chart is given to health information management, which is directed or managed by a registered health information administrator (RHIA) or registered health information technician (RHIT). In some situations, an RHIA/RHIT may act as a consultant to several hospitals and may not be employed by one hospital. This department is also composed of discharge analysts, coding specialists, and clerical staff. A *medical record number* is assigned at the time of admission. The medical record number never changes (even on future admits), and all records are compiled under this number.

An HIM coder abstracts procedures and diagnoses from the patient's health record and assigns the appropriate codes for the services given. It is possible that the coder may use an encoder to perform this function. As learned, an encoder is a computer software program that assigns a code to represent data. See Chapter 8 for detailed information.

Coding Credentials

Accuracy of coding affects the financial viability of acute care hospitals. The coder, whose job is highly analytical, should not only abstract information from the medical record and assign the correct code but also guard against the most common errors of transposing numbers and leaving off fourth and fifth digits from diagnostic codes. A majority of coders in the hospital setting have credentials and have earned a certificate or degree from an educational institute. A number of different professional organizations that offer certification for coders are mentioned in Chapter 18.

Insurance Billing Editor

The 837i (CMS-1450/UB-04) electronic claim form is put through software that has editing capabilities (e.g., outpatient coding edits [OCE] and Medicare coding edits [MCE]). It is then generated and reviewed by an insurance billing editor before it is generated as a paper claim or transmitted electronically to the appropriate insurance company to obtain payment. Editing claims is a vital skill that is gained from hands-on experience. Information from the patient's financial data may be compared to verify insurance information. The CMS-1450 (UB-04) is considered a *summary statement*, which compiles all charges, and is accompanied by a *detailed statement*, which shows itemized charges. The detailed statement, which is sent to the patient, lists dates of services, codes, descriptions, and fees for individual services. The CMS-1500 (08-05) claim form is used for physicians' professional outpatient claims.

A systematic approach should be established when editing a claim, and the same procedure should be used each time. The procedure of learning to edit a CMS-1450 (UB-04) is presented at the end of this chapter. This helps train the editor to notice errors or omitted information. Insurance personnel should understand coding, but in a hospital setting it is not their job to assign codes. Final code selection is done by clinical coding specialists. Reviewing form locators (FL) 42 through 47 is the most time-consuming portion of the editing process and the area that requires experience to master. This is the area where most of the errors and omissions occur.

Refer to the procedure at the end of this chapter for a suggested sequence of steps in editing a CMS-1450 (UB-04) claim.

The claim form may go back to the health information management department after it is edited (where the coder verifies all codes) and to the contract department (where a contractor matches the bill with the insurance type). An adjustment to the account is posted, indicating the dollar amount above that which the insurance carrier will pay according to the contract. This adjustment is done after the insurance payment is received in the majority of hospitals. However, a small number of hospitals are able to write off the portion of the bill that is not covered by the insurance plan before receipt of payment. This transaction is referred to as *relieving the accounts receivable on the front end* and is desirable because the accounts receivable does not appear inflated.

Electronically transmit or mail all claim forms to the insurance carrier for payment and retain computer files or copies for the office files. Document the patient's file with the date mailed and the address to which the insurance claim was filed. The claim may be rejected or delayed if errors are not caught, leading to slow payment or nonpayment. See Chapter 7 for a list of common reasons why claims are rejected or delayed.

Nurse Auditor

Registered nurses (RNs) work as nurse auditors and verify the doctor's orders and the medical record against each charge item on the bill. They may be onsite employees or hired offsite to come in periodically. The nurse must have clinical and financial expertise. A *clean bill* has no errors. An *under bill* has services that have been provided and not billed. An *over bill* has charged items that have not been documented in the chart. A report goes to the health information management department if a coding error or omission occurs. All such accounts have coding priority. Several types of audits follow:

- *Random internal audit.* This occurs continually. Blind charts are pulled and audited to maintain quality control.
- *Audit by request.* The patient can request an audit to verify charges.
- *Defense audit.* The insurance company requests an audit. The insurance auditor may or may not (but should) meet with a hospital auditor, depending on the circumstances. Charts are pulled and audited.

REIMBURSEMENT PROCESS

Generally, a hospital bill for inpatient care is much larger than the bill for services rendered in a physician's office. Individuals are admitted to hospitals for severe health problems, and many require major surgery, resulting in considerable expense to the patient. Hospitals use and maintain highly sophisticated, expensive equipment; are located in large facilities; and employ large numbers of personnel, many of whom are state licensed and specialized. Salaries and operating costs must be recovered through patient billing. The majority of hospital reimbursement is from insurance companies. However, working parents with families, elderly people, and jobless persons (even those who have insurance) have found it increasingly difficult to pay their share of the hospital bills. Consequently, accurate and timely hospital billing and good follow-up and collection techniques are in demand. In Chapter 10, you learned that a patient seeking medical care who is unable to pay for services and is ineligible for state aid should be directed to the local hospital that services recipients under the Hill-Burton Act of 1946. These hospitals obtained federal construction grants to enlarge their facilities in exchange for their provision of health care for needy patients. The Department of Health and Human Services will furnish the names of local hospitals that participate in this service. Patients must complete financial applications to determine eligibility before care is rendered.

Reimbursement Methods

Growing numbers of the population are being served by a variety of managed health care programs. All of these programs operate under varying contracts, policies, and guidelines, depending on individual state and federal laws. In negotiating a reimbursement arrangement, the managed care plan administrator tries to obtain discount rates for participation by a hospital in the plan in exchange for an increased volume of patients. These programs use any one or a combination of various payment methods. However, as health care costs escalate, some of these payment methods have been discontinued. See Chapter 11 for definitions on types of managed care plans. A brief description of some reimbursement methods follows:

- *Ambulatory payment classifications.* An outpatient classification system developed by Health Systems International is **ambulatory payment classifications (APCs).** This method is based on procedures rather than diagnoses. For Medicare patients, services associated with a specific procedure or visit are bundled into the APC reimbursement. More than one APC may be billed if more than one procedure is performed, but discounts may be applied to any additional APCs. This topic is discussed in detail at the end of this chapter.
- *Bed leasing.* A managed care plan leases beds from a facility (e.g., payment to the hospital of $300 per bed for 20 beds, regardless of whether those beds are used).
- *Capitation or percentage of revenue.* **Capitation** means reimbursement to the hospital on a per-member, per-month basis regardless of whether the patient is hospitalized. **Percentage of revenue** means a fixed percentage paid to the hospital to cover charges.
- *Case rate.* **Case rate** is an averaging after a flat rate (set amount paid for a service) has been given to certain categories of procedures (e.g., normal vaginal delivery is $1800 and cesarean section is $2300). Utilization is expected to be 80% vaginal deliveries and 20% cesarean section; therefore the case rate is $1900 for all deliveries. Specialty procedures may also be given a case rate (e.g., coronary artery bypass graft surgery or heart transplantation). *Bundled case rate* means an all-inclusive rate is paid for both institutional and professional services; for example, for coronary artery bypass graft surgery, a rate is used to pay all who provide services connected with that procedure. Bundled case rates are seen in teaching facilities in which a faculty practice plan works closely with the hospital.

- *Contract rate.* A set amount for payment to the hospital is established in the contract between the hospital and the managed care plan.
- *Diagnosis-related groups.* A classification system called **diagnosis-related groups (DRGs)** categorizes patients who are medically related with respect to diagnosis and treatment and are statistically similar in length of hospital stay. Medicare and some private hospital insurance payments are based on fixed dollar amounts determined by DRGs. DRGs are discussed in detail later in the chapter.
- *Differential by day in hospital.* The first day of the hospital stay is paid at a higher rate (e.g., the first day may be paid at $1000 and each subsequent day at $500). Most hospitalizations are more expensive on the first day. This type of reimbursement method may be combined with a per diem arrangement.
- *Differential by service type.* The hospital receives a flat per-admission reimbursement for the service to which the patient is admitted. A prorated payment may be made (e.g., 50% for intensive care and 50% medicine) if services are mixed. Service types are defined in the contract (e.g., medicine, surgery, intensive care, neonatal intensive care, psychiatry, obstetrics).
- *Fee-for-service.* The hospital is paid for each medical service provided on the basis of an established schedule of fees.
- *Fee schedule.* A comprehensive listing of charges based on procedure codes, under a fee-for-service (FFS) arrangement, or discounted FFS, states fee maximums paid by the health plan within the period of the managed care contract. Usually the fee schedule is based on CPT codes. For industrial cases, whether managed care or not, this listing may be called a workers' compensation fee schedule. This document is also known as a *fee maximum schedule* or *fee allowance schedule* as established by the state.
- *Flat rate.* A set amount (single charge) per hospital admission is paid by the managed care plan, regardless of the cost of the actual services the patient receives.
- *Per diem.* **Per diem** is a single charge for a day in the hospital regardless of actual charges or costs incurred (e.g., a plan that pays $800 for each day regardless of the actual cost of service).
- *Percentage of accrued charges.* Payment calculates reimbursement on the basis of a percentage of total approved charges accrued during a hospital stay and submitted to the insurance plan.
- *Periodic interim payments (PIPs) and cash advances.* These are methods in which the plan advances cash to cover expected claims to the hospital. The fund is replenished periodically. Insurance claims may be applied to the cash advance or may be paid outside it. Generally this is done by Medicare.
- *Relative value studies (scale) (RVS).* A list of procedure codes for professional services and procedures are assigned unit values that indicate the relative value of one procedure over another.
- *Resource-based relative value scale (RBRVS).* This payment system is implemented under the prospective payment system for Medicare and other government programs and provides reimbursement for outpatient services. It is based on a formula. The formula is the relative value unit of each service must equal the sum of relative value units representing physicians' work, practice expenses, and cost of professional liability insurance.
- *Usual, customary, and reasonable (UCR).* This method is used by third-party payers to establish their fee schedules in which three fees are considered in calculating payment: (1) the usual fee is the fee typically submitted by the provider; (2) the customary fee falls within the range of usual fees charged by the provider in a geographic area; and (3) the reasonable fee meets the aforementioned criteria or is considered justifiable because of special circumstances.
- *Withhold.* In this method, part of the plan's payment to the hospital may be withheld or set aside in a bonus pool. If the hospital meets or exceeds the criteria set down, the hospital receives its withhold or bonus; other terms used are bonus pools, capitation, risk pools, and withhold pools.
- *Managed care stop loss outliers.* **Stop loss** is a form of guarantee that may be written into a contract using one of a variety of methods. The purpose is to limit the exposure of cost to a reasonable level to prevent excessive loss. Stop loss is the least understood of reimbursement issues and can leave many thousands of dollars uncollected. There are a number of different ways stop loss can be applied; each contract is different. Become familiar with each contract and the stop loss provisions in it. Following are some methods that may be encountered.
  - *Case-based stop loss.* This is the most common stop loss and can apply to the physician, on a smaller case basis, as well as to the individual hospital claim. For example, the hospital bill may run more than $1 million in cases of premature infants of extremely low birth weight. The contract may pay $2000 to $3000 per day, which may reimburse the hospital several hundred thousand dollars, but the hospital must absorb the excess. Stop loss provisions may pay 65% of the excess over $100,000. Thus the hospital and the insurance carrier share the loss.
  - *Reinsurance stop loss.* The hospital buys insurance to protect against lost revenue and receives less of a capitation fee; the amount they do not receive helps pay for the insurance. For example, if a case has one or more claims that exceeds $100,000 in a calendar year, the plan may receive 80% of expenses in excess of $100,000 from the reinsurance company for the remainder of the year.

- *Percentage stop loss.* Some managed care contracts pay a percentage of charges when the total charge exceeds a listed contracted amount.
- *Medicare stop loss.* Medicare provides stop loss called *outliers* in its regulations. The *day outliers* for patients who remain in the hospital for long spells of illness no longer apply. Medicare provides cost outliers for those cases in which charges exceed the DRG or $30,000. DRGs are discussed at the end of this chapter.

Some reimbursement methods that are not used very much follow:

- *Charges.* In a managed care plan, **charges** are the dollar amounts owed to a participating provider for health care services rendered to a plan member, according to a fee schedule set by the managed care plan. This is the most expensive and least desirable type of reimbursement contract, so not many of these contracts exist.
- *Discounts in the form of sliding scale.* This is a form of discount with a limit in which the percentage amount increases, based on hospital numbers (e.g., a 10% reduction in charges for 0 to 500 total bed days per year with incremental increases in the discount up to a maximum percentage.
- *Sliding scales for discounts and per diems.* Based on total volume of business generated, this is a reimbursement method in which an interim per diem is paid for each day in the hospital. For example, a lump sum is either added to or withheld from the payment due at the end of each year to adjust for actual hospital usage. This is difficult to administer because it can be done either monthly or annually.

Electronic Data Interchange

As early as the 1980s, large hospitals began submitting electronic claims for payment to third-party payers instead of printing the CMS-1450 (UB-82) claim form. Just as in the health care provider's office, the use of electronic data interchange (EDI) allows the claim to arrive at the insurance company the same day it is generated to allow for an expeditious payment. Confirmation of claim transmission and receipt is received within minutes or hours and must be recorded in the hospital financial records. Use of computer software assists the insurance billing editor in checking for errors before forwarding the claim to the proper claims office. This is called **scrubbing** or *cleaning the bill*. Medicare, Medicaid, group health carriers, many managed care plans, and some workers' compensation carriers mandate use of EDI. All hospital electronic billing goes through a clearinghouse, where additional edits are made and claims are batched and sent electronically to insurance companies.

Billing can be set up according to days or dollar amounts, typically every 30 days. If a Medicare patient remains in an acute care hospital, he or she may be billed on the 60th day and not again until discharge. Refer to Chapter 8 for detailed information on this topic.

Hard Copy Billing

A printed paper copy of the CMS-1450 (UB-04) that is generated from the computer system is referred to as a *hard copy*. The same edits are made and the claim is cleaned (scrubbed) before it is sent. Some insurance companies are not capable of receiving electronic claims, so billing by hard copy is mandatory. All secondary insurance companies and claims that require attachments also fit into this category.

Receiving Payment

Timeliness of payment may be included in a contract to encourage a hospital to join a plan (e.g., an additional 4% discount for paying a clean claim within 14 days of receipt), or a hospital may demand a penalty for clean claims not processed within 30 days. Some states require this payment by law.

After receipt of payment from insurance and managed care plans, the patient is sent a net bill that lists any owed deductible, coinsurance amount, and charges for services not covered under the insurance policy. Standard bookkeeping procedures are used to post entries showing payments and adjustments. Financial management for managed care programs is discussed and shown in figures in Chapter 11.

OUTPATIENT INSURANCE CLAIMS

The term **outpatient** is used when an individual receives medical service in a section or department of the hospital and goes home the same day or receives care in a physician's office. In addition, outpatient services may occur in a clinic, imaging center, laboratory, emergency department, rehabilitation center, urgent care clinic, or ambulatory surgery center. If an individual has an accident, injury, or acute illness, he or she may seek the services of medical personnel in the emergency department of the hospital. When seen in this department, a patient is considered an outpatient unless he or she is admitted for overnight hospital stay. Many elective surgeries are done on an outpatient surgery basis. **Elective surgery** indicates a surgical procedure that can be scheduled in advance, is not an emergency, and is discretionary on the part of the physician and patient. Elective procedures are those that are deferrable, which means that the patient will not experience serious consequences if the operation is postponed or there is failure to undergo the operation.

Some insurance policies require a second opinion for elective surgery. The insurance company may not pay if the patient does not seek a second opinion and chooses to undergo surgery. See Chapter 12 for elective surgery in regard to the Medicare program. Patients may receive certain types of therapy and diagnostic testing services on an outpatient basis.

Hospital Professional Services

Although physicians make daily hospital visits to their patients, perform surgeries, discharge patients from the hospital, and are called to the hospital to provide consultations and emergency department treatment, their professional services are submitted on the CMS-1500 (08-05) insurance claim form by the physician and not by the hospital billing department. Only services provided by the hospital should be submitted by the hospital unless the hospital is billing for physicians who are on the hospital payroll. Such hospital services include the following:

- ED facility fee (supplies)
- Laboratory (technical component)
- Radiology (technical component)
- Physical and occupational therapy facility fee

Personnel who work in these departments (e.g., ED physician, pathologist, radiologist, and physical therapist) might be employees of the hospital. The hospital submits bills for professional services in that situation. The professional charges are billed independently if the physician is not an employee.

Using the hospital for surgical or medical consultations that could be done in a specialist's office should be avoided unless the patient physically requires admission. This necessity should be documented. If a patient is admitted for consultation only, the entire payment for hospital admission will be denied, as will any physician fees involved.

BILLING PROBLEMS

Most hospitals routinely send the patient an itemized list of all charges. Many times, patients are stunned by the total balance due and are unable to make sense of specific items, abbreviations, or codes on the statement. A bill should never show unexplained codes or items without descriptions. A brief hospital stay may translate into hundreds of individual charges. A patient has the right to request, examine, and question a detailed statement, as mentioned in the Patient's Bill of Rights—a nationally recognized code of conduct published by the American Hospital Association. If the bill lumps charges together under broad categories, such as pharmacy, surgical supplies, and radiology, and the patient requests an itemized

invoice, it should be provided at no cost to the patient. In fact, consumer advocates and policies governing the Medicare program encourage consumers to scrutinize their hospital bills for mistakes. The hospital may receive a call or letter from the patient asking for an explanation of the charges if the charges seem exorbitant. Sometimes, hospital billing personnel, a hospital patient representative or advocate, the attending physician, and his or her staff may be able to satisfactorily explain a confusing charge.

Medicare, Medicaid, and some insurance companies have begun to stop reimbursing hospitals for never events. *Never events* are surgical procedures that are performed on the wrong side, wrong site, wrong body part, or wrong person (e.g., an object left inside a patient during surgery, use of the wrong blood type during a transfusion, or infection from a urinary catheter). Some hospitals do not charge for never events, whereas other facilities may charge for certain ones.

Common billing errors are as follows:

- Incorrect name; use of maiden name instead of married name
- Wrong subscriber; patient's name listed in error
- Covered days versus noncovered days

Duplicate Statements

Duplicate billings, which may confuse the patient, can occur when a patient receives inpatient and outpatient preadmission tests or services. Perhaps a test was canceled and rescheduled and a charge is shown for the canceled test, or several physicians may have consulted on a case and each ordered the same test or therapy. Possibly, a technician took the incorrect amount of blood or produced an unclear radiograph, submitted a charge for the service performed in error, as well as for the correct service, and thereby generated two charges for one test. These examples are hospital personnel errors.

Double Billing

Another example involving a violation of Medicare policy is double billing, which results when a patient undergoes routine outpatient testing for a specific diagnosis and then develops unanticipated problems related to that diagnosis that require hospital admission. Outpatient personnel may not be aware that the patient was later admitted, and inpatient personnel may not know that the patient had undergone outpatient testing within the previous 72 hours. A hospital that bills for such services may be fined because it is in violation of the Medicare 3-day window rule. Such charges must be bundled into the inpatient DRG payment. Therefore it is imperative that the hospital billing department develop procedures to check for potential double-billing problems.

Phantom Charges

Physicians order admission procedures for each patient who enters the hospital. If a patient refuses some of these tests, the charges should be deleted from the financial records before the bill is sent out. Similarly, a patient should not be charged for refused medication. The hospital may offer a standard kit of supplies on admission or a new-mother packet when appropriate. A patient should not have to pay for supplies that he or she refuses. If a patient requests a semiprivate room but is sent to a private room because all semiprivate rooms are occupied, the patient should not be billed at the higher rate. Phantom charges may appear if a scheduled test is canceled by a physician or the patient is released early, making it imperative to check the dates and times of admission and discharge. Charges that should appear on a patient's itemized statement may be missing because the charges were transferred to the wrong patient's bill. This requires a review of the patient's medical records. The charge should be deleted from the bill when a charge cannot be accounted for by a review of the patient's medical record or by talking to the attending physician.

HOSPITAL BILLING CLAIM FORM

Uniform Bill Inpatient and Outpatient Paper or Electronic Claim Form

In 1982 the UB-82 claim form was developed for hospital claims and printed in green ink. A revision was issued in 1992, which became known as the Uniform Bill (UB-92). Because it was determined that an update of this form was necessary, a new form made its appearance in 2007 called the UB-04 claim form. The **Uniform Bill (UB-04) paper** or **electronic claim form** is also known as the **CMS-1450.** This form is considered a summary document supported by an itemized or detailed bill. It is used by institutional facilities (e.g., inpatient and outpatient departments, rural health clinics, chronic dialysis services, or adult day health care) to submit claims for inpatient and outpatient services. The UB-04 has 81 form locators (fields) and its four sections are divided as follows: provider information (form locators 1-7), patient information (form locators 8-38), billing information (form locators 39-49 and claim line 23), payer information (form locators 50-65), and diagnostic information (form locators 66-81). This paper claim form is printed in red ink on white paper for processing with optical scanning equipment. Figure 17-5 illustrates a completed CMS-1450 (UB-04) paper claim form. Dates of service and monetary values are entered without spaces or decimal points (e.g., $200 should be shown as 20000, and June

23, 2007, should be shown as 062307). Dates of birth are entered using two sets of two-digit numbers for the month and day and a four-digit number for the year (e.g., June 23, 1995, should be shown as 06231995). See Chapter 6 for information on how to complete the CMS-1500 (08-05) Claim Form for professional services.

DIAGNOSIS-RELATED GROUPS

History

The concept of DRGs was developed by Professors John D. Thompson and Robert B. Fetter at Yale University and tested in New Jersey from 1977 to 1979. The goal was to develop a scheme of patient classification to be used in UR.* Soon, other applications were found in such areas as budgeting, planning, and reimbursement.

Because of inconsistencies and inadequacies in the original concept, a second set of DRGs was developed and was used in New Jersey since 1982. Under the Medicare PPS, the DRGs were implemented nationwide for all hospitalizations after the Tax Equity and Fiscal Responsibility Act of 1982 (TEFRA) was passed. The purpose of a DRG-based two-tiered system used for Medicare reimbursement was to hold down rising health care costs. Therefore Medicare reimbursement as a whole was expected to and did decrease significantly under the original DRG payment system. In 2008, the system was renamed Medicare Severity Diagnosis-Related Group (MS-DRG), which is a more complex three-tiered system. Extensive changes were made to the program, and this system is designed to increase reimbursement for sicker patients.

The Medicare Severity Diagnosis-Related Group System

The original DRG system was a patient classification method that categorized patients who were medically related with respect to diagnosis and treatment and who were statistically similar in length of stay. It was used to both classify past cases to measure the relative resources hospitals have expanded to treat patients with similar illnesses and to classify current cases to determine payment. This system changed hospital reimbursement from a fee-for-service system to a lump sum, fixed-fee payment on the basis of the diagnoses rather than on time or services rendered. The fees were fixed by a research team, which determined a national "average" fee for each of the principal discharge diagnoses. The classifications were formed from more than 10,000 ICD-9-CM codes that were divided into 25 basic **major diagnostic categories (MDCs).**

---

*Review of hospital admissions to determine whether they are justified; this is discussed at the beginning of the chapter.

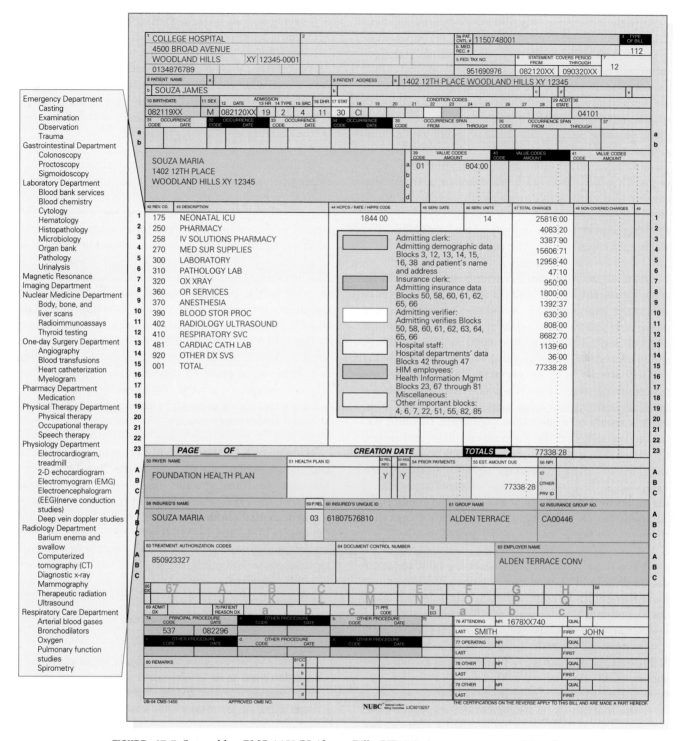

FIGURE 17-5 Scannable CMS-1450/Uniform Bill (UB-04) insurance paper claim form completed for an inpatient showing hospital departments that input data for hospital services. Colored blocks indicate data obtained by various hospital personnel. Job titles and the exact data each person obtains may vary from facility to facility. Form locator guidelines vary and may not always follow the visual guide presented here.

As of the printing of this edition, Medicare's Inpatient Prospective Payment System (IPPS) has 745 MS-DRGs. These diagnoses were assigned specific values commensurate with severity of illness, whereas the original DRGs were assigned values based on geographic areas, types of hospitals, depreciation values, teaching status, and other specific criteria. MS-DRGs are split into a maximum of three payment tiers on the basis of patient severity as determined by the presence of a major complication/comorbidity (MCC), a complication/comorbidity (CC), or no CC. TRICARE and other private insurers that employ DRGs use DRG numbers 600 to 900. To obtain MS-DRG information, go to the *Federal Register's* website each September for the update, which is mentioned in the Internet Resources at the end of this chapter.

Hospital facilities contract with Medicare to supply acute inpatient care and agree to accept a predetermined amount of reimbursement based on the diagnoses and procedures related to the patient during their inpatient hospital stay. The diagnoses stated on the discharge summary and the procedures that were performed during the stay are the basis for payment. Each diagnosis and procedure is grouped into MS-DRGs that contain similar amounts and types of hospital resources. Using a computer software program called a **grouper,** this information is keyed in and the program calculates and assigns the MS-DRG payment group. These MS-DRGs are weighted to reflect the average costs for inpatient care. **Looping** is the grouper process of searching all listed diagnoses for the presence of any comorbid condition or complication or searching all procedures for operating room procedures or more specific procedures.

When the ICD-10 is implemented, a reimbursement crosswalk should be used that identifies ICD-9 and corresponding ICD-10 codes and MS-DRGs. If an ICD-10 code combines the descriptions of two separate ICD-9 codes, then the ICD-10 code replaces the more commonly used ICD-9 code. In some cases, several general ICD-9 codes in a "cluster" may be replaced with one specific ICD-10 code.

A case that cannot be assigned to an appropriate DRG because of an atypical situation is called a **cost outlier.** These atypical situations are as follows:

1. **Clinical outliers:**
   a. Unique combinations of diagnoses and surgeries causing high costs
   b. Very rare conditions
2. Long length of stay, or day outliers, no longer apply
3. Low-volume DRGs
4. Inliers (hospital case falls below the mean average or expected length of stay)
5. Death

6. Leaving against medical advice (AMA)
7. Admitted and discharged on the same day

The current federal plan for outliers is the full DRG rate plus an additional payment for the services provided. An unethical practice, **DRG creep,** is to code a patient's DRG category for a more severe diagnosis than indicated by the patient's condition. This is also called *upcoding.*

In hospital billing, *downcoding* can also erroneously occur when sequencing several diagnoses (e.g., listing a normal pregnancy as the primary diagnosis for payment and complications in the secondary position when the patient remained in the hospital for an extended number of days). Additional examples are discussed in Chapter 6.

The amount of payment may be increased by documenting in the patient's medical record any comorbid conditions or complications. When referring to DRGs, the abbreviation CC is used to indicate such complications or comorbidities (not the more common interpretation found in patient charting, chief complaint). **Comorbidity** is defined as a preexisting condition that, because of its effect on the specific principal diagnosis, will require more intensive therapy or cause an increase in length of stay by at least 1 day in approximately 75% of cases.

If a patient is discharged with two or more conditions and the physician fails to indicate the "most resource-intensive" or "most specific" diagnosis as the principal diagnosis, the DRG assessment will be incorrect, resulting in decreased reimbursement to the health care facility (Examples 17-12 and 17-13). It is the responsibility of the attending physician to certify the sequencing of the principal diagnosis and other diagnoses on the basis of his or her best judgment.

Example 17-12 Comorbid Condition and Complication

A patient has had congestive heart failure for several years and is admitted with an admitting diagnosis of chest pain and principal diagnosis of anterior wall myocardial infarction (MI). While hospitalized, the patient experiences atrial fibrillation.

ICD-9-CM

Principal diagnosis:	410.11 anterior wall myocardial infarction, initial episode
Comorbid condition (CC):	428.0 congestive heart failure
Complication:	427.31 atrial fibrillation

ICD-10-CM

Principal diagnosis:	I21.09 acute transmural myocardial infarction of anterior wall
Comorbid condition (CC):	I50.9 Congestive heart failure NOS
Complication:	I48.0 atrial fibrillation

Example 17-13 **Comorbid Condition and Complication**

A patient has had chronic obstructive pulmonary disease (COPD) for the past 6 months and is admitted with an admitting diagnosis of chest pain and a principal diagnosis of anterior wall myocardial infarction (MI). While hospitalized, the patient experiences respiratory failure.

ICD-9-CM

Principal diagnosis:	410.11 anterior wall myocardial infarction
Comorbid condition:	496 chronic obstructive pulmonary disease
Complication:	799.1 respiratory failure

ICD-10-CM

Principal diagnosis:	I21.09 acute transmural myocardial infarction of anterior wall
Comorbid condition:	J44.9 chronic obstructive pulmonary disease, unspecified
Complication:	J96.9 respiratory failure, unspecified

Both examples warrant additional payment because of comorbid conditions and complications.

Diagnosis-Related Groups and the Physician's Office

Even though DRGs affect Medicare hospital payments, the individual in a physician's office who communicates the admitting diagnosis to the hospital can greatly affect the DRG assignment. Remember the following points:

1. Give all of the diagnoses authorized by the physician, if there are more than one, when calling the hospital to admit a patient so that the hospital personnel can use their expertise in listing the primary and secondary diagnoses.
2. Ask the physician to review the treatment or procedure in question when a hospital representative calls about a test, length of stay, or treatments ordered by the attending physician. The hospital needs this information to justify a higher-than-average bill to Medicare.
3. Get to know the hospital personnel on a first-name basis so that when the physician or patients have DRG-related questions, you can call on this hospital expert.

OUTPATIENT CLASSIFICATION

In late 2000, under the requirements of the Balanced Budget Act of 1997, the CMS implemented a PPS for Medicare beneficiaries. This was a move from a cost-based reimbursement system to a line-item billing system for ambulatory surgery centers and hospital outpatient services. The CMS has categorized outpatient services into an ambulatory payment classification system. Some Medicaid programs and private payers have embraced this system because of the escalation of outpatient costs.

Ambulatory Payment Classification System

Originally, ambulatory visit groups (AVGs) and then ambulatory patient groups (APGs) were developed as outpatient classification systems by Health Systems International (HSI). These groups were based on patient classifications (ICD-9-CM diagnoses, CPT and HCPCS procedures, age, and gender) rather than disease classifications. Ambulatory surgery categories (ASCs) were then adopted, replacing APGs for outpatient or 1-day surgery cases that were derived from the surgery section of the CPT. ASCs used disease and procedural coding classification systems to supply the input to the computer program to assign ASCs.

Recently, the General Accounting Office (GAO) ordered Congress to begin conversion of surgical, radiologic, and other diagnostic services to an APC system effective August 1, 2000, which replaced ASCs. The more than 500 APCs are continually being modified (added to) and deleted. Because of this constant state of change, APC information is updated and released twice a year in *The Federal Register.*

APCs are applied to the following:

● Ambulatory surgical procedures
● Chemotherapy
● Clinic visits
● Diagnostic services and diagnostic tests
● Emergency department visits
● Implants
● Outpatient services furnished to nursing facility patients not packaged into nursing facility consolidated billing (services commonly furnished by hospital outpatient departments that nursing facilities are not able to provide [computed tomography, magnetic resonance imaging, or ambulatory surgery])
● Partial hospitalization services for community mental health centers (CMHCs)
● Preventive services (colorectal cancer screening)
● Radiology including radiation therapy
● Services for patients who have exhausted Part A benefits
● Services to hospice patient for treatment of a nonterminal illness
● Surgical pathology

Hospital Outpatient Prospective Payment System

The development process for APCs is similar to that used for DRGs; however, the procedure code is the primary axis of classification, not the diagnosis code. The reimbursement methodology is based on median costs of services and facility cost to determine charge ratios in addition to copayment amounts. There is also an adjustment for area wage differences, which is based on the hospital wage index currently used for inpatient services. This hospital Outpatient Prospective Payment System (OPPS) may be updated annually, not periodically. An APC group may have a number of services or items packaged within it so that separate payment cannot be obtained.

Ambulatory Payment Classification Status

Categories of services have payment status indicators consisting of alpha code letters or symbols. These are the following:

Category	Payment Status Indicator
A	Durable medical equipment, prosthetics and orthotics
A	Physical, occupational and speech therapy
A	Ambulance
A	Erythropoietin (EPO) for end-stage renal disease (ESRD) patients
A	Clinical diagnostic laboratory services
A	Physician services for ESRD patients
A	Screening mammography
C	Inpatient procedures
E	Noncovered items and services
F	Acquisition of corneal tissue
G	Drug/biologic pass-through payment
H	Device pass-through payment
K	Non–pass-through drug/biologic
N	Incidental services, packaged into APC rate
P	Partial hospitalization
S	Significant procedure, not discounted when multiple
T	Significant procedure, multiple procedure reduction applies
V	Visit to clinic or emergency department
X	Ancillary service

Partial hospitalization refers to a distinct and organized intensive psychiatric outpatient day treatment program designed to provide patients with profound and disabling mental health conditions with an individual, coordinated, comprehensive, and multidisciplinary treatment program.

Types of APCs

The four types of APCs are as follows:

1. *Surgical procedure APCs.* These are surgical procedures for which payment is allowed under the PPS (e.g., cataract removal, endoscopies, biopsies). Surgical APCs are assigned on the basis of CPT codes.
2. *Significant procedure APCs.* These consist of nonsurgical procedures that are the main reason for the visit and account for the majority of the time and services used during the visit (e.g., psychotherapy, computed tomography and magnetic resonance imaging, radiation therapy, chemotherapy administration, or partial hospitalization). Significant procedure APCs are selected on the basis of CPT codes.
3. *Medical APCs.* These include encounters with a health care professional for evaluation and management services. The medical APC is determined by site of service (clinic or ED), level of the evaluation and management service (CPT code), and diagnosis from one of 20 diagnostic categories (ICD-9-CM code).
4. *Ancillary APCs.* These involve diagnostic tests or treatments not considered to be significant procedure APCs (e.g., plain x-ray film, ECGs, or cardiac rehabilitation). Ancillary APCs are assigned on the basis of CPT codes.

It is possible that multiple APCs can be used when billing for a visit. Use of CPT modifiers for hospital outpatient visits affects APC payments; therefore it is important to accurately apply correct modifiers when applicable.

Most hospitals use a type of computer encoder program in which the CPT code is input and an APC group code number is assigned. For example, if CPT code number 99282 is input for a low-level emergency department visit, the encoder assigns APC Group 610. Use of an unbundling reference book may be helpful in assigning a CPT code; it is preferable to use the code that will generate the highest APC payment.

The data that hospitals submit during the first years of implementation of the APC system are vitally important to the revision of weights and other adjustments that affect payment in future years. The APC data that appear on the CMS-1450 (UB-04) paper claim form are shown in Figure 17-6.

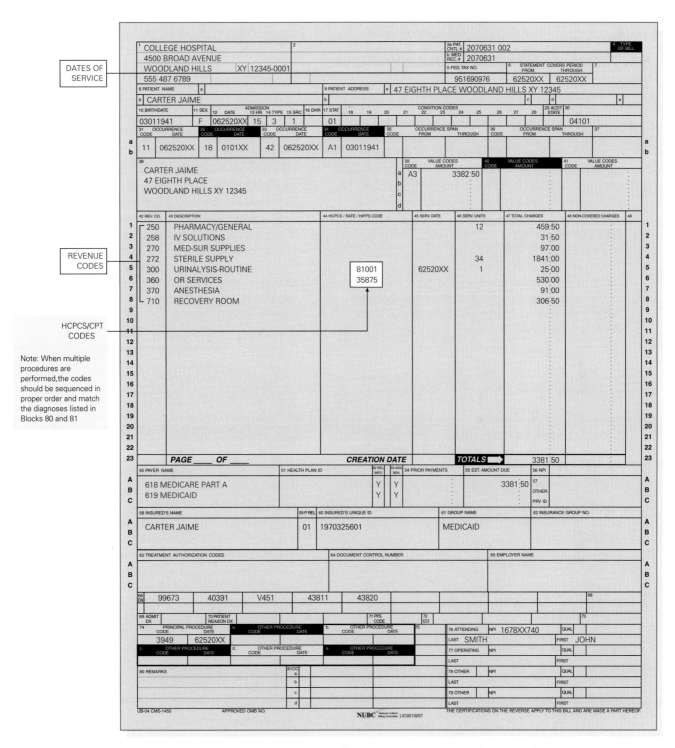

FIGURE 17-6 Scannable CMS-1450/Uniform Bill (UB-04) insurance paper claim form showing placement of APC data for an outpatient for submission to insurance company.

PROCEDURE 17-1

New Patient Admission and Insurance Verification

1. Interview the patient and obtain complete and accurate information during initial registration. If an emergency inpatient admission, the managed care program should be notified the next working day or within 48 hours to obtain an authorization number.
2. Write down the information from the physician's office who has telephoned for admittance of the patient.
3. Make photocopies of the front and back of all insurance cards.
4. Contact the insurance company or the insured individual's employer to verify the type of health insurance or telephone the insurance company to verify eligibility and benefits and determine whether prior authorization is necessary.
5. Obtain an approved signed treatment authorization request for elective admissions for a Medicaid or TRICARE patient.
6. Collect any copayment or deductible.
7. Obtain information relating to the injured patient, industrial accident, insurance carrier, and employer for a patient injured on the job.
8. Get an authorization for admission, length of stay, and all surgical procedures for an elective admission of a patient injured on the job from the workers' compensation insurance adjuster.
9. Ask the patient to read and sign the necessary hospital admitting documents (e.g., Notice of Privacy document, surgical consent form, and financial agreement).

PROCEDURE 17-2

Coding from ICD-9-CM Volume 3

Basic steps in coding from volume 3 of ICD-9-CM code book are as follows:

1. Locate the main term (procedure) in the Alphabetical Index.
2. Read all modifiers (descriptive notations relating to the condition).
3. Obtain the code number and refer to the Tabular List (volume 3) to verify that the code number selected matches the description of the procedure. Never code using only the Alphabetical Index because important instructions may appear in the Tabular List.
4. Note any exclusions, inclusions, remarks concerning fourth digits, colons, and any other information that may affect the choice of codes. Notice "code also" and "omit code" instructions.
5. Select the appropriate code number. Use fourth digit codes and, if necessary, apply two or more code numbers to completely describe a procedure (Example 17-14).
6. The *DRG/ICD-9-CM Code Book* is a good reference and code book presented in an easy-to-use binder and containing volumes 1, 2, and 3 of ICD-9-CM. Sections are color-highlighted for maximum payment. Refer to the Appendix to locate publishers of ICD-9-CM code books.

Example 17-14	Procedure: Complete Vaginal Hysterectomy with Bilateral Salpingectomy

Code	Description
68.5	Vaginal hysterectomy
66.51	Removal of both fallopian tubes at same operative episode

PROCEDURE 17-3

Editing a UB-04 (CMS-1450) Paper or Electronic Claim Form

Each field or block is called a form locator (FL).

1. Review the top left corner to determine if the facility information is printed (FL 1 and 5).
2. Determine whether it is an inpatient (11X) or outpatient (13X) type of bill (FL 4).
3. Scan the UB-04 (CMS-11450) claim form to determine who the patient is (FL 8b), the responsible party (FL 38), the insured (FL 58), and the patient's relationship to the insured (FL 59).
4. Check the birth date of the patient (FL 10); it should be printed in eight digits.
5. Confirm the gender of the patient (FL 11), comparing it with the patient's name (FL 8). If the patient's name could be used for either gender, verify the sex by reviewing the patient's insurance identification card, patient's medical record, or handwritten admitting record.
6. Verify the insurance information including the payer (FL 50), certificate, Social Security, or insured's unique identification number (FL 60), group name (FL 61), insurance group number (FL 62), and employer name (FL 65). FLs 50 and 60 are mandatory.
7. Confirm that data are present by reviewing the following: principal diagnostic code (FL 67) and admitting diagnostic code (FL 69), if applicable.
8. Verify that there is a principal procedure code with date (FL 74) and all other procedures with date(s) or service (FL 74a-e). These should match the sequence and services provided.
9. Verify that there is an attending, referring, or prescribing physician with identification number listed (FL 76). A physician other than the attending physician should be listed (FL 77).
10. Cross-check the third digit in FL 4, indicating the bill type with statement from and through dates (FL 6), admission date (FL 12), and occurrence date (FL 31) to determine whether this is the first bill. If it is not, look at the original bill so that all entries are understood.
11. Inpatient: Verify the number of hospital days for semiprivate or coronary care unit (CCU) room charges (FL 42 through 47). These should match. Look at the hour the patient was admitted (FL 13) and the hour of discharge (FL 16) if there is a discrepancy.
12. Correlate the room rates (FL 47) with the preceding services, making sure the per diem is based on the revenue. The computer software program takes the number of days and multiplies that by the room rate, and this figure equals the amount of the revenue shown.
13. Review all of the patient's services listed (FL 42) line by line. Each service listed must show a unit value (FL 46). Search for any revenue codes that may be used for a special type of service that may be itemized and charged separately (e.g., 0274 through 0279 implants or 0258 through 0259 special drugs).
14. Outpatient: Verify that each service described (FL 43) has a CPT or HCPCS code (FL 44) and a date of service listed (FL 45).
15. Check the detailed patient's health record (chart) if there is a question about a service listed. All services must be listed by hospital department.
16. Verify the total amount due by adding all amounts (FL 47) and comparing them with the last line item in FL 42 (0001), FL 43 (Total), and final totaled amount as the last line entry in FL 47.
17. Determine whether the estimated amount due from the insurance company is calculated and shown (FL 55).

PROCEDURE 17-4

Completing the UB-04 (CMS-1450) Paper or Electronic Claim Form

Only general guidelines for completing the UB-04 (CMS-1450) claim form are mentioned here. The medical hospital manual and the local UB-04 (CMS-1450) manual if available should always be consulted to determine whether billing guidelines pertain to a particular region. No guidelines had been published about insertion of the APC group number for outpatient claims at the time this edition was printed. The recommendation is to use either FL 75 or 84 for this purpose. Some facilities are grouping claims in-house that relate to APCs before submitting them to the fiscal intermediaries. The following color screens, item numbers, and descriptions correspond to FL 5, which shows a completed UB-04 (CMS-1450) paper claim form for inpatient claims.

FL 1.

Billing Provider Name, Address, and Telephone Number.

Enter the provider name, address, city, state, and ZIP code on the first three lines. Enter telephone number, fax number, or county code applicable to the provider on the fourth line. Medicaid and Medicare: The fourth line is optional. TRICARE: The fourth line is required.

FL 2.

Pay-to Name and Address.

(When different from provider in FL 1): Enter pay-to name on the first line. Enter street address on second line. Enter city, state, and ZIP code on third line. Leave fourth line blank.

FL 3a.

Patient Control Number.

This is an optional form locator that can be used to identify an individual patient account. It is the patient's medical record number or account number in some facilities. Medicare: Required.

FL 3b.

Enter the number assigned by the provider to the patient's health record.

FL 4.

Type of Bill (TOB).

Enter the appropriate facility code preceded by a leading zero as specified in the UB-04 (CMS-1450). Manual Billing Procedures. The digits indicate the following:

Second digit (type of facility)

Third digit is the type of care billed.

Fourth digit is the sequence of the bill for a specific episode of care. 011X = Hospital inpatient (including Medicare Part A)

    012X = Hospital inpatient (Medicare Part B only)

    013X, 014X = Hospital outpatient

    018X = Hospital swing beds

021X = Skilled nursing facility (inpatient Medicare Part A)

022X = Skilled nursing facility (inpatient Medicare Part B)

023X = Skilled nursing outpatient

032X = Home health inpatient (Medicare Part B only)

033X = Home health outpatient (includes HHA visits under a Part A plan of treatment including DME under Part A)

034X = Home health laboratory services provided to nonpatients or home health not under a plan of treatment)

041X = Religious nonmedical health care institutions hospital inpatient (including Medicare Part A)

043X = Religious nonmedical health care institutions (RNHCI) hospital outpatient

071X = Rural health clinic

072X = Renal Dialysis Facility

073X = Federally Qualified Health Center

074X = Outpatient Rehabilitation Facility (ORF)

075X = Comprehensive ORF

076X = Community Mental Health Center

081X, 082X = Hospice (Medicare Part A only)

083X = Outpatient surgery (subject to ASC payment limits)

085X = Critical Access Hospital

FL 5.

Federal Tax Number.

Enter the facility's provider federal tax number. This number is also called a *tax identification number* (TIN) or *employer identification number* (EIN). Medicare: Required. Private payers and TRICARE: Required. Some Medicaid programs: A number in this field may be required.

FL 6.

Statement Covers Period.

Enter beginning and ending dates of service for the period shown on the bill (e.g., 011820XX to 012020XX). The electronic version requires an eight-character date listing year, month, and day: 20XX0118 to 20XX0120. Medicare and Private payers: Required.

FL 7.

Reserved.

This field is reserved for assignment by the National Uniform Billing Committee (NUBC).

FL 8a.

Patient Name/Identifier.

Insert only if the patient's identification number differs from the insured's number in FL 60 (insured's unique ID). Some national health plans have unique ID numbers for each patient that differ from their subscriber number.

FL 8b.

Insert the patient's name.

PROCEDURE 17-4—cont'd

Completing the UB-04 (CMS-1450) Paper or Electronic Claim Form

FL 9.

Patient's Address.

Enter the patient's street address, city, state, and ZIP code. Private payers, some Medicaid programs, Medicare, and TRICARE: Required. Medi-Cal: Not required.

FL 10.

Patient's Birth Date.

Enter the patient's date of birth in an eight-digit format (e.g., June 1, 20XX, becomes 060120XX). If birth date is unknown, insert eight zeros. Private payers and Medicare: Required.

FL 11.

Patient's Sex.

Enter a capital "M" for male, "F" for female, or "U" for unknown. Private payers and Medicare: Required.

FL 12.

Admission/Start of Care Date.

Enter admission or start of care date. The electronic version requires an eight-character date in this format: 20XX 0710. Medicaid, Medicare, third-party payers, and TRICARE: Required.

FL 13.

Admission Hour.

Enter the hour during which the patient was admitted for inpatient or outpatient care in two numeric characters using the 24-hour clock (e.g., midnight is 00 and noon is 12, 1 to 1:59 AM is 01, 1 to 1:59 PM is 13, 11:59 PM is shown as 23; Figure 17-7). Private payers and TRICARE: Required. Medicare: Not required.

FL 14.

Priority (Type) of Admission/Visit.

Enter the code indicating the priority of the inpatient admission. Coding structure: 1 = indicates emergency; 2 = urgent; 3 = elective; 4 = newborn; 5 = trauma center, 6-8 = reserved for national assignment, and 9 = information not available. Private payers, some

Medicaid programs, Medicare, and TRICARE: Required when inpatient claim submitted.

FL 15.

Point of Origin for Admission or Visit.

Enter the code identifying the point of patient origin for this admission or visit. Medicare, private payers, and TRICARE: Required. Medicaid: Not required. Code as follows:

Point of Origin for Admission or Visit Codes

1	Non–health care facility point of origin
2	Clinic
3	Discontinued
4	Transfer from a hospital (different facility)
5	Transfer from a skilled nursing facility (SNF) or intermediate care facility (ICF)
6	Transfer from another healthcare facility
7	Emergency department
8	Court/law enforcement
9	Information not available
A	Reserved
B	Transfer from another home health agency
C	Readmission to same home health agency
D	Transfer from one distinct unit of the hospital to another distinct unit of the same hospital resulting in a separate claim to the payer
E	Transfer from ambulatory surgery center
F	Transfer from hospice and is under a hospice plan of care or enrolled in a hospice program
G-Z	Reserved for national assignment

Newborn Codes

1	Normal delivery
2	Premature delivery
3	Sick baby
4	Extramural birth
5-8	Reserved for national assignment
9	Information not available

FL 16.

Discharge Hour.

Enter hour when patient was discharged from inpatient care. Hours are indicated by two numeric characters using the 24-hour clock (e.g., midnight is 00 and noon is 12, 1 to 1:59 AM is 01, 1 to 1:59 PM is 13, 11:59 PM is 23; see FL 8). Required on inpatient claims with a frequency code of 1 or 4 except for SNF inpatient, TOB 21X.

FL 17.

Patient Discharge Status.

Enter a code indicating the patient's disposition as of the ending date of service for the period of care reported. Private payers, Medicaid, Medicare, and TRICARE: Required for inpatient claims.

FIGURE 17-7 Clock face depicting standard am time and clock face depicting pm military time.

Continued

PROCEDURE 17-4—cont'd

Completing the UB-04 (CMS-1450) Paper or Electronic Claim Form

Patient Status Codes

01	Discharged to home or self-care (routine discharge)
02	Discharged/transferred to a short-term general hospital for inpatient care
03	Discharged or transferred to SNF with Medicare certification in anticipation of covered skilled care
04	Discharged/transferred to an ICF
05	Discharged/transferred to another type of health care institution not defined elsewhere in this code list
06	Discharged/transferred to home under care of organized home health service organization in anticipation of covered skilled care
07	Left against medical advice or discontinued care
08	Reserved for national assignment
09	Admitted as an inpatient to this hospital
10-19	Reserved for national assignment
20	Expired
21-29	Reserved for national assignment
30	Still a patient
31-39	Reserved for national assignment
40	Expired at home (for hospice care)
41	Expired in a medical facility such as a hospital, SNF, ICF, or freestanding hospice (for hospice care)
42	Expired, place unknown (for hospice care)
43	Discharged/transferred to a federal health care facility
44-49	Reserved for national assignment
50	Discharged to hospice or home
51	Discharged to hospice or medical facility
52-60	Reserved for national assignment
61	Discharged/transferred within this institution to a hospital-based, Medicare-approved swing bed
62	Discharged/transferred to an inpatient rehabilitation facility (IRF), including rehabilitation distinct part units of a hospital
63	Discharged/transferred to a Medicare-certified long-term care hospital (LTCH)
64	Discharged/transferred to a nursing facility certified under Medicaid but not certified under Medicare
65	Discharged/transferred to a psychiatric hospital or psychiatric distinct part unit of a hospital
66	Discharges/transfers to a critical access hospital
67-69	Reserved for national assignment
70	Discharged/transferred to another type of health care institution not defined elsewhere in this code list
71-99	Reserved for national assignment

FLS 18-28.
Condition Codes.
The codes help determine patient eligibility and benefits from primary or secondary insurance coverage and may affect payer processing.

Condition Codes

01	Military service related
02	Condition is employment related
03	Patient is covered by insurance not reflected here
04	Information-only bill
05	Lien has been filed
06	ESRD patient in first 18 months of entitlement covered by employer group health insurance
07	Treatment of nonterminal condition for hospice patient
08	Beneficiary will not provide information concerning other insurance coverage
09	Neither patient nor spouse is employed
10	Patient or spouse is employed but no employer group health plan (EGHP) coverage exists
11	Disabled beneficiary but no large group health plan (LGHP) coverage
12-16	Reserved for payer use only
17	Patient is homeless
18	Maiden name retained
19	Child retains mother's name
20	Beneficiary requested billing
21	Billing for denial notice
22	Patient is on multiple-drug regimen
23	Home caregiver is available
24	Home intravenous therapy patient also receiving home health agency (HHA) services
25	Patient is a non-US resident
26	VA–eligible patient chooses to receive services in Medicare-certified facility
27	Patient is referred to a sole community hospital for a diagnostic laboratory test
28	Patient's or spouse's EGHP is secondary to Medicare
29	Disabled beneficiary's or family member's LGHP is secondary to Medicare
30	Nonresearch services provided to patients enrolled in a qualified clinical trial
31	Patient is student (full-time day)
32	Patient is student (cooperative or work study program)
33	Patient is student (full-time night)
34	Patient is student (part-time)
35	Reserved for national assignment
36	General care patient is in a special unit
37	Ward accommodation at patient's request
38	Semiprivate room is not available
39	Private room is medically necessary
40	Same-day transfer
41	Partial hospitalization

PROCEDURE 17-4—cont'd

Completing the UB-04 (CMS-1450) Paper or Electronic Claim Form

Condition Codes—cont'd

42	Continuing care is not related to inpatient admission
43	Continuing care is not provided within prescribed postdischarge window
44	Inpatient admission changed to outpatient
45	Ambiguous gender category
46	TRICARE Nonavailability Statement on file
47	Reserved for national assignment
48	Psychiatric residential treatment centers (RTCs) for children and adolescents
49	Product replacement within product life cycle
50	Product replacement for known recall of a product
51-54	Reserved for national assignment
55	SNF bed is not available
56	Medical appropriateness; SNF admission was delayed more than 30 days after hospital discharge
57	SNF readmission
58	Terminated Medicare Advantage enrollee
59	Nonprimary ESRD facility
60	Day outlier
61	Cost outlier
62-65	Payer-only codes
66	Provider does not wish cost outlier payment
67	Beneficiary elects not to use lifetime reserve (LTR) days
68	Beneficiary elects to use LTR days
69	Indirect medical education (IME), direct graduate medical education (DGME), and nursing and allied health (N & AH) payment only
70	Self-administered anemia management drug
71	Full care in dialysis unit
72	Self-care in dialysis unit
73	Self-care in dialysis training
74	Patient receiving dialysis services at home
75	Home dialysis—100% payment
76	Backup in-facility dialysis
77	Provider accepts or is obligated or required because of a contractual arrangement or law to accept payment by a primary payer as payment in full
78	New coverage not implemented by managed care plan
79	Comprehensive ORF (CORF) services provided offsite
80	Home dialysis—nursing facility
81-99	Reserved for state assignment
A0	TRICARE External Partnership Program
A1	Early Periodic Screening Diagnosis Treatment/Child Health Assurance Program (EPSDT/CHAP)
A2	Physically handicapped children's program
A3	Special federal funding
A4	Family planning
A5	Disability
A6	Vaccines/Medicare 100% payment
A7-A8	Reserved for national assignment
A9	Second-opinion surgery
AA	Abortion performed because of rape
AB	Abortion performed because of incest
AC	Abortion performed because of serious fetal genetic defect, deformity, or abnormality
AD	Abortion performed because of a life-endangering physical condition caused by, arising from, or exacerbated by the pregnancy itself
AE	Abortion performed because of physical health of mother that is not life endangering
AF	Abortion performed because of emotional or psychologic health of the mother
AG	Abortion performed because of social or economic reasons
AH	Elective abortion
AI	Sterilization
AJ	Payer responsible for copayment
AK	Air ambulance required
AL	Specialized treatment or bed unavailable
AM	Nonemergency medically necessary stretcher transport required
AN	Preadmission screening not required
AO-AZ	Reserved for national assignment
B0	Medicare coordinated care demonstration claim
B1	Beneficiary ineligible for demonstration program
B2	Critical access hospital ambulance attestation
B3	Pregnancy indicator
B4	Admission unrelated to discharge on same day
B5-BZ	Reserved for national assignment
C0	Reserved for national assignment
C1	Approved as billed
C2	Automatic approval as billed based on focused review
C3	Partial approval
C4	Admission or services denied
C5	Postpayment review applicable
C6	Admission preauthorization
C7	Extended authorization
C8-CZ	Reserved for national assignment
D0	Change to services dates
D1	Change to charges
D2	Changes in revenue codes or HCPCS or Health Insurance Prospective Payment System (HIPPS) rate codes
D3	Second or subsequent interim prospective payment system bill
D4	Change in ICD-9-CM diagnosis and/or procedure codes
D5	Cancel to correct health insurance claim number (HICN) or provider identification number

Continued

PROCEDURE 17-4—cont'd

Completing the UB-04 (CMS-1450) Paper or Electronic Claim Form

Condition Codes—cont'd

D6	Cancel only to repay a duplicate or OIG overpayment
D7	Change to make Medicare the secondary payer
D8	Change to make Medicare the primary payer
D9	Any other change
DA-DQ	Reserved for national assignment
DR	Disaster related
DS-DZ	Reserved for national assignment
E0	Change in patient status
E1-FZ	Reserved for national assignment
G0	Distinct medical visit
GI-GZ	Reserved for national assignment
HO	Delayed filing, statement of intent submitted
H1-LZ	Reserved for national assignment
MO-MZ	Reserved for payer assignment
NO-OZ	Reserved for national assignment
PO	Reserved for national assignment for public health reporting only
P1	Do not resuscitate (DNR) order for public health reporting only
P2-PZ	Reserved for national assignment for public health reporting only
Q0-VZ	Reserved for national assignment
W0	United Mine Workers of America (UMWA) demonstration indicator
W1-ZZ	Reserved for national assignment

FL 29.

Accident state.

Enter two-digit code for where the accident occurred, if applicable.

AA	automobile accident
AB	abuse
AP	another party responsible
EM	employment
OA	other accident

FL 30.

Reserved.

This field is reserved for national assignment.

FL 31-34.

Occurrence Codes and Dates.

Occurrence codes and dates are used to identify significant events relating to a bill that may affect payer processing (e.g., determination of liability, coordination of benefits, or administration of subrogation clauses in benefit programs). The electronic version requires an eight-character date listing year, month, and day: 20XX0328. A total of eight occurrence codes and dates may be reported on a CMS-1450 (UB-04). Private payers or Medicare: Required.

Occurrence Codes and Dates

01	Auto accident or medical coverage
02	No-fault insurance involved including auto accident or other
03	Accident—tort liability
04	Accident—employment related
05	Accident or no medical or liability coverage
06	Crime victim
07-08	Reserved for national assignment
09	Start of infertility treatment cycle
10	Last menstrual period
11	Onset of symptoms or illness
12	Date of onset for a chronically dependent individual (CDI) (HHA claims only)
13-15	Reserved for national assignment
16	Date of last therapy
17	Date outpatient occupational therapy plan established or last reviewed
18	Date of retirement of patient and beneficiary
19	Date of retirement of spouse
20	Guarantee of payment began
21	UR notice received
22	Date active care ended
23	Date of cancellation of hospice election period
24	Date insurance denied
25	Date benefits terminated by primary payer
26	Date SNF bed became available
27	Date of hospice certification or recertification
28	Date comprehensive outpatient rehabilitation plan established or last reviewed
29	Date outpatient physical therapy plan established or last reviewed
30	Date outpatient speech pathology plan established or last reviewed
31	Date beneficiary notified of intent to bill (accommodations)
32	Date beneficiary notified of intent to bill (procedures or treatments)
33	First day of the Medicare coordination period for ESRD beneficiaries covered by an EGHP
34	Date of election of extended care services
35	Date treatment started for physical therapy
36	Date of inpatient hospital discharge for covered transplant patient
37	Date of inpatient hospital discharge for noncovered transplant patient
38	Date treatment started for home intravenous therapy
39	Date discharged on a continuous course of intravenous therapy
40	Scheduled date of admission
41	Date of first test for preadmission testing
42	Date of discharge (hospice only)
43	Scheduled date of canceled surgery

PROCEDURE 17-4—cont'd

Completing the UB-04 (CMS-1450) Paper or Electronic Claim Form

Occurrence Codes and Dates—cont'd

44	Date treatment started for occupational therapy
45	Date treatment started for speech therapy
46	Date treatment started for cardiac rehabilitation
47	Date cost outlier status begins
48-49	Payer codes
50-69	Reserved for national assignment
70-99	Reserved for occurrence span codes
A0	Reserved for national assignment
A1	Birthdate—insured A
A2	Effective date—insured A policy
A3	Benefits exhausted
A4	Split bill date
A5-AZ	Reserved for national assignment
B0	Reserved for national assignment
B1	Birthdate—insured B
B2	Effective date—insured B policy
B3	Benefits exhausted
B4-BZ	Reserved for national assignment
C0	Reserved for national assignment
C1	Birthdate—insured C
C2	Effective date—insured C policy
C3	Benefits exhausted
C4-CZ	Reserved for national assignment
D0-DQ	Reserved for national assignment
DR	Reserved for disaster related occurrence code
DS-DZ	Reserved for national assignment
E0	Reserved for national assignment
E1-E3	Discontinued March 1, 2007
E4-EZ	Reserved for national assignment
F0	Reserved for national assignment
F1-F3	Discontinued March 1, 2007
F4-FZ	Reserved for national assignment
G0	Reserved for national assignment
G1-G3	Discontinued March 1, 2007
G4-GZ	Reserved for national assignment
H0-IZ	Reserved for national assignment
J0-LZ	Reserved for national assignment
M0-ZZ	See FL occurrence span codes

FL 35-36.

Occurrence Span Codes and Dates.

Enter code-identifying occurrence that happened over a span of time. The electronic version requires an eight-character date listing year, month, and day (20XX0812). Medicaid: Complete when required. Private payer, Medicare, and TRICARE: Required.

Qualifying Span Codes

70	Qualifying stay dates (for SNF use only)
71	Prior stay dates
72	First and last visits
73	Benefit eligibility period
74	Noncovered level of care or leave of absence (LOA)
75	SNF level of care
76	Patient liability period
77	Provider liability period
78	SNF prior stay dates
79	Payer code
80-99	Reserved for national assignment
MO	QIO/UR approved stay dates (partial approval)
M1	Provider liability—no utilization
M2	Dates of inpatient respite care
M3	ICF level of care
M4	Residential level of care
M5-MQ	Reserved for national assignment
MR	Reserved for disaster-related occurrence span code
MS-WZ	Reserved for national assignment
XO-ZZ	Reserved for national assignment

FL 37.

Reserved (not used).

FL 38.

Responsible Party Name and Address.

Enter the name and address of the party responsible for the bill. Private payers: Required. Medicaid, Medicare, or TRICARE: Not required.

FL 39-41.

Value Codes and Amounts.

Enter codes that have related dollar amounts that identify monetary data required for processing claims. If more than three codes are necessary, enter A4 and the value code and amount in Field 74. Medicaid: May be required depending on state policy. Private payer, Medicare, and TRICARE: Complete when applicable. Enter the value codes as described in the following:

Value Codes

01	Most common semiprivate room rate
02	Hospital has no semiprivate rooms
03	Reserved for national assignment
04	Inpatient professional component charges that are combined billed
05	Professional component included in charges and also billed separately to carrier
06	Medicare blood deductible amount
07	Reserved for national assignment
08	Medicare lifetime reserve amount in the first calendar year
09	Medicare coinsurance amount in the first calendar year in billing period
10	Medicare lifetime reserve amount in the second calendar year
11	Medicare coinsurance amount for second calendar year
12	Working aged beneficiary or spouse with EGHP
13	ESRD in a Medicare coordination period with an EGHP

Continued

PROCEDURE 17-4—cont'd

Completing the UB-04 (CMS-1450) Paper or Electronic Claim Form

Value Codes—cont'd

14	No-fault insurance, including auto or other
15	Workers' compensation
16	Public health service (PHS) or other federal agency
17	Outlier amount
18	Disproportionate share amount
19	Indirect medical education amount
20	Total prospective payment system capital payment amount
21	Catastrophic (Medicaid-specific code)
22	Surplus (Medicaid-specific code)
23	Recurring monthly income (Medicaid-specific code)
24	Medicaid rate code
25	Offset to the patient-payment amount—prescription drugs
26	Offset to the patient-payment amount—hearing and ear services
27	Offset to the patient-payment amount—vision and eye services
28	Offset to the patient-payment amount—dental services
29	Offset to the patient-payment amount—chiropractic services
30	Preadmission testing
31	Patient liability amount
32	Multiple patient ambulance transport
33	Offset to the patient-payment amount—podiatric services
34	Offset to the patient-payment amount—other medical services
35	Offset to the patient-payment amount—health insurance premiums
36	Reserved for national assignment
37	Pints of blood furnished
38	Blood deductible pints
39	Pints of blood replaced
40	New coverage not implemented by HMO (for inpatient claims only)
41	Black lung
42	Veterans affairs
43	Disabled beneficiary younger than age 65 with LGHP
44	Amount provider agreed to accept from primary insurer when this amount is less than total charges but higher than payment received
45	Accident hour
46	Number of grace days
47	Any liability insurance
48	Hemoglobin reading
49	Hematocrit reading
50	Physical therapy visits
51	Occupational therapy visits
52	Speech therapy visits
53	Cardiac rehabilitation visits
54	Newborn birth weight in grams
55	Eligibility threshold for charity care
56	Skilled nurse—home visit hours (HHA only)
57	Home health aide—home visit hours (HHA only)
58	Arterial blood gas (PO_2/PA_2)
59	Oxygen saturation (O_2 SAT/oximetry)
60	HHA branch metropolitan statistical area (MSA)
61	Location where service is furnished (HHA and hospice)
62	HHA visits—Part A
63	HHA visits—Part B
64	HHA reimbursement—Part A
65	HHA reimbursement—Part B
66	Medicaid spend down amount
67	Peritoneal dialysis
68	EPO—drug
69	State charity care percent
70-72	Payer codes
73	Drug deductible; payer code
74	Drug coinsurance; payer code
75-76	Payer codes
77	Payer code; new technology add-on payment
78-79	Payer codes
80	Covered days
81	Noncovered days
82	Coinsurance days
83	Lifetime reserve days
84-99	Reserved for national assignment
A0	Special zip code reporting
A1	Deductible payer A
A2	Coinsurance payer A
A3	Estimated responsibility payer A
A4	Covered self-administrable drugs—emergency
A5	Covered self-administrable drugs—not self-administered in form and situation furnished to patient
A6	Covered self-administrable drugs—diagnostic study and other
A7	Copayment payer A
A8	Patient weight
A9	Patient height
AA	Regulatory surcharges, assessments, allowances, or health care–related taxes payer A
AB	Other assessments or allowances (e.g., medical education) payer A
AC-AZ	Reserved for national assignment
B0	Reserved for national assignment
B1	Deductible payer B
B2	Coinsurance payer B
B3	Estimated responsibility payer B
B4-B6	Reserved for national assignment
B7	Copayment payer B
B8-B9	Reserved for national assignment
BA	Regulatory surcharges, assessments, allowances, or health care–related taxes payer B

PROCEDURE 17-4—cont'd

Completing the UB-04 (CMS-1450) Paper or Electronic Claim Form

Value Codes—cont'd

BB	Other assessments or allowances (e.g., medical educational) payer B
BC-C0	Reserved for national assignment
C1	Deductible payer C
C2	Coinsurance payer C
C3	Estimated responsibility payer C
C4-C6	Reserved for national assignment
C7	Copayment payer C
C8-C9	Reserved for national assignment
CA	Regulatory surcharges, assessments, allowances, or health care–related taxes payer C
CB	Other assessments or allowances (e.g., medical education) payer C
CC-CZ	Reserved for national assignment
D0-D2	Reserved for national assignment
D3	Estimated responsibility patient
D4	Clinical trial number assigned by the National Library of Medicine or National Institutes of Health
D5–DQ	Reserved for national assignment
DR	Disaster related value (code is pending)
DS-DZ	Reserved for national assignment
E0-EZ	Reserved for national assignment
F0-FB	Reserved for national assignment
FC	Patient paid amount
FD	Credit received from the manufacturer for a replaced medical device
FE-FZ	Reserved for national assignment
G0-G7	Reserved for national assignment
G8	Facility where inpatient hospice service is delivered
G9-GZ	Reserved for national assignment
H0-OZ	Reserved for national assignment
PO-PZ	Reserved for national assignment for public health data reporting only
Q0-YO	Reserved for national assignment
Y1	Part A demonstration payment
Y2	Part B demonstration payment
Y3	Part B coinsurance
Y4	Conventional provider payment for non-demonstration claims
Y5-ZZ	Reserved for national assignment

FL 42.

Revenue Code.

Enter a four-digit code corresponding to each narrative description or standard abbreviation that identifies a specific accommodation, ancillary service, or billing calculation related to services billed. Revenue code 0001 indicating a total must be the final entry on all bills. Revenue codes are an important factor when payment is considered by managed care contractors or private payers. Billing guidelines for revenue codes are extensive, so refer to the UB-04 (CMS-1450) manual for detailed information. Managed care: Required because payment may be based on diagnosis, procedure, and revenue codes. For example, codes 0274, 0275, 0276, and 0278 relate to implant of a pacemaker, lens, pin, or bolt. If the correct code is not used, payment will not be made for implant item if the cost is buried in supplies. Other items to be sure to code are special drugs for chemotherapy, cardiac balloons, cardiac catheters, and so on. Medicare: Required. All revenue codes from 001 to 999 must be preceded with a "0." The leading "0" is added automatically for electronic claims. Basic revenue codes end in "0." Detailed revenue codes end in 1 through 9. List revenue codes in ascending order. Do not repeat revenue codes on the same claim except when required by field or for coding more than one HCPCS code for the same revenue code item.

FL 43.

Revenue Description.

This optional form locator helps separate and identify descriptions of each service. The description must identify the particular service code indicated in FL 44, the HCPCS/Rates form locator. Third-party payers and TRICARE: Required Medicare: Not required. Medicaid: May be required depending on contract.

FL 44.

HCPCS/Rates/HIPPS Rate Codes.

Enter the applicable CPT or HCPCS code number and modifier (applicable to ancillary services for outpatient claims), HIPPS rate code, and two-digit modifier, or the accommodation rate for inpatient claims. Dollar values must include whole dollars, the decimal, and cents (e.g., $999.99). Medicare: Required. Medicaid and private payers: May be required depending on contract.

FL 45.

Service Date.

Enter the date the service was rendered for outpatient services in eight digits (e.g., 062320XX). See the patient's itemized bill for dates. The electronic version requires an eight-character date listing year, month, and day (e.g., 20XX0128). Inpatient dates are not required in this form locator. Medicare: Required. Medicaid and private payers: May be required depending on contract.

FL 46.

Service Units.

Enter the number of accommodation days, ancillary units, or visits when appropriate for each revenue code. This is itemized on the patient's detail bill. Medicare and private payers: Required.

FL 47.

Total Charges.

Enter the total charge pertaining to the related revenue codes (Example 17-15). Medicare and private payers: Required.

Continued

PROCEDURE 17-4—cont'd

Completing the UB-04 (CMS-1450) Paper or Electronic Claim Form

Example 17-15

	42 Rev. CD.	43 Description	44 HCPCS/ Rates	45 Serv Date	46 Serv Units	47 Total Charges	48 Noncovered Charges	49
1	0175	Neonatal ICU	1844.00		14	25816.00		1
2	0250	Pharmacy				4083.20		2
3	0258	IV Solutions—Pharmacy				3387.90		3
4	0270	Med-Sur Supplies				15606.71		4
5	0300	Laboratory				12958.40		5
6	0310	Pathology Lab				47.10		6
7	0320	OX X-Ray				950.00		7
8	0360	OR Services				1800.00		8
9	0370	Anesthesia				1392.37		9
10	0390	Blood/Stor-Proc				630.30		10
11	0402	Radiology Ultrasound				808.00		11
12	0410	Respiratory SVC			22	8682.70		12
13	0481	Cardiac Cath Lab				1139.60		13
14	0920	Other DX SVS				36.00		14
15								15
16								16
17								17
18								18
19								19
20								20
21								21
22								22
23	001	TOTAL				77338.28		23

PROCEDURE 17-4—cont'd

Completing the UB-04 (CMS-1450) Paper or Electronic Claim Form

FL 48.
Noncovered Charges.
Enter total noncovered charges for the primary payer pertaining to a particular revenue code. Personal items are not covered. Medicaid, Medicare, and private payers: Required. TRICARE: Not required.

FL 49.
Reserved.
This field is reserved for national assignment by the NUBC.

FL 50.
Payer Name.
Enter name and number identifying each payer organization from which the provider may expect some payment for the bill. Line 50A is used to report the primary payer. Line 50B is used for the secondary payer. Line 50C is used for the tertiary payer. Medicaid, Medicare, private payers, and TRICARE: Required.

FL 51.
Health Plan Identification Number.
Enter the number assigned to the health plan. Contact payer to obtain health plan identifier. Medicaid, Medicare, and private payers: Required. TRICARE: Requires the ZIP code of the physical location of the provider plus the four-digit subidentification number.

FL 52.
Release of Information Certification Indicator.
Enter code indicating if provider has patient's signature on file permitting release of data. A (appropriate release of information on file at health care service provider or at utilization review organization); I (informed consent to release of medical information for conditions or diagnoses regulated by federal statutes); Y (yes); M (restricted or modified release); O (signature on file); and N (no release). Medicaid: May be required depending on contract. Medicare, private payers, and TRICARE: Required.

FL 53.
Assignment of Benefits Certification Indicator.
Enter Y (yes, benefits assigned), N (no, benefits not assigned), or W (not applicable). Private payers and TRICARE: Required. Medicaid, Medicare: Not required.

FL 54.
Prior Payments/Payers.
Enter the amount of payment received on this bill before the billing date. If payment has been received from other coverage, enter the amount on the same line as the other coverage "payer" listed in FL 50 (e.g., $100 should be entered as 100 00). Do not enter Medicare payments in this form locator; leave blank if not applicable. Medicaid and Medicare: Required.

FL 55.
Estimated Amount Due Payer.
Enter the estimated amount due from the indicated payer according to the contract. Medicaid, Medicare, private payers, and TRICARE: Not required.

FL 56.
National Provider Identifier–Billing Provider.
This field contains the unique identification number assigned to the provider submitting the bill.

FL 57.
Other (Billing) Provider Identifier.
This field contains the unique identification number assigned to the provider submitting the bill by the health plan.

FL 58.
Insured's Name.
Enter name of the patient or insured individual in whose name the insurance is issued. If billing for an infant, use the mother's name. If billing for an organ donor, enter the recipient's name and the patient's relationship to the recipient in FL 59. Otherwise leave blank. Medicaid, Medicare, private payers, and TRICARE: Required.

FL 59.
Patient's Relationship to Insured.
Enter code number indicating relationship of the patient to the insured individual identified in FL 58. Medicaid, Medicare, private payers, and TRICARE: Required.

Patient Relationship Codes

01	Spouse
04	Grandfather or grandmother
05	Grandson or granddaughter
07	Nephew or niece
10	Foster child
15	Ward
17	Stepson or stepdaughter
18	Self
19	Child
20	Employee
21	Unknown
22	Handicapped dependent
23	Sponsored dependent
24	Dependent or a minor dependent
29	Significant other
32	Mother
33	Father
36	Emancipated minor
39	Organ donor
40	Cadaver donor
41	Injured plaintiff
43	Child—insured does not have financial responsibility
53	Life partner
G8	Other relationship

Continued

PROCEDURE 17-4—cont'd

Completing the UB-04 (CMS-1450) Paper or Electronic Claim Form

FL 60.

Insured's Unique Identifier.

Enter the insured's unique identification number assigned by the payer organization.

FL 61.

Insured Group Name.

Enter the group name or plan through which the health insurance coverage is provided to the insured. Medicare and private payers: Required. TRICARE: Enter the sponsor's branch of service (e.g., USAF).

FL 62.

Insurance Group Number.

Enter the insurance group number. Private payers: Required. Medicare: Not required. TRICARE: Enter the sponsor's military status and pay grade codes. CHAMPVA: Enter the veteran's military status code (e.g., "ACT" for active or "RET" for retired).

FL 63.

Treatment Authorization Code.

Enter the treatment authorization request (TAR) number provided by the payer. Medicare, private payers, and TRICARE: Required.

FL 64.

Document Control Number (DCN).

Enter the control number assigned to the claim by the payer.

FL 65.

Employer Name (of the Insured).

Enter the employer's name for the individual listed in FL 58. Medicaid: May be required. Medicare, private payers, and TRICARE: Required.

FL 66.

Diagnosis and Procedure Code Qualifier (ICD version).

This code indentifies the version of ICD being reported. Enter "9" for the ninth revision or enter "0" (zero) for the tenth revision.

FL 67.

Principal Diagnosis Code.

Enter all numbers and letters of the ICD-9-CM code for the principal diagnosis, including fourth and fifth digits. Do not insert a decimal point. Required for all programs. For reporting Medicare inpatients' claims, a present-on-admission indicator code—eighth digit—that is attached to the diagnostic code is required for specific types of conditions. It is to be reported in diagnostic coding fields 67, 67A-Q, and 72. For electronically transmitted claims, the POA is reported in loop 2300, data element K301, which should contain the letters "POA" followed by the assigned value for the code.

FL 67A-Q.

Other Diagnosis Codes.

Enter all numbers and letters of the ICD-9-CM codes that correspond to the patient's additional conditions that coexist at the time of admission or develop subsequently and have an effect on the treatment received or length of stay. Required for all programs. Allows for a flag to indicate whether the diagnosis was present at admission; see field on far right following the code. Medicare allows 8 additional diagnoses in claims processing. Electronic claims 837i allow 12 other diagnosis codes.

FL 68.

Reserved.

This field is reserved for national assignment.

FL 69.

Admitting Diagnosis.

Enter admitting diagnosis code including fourth and fifth digits as stated by the physician at the time of admission for inpatient claims. For outpatient claims, enter the patient's stated reason for seeking care. Required for all programs.

PROCEDURE 17-4—cont'd

Completing the UB-04 (CMS-1450) Paper or Electronic Claim Form

FL 70 A-C.
Patient's Reason for Visit.
Enter the ICD code that describes the patient's condition at outpatient registration.

FL 71.
PPS Code.

FL 72 A-C.
External Cause of Injury (E Code).

If there is an external cause of injury, poisoning, or adverse effect, enter the diagnostic E code including the third and fourth digits. Medicare and private payers: Not required.

FL 73.
Reserved.
This field is reserved for assignment by the NUBC.

FL 74.
Principal Procedure Codes and Date.
Enter the procedure code for the principal procedure and date performed. The electronic version requires an eight-character date listing year, month, and day (20XX0425). Medicaid, Medicare, private payers, and TRICARE: Required.

FL 74 A-E.
Other Procedure Codes and Dates.
Enter one or two additional major procedure codes and dates performed to identify significant procedures other than the principal procedure and corresponding dates when procedures were performed. The electronic version requires an eight-character date listing year, month, and day (20XX0215). Medicare, private payers, and TRICARE: Required. Medicaid: May be required depending on contract.

FL 75.
Reserved.
This field is reserved for national assignment.

FL 76.
Attending Provider Name and Identifier.
Enter the name or provider number for the physician who has primary responsibility for the patient's care and treatment. This form locator is mandatory for radiologists. If the physician is a Medicaid provider, enter the state license number. Do not use a group provider number. Required by all programs.

FL 77.
Operating Physician Name and Identifiers.
This field identifies the name and identification number of the person with primary responsibility for performing the surgery.

FL 78-79.
Other Provider Names and Identifiers.
These fields show the name and identification number of the provider that corresponds to the indicated provider type on this claim.

FL 80.
Remarks.
Use this area to fulfill any reporting requirements such as procedures that require additional information, justification for services, an emergency certification statement, or as an optional form locator for DRG group number for inpatient claims if not entered in FL 75. If it will not fit in this area, attach the statement to the claim. Required for all programs.

FL 81.
Code-code.
Enter if additional condition or occurrence codes are necessary to describe more information.

Taking the hospital billing process a step further, FL 5 illustrates which form locator of the UB-04 (CMS-1450) claim form is affected by the hospital department and employee. To become familiar with the UB-04 (CMS-1450) claim form, an assignment is presented in the *Workbook* asking that the 81 form locators of information be divided into six categories according to departmental input.

KEY POINTS

This is a brief chapter review or summary of the key issues presented. To further enhance your knowledge of the technical subject matter, review the key terms and key abbreviations for this chapter by locating the meanings in the glossary at the end of this book that appear in a section before the index.

1. A primary job function of a patient service representative is to promptly file hospital inpatient and outpatient claims with third-party payers, following up in a timely and efficient manner, to ensure maximum reimbursement is received for services provided.

2. Under the HIPAA, patients' financial and medical records, verbal communications, and computer security in a hospital must be confidential.

3. A patient is considered an inpatient on admission to the hospital for an overnight stay for medical services.

4. To obtain necessary diagnostic information, reduce inpatient expenses, and eliminate extra hospital days, a patient is usually sent to the hospital for PAT.

5. Medicare policy that states if a patient receives diagnostic tests and hospital outpatient services within 72 hours of admission to a hospital, then all such tests and services are combined (bundled) with inpatient services only if services are related to the admission.

6. The CMS administers the QIO program, which is responsible for the following types of reviews: admissions, readmissions, procedures, day outliers, cost outliers, DRG validations, and transfers.

7. For coding and billing outpatient claims, CPT and HCPCS codes are used for procedures and ICD-9-CM volumes 1 and 2 for diagnoses.

8. For coding and billing inpatient claims, ICD-9-CM volumes 1 and 2 are used for diagnoses and volume 3 for procedures. In 2013 ICD-10-PCS will replace volume 3 of ICD-9-CM.

9. The principal diagnosis is the condition that is assigned a code representing the diagnosis established after study that is chiefly responsible for the admission of the patient to the hospital.

10. The diagnostic code sequence is important in billing of hospital inpatient cases because maximum payment is based on the DRG system.

11. After an admitting clerk registers and admits a patient, an insurance verifier must confirm the insurance coverage.

12. All hospital services are coded with an internal code and link various hospital departments via a computer system called a CDM. It contains the charges for items and services provided to each patient.

13. The UB-04 claim form, also known as CMS-1450, is the institutional uniform claim form developed by the NUBC for hospital inpatient and outpatient billing and payment transactions.

14. Managed health care programs operate under varying contracts, policies, and guidelines and they use any one or a combination of various payment methods to reimburse hospital facilities for their services.

15. After receiving payment from insurance and managed care plans, the patient is sent a net bill that lists any owed deductible, coinsurance amount, and charges for services not covered under the insurance policy.

16. When an individual receives medical service in a section or department of the hospital and goes home the same day, he or she is classified as an outpatient.

17. A patient classification system that categorizes patients who are medically related with respect to principal diagnosis, presence of a surgical procedure, age, presence or absence of significant complications, treatment, and statistically similar in length of hospital stay is referred to as a DRG. Medicare hospital insurance payments are based on fixed dollar amounts for a principal diagnosis as listed in DRGs.

18. A method developed by the CMS for outpatient hospital reimbursement based on procedures that have similar clinical characteristics and similar costs rather than on diagnoses is known as the APC system.

℮volve INTERNET RESOURCES

For active links to the following resources, visit the Evolve website at
http://evolve.elsevier.com/fordney/handbook

- Official Coding Guidelines
- The American Hospital Association (AHA)
- The American Medical Association
- The Centers for Medicare and Medicaid Services (CMS)

- Hospital Accreditation Regulations
- National Uniform Billing Committee (NUBC)
- Managing Claim Forms
- Third-Party Payers
- Government Payers
- HIPAA Compliance Issues
- ICD-10-CM PCS 2009 rough draft version

STUDENT ASSIGNMENT

✓ Study Chapter 17.

✓ Answer the fill-in-the-blank, multiple choice, true/false, and mix and match review questions and assignments in the *Workbook* to reinforce the theory learned in this chapter and to help prepare you for a future test.

✓ Complete the assignments in the *Workbook* to gain hands-on experience in analyzing and editing information from computer-generated UB-04 (CMS-1450) claim forms for inpatient and outpatient

hospital billing. One of the assignments will assist you in further enhancing your diagnostic coding skills in relation to DRGs. These problems point out the value of coding properly in terms of proper diagnostic sequence, indicating the variance in payment.

✓ Turn to the glossary at the end of this textbook for a further understanding of the key terms and key abbreviations used in this chapter.

UNIT 5
Employment

KEY TERMS*

alien
application form
blind mailing
business associate agreement
certification
Certified Coding Specialist
Certified Coding
  Specialist-Physician
Certified Medical Assistant
Certified Medical Billing
  Specialist
Certified Professional Coder

chronologic résumé
claims assistance professional
combination résumé
continuing education
cover letter
employment agencies
functional résumé
interview
mentor
National Certified Insurance and
  Coding Specialist
networking

portfolio
Professional Association of
  Health Care Office Managers
Registered Medical Assistant
Registered Medical Coder
registration
résumé
self-employment
service contract

KEY ABBREVIATIONS*

AAPC	CCS-P	CPC, CPC-A, CPC-H	NCICS
AHIMA	CECP	ECP	PAHCOM
CAP	CMA	EEOC	RMA
CCAP	CMBS	HRS	RMC
CCS	CMRS	INS	

*Definitions for the key terms and key abbreviations are located near the back of this textbook in the glossary.

CHAPTER 18

Seeking a Job and Attaining Professional Advancement

OBJECTIVES

After reading this chapter, you should be able to:

- Prepare to find a position as an insurance billing specialist, claims assistance professional, or electronic claims processor.
- State types of certification and registration available to insurance billers and coders.
- State various actions to take to search for a job.
- Contact computerized job search databases for online services.
- Search online for employment opportunities.

- List guidelines for completing a job application form.
- Compose a letter of introduction to accompany the résumé.
- Analyze education and experience to prepare a résumé.
- Prepare responses to interview questions.
- Identify illegal interview questions.
- Explore the business aspects of self-employment.
- Name the items to assemble for a job portfolio.

Service to Patients

An insurance billing specialist has other service-oriented positions, such as collection manager, claims assistant professional for elderly patients, and insurance counselor, that focus on attention to patient needs. Whatever you decide to specialize in as far as a career related to insurance billing and coding is concerned, remember that the most important aspect of your job is patient care.

EMPLOYMENT OPPORTUNITIES

Insurance Billing Specialist

Employment opportunities are available throughout the United States (US) for insurance billing specialists who attain coding skills, knowledge of insurance programs, and expertise in completing insurance claims accurately. In addition to the skills necessary for performance on the job, ask yourself the following questions to determine

whether you need to sharpen your job-seeking techniques:

- Are you motivated and interested in finding a job?
- Can you communicate effectively in an interview?
- Do you enjoy good health?
- Are you mature?
- Do you have good grooming and manners?

The increase in the knowledge necessary and volume of paperwork associated with insurance claims, medical record keeping, and state and government agencies means a corresponding increase in the need for an insurance billing specialist. Because an individual can choose a number of different types of positions, this chapter provides information on each.

You can work in one of two ways: either employed by someone or self-employed after a number of years of

---

Performance objectives, testing and review material, and hands-on practical exercises for this chapter are available in these resources

 The Insurance Handbook Student Workbook   The Insurance Handbook Evolve Site

613

experience (Figure 18-1). The following are some of the choices in this career field:

- Insurance billing specialist
- Electronic claims processor (ECP)
- Medicare or Medicaid billing specialist
- Claims assistance professional
- Coding specialist (freelance or employed)
- Physician Coding Specialist (PCS)

Some hospital facilities and physicians prefer credentialed coders or insurance billers and advertise for the following:

- Certified medical billing specialist (CMBS)
- Certified medical reimbursement specialist (CMRS)
- Certified professional coder (CPC)
- Certified professional coder-apprentice (CPC-A)
- Certified professional coder-hospital (CPC-H)
- Certified coding specialist (CCS)
- Certified coding specialist-physician (CCS-P)
- Certified electronic claims processor (CECP)
- Certified claims assistance professional (CCAP)
- Facility Coding Specialist (FCS)
- Health care reimbursement specialist (HRS)
- National certified insurance and coding specialist (NCICS)
- **Registered medical coder (RMC)**

Becoming certified is certainly an essential goal if one seeks career advancement, and the steps to accomplish this, as well as certification in other careers allied to this one, are detailed at the end of this chapter.

Claims Assistance Professional

Contact local hospitals to determine whether they have patients who require insurance help if you want to establish yourself as a self-employed **claims assistance professional (CAP)** (in addition to some of the aforementioned positions). You can also call on small employers to determine whether they need assistance explaining their health insurance policies or enhancing insurance benefits.

JOB SEARCH

You can seek employment in several ways. You may wish to be employed by a physician, hospital, medical facility, insurance company, or managed care organization. You may choose to be self-employed if you have had a number of years of experience or you may even choose some type of combination situation. The following lists suggested actions to take to search for a job.

1. Join a professional organization, as mentioned later in this chapter, to network with others in the same career field and to hear about job openings (Figure 18-2). Put a notice about your availability in the chapter newsletter.
2. Attend meetings and workshops in this career field to keep up to date and network with others.
3. Contact the school placement personnel, complete the necessary paperwork, and leave a résumé on file if you have just completed a course at a community college or trade school.
4. Spread the word to those who work in medical settings and those who might hear of openings in medical facilities such as classmates, instructors, school counselors, relatives, and friends. If you are introducing yourself to a hiring manager identified via a professional colleague, type the colleague's name in the e-mail subject line (e.g., "John Doe referred me") so the manager is less likely to delete your e-mail.

FIGURE 18-1 Staff conference discussing applicants for potential interviews.

FIGURE 18-2 Student scanning a professional journal for job leads.

5. Contact pharmaceutical representatives who visit physicians' offices and hospitals for employment information or leads.
6. Visit public and private **employment agencies,** including temporary and temporary to permanent agencies. Before signing up with an agency, ask whether the employer or applicant pays the agency fee.
7. Inquire at state and federal government offices and their employment agencies.
8. Look for part-time employment that might lead to a permanent full-time position.
9. Check bulletin boards frequently in personnel offices of hospitals and clinics for posted job offerings.
10. Go to your local medical society to determine whether it has a provision for supplying job leads.
11. Consult the Yellow Pages of the telephone directory or medical society roster for names of professional offices and hospitals to contact with an introductory telephone call, letter, or e-mail message.
12. Send a **blind mailing** of the résumé, including a cover letter, to possible prospects. A blind mailing means to send information to employers whom you do not know personally and who have not advertised for a job opening. This may result in a positive response with either a request to complete an application form or an invitation for an interview.
13. Go to the local library and look through Dun and Bradstreet's *Million Dollar Directory* or go online to the *Million Dollar Database* for information on potential employers in many cities.
14. Visit the chamber of commerce and ask for some of their publications that contain membership directories, names of major professional employers in specific areas, and brochures describing regional facts.
15. Subscribe to the principal newspaper of the city where employment is desired. Read help wanted advertisements in the classified section, especially in the Sunday newspaper. Positions of interest might be listed as insurance billing specialist, reimbursement manager, insurance claims manager, insurance coordinator, insurance biller, coding/reimbursement specialist, reimbursement coordinator, coder/abstracter, electronic claims processor, and so on. Do not be discouraged by specific requirements in an advertisement; apply anyway. Send your résumé and a cover letter the next day. Some employers give priority to candidates who respond within the first 3 or 4 days after a job announcement because they believe it is an indication that someone is truly interested in the position. Many jobs are not advertised and there could be an opening available for which you qualify.
16. E-mail or telephone job hot lines of large medical clinics in your area.
17. Visit job locations unannounced (referred to as "cold calling").
18. Explore the Internet. See Internet Resources at the end of this chapter, and go to the Evolve website, which has links to many search engines.
19. Upload your résumé to as many databases as possible.

Online Job Search

Because of vast communication available via the Internet, newspaper and magazine classified advertisements may become resources of the past. An individual with a computer and modem can access online services. Many websites on the Internet incorporate text, sound, graphics, animation, and video. It is possible to locate potential employers at their websites who are offering jobs to health care workers by using various search engines. At some sites, you can find detailed descriptions of posted positions and locate opportunity postings by location or employer. You may be able to find and respond to a specific job of interest by delivering an online résumé, attaching a cover letter, and updating your posting as often as needed. Some websites allow you to receive e-mailed job alerts. Employers may use automated résumé scanning to sort e-mailed résumés for key words. Use standard typefaces and font sizes between 10 to 14 points. Keep text lines under 74 characters, and use bold face for section headings. You need to have a 95% to 100% key word match for the position, therefore sprinkle your résumé and cover letter with the verbiage used in the job advertisement. Key words can be entered at the end of the document. To make them unnoticeable, select the words and make the font color white; thus they will not appear when printed or viewed on the monitor, but the electronic scan will see them when sorting.

You can gain Internet access in several ways. Your school may allow you to access the Internet on campus. Many libraries have computers with free Internet service. If you have a computer at home, you may wish to subscribe to either a commercial online service (e.g., America Online) with Internet access or an Internet service in your locale (Figure 18-3).

Internet

Once online, go to a Web index to locate a search engine, such as Yahoo (www.yahoo.com), Google (www.google.com), or Alta Vista (www.altavista.com), that lists different options to explore. One of the resources is *Career Magazine* (www.careermag.com), which lets you browse through hundreds of national job openings in a variety of fields. Check out America's Job Bank, which has job postings that you can browse according to field, location, and career type. Go to PracticeNet (www.practice-net.com), which provides descriptions of medical practice opportunities. This 24-hour service

FIGURE 18-3 Student doing an online job search.

names the recruiter, location, and a toll-free telephone number to contact. MedSearch America is another health employment service that posts jobs for hospitals, managed care organizations (MCOs), and pharmaceutical companies. MedSearch, Monster Board, and Online Career Center combined to form monster.com. Job seekers can send their résumés via e-mail for free online posting by going to www.monster.com.

If you subscribe monthly to a commercial online service, you can network by posting a notice on a bulletin board with your résumé or a note that you are looking for a particular type of position in a given locale.

Career options on the Internet are discussed in Joyce Lain Kennedy's book *Hook Up, Get Hired! The Internet Job Search Revolution*, published by John Wiley & Sons, New York.

Job Fairs

Annual community events feature job fairs at community colleges and technical trade schools. Some job fairs are sponsored by professional associations. Job recruiters set up booths with information about their companies and available positions; however, they do not have much time to spend with each job seeker. Thus it is wise to go prepared and practice a 30-second introduction before attending. This introduction should consist of a quick overview of your career goals, experience, skills, training, education, and personal strengths. Be sure to explain what you can offer the employer. These are usually day-long events and you may want to investigate a number of participating employers' booths.

Go prepared by dressing professionally and carrying a binder or folder with plenty of copies of your résumé to give to the company representatives you meet. Résumés should be neat, clean, and not folded, wrinkled, or coffee stained. Take a pen, pencil, and notepad to obtain information. Research the employers attending so that you know which ones you will visit. Keep a positive attitude and approach each employer with confidence and enthusiasm. Show that you are interested and knowledgeable to the job recruiter.

Take home the business card and brochure of anyone you talk to who genuinely interests you. After the fair, send that person a follow-up letter or e-mail message to reaffirm your interest.

Application

When visiting a potential employer, ask for an **application form** to complete and inquire whether the facility keeps potential job applicants on file and for how long (Figure 18-4). Study each question carefully before answering because the employer may evaluate the application itself to determine whether the applicant can follow instructions. Furnish as much information as possible, and if a question does not apply or cannot be answered, insert "no," "none," "NA" (not applicable), or "DNA" (does not apply). Some application forms may request information that may be considered discriminatory. If this situation should occur, use your best judgment on whether to insert or omit an answer. When visiting a potential employer for an application form, be sure you have prepared in advance for an interview in case an opportunity arises on that first visit.

Follow these guidelines when completing an application form:

1. Read the whole application form because some instructions may appear on the last page or last line.
2. Read the fine print and instructions: "Please print," "Put last name first," or "Complete in your own handwriting." This indicates ability to follow directions or instructions.
3. Print if your handwriting is poor, and abbreviate only when there is lack of space.
4. Complete the application in black ink unless pencil is specified.
5. Refer to data from a portfolio, sample application form, or résumé that has been checked for accuracy;

APPLICATION FOR POSITION / Medical or Dental Office
AN EQUAL OPPORTUNITY EMPLOYER

(In answering questions, use extra blank sheet if necessary)

No employee, applicant, or candidate for promotion, training or other advantage shall be discriminated against (or given preference) because of race, color, religion, sex, age, physical handicap, veteran status, or national origin.

PLEASE READ CAREFULLY AND WRITE OR PRINT ANSWERS TO ALL QUESTIONS. DO NOT TYPE.

Date of application *7-2-20XX*

A. PERSONAL INFORMATION

Name - Last *Valasquez*　First *Jennifer*　Middle *M*

Home Tel. (555) *439-4800*
Bus. Tel. (　)
E-mail (optional) *valasquezj@gmail.com*
Cell Phone (optional) *555-301-2612*

Present address: Street *1234 Martin Street*　(Apt.#)　City *Woodland Hills*　State *XY*　Zip *12345*

Person to notify in case of emergency or accident - name: *Elena Sanchez*
Address: *20 South M Street Woodland Hills, XY 12345*　Telephone: *555-261-0707*

B. EMPLOYMENT INFORMATION

Position desired: *insurance biller*

X Full-time　Part-time　Either

Date available for employment: *7-6-20XX*

Wage/salary expectations: *negotiable*

List hrs./days you prefer to work: *M-F 8-5 PM*

List any hrs./days you are not available: (Except for times required for religious practices or observances)

Can you work overtime, if necessary?　X Yes　No

Are you employed now?:　Yes　X No

If so, may we inquire of your present employer?:　No　Yes, if yes:
Name of employer:　　Phone number: (　)

Have you applied for a position with this office before?　X No　Yes　If Yes, when?: Month and year _____ Location _____

Are you able to perform the essential functions of the job for which you are applying? . . . . X Yes　No

If no, describe the functions that cannot be performed _____

(Note: We comply with the ADA and consider reasonable accommodation measures that may be necessary for eligible applicants/employees to perform essential functions. Hire may be subject to passing a medical examination, and to skill and agility tests.)

Have you ever been convicted of a criminal offense (felony or serious misdemeanor)? *(Convictions for marijuana-related offenses that are more than two years old need not be listed.)*　Yes　No

If yes, state nature of the crime(s), when and where convicted and disposition of the case _____

(Note: No applicant will be denied employment solely on the grounds of conviction of a criminal offense. The nature of the offense, the date of the offense, the surrounding circumstances and the relevance of the offense to the position(s) applied for may, however, be considered.)

Referred by/or where did you learn of this job?: *Read advertisement in newspaper*

Can you, upon employment, submit verification of your legal right to work in the United States?　X Yes　No
Submit proof that you meet legal age requirement for employment?　X Yes　No

Language(s) applicant speaks or writes (if use of a language other than English is relevant to the job for which the applicant is applying: *Spanish*

C. EDUCATION HISTORY

	Name and address of schools attended (include current)	Number of months/years attended	Highest grade/level completed	Diploma/degree(s) obtained/areas of study
High school	*ABC High School, Woodland Hills, XY*	*2000-2004*	*12*	*Diploma*
College	*Vocational-Tech School, Woodland Hills, XY*	*2005*		Degree/major *Certificate*
Post graduate	*Montana State Univ., Woodland Hills, XY*	*2005-2007*		Degree/major *24 credits*
Business/trade/technical				Course/diploma/license/certificate
Other				Course/diploma/license/certificate

Specific training, skills, education, or experiences which will assist you in the job for which you have applied. *See resume*

Membership/professional or civic organizations (excluding those that disclose race, color, religion or national origin) *Amer. Acad. of Professional Coders*

Future educational plans *Continuing education—preparing for certification in coding*

Military - did you serve in the armed forces　X No　Yes, if yes, branch?:_____
Training relevant to position for which you are applying:

D. SPECIAL SKILLS (Check below the kinds of work you have done)

Front Office		Back Office	
X Accounts receivable	X Filing	Blood counts	Phlebotomy
Bookkeeping	X Medical terminology	Dental assistant	Urinalysis
X Collections	Medical transcription	Dental hygienist	X-ray
X Data entry	Receptionist	Injections	Other:
X Electronic/medical billing	Other:	Nursing/assisting	Other:

Other kinds of tasks performed or skills that may be applicable to position:

Office equipment/machines used: *computer, calculator, printer*

Keyboarding/typing speed *65 wpm*

Computer programs used: *Word, Excel*

FIGURE 18-4 Application for Position/Medical or Dental Office form. (Courtesy Bibbero Systems, Inc., Petaluma, CA. Telephone: (800) 242-2376; fax: (800) 242-9330; website: www.bibbero.com.)

Continued

E. EMPLOYMENT RECORD

☐ INFORMATION SUPPLIED ON ATTACHED RESUME

LIST MOST RECENT EMPLOYMENT FIRST (Full or Part-Time) May we contact your previous employer(s) for a reference? ☒ Yes ☐ No

1) Employer/Company name *St. John's Outpatient Clinic*

Type of business: *Hospital outpatient medical clinic*

Address Street *24 Center St.* City *Woodland Hills,* State *XY* Zip code *12345*

Worked performed. Be specific:

Phone number *(555) 782-0155*

Your position *Insurance billing specialist* | Dates From Mo. *6* Yr. *07* To Mo. *6* Yr. *09*

Supervisor's name *Candice Johnson* | Hourly rate/salary Starting *$12/hr* Final *$15/hr*

Reason for leaving *Professional advancement*

2) Employer/Company name *Eastern Airlines*

Type of business: *Airline transportation*

Address Street City *Orlando* State *FL* Zip code

Worked performed. Be specific:

Phone number *(555) 350-7000*

Your position *Receptionist* | Dates From Mo. *1* Yr. *99* To Mo. *1* Yr. *2000*

Supervisor's name *Gary Stevens* | Hourly rate/salary Starting *$9/hr* Final *$11.50/hr*

Reason for leaving *Career change*

3) Employer/Company name

Type of business:

Address Street City State Zip code

Worked performed. Be specific:

Phone number ( )

Your position | Dates From Mo. Yr. To Mo. Yr.

Supervisor's name | Hourly rate/salary Starting Final

Reason for leaving

F. REFERENCES — List below two persons NOT related to you who have knowledge of your work performance within the last three years.

(1) *Furnished upon request*

Name | Address | Telephone number | (☐ Work ☐ Home) | Occupation | Years acquainted

(2)

Name | Address | Telephone number | (☐ Work ☐ Home) | Occupation | Years acquainted

Please feel free to add any information which you feel will help us consider you for employment

DO NOT ANSWER ANY QUESTIONS IN THIS SECTION UNLESS THE BOXES ARE CHECKED - If the employer has checked the box next to the question, the information requested is needed for a legally permissible reason, including, without limitation, national security considerations, a legitimate occupational qualification or business necessity. The Civil Rights Act of 1964 prohibits discrimination in employment because of race, color, religion, sex or national origin. Federal law also prohibits discrimination based on age, citizenship and disability. The laws of most States also prohibit some or all of the above types of discrimination as well as some additional types such as discrimination based upon ancestry, marital status and sexual preference.

☐ Provide dates you attended school: | Elementary From To | ☐ Number of dependents, including yourself

☐ High School From To | College From To | ☐ Are you a Vietnam veteran? ☐ Yes ☐ No

Other (give name and dates) | ☐ Sex ☐ Male ☐ Female

☐ Marital status ☐ Single ☐ Engaged ☐ Married ☐ Separated ☐ Divorced ☐ Widowed ☐ Date of marriage | ☐ Are you a U.S. citizen? ☐ Yes ☐ No

☐ What was your previous address? | ☐ How long at previous address? _____ years

☐ State names of relatives and friends working for us, other that your spouse. | ☐ How long at present address? _____ years

☐ Have you ever been bonded? ☐ Yes ☐ No If "Yes," with what employers? | ☐ Are you over 18 years of age? ☐ Yes ☐ No If not, employment is subject to verification of age.

READ THE FOLLOWING CAREFULLY, THEN SIGN AND DATE THE APPLICATION

The information provided in this Application for Employment is true, correct, and complete. If employed, any misstatement or omission of fact on this application may result in my dismissal. I understand that acceptance of an offer of employment does not create a contractual obligation upon the employer to continue to employ me in the future. If you decide to engage an investigative consumer reporting agency to report on my credit and personal history I authorize you to do so. If a report is obtained you must provide, at my request, the name of the agency so I may obtain from them the nature and substance of the information contained in the report.

If requested, I hereby agree to submit to binding arbitration all disputes and claims arising out of the submission of this application. I further agree, in the event that I am hired by the company, that all disputes that cannot be resolved by informal internal resolution which might arise out of my employment with the company, whether during or after that employment, will be submitted to binding arbitration. I agree that such arbitration shall be conducted under the rules of the American Arbitration Association. This application contains the entire agreement between the parties with regard to dispute resolution, and there are no other agreements as to dispute resolution, either oral or written.

Date: *7-2-20XX* Signature: *Jennifer M. Valasquez*

FIGURE 18-4, cont'd

use this information to copy onto each new application form. Be neat.

6. List correct dates of previous employment so that it will be accurate if the employer seeks verification. If a question is presented asking the reason for leaving a position, leave it blank and discuss this during the interview.

7. Name specific skills such as procedural coding, diagnostic coding, knowledge of insurance programs, ability to complete and/or transmit the CMS-1500 (08-05) claim form, typing or keyboarding (number of words per minute), fluency in a second language, knowledge of medical terminology, and knowledge and use of computer software.

8. When a question is asked about salary amount, write in "negotiable" or "flexible" and then discuss this during the interview.

9. Sign the application after completion.

10. Reread the entire form, word for word, to find any errors of omission or commission. This avoids having to apologize during an interview for a mistake.

Letter of Introduction

Individuals spend days perfecting a résumé but throw together a letter of introduction or **cover letter** in minutes. This is a mistake. The main goal of the cover letter is to get the employer to take notice of the potential employee and résumé so that an interview appointment can be made. Letters should be typed, addressed to a specific person, and customized to each potential employer. If the advertisement gives a telephone number, call and ask for the name of the person doing the interviewing so that the letter can include that person's name. When the name is unknown, use "Dear Sir or Madam" or "To Whom It May Concern," or a less formal "Hello" or "Good Morning."

Do not repeat everything in the résumé. Begin with an attention grabber, and get right to the point so that the employer knows what you want and why. The letter should explain how the applicant's qualifications and skills would benefit the employer. Use key words that appear in the "position wanted" advertisement. End the letter by requesting an interview and be sure to enclose a résumé. Always include telephone numbers (home and cell) and the time of day when you are available.

Reread the letter for typos and errors in grammar, punctuation, and spelling. Avoid the use of "I" in the sentence structure (Figure 18-5).

Résumé

A **résumé** is a data sheet designed to sell job qualifications to prospective employers. A résumé should be created with information highlighted that relates to the position the applicant is trying to obtain and therefore would differ for each job. There are several formats from which to choose:

- A **chronologic résumé** gives recent experiences first with dates and descriptive data for each job.
- A **functional résumé** states the qualifications or skills an individual is able to perform.
- A **combination résumé** summarizes the applicant's job skills, as well as educational and employment history. The combination style is the best choice for an insurance billing specialist (Figure 18-6).

A results-oriented résumé focuses on results, not characteristics. It helps prospective employers reduce the risks that are associated with hiring because it shows what the job seeker has accomplished and his or her attitude toward work.

The ideal length for a résumé is one page. It can be typed on an $8\frac{1}{2} \times 14$-inch page and reduced to letter size. The résumé should be keyed or typed, not handwritten, on high-quality, wrinkle-free bond off-white or white paper; single spaced internally with double spacing between main headings; and balanced spacing for all four margins. Laser-printed résumés give a professional appearance. You might want to have a longer (two-page maximum) résumé on hand to offer during an interview.

Under the Civil Rights Act of 1964, enforced by the Equal Employment Opportunity Commission, information about height, weight, birth date, marital status, Social Security number, and physical condition may be omitted. Additional items to omit are salary requirements, reason for leaving jobs, date of résumé preparation, date available to begin work, references, and vague references to time gaps. Questions about these items might be asked by the interviewer during an interview. If you get laid off and have a gap between jobs, get actively involved in volunteer projects or consulting opportunities, even if you do the work free. This allows you to use your skills that may be described on your résumé. Hobbies and outside interests that relate to the profession might be included. Membership or leadership positions held in professional organizations related to the medical field might be mentioned. A photograph is not necessary but might be included if it will be of value to the interviewer for recall purposes.

The format may include the following:

- Title. Résumé, personal data sheet, biographic sketch, or curriculum vitae.
- Heading. At the beginning of the résumé, the applicant's name, address, e-mail address, and telephone (home and cell) and fax numbers.

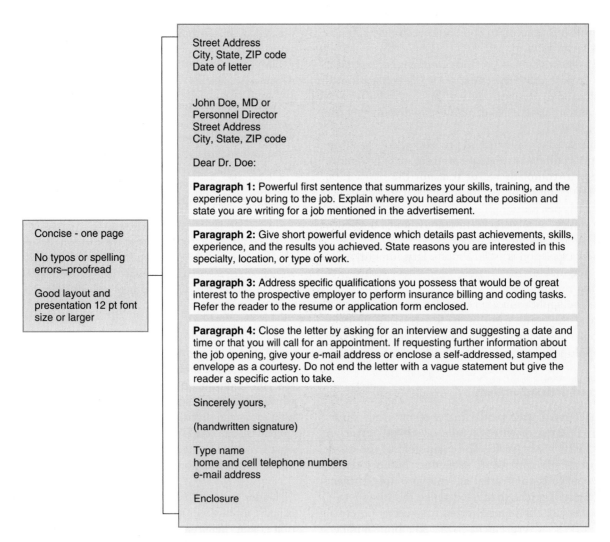

Street Address
City, State, ZIP code
Date of letter

John Doe, MD or
Personnel Director
Street Address
City, State, ZIP code

Dear Dr. Doe:

Paragraph 1: Powerful first sentence that summarizes your skills, training, and the experience you bring to the job. Explain where you heard about the position and state you are writing for a job mentioned in the advertisement.

Paragraph 2: Give short powerful evidence which details past achievements, skills, experience, and the results you achieved. State reasons you are interested in this specialty, location, or type of work.

Paragraph 3: Address specific qualifications you possess that would be of great interest to the prospective employer to perform insurance billing and coding tasks. Refer the reader to the resume or application form enclosed.

Paragraph 4: Close the letter by asking for an interview and suggesting a date and time or that you will call for an appointment. If requesting further information about the job opening, give your e-mail address or enclose a self-addressed, stamped envelope as a courtesy. Do not end the letter with a vague statement but give the reader a specific action to take.

Sincerely yours,

(handwritten signature)

Type name
home and cell telephone numbers
e-mail address

Enclosure

Concise - one page

No typos or spelling errors–proofread

Good layout and presentation 12 pt font size or larger

FIGURE 18-5 Suggested content for a letter of introduction to accompany a résumé.

- Summary. This may be a statement as to why the employer should be interested in this applicant. Use action words as shown in Figure 18-6 and avoid the personal pronoun.
- Education. Name high school, college, any business school attended, and **continuing education** classes, city and state, degree, and date received. List in reverse chronologic order. Grade average and awards or scholastic honors may be included.
- Professional experience. Name all employers in reverse chronologic order with addresses, telephone numbers, and dates of employment. Include summer, full-time, part-time, and temporary jobs, as well as externship and volunteer work. Detail achievements, not duties (e.g., "possess strong communication, service to patients, and organizational skills" or "consistently surpassed collection goals by 10 percent or more each year").
- Skills. List typing or keyboarding words per minute, computer equipment operated, experience in medical practice management software programs, accurate procedure and diagnostic coding including knowledge of modifiers, expertise in insurance claims completion and submission, knowledge of medical terminology and insurance terminology, bookkeeping (posting charges, payments, and adjustments to accounts receivable journal), experience in preparing appeals for denied claims, resubmittal of delinquent claims, ability to explain insurance programs and plans (e.g., benefits, requirements, and submission of claims), ability to abstract information from patients' medical and financial records, and ability to review insurance payments from explanation of benefit documents. If you are fluent in another language, provide this information. Telephone and reception skills also might be mentioned.
- References. Type in the phrase "Furnished on request." Prepare approximately five references on a separate sheet and be sure to contact the persons referenced before an interview.

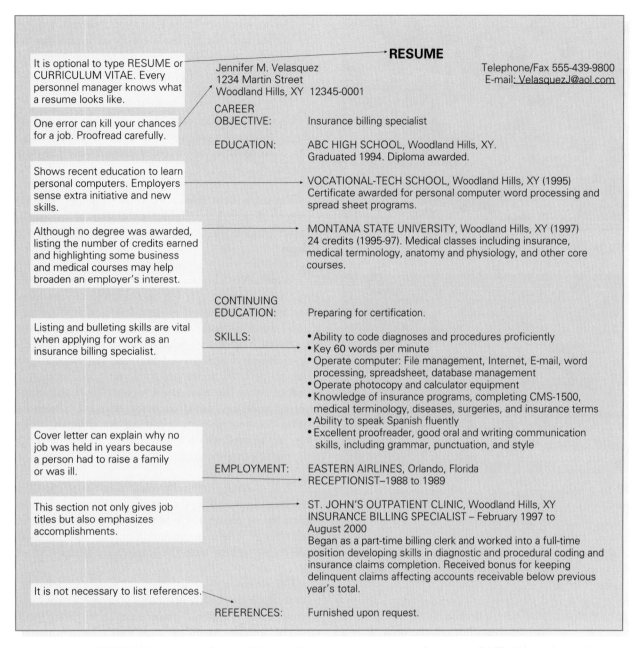

It is optional to type RESUME or CURRICULUM VITAE. Every personnel manager knows what a resume looks like.

One error can kill your chances for a job. Proofread carefully.

Shows recent education to learn personal computers. Employers sense extra initiative and new skills.

Although no degree was awarded, listing the number of credits earned and highlighting some business and medical courses may help broaden an employer's interest.

Listing and bulleting skills are vital when applying for work as an insurance billing specialist.

Cover letter can explain why no job was held in years because a person had to raise a family or was ill.

This section not only gives job titles but also emphasizes accomplishments.

It is not necessary to list references.

RESUME

Jennifer M. Velasquez
1234 Martin Street
Woodland Hills, XY 12345-0001

Telephone/Fax 555-439-9800
E-mail: VelasquezJ@aol.com

CAREER OBJECTIVE: Insurance billing specialist

EDUCATION: ABC HIGH SCHOOL, Woodland Hills, XY.
Graduated 1994. Diploma awarded.

VOCATIONAL-TECH SCHOOL, Woodland Hills, XY (1995)
Certificate awarded for personal computer word processing and spread sheet programs.

MONTANA STATE UNIVERSITY, Woodland Hills, XY (1997)
24 credits (1995-97). Medical classes including insurance, medical terminology, anatomy and physiology, and other core courses.

CONTINUING EDUCATION: Preparing for certification.

SKILLS:
• Ability to code diagnoses and procedures proficiently
• Key 60 words per minute
• Operate computer: File management, Internet, E-mail, word processing, spreadsheet, database management
• Operate photocopy and calculator equipment
• Knowledge of insurance programs, completing CMS-1500, medical terminology, diseases, surgeries, and insurance terms
• Ability to speak Spanish fluently
• Excellent proofreader, good oral and writing communication skills, including grammar, punctuation, and style

EMPLOYMENT: EASTERN AIRLINES, Orlando, Florida
RECEPTIONIST–1988 to 1989

ST. JOHN'S OUTPATIENT CLINIC, Woodland Hills, XY
INSURANCE BILLING SPECIALIST – February 1997 to August 2000
Began as a part-time billing clerk and worked into a full-time position developing skills in diagnostic and procedural coding and insurance claims completion. Received bonus for keeping delinquent claims affecting accounts receivable below previous year's total.

REFERENCES: Furnished upon request.

FIGURE 18-6 Example of the combination-format résumé stressing education and skills. Personal data may be excluded as a result of the Civil Rights Act of 1964, enforced by the EEOC.

● Final details. It is acceptable to e-mail or fax a résumé to an employer who advertises a job opening but gives no guidelines on how to submit the résumé. It is wise to use every advantage possible in a competitive employment market in which time is of the essence (Figure 18-7).

Proofread the résumé carefully for spelling, punctuation, grammar, and typographic errors. Ask a friend or professional individual with excellent English skills to read and critique it. Remember that the résumé is only a foot in the door and not what is going to land that job for you—you are!

Interview

After looking for a potential employer, preparing a résumé, and completing an application, the final step in landing a job is the face-to-face interview. An **interview**

FIGURE 18-7 Insurance billing student at an externship site.

FIGURE 18-8 Student being interviewed for an insurance billing position.

is a formal consultation with questions by an employer to evaluate the qualifications of a prospective job applicant (Figure 18-8).

Make the best impression possible on the prospective employer as soon as you walk through the door. It is a well-known fact that the first 30 seconds makes either a positive or negative impression. Hiring depends on positive qualities. Concentrate on good grooming and a fresh, relaxed appearance. Display a warm, positive attitude. Use proper grammar, avoid using slang, and maintain eye contact.

A female applicant should wear a clean skirt, dress, or tailored suit and nylon stockings with low-heeled pumps. A male applicant should wear a clean dark suit or sport coat, conservative necktie, white shirt, plain slacks, plain socks, and well-shined shoes. A man should avoid a lot of facial hair, long hair, earrings, and heavy aftershave lotion. A woman should have a conservative hairstyle, wear jewelry sparingly, and avoid heavy makeup, a low-cut neckline, a sleeveless dress, strong perfume, and dark or bright nail polish.

Do not smoke or chew gum. Use a proper deodorant. Eliminate nervous habits. It has been found that when applicants have similar skills and education, the decision to hire has been based on physical appearance at the interview.

Figure 18-9 is an example of an interview evaluation and reference investigation form. This form points out the areas an interviewer observes and how impressions are rated.

Research beforehand to know whether the salary (when offered) is acceptable. If you want to ask questions about benefits, do not appear to be overly interested in them.

If possible, choose a good time for the interview and arrive promptly. It has been found that late Monday and Friday afternoons between 4:00 and 5:00 PM are not good times for interviews because Mondays are usually catch-up, heavily scheduled days and Fridays are getaway days. Research has proved that the likelihood of hiring the last person interviewed for a position is greater than that of hiring those interviewed first. Carry something in your hand (e.g., portfolio with notepad, résumé, and other documents) so that you are not showing nervousness or anxiety, which might detract and be detrimental during the interview.

Role-playing is a good method to use to prepare for an interview. Give a friend a list of questions to ask you and then try to answer the questions spontaneously without stumbling. Videotape or audiotape the session, if possible, to see or hear what the employer will experience.

Questions an interviewer might ask about personal life (marital status), family planning, pregnancy, provision for child care, religious preference, club memberships, height, weight, dependents, age (birth date), ethnic background, maiden name, native language, physical or psychiatric problems, spouse's employment and earnings, credit rating, and home and automobile ownership are illegal and do not have to be answered. (It is not considered discriminatory if an employer wants to know whether an applicant smokes.) Three suggestions for handling an illegal question follow:

1. Answer the question and ignore the fact that you know it is illegal.
2. Answer with, "I think the question is not relevant to the requirements of this position."
3. Refuse to answer and contact the nearest Equal Employment Opportunity Commission (EEOC) office.

Shake the interviewer's hand at the conclusion of the meeting (Figure 18-10). Ask how long it will be before a

INTERVIEW EVALUATION AND REFERENCE INVESTIGATION FORM, MEDICAL or DENTAL OFFICE

SUMMARY OF EVALUATION	
POINTS FROM APPLICATION AND INTERVIEW	
POINTS FROM REFERENCES	
TOTAL POINTS	

NAME OF APPLICANT	DATE	OVERALL IMPRESSION	

RATING: GOOD – 2 POINTS
FAIR – 1 POINT
POOR – 0 POINTS

POSITION APPLIED FOR:

FROM APPLICATION FOR POSITION, GAUGE APPLICANT IN FOLLOWING AREAS	GOOD	FAIR	POOR
1. STABILITY (REMAINED IN ONE PLACE OF RESIDENCE AND ONE JOB FOR A REASONABLE LENGTH OF TIME)?			
2. HEALTH?			
3. THE PROPER EDUCATIONAL BACKGROUND TO FILL THE POSITION?			
4. LEGIBLE HANDWRITING?			
5. AN EMPLOYMENT HISTORY THAT POINTS TOWARD DEPENDABILITY?			
6. LIMITATION ON WORKING HOURS?			
7. THE PROPER EXPERIENCE AND / OR SKILLS TO FILL THE POSITION?			
8. SALARY REQUIREMENT COMMENSURATE WITH POSITION?			
FROM THE PERSONAL INTERVIEW – (SHOULD BE SPECIFIC QUALITIES – OBJECTIVE)			
9. SUFFICIENT CAPABILITY TO HANDLE ANY SITUATION THAT MAY ARISE WHEN ALONE IN OFFICE?			
10. AN APPROPRIATE ATTITUDE TOWARD WORK?			
11. AN APPROPRIATE VOICE, DICTION, GRAMMAR?			
12. POISE?			
13. SELF CONFIDENCE (NOT OVER-CONFIDENCE)?			
14. TACT?			
15. SUFFICIENT MATURITY FOR JOB?			
16. AN ABILITY TO EXPRESS ONESELF WELL?			
17. AN INITIATIVE OR INTEREST IN LEARNING?			
18. APPROPRIATE APPEARANCE (NEAT, CLEAN; SUITABLE TO BUSINESS)			
19. ENERGY, VITALITY AND PERCEIVED ABILITY TO HANDLE PRESSURE OF POSITION?			
20. EAGERNESS TO OBTAIN THE POSITION IN QUESTION?			
COLUMNAR TOTALS			
GRAND TOTAL			

(Left margin vertical label: APPLICATION SECTION REFERENCE)

DIRECTIONS FOR USE OF FORM:

1. Look over your ratings. A zero score on any one VITAL question should automatically eliminate applicant. Add up the total rating points and enter in the SUMMARY OF EVALUATION BLOCK in the upper right-hand corner of this page.
2. After finishing all interviews, choose the "best bets" and check their references using the reverse side of this form.
3. Enter, as above, the results of your reference check and then your overall impression. (E – Excellent, G – Good, F – Fair, P – Poor)

FIGURE 18-9 Example of an interview evaluation and reference investigation form. (Courtesy Bibbero Systems, Inc., Petaluma, CA. Telephone: (800) 242-2376; fax: (800) 242-9330; website: www.bibbero.com.)

Continued

NOTES:

REFERENCE INVESTIGATION

1.

OFFICE CONTACTED	PHONE: ( )	DATE

PERSON CONTACTED

HOW LONG HAVE YOU KNOWN THIS PERSON?

BETWEEN WHAT DATES WAS THIS PERSON EMPLOYED BY YOU?	FROM	TO

WHAT TYPE OF WORK DID THIS PERSON DO FOR YOU?	TITLE OF POSITION:	SATISFACTORILY?

WAS THIS PERSON CONSISTENTLY COOPERATIVE?	WHAT WERE SHORTCOMINGS?

DID THIS PERSON GET ALONG WELL WITH OTHERS?

WAS THIS PERSON TRUSTWORTHY / DEPENDABLE?	ATTENDANCE RECORD:

WHY DID THIS PERSON LEAVE YOUR EMPLOY?	SALARY LEVEL:

WOULD YOU REHIRE THIS PERSON?

NOTES:

RATING:

2.

OFFICE CONTACTED	PHONE: ( )	DATE

PERSON CONTACTED

HOW LONG HAVE YOU KNOWN THIS PERSON?

BETWEEN WHAT DATES WAS THIS PERSON EMPLOYED BY YOU?	FROM	TO

WHAT TYPE OF WORK DID THIS PERSON DO FOR YOU?	TITLE OF POSITION:	SATISFACTORILY?

WAS THIS PERSON CONSISTENTLY COOPERATIVE?	WHAT WERE SHORTCOMINGS?

DID THIS PERSON GET ALONG WELL WITH OTHERS?

WAS THIS PERSON TRUSTWORTHY / DEPENDABLE?	ATTENDANCE RECORD:

WHY DID THIS PERSON LEAVE YOUR EMPLOY?	SALARY LEVEL:

WOULD YOU REHIRE THIS PERSON?

NOTES:

RATING:

3.

OFFICE CONTACTED	PHONE: ( )	DATE

PERSON CONTACTED

HOW LONG HAVE YOU KNOWN THIS PERSON?

BETWEEN WHAT DATES WAS THIS PERSON EMPLOYED BY YOU?	FROM	TO

WHAT TYPE OF WORK DID THIS PERSON DO FOR YOU?	TITLE OF POSITION:	SATISFACTORILY?

WAS THIS PERSON CONSISTENTLY COOPERATIVE?	WHAT WERE SHORTCOMINGS?

DID THIS PERSON GET ALONG WELL WITH OTHERS?

WAS THIS PERSON TRUSTWORTHY / DEPENDABLE?	ATTENDANCE RECORD:

WHY DID THIS PERSON LEAVE YOUR EMPLOY?	SALARY LEVEL:

WOULD YOU REHIRE THIS PERSON?

NOTES:

RATING:

INTERVIEWER _____   DATE: _____

FIGURE 18-9, cont'd

job offer or denial is forthcoming, and then leave with a "thank you." If the job is offered at the interview and you are not sure about accepting, ask, "How soon do you need to know?" This will allow time to think and compare job offers before making a commitment.

Portfolio

Prepare in advance for the interview by organizing a **portfolio.** Assemble letters of recommendation (from former employers, teachers, family physician, professional friends, or community leaders), school diplomas or degrees, transcripts, certificates, names and addresses of

FIGURE 18-10 Job applicant concluding an interview with an office manager.

references, extra copies of the résumé, timed typing test certified by an instructor, some neatly typed insurance claim forms with evidence of coding skills, and any other items related to prior education and work experience.

Alien

Any **alien** employee must have an Employment Eligibility Verification Form I-9 on file with his or her employer. As presented in Chapter 12, an alien is an individual who is not a citizen or national of the United States but belongs to another country or people; also referred to as an immigrant or foreigner. Form I-9 can be obtained by writing to the Department of Homeland Security, Immigration and Naturalization Service (INS) at 425 I Street, NW, Washington, DC 20536. Within 3 days of being hired, an employee must show one of the following: a naturalization certification (citizen papers), an alien registration receipt card, a temporary resident receipt card, or an employment authorization card. One of these items should be available in the event it is requested by the prospective employer during the interview.

Follow-Up Letter

Write a follow-up letter or send an e-mail message within 24 hours of the interview. Indicate a thank you for the interview and restate interest in the position (Figure 18-11). This keeps the applicant's name before the potential employer. Telephone to express continued interest in the position if no response is heard within the time frame given.

Street Address
City, State, ZIP code
Date of letter

John Doe, MD or
Personnel Director
Street Address
City, State, ZIP code

Dear Dr. Doe:

Thank you for spending your valuable time yesterday to interview me for the insurance billing specialist position in your clinic.

I hope that you will allow me the opportunity to prove my abilities as I feel that I am able to perform the work with expertise. Meeting your staff was most enjoyable, and it would certainly be pleasurable working with them as a team.

I am looking forward to hearing from you in the near future.

Sincerely yours,

(handwritten signature)

Type name

FIGURE 18-11 Example of a thank-you letter sent after an interview.

SELF-EMPLOYMENT

Setting Up an Office

When an individual wants to be his or her own boss (self-employment), it is usually wise to become educated and have some experience in the chosen career before undertaking this task. Having a positive and effective rapport with the public, as well as a strong background in insurance, is desirable for the individual who wants to work independently as a billing specialist. Outpatient hospital and physician billing experience in several specialties is important if you choose to focus on outpatient billing/coding services. If you specialize in hospital services billing/coding, experience is necessary, especially because it is not common for a hospital to outsource these services to a small billing company. If coding services are to be part of the billing company's offerings, the coding professional should be certified by a reputable professional organization such as the American Academy of Professional Coders (AAPC) or American Health Information Management Association (AHIMA).

The Health Insurance Portability and Accountability Act (HIPAA) security rules indicate that working from home requires security policies and practices the same as working in the office. However, there are no specific policies given. It is up to each covered entity to establish these documents on the basis of their security risk assessment. Security measures should address the technical setup. For example, typical security policy might stipulate that the telecommuter use a dedicated computer with a virtual private network solution, antivirus software, and a firewall if the computer is connected to the Internet and the office. Management of work papers and disks and the computer work environment (protected from family and visitors) might also be indicated. Additionally, privacy compliance policies apply at home just as they do when working in an office.

One must have something to offer clients when marketing and selling one's services and skills. This knowledge and expertise can only be gained with years of experience and persistence. Full-time commitment, hard work, dedication, and many long hours to obtain clients are encountered when beginning a business. Be cautious when purchasing billing service software and obtain a complete picture of what hardware is necessary, how the program works, and the benefits it offers to your clients.

If you work awhile before striking out independently, you will make contacts on the job that may help build clientele. Networking is extremely important and may open up many opportunities when starting and growing a successful business. Many times it is who the individual knows that may get a foot in the potential client's door.

An insurance billing specialist can work as an independent contractor to have flexible hours, work from home, and reduce a medical practice's overhead. Some communities prohibit residents from telecommuting or operating a home-based business, although most allow it with restrictions. Working at home requires self-discipline, and one must develop a schedule and stick to it. Good time management is essential. It takes additional hours to advertise, obtain clients, bill, and perform the bookkeeping tasks. Box 18-1 is a checklist of tasks that must be done to establish a new business.

Planning Your Business

Every successful business endeavor begins with a smart business plan. This is a roadmap that can guide your business from start-up to continuous success. A business plan addresses facts and figures pertinent to your business and financial abilities and assesses your objectives and goals. Visit website http://www.entrepreneur.com/howto/bizplan/ for a complete guide on writing a business plan.

Professional Mailing Address

No doubt you will receive mail, so it is important to establish a professional address. It is always wise to rent a post office box. Doing this creates a business-oriented mailing address, helps maintain confidentiality in mailings you receive about clients and patient accounts, and protects you from unwanted visitors to your home. Visit the website of the Internal Revenue Service (IRS) at http://www.irs.gov/businesses/small/ for self-employed and small business resources.

Finances to Consider
Taxes

You must decide on what form of business entity you will be (i.e., sole proprietor, partnership, or corporation). It is advisable to seek the services of a lawyer, accountant, or both before legally establishing a business and making appropriate selection of the tax options involved. Set up detailed financial records from the beginning, even if an accountant is to be hired. Obtain simplified bookkeeping software for use on the computer. Expert advice is essential and helps develop a successful business; a business could fail without it.

Box 18-1   New Business Checklist

The following is a checklist to help you in starting a new home business. This is not a complete list of items to consider nor the exact order to accomplish them in; however, important points are covered in this list.

- Define your services and construct a business plan. Make sure you forecast for success. Will this business be viable? Can you accomplish the services you will promise to carry out? Can you financially afford this endeavor?
- Research whether you need to obtain a business license from the business license section of your city hall. Regulations vary in each city licensing office. You might have to obtain a home occupation permit from the planning department and have it signed by your landlord if you are renting. The city may have guidelines on hours of business, pedestrian and vehicular activity, noise, and so on in the residential area. Determine whether your county has rules on operating a small business from home.
- Consider a name for your business. File a fictitious business name (doing business as [DBA]) at the county clerk's office by obtaining the proper form for completion. If you use your given name, you do not have to file a fictitious business name.
- Decide what address to use. You may want to obtain a post office box number instead of using your home address. This will help with a professional mailing address, as well as protect you from unexpected visitors to your home.
- Consult with an accountant for advice on tax structure of your company (e.g., sole proprietor, corporation). Learn about what expenses are deductible. Depending on how you set up your business, some possible tax breaks are depreciation of office equipment; declaring a room of your home as an office; subscriptions to professional publications; dues to professional associations; expenses associated with your automobile; telephone, photocopying, and office supplies (e.g., stationery, books, and photocopy and fax paper); promotion and advertising (e.g., postage, meals with business associates, and website development and fees); and any expenses pertaining to meetings, conventions, workshops, or seminars (e.g., registration fees, lodging, meals, transportation, and parking). Visit the website http://www.irs.gov to learn more about how taxes can affect your business.

- Obtain the insurance that you need: health insurance, disability insurance, life insurance, liability insurance, workers' compensation (if you have employees), and so on. Insurance called "release of information insurance" or "errors and omissions insurance" with a "hold harmless" clause is available to protect you against loss of material. Consider a retirement plan such as an individual retirement account or a Keogh plan.
- Obtain a separate telephone number and possibly fax number to separate "home" from "business." However, you might consider using your existing telephone number and switching to a business listing. Having a business listing allows you to be listed in the Yellow Pages of your telephone directory. Remember that advertising can be expensive, so be sure this falls within your budget.
- Create a website advertising your services.
- Open a bank account. Many banks offer small business accounts with nominal monthly fees. For example, you can open an account "Jane Doe DBA 123 Claims Service."
- Create a professional image through business cards, stationery, and invoice billing forms. You can find resources on the Internet or in software programs to print your own.
- Stay current in the industry with up-to-date reference books. Begin to assemble a library to include a good medical dictionary, procedural and diagnostic code books, compliance handbooks, trade journals, and so on.
- Start a contact database and begin to advertise your business by some of the following methods: visiting offices, mailing flyers, advertising in trade journals or your local newspaper, sending announcements, putting up signs (be sure to get permission), and sending personalized letters to prospects (hospitals, clinics, and physician's offices).
- If you have opened an office at a location outside of your home, make sure you have reviewed a proper lease before signing it and consider the finances needed for items such as utility deposits (i.e., water, gas, and electricity). Rent, renovation, and janitorial or trash services must also be considered.
- Some contracts may include a statement on confidentiality assuring the contracting facility that all patient data are handled in a confidential manner.

Establishing a business in a home may result in some deductions, so obtain all the information you can from your accountant and the IRS regarding important laws concerning small business and self-employment taxes. Keep receipts and complete records of income and expenses because these are extremely important for IRS purposes.

Check stubs, copies of hours worked, and identifying data on clients must be retained for the period of time stipulated by the IRS. The following is a record retention schedule.

- Bank statements and canceled checks: 7 years
- Expired contracts: 7 years
- Financial statements: permanently
- General correspondence: 1 to 5 years
- Payroll records and summaries: 7 years

- Income tax returns: permanently
- Worksheets and supporting documents: 7 years

Keep a record of business travel expenses and document mileage. Travel log books are available at stationery stores.

Start-Up Expenses

In addition, money is necessary for equipment, computer software, overhead, taxes, stationery, preprinted statements and forms, and a myriad of other expenses. It is vital to have sufficient funds to run the business for a period of 1 year or more. It is imperative that this be accrued before vacating a full-time job. This will help eliminate a lot of fear and anxiety over not having enough business clients. A common reason for business failure is running out of the money necessary to keep the business going. It may take a year or more to begin seeing a profit, so one must be patient. This is where the business plan becomes a useful resource!

If an individual has had no business management experience, courses may be taken to gain knowledge and instill confidence in these areas before beginning a business. Attend workshops and lectures on starting a business that are offered by financial institutions, universities, community colleges, or private institutions.

Bank Account

Open a bank account that is separate from your own personal checking account. This smart approach saves a lot of time in the future when it comes to sorting out expenses and working on taxes. Also, think about the professional image that a business check will convey. Most banks have small business account services, including those for the self-employed. Shop around and visit several banks, if you do not already have a preference, and compare monthly fees and transaction capabilities.

Business Name, Plan, and License

Some towns or counties require a business license to operate a business. This may include working from your home office. Check with your local offices to determine whether an application or fee is required. This is the time to choose an appropriate business name and get applicable town and county licenses.

A business name should be easy to remember and explain what your company does. For example, ABC's #1 Medical Billing Service tells potential clients that the company works with health care related to billing and insurance claims.

A successful business must start with a smart business plan. This guides and helps your small business with financial and business strategies. It would be wise to meet with an accountant, an attorney, or a business consultant to help get your start-up company off in the right direction.

For more information about business planning, visit the US Small Business Association (SBA) website at http://www.sba.gov.

Insurance

It may be necessary and sometimes required that business owners protect income and property from unexpected loss. The following are types of insurance to investigate:

- Professional liability/errors and omissions protects you and your company from claims if your client holds you responsible for errors, or the failure of your work to perform as promised in your service contract. Coverage can include legal costs and may pay for resulting judgments against you.
- Business interruption insurance and property insurance in case of fire, theft, or disaster protects your assets and may help you in the recovery of data.
- Disability insurance if one becomes unable to work because of illness or injury can include yourself and/or an employee.
- Health and life insurance covers health care for yourself and/or employee, as well as life insurance.

Business Associate Under the Health Insurance Portability and Accountability Act

HIPAA rules apply to most billing companies as a business associate when a relationship is formed with one or more health care providers for whom you perform billing services.

Business associate: (Sect: 160.103)

A person (or organization) who, on behalf of such covered performs, or assists in the performance of a function or activity involving the use or disclosure of individually identifiable health information, including claims processing or administration, data analysis, processing or administration, utilization review, quality assurance, billing, benefit management, practice management, and repricing;

or

(ii) Provides, other than in the capacity of a member of the workforce of such covered entity, legal, actuarial, accounting, consulting, data aggregation, management, administrative, accreditation, or financial services, where the provision of the service involves the disclosure of individually identifiable health information from such covered entity or arrangement, or from another business associate of such covered entity or arrangement, to the person.

Therefore, if your billing company gets personal health information from a covered entity to perform a function or activity on behalf of that covered entity, your relationship is likely that of a business associate and your responsibilities must be defined with a Business Associate Agreement.

The Business Associate Agreement and the Service Contract

The **business associate agreement** must give "satisfactory assurances" to the covered entity on whose behalf it performs services and must include, according to HIPAA rule, the following terms as set forth in the regulation:

Obligations and Activities of Business Associate

- Business Associate agrees to not use or disclose Protected Health Information other than as permitted or required by the Agreement or as Required by Law.
- Business Associate agrees to use appropriate safeguards to prevent use or disclosure of the Protected Health Information other than as provided for by this Agreement.
- Business Associate agrees to mitigate, to the extent practicable, any harmful effect that is known to Business Associate of a use or disclosure of Protected Health Information by Business Associate in violation of the requirements of this Agreement. (This provision may be included if it is appropriate for the Covered Entity to pass on its duty to mitigate damages to a Business Associate.)
- Business Associate agrees to report to Covered Entity any use or disclosure of the Protected Health Information not provided for by this Agreement of which it becomes aware.
- Business Associate agrees to ensure that any agent including a subcontractor, to whom it provides Protected Health Information received from, or created or received by Business Associate on behalf of, Covered Entity agrees to the same restrictions and conditions that apply through this Agreement to Business Associate with respect to such information.
- Business Associate agrees to provide access, at the request of Covered Entity, and in the time and manner [Insert negotiated terms], to Protected Health Information in a Designated Record Set, to Covered Entity or, as directed by Covered Entity, to an Individual in order to meet the requirements under 45 CFR § 164.524. (Not necessary if business associate does not have protected health information in a designated record set.)
- Business Associate agrees to make any amendment(s) to Protected Health Information in a Designated Record Set that the Covered Entity directs or agrees to pursuant to 45 CFR § 164.526 at the request of Covered Entity or an Individual, and in the time and manner [Insert negotiated terms]. (Not necessary if business associate does not have protected health information in a designated record set.)
- Business Associate agrees to make internal practices, books, and records, including policies and procedures and Protected Health Information, relating to the use and disclosure of Protected Health Information received from, or created or received by Business Associate on behalf of, Covered Entity available [to the Covered Entity, or] to the Secretary, in a time and manner [Insert negotiated terms] or designated by the Secretary, for purposes of the Secretary determining Covered Entity's compliance with the Privacy Rule.
- Business Associate agrees to document such disclosures of Protected Health Information and information related to such disclosures as would be required for Covered Entity to respond to a request by an Individual for an accounting of disclosures of Protected Health Information in accordance with 45 CFR § 164.528.
- Business Associate agrees to provide to Covered Entity or an Individual, in time and manner [Insert negotiated terms], information collected in accordance with Section [Insert section number in contract where provision (i) appears] of this Agreement, to permit Covered Entity to respond to a request by an Individual for an accounting of disclosures of Protected Health Information in accordance with 45 CFR § 164.528.

Service Contract

The **service contract** is a separate document from the business associate agreement. The service contract is a necessary document that defines the duties and obligations of each party involved in the business relationship as far as who is responsible for what duty or task that carries out the purpose of the service contract agreement. Contracts or agreements should be made in writing, signed, and notarized. For example, a contract should define the following:

- Who is responsible for the coding (the physician or the billing service)?
- What will be the routine for claim submission?
- Is there a per-claim processing fee or is there a flat monthly fee?
- Who is responsible for follow-up on collection procedures (telephone calls or letters)?
- Who pays for rebilling, photocopying of records, mailing fees, and clearinghouse charges? Is this included in a flat monthly service fee?
- Under whose name will bills be sent to patients (the physician or the billing service)?
- Will the billing service telephone number appear on the statement, or will a toll-free or local number be used?
- How will the telephone be answered?
- What are the charges for coding consultation services?
- What are the coverage arrangements for absence or illness?
- How will information be protected and handled between client and billing company?

If there is any change in the terms of the agreements, write an addendum to the original agreement and have both parties sign to acknowledge the change. Be sure all agreements and contracts have proper effective and termination dates. Remember that renegotiation is in order when the contract expires.

Some contracts may include a statement on confidentiality assuring the contracting facility that all patient data will be handled in a confidential manner.

Pricing Your Services

Define your services and work out a structured fee schedule, making sure to review state laws regarding percentage billing (it is illegal in some states). It is imperative to get legal advice when creating contracts and agreements.

A variety of methods are used to price services such as a percentage of reimbursement or an annual, hourly, or per-claim fee. Deciding on which method depends on the type of client being served and the work to be done. For example, a claims assistance professional may bill in 15-minute increments. Telephone other billing and insurance services, preferably outside the area, to learn what they are charging because in-area competitors may be reluctant to divulge that information.

Setting Up Your Office

The most important consideration is privacy and security of the health information and business documents you will handle and be responsible for. Review the security suggestions as outlined in Chapter 8.

An initial equipment checklist may include the following:

- Computer
- Laser and/or ink jet printer
- Paper
- Current billing and coding manuals and books
- Desk supplies such as stapler, paper clips, and self-adhesive notes
- Locking file cabinets
- Fax machine

Also consider using separate computer backup protection (e.g., a surge protector with battery power) to guard against faulty wiring or power failure. This gives more than 10 minutes to back up your current project and then shut down. These are available at office stores for about $100.

Shop smart. Research upcoming sales and lease programs, rebates, upgrade trade-ins, and service plans.

Research the various medical billing software programs asking for demo software before purchasing. Also,

look for a reputable clearinghouse. Compare functionality, customer service, technical support, and prices.

Marketing, Advertising, Promotion, and Public Relations

Marketing refers to how a business is presented or advertised to promote sales. Marketing strategies vary, depending on the section of the public that is targeted. When promoting a medical billing service, develop a well-organized marketing plan and follow basic guidelines to reach a specific target audience.

Ways to market a business and the reasons for marketing strategies are presented in Table 18-1.

At this point you should be ready to start marketing your business. If you are creative, you can certainly design your own business cards and get them printed. A classic white card with black font (print) depicts professionalism. You can also find matching stationery sets, and create flyers, brochures, newsletters, surveys, and so on. Obtain financial data to help convince clients that the service you are offering is better and can do more for their business than what they presently have. Save them time and money! Stress being honest, reliable, committed, efficient, and professional, and offer them something they cannot do for themselves.

Put yourself in front of the office managers and health care providers to advertise your services. Consider visiting the health care offices in your area and be sure to follow-up with visits and calls. Be careful with offices that have a sign stating "No Soliciting." If you see this sign, respect it and jot the address down to mail them literature instead. Also, note that solicitation by fax is illegal according to the Federal Communications Commission: "Enacted by Congress in 1991, the Telephone Consumer Protection Act (TCPA) restricts the use of the telephone and facsimile machine to deliver unsolicited advertisements. Under the TCPA, one may not send an unsolicited advertisement to a fax machine. In addition, those sending fax messages or transmitting artificial or prerecorded voice messages are subject to certain identification requirements."

Marketing can be tough and intimidating. Networking with other colleagues and professions along with persistence will pay off.

Documentation

Besides keeping documentation received from your client, keep written records of the numbers of hours worked, the quantity of work done each day, and the corrections applied to the work by officials in the

Table 18-1 Business Marketing and Strategies	
STRATEGY	**REASON**
Obtain professionally printed stationery and business cards.	Enhances professional image.
Pass out business cards at professional meetings.	Advertises availability and services. Helps with networking.
Develop a business name and logo for the company.	Enables potential clients to identify that you are in business.
Ensure accuracy of all printed materials.	When items are not professionally assembled or proofread to eliminate typographical errors, a potential client receives a doubtful or negative image of the company.
Develop a professional flyer and distribute it to medical facilities and physicians' offices.	Introduces company name, advertises services, and describes benefits.
Follow up with a personal visit or telephone call.	A friendly voice and professional image offer personal services and let potential clients know you are available and interested.
Advertise in the journal or newsletter of the country medical society and state medical association.	Potential clients read such publications and advertisements of this nature lend to your credibility.
Place an ad in the newspaper or on cable television.	Circulates business within the county.
Put an ad in the Yellow Pages.	Solicits wider range of prospective clients.
Network with members of professional organizations.	Word-of-mouth advertising can be the best public relations tool, especially if done by professional peers.
Network via computer using the Internet's discussion and career boards such as America Online and Yahoo.	Offers wide range of contacts.
Promote your business with a professionally developed website.	Search engines will help find you. Websites deliver immediate, detailed information about your company.
Check with established businesses to determine whether they are overloaded with work, the owner needs a vacation, or they need help in a temporary situation because of illness.	Present your services as a help not a threat to current office staff.

contracting facility or hospital. Retain any written coding guideline from the contracting facility or hospital.

Trends for Success with Professional Associations, Certification, and Registration

More exacting professional requirements have evolved because of specialization in the allied health careers. Certification and registration are two ways of exhibiting professional standards (Table 18-2). **Certification** is a statement issued by a board or association verifying that a person meets professional standards. **Registration** may be accomplished in two methods, as an entry in an official registry or record that lists names of persons in an occupation who have satisfied specific requirements or by attaining a certain level of education and paying a registration fee. In the latter, if there are certain requirements for registration, then an unregistered person may be prevented from working in a career for which he or she is otherwise qualified.

Membership in professional organizations helps in keeping up to date. Most of these associations have student, as well as active and associate membership, categories. You can inquire whether there is a local chapter or state organization affiliated with the national association. Benefits of belonging to a professional organization, in addition to certification and recertification, include problem solving, continuing education, and employment opportunities. Local meetings can keep you

knowledgeable by providing guest speakers on topics of current interest. The newsletters and journals published by these organizations keep you abreast of current trends either as a subscriber or as a benefit when becoming a member.

Mentor and Business Incubator Services

A valuable vehicle for career development is to find a mentor in the business. A **mentor** is a guide or teacher who offers advice, criticism, wisdom, guidance, and perspective to an inexperienced but promising protégé to help reach a life goal. Decide what kind of help you want (e.g., technical, general feedback, or managerial), then look for a mentor whose background, values, and style are similar to yours. Be willing to face criticism with a positive attitude and express gratitude when excellence is praised.

Another way to develop a business and obtain management assistance is to seek the services of a business incubator. A *business incubator* is an environment that grows and nurtures small businesses through their early years of existence by offering an array of business assistance services, shared resources, and networking. An incubator facility can be an actual building that has several small business tenants. It is run by managers and staff who offer business advice and referral services to tenants and many additional services, such as high-speed Internet; conference rooms; secretarial, mail, and courier service; fax;

Text continued on p. 636

Table 18-2 Certification and Registration

TITLE/ABBREVIATION	DESCRIPTION TO OBTAIN CERTIFICATION OR REGISTRATION	PROFESSIONAL ASSOCIATION MAILING ADDRESS	TELEPHONE NUMBER	WEBSITE	E-MAIL ADDRESS
Advanced Coding Specialist (ACS) Specialty Coding Professional (SCP) Certified Compliance Professional-Physician (CCP-P)	2-3 yrs' experience and working knowledge of coding in the specialty	Board of Medical Specialty Coding 9737 Washington Blvd. Suite 100 Gaithersburg, MD 20878	(800) 897-4509	www.advanced medical coding.com	info@medicalspecialty coding.com
Certified Billing and Coding Specialist (CBCS)	Graduate of health care training program or 1+ yrs' full-time job experience; exam or home study certification program	National Healthcare Association 7500 West 160th Street Stilwell, KS 66085	(800) 499-9092	www.nhanow.com	info@nhanow.com
Certified Bookkeeper (CB)	Self-study program and employment experience; pass three tests	American Institute of Professional Bookkeepers 6001 Montrose Road Suite 500 Rockville, MD 20852	(800) 622-0121	www.aipb.org	info@aipb.org
Certified Coding Associate (CCA) Certified Coding Specialist (CCS) Certified Coding Specialist-Physician (CCS-P) Certified in Healthcare Privacy (CHP)	Self-study program; pass certification examination	American Health Information Management Association (AHIMA) 233 N. Michigan Ave. 21st Floor Chicago, IL 60601-5809	(800) 335-5535	www.ahima.org	info@ahima.org
Certified Cardiology Coding Specialist (CCCS) Certified ENT Coding Specialist (CENTCS) Certified Family Practice Coding Specialist (CFPCS) Certified Gastroenterology Coding Specialist (CGCS) Certified General Surgery Coding Specialist (CGSCS) Certified Internal Medicine Coding Specialist (CIMCS) Certified Nephrology Coding Specialist (CNCS) Certified OB/GYN Coding Specialist (COBGCS) Certified Orthopedics Coding Specialist (COPCS) Certified Pediatrics Coding Specialist (CPCS) Certified Podiatry Coding Specialist (CPODCS) Certified Pulmonary Medicine Coding Specialist (CPMCS)	Active member of Professional Association of Healthcare Coding Specialists, employed as a coder with 2 yrs' experience, 6 college credit course hours in coding	Professional Association of Healthcare Coding Specialists (PAHCS) 218 E. Bearss Ave. #354 Tampa, FL 33613	(888) 708-4707	www.pahcs.org	info@pahcs.org

Continued

Certified Urology Coding Specialist (**CUCS**) Certified Multi-Specialty Coding Specialist (**CMSCS**)				
Certified Healthcare Financial Professional (**CHFP**)	60 hrs' college/university and complete core exam and one specialty exam within 2-yr period	Healthcare Financial Management Association (HFMA) 2 Westbrook Corporate Center Suite 700 Westchester, IL 60154-5700	(800) 252-4362	www.hfma.org	webmaster@Financial Professionalhfma.com
Certified Electronic Claims Professional (**CECP**) Certified Claim Assistant Professional (**CCAP**)	Self-study program; pass certification examination	Alliance of Claims Assistance Professionals (ACAP) 9600 Escarpment Suite 745-65 Austin, TX 78749	(888) 394-5163	www.claims.org	capinfo@claims.org
Certified Healthcare Billing and Management Executive (**CHBME**)	Complete comprehensive program; pass proficiency test	Healthcare Billing and Management Association (HMBA) 1540 South Coast Highway Suite 203 Laguna Beach, CA 92651	(877) 640-4262	www.hbma.com	info@hbma.com
Certified in Healthcare Compliance (**CHC**)	Have work experience, continuing education, and pass examination	Healthcare Compliance Assn 6500 Barrie Road Suite 250 Minneapolis, MN 55435	(888) 580-8373	www.hcca-info.org	info@hcca-info.org
Certified in Healthcare Privacy (**CHP**) Certified in Healthcare Privacy and Security (**CHPS**) Certified in Healthcare Security (**CHS**) Certified Health Data Analyst (**CHDA**)	Eligibility requirements and pass examination Pass CHP and CHS examinations	American Health Information Management Association (AHIMA) 233 N. Michigan Ave. 21st Floor Chicago, IL 60601-5809	(800) 335-5535	www.ahima.org	info@ahima.com
Certified Information Systems Security Professional (**CISSP**) Systems Security Certified Practitioner (**SSCP**)	Pass examination and submit endorsement form	International Information Systems Security Certifications Consortium, Inc. 1964 Gallows Road Suite 210 Vienna, VA 22182	(866) 462-4777	www.isc2.org	isc2@asestores.com
Certified Medical Assistant (**CMA**)	Graduate from accredited medical assisting program; apply to take national certifying examination	American Association of Medical Assistants (AAMA) 20 North Wacker Drive, Suite 1575 Chicago, IL 60606	(800) 228-2262	www.aama-ntl.org	Visit website
Certified Medical Billing Specialist (**CMBS**)	Complete 6 courses and provide evaluation of billing performance by supervisor	Medical Association of Billers (MAB) 2620 Regatta Dr. Suite 102 Las Vegas, NV 89128	(702) 240-8519	www.physicians websites.com	medassocb@aol.com

Table 18-2 Certification and Registration—cont'd

TITLE/ABBREVIATION	DESCRIPTION TO OBTAIN CERTIFICATION OR REGISTRATION	PROFESSIONAL ASSOCIATION MAILING ADDRESS	TELEPHONE NUMBER	WEBSITE	E-MAIL ADDRESS
Certified Medical Office Manager (CMOM)	Examination for supervisors or managers of small-group and solo practices	Professional Association of Health Care Office Managers (PAHCOM) 1576 Bella Cruz Dr. Suite 360 Lady Lake, FL 32159	(800) 451-9311	www.pahcom.com	pahcom@pahcom.com
Certified Medical Practice Executive (CMPE) Nominee 1st level Certification 2nd level Fellow 3rd level	First level—Eligible Group managers join; membership/nominee Second level—Complete 6- to 7-hr examination Third level—Mentoring project of thesis	Medical Group Management Association (MGMA), American College of Medical Practice Executives (affiliate) 104 Inverness Terrace East Englewood, CO 80112-5306	(877) 275-6462	www.mgma.com	acmpe@mgma.com
Certified Medical Coder (CPC)	Self-study program and successfully pass exam	Practice Management Institute 9501 Console Drive Suite 100 San Antonio, TX 78229-2033	(800) 259-5562	www.pmimd.com	info@pmimd.com
Certified Medical Insurance Specialist (CMIS) Certified Medical Reimbursement Specialist (CMRS)	Self-study program; successfully pass 18 sections of examination	American Medical Billing Association (AMBA) 2465 E. Main, Davis, OK 73030	(580) 369-2700	www.ambanet.net/cmrs.htm	larry@brightok.net
Certified Medical Transcriptionist (CMT)	Self-study program and successfully pass written and practical examinations offered by Medical Transcription Certification Commission (MTCC)	Association for Healthcare Documentation Integrity (AHDI) 4230 Kiernan Avenue Suite 130 Modesto, CA 95356	(800) 982-2182	www.ahdionline.org	ahdi@ahdionline.org
Certified Patient Account Technician (CPAT) Certified Clinic Account Technician (CCAT) Certified Clinic Account Manager (CCAM)	Complete self-study course; pass standard examination administered twice yearly	American Association of Healthcare Administrative Mgmt (AAHAM) National Certification Examination Program 11240 Waples Mill Road Suite 200 Fairfax, VA 22030	(703) 281-4043	www.aaham.org	moayad@aaham.org
Certified Professional Coder (CPC) Certified Professional Coder Apprentice (CPC-A) Certified Professional Coder–Hospital (CPC-H)	Independent study program; examination approximately 5 hrs (CPC) and 8 hrs (CPC-H) in length	American Academy of Professional Coders (AAPC) 2480 South 3850 West Suite B Salt Lake City, UT 84120	(800) 626-CODE	www.aapc.com	info@aapc.com

Certification	Requirement	Organization/Address	Phone	Website	Email
Facility Coding Specialist (FCS) Physician Coding Specialist (PCS) Coding Specialist for Payers (CSP)		American College of Medical Coding Specialists (ACMCS) 1540 South Coast Highway Suite 203 Laguna Beach, CA 92651	(800) 946-9402	www.acmcs.org	info@acmcs.org
Healthcare Reimbursement Specialist (HRS)	Successfully complete open-book examination	National Electronic Biller's Alliance (NEBA) 2226-A Westborough Blvd. #504 South San Francisco, CA 94080	(650) 359-4419	www.nebazone.com	mmedical@aol.com
National Certified Insurance and Coding Specialist (NCICS)	Graduate from an insurance program; sit for certification examination given by independent testing agency at many school sites across the nation	National Center for Competency Testing 7007 College Blvd. Suite 705 Overland Park, KS 66211	(800) 875-4404	www.ncctinc.com	staff@ncctinc.com
Registered Medical Assistant (RMA)	Sit for certification exam	American Medical Technologists (AMT) 10700 West Higgins Road Suite 150 Rosemont, IL 60018	(800) 275-1268	www.amt1.com	amtmail@aol.com
Compliance various designations for URAC Accredited Consultant	Application	Utilization Review Accreditation Commission 1220 L Street, NW Suite 400 Washington, DC 20005	(202) 216-9010	www.urac.org	ita@urac.org
Certified in Healthcare Compliance (CHC)	Examination, work experience, and continuing education	Health Care Compliance Association 6500 Barrie Road Suite 250 Minneapolis, MN 55435	(888) 580-8373	www.hcca-info.org	info@hcca-info.org
Systems Security Certified Practitioner (SSCP)	Pass examination and submit endorsement form	International Information Systems Security Certifications Consortium, Inc. 1964 Gallows Road Suite 210 Vienna, VA 22182	(866) 462-4777	www.isc2.org	isc2@asestores.com

copier; printer; TV/DVD/VCR; break room; and free parking.

Networking

Another avenue to pursue for career development is to network. **Networking** is the exchange of information or services among individuals, groups, or institutions and making use of professional contacts. To do this, join as many organizations as possible because it can be difficult to keep abreast of ongoing changes in the insurance industry when you are self-employed. Many of the professional organizations publish monthly newsletters or quarterly journals, offer certification, and plan national conventions, state conferences, and regional meetings.

Claims assistance professionals should attend local meetings for Medicare recipients. Join local volunteer service organizations and the chamber of commerce to network with others. Contact the LEADS Club at (800) 783-3761 or the National Association for Female Executives at (800) 927-6233 for potential client leads and networking.

Reassess and Continue with Success

Once your billing service is under way, you will find it necessary to routinely assess the overall health of the business. Review your business plans and make sure you are following the guidelines. Make changes where applicable and revise strategies and goals. Running your own successful business is challenging and highly rewarding both emotionally and financially. Good luck!

HIPAA security rules indicate that working from home requires security policies and practices the same as working in an office. However, there are no specific policies given. It is up to each covered entity to establish these documents on the basis of their security risk assessment. Security measures should address the technical setup. For example, typical security policy might stipulate that the telecommuter use a dedicated computer with a virtual private network solution, antivirus software, and a firewall if the computer is connected to the Internet and the office. Management of work papers and disks and the computer work environment (protected from family and visitors) might also be indicated. Additionally, privacy compliance policies apply at home just as they do when working in an office.

PROCEDURE 18-1

Creating an Electronic Résumé

Once a medical position has been discovered, a résumé may be e-mailed or a hard copy may be faxed. The basic steps for creating a résumé are as follows:

1. Compose a résumé using a word processor with accurate spelling features and be sure to keep it simple. Each line should be no more than 65 characters in length.
2. Discard traditional résumé-writing techniques such as focusing on action verbs. Instead, think of descriptive nouns such as medical biller, education, experience, skills, knowledge, and abilities.
3. Avoid the use of decorative graphics and complex typefaces, bulleted lists, complicated page formatting, symbols, underlining, or italics. These features may not appear the same on an employer's computer online.
4. Forget the one-page rule; electronic résumés may be three to four pages.
5. Proofread the résumé and save the electronic résumé in a job search file. Or refer to the word processor manual to convert the cover letter and résumé to ASCII (American Standard Code for

Information Interchange; pronounced AS-kee), or plain text, which can be read by most personal computers.

6. Study online guides presenting special procedures for sending e-mail and files. Some e-mail programs allow binary files to be sent, whereas others only allow ASCII text files.
7. Use the word processing software's "copy and paste" feature and enter the information into e-mail, or if you save it as an electronic file, it can be transmitted as an attachment to an e-mail message.
8. Do not post a letter of introduction when posting a résumé to a bulletin board.
9. Upload the résumé to post online using the file transfer feature of the software following the computer manual directions. The ASCII file is all that is necessary when sending the résumé over an online service or from a computer to a dial-direct bulletin board.
10. After you send a résumé electronically, mail a hard copy and call the hiring manager directly to follow up. Be assertive.

KEY POINTS

This is a brief chapter review or summary of the key issues presented. To further enhance your knowledge of the technical subject matter, review the key terms and key abbreviations for this chapter by locating the meanings in the glossary at the end of this book that appear in a section before the index.

1. Use many ways to search for a job as an insurance billing specialist.
2. Access the Internet and use a search engine to locate job offers by potential employers.
3. Prepare for and attend a job fair to make contact and network with potential employers.
4. Visit potential employers and complete job application forms.
5. Compose a letter of introduction and an updated résumé focused on the type of job you wish to obtain.
6. Prepare yourself for an interview so that you make a positive impression.
7. Organize a portfolio by assembling documents related to education, prior work experience, and skills.
8. Research thoroughly and begin steps in establishing a billing service.
9. Under the HIPAA, know all security and confidentiality policy and practice requirements when working from a home-based business.
10. Pursue becoming certified or registered to exhibit a higher level of professionalism.
11. Become a member of a professional organization to network and keep current on technical data and federal regulations.

evolve INTERNET RESOURCES

For active links to the following resources, visit the Evolve website at
http://evolve.elsevier.com/fordney/handbook
Advance for Careers is a website designed to assist the job-seeking process. Go to the website and click on "Need to find a job."

- Google (search engine)
- Yahoo (search engine)
- Alta Vista (search engine)
- Ask.com (search engine)
- Kanoodle (search engine)
- Lycos (search engine)
- *Career Magazine*
- America's Job Bank
- Monster.com

See Table 18-2 for professional organization websites.

STUDENT ASSIGNMENT

✓ Study Chapter 18.
✓ Answer the fill-in-the-blank, multiple choice, and true/false review questions in the *Workbook* to reinforce the theory learned in this chapter and help prepare you for a future test.
✓ Complete the assignments in the *Workbook* to give you hands-on experience in completing an application for a position as an insurance billing specialist, preparing and typing a résumé, composing a cover letter to go with the résumé, having someone evaluate you during an interview, and typing a follow-up thank-you letter after being interviewed.
✓ Turn to the glossary at the end of this textbook for a further understanding of the key terms and key abbreviations used in this chapter.

Appendix

RESOURCES FOR AUDIOTAPES, BOOKS, NEWSLETTERS, PERIODICALS, SOFTWARE, AND VIDEOTAPES

Technical data change quickly in the field of insurance billing and coding, so the need for current editions and titles is imperative. From the following list, either telephone the toll-free numbers or go to the websites to access the most up-to-date information on audiotapes, books, certification, newsletters, periodicals, software, and videotapes.

Alliance of Claims Assistance Professionals (resource for patients on insurance claims issues)
Website: www.claims.org

American Academy of Orthopaedic Surgeons (diagnostic and procedural books)
6300 N. River Road, Rosemont, IL 60018-4262
Phone: (800) 346-AAOS or (847) 823-7186
Fax: (847) 823-8125
Website: www.aaos.org

American Academy of Pediatrics (diagnostic and procedural books)
141 N.W. Point Boulevard, Elk Grove Village, IL
    60007-1098
(847) 434-4000
Website: www.aap.org

American Academy of Professional Coders (books, certification study guides)
2480 South 3850 West, Suite B, Salt Lake City, UT
    84120
(800) 626-CODE (2633)
Website: www.aapc.com

American Association of Medical Assistants (education and training code books)
20 N. Wacker Drive, Suite 1575, Chicago, IL 60606
(800) 228-2262
Website: www.aama-ntl.org

American College of Emergency Physicians (diagnostic and procedural books)
P.O. Box 619911, Dallas, TX 75261-9911
(800) 798-1822
Website: www.acep.org

American College of Radiology (radiology coding books)
1891 Preston White Drive, Reston, VA 20191
(703) 648-8900
Website: www.acr.org

American College of Rheumatology (diagnostic and procedural books)
2200 Lake Boulevard NE, Atlanta, GA 30319
(404) 633-3777
Website: www.rheumatology.org

American Health Information Management Association (books, certification information, medical documentation, publications, education and training code books and seminars)
233 North Michigan Avenue, 21st Floor, Chicago, IL
    60601-5809
(312) 233-1100 or (800) 335-5535
Website: www.ahima.org

American Hospital Association (books)
AHA Resource Center
155 North Wacker Drive, Suite 400, Chicago, IL
    60606
(312) 422-2050
Website: http://aharc.library.net

American Medical Association (diagnostic and procedural books, code journals, code software, fraud and abuse compliance book, law and ethics books)
515 N. State Street, Chicago, IL 60654-0946
(800) 621-8335
Website: www.ama-assn.org

American Psychiatric Publishing, Inc. (diagnostic and procedural books)
1000 Wilson Boulevard, Suite 1825, Arlington, VA
    22209-3901
(800) 368-5777 or (703) 907-7322
Website: www.appi.org

America's Health Insurance Plans (health insurance glossary book, disability income insurance book, audiocassette tapes for education and training)
601 Pennsylvania Avenue, NW, South Building, Suite 500, Washington DC 20004
(202) 778-3200
Website: www.ahip.org

Appeal Solutions (collection software)
P.O. Box 191, League City, TX 77574
(888) 399-4925
Website: www.appealsolutions.com

Aspen Publishers, Inc. (books, newsletters, compliance books, medical documentation book, healthcare software source book, reference guides)
7201 McKinney Circle (21704), P.O. Box 990, Frederick, MD 21705-9727
(800) 638-8437
Website: www.aspenpublishers.com

California Health Information Association (education and training code books)
1915 North Fine Avenue, Suite 104, Fresno, CA 93727-1565
(800) 247-8907
Website: www.californiahia.org

CCH (disability, unemployment, and managed care newsletters; Medicare and Medicaid books and newsletters; CDs)
4025 West Peterson Avenue (60646), P.O. Box 5490, Chicago, IL 60680-9882
(800) 248-3248
Website: www.cch.com

Cengage Learning, Inc. (formerly Thomson Delmar Learning) (education and training code and insurance books, law and ethics books)
P.O. Box 6904, Florence, KY 41022-6904
(800) 354-9706
Website: www.cengage.com

Channel Publishing, Ltd. (diagnostic and procedural books, code software)
4750 Longley Lane, Suite 110, Reno, NV 89502
(800) 248-2882 or (777) 825-0880 (Nevada)
Website: www.channelpublishing.com

ChartCare, Inc. (diagnostic and procedural books)
140 Broadway, New York, NY 10005
(800) 438-1277
Website: www.chartcare.com

Conomikes Associates, Inc. (collection handbook, Medicare RVU Scale handbook, newsletters, and seminars)
990 Highland Avenue, Suite 110A, San Diego, CA 92075
(800) 421-6512
Website: www.conomikes.com

Contexo Media (formerly Medical Management Institute) (diagnostic and procedural books, compliance books, seminars)
P.O. Box 25128, Salt Lake City, UT 84125
(800) 334-5724 ext. 1
Website: www.codingbooks.com

DecisionHealth (billing books, newsletters, RBRVS code book, code software)
Two Washingtonian Center, 9737 Washington Blvd., Ste 100, Gaithersburg, MD 20878-7364
(877) 602-3835
Website: www.decisionhealth.com

Elsevier/Mosby/Saunders (diagnostic and procedural books, education and training code and insurance books, medical dictionaries)
3251 Riverport Lane, Maryland Heights, MO 63043
(800) 545-2522
Fax: (800) 535-9935
Website: www.elsevier.com

EMC Captiva Context (code software)
176 South Street, Hopkinton, MA 01748
(866) 438-3622
Website: www.emc.com

F.A. Davis Company/Publishers (medical dictionaries)
1915 Arch Street, Philadelphia, PA 19103
(800) 323-3555
Website: www.fadavis.com

Glencoe/McGraw-Hill (education and training code and insurance books, law and ethics books)
P.O. Box 543, Blacklick, OH 43004-0544
(800) 334-7344
Website: www.glencoe.com

Ingenix Publishing Group (diagnostic and procedural code books, RVS code books, newsletters, research and review services, code hotlines, compliance books, DRG books, medical documentation book, education and training books, fee schedules for specialties, hospital insurance claims, DRG, RBRVS fee schedule, APC, insurance directory)
2525 Lake Park Boulevard, Salt Lake City, UT 84120
Phone: (800) 464-3649
Fax: (801) 982-4033
Website: www.ingenixonline.com

Ingenix seminars
Website: www.ingenix.com

Lexi-Comp (diagnostic and procedure handbooks for terminology)
1100 Terex Road, Hudson, OH 44236
(800) 837-5394 (sales)
Website: www.lexi.com

Lippincott Williams & Wilkins (medical dictionaries)
P.O. Box 1620, Hagerstown, MD 21741
(800) 638-3030
Website: www.lww.com

MAG Mutual HealthCare Solutions (specialty software for fees, fee and coding guide)
3525 Piedmont Road NE Bldg 7-601, Atlanta, GA
   30305-7041
Phone: (800) 253-4945
Website: www.coderscentral.com

McGraw-Hill Healthcare Management Group (diagnostic and procedural books)
Order Services, P.O. Box 182604, Columbus, OH
   43272-3031
(877) 833-5524
Website: http://books.mcgraw-hill.com

MedBooks (education and training code books)
101 West Buckingham Road, Richardson, TX
   75081-4802
(800) 443-0397
Website: www.medbooks.com

Medical Economics Publishing (practice management articles)
24950 Country Club Blvd., Suite 200, North Olmstead,
   OH 44070
(440) 243-8100
Website: www.memag.com (click on "practice
   management" to get to billing topics)

Medical Learning Incorporated (diagnostic and procedural books)
287 East Sixth Street, Suite 400, St. Paul, MN 55101
(800) 252-1578
Website: www.medlearn.com

Opus Communications (newsletters, code software)
200 Hoods Lane, P.O. Box 1168, Marblehead, MA
   01945
(800) 650-6787
Website: www.hcpro.com

Practice Management Information Corporation (diagnostic and procedural books, collection books, fee books, insurance directory)
4727 Wilshire Boulevard, #300 Los Angeles, CA 90010
(800) MED-SHOP
Website: http://pmiconline.com

Rayve Productions, Inc. (independent medical coding book)
P.O. Box 726, Windsor, CA 95492
(800) 852-4890
Website: www.rayvepro.com

Society of Interventional Radiology (diagnostic and procedural books)
3975 Fair Ridge Drive, Suite 400 North, Fairfax, VA
   22033
(800) 488-7284 or (703) 691-1805
Website: www.sirweb.org

The Society of Thoracic Surgeons (diagnostic and procedural books)
633 N. Saint Clair St., Suite 2320, Chicago, IL
   60611-3658
(312) 202-5800
Website: www.sts.org

State of California, Department of Industrial Relations, Division of Workers' Compensation (California Medical Fee Schedule)
455 Golden Gate Avenue, Room 5182, San Francisco,
   CA 94102
http://www.dir.ca.gov/

Thomson West (fee manual, law and ethics books and software)
610 Opperman Drive, P.O. Box 64526, Eagan, MN
   55123-1396
(800) 344-5008
Website: www.west.thomson.com

Unicor Medical, Inc. (diagnostic and procedural books, code newsletters, code software)
4160 Carmichael Road, Suite 101, Montgomery, AL
   36106
(800) 825-7421
Website: www.unicormed.com

United States Government Printing Office (books on fraud and abuse, Medicare, and RBRVS fee schedule in Federal Register)
Superintendent of Documents, 732 N. Capitol Street,
   NW, Washington, DC 20401
(866) 512-1800
Website: http://bookstore.gpo.gov

Wasserman Medical Publishers, Limited (physicians' fee reference book and disk, HCPCS code books, insurance directory)
P.O. Box 510949, Milwaukee, WI 53203
(800) 669-3337
Website: www.medfees.com

ZHealth Publishing (code books on interventional radiology and cardiology)
330 Franklin Road, Suite 135A, #232, Brentwood, TN 37027
(877) 873-9893 or (615) 807-1152
Website: www.zhealthpublishing.com

Karen Zupko & Associates (forms and downloads)
625 N. Michigan Avenue, Suite 2225, Chicago, IL 60611
(312) 642-5616
Website: www.karenzupko.com

Glossary

Chapter number(s) is(are) shown in parentheses after each term.

Abuse (2): Incidents or practices, not usually considered fraudulent, that are inconsistent with accepted sound medical business or fiscal practices.

Accident (15): An unexpected happening, causing injury traceable to a definite time and place.

Accidental death and dismemberment (16): An insurance policy provision that protects the insured if he or she suffers loss of sight or loss of limb(s) or death by accident.

Accounts receivable (A/R) (10): The total amount of money owed for professional services rendered.

Accounts receivable management (3): The organization and administration of coding and billing in a medical practice.

Accredited Standards Committee X12 (ASC X12) (8): The U.S. standards body formed by the American National Standards Institute (ANSI) for cross-industry development, maintenance, and publication of electronic data exchange standards.

Active duty service member (ADSM) (14): An active member of the United States government military services (e.g., Army, Navy, Air Force, Marines, or Coast Guard).

Acute (4): A medical condition that runs a short but relatively severe course.

Adjudication (15): The final determination of the issues involving settlement of an insurance claim; also known as a *claim settlement*.

Admission review (17): A review for appropriateness and necessity of admissions.

Advance beneficiary notice of noncoverage (ABN) (12): An agreement given to the patient to read and sign before rendering a service if the participating physician thinks that it may be denied for payment because of medical necessity or limitation of liability by Medicare. The patient agrees to pay for the service; also known as a *waiver of liability agreement* or *responsibility statement*.

Adverse effect (5): An unfavorable, detrimental, or pathologic reaction to a drug that occurs when appropriate doses are given to humans for prophylaxis (prevention of disease), diagnosis, and therapy.

Age analysis (10): The procedure of systematically arranging the accounts receivable, by age, from the date of service.

Alien (18): An individual belonging to another country or people; a foreigner. Referred to as an *immigrant* when a person from another country comes to settle.

Allowable charge (14): An amount on which TRICARE figures the patient's cost-share for covered care. This is based on 75% to 80% of the allowable charge.

Alternative billing codes (ABCs) (6): A code system for integrative health care products and services consisting of five-character alphabetic symbols with appended two-character practitioner modifiers that represent the practitioner type.

AMA Code of Medical Ethics (10): A code of medical ethics formulated by the American Medical Association and adopted in 1847.

Ambulatory payment classifications (APCs) (17): A system of outpatient hospital reimbursement based on procedures rather than diagnoses.

American Health Information Management Association (AHIMA) (1): A national professional organization for promoting the art and science of medical record management and improving the quality of comprehensive health information for the welfare of the public.

American Medical Association (AMA) (1): A national professional society of physicians.

Ancillary services (11): Supportive services other than routine hospital services provided by the facility, such as x-ray films and laboratory tests.

Appeal (9): A request for a review of an insurance claim that has been underpaid or denied by an insurance company to receive additional payment.

Applicant (3): A person applying for insurance coverage.

Application form (18): A request form to be completed with pertinent data when applying for employment.

Application service provider (ASP) (8): A practice management system available over the Internet in which data are housed on the server of the ASP but the accounts are managed by the health care provider's staff.

Appropriateness evaluation protocols (AEPs) (17): Nineteen criteria for admission under the prospective payment system, separated into two categories: severity and intensity of illness. To allow a patient admission to an acute care facility, one criterion from each category must be met.

Approved charges (12): A fee that Medicare decides the medical service is worth, which may or may not be the same as the actual amount billed. The patient may or may not be responsible for the difference.

Armed Services Disability (16): A disability occurring or aggravated while the patient is in military service.

Assignment (3, 12): A transfer, after an event insured against, or an individual's legal right to collect an amount payable under an insurance contract. When related to Medicare this is an agreement in which a patient assigns the right to receive payment from the Medicare administrative contractor to the physician. Under this agreement, the physician must agree to accept 80% of the allowed amount as payment in full once the deductible has been met. For TRICARE, providers who accept assignment agree to accept 75% or 80% of the TRICARE allowable charge as the full fee, collecting the deductible and 20% or 25% of the allowable charge from the patient. With other carriers, accepting assignment means that, in return for payment of the claim, the provider accepts the terms of the contract between the patient and carrier.

Attending physician (4): A medical staff member who is legally responsible for the care and treatment given to a patient.

Authorization (2): Under the Health Insurance Portability and Accountability Act (HIPAA) privacy rule, an individual's formal, written permission to use or disclose his or her personally identifiable health information for purposes other than treatment, payment, or health care operations.

Authorization form (2): A document signed by the patient that is needed for use and disclosure of protected health information that is not included in any existing consent form agreements.

Authorized provider (14): A physician or other individual authorized provider of care or a hospital or supplier approved by TRICARE to provide medical care and supplies.

Automatic stay (10): A court order that goes into effect once a bankruptcy petition is filed; all other legal actions such as attachments and foreclosures, are halted.

Backup (8): A duplicate data file, such as tape, CD-ROM, disk, or zip disk, used to record data; it may be used to complete or redo the operation if the primary equipment fails.

Balance (10): An amount owed on a credit transaction; also known as the *outstanding or unpaid balance.*

Bankruptcy (10): A condition under which a person or corporation is declared unable to pay debts.

Batch (8): A group of claims for different patients from one office submitted in one computer transmission.

Beneficiary (14): An individual entitled to receive insurance policy or government program health care benefits. Also known as *participant, subscriber, dependent, enrollee,* or *member.*

Benefit period (12, 16): A period of time during which payments for Medicare inpatient hospital benefits are available. A benefit period begins the first day an enrollee is given inpatient hospital care (nursing care or rehabilitation services) by a qualified provider and ends when the enrollee has not been an inpatient for 60 consecutive days. In workers' compensation cases, it is the maximum amount of time that benefits will be paid to the injured or ill person for the disability. For disability insurance, it is the maximum amount of time that benefits will be paid to the injured or ill person for a disability.

Benign tumor (5): An abnormal growth that does not have the properties of invasion and metastasis and is usually surrounded by a fibrous capsule; also called a *neoplasm.*

Bilateral (6): When coding surgical procedures, this term refers to both sides of the body.

Blanket contract (3): Comprehensive group insurance coverage through plans sponsored by professional associations for their members.

Blind mailing (18): To send a résumé with cover letter to possible prospects whom the individual does not know personally and who have not advertised for a job opening.

Bonding (10): An insurance contract by which, in return for a stated fee, a bonding agency guarantees payment of a certain sum to an employer in the event of a financial loss to the employer by the act of a specified employee or by some contingency over which the employer has no control.

Breach of confidential communication (2): *Breach* means "breaking or violation of a law or agreement." In the context of the medical office it means the unauthorized release of information about the patient.

Buffing (11): A physician's justifying the transference of sick, high-cost patients to other physicians in a managed care plan.

Bundled codes (6): To group more than one component (service or procedure) into one *Current Procedural Terminology* (CPT) code.

Business associate (2): A person who, on behalf of the covered entity, performs or assists in the performance of a function or activity involving the use or disclosure of individually identifiable health information, including claims processing or administration, data analysis, processing or administration, utilization review, quality assurance, billing, benefit management, practice management, and repricing.

Business associate agreement (8, 18): Contract between the provider and a clearinghouse that submits the electronic claims on behalf of the provider.

By report (BR) (15): A report must be submitted with the claim when the notation "BR" follows the procedure code description. This term is sometimes seen in workers' compensation fee schedules.

Cable modem (8): A modem used to connect a computer to a cable television system that offers online services.

Cancellable (3): A renewal provision in an insurance agreement that grants the insurer the right to cancel the policy at any time and for any reason.

Capitation (3, 11, 17): A system of payment used by managed care plans in which physicians and hospitals are paid a fixed per capita amount for each patient enrolled over a stated period of time, regardless of the type and number of services provided; reimbursement to the hospital on a per-member/per-month basis to cover costs for the members of the plan. Capitation can also mean a set amount to be paid per claim.

Carve outs (11): Medical services not included within the capitation rate as benefits of a managed care contract and may be contracted for separately.

Case rate (17): An averaging after a flat rate is given to certain categories of procedures.

Cash flow (1, 10): In a medical practice, the amount of actual cash generated and available for use by the medical practice within a given period of time.

Catastrophic cap (14): The maximum dollar amount that a member has to pay under TRICARE or CHAMPVA in any fiscal year or enrollment period for covered medical bills.

Catchment area (14): In the TRICARE program, an area, defined by ZIP codes, that is approximately 40 miles in radius surrounding each United States military treatment facility.

Categorically needy (13): Aged, blind, or disabled individuals or families and children who meet financial eligibility requirements for Aid to Families with Dependent Children, Supplemental Security Income, or an optional state supplement.

Centers for Medicare and Medicaid Services (CMS) (12): Formerly known as the Health Care Financing Administration (HCFA), CMS divides responsibilities among three divisions: the Center for Medicare Management, the Center for Beneficiary Choices, and the Center for Medicaid and State Operations.

Certification (18): A statement issued by a board or association verifying that a person meets professional standards.

Certified Coding Specialist (CCS) (18): A title received by a person after appropriate training and by passing a certification examination administered by the American Health Information Management Association for hospital-based coding.

Certified Coding Specialist-Physician (CCS-P) (18): A title received by a person after appropriate training and by passing a certification examination administered by the American Health Information Management Association for physician-based coding.

Certified Medical Assistant (CMA) (18): A title received by a person after appropriate training and by passing a certification examination administered by the American Association of Medical Assistants, Inc.

Certified Medical Billing Specialist (CMBS) (18): A title received by a person after appropriate training and by passing a certification examination administered either by the American Association of Medical Billers in Los Angeles or the Medical Association of Billers in Las Vegas.

Certified Professional Coder (CPC) (18): A title received by a person after appropriate training and the passing of a certification examination administered by the American Academy of Professional Coders.

CHAMPVA (3, 14): See the *Civilian Health and Medical Program of the Department of Veterans Affairs*.

Charge description master (CDM) (17): A computer program that is linked to various hospital departments and includes procedure codes, procedure descriptions, service descriptions, fees, and revenue codes; also known as *charge master* or *procedure code dictionary*.

Charges (17): The dollar amount a hospital bills an outlier case on the basis of the itemized bill.

Chief complaint (CC) (4, 5): A patient's statement describing symptoms, problems, or conditions as the reason for seeking health care services from a physician.

Chronic (4): A medical condition persisting over a long period of time.

Chronologic résumé (18): A data sheet that outlines experience and education by dates.

Churning (11): When physicians see a high volume of patients—more than medically necessary—to increase revenue. May be seen in fee-for-service or managed care environments.

Civil Service Retirement System (CSRS) (16): A program for federal employees hired before 1984.

Civilian Health and Medical Program of the Department of Veterans Affairs (CHAMPVA) (3, 14): The Civilian Health and Medical Program of the Department of Veterans Affairs, a program for veterans with total, permanent, service-connected disabilities or surviving spouses and dependents of veterans who died of service-connected disabilities.

Claim (3): A bill sent to an insurance carrier requesting payment for services rendered; also known as *encounter record*.

Claims assistance professional (CAP) (1, 18): A practitioner who works for the consumer and helps patients organize, complete, file, and negotiate health insurance claims of all types to obtain maximum benefits, as well as tell patients what checks to write to providers to eliminate overpayment.

Claims examiner (15): In industrial cases, a representative of the insurer who authorizes treatment and investigates, evaluates, and negotiates the patient's insurance claim and acts for the company in the settlement of claims; also known as *claims adjuster, claims representative,* and *claims administrator.*

Claims-review type of foundation (11): A type of foundation that provides peer review by physicians to the numerous fiscal agents or carriers involved in its area.

Clean claim (7): A completed insurance claim form submitted within the program time limit that contains all the necessary information without deficiencies so that it can be processed and paid promptly.

Clearinghouse (2, 8): An independent organization that receives insurance claims from the physician's office, performs software edits, and redistributes the claims electronically to various insurance carriers.

Clinical outliers (17): Cases that cannot adequately be assigned to an appropriate diagnosis-related group (DRG), owing to unique combinations of diagnoses and surgeries, rare conditions, or other unique clinical reasons. Such cases are grouped together into clinical outlier DRGs and therefore considered outliers.

Closed panel program (11): A form of health maintenance organization (HMO) that limits the patient's choice of personal physicians to only those doctors practicing in the HMO group practice within the geographic location or facility. A physician must meet narrow criteria to join a closed panel.

Code of Medical Ethics (10): A code of medical ethics written by Thomas Percival in 1803.

Code sequence (17): The correct order of diagnostic codes (1, 2, 3, 4) when submitting an insurance claim that affects maximum reimbursement. Other factors affecting maximum reimbursement are accurate diagnostic code selection and linking the proper service or procedures provided to the patient.

Code set (2, 8): Any set of codes with their descriptions used to encode data elements such as tables of terms, medical concepts, medical diagnostic codes, or medical procedure codes.

Coinsurance (3, 13): (A) A cost-sharing requirement under a health insurance policy providing that the insured will assume a percentage of the costs for covered services. (B) For Medicare, after application of the yearly cash deductible, the portion of the reasonable charges (20%) for which the beneficiary is responsible. (C) In the Medicaid Qualified Medicare Beneficiary program, the amount of payment that is above the rate that Medicare pays for medical services. The state assumes responsibility for payment of this amount.

Collateral (10): Any possession, such as an automobile, furniture, stocks, or bonds, that secures or guarantees the discharge of an obligation.

Collection ratio (10): The relationship between the amount of money owed and the amount of money

collected in reference to the doctor's accounts receivable.

Combination code (5): A code from one section of the procedural code book combined with a code from another section that is used to completely describe a procedure performed; in diagnostic coding, a single five-digit code used to identify etiology and secondary process (manifestation) or complication of a disease.

Combination résumé (18): A data sheet that combines specific dates or work experience with educational skills.

Comorbidity (4, 17): An ongoing condition that exists along with the condition for which the patient is receiving treatment; in regard to DRGs, a preexisting condition that, because of its presence with a certain principal diagnosis, causes an increase in length of stay by at least 1 day in approximately 75% of cases. Also known as *substantial comorbidity.*

Competitive Medical Plan (CMP) (3): A state-licensed health plan similar to a HMO that delivers comprehensive, coordinated services to voluntarily enrolled members on a prepaid capitated basis. CMP status may be granted by the federal government for the enrollment of Medicare beneficiaries into managed care plans, without having to qualify as an HMO.

Compliance (2): A process of meeting regulations, recommendations, and expectations of federal and state agencies that pay for health care services and regulate the industry.

Compliance plan (2): A management plan composed of policies and procedures to accomplish uniformity, consistency, and conformity in medical record keeping that fulfills official requirements.

Complication (5): A disease or condition arising during the course of, or as a result of, another disease modifying medical care requirements; for DRGs, a condition that arises during the hospital stay that prolongs the length of stay by at least 1 day in approximately 75% of cases. Also known as *substantial complication.*

Comprehensive (4): A term used to describe a level of history or physical examination.

Comprehensive code (6): A single procedural code that describes or covers two or more CPT component codes that are bundled together as one unit.

Comprehensive type of foundation (11): A type of foundation that designs and sponsors prepaid health programs or sets minimum benefits of coverage.

Compromise and release (C and R) (15): An agreement arrived at, whether in or out of court, for settling a workers' compensation case after the patient has been declared permanent and stationary.

Computer-assisted coding (CAC) (5): Use of computer software that automatically generates a set of medical codes for review, validation, and use based on clinical documentation provided by health care practitioners. CAC uses two technology options: natural language processing (NLP) and structured input.

Concurrent care (4): The provision of similar services (e.g., hospital visits) to the same patient by more than one physician on the same day. Usually a separate physical disorder is present.

Conditionally renewable (3): An insurance policy renewal provision that grants the insurer a limited right to refuse to renew a health insurance policy at the end of a premium payment period.

Confidential communication (2): A privileged communication that may be disclosed only with the patient's permission.

Confidentiality (2): The state of treating privately or secretly, and not disclosing to other individuals or for public knowledge, the patient's conversations or medical records.

Consent (2): Verbal or written agreement that gives approval to some action, situation, or statement.

Consent form (2): A document that is not required before physicians use or disclose protected health information for treatment, payment, or routine health care operations of the patient. For other purposes, see *Authorization form.*

Consultation (4): Services rendered by a physician whose opinion or advice is requested by another physician or agency in the evaluation or treatment of a patient's illness or suspected problem.

Consultative examiner (CE) (16): A physician who is paid a fee to examine or test a person for disability under either the SSDI or SSI program.

Consulting physician (4): A provider whose opinion or advice about evaluation or management of a specific problem is requested by another physician.

Continuing education (CE) (18): Formal education pursued by a working professional and intended to improve or maintain professional competence.

Continuity of care (4): When a physician sees a patient who has received treatment for a condition and is referred by the previous doctor for treatment of the same condition.

Contract (3): A legally enforceable agreement when relating to an insurance policy; for workers' compensation cases, an agreement involving two or more parties in which each is obligated to the other to fulfill promises made. (The contract exists between the physician and the insurance carrier.)

Conventions (5): Rules or principles for determining a diagnostic code when using diagnostic code books such as each space, typefaces, indentations, punctuation marks, instructional notes, abbreviations, cross-reference notes, and specific usage of the words *and, with,* and *due to.* These rules assist in the selection of correct codes for the diagnoses encountered.

Conversion factor (6): The dollars and cents amount that is established for one unit as applied to a procedure or service rendered. This unit is then used to convert various procedures into fee-schedule payment amounts by multiplying the relative value unit by the conversion factor.

Cooperative care (14): A term used when a patient is seen by a civilian physician or hospital for services cost-shared by TRICARE.

Coordination of benefits (3, 14): Two insurance carriers working together and coordinating the payment of their benefits so that there is no duplication of benefits paid between the primary and secondary insurance carriers. In TRICARE, the coordination of the payment of TRICARE benefits with the payment of benefits made by the double coverage plan so that there is no duplication of benefits paid between the double coverage plan and TRICARE; likewise applied to disability programs.

Copayment (copay) (11, 13): (A) A patient's payment (e.g., 20% of a bill or flat fee of $10 per visit) of a portion of the cost at the time the service is rendered; sometimes referred to as *coinsurance.* (B) In the Medicaid program, a required specific dollar amount that must be collected at each office visit for medical services received by an individual. Different copayment amounts may be set for each patient type and for certain medical procedures.

Correct coding initiative (CCI) (12): Federal legislation that attempts to eliminate unbundling or other inappropriate reporting of procedural codes for professional medical services rendered to patients.

Cost-of-living adjustment (16): A disability insurance provision to increase monthly benefits.

Cost outlier (17): A typical case that has an extraordinarily high cost when compared with most discharges classified to the same DRG.

Cost outlier review (17): A review by a professional review organization (PRO) for the necessity of a patient's hospital admission and to determine whether all services rendered were medically necessary. Cost outlier cases are recognized only if the case is not eligible for day outlier status.

Cost-share (14): The portion of the allowable charges (20% or 25%) after the deductible has been met that the TRICARE patient is responsible for.

Counseling (4): A discussion between the physician and a patient, family, or both concerning the diagnosis, recommended studies or tests, prognosis, risks, and benefits of treatment, treatment options, patient and family education, and so on.

Cover letter (18): A letter of introduction prepared to accompany a résumé when seeking a job.

Covered entity (CE) (2, 8): An entity that transmits health information in electronic form in connection with a transaction covered by HIPAA. The covered entity may be (1) a health care coverage carrier such as Blue Cross/Blue Shield, (2) a health care clearinghouse through which claims are submitted, or (3) a health care provider such as the primary care physician.

Covered services (13): Specific services and supplies for which Medicaid will provide reimbursement; these consist of a combination of mandatory and optional services stated in the plan.

CPT (6): See *Current Procedural Terminology* (CPT).

Credit (10): (A) From the Latin *credere,* meaning "to believe" or "to trust"; trust in regard to financial obligation. (B) Accounting entry reflecting payment by a debtor (patient) of a sum received on his or her account.

Credit card (10): A card issued by an organization and devised for the purpose of obtaining money, property, labor, or services on credit.

Creditor (10): A person to whom money is owed.

Critical care (4): In reference to coding professional services, this phrase relates to intensive care provided in a variety of acute life-threatening conditions requiring constant bedside attention by a physician.

Crossover claim (12): A bill for services rendered to a patient receiving benefits simultaneously from Medicare and Medicaid or from Medicare and a Medigap plan. Medicare pays first and then determines the amounts of unmet Medicare deductible and coinsurance to be paid by the secondary insurance carrier. The claim is automatically transferred (electronically) to the secondary insurance carrier for additional payment. Also known as *claims transfer.*

***Current Procedural Terminology* (CPT) (6):** A reference procedural code book using a five-digit numerical system to identify and code procedures established by the American Medical Association.

Customary fee (6): The amount that a physician usually charges most of her or his patients.

Cycle billing (10): A system of billing accounts at spaced intervals during the month based on breakdown of accounts by alphabet, account number, insurance type, or date of first service.

Data elements (8): Medical code sets used uniformly to document why patients are seen (diagnosis, ICD-9-CM) and what is done to them during their encounter (procedure, CPT-4, HCPCS).

Day outlier review (17): A review of potential day outliers (short or unusually long length of hospital stay) to determine the necessity of admission and number of days before the day outlier threshold is reached, as well as the number of days beyond the threshold. The PRO determines the certification of additional days.

Daysheet (3): A register for recording daily business transactions (charges, payments, or adjustments); also known as *daybook, daily log,* or *daily record sheet.*

Debit card (10): A card permitting bank customers to withdraw from any affiliated automated teller machine (ATM) and make cashless purchases from funds on deposit without incurring revolving finance charges for credit.

Debt (10): A legal obligation to pay money.

Debtor (10): A person owing money.

Deductible (2, 11): A specific dollar amount that must be paid by the insured before a medical insurance plan or government program begins covering health care costs.

Defense Enrollment Eligibility Reporting System (DEERS) (14): An electronic database used to verify beneficiary eligibility for those individuals in the TRICARE programs.

Deleted claim (7): Insurance claim that has been canceled, deleted, or voided by a Medicare fiscal intermediary for the following reasons: CMS-1500 (08-05) or current CMS-1450 is not used, itemized charges are not provided, more than six line items are submitted on the CMS-1500 (08-05) claim form, patient's address is missing, internal clerical error was made, Certificate of Medical Necessity (CMN) was not with the Part B claim or was incomplete or invalid, and name of the store is not on the receipt that includes the price of the item.

Delinquent claim (9): An insurance claim submitted to an insurance company, for which payment is overdue.

Denied paper or electronic claim (9): An insurance claim submitted to an insurance company in which payment has been rejected owing to a technical error or because of medical coverage policy issues.

Deposition (15): The process of taking sworn testimony from a witness out of court. This is usually done by an attorney.

Detailed (4): A term used to describe a level of history or physical examination.

Diagnosis-related groups (DRGs) (17): A patient classification system that categorizes patients who are medically related with respect to diagnosis and treatment and statistically similar in length of hospital stay. Medicare hospital insurance payments are based on fixed dollar amounts for a principal diagnosis as listed in DRGs.

Diagnostic cost groups (DCGs) (12): A system of Medicare reimbursement for HMOs with risk contracts in which enrollees are classified into various DCGs on the basis of each beneficiary's prior 12-month hospitalization history.

Diagnostic creep (17): See *DRG creep.*

Direct data entry (DDE) (8): Keying claim information directly into the payer system by accessing over modem dial-up or DSL. This is a technology to directly enter the information into the payer system via the access whether it is dial-up or DSL.

Digital subscriber line (DSL) (8): A high-speed connection through a telephone line jack and usually a means of accessing the Internet.

Direct referral (11): Certain services in a managed care plan may not require preauthorization. The authorization request form is completed and signed by the physician and handed to the patient (e.g., obstetric care or dermatology) to be done directly.

Dirty claim (7): A claim submitted with errors or one that requires manual processing to resolve problems or is rejected for payment.

Disability Determination Services (DDS) (16): A state Social Security division office that assesses a case for disability benefits.

Disability income insurance (3, 16): A form of health insurance that provides periodic payments to replace income when the insured is unable to work as a result of illness, injury, or disease—not as a result of a work-related accident or condition.

Disabled (12): For purposes of enrollment under Medicare, individuals younger than 65 years of age who have been entitled to disability benefits under the Social Security Act or the Railroad Retirement system for at least 24 months are considered disabled and are entitled to Medicare.

Disclosure (2): The release, transfer, provision of access to, or divulging in any other manner of information outside the entity holding the information.

Discount (10): A reduction of a normal charge based on a specific amount of money or a percentage of the charge.

Disenrollment (11): A member's voluntary cancellation of membership in a managed care plan.

Documentation (4): A chronologic detailed recording of pertinent facts and observations about a patient's health as seen in chart notes and medical reports; entries in the medical record such as prescription refills, telephone calls, and other pertinent data. For computer software, a user's guide to a program or piece of equipment.

Double indemnity (16): A feature in some life and disability insurance policies that provides for twice the face amount of the policy to be paid if death results to the insured from accidental causes.

Downcoding (6): This occurs when the coding system used by the physician's office on a claim does not match the coding system used by the insurance company receiving the claim. The insurance company computer system converts the code submitted to the closest code in use, which is usually down one level from the submitted code, generating decreased payment.

DRG creep (17): Coding that is inappropriately altered to obtain a higher payment rate; also known as *coding creep, diagnostic creep,* or *upcoding.*

DRG validation (17): To find out whether the diagnostic and procedural information affecting DRG assignment is substantiated by the clinical information in the patient's chart.

Dun message (10): A message or phrase to inform or remind a patient about a delinquent account.

Durable medical equipment (DME) number (7): A group or individual provider number used when submitting bills for specific medical supplies, devices, and equipment to the Medicare fiscal intermediary for reimbursement.

E codes (5): A classification of ICD-9-CM coding used to describe environmental events, circumstances, and conditions as the external cause of injury, poisoning, and other adverse effects. E codes are also used in coding adverse reactions to medications.

Early and Periodic Screening, Diagnosis, and Treatment (EPSDT) (13): The EPSDT program covers screening and diagnostic services to determine physical or mental defects in recipients younger than 21 years of age and health care, treatment, and other measures to correct or ameliorate any defects and chronic conditions discovered. In New York, this is called the Child Health Assurance Program (CHAP).

E-Health information management (e-HIM) (2): A term coined by the AHIMA's eHealth Task Force to describe any and all transactions in which health care information is accessed, processed, stored, and transferred using electronic technologies.

Elective surgery (17): A surgical procedure that may be scheduled in advance, is not an emergency, and is discretionary on the part of the physician and patient.

Electronic claim (7): An insurance claim submitted to the insurance carrier via a central processing unit (CPU), tape, diskette, direct data entry, direct wire, dial-in telephone, digital fax, or personal computer download or upload.

Electronic claims processor (ECP) (18): An individual who converts insurance claims to standardized electronic format and transmits electronic insurance claims data to the insurance carrier or clearinghouse to help the physician receive payment. Sometimes referred to as *electronic claims professional.*

Electronic data interchange (EDI) (8): The process by which understandable data items are sent back and forth via computer linkages between two or more entities that function alternatively as sender and receiver.

Electronic funds transfer (EFT) (8): A paperless computerized system enabling funds to be debited, credited, or transferred, eliminating the need for personal handling of checks.

Electronic health record (EHR) (4): A patient record that is created using a computer with software. A template is brought up and by answering a series of questions data are entered.

Electronic media (2): The mode of electronic transmission (e.g., Internet, Extranet, leased phone or dial-up phone lines, or fax modems).

Electronic remittance advice (ERA) (8): An online transaction about the status of a claim.

Electronic signature (3): An individualized computer access and identification system (e.g., a series of numbers, letters, electronic writing, voice, computer key, and fingerprint transmission [biometric system]) accepted by both parties to show intent, approval of, or responsibility for computer document content.

Eligibility (3): Qualifying factors that must be met before a patient receives benefits (medical services) under a specified insurance plan, government program, or managed care plan.

Emancipated minor (3): A person younger than 18 years of age who lives independently, is totally self-supporting, and possesses decision-making rights.

Embezzlement (2, 10): A willful act by an employee of taking possession of an employer's money.

Emergency (14): A sudden and unexpected medical condition, or the worsening of a condition, that poses a threat to life, limb, or sight and requires immediate treatment to alleviate suffering (e.g., shortness of breath, chest pain, drug overdose).

Emergency care (4): Health care services provided to prevent serious impairment of bodily functions or serious dysfunction to any body organ or part. Advanced life support may be necessary. Not all care provided in an emergency department of a hospital can be termed "emergency care."

Employer identification number (EIN) (7): An individual's federal tax identification number issued by the Internal Revenue Service for income tax purposes.

Employment agency (18): A business organization that refers job applicants to potential employers.

Encoder (8): An add-on software to practice management systems that can reduce the time it takes to build or review insurance claims before batch transmission to the carrier.

Encounter form (3): An all-encompassing billing form personalized to the practice of the physician, it may be used when a patient submits an insurance billing; also called *charge slip, communicator, multipurpose billing form, fee ticket, patient service slip, routing form, superbill,* and *transaction slip.*

Encryption (8): To assign a code to represent data. This is done for security purposes.

End-stage renal disease (ESRD) (12): Individuals who have chronic kidney disease requiring dialysis or kidney transplant are considered to have ESRD. To qualify for Medicare coverage, an individual must be fully or currently insured under Social Security or the Railroad Retirement system or be the dependent of an insured person. Eligibility for Medicare coverage begins with the third month after beginning a course of renal dialysis. Coverage may commence sooner if the patient participates in a self-care dialysis training program or receives a kidney transplant without dialysis.

Eponym (4, 5): The name of a disease, anatomic structure, operation, or procedure, usually derived from the name of a place where it first occurred or a person who discovered or first described it.

Ergonomic (15): Science and technology that seek to fit the anatomic and physical needs of the worker to the workplace.

Established patient (4): An individual who has received professional services within the past 3 years from the physician or another physician of the same specialty who belongs to the same group practice.

Estate administrator (10): One who takes possession of the assets of a decedent, pays the expenses of administration and the claims of creditors, and disposes of the balance of an estate in accordance with the statutes governing the distribution of decedents' estates.

Estate executor (10): One who takes possession of the assets of a decedent, pays the expenses of administration and the claims of creditors, and disposes of the balance of an estate in accordance with the decedent's will.

Ethics (1): Standards of conduct generally accepted as a moral guide for behavior by which an insurance billing or coding specialist may determine the appropriateness of his or her conduct in a relationship with patients, the physician, co-workers, the government, and insurance companies.

Etiology (5): The cause of disease; the study of the cause of a disease.

Etiquette (1): Customs, rules of conduct, courtesy, and manners of the medical profession.

Exclusion(s) (3, 16): Provisions written into the insurance contract denying coverage or limiting the scope of coverage.

Exclusive provider organization (EPO) (3, 11): A type of managed health care plan that combines features of HMOs and PPOs. It is referred to as "exclusive" because it is offered to large employers who agree not to contract with any other plan. EPOs are regulated under state health insurance laws.

Expanded problem focused (EPF) (4): A phrase used to describe a level of history or physical examination.

Explanation of benefits (EOB) (9): A document detailing services billed and describing payment determinations; also known in Medicare, Medicaid, and some other programs as a *remittance advice.* In the TRICARE program, it is called a *summary payment voucher.*

Explanation of Medicare benefits (EOMB): See *Remittance advice (RA).*

Expressed contract (3): A verbal or written agreement.

Extended (3): To carry forward the balance of an individual financial accounting record.

External audit (4): A review done after claims have been submitted (retrospective review) of medical and financial records by an insurance company or Medicare representative to investigate suspected fraud or abusive billing practices.

Extraterritorial (15): State laws effective outside the state by either specific provision or court decision. In workers' compensation cases, benefits under the state law that apply to a compensable injury of an employee hired in one state but injured outside that state.

Facility provider number (7): A facility's (hospital, laboratory, radiology office, or nursing facility) provider number to be used by the facility to bill for services, or by the performing physician to report services done at that location.

Facsimile (4): An electronic process for transmitting graphic and written documents over telephone lines; also referred to as *fax*.

Family history (FH) (4): A review of medical events in the patient's family including diseases that may be hereditary or place the patient at risk.

Federal Employees' Compensation Act (FECA) (15): An act instituted in 1908 providing benefits for on-the-job injuries to all federal employees.

Federal Employees Retirement System (FERS) (16): A program for federal employees hired after 1984 or those hired before 1984 who switched from CSRS to FERS.

Fee for service (11): A method of payment in which the patient pays the physician for each professional service performed from an established schedule of fees.

Fee schedule (6, 10, 15): A list of charges or established allowances for specific medical services and procedures. See also *Relative value studies (RVS)*.

Financial accounting record (3, 10): An individual record indicating charges, payments, adjustments, and balances owed for services rendered; also known as a *ledger*.

Fiscal agent (13): An organization under contract to the state to process claims for a state Medicaid program; insurance carrier handling claims from physicians and other suppliers of service for Medicare Part B; also referred to as *Medicare administrative contractor* (MAC), formerly fiscal intermediary.

Formal referral (11): An authorization request (telephone, fax, or completed form) required by the managed care organization contract to determine medical necessity and grant permission before services are rendered or procedures performed.

Formulary (12): List of drugs that a health insurance plan covers as a benefit.

Foundation for medical care (FMC) (3, 11): An organization of physicians sponsored by a state or local medical association concerned with the development and delivery of medical services and the cost of health care.

Fraud (2): An intentional misrepresentation of the facts to deceive or mislead another.

Functional résumé (18): A data sheet that highlights qualifications and skills.

Future purchase option (16): See *Cost-of-living adjustment*.

Garnishment (10): A court order attaching a debtor's property or wages to pay off a debt.

Gatekeeper (11): In the managed care system, this is the physician who controls patient access to specialists and diagnostic testing services.

Global surgery policy (6): A Medicare policy relating to surgical procedures in which preoperative and postoperative visits (24 hours before [major] and day of [minor]), usual, intraoperative services, and complications not requiring additional trips to the operating room are included in one fee.

Group national provider number (group NPI) (7): A number assigned to a group of physicians submitting insurance claims under the group name and reporting income under one name.

Grouper (17): The computer software program that assigns DRGs of discharged patients using the following information: patient's age, sex, principal diagnosis, complications/comorbid conditions, principal procedure, and discharge status.

Guaranteed renewable (3, 16): A clause in an insurance policy that means the insurance company must renew the policy as long as premium payments are made. However, the premium may be increased when it is renewed. These policies may have age limits of 60, 65, or 70 years or may be renewable for life.

Guarantor (3): An individual who promises to pay the medical bill by signing a form agreeing to pay or who accepts treatment, which constitutes an expressed promise.

Health benefits advisor (HBA) (14): An individual at military hospitals or clinics who is there to help TRICARE beneficiaries obtain medical care through the military and through TRICARE.

Health Care Financing Administration (HCFA) (12): See *Centers for Medicare and Medicaid Services (CMS)*.

Health care finder (HCF) (14): Health care professionals, generally registered nurses, who are located at TRICARE Service Centers to act as liaison between military and civilian providers, verify eligibility, determine availability of services, coordinate care, facilitate the transfer of records, and perform first level medical review. HCFs help TRICARE beneficiaries and providers with preauthorization of medical services.

Healthcare Common Procedure Coding System (HCPCS) (6): The CMS's Common Procedure Coding System. A three-tier national uniform coding system developed by the Centers for Medicare and Medicaid Services (CMS), formerly HCFA, used for reporting physician or supplier services and procedures under the Medicare program. Level I codes are national CPT codes. Level II codes are HCPCS national codes used to report items not covered under CPT. Level III codes are HCPCS regional or local codes used to identify new procedures or items for which there is no national code. Pronounced "hick-picks."

Health care provider (2): A provider of medical or health services and any other person or organization who furnishes bills or is paid for health care in the normal course of business.

Health insurance (3): A contract between the policyholder or member and insurance carrier or government program to reimburse the policyholder or member for all or a portion of the cost of medical care rendered by health care professionals; generic term applying to lost income arising from illness or injury; also known as *accident and health insurance* or *disability income insurance.*

Health Insurance Claim Form (CMS-1500 [08-05]) (7): Known as CMS-1500. A universal insurance claim form developed and approved by the AMA Council on Medical Service and the Centers for Medicare and Medicaid Services. It is used by physicians and other professionals to bill outpatient services and supplies to TRICARE, Medicare, and some Medicaid programs, as well as some private insurance carriers and managed care plans.

Health maintenance organization (HMO) (3, 11): The oldest of all prepaid health plans. A comprehensive health care financing and delivery organization that provides a wide range of health care services with an emphasis on preventive medicine to enrollees within a geographic area through a panel of providers. Primary care physician "gatekeepers" are usually reimbursed via capitation. In general, enrollees do not receive coverage for the services from providers who are not in the HMO network, except for emergency services.

Health record (4): Written or graphic information documenting facts and events during the rendering of patient care. Also known as *medical record.*

Hearing (16): The second level of the appeal process for an individual applying for SSDI or SSI. This is a hearing before an administrative law judge who had no part in the initial or reconsideration disability determination.

High complexity (HC) (4): A phrase used to describe a type of medical decision making when a patient is seen for an E/M service.

High risk (3): A high chance of loss.

HIPAA Transaction and Code Set (TCS) rule (8): This regulation under HIPAA defines the standardized methods for transmitting electronic health information. The TCS process includes any set of HIPAA-approved codes with their descriptions used to encode data elements such as tables of terms, medical concepts, medical diagnostic codes, or medical procedure codes. TCS regulations were implemented to streamline electronic data interchange.

History of present illness (HPI) (4): A chronologic description of the development of the patient's present illness from the first sign or symptom or from the previous encounter to the present.

Hospice (12): A public agency or private organization primarily engaged in providing pain relief, symptom management, and supportive services to terminally ill patients and their families in their own homes or in a homelike center.

Hospital insurance (12): Known as *Medicare Part A.* A program providing basic protection against the costs of hospital and related after-hospital services for individuals eligible under the Medicare program.

Implied contract (3): A contract between physician and patient not manifested by direct words but implied or deduced from the circumstance, general language, or conduct of the patient.

In-area (11): Within the geographic boundaries defined by an HMO as the area in which it will provide medical services to its members.

Incomplete claim (7): Any Medicare claim missing necessary information; such claims are identified to the provider so that they may be resubmitted.

Indemnity (3): Benefits paid to an insured while disabled; also known as *reimbursement.*

Independent (or Individual) Practice Association (IPA) (3, 11): A type of HMO in which a program administrator contracts with a number of physicians who agree to provide treatment to subscribers in their own offices. Physicians are not employees of the managed care organization (MCO) and are not paid salaries. They receive reimbursement on a capitation or fee-for-service basis; also referred to as a *medical capitation plan.*

Individually identifiable health information (IIHI) (2): Any part of an individual's health information including demographic information (e.g., address, date of birth) collected from the individual that is created or received by a covered entity.

Injury (15): In a workers' compensation policy, this term signifies any trauma or damage to a body part or disease sustained, arising out of, and in the course of employment, including injury to artificial members and medical braces of all types.

Inpatient (17): A term used when a patient is admitted to the hospital for overnight stay.

Inquiry (9): See *Tracer.*

In situ (5): A description applied to a malignant growth confined to the site of origin without invasion of neighboring tissues.

Insurance adjuster (15): An individual at the workers' compensation insurance carrier overseeing an industrial case, authorizing diagnostic testing and medical treatment, and communicating with the provider of medical care.

Insurance balance billing (10): A statement sent to the patient after his or her insurance company has paid its portion of the claim.

Insurance billing specialist (1): A practitioner who carries out claims completion, coding, and billing responsibilities and may or may not perform managerial and supervisory functions; also known as an *insurance claims processor, reimbursement specialist, medical billing representative,* or *senior billing representative.*

Insured (3): An individual or organization protected in case of loss under the terms of an insurance policy.

Intelligent character recognition (ICR) (7): Same as *Optical character recognition.*

Intermediate care facilities (ICFs) (12): Institutions furnishing health-related care and services to individuals who do not require the degree of care provided by acute care hospitals or nursing facilities.

Internal review (4): The process of going over financial documents before and after billing to insurance carriers to determine documentation deficiencies or errors.

***International Classification of Diseases, Ninth Revision, Clinical Modification* (ICD-9-CM) (5, 17):** A diagnostic code book that uses a system for classifying diseases and operations to assist collection of uniform and comparable health information. A code system to replace this is ICD-10, which is being modified for use in the United States.

***International Classification of Diseases, Tenth Revision, Clinical Modification* (ICD-10-CM) (5, 17):** Diagnostic code book that uses a system for classifying diseases and operations to assist collection of uniform and comparable health information. It has been modified, will be implemented on October 1, 2013, and will replace ICD-9-CM Volumes 1 and 2 when submitting insurance claims for billing hospital and physician office medical services.

***International Classification of Diseases, Tenth Revision, Procedural Coding System* (ICD-10-PCS) (5, 17):** Procedural code system developed by 3M Health Information Systems (HIS) under contract with the Centers for Medicare and Medicaid Services (CMS). When implemented on October 1, 2013, it will replace ICD-9-CM Volume 3 for hospital inpatient procedure reporting in the United States.

Interview (18): Meeting an individual face-to-face for evaluating and questioning a job applicant.

Intoxication (5): A diagnostic coding term that relates to an adverse effect rather than a poisoning when drugs such as digitalis, steroid agents, and so on are involved.

Invalid claim (7): Any Medicare claim that contains complete, necessary information but is illogical or incorrect (e.g., listing an incorrect provider number for a referring physician). Invalid claims are identified to the provider and may be resubmitted.

Italicized code (5): A diagnostic code in ICD-9-CM, volume 1, Tabular List, that may never be sequenced as the principal diagnosis.

Itemized statement (10): A detailed summary of all transactions of a patient's account: dates of service, detailed charges, payments (copayments and deductibles), date the insurance claim was submitted, adjustments, and account balance.

Late effect (5): An inactive residual effect or condition produced after the acute phase of an illness or injury has ended.

Ledger card (3, 10): See *Financial accounting record.*

Lien (10, 15): A claim on the property of another as security for a debt. In litigation cases, it is a legal promise to satisfy a debt owed by the patient to the physician out of any proceeds received on the case.

Limiting charge (12): A percentage limit on fees, specified by legislation, that nonparticipating physicians may bill Medicare beneficiaries above the fee schedule amount.

List service (listserv) (1): An online computer service run from a website where questions may be posted by subscribers.

Long-term disability insurance (16): A provision to pay benefits to a covered disabled person to age 65.

Looping (17): The automated grouper (computer software program that assigns DRGs) process of searching all listed diagnoses for the presence of any comorbid condition or complication, or searching all procedures for operating room procedures or other specific procedures.

Lost claim (9): An insurance claim that cannot be located after sending it to an insurer.

Low complexity (LC) (4): Phrase used to describe a type of medical decision making when a patient is seen for an E/M service.

Major diagnostic categories (MDCs) (17): A broad classification of diagnoses. There are 83 coding system–oriented MDCs in the original DRGs and 23 body system–oriented MDCs in the revised set of DRGs.

Major medical (3): A health insurance policy designed to offset heavy medical expenses resulting from catastrophic or prolonged illness or injury.

Malignant tumor (5): An abnormal growth that has the properties of invasion and metastasis (e.g., transfer of diseases from one organ to another). The word *carcinoma* (CA) refers to a cancerous or malignant tumor.

Managed care organizations (MCOs) (11): A generic term applied to a managed care plan. May apply to EPO, HMO, PPO, integrated delivery system, or other different managed care arrangement. MCOs are usually prepaid group plans, and physicians are typically paid by the capitation method.

Manual billing (10): Processing statements by hand; may involve typing statements or photocopying the patient's financial accounting record and placing it in a window envelope, which then becomes the statement.

Maternal and Child Health Program (MCHP) (3, 13): A state service organization to assist children younger than 21 years of age who have conditions leading to health problems.

Medicaid (MCD) (3, 13): A federally aided, state-operated, and state-administered program that provides medical benefits for certain low-income persons in need of health and medical care. California's Medicaid program is known as Medi-Cal.

Medi-Cal (13): California's version of the nationwide program known as Medicaid. See *Medicaid*.

Medical billing representative (1): See *Insurance billing specialist*.

Medical decision making (MDM) (4): Health care management process done after performing a history and physical examination on a patient that results in a plan of treatment. It is based on establishing one or more diagnoses and/or selecting a management or treatment option, amount of data or complexity of data reviewed, and complications and/or morbidity or mortality.

Medical necessity (4, 12): The performance of services and procedures that are consistent with the diagnosis in accordance with standards of good medical practice, performed at the proper level, and provided in the most appropriate setting. Medical necessity must be established (via diagnostic or other information presented on the individual claim under consideration) before the carrier may make payment.

Medical record (4): See *Health record*.

Medical report (4): A permanent, legal document (letter or report format) that formally states the consequences of the patient's examination or treatment.

Medical service order (15): An authorization given to the physician, either written or verbal, to treat the injured or ill employee.

Medically (or psychologically) necessary (14): Medical or psychologic services considered appropriate care and generally accepted by qualified professionals to be reasonable and adequate for the diagnosis and treatment of illness, injury, pregnancy, and mental disorders, or that are reasonable and adequate for well-baby care.

Medically needy (MN) (13): Persons in need of financial assistance or whose income and resources will not allow them to pay for the costs of medical care; also called *medically indigent* in some states.

Medicare (3, 12): A nationwide health insurance program for persons age 65 years of age and older and certain disabled or blind persons regardless of income, administered by CMS. Local Social Security offices take applications and supply information about the program.

Medicare administrative contractor (MAC) (12): Insurance carrier that receives and processes claims from physicians and other suppliers of service for Medicare Part B; formerly referred to as *fiscal intermediary, Medicare carrier, fiscal agent, Medicare Part B carrier,* or *contractor*.

Medicare/Medicaid (Medi-Medi) (3, 12): Refers to an individual who receives medical or disability benefits from both Medicare and Medicaid programs; sometimes referred to as a *Medi-Medi case* or a *crossover*.

Medicare Part A (12): Hospital benefits of a nationwide health insurance program for persons age 65 years of age and older and certain disabled individuals regardless of income, administered by CMS. Local Social Security offices take applications and supply information about the program.

Medicare Part B (12): Medical insurance of a nationwide health insurance program for persons age 65 years of age and older and certain disabled individuals regardless of income, administered by CMS. Local Social Security offices take applications and supply information about the program.

Medicare Part C (12): Medicare Plus (+) Choice plans offer a number of health care options in addition to those available under Medicare Part A and Part B. Plans may include health maintenance organizations, fee-for-service plans, provider-sponsored organizations, religious fraternal benefit societies, and Medicare medical savings accounts.

Medicare Part D (12): Stand-alone prescription drug plan, presented by insurance and other private companies that offer drug coverage that meets the standards established by Medicare. Other names for these plans are *Part D private prescription drug plans (PDPs)* or *Medicare Advantage prescription drug plans (MA-PDs)*.

Medicare Secondary Payer (MSP) (12): The primary insurance plan of a Medicare beneficiary that must pay for any medical care or services first before Medicare is sent a claim.

Medicare Summary Notice (MSN) (12): A document received by the patient explaining amount charged, Medicare approved, deductible, and coinsurance for medical services rendered.

Medigap (MG) (12): A specialized supplemental insurance policy devised for the Medicare beneficiary that covers the deductible and copayment amounts typically not covered under the main Medicare policy written by a nongovernmental third-party payer. Also known as *Medifill*.

Member (3): Person covered under an insurance program's contract, including (1) the subscriber or contract holder who is the person named on the membership identification card and (2) in the case of (a) two-person coverage, (b) one adult–one child coverage, or (c) family coverage, the eligible family dependents enrolled under the subscriber's contract.

Mentor (18): Guide or teacher who offers advice, criticism, wisdom, guidance, and perspective to an inexperienced but promising protégé to help reach a life goal.

Metastasis (5): Process in which tumor cells spread and transfer from one organ to another site.

Military treatment facility (MTF) (14): All uniformed service hospitals or health clinics; also known as *military hospitals* or *uniformed service hospitals*.

Moderate complexity (MC) (4): A phrase used to describe a type of medical decision making when a patient is seen for an E/M service.

Modifier (6): In CPT coding, a two-digit add-on number placed after the usual procedure code number to indicate a procedure or service has been altered by specific circumstances. The two-digit modifier may be separated by a hyphen. In HCPCS level II coding, one-digit or two-digit add-on alpha characters, placed after the usual procedure code number (Example G-1).

Example G-1

27372-51 (typed on one line)

Multipurpose billing form (3): See *Encounter form*.

Multiskilled health practitioner (MSHP) (1): An individual cross-trained to provide more than one function, often in more than one discipline. These combined functions can be found in a broad spectrum of health-related jobs, ranging in complexity including both clinical and administrative functions. The additional skills added to the original health care worker's job may be of a higher, lower, or parallel level. The terms *multiskilled, multicompetent*, and *cross-trained* can be used interchangeably.

National alphanumeric codes (12): Alphanumeric codes developed by HCFA. See *Health Care Financing Administration Common Procedure Coding System (HCPCS)*.

National Certified Insurance and Coding Specialist (NCICS) (18): An insurance and coding certification that is awarded by an independent testing agency, the National Center for Competency Testing (NCCT).

National provider identifier (NPI) (7): A Medicare lifetime 10-digit number issued to providers. When adopted, it will be recognized by Medicaid, Medicare, TRICARE, and CHAMPVA programs and eventually may be used by private insurance carriers.

National standard format (NSF) (8): The name of the standardization of data to reduce paper and have more accurate information and efficient organization.

Neoplasm (5): Benign or malignant tumor.

Netback (10): Evaluating a collection agency's performance by taking the amount of monies collected and subtracting the agency's fees.

Networking (18): Exchanging information or services among individuals, groups, or institutions and making use of professional contacts.

Never event (6): Incident related to either a wrong surgical device, patient protection, care management, environment, or criminal occurrence that results in injury or death due to error in health care management or failure to follow standard care or institutional practices or policies. Also referred to as *serious reportable event* (SRE).

New patient (NP) (4): An individual who has not received any professional services from the physician or another physician of the same specialty who belongs to the same group practice within the past 3 years.

No charge (NC) (10): Waiving the entire fee owed for professional care.

Noncancelable clause or policy (3, 16): An insurance policy clause that means the insurance company cannot increase premium rates and must renew the policy until the insured reaches the age stated in the contract. Some disability income policies have noncancelable terms.

Nondisability (ND) claim (15): A claim for an on-the-job injury that requires medical care but does not result in loss of working time or income.

Nonexempt assets (10): One's total property (in bankruptcy cases) not falling in the exemption category; including money, automobile equity, and property, more than a specified amount, depending on the state in which the person lives.

Nonparticipating physician (nonpar) (12): A provider who does not have a signed agreement with Medicare and has an option about assignment. The physician may not accept assignment for all services or has the option of accepting assignment for some services and collecting from the patient for other services performed at the same time and place.

Nonparticipating provider (nonpar) (3, 14): A provider who decides not to accept the determined allowable charge from an insurance plan as the full fee for care. Payment goes directly to the patient in this case, and the patient is usually responsible for paying the bill in full.

Non-physician practitioner (NPP) (4): Health care provider who meets state licensing requirements to provide specific medical services. Medicare allows payment for services furnished by non-physician practitioners including, but not limited to, advance registered nurse practitioners (ARNPs), certified registered nurse practitioners, clinical nurse specialists (CNSs), licensed clinical social workers (LCSWs), physician assistants (PAs), nurse midwives, physical therapists, speech therapists, and audiologists. Also referred to as *midlevel practitioner, midlevel provider (MLP),* or *physician extender (PE).*

Nonprivileged information (2): Information consisting of ordinary facts unrelated to the treatment of the patient. The patient's authorization is not required to disclose the data unless the record is in a specialty hospital or in a special service unit of a general hospital such as the psychiatric unit.

Not elsewhere classifiable (NEC) (5): This term is used in the ICD-9-CM diagnostic coding system when the code lacks the information necessary to code the term in a more specific category.

Not otherwise specified (NOS) (5): Unspecified. Used in ICD-9-CM numeric code system for coding diagnoses.

Notice of Privacy Practices (NPP) (2): Under HIPAA, a document given to the patient at the first visit or at enrollment explaining the individual's rights and the physician's legal duties in regard to protected health information (PHI).

Nursing facility (NF) (12): A specially qualified facility that has the staff and equipment to provide skilled nursing care and related services that are medically necessary to a patient's recovery; formerly known as a *skilled nursing facility.*

Occupational illness (or disease) (15): An abnormal condition or disorder caused by environmental factors associated with employment. It may be caused by inhalation, absorption, ingestion, or direct contact.

Occupational Safety and Health Administration (OSHA) (15): A federal agency that regulates and investigates safety and health standards in work locations.

Optical character recognition (OCR) (7): A device that can read typed characters at very high speed and convert them to digitized files that can be saved on disk. Also known as *intelligent character recognition (ICR).*

Optionally renewable (3): An insurance policy renewal provision in which the insurer has the right to refuse to renew the policy on a date and may add coverage limitations or increase premium rates.

Ordering physician (4): The physician ordering nonphysician services for a patient (e.g., diagnostic laboratory tests, pharmaceutical services, or durable medical equipment) when an insurance claim is submitted by a nonphysician supplier of services. The ordering physician also may be the treating or performing physician.

"Other" claims (7): Medicare claims not considered "clean" claims that require investigation or development on a prepayment basis to determine if Medicare is the primary or secondary carrier.

Other health insurance (OHI) (14): Health care coverage for TRICARE beneficiaries through an employer, an association, or a private insurer. A student in the family may have a health care plan through school.

Outpatient (17): A patient who receives services in a health care facility, such as a physician's office, clinic, urgent care center, emergency department, or ambulatory surgical center, and goes home the same day.

Overpayment (9): Money paid over and above the amount due by the insurer or patient.

Paper claim (7): An insurance claim submitted on paper, including those optically scanned and converted to an electronic form by the insurance carrier.

Partial disability (16): A disability from an illness or injury that prevents an insured person from performing one or more of the functions of his or her regular job.

Participating physician (11): (A) A physician who contracts with an HMO or other insurance company to provide services. (B) A physician who has agreed to accept a plan's payments for services to subscribers (e.g., some Blue plans). Eighty percent of practicing American physicians are participating physicians.

Participating physician (par) (12): A physician who agrees to accept payment from Medicare (80% of the approved charges) plus payment from the patient (20% of approved charges) after the $100 deductible has been met.

Participating provider (par) (3, 14): One who accepts TRICARE assignment. Payment in this case goes directly to the provider. The patient must still pay the cost-share outpatient deductible and the cost of care not covered by TRICARE. See *Assignment.*

Partnership program (14): A program that lets TRICARE-eligible individuals receive inpatient or outpatient treatment from civilian providers of care in a military hospital or from uniformed services providers of care in civilian facilities.

Password (8): A combination of letters and numbers that each individual is assigned to access computer data.

Past history (PH) (4): A patient's past experiences with illnesses, operations, injuries, and treatments.

Patient registration form (3): A questionnaire designed to collect demographic data and essential facts about medical insurance coverage for each patient seen for professional services; also called *patient information form.*

Peer review (9): The review of a patient's case by one or more physicians using federal guidelines to evaluate another physician in regard to the quality and efficiency of medical care. This is done to discover overutilization or misutilization of a plan's benefits.

Pending claim (7): An insurance claim held in suspense because of review or other reason. These claims may be cleared for payment or denied.

Per capita (11): See *Capitation.*

Percentage of revenue (17): The fixed percentage of the collected premium rate that is paid to the hospital to cover services.

Per diem (17): A single charge for a day in the hospital regardless of any actual charges or costs incurred.

Permanent and stationary (P and S) (15): A phrase used when a workers' compensation patient's condition has become stabilized and no improvement is expected. It is only after this declaration that a case can be rated for a compromise and release.

Permanent disability (PD) (15): An illness or injury (impairment of the normal use of a body part) expected to continue for the lifetime of the injured worker that prevents the person from performing the functions of his or her regular occupation, therefore impairing his or her earning capacity.

Personal insurance (3): An insurance plan issued to an individual (or his or her dependents); also known as *individual contract.*

Petition (15): A formal written request commonly used to indicate an appeal; also means any request for relief other than an application.

Phantom billing (2): Billing for services not performed.

Physical examination (PE or PX) (4): Objective inspection or testing of organ systems or body areas of a patient by a physician.

Physically clean claim (7): Insurance claims with no staples or highlighted areas. The bar code area has not been deformed.

Physician provider group (PPG) (11): A physician-owned business that has the flexibility to deal with all forms of contract medicine and still offer its own packages to business groups, unions, and the general public.

Physician Quality Reporting Initiative (PQRI) (12): Voluntary pay-for-reporting program for providers who successfully report quality information related to services provided to patients under Medicare Part B between July 1 and December 31, 2007.

Physician's fee profile (5): A compilation of each physician's charges and the payments made to him or her over a given period of time for each specific professional service rendered to a patient.

Point-of-service (POS) option (14): Individuals under the TRICARE program can choose to get TRICARE-covered nonemergency services outside the prime network of providers without a referral from the primary care manager and without authorization from a health care finder.

Point-of-service (POS) plan (3, 11): A managed care plan in which members are given a choice as to how to receive services, whether through an HMO, PPO, or fee-for-service plan. The decision is made at the time the service is necessary (e.g., "at the point of service"); sometimes referred to as *open-ended HMOs, swing-out HMOs, self-referral options,* or *multiple option plans.*

Poisoning (5): A condition resulting from an overdose of drugs or chemical substances or from the wrong drug or agent given or taken in error.

Portfolio (18): A compilation of items that represents a job applicant's skills.

Posted (3): To record or transfer financial entries, debit or credit, to an account (e.g., daysheet, financial account record [ledger], bank deposit slip, check register, journal).

Preadmission testing (PAT) (17): Treatment, tests, and procedures done 48 to 72 hours before admission of a patient into the hospital. This is done to eliminate extra hospital days.

Preauthorization (3, 14): A requirement of some health insurance plans to obtain permission for a service or procedure before it is done and to see whether the insurance program agrees it is medically necessary.

Precertification (3): A procedure done to determine whether treatment (surgery, tests, or hospitalization) is covered under a patient's health insurance policy.

Predetermination (3): A financial inquiry done before treatment to determine the maximum dollar amount the insurance company will pay for surgery, consultations, postoperative care, and so forth.

Preexisting conditions (3): Illnesses or injuries acquired by the patient before enrollment in an insurance plan. In some insurance plans, preexisting conditions are excluded from coverage temporarily or permanently or may disqualify membership in the plan.

Preferred provider organization (PPO) (3, 11): A type of health benefit program in which enrollees receive the highest level of benefits when they obtain services from a physician, hospital, or other health care provider designated by their program as a "preferred provider." Enrollees may receive substantial, although reduced, benefits when they obtain care from a provider of their own choosing who is not designated as a "preferred provider" by their program.

Premium (3, 12): The cost of insurance coverage paid annually, semiannually, or monthly to keep the policy in force. In the Medicare program, monthly fee that enrollees pay for Medicare Part B medical insurance. This fee is updated annually to reflect changes in program costs.

Prepaid group practice model (11): A plan under which specified health services are rendered by participating physicians to an enrolled group of persons, with fixed periodic payments made in advance, by or on behalf of each person or family. If a health insurance carrier is involved, it contracts to pay in advance for the full range of health services to which the insured is entitled under the terms of the health insurance contract. Such a plan is one form of a health maintenance organization.

Primary care manager (PCM) (14): A physician who is responsible for coordinating and managing all of the TRICARE beneficiary's health care unless there is an emergency.

Primary care physician (PCP) (4, 11): A physician (e.g., family practitioner, general practitioner, pediatrician, obstetrician/gynecologist, or general internist) who oversees the care of patients in a managed health care plan (HMO or PPO) and refers patients to see specialists (e.g., cardiologists, oncologists, or surgeons) for services as needed. Also known as a *gatekeeper.*

Primary diagnosis (5): Initial identification of the condition or chief complaint for which the patient is treated for outpatient medical care.

Principal diagnosis (5, 17): A condition established after study that is chiefly responsible for the admission of the patient to the hospital.

Prior approval (13): The evaluation of a provider request for a specific service to determine the medical necessity and appropriateness of the care requested for a patient. Also called *prior authorization* in some states.

Privacy (2): The condition of being secluded from the presence or view of others.

Privacy officer, privacy official (2): An individual designated to help the provider remain in compliance by setting policies and procedures in place, and by training and managing the staff regarding HIPAA and patient rights; usually the contact person for questions and complaints.

Privileged information (2): Data related to the treatment and progress of the patient that can be released only when written authorization of the patient or guardian is obtained.

Problem focused (PF) (4): A phrase used to describe a type of medical decision making when a patient is seen for an E/M service.

Procedure code numbers (6): Five-digit numeric codes that describe each service the physician renders to a patient.

Procedure review (17): A review of diagnostic and therapeutic procedures to determine appropriateness.

Professional Association of Health Care Office Managers (PAHCOM) (18): A nationwide organization dedicated to providing a strong professional network for health care office managers.

Professional component (PC) (6): That portion of a test or procedure (containing both a professional and

technical component) which the physician performs (e.g., interpreting an electrocardiogram [ECG], reading an x-ray, or making an observation and determination using a microscope).

Professional courtesy (10): A discount or exemption from charges given to certain people at the discretion of the physician rendering the service. It is rarely used in current medicine.

Prospective payment system (PPS) (12): A method of payment for Medicare hospital insurance based on DRGs (a fixed dollar amount for a principal diagnosis).

Prospective review (4): The process of going over financial documents before billing is submitted to the insurance company to determine documentation deficiencies and errors.

Protected health information (PHI) (2): Any data that identify an individual and describe his or her health status, age, sex, ethnicity, or other demographic characteristics, whether or not that information is stored or transmitted electronically.

Quality assurance program (14): A plan that continually assesses the effectiveness of inpatient and outpatient care in the TRICARE and CHAMPVA programs.

Quality improvement organization (QIO) program (12, 17): A program that replaces the peer review organization (PRO) program and is designed to monitor and improve the usage and quality of care for Medicare beneficiaries.

Qui tam action (12): An action to recover a penalty brought on by an informer in a situation in which one portion of the recovery goes to the informer and the other portion to the state or government.

Readmission review (17): A review of patients readmitted to a hospital within 7 days with problems related to the first admission, to determine whether the first discharge was premature or the second admission is medically necessary.

Real time (8): Online interactive communication between two computer systems allowing instant transfer of information.

Reasonable fee (6, 12): A charge is considered reasonable if it is deemed acceptable after peer review even though it does not meet the customary or prevailing criteria. This includes unusual circumstances or complications requiring additional time, skill, or experience in connection with a particular service or procedure. In Medicare, the amount on which payment is based for participating physicians.

Rebill (resubmit) (9): To send another request for payment for an overdue bill to either the insurance company or patient.

Recertification (18): A renewal of certification after a specified time.

Recipient (13): A person certified by the local welfare department to receive the benefits of Medicaid under one of the specific aid categories; an individual certified to receive Medicare benefits.

Reconsideration (16): The first level of appeal process for an individual applying for SSDI or SSI. It is a complete review of the claim by a medical or psychologic consultant or disability examiner team who did not take part in the original disability determination.

Recovery Audit Contractor (RAC) Initiative (12): Proposal of legislation that originally created a demonstration program that became permanently implemented when Congress enacted the Tax Relief and Health Care Act of 2006 (TRHCA). This extended the RAC program to all fifty states by 2010. Its goals are to identify Medicare underpayments and overpayments and recover overpayments using automated review and complex review. An automated review is done electronically without human review and complex review is done using human review of the medical record.

Referral (4): The transfer of the total or specific care of a patient from one physician to another. In managed care, a request for authorization for a specific service.

Referring physician (4): A physician who sends the patient for testing or treatment noted on the insurance claim when it is submitted by the physician performing the service.

Regional contractor (14): For TRICARE and CHAMPVA, the insurance company that handles the claims for care received within a particular state or country. Also known as *claims processor* and formerly known as *fiscal agent, fiscal carrier,* or *fiscal intermediary.* For Medicare, see *Medicare administrative contractor (MAC).*

Regional office (RO) (16): A Social Security state office.

Registered Medical Assistant (RMA) (18): A title earned by completing appropriate training and passing a registry examination administered by the American Medical Technologists (AMT).

Registered Medical Coder (RMC) (18): A registered title awarded after completion of coursework given by the Medical Management Institute (MMI) with recertification requirements.

Registration (18): Entry in an official registry or record that lists names of persons in an occupation who have satisfied specific requirements or by attaining a certain level of education and paying a registration fee.

Reimbursement (10): Repayment; the term used when insurance payment is pending.

Reimbursement specialist (1): See *Insurance billing specialist.*

Rejected claim (7, 9): An insurance claim submitted to an insurance carrier that is discarded by the system because of a technical error (omission or erroneous information) or because it does not follow Medicare instructions. It is returned to the provider for correction or change so that it may be processed properly for payment.

Relative value studies (scale) (RVS) (6): A list of procedure codes for professional services and procedures that are assigned unit values that indicate the relative value of one procedure over another.

Relative value unit (RVU) (6, 12): A monetary value assigned to each service on the basis of the amount of physician work, practice expenses, and cost of professional liability insurance. These three RVUs are then adjusted according to geographic area and used in a formula to determine Medicare fees.

Remittance advice (RA) (9, 12): A document detailing services billed and describing payment determination issued to providers of the Medicare or Medicaid program; also known in some programs as an *explanation of benefits.*

Resident physician (4): A physician who has finished medical school and is performing one or more years of training in a specialty area on the job at a hospital (medical center).

Residual benefits (16): A term used in disability income insurance for disability that is not work related. It is the payment of partial benefits when the insured is not totally disabled.

Residual disability (16): A disability from an illness or injury that prevents an insured person from performing one or more of the functions of his or her regular job. This is sometimes referred to as *partial disability.* See also *Partial disability.*

Resource-based relative value scale (RBRVS) (6, 12): A system that ranks physician services by units and provides a formula to determine a Medicare fee schedule.

Respite care (12): A short-term hospice inpatient stay for a terminally ill patient to give temporary relief to the person who regularly assists with home care of a patient.

***Respondeat superior* (1):** "Let the master answer." Refers to a physician's liability in certain cases for the wrongful acts of his of her assistant(s) or employee(s).

Résumé (18): A summary of education, skills, and work experience, usually in outline form.

Retrospective review (4): The process of going over financial documents after billing an insurance carrier to determine documentation deficiencies and errors.

Review (9): To look over a claim to assess how much payment should be made.

Review of systems (ROS) (4): An inventory of body systems obtained through a series of questions used to identify signs or symptoms that the patient might be experiencing or has experienced.

Running balance (3): An amount owed on a credit transaction; also known as *outstanding or unpaid balance.*

Scrubbing (17): The process in which computer software checks for errors before a claim is submitted to an insurance carrier for payment; also known as *edit check* or *cleaning the bill.*

Second-injury fund (15): See *Subsequent injury fund.*

Secondary diagnosis (5): A reason subsequent to the primary diagnosis for an office or hospital encounter that may contribute to the condition or define the need for a higher level of care but is not the underlying cause. There may be more than one secondary diagnosis.

Secured debt (10): A debt (an amount owed) in which a debtor pledges certain property (collateral), in a written security agreement, to the repayment of the debt.

Security officer (2): A person who protects the computer and networking systems within the practice and implements protocols such as password assignment, backup procedures, firewalls, virus protection, and contingency planning for emergencies.

Security Rule (2): Under HIPAA, regulations related to the security of electronic protected health information (ePHI) that, along with regulations related to electronic transactions and code sets, privacy, and enforcement, compose the Administrative Simplification provisions.

Self-employment (18): Working for oneself, with direct control over work, services, and fees.

Self-referral (11): A patient in a managed care plan that refers himself or herself to a specialist. The patient may be required to inform the primary care physician.

Senior billing representative (1): See *Insurance billing specialist.*

Sequelae (15): Diseased conditions after and usually resulting from a previous disease.

Service area (11): The geographic area defined by an HMO as the locale in which it will provide health care services to its members directly through its own resources or arrangements with other providers in the area.

Service benefit program (14): A program (e.g., TRICARE) that provides benefits without a contract guaranteeing the indemnification of an insured party against a specific loss; there are no premiums. TRICARE Standard is considered a service benefit program.

Service-connected injury (14): Injury incurred by a service member while on active duty or incurred during reserve duty with a military unit.

Service contract (18): A document that enumerates the obligations of a billing service and a medical practice stating the responsible party for each specific duty and task.

Service retiree (14): An individual who is retired from a career in the armed forces; also known as a *military retiree.*

Share of cost (13): The amount the patient must pay each month before he or she can be eligible for Medicaid; also known as *liability* or *spend down.*

Short-term disability insurance (16): A provision to pay benefits to a covered disabled person as long as he or she remains disabled, up to a specified period not exceeding 2 years.

Skip (10): A debtor who has moved and neglected to give a forwarding address (e.g., skipped town).

Slanted brackets (5): A symbol used with a diagnostic code in ICD-9-CM, volume 2, Alphabetic Index, indicating the code may never be sequenced as the principal diagnosis.

Social history (SH) (4): An age-appropriate review of a patient's past and current activities (e.g., smoking, diet intake, or alcohol use).

Social Security Administration (SSA) (16): Administers SSDI and SSI programs for disabled persons.

Social Security Disability Insurance (SSDI) (16): Entitlement program for disabled workers or self-employed individuals.

Social Security Disability Insurance (SSDI) program (16): A federal entitlement program for long-term disability under Title II of the Social Security Act. It provides monthly benefits to workers and those self-employed who meet certain conditions.

Social Security number (SSN) (7): An individual's tax identification number issued by the federal government.

Sponsor (14): For the TRICARE program, the service person (active duty, retired, or deceased) whose relationship makes the patient (dependent) eligible for TRICARE.

Staff model (11): The type of HMO in which the health plan hires physicians directly and pays them a salary.

Standard (2): A rule, condition, or requirement.

Standard transactions (8): The electronic files in which medical data are compiled to produce a specific format.

State Children's Health Insurance Program (SCHIP) (13): A state child health program that operates with federal grant support under Title V of the Social Security Act. In some states this program may be known as *Maternal and Child Health Program (MCHP)* or *Children's Special Health Care Services (CSHCS).*

State Disability Insurance (SDI) (3, 16): See *Unemployment Compensation Disability.*

State license number (7): A number issued to a physician who has passed the state medical examination indicating his or her right to practice medicine in the state where issued.

State preemption (2): A complex technical issue not within the scope of the health care provider's role; refers to instances when state law takes precedence over federal law.

Statute of limitations (10): A time limit established for filing lawsuits; may vary from state to state.

Stop loss (11, 17): An agreement between a managed care company and a reinsurer in which absorption of prepaid patient expenses is limited; or limiting losses on an individual expensive hospital claim or professional services claim; form of reinsurance by which the managed care program limits the losses of an individual expensive hospital claim.

Straightforward (SF) (4): Phrase used to describe a type of medical decision making when a patient is seen for an E/M service.

Subpoena (4): "Under penalty." A writ that commands a witness to appear at a trial or other proceeding and give testimony.

Subpoena duces tecum (4): "In his possession." A subpoena that requires the appearance of a witness with his or her records. Sometimes the judge permits the mailing of records and it is not necessary for the physician to appear in court.

Sub rosa films (15): Videotapes made without the knowledge of the subject; used to investigate suspicious claims in workers' compensation cases.

Subscriber (3): The contract holder covered by an insurance program or managed care plan, who either has coverage through his or her place of employment or has purchased coverage directly from the plan or affiliate. This term is used primarily in Blue Cross and Blue Shield plans.

Subsequent-injury fund (SIF) (15): A special fund that assumes all or part of the liability for benefits provided to a worker because of the combined effect of a work-related impairment and a preexisting condition; also known as *second-injury fund.*

Summary payment voucher (14): The document the fiscal agent sends to the provider or beneficiary, showing the service or supplies received, allowable charges, amount billed, the amount TRICARE paid, how much deductible has been paid, and the patient's cost-share.

Supplemental benefits (16): Disability insurance provisions that allow benefits to the insured to increase the monthly indemnity or receive a percentage of the policy premiums if an individual keeps a policy in force for 5 or 10 years or does not file any claims.

Supplemental Security Income (SSI) (12, 13, 16): A program of income support for low-income aged, blind, and disabled persons established by Title XVI of the Social Security Act.

Supplementary medical insurance (SMI) (12): Part B—medical benefits of Medicare program.

Surgical package (6): Surgical procedure code numbers include the operation; local infiltration, digital block, or topical anesthesia; and normal, uncomplicated postoperative care. This is referred to as a *package,* and one fee covers the whole package.

Suspended claim (9): An insurance claim that is processed by the insurance carrier but held in an indeterminate (pending) state about payment either because of an error or the need for additional information.

Suspense (9): The pending indeterminate state of an insurance claim because of an error or need for more information.

Syndrome (5): Another name for a symptom complex (a set of complex signs, symptoms, or other manifestations resulting from a common cause or appearing in combination, presenting a distinct clinical picture of a disease or inherited abnormality).

T-1 (8): A T-carrier channel that can transmit voice or data channels quickly.

Taxonomy codes (8): Numeric and alpha provider specialty codes that are assigned and classify each health care provider when transmitting electronic insurance claims.

Teaching physician (4): A physician who is responsible for training and supervising medical students, interns, or residents and who takes them to the bedsides of patients in a teaching hospital to review course and treatment.

Technical component (6): Portion of a test or procedure (containing both a technical and a professional component) that pertains to the use of the equipment and the operator who performs it (e.g., ECG machine and technician, radiography machine and technician, or microscope and technician).

Temporary disability (TD) (15, 16): The recovery period after a work-related injury during which the employee is unable to work and the condition has not stabilized; a schedule of benefits payable for the temporary disability.

Temporary disability insurance (TDI) (16): See *Unemployment Compensation Disability.*

Tertiary care (11): Services requested by a specialist from another specialist (e.g., neurosurgeons, thoracic surgeons, and intensive care units).

Third-party liability (15): Third-party liability exists if an entity is liable to pay the medical cost for injury, disease, or disability of a person hurt during the performance of his or her occupation and the injury is caused by an entity not connected with the employer.

Third-party subrogation (15): The legal process by which an insurance company seeks from a third party, who has caused a loss, recovery of the amount paid to the policyholder.

Total disability (16): A term that varies in meaning from one disability insurance policy to another. For example, a liberal definition might read, "The insured must be unable to perform the major duties of his or her specific occupation."

Total, permanent service-connected disability (14): A total permanent disability incurred by a service member while on active duty.

Tracer (9): An inquiry made to an insurance company to locate the status of an insurance claim (e.g., claim in review, claim never received).

Trading partner agreement (TPA) (8): See *Business associate agreement.*

Transaction (2): The transmission of information between two parties to carry out financial or administrative activities related to health care.

Transfer review (17): Review of transfers to different areas of the same hospital that are exempted from prospective payment.

Treating or performing physician (4): A provider who renders a service to a patient.

TRICARE (3): A three-option managed health care program offered to spouses and dependents of service personnel with uniform benefits and fees implemented nationwide by the federal government.

TRICARE Extra (14): A PPO-type of TRICARE option in which the individual does not have to enroll or pay an annual fee. On a visit-by-visit basis, the individual may seek care from an authorized network provider and receive a discount on services and reduced cost-share (copayment).

TRICARE for Life (14): A health care program that offers additional TRICARE benefits as a supplementary payer to Medicare for uniformed service retirees, their spouses, and survivors age 65 years of age or older.

TRICARE Prime (14): A voluntary HMO-type option for TRICARE beneficiaries.

TRICARE Service Center (14): An office staffed by TRICARE Health Care Finders and beneficiary service representatives.

Turfing (11): Transferring the sickest, high-cost patients to other physicians so that the provider appears as a "low-utilizer" in a managed care setting.

Unbundling (6): The practice of using numerous CPT codes to identify procedures normally covered by a single code; also known as *itemizing, fragmented billing, exploding,* or *a la carte medicine;* billing under Medicare Part B for nonphysician services to hospital inpatients furnished to the hospital by an outside supplier or another provider. Under the new law, unbundling is prohibited and all nonphysician services provided in an inpatient setting will be paid as hospital services.

Unemployment Compensation Disability (UCD) (3, 16): Insurance that covers off-the-job injury or sickness and is paid for by deductions from a person's paycheck. This program is administered by a state agency and is sometimes also known as State Disability Insurance (SDI) or temporary disability insurance (TDI).

Uniform Bill (UB-04) paper or electronic claim form (17): A Uniform Bill insurance claim form developed by the National Uniform Billing Committee for hospital inpatient billing and payment transactions.

Unsecured debt (10): Any debt (amount owed) that is not secured or backed by any form of collateral.

Upcoding (6): Deliberate manipulation of CPT codes for increased payment.

Urgent care (14): Medically necessary treatment that is required for illness or injury that would result in further disability or death if not treated immediately.

Use (2): The sharing, employment, application, utilization, examination, or analysis of individually identifiable health information (IIHI) within an organization that holds such information.

Usual, customary, and reasonable (UCR) (6): A method used by insurance companies to establish their fee schedules in which three fees are considered in calculating payment: (1) the usual fee is the fee typically submitted by the physician, (2) the customary fee falls within the range of usual fees charged by providers of similar training in a geographic area, and (3) the reasonable fee meets the aforementioned criteria or is considered justifiable because of special circumstances. UCR uses the conversion factor method of establishing maximums; the method of reimbursement used under Medicaid by which state Medicaid programs set reimbursement rates using the Medicare method or a fee schedule, whichever is lower.

Utilization review (UR) (11, 17): A process, based on established criteria, of reviewing and controlling the medical necessity for services and providers' use of medical care resources. Reviews are carried out by allied health personnel at predetermined times during the hospital stay to assess the need for the full facilities of an acute care hospital. In managed care systems such as an HMO, reviews are done to establish medical necessity, thus curbing costs. Also called *utilization* or *management control.*

V codes (5): A subclassification of ICD-9-CM coding used to identify health care encounters that occur for reasons other than illness or injury and to identify patients whose injury or illness is influenced by special circumstances or problems.

Verbal referral (11): A primary care physician informs the patient and telephones to the referring physician that the patient is being referred for an appointment.

Veteran (14): Any person who has served in the armed forces of the United States, especially in time of war; is no longer in the service; and has received an honorable discharge.

Veterans Affairs (VA) disability program (16): A program for honorably discharged veterans who file claim for a service-connected disability.

Veterans Affairs (VA) outpatient clinic (3): A facility where medical and dental services are rendered to a veteran who has a service-related disability.

Veterans Affairs (VA) outpatient clinic card (16): An identification card belonging to a retired member of the armed forces that is shown when receiving medical or dental services for service-related disabilities from a clinic.

Volume performance standard (VPS) (12): The desired growth rate for spending on Medicare Part B physician services, set each year by Congress.

Voluntary disability insurance (16): A majority of employees of an employer voluntarily consent to be covered by an insured or self-insured disability insurance plan instead of a state plan.

Waiting period (WP) (15, 16): For disability insurance, the initial period of time when a disabled individual is not eligible to receive benefits even though unable to work; for workers' compensation, the days that must elapse before workers' compensation weekly benefits become payable. Also known as *elimination period.*

Waiver of premium (16): A disability insurance policy provision that an employee does not have to pay any premiums while disabled.

Whistleblowers (12): Informants who report physicians suspected of defrauding the federal government.

Withhold (11): A portion of the monthly capitation payment to physicians retained by the HMO until the end of the year to create an incentive for efficient care. If the physician exceeds utilization norms, he or she will not receive it.

Workers' Compensation Appeals Board (WCAB) (15): The board that handles workers' compensation liens and appeals.

Workers' compensation (WC) insurance (3, 15): A contract that insures a person against on-the-job injury or illness. The employer pays the premium for his or her employees.

Work hardening (15): An individualized program of therapy using simulated or real job duties to build up strength and improve the worker's endurance to be able to work up to 8 hours per day. Sometimes work site modifications are instituted to get the employee back to gainful employment.

Write-off (10): Assets or debts that have been determined to be uncollectable and are therefore adjusted off the accounting books as a loss.

Key Abbreviations

AAMA (American Association of Medical Assistants)

AAMB (American Association of Medical Billers)

AAPC (American Academy of Professional Coders)

ABCs (alternative billing codes)

ABN (advance beneficiary notice)

ACA (American Collectors Association)

ADSM (active duty service member)

AEPs (appropriateness evaluation protocols)

AHA (American Hospital Association)

AHIMA (American Health Information Management Association)

AIDS (acquired immunodeficiency syndrome)

ALJ (administrative law judge)

AMA (American Medical Association)

AME (agreed medical evaluator)

ANSI (American National Standards Institute)

APCs (ambulatory payment classifications)

APGs (ambulatory patient groups)

A/R (accounts receivable)

ARRA (American Recovery and Reinvestment Act)

ASCs (ambulatory surgery categories)

ASCVD (arteriosclerotic cardiovascular disease)

ASET (administrative simplification enforcement tool)

ASHD (arteriosclerotic heart disease)

ASP (application service provider)

ASC X (Accredited Standards Committee X)

ATM (automated teller machine)

AVGs (ambulatory visit groups)

BR (by report)

C (comprehensive) level of history or examination

C and R (compromise and release)

CAC (computer-assisted coding)

CAP (claims assistance professional)

CC (chief complaint)

CC (complication/comorbidity)

CCAP (certified claims assistance professional)

CCI (Correct Coding Initiative)

CCS (certified coding specialist)

CCS-P (certified coding specialist-physician)

CCU (coronary care unit)

CD (compact disk)

CDM (charge description master)

CDT (Code on Dental Procedures and Nomenclature)

CE (consultative examiner)

CECP (certified electronic claims processor)

CF (conversion factor)

CHAMPVA (Civilian Health and Medical Program of the Department of Veterans Affairs)

CHEDDAR (chief complaint history of present illness examination details drugs and dosages assessment return visit information or referral)

CLIA (Clinical Laboratory Improvement Amendments)

CMA (certified medical assistant)

CMBS (certified medical billing specialist)

CMHCs (community mental health centers)

CMP (civil monetary penalty)

CMP (competitive medical plan)

CMRS (certified medical reimbursement specialist)

CMS (Centers for Medicare and Medicaid Services)

CMS-1450 (Centers for Medicare and Medicaid Services UB-4 insurance claim form)

CMS-1500 (Centers for Medicare and Medicaid Services Health Insurance Claim Form)

COB (coordination of benefits)

COBRA (Consolidated Omnibus Budget Reconciliation Act)

copay (copayment)

CPC (certified procedural coder)

CPC-A CPC-H (certified professional coder)

CPT *(Current Procedural Terminology)*

CSRS (civil service retirement system)

D (detailed) level of history or examination

DAB (Departmental Appeal Board)

DC (doctor of chiropractic)

DCGs (diagnostic cost groups)

DDE (direct data entry)

DDS (Disability Determination Services)

DEERS (Defense Enrollment Eligibility Reporting System)

DEFRA (Deficit Reduction Act)

DHHS (U.S. Department of Health and Human Services)

DME (durable medical equipment)

DME (durable medical equipment) number

DNA (does not apply)

DoD (Department of Defense)

DOJ (Department of Justice)

DOS (date of service)

DRG (diagnosis related group)

DSL (digital subscriber liner)

DSM-IV *(Diagnostic and Statistical Manual of Mental Disorders Fourth Edition)*

dx Dx (diagnosis)

E codes

EBP (employee benefit plan)

ECG (electrocardiogram)

e-check (electronic check)

ECP (electronic claims processor)

ED or ER (emergency department or emergency room)
EDI (electronic data interchange)
EEOC (Equal Employment Opportunity Commission)
EFT (electronic funds transfer)
EGHP (employee group health plan)
eHIM (electronic health information management)
EHR (electronic health record)
EIN (employer identification number)
E/M (evaluation and management) service
e-mail (electronic mail)
EMC (electronic medical claim)
EMG (emergency)
EMR (electronic medical record)
EMTALA (Emergency Medical Treatment and Active Labor Act)
EOB (explanation of benefits)
EOMB (explanation of Medicare benefits)
EPF (expanded problem focused) level of history or examination
ePHI (electronic protected health information)
EPO (exclusive provider organization)
EPSDT (early periodic screening diagnosis and treatment)
ERA (electronic remittance advice)
ERISA (Employee Retirement Income Security Act)
ESI (electronically stored information)
ESRD (end-stage renal disease)
FACT (Fair and Accurate Credit Transactions Act)
fax (facsimile)
FBI (Federal Bureau of Investigation)
FCA (False Claims Act)
FCBA (Fair Credit Billing Act)
FCRA (Fair Credit Reporting Act)
FDA (Food and Drug Administration)
FDCPA (Fair Debt Collection Practices Act)
FDIC (Federal Deposit Insurance Corporation)
FECA (Federal Employees' Compensation Act)
FEHBA (Federal Employee Health Benefit Act)
FERS (Federal Employees Retirement System)
FH (family history)
FL (field locator)
FMC (foundation for medical care)
FPL (federal poverty level)
FSA (flexible spending account)
FTC (Federal Trade Commission)
FTM (full-time manager)
FTP (file transfer protocol)
GAF (geographic adjustment factor)
GAO (General Accounting Office)
GED (general equivalency diploma)
GPCIs (geographic practice cost indices)
HAC (health administration center)
HBA (health benefits advisor)
HBMA (Healthcare Billing and Management Association)
HC (high complexity) medical decision making
HCF (health care finder)
HCFAP (Health Care Fraud and Abuse Control Program)

HCPCS (Healthcare Common Procedure Coding System)
HDHP (high deductible health plan)
HEDIS (Health Plan Employer Data Information Set)
HFMA (Healthcare Financial Management Association)
HHA (home health agency or hospice health agency)
HHS (U.S. Department of Health and Human Services)
HIM (health information management)
HIPAA (Health Insurance Portability and Accountability Act)
HIV (human immunodeficiency virus)
HL (Health Level Seven)
HMO (health maintenance organization)
HO (hearing officer)
HPI (history of present illness)
HRA (Health Reimbursement Account)
HRS (health care reimbursement specialist)
HSA (health savings account)
HSI (Health Systems International)
IAIABC (International Association of Industrial Accident Boards and Commissions)
ICD-9-CM (*International Classification of Diseases Ninth Revision Clinical Modification*)
ICD-10-CM (*International Classification of Diseases Tenth Revision Clinical Modification*)
ICD-10-PCS (*International Classification of Diseases Tenth Revision Procedural Coding System*)
ICFs (intermediate care facilities)
ICR (intelligent character recognition or image copy recognition)
ICU (intensive care unit)
IDDM (type I diabetes)
IDE (investigational device exemption)
IIHI (individually identifiable health information)
IME (independent medical evaluator)
imp (impression)
INS (Immigration and Naturalization Service)
IPA (independent or individual practice association)
IRS (Internal Revenue Service)
LC (low complexity) medical decision making
LCD (local coverage decision)
LGHP (large group health plan)
LHWCA (Longshoremen's and Harbor Workers' Compensation Act)
listserv (list service)
LLQ (left lower quadrant)
LMP (last menstrual period)
LMRP (local medical review policy)
LOS (length of stay)
LUQ (left upper quadrant)
MAAC (maximum allowable actual charge)
MAB (Medical Association of Billers)
MAC (Medicare administrative contractor)
MC (moderate complexity) medical decision making
MCC (major complication/comorbidity)
MCD (Medicaid)
MCE (Medicare coding edits)

MCHP (Maternal and Child Health Program)
MCO (managed care organization)
MDCs (major diagnostic categories)
MDM (medical decision making)
Medi-Medi (Medicare/Medicaid)
MG (Medigap)
MGMA (Medical Group Management Association)
MHS (Military Health System)
MIP (Medicare Integrity Program)
MMA (Medicare Prescription Drug Improvement and
    Modernization Act)
MN (medically needy)
MQMB (Medicaid Qualified Medicare Beneficiary)
MRI (magnetic resonance imaging)
MSA (medical savings account)
MS-DRGs (Medicare-Severity Diagnostic Related Groups)
MSDS (material safety data sheets)
MSHP (multiskilled health practitioner)
MSN (Medicare summary notice)
MSO (management services organization)
MSP (Medicare Secondary Payer)
MTF (military treatment facility)
MTS (Medicare Transaction System)
NA N/A (not applicable)
NAS (nonavailability statement)
NC (no charge)
NCCI (National Correct Coding Initiative) edits
NCDs (national coverage determinations)
NCHS (National Center for Health Statistics)
NCICS (National Certified Insurance and Coding Specialist)
NCQA (National Committee for Quality Assurance)
NCVHS (National Committee on Vital and Health Statistics)
ND (nondisability) claim
NDC (National Drug Code)
NEC (not elsewhere classifiable)
NEMB (Notice of Exclusions from Medicare Benefits)
NF (nursing facility)
NHII (National Health Information Infrastructure)
NIDDM (type II diabetes)
NLP (natural language processing)
NOC (not otherwise classified)
nonpar (nonparticipating) provider or physician
NOS (not otherwise specified)
NP (new patient)
NPI (National Provider Identifier) number
NPP (nonphysician practitioner)
NPP (Notice of Privacy Practices)
NSF (nonsufficient funds or not sufficient funds)
NSF (National Standard Format)
OASDI (Old Age Survivors and Disability Insurance)
OASDHI (Old-Age Survivors Disability and Health
    Insurance)
OBRA (Omnibus Budget Reconciliation Act)
OCE (outpatient coding edits)
OCNA (other carrier name and address) key
OCR (optical character recognition)

OCR (Office for Civil Rights)
OHI (other health insurance)
OIG (Office of the Inspector General)
OOY (over-one-year) claims
OPPS (Outpatient Prospective Payment System)
ORT (Operation Restored Trust)
OSHA (Occupational Safety and Health Administration)
P & P (policies and procedures)
P and S (permanent and stationary)
PAHCOM (Professional Association of Health Care Office
    Management)
par (participating) provider
PAT (preadmission testing)
PAYERID (payer identification)
PC (professional component)
PCM (primary care manager)
PCP (primary care physician)
PD (permanent disability)
PE or PX (physical examination)
PF (problem focused) level of history or examination
PFFS (private fee-for-service) plan
PFSH (past history family or social history)
PH (past history)
PHI (protected health information)
PHP (prepaid health plan)
PIN (provider identification number)
PMS (practice management software or practice
    management system)
PO (privacy officer or privacy official; postoperative)
POR (problem-oriented record) system
POS (place of service)
POS (point of service)
POS (point-of-service) machine
POS (point-of-service) option
POS (point-of-service) plan
PPG (physician provider group)
PPO (preferred provider organization)
PPS (prospective payment system)
PPS (physician or provider service)
PQRI (physician quality reporting initiative)
PRO (peer review organization or professional review
    organization)
PSO (provider-sponsored organization)
QI (qualifying individuals) program
QIO (Quality Improvement Organization) program
QISMC (Quality Improvement System for Managed Care)
QMB (qualified Medicare beneficiary)
QME (qualified medical evaluator)
RA (remittance advice)
RAC (recovery audit contractor)
RBRVS (resource-based relative value scale)
RCU (respiratory care unit)
RFBS (religious fraternal benefit society)
RHIA (registered health information administrator)
RHIT (registered health information technician)
RLQ (right lower quadrant)

RMA (registered medical assistant)
RMC (registered medical coder)
RN (registered nurse)
RO (regional office)
R/O (rule out)
ROA (received on account)
ROM (range of motion)
ROS (review of systems)
RUQ (right upper quadrant)
RVS (relative value studies)
RVU (relative value unit)
SCHIP (State Children's Health Insurance Program)
SDI (State Disability Insurance)
SF (straightforward) medical decision making
SH (social history)
SHCP (Supplemental Health Care Program)
SIF (second injury fund or subsequent injury fund)
SLMB (specified low-income Medicare beneficiary)
SMI (supplementary medical insurance)
SNOMED (Systematized Nomenclature of Human and
   Veterinary Medicine)
SOAP (subjective objective assessment plan) style
SOF (signature on file)
SOR (source-oriented record) system
SSA (Social Security Administration)
SSDI (Social Security Disability Insurance) program
SSI (Supplemental Security Income)
SSN (Social Security number)
TANF (Temporary Assistance to Needy Families)

TC (technical component)
TCS (HIPAA transaction and code set)
TD (temporary disability)
TDI (temporary disability insurance)
TEFRA (Tax Equity and Fiscal Responsibility Act)
TFL (TRICARE for Life)
TILA (Truth in Lending Act)
TJC The Joint Commission
TMA (TRICARE management activity)
TPA (third-party administrator)
TPO (treatment payment and health care operations)
TPR (TRICARE Prime Remote)
TPRADFM (TRICARE Prime Remote for Active Duty Family
   Members)
TSC (TRICARE service center)
UB- (Uniform Bill) paper or electronic claim form
UCD (unemployment compensation disability)
UCR (usual, customary, and reasonable)
USFHP (Uniformed Services Family Health Plan)
UPS (uninterruptible power supply)
UR (utilization review)
V codes
VA (Veterans Affairs)
VPS (volume performance standard)
W2 (wage and tax statement)
WC (workers' compensation)
WCAB (Workers' Compensation Appeals Board)
WNL (within normal limits)
WP (waiting period)

Note: Page numbers followed by b, f, and t indicate boxes, figures, and tables, respectively.